REVIEW QUESTIONS *and* ANSWERS *for* VETERINARY TECHNICIANS

SIXTH EDITION

REVIEW QUESTIONS *and* ANSWERS *for* VETERINARY TECHNICIANS

Heather Prendergast, RVT, CVPM, SPHR
President
Synergie Consulting
Las Cruces, New Mexico

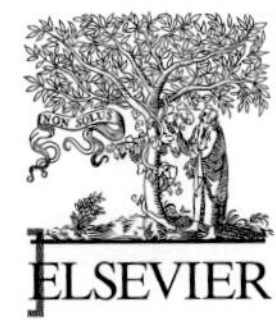

ELSEVIER

3251 Riverport Lane
St. Louis, Missouri 63043

REVIEW QUESTIONS AND ANSWERS FOR VETERINARY TECHNICIANS, SIXTH EDITION ISBN: 978-0-323-75987-8

Notices

Practitioners and researchers must always rely on their own experience and knowledge in evaluating and using any information, methods, compounds or experiments described herein. Because of rapid advances in the medical sciences, in particular, independent verification of diagnoses and drug dosages should be made. To the fullest extent of the law, no responsibility is assumed by Elsevier, authors, editors or contributors for any injury and/or damage to persons or property as a matter of products liability, negligence or otherwise, or from any use or operation of any methods, products, instructions, or ideas contained in the material herein.

ISBN: 9780323759878

Content Strategist: Brandi Graham
Content Development Manager: Ellen Wurm-Cutter
Content Development Specialist: Dominque McPherson
Publishing Services Manager: Shereen Jameel
Project Manager: Nadhiya Sekar
Design Direction: Margaret Reid

Printed in India

Last digit is the print number: 9 8 7 6 5 4 3

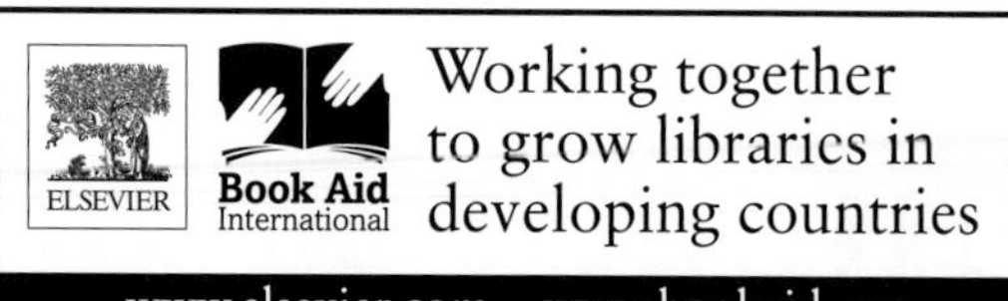

Contributors

Mary Ellen Goldberg AS, BS, LVT, CVT, SRA, CCRVN, CVPP, VTS (Physical Rehabilitation, Lab Animal Medicine–Research Anesthesia)
Veterinary Medical Technologist
Independent Contractor
Boynton Beach, Florida

Brooke Lockridge, RDMS, RVT
Diagnostic Medical Sonographer
Department of Radiology
University Medical Center
El Paso, Texas

Jody Nugent-Deal, RVT, VTS (Anesthesia/Analgesia, Clinical Practice–Exotic Companion Animal)
Anesthesia Service Supervisor
Small and Large Animal Anesthesia
University of California Davis Veterinary Medical Teaching Hospital
Davis, California

Jeanne Perrone, MS, CVT, VTS (Dentistry)
Veterinary Technician Specialist in Dentistry
VT Dental Training
Plant City, Florida

Rachel Poulin, RVT, VTS (SAIM)
Regional Recruiting Manager
Amerivet Veterinary Partners
San Antonio, Texas

Nicholas Raimondi, BS, CVT
Instructor
Veterinary Technology
New England Institute of Technology
East Greenwich, Rhode Island

Brandy Tabor, BS, CVT, VTS (ECC)
Senior Emergency/Critical Care Technician
Director of Clinical Education
Department of Emergency/Critical Care
Animal Emergency & Specialty Center
Parker, Colorado

To my mother
~the wind beneath my wings~
who has guided and given me inspiration, motivation, and empowerment.
You have been a truly amazing woman.
I miss you dearly.

Preface

The content of the book is arranged to allow intuitive review for the Veterinary Technician National Examination (VTNE). The main subject areas in the ***VTNE Review*** section represent the "domains" of the VTNE that were in effect when this was written. The subjects included in the ***Foundation Knowledge Review*** section represent general knowledge that is included in all of the VTNE domains.

The 5000 questions in this book resulted from a process that began with a rigorous review of each of the questions from the fifth edition. To meet the criteria for inclusion in this edition, each question, answer, and rationale had to reflect accurate, contemporary, entry-level veterinary technology knowledge.

The questions in *Review Questions and Answers for Veterinary Technicians* test factual knowledge, reasoning skills, and clinical judgment. To the best of our knowledge, none of the questions in this book have come directly from any current or previous credentialing examination. When properly used, however, the questions can help identify an individual's strengths and weaknesses in various subject areas. The rationales have been developed to serve as a learning tool and are very descriptive as to why an option is correct or incorrect. Take the time to read through the answers and apply critical thinking and practical analysis.

Heather Prendergast, RVT, CVPM, SPHR

Acknowledgments

This book is the result of the hard work of a veterinary technician team. I am honored to work with these skilled professionals, all of whom teach or work in practice.

I am grateful for the hard work and dedication given by Jody Nugent-Deal, RVT, VTS (Anesthesia/Analgesia, Clinical Practice–Exotic Companion Animal); Mary Ellen Goldberg, AS, BS, LVT, CVT, SRA, CCRVN, CVPP, VTS (Physical Rehabilitation, Lab Animal Medicine–Research Anesthesia); Brooke Lockridge, RDMS, RVT; Jeanne Perrone, CVT, VTS (Dentistry); Rachel V. Poulin, RVT, VTS (SAIM); Nicholas Raimondi, BS, CVT; and Brandy Tabor, BS, CVT, VTS (ECC). Without their skills and knowledge, the revision would not have been possible.

Last, and certainly not least, this book would not have been possible without the support from Clint. Hats off to an awesome man who can hold down the fort while I continue to pursue my dream, and carry out an awesome career, and still have welcome arms every time I come home from another trip. I love you.

Credentialing of Veterinary Technicians

In most states and Canadian provinces, individuals who wish to work as veterinary technicians must demonstrate their knowledge and competence by completing a credentialing process that is administered by an appropriate regulatory agency. Successful completion of this credentialing process generally confers the title of Licensed Veterinary Technician (LVT), Licensed Veterinary Medical Technician (LVMT), Certified Veterinary Technician (CVT), or Registered Veterinary Technician (RVT) on the individual, depending on the terminology used in each state.

Nearly all states and provinces that regulate the veterinary technology profession use the Veterinary Technician National Examination (VTNE) as the main component of their credentialing process, although some jurisdictions have additional requirements. Candidates should contact the appropriate regulatory agency in the state or province in which they desire credentialing to obtain information on processes, requirements, and deadlines. Contact information can be found on the website of the American Association of Veterinary State Boards (AAVSB) at http://www.aavsb.org.

The VTNE is offered by the AAVSB under a contractual agreement with the Professional Examination Service (PES). It is designed to evaluate essential job-related knowledge at entry level, and it consists of 150 multiple-choice questions and 20 pilot questions in primary subject areas called "domains." The current VTNE domains are:

- Pharmacy and Pharmacology
- Surgical Nursing
- Dentistry
- Laboratory Procedures
- Animal Care and Nursing
- Diagnostic Imaging
- Anesthesia
- Emergency Medicine and Critical Care
- Pain Management and Analgesia

After a student passes the VTNE in a state or province, the examination score can be transferred to other states or provinces. Information on this process is also available on the AAVSB website.

How to Use This Book

Review Questions and Answers for Veterinary Technicians, Sixth Edition, covers every major aspect of veterinary technology. It contains 5000 questions and answers. An accompanying Evolve website contains all of the book's content in practice and exam modes. The rationales and sources are now included in the Answer Key located in the back of the book. A 170-question practice test can be taken in the simulated exam mode. The questions are divided by section for the study mode. In exam mode, questions are organized according to VTNE domains of practice and pulled according to percentages comparable to the actual VTNE format.

The subjects covered in the ***Foundation Knowledge Review*** section represent general knowledge that is included in all of the VTNE domains. They are:

- Anatomy and Physiology
- Hospital Management
- Medical Calculations
- Terminology

The foundation subjects are particularly important because questions in the second section, ***VTNE Review,*** are built on the foundational knowledge in the first section. It may be helpful to complete the ***Foundation Knowledge Review*** section before beginning the ***VTNE Review*** section.

The VTNE Review section covers subjects related to the VTNE domains that were in effect when this edition was written. The subjects are:

- Pharmacology
- Surgical Nursing
- Dentistry
- Laboratory Procedures
- Animal Nursing
- Diagnostic Imaging
- Anesthesia
- Emergency and Critical Care
- Pain Management and Analgesia
- Exotic Animals

The primary intent of this book is to help students and graduate veterinary technicians prepare for examinations—either in academic programs or for credentialing purposes. Before beginning a section, the student should review textbooks and course notes pertaining to that subject area, and then approach each section as though it were an actual examination.

- *Carefully read each question.* Look for key words such as "most," "best," "least," "always," "never," and "except." Consider only the facts presented in the question. Do not make assumptions and inferences that may not be true.
- *Carefully evaluate each answer choice.* Each question has only one correct answer. The other three choices are incorrect "distractors." If more than one answer choice appears to be correct, closely examine each one for clues that would eliminate it from being correct.
- *Select an answer for each question.*
- *Compare your answers with the correct answers.* The correct answers are listed in the answer key at the end of this book.
- *Identify "weak" areas.* Subject areas with many incorrect answers may indicate the need for further review.

The Evolve website is set up in two different modes to better help the student study for the VTNE.

The *practice mode* includes all of the multiple-choice questions available in the book divided by section. The student chooses the specific sections he or she wishes to study, and he or she can select any number of questions to review. The student receives instant feedback as to whether the question was answered correctly or incorrectly, along with rationales and source information.

Simulated exam mode, similar to the format of the actual VTNE exam, contains 170 questions that are selected across all sections. The exam is timed and scored. After the student completes it, the results are available for viewing. The student may then review the exam in its entirety with answers and rationales.

Table of Contents

SECTION 1

Anatomy and Physiology

Brooke Lockridge

QUESTIONS

1. Where are striated muscles located?
   a. Stomach wall and uterus
   b. Urinary bladder and intestine
   c. Ciliary body of the eye
   d. Heart and skeletal muscles
2. Systemic circulation is under:
   a. High pressure
   b. Low pressure
   c. Partial pressure
   d. Equilibrium
3. A pregnant mare has what kind of placentation?
   a. Zonary
   b. Cotyledonary
   c. Diffuse
   d. Discoid
4. The pressure in the systemic arteries during ventricular contraction is:
   a. Diastolic blood pressure
   b. Osmotic pressure
   c. Systolic blood pressure
   d. Low pressure
5. Which hormone contracts the female reproductive tract to help move spermatozoa into the oviducts?
   a. Estrogen
   b. Progesterone
   c. Prolactin
   d. Oxytocin
6. Cardiac muscle is considered a:
   a. Nonstriated involuntary muscle
   b. Striated involuntary muscle
   c. Nonstriated voluntary muscle
   d. Striated voluntary muscle
7. In what order does the impulse for depolarization travel through the heart?
   a. AV node, SA node, bundle of His, Purkinje fibers
   b. SA node, AV node, bundle of His, Purkinje fibers
   c. SA node, AV node, Purkinje fibers, bundle of His
   d. AV node, SA node, Purkinje fibers, bundle of His
8. A pregnant queen has what kind of placentation?
   a. Zonary
   b. Cotyledonary
   c. Diffuse
   d. Discoid
9. The control of color changes in the pigment cells of reptiles, fish, and amphibians is associated with which hormone?
   a. FSH
   b. LH
   c. MSH
   d. TSH
10. The wave on an electrocardiogram that is associated with the atrial wall depolarization is the:
    a. PR interval
    b. T wave
    c. QRS complex
    d. P wave
11. The SA node is located in the wall of which chamber?
    a. Left atrium
    b. Left ventricle
    c. Right atrium
    d. Right ventricle
12. The muscular sphincter located between the stomach and the duodenum is the:
    a. Pylorus
    b. Cardia
    c. Chyme
    d. Rugae
13. The type of cell responsible for the transmission of impulses through the nervous system is the:
    a. Neuroglia
    b. Schwann
    c. Neuron
    d. Oligodendrocyte
14. Dogs demonstrate what type of estrous cycle?
    a. Polyestrous
    b. Seasonally polyestrous
    c. Diestrous
    d. Monoestrous
15. Which system is anatomically composed of the brain and spinal cord?
    a. Central nervous system
    b. Peripheral nervous system
    c. Parasympathetic nervous system
    d. Sympathetic nervous system

16. Functions that an animal does *not* have to control consciously, such as peristalsis in the intestine, are influenced by the:
    a. Somatic nervous system
    b. Central nervous system
    c. Peripheral nervous system
    d. Autonomic nervous system
17. The cranial nerves and the spinal nerves are anatomically part of what system?
    a. Central nervous system
    b. Peripheral nervous system
    c. Parasympathetic nervous system
    d. Sympathetic nervous system
18. Sensory nerves are considered:
    a. Efferent motor nerves
    b. Motor nerves
    c. Efferent nerves
    d. Afferent nerves
19. When a stimulus is strong enough to cause complete depolarization, it has reached:
    a. Threshold
    b. Repolarization
    c. Refractory period
    d. Action potential
20. What happens within the neuron that allows local anesthetics to be effective?
    a. Potassium gates open
    b. The charge within the cell becomes positive
    c. The charge within the cell becomes negative
    d. Sodium channels become blocked
21. Smooth muscles can be found in the:
    a. Heart
    b. Stomach
    c. Pelvic limb
    d. Diaphragm
22. Which muscle cells have single nuclei?
    a. Skeletal and cardiac
    b. Skeletal and smooth
    c. Smooth and cardiac
    d. Skeletal only
23. Cattle and swine display what type of estrous cycle?
    a. Polyestrous
    b. Seasonally polyestrous
    c. Diestrous
    d. Monoestrous
24. Which species is an induced ovulator?
    a. Bovine
    b. Equine
    c. Canine
    d. Feline
25. In which stage of the estrous cycle does the corpus luteum develop?
    a. Proestrus
    b. Estrus
    c. Metestrus
    d. Diestrous
26. Which reaction is the result of sympathetic nervous system stimulation?
    a. Decreased heart rate
    b. Dilated pupils
    c. Increased GI activity
    d. Increased salivation
27. The hormone produced by a developing ovarian follicle is:
    a. Estrogen
    b. Progesterone
    c. Prolactin
    d. Oxytocin
28. To achieve a normal pregnancy, the blastocyst attaches to what structure?
    a. Endometrium
    b. Placenta
    c. Oviduct
    d. Cervix
29. Giving birth is known as:
    a. Parturition
    b. Gestation
    c. Lactation
    d. Estrous
30. From the estrous cycle to parturition, in which order are the following hormones released?
    a. Estrogen, oxytocin, progesterone
    b. Oxytocin, estrogen, progesterone
    c. Estrogen, progesterone, oxytocin
    d. Progesterone, estrogen, oxytocin
31. All of the following are types of chorion attachments *except*:
    a. Diffuse
    b. Cotyledonary
    c. Zonary
    d. Polycyton
32. A pregnant bitch has what kind of placentation?
    a. Zonary
    b. Cotyledonary
    c. Diffuse
    d. Discoid
33. The canine uterus is shaped like the letter:
    a. U
    b. Y
    c. J
    d. V
34. How many mammary glands are typically found on a bitch?
    a. 8–12
    b. 12–14
    c. 4–6
    d. 10–16
35. Which reaction is the result of parasympathetic nervous system stimulation?
    a. Bronchodilation
    b. Pupil dilation
    c. Decreased GI motility
    d. Decreased heart rate
36. The neurotransmitter that is most responsible for the "flight or fight" reaction is:
    a. Epinephrine
    b. Acetylcholine
    c. Dopamine
    d. Serotonin
37. In the healthy heart, the heartbeat is initiated by the:
    a. SA node
    b. Purkinje fibers
    c. Vagus nerve
    d. AV node

38. On an electrocardiogram, the T wave is most closely associated with:
   a. Atrial depolarization
   b. Atrial repolarization
   c. Ventricular depolarization
   d. Ventricular repolarization
39. On inspiration, the pressure in the thoracic cavity, compared with ambient air pressure, is:
   a. Negative
   b. Positive
   c. Same as the ambient air pressure
   d. Fluctuating
40. In the healthy awake cat, the primary stimulus within blood for respiration is:
   a. Increased CO_2
   b. Decreased O_2
   c. Increased lactic acid
   d. Increased K+
41. An increased packed cell volume (PCV) could be indicative of:
   a. Liver disease
   b. Anemia
   c. Leukocytosis
   d. Dehydration
42. Apnea will cause:
   a. Metabolic acidosis
   b. Metabolic alkalosis
   c. Respiratory acidosis
   d. Respiratory alkalosis
43. Which of the following nutrients can be used for gluconeogenesis?
   a. Long-chain fatty acids
   b. Amino acids
   c. Vitamin C
   d. Iron
44. Cataracts result from a problem with transparency of the:
   a. Cornea
   b. Vitreous humor
   c. Lens
   d. Aqueous humor
45. Within the eye, the choroid is located between which two structures?
   a. Sclera and retina
   b. Iris and pupil
   c. Lens and cornea
   d. Optic nerve and fovea centralis
46. Which of the following are considered to be a category of lipids?
   a. Neutral fats
   b. Steroids
   c. Phospholipids
   d. All of the above
47. Which of the following processes is *not* a function of insulin?
   a. Increased glucose transport into muscle
   b. Lipogenesis
   c. Fatty acid synthesis
   d. Increased blood pressure
48. Which endocrine cells of the pancreatic islets produce the hormone glucagon?
   a. Alpha cells
   b. Beta cells
   c. Delta cells
   d. Somatostatin
49. Long-term use of glucocorticoids will:
   a. Increase lymphocyte production
   b. Increase plasma protein levels
   c. Suppress the immune system
   d. Decrease blood glucose levels
50. Nociceptors are important for detecting:
   a. Color
   b. Warmth
   c. Lactic acid
   d. Pain
51. The sensation of hunger falls under which general sense?
   a. Tactile sensation
   b. Pain sensation
   c. Proprioception
   d. Visceral sensation
52. The vagus nerve is cranial nerve ________.
   a. X
   b. XII
   c. V
   d. VI
53. The cranial nerves originate from the:
   a. Cerebellum
   b. Spinal cord
   c. Brainstem
   d. Cerebrum
54. Glaucoma is:
   a. Decreased pressure in the posterior chamber of the eye
   b. Increased pressure in the posterior chamber of the eye
   c. Increased pressure in the anterior chamber of the eye
   d. Decreased pressure in the anterior chamber of the eye
55. Aqueous humor is formed in which chamber of the eye?
   a. Posterior chamber
   b. Anterior chamber
   c. Canal of Schlemm
   d. Cornea
56. Clients should be cautioned against sticking Q-tips in the ears of their pets because they could rupture the:
   a. Oval window
   b. Round window
   c. Cochlea
   d. Tympanic membrane
57. Which condition would be typical of hypothyroidism?
   a. Decreased water consumption
   b. Oily hair coat
   c. Very active
   d. Weight gain
58. In dairy cattle, the teats and udder are gently washed before milking to stimulate milk letdown by releasing one of the following:
   a. Adrenalin
   b. Norepinephrine
   c. Dopamine
   d. Oxytocin

59. Which hormone helps to trigger and maintain lactation?
a. FSH
b. Prolactin
c. LH
d. TSH

60. Lymph nodes that are found medial to the caudal part of the jaw are the:
a. Popliteal nodes
b. Inguinal nodes
c. Mandibular nodes
d. Prescapular nodes

61. A pregnant rodent has what kind of placentation?
a. Zonary
b. Cotyledonary
c. Diffuse
d. Discoid

62. The neurohypophysis is an anatomic section of which of the following?
a. Hypothalamus
b. Adrenal gland
c. Pancreas

63. The portal vein:
a. Carries blood from the spleen to the heart
b. Delivers blood to the liver
c. Delivers blood to the kidney
d. Carries blood from the lungs to the heart

64. To proceed from a point between the eyes to the tip of a dog's nose, you would move
a. Rostrally
b. Cranially
c. Caudally
d. Laterally

65. Typically, what percentage of an animal's body weight consists of blood?
a. 0.10%
b. 1%
c. 8%
d. 30%

66. A dog that weighs 10 kg would have approximately how much blood?
a. 50 mL
b. 800 mL
c. 1.5 L
d. 2 L

67. Which of the following dissections could be made without cutting through a bone-to-bone joint?
a. Forelimb from the body
b. Hind limb from the body
c. Head from the neck
d. Tail from the body

68. If you were to grasp your hands behind your head at the base of your skull, your hands would be over which bone of the skull?
a. Occipital
b. Frontal
c. Temporal
d. Parietal

69. The glucose absorbed from the GI tract may be stored in the liver as glycogen through a process known as what?
a. Glycogenesis
b. Gluconeogenesis
c. Glycogenolysis
d. Fatty acid synthesis

70. The process of voice production usually begins in which location?
a. Pharynx
b. Larynx
c. Thorax
d. Trachea

71. Essential nutrients can be divided into how many categories?
a. 3
b. 4
c. 6
d. 10

72. Efferent nerves carry nerve impulses:
a. To the body from the central nervous system
b. To the body from the spinal cord
c. From the body to the central nervous system
d. From one part of a limb to another part of the same limb

73. The name for the bile acid–lipid units that carry fat within the gut is:
a. LPL
b. Micelles
c. VLDL
d. Chylomicrons

74. Which type of RNA copies the information in the DNA?
a. Messenger RNA
b. Ribosomal RNA
c. Copy RNA
d. Transfer RNA

75. Bile acids are important in the digestion of:
a. Carbohydrates
b. Electrolytes
c. Fats
d. Proteins

76. Which of the following lowers blood glucose?
a. Insulin
b. Glucagon
c. Epinephrine
d. Glucocorticoids

77. Which system is considered to be the largest and most extensive organ system in the body?
a. Integument
b. Cardiovascular
c. Digestive
d. Central nervous system

78. Different nitrogen bases are found in both DNA and RNA nucleotides. Which nucleotide is only found in DNA?
a. Adenine (A)
b. Cytosine (C)
c. Guanine (G)
d. Thymine (T)

79. The P wave component of a QRS complex usually corresponds to:
a. Atrial contraction
b. Ventricular contraction
c. Atrial relaxation
d. Electrical conduction in Purkinje fibers

80. The islets of Langerhans are found in the:
a. Spleen
b. Pancreas
c. Liver
d. Kidney

81. Which of the following is the basic functional unit of the kidney?
a. Nephron
b. Calyces
c. Hilus
d. Medulla

82. The kidneys are located in which cavity?
a. Peritoneal cavity
b. Pelvic cavity
c. Retroperitoneal cavity
d. Abdominal cavity

83. Which circulatory system is under the highest pressure?
a. Pulmonary
b. Coronary
c. Systemic
d. Capillaries

84. Fat in the lymph would most likely be associated with:
a. Micelles
b. Chylomicrons
c. VLDL cholesterol
d. LDL cholesterol

85. The mesovarium ligament supports which organ?
a. Testicles
b. Ovaries
c. Oviduct
d. Uterus

86. Milk fever in dairy cows is typically treated with:
a. IV glucose
b. IV calcium
c. Atropine
d. Antibiotics

87. For an animal that had lost RBCs to a moderate hookworm infection, the capillary refill time would be expected to be:
a. Less than 2 seconds
b. Greater than 4 seconds
c. Greater than 2 minutes
d. Greater than 4 minutes

88. A pulse taken from the inguinal area of a dog would be from the:
a. Femoral artery
b. Axillary artery
c. Popliteal artery
d. Saphenous artery

89. The "knee" in the forelimb of a horse would be called the ______ in the human.
a. Hip joint
b. Wrist joint
c. Finger joint
d. Knee joint

90. The linea alba on a standing cat is ____________ to the spinal cord.
a. Ventral
b. Dorsal
c. Medial
d. Contralateral

91. Arteries have relatively thick walls composed of three layers. Which layer is the outermost layer?
a. Tunica intima
b. Tunica adventitia
c. Tunica media
d. Arteries only have one layer

92. Yellow mucous membranes would suggest:
a. Renal disease
b. Hepatic disease
c. Shock
d. Dehydration

93. A capillary refill time of 2 seconds would suggest which of the following?
a. Shock
b. Anemia
c. A healthy animal
d. Dehydration

94. What is the name of the large, flat projection located lateral to the head of the femur?
a. Lesser trochanter
b. Greater trochanter
c. Trochanteric fossa
d. Tubercle

95. The femur articulates distally with the tibia, forming the:
a. Hip joint
b. Stifle joint
c. Tarsal joint
d. Shoulder joint

96. What is the term for a part closer to a point of attachment or to the trunk?
a. Distal
b. Lateral
c. Proximal
d. Superficial

97. What is the term used below the carpus for the surface directed caudally or ventrally?
a. Plantar
b. Sagittal
c. Palmar
d. Longitudinal

98. In growing bone, where does lengthening take place?
a. Epiphyseal plate
b. Metaphysis
c. Diaphysis
d. Periosteal plane

99. Which layer of bone tissue is necessary for the attachment of ligaments and tendons?
a. Periosteum
b. Endosteum
c. Cartilage
d. Meniscus

100. The fibrous covering around the part of the bone *not* covered by articular cartilage is:
a. Endosteum
b. Ligament
c. Tendon
d. Periosteum

101. Which two valves comprise the atrioventricular valves?
a. Mitral valve, pulmonic valve
b. Aortic valve, pulmonic valve
c. Mitral valve, tricuspid valve
d. Pulmonic valve, tricuspid valve

102. What two valves comprise the semilunar valves?
a. Mitral valve, pulmonic valve
b. Pulmonic valve, aortic valve
c. Mitral valve, tricuspid valve
d. Pulmonic valve, tricuspid valve

103. The normal dentition pattern for an adult cat is:
a. Incisor 3/3, Canine 1/1, Premolar 3/2, Molar 1/1
b. Incisor 3/3, Canine 1/1, Premolar 4/3, Molar 2/2
c. Incisor 2/2, Canine 1/1, Premolar 3/2, Molar 2/1
d. Incisor 2/2, Canine 1/1, Premolar 4/4, Molar 1/1

104. In the avian species, the ventral wall of the esophagus is greatly expanded to form the:
a. Proventriculus
b. Crop
c. Gizzard
d. Duodenum

105. What is the average number of air sacs that birds have?
a. 4
b. 6
c. 8
d. 9

106. In birds, the cloaca is:
a. An appendage suspended from the head
b. A blind sac at the distal end of the jejunum
c. A cleft in the hard palate
d. A common passage for fecal, urinary, and reproductive systems

107. In the avian species, the gizzard is also referred to as the:
a. Proventriculus
b. Ventriculus
c. Crop
d. Colon

108. Which muscle is the main muscle for inspiration?
a. Epaxial muscle
b. Diaphragm
c. Internal abdominal oblique
d. Hypaxial muscles

109. The uvea consists of the iris, ciliary body, and:
a. Neural tunic
b. Fibrous tunic
c. Anterior chamber
d. Choroid

110. The front surface of the lens is in contact with which of the following?
a. Vitreous humor
b. Aqueous humor
c. Retina
d. Sclera

111. The muscular structure that separates the right and left ventricles is called the interventricular:
a. Sternum
b. Coronary muscle
c. Septum
d. Myocardium

112. The muscular layer that makes up the majority of the heart mass is the:
a. Myocardium
b. Endocardium
c. Myometrium
d. Pericardium

113. The major artery that carries blood out of the left ventricle is the:
a. Subclavian artery
b. Carotid artery
c. Pulmonary artery
d. Aorta

114. All of the following major vessels contribute to blood flowing into the cranial vena cava *except* the:
a. Brachiocephalic vein
b. Thoracic duct
c. Azygos vein
d. Femoral vein

115. Which structure drains blood from the stomach, intestine, and pancreas and flows directly to the liver?
a. Hepatic veins
b. Hepatic portal vein
c. Hepatic artery
d. Portosystemic shunt

116. The coronary veins empty blood via the coronary sinus into the:
a. Left atrium
b. Right atrium
c. Left ventricle
d. Right ventricle

117. The pulmonary circulation is under:
a. High pressure
b. Low pressure
c. Partial pressure
d. Equilibrium

118. How many teeth does an adult dog have?
a. 28
b. 32
c. 42
d. 50

119. Which of these is *not* a division of the small intestine?
a. Duodenum
b. Ilium
c. Ileum
d. Jejunum

120. Which abdominal organ is absent in the horse and rat?
a. Right kidney
b. Gallbladder
c. Pancreas
d. Cecum

121. What is unique about the ruminant oral cavity?
a. Presence of a dental pad
b. Absence of salivary glands
c. Absence of molars
d. Presence of needle teeth

122. What is the actual true stomach called in ruminants?
a. Abomasum
b. Reticulum
c. Rumen
d. Omasum

123. What is the most common site of feed impactions in a horse?
a. Sternal flexure
b. Diaphragmatic flexure
c. Stomach
d. Pelvic flexure

124. Food is moved along the digestive tract by the process known as:
a. Mastication
b. Prehension
c. Peristalsis
d. Elimination

125. The most distal portion of the monogastric stomach is the:
a. Fundus
b. Antrum
c. Cardia
d. Pylorus

126. Which one of the following are *not* found in the fundus and body of the stomach:
a. Parietal cells
b. Chief cells
c. G cells
d. Mucous cells

127. Which of the following is *not* a hormone produced or released by the pituitary gland?
a. Luteinizing hormone
b. Oxytocin
c. Growth hormone
d. Calcitonin

128. Which of the following is a ductless system?
a. Exocrine system
b. Endocrine system
c. Lymphatic system
d. All of the above systems contain ducts

129. The hormone responsible for maintaining pregnancy is:
a. Oxytocin
b. Luteinizing hormone
c. Estrogen
d. Progesterone

130. The structure produced immediately after an ovarian follicle has ruptured and released its ovum is the:
a. Corpus callosum
b. Corpus luteum
c. Corpus albicans
d. Graafian follicle

131. A deficiency in antidiuretic hormone causes:
a. Diabetes insipidus
b. Diabetes mellitus
c. Cushing disease
d. Pancreatic insufficiency

132. The kidney produces what hormone?
a. Antidiuretic hormone
b. Adrenocorticotropic hormone
c. Erythropoietin
d. Adrenal cortex hormone

133. Which hormone is produced by the beta cells in the pancreas?
a. Insulin
b. Glucagon
c. Glycogen
d. Somatostatin

134. Which hormone stimulates the growth and development of the cortex of the adrenal gland and the release of some of its hormones?
a. Thyroid-stimulating hormone
b. Adrenocorticotropic hormone
c. Prolactin
d. Follicle-stimulating hormone

135. The endocrine structure responsible for secreting melatonin is:
a. Pituitary gland
b. Spleen
c. Thymus
d. Pineal gland

136. The lymphatic system is *not* involved in:
a. Waste material transport
b. Protein transport
c. Carbohydrate transport
d. Fluid transport

137. Lymph from the digestive system is known as what?
a. GALT
b. Haustra
c. Chylomicrons
d. Chyle

138. The lymphatic structure found in the small intestines responsible for the transport of fats and fat-soluble vitamins is:
a. Afferent lymphatic vessels
b. Lacteals
c. Trabeculae
d. Spleen

139. Which of the following is a lymphatic structure?
a. Bile duct
b. Islets of Langerhans
c. Thyroid
d. Tonsil

140. Which structure is *not* found in the brainstem?
a. Midbrain
b. Pons
c. Hypothalamus
d. Medulla oblongata

141. The point at which blood vessels, nerves, and ureters enter and leave the kidneys is known as:
a. Medulla
b. Hilus
c. Cortex
d. Pelvis

142. How much urine do horses produce a day?
a. 10 mL/kg/day
b. 20 mL/kg/day
c. 40 mL/kg/day
d. 60 mL/kg/day

143. Ruminants have what type of placentation?
a. Cotyledonary
b. Zonary
c. Diffuse
d. Discoid

144. Which of the following is a posterior pituitary hormone?
a. Luteinizing hormone
b. Growth hormone
c. Oxytocin
d. Follicle-stimulating hormone

145. Sperm cells are produced by the:
a. Seminiferous tubule
b. Epididymis
c. Vas deferens
d. Seminal vesicles

146. Which domestic species lacks the bulbourethral gland, also called Cowper's gland?
a. Equine
b. Feline
c. Canine
d. Bovine

147. All of the following are induced ovulators *except*:
a. Rabbit
b. Rat
c. Cat
d. Ferret

148. The time period from the beginning of one heat cycle to the beginning of the next is called:
a. Estrous
b. Estrus
c. Ovulation
d. The mating cycle

149. Which muscle is responsible for pulling the testicles closer to the body?
a. Retractor penis muscle
b. Cremaster muscle
c. Kegel muscle
d. Retractor testicle muscle

150. Not all follicles activated in a particular ovarian cycle develop fully and ovulate. This is known as:
a. Ovulation
b. Follicular atresia
c. Graafian follicle
d. Corpus albicans

151. Which primary ovarian structure is responsible for the release of estrogen?
a. Follicle
b. Placenta
c. Corpus hemorrhagicum
d. Corpus luteum

152. What is the normal gestational period for dogs?
a. 36 days
b. 54 days
c. 63 days
d. 120 days

153. The average gestational length in the ferret is:
a. 69 days
b. 42 days
c. 151 days
d. 20 days

154. The condition known as pseudopregnancy can result from an exaggerated:
a. Anestrus
b. Metestrus
c. Diestrus
d. Proestrus

155. The thorax is normally under:
a. Partial pressure
b. Positive pressure
c. Equilibrium
d. Negative pressure

156. Skeletal muscles are:
a. Under voluntary control
b. Nonstriated
c. Under involuntary control
d. Found in the walls of hollow organs

157. The two main minerals that make up bone are:
a. Calcium and magnesium
b. Sodium and potassium
c. Calcium and phosphorus
d. Calcium and potassium

158. Basic functions of bones include all of the following *except*:
a. Protection
b. Storage
c. Leverage
d. Metabolism

159. The hormone primarily responsible for preventing hypocalcemia is:
a. T4
b. Parathyroid hormone
c. Calcitonin
d. Vitamin D

160. The bone cells responsible for the removal of bone are:
a. Osteoclasts
b. Osteoblasts
c. Chondroblasts
d. Chondroclasts

161. The periosteum:
a. Covers joint cavities
b. Lines the heart
c. Lines the marrow cavity of bones
d. Covers the outer surface of bones

162. Bones come in all of the following shapes *except*:
a. Flat
b. Short
c. Regular
d. Long

163. The shaft of the bone is also called the:
a. Trunk
b. Epiphysis
c. Periosteum
d. Diaphysis

164. An example of a short bone would be a:
a. Vertebra
b. Tarsal bone
c. Scapula
d. Patella

165. The skull bone that articulates with the first cervical vertebra is the:
a. Parietal bone
b. Temporal bone
c. Occipital bone
d. Frontal bone

166. The bones known collectively as the ossicles include all of the following *except* the:
a. Sphenoid
b. Malleus
c. Stapesus
d. Incus

167. How many cervical vertebrae does a cat have?
a. 13
b. 7
c. 3
d. 10

168. The first cervical vertebra, C1, is referred to as the:
a. Axis
b. Atlas
c. Arch
d. Auricle

169. The breastbone is the:
a. Hyoid
b. Septum
c. Tubercle
d. Sternum

170. The most caudal portion of the sternum is called the:
a. Xiphoid
b. Coccyx
c. Manubrium
d. Costal

171. Claws, hooves, and horns are made up of which type of cell?
a. Keratinized
b. Agglutinated
c. Calcified
d. Crystallized

172. Which of the following is considered a part of the external structure of the equine hoof?
a. Digital cushion
b. Corium
c. Lateral cartilage
d. Frog

173. Adult cattle have how many upper incisors?
a. 6
b. 4
c. 0
d. 5

174. The anatomic term for synovial joints is:
a. Fibroarthroses
b. Amphiarthroses
c. Synarthroses
d. Diarthroses

175. Which joint is *not* a synovial joint?
a. Hinge joint
b. Gliding joint
c. Swinging joint
d. Pivot joint

176. The area of the kidney where urine collection occurs before entering the ureter is known as the:
a. Renal pelvis
b. Hilus
c. Cortex
d. Medulla

177. In the kidney, the primary site of action for ADH is in the:
a. Loop of Henle
b. Proximal convoluted tubule
c. Glomerulus
d. Collecting ducts

178. The renal corpuscle is located in the:
a. Renal pelvis
b. Hilus
c. Medulla
d. Cortex

179. The renal corpuscle is comprised of the:
a. Glomerulus and Bowman's capsule
b. Collecting ducts and proximal convoluted tubule
c. Descending and ascending loops of Henle
d. Collecting ducts and afferent arteriole

180. The urinary bladder is *not* responsible for:
a. Urine storage
b. Urine filtration
c. Urine collecting
d. Urine release

181. The trunk of an animal is defined as:
a. The front half of the animal
b. The back half of the animal
c. The thorax of the animal
d. The thorax and abdomen of the animal

182. The middle phalanx is located:
a. Lateral to the distal phalanx
b. Distal to the distal phalanx
c. Medial to the distal phalanx
d. Proximal to the distal phalanx

183. The humeroradioulnar joint is located:
a. Lateral to the carpus
b. Distal to the left of the carpus
c. Medial to the carpus
d. Proximal to the carpus

184. Which organ is the largest abdominal organ in the body?
a. Stomach
b. Pancreas
c. Kidney
d. Liver

185. The leg bone responsible for minimal support is the:
a. Fibula
b. Femur
c. Tibia
d. Humerus

186. The large muscle of the caudal aspect of the canine lower hind leg is the:
a. Tibialis anterior
b. Gracilis
c. Semimembranosus
d. Gastrocnemius

187. Which of the following is *not* a muscle in the abdominal group?
a. External oblique
b. Rectus abdominis
c. Latissimus dorsi
d. Internal oblique

188. How many muscle heads are in the canine triceps brachii group?
a. 4
b. 3
c. 2
d. 1

189. Fascia is described as:
a. The facial muscular surface
b. A tough sheet of fibrous connective tissue
c. A broad band of muscle fiber
d. A lacy network of connective tissue

190. The deltoid muscles allow fine movements of the:
a. Shoulder
b. Hip
c. Elbow
d. Jaw

191. Which of the following structures suspends the larynx from the skull?
a. Pharynx
b. Epiglottis
c. Hyoid apparatus
d. Mediastinum

192. The two gastric sphincters of the canine are:
a. Rectal and cecal
b. Cardiac and pyloric
c. Cardiac and rectal
d. Pyloric and rectal

193. The dorsal plane divides the:
a. Upper and lower halves of the body
b. Front and back halves of the body
c. Head from the rest of the body
d. Right and left sides of the body

194. The middle portion of the small intestine is the:
a. Jejunum
b. Jejunem
c. Jajunem
d. Jujunem

195. The __________ pleura overlays organs in the body.
a. Parietal
b. Viscous
c. Partial
d. Visceral

196. Which sinus is *not* considered to be a "true" sinus of the dog?
a. Frontal sinus
b. External nares
c. Paranasal sinuses
d. Maxillary sinus

197. The triangular-shaped muscle that originates from the dorsal midline and inserts on the spin of the scapula is which of the following?
a. Latissimus dorsi
b. Brachiocephalicus
c. External intercostals
d. Trapezius

198. The cardiovascular system has four components. Which of the following is *not* part of the system?
a. Heart
b. Blood circulation
c. Blood vessels
d. Lungs

199. The appendicular skeleton includes the:
a. Os cordis
b. Ribs
c. Pelvic girdle
d. Clavicles

200. Which animal does *not* have an os penis?
a. Dog
b. Cat
c. Wolf
d. Pig

201. Which statement best describes short bones?
a. Greater size in one dimension than another
b. Filled with spongy bone and marrow spaces
c. Thick outer layer of compact bone
d. Irregularly shaped bones that make up the spinal column

202. The scapula is an example of a:
a. Long bone
b. Short bone
c. Flat bone
d. Irregular bone

203. An example of an irregular bone is:
a. Cervical vertebra 1
b. Metacarpal 3
c. Ulna
d. Scapula

204. Which of the following is *not* part of the axial skeleton?
a. Cervical vertebra 3
b. Scapula
c. Skull
d. Thoracic vertebra 1

205. A skull suture is an example of what type of joint?
a. Diarthrosis
b. Synarthrosis
c. Amphiarthrosis
d. Cartilaginous

206. The only true pivot joint in the body is the:
a. Spheroidal
b. Elbow
c. Carpal
d. Atlantoaxial

207. Muscles and ligaments attach to structures on bony surfaces. Which of the following is *not* found in the forelimb?
a. Trochanter
b. Tuberosity
c. Spine
d. Epicondyle

208. Which structure will *not* allow blood vessels and nerves to pass through?
a. Meatus
b. Sinus
c. Foramen
d. Facet

209. The joint between the bony rib and cartilaginous portion of the rib is called the:
a. Cartilaginous junction
b. Chondralcartilaginous junction
c. Costochondral junction
d. Costicartilaginous junction

210. Dogs have how many cervical, thoracic, and lumbar vertebrae?
a. 7, 13, 6
b. 7, 12, 7
c. 6, 13, 7
d. 7, 13, 7

211. Horses have how many cervical, thoracic, and lumbar vertebrae?
a. 7, 13, 7
b. 7, 18, 7
c. 6, 7, 18
d. 7, 18, 4

212. What is the value of X in this cow's dentition chart? I 0/3; C 0/1; P 3/3; M X/3
a. 4
b. 3
c. 2
d. 1

213. The valves that prevent backflow of blood from the arteries to the ventricles are called the:
a. Tricuspid
b. Bicuspid
c. Mitral
d. Semilunar

214. Which structures disseminate electrical impulses across the ventricles?
a. Perkinje fibers
b. Purkinje fibers
c. Purkinge fibers
d. Perkingi fibers

215. Systole is:
a. Contraction of the atria and ventricles
b. Relaxation of the atria and ventricles
c. Contraction of the atria and relaxation of the ventricles
d. Relaxation of the atria and contraction of the ventricles

216. The aorta leaves the heart from the:
a. Left ventricle
b. Right ventricle
c. Left atrium
d. Right atrium

217. Blood enters the heart from the pulmonary veins in the:
a. Left ventricle
b. Right ventricle
c. Left atrium
d. Right atrium

218. Which circulation system is under the highest pressure?
a. Coronary circulation
b. Systemic circulation
c. Pulmonary circulation
d. All of the circulatory systems are under the same pressure

219. The name of the hole between the cardiac atria that closes at birth in the mammal is:
a. Aortic hiatus
b. Foramen
c. Fossa
d. Foramen ovale

220. Which of these is *not* a characteristic of lymph?
a. Tissue fluids
b. A large number of neutrophils
c. B cells
d. Part of the circulatory system

221. The tricuspid valve controls the flow of blood:
a. Into the left ventricle
b. Out of the left ventricle
c. Into the right ventricle
d. Out of the right ventricle

222. The thymus:
a. Is another name for the thyroid gland
b. Produces cells that destroy foreign substances
c. Is more prominent in adults than in young animals
d. Is located in the cranial abdomen

223. The eardrum is also called the:
a. Pinna
b. Tympanic membrane
c. Eustachian tubes
d. Cochlea

224. Which organ is most commonly associated with the capacity for extramedullary hematopoiesis if necessary?
a. Spleen
b. Pancreas
c. Lung
d. Prostate

225. Efferent neurons are part of what system?
a. Motor
b. Interneuron
c. Sensory
d. Extraneuron

226. Afferent neurons are part of what system?
a. Motor
b. Interneuron
c. Sensory
d. Extraneuron

227. The function of the red blood cell is to:
a. Provide defense from foreign invaders
b. Act as a phagocyte
c. Carry oxygen to the tissues
d. Respond to the need for clotting

228. Which artery carries deoxygenated blood?
a. Aorta
b. Pulmonary
c. Coronary
d. Carotid

229. Albumin is found in the blood and is a type of:
a. Lipoprotein
b. Phospholipid
c. Enzyme
d. Protein

230. Albumin is produced in the:
a. Liver
b. Red bone marrow
c. Lymph nodes
d. Pancreas

231. The production of platelets is known as:
a. Hemostasis
b. Thrombopoiesis
c. Homeostasis
d. Coagulation

232. What cells are involved in antibody production?
a. Monocytes
b. Neutrophils
c. Lymphocytes
d. Basophils

233. An increase in WBCs is referred to as which of the following?
a. Leukopenia
b. Anemia
c. Leukocytosis
d. Thrombocytopenia

234. Which of the following is known as the largest gland in the body?
a. Pancreas
b. Thyroid
c. Liver
d. Spleen

235. Bile is produced by which of the following organs?
a. Gallbladder
b. Liver
c. Pancreas
d. Spleen

236. What causes the gallbladder to contract?
a. The release of CCK
b. The release of glucagon
c. The production of bile
d. The gallbladder contracts involuntarily after it is filled

237. Red blood cell production is stimulated by:
a. Hypoxia and erythropoietin
b. Erythropoietin and thrombocytes
c. Fibrinogen and acetylcholine
d. Leukocytes

238. What structure is the pacemaker of the heart?
a. Bundle of His
b. Purkinje fibers
c. Atrioventricular node
d. Sinoatrial node

239. What is meant by cardiac output?
a. Strokes (beats) per minute
b. Volume of blood pumped per stroke (beat)
c. Volume of blood pumped per minute
d. Strokes (beats) per volume

240. In the normal heart ECG, the QRS complex corresponds to what portion of the cardiac cycle?
a. The QRS complex is the entire ECG cycle
b. Atrial depolarization
c. Ventricular depolarization
d. Ventricular repolarization

241. The term for accumulation of fluid in the abdominal cavity is:
a. Pleural effusion
b. Ascites
c. Abscess
d. Pneumothorax

242. Which of the following mammals does *not* have a gallbladder?
a. Dogs
b. Cats
c. Horses
d. Animals cannot function without a gallbladder

243. Which organ is considered both an exocrine and endocrine organ?
a. Small intestine
b. Thyroid
c. Pancreas
d. Kidneys

244. The islets of Langerhans are associated with which organ?
a. Pancreas
b. Liver
c. Kidneys
d. Adrenal glands

245. Which cells within the pancreas produce insulin?
a. Alpha cells
b. Beta cells
c. Delta cells
d. All of the cells within the pancreas produce insulin

246. Which of the following hormones is produced by the ovaries late in pregnancy?
a. Estrogen
b. Progesterone
c. Relaxin
d. Testosterone

247. Which of the following are clinical signs of diabetes mellitus?
a. Polyuria
b. Polydipsia
c. Polyphagia
d. All of the above

248. Which body system is the most important route of waste-product removal?
a. Respiratory system
b. Urinary system
c. Digestive system
d. All of the systems are equal in importance for waste-product removal

249. Which of the following is the correct path for urine elimination?
a. Ureter, kidneys, urethra, bladder
b. Kidneys, urethra, bladder, ureter
c. Kidney, ureters, bladder, urethra
d. Urethra, bladder, ureter, kidneys

250. Which organ(s) is/are responsible for acid-base balance regulation?
a. Lungs
b. Kidneys
c. Liver
d. Spleen

251. The indented area on the medial side of the kidney is known as the:
a. Porta hepatis
b. Hilum
c. Convex
d. Cortex

252. What is the basic functional unit of the kidney?
a. Cortex
b. Nephron
c. Bowman's capsule
d. Loop of Henle

253. Approximately how many nephrons are in each kidney of the cow?
  a. 700,000
  b. 100,000
  c. 1,000,000
  d. 4,000,000
254. In which portion of the kidney is the renal corpuscle located?
  a. Cortex
  b. Medulla
  c. Renal sinus
  d. Hilum
255. Approximately what percentage of blood, pumped by the heart, goes to the kidneys?
  a. 5%
  b. 10%
  c. 25%
  d. 60%
256. Which of the following is considered the main mechanism in which the kidneys perform waste elimination?
  a. Filtration
  b. Reabsorption
  c. Secretion
  d. All of the above
257. Which of the following hormones are responsible for urine volume regulation?
  a. ADH
  b. Aldosterone
  c. Glucagon
  d. Both a and b
258. The ureters are composed of how many layers?
  a. 1
  b. 2
  c. 3
  d. 4
259. Which of the following conditions can cause prerenal uremia?
  a. Dehydration
  b. Congestive heart failure
  c. Shock
  d. All of the above
260. Which of the following is/are considered functions of the male testes?
  a. Spermatogenesis
  b. Hormone production
  c. Urine formation
  d. Both a and b
261. Which of the following best defines the term cryptorchidism?
  a. Torsion of one or both testicles
  b. One or both testes do not fully descend into the scrotum
  c. The surgical removal of both testicles
  d. An inflammatory condition of the testis
262. A flat ribbon-like structure that lies along the surface of the testis is known as:
  a. Cremaster muscle
  b. Vas deferens
  c. Epididymis
  d. Seminiferous tubule
263. All of the following common domestic animals have a bulbourethral gland (Cowper's gland) *except*:
  a. Cat
  b. Dog
  c. Horse
  d. Cow
264. The mesosalpinx ligament within the female reproductive tract supports which of the following structures?
  a. Uterus
  b. Ovaries
  c. Oviduct
  d. Vagina
265. Which of the following species is *not* considered to be multiparous?
  a. Dogs
  b. Sows
  c. Cattle
  d. Cats
266. When an animal is said to be in a period of temporary ovarian inactivity, this is known as:
  a. Anestrus
  b. Diestrus
  c. Pseudocyesis
  d. Heat
267. During pregnancy, what provides the life-support system for the developing fetus?
  a. Ovum
  b. Uterus
  c. Amnion
  d. Placenta
268. What is the gestational period for cats?
  a. 56–69 days
  b. 271–291 days
  c. 42 days
  d. 19–20 days
269. Which of the following animals has the longest gestational period?
  a. Horses
  b. Sheep
  c. Elephants
  d. Cattle
270. Which of the following conditions does the term mastitis refer to?
  a. The production of colostrum from the mammary gland
  b. An infection of a mammary gland
  c. The mammary glands in male species only
  d. A hormone produced to allow for the production of milk
271. Which endocrine gland produces the hormone prolactin?
  a. Posterior pituitary
  b. Thyroid
  c. Anterior pituitary
  d. Ovaries
272. The testes are responsible for producing which of the following hormones?
  a. Estrogen
  b. Androgen
  c. Progestin
  d. Sex hormones

273. Which hormone is responsible for the movement of glucose into cells and its use for energy?
   a. Progestin
   b. Insulin
   c. Glucagon
   d. Calcitonin
274. Which organ is part of the endocrine system?
   a. Pancreas
   b. Kidneys
   c. Stomach
   d. All of the above
275. Which hormone is secreted by the anterior pituitary gland?
   a. Melanocyte-stimulating hormone
   b. Adrenocorticotropic hormone
   c. Prolactin
   d. Follicle-stimulating hormone
276. Which hormone is responsible for triggering and maintaining lactation?
   a. Follicle-stimulating hormone
   b. Luteinizing hormone
   c. Mineralocorticoid hormone
   d. Prolactin hormone
277. Waste excretion is a requirement for maintaining homeostasis and can be achieved through which route of excretion?
   a. Urinary system
   b. Respiratory system
   c. Digestive system
   d. All of the above are routes of waste excretion
278. The kidneys are located in which cavity?
   a. Abdominal cavity
   b. Retroperitoneal cavity
   c. Pelvic cavity
   d. Thoracic cavity
279. Which species does *not* have a smooth outer surface of the kidneys?
   a. Cats
   b. Dogs
   c. Cattle
   d. Horses
280. Which of the following arteries enters the kidney at this hilus?
   a. Aorta
   b. Renal artery
   c. Interlobar artery
   d. Iliac artery
281. The renal vein leaves the hilum of the kidney to join which vessel?
   a. Aorta
   b. Vena cava
   c. Hepatic vein
   d. Portal vein
282. How many types of white blood cells are there?
   a. 1
   b. 2
   c. 4
   d. 5
283. Which of the following white blood cells does *not* contain cytoplasmic granules?
   a. Eosinophls
   b. Neutrophils
   c. Monocytes
   d. Basophils
284. Birds contain an uropygial or preen gland located on the dorsal surface at the upper base of the tail. For what is this structure responsible?
   a. It secretes an oily, fatty substance that spreads throughout the feathers to clean and waterproof them
   b. It is responsible for the mating process
   c. It is responsible for the growth of feathers
   d. It is a scent gland
285. The vane is which part of the feather?
   a. The flattened weblike part of each side of the rachis
   b. The main feather shaft
   c. The opening of the feather shaft
   d. The opening at the base of the feather
286. Flight feathers within the wings of birds are known as:
   a. Retrices
   b. Remiges
   c. Auriculars
   d. Down feathers
287. Which portion of the digestive system in birds is responsible for grinding food products?
   a. Gizzard
   b. Proventriculus
   c. Atrioventricular node
   d. All of the above
288. The restrained heart rate of a small bird, approximately 25 g in body weight, is:
   a. 100–150 bpm
   b. 110–175 bpm
   c. 400–600 bpm
   d. 300–500 bpm
289. Where is the cloaca located in birds?
   a. The end of the digestive tract
   b. Distal to the stomach
   c. The throat
   d. At the base of the tail
290. Which layer of the skin is the most superficial?
   a. Dermis
   b. Epidermis
   c. Hypodermis
   d. None of these
291. Which layer of skin is composed of multiple layers of cells that are continually renewed?
   a. Dermis
   b. Epidermis
   c. Hypodermis
   d. All of the above
292. Which layer of skin contains the hair follicles, sebaceous glands, and sweat glands?
   a. Dermis
   b. Epidermis
   c. Hypodermis
   d. Both a and b

293. How many different cell shapes are found within the epithelial cells?
a. 1
b. 2
c. 3
d. 4

294. Squamous cells describe what shaped cells?
a. Column shaped
b. Square or cube shaped
c. Flattened in shape
d. Circular shaped

295. Epithelial cells that contain tiny hair-like projections that move foreign particles along the epithelial surface are known as:
a. Simple columnar epithelium
b. Ciliated epithelium
c. Stratified epithelium
d. Transitional epithelium

296. Which of the following connective tissues contains the highest density?
a. Blood
b. Cartilage
c. Fibrous connective tissue
d. Bone

297. Which tissue is responsible for forming bone marrow within the long bones and for the formation of the blood cells?
a. Hemopoietic tissue
b. Areolar tissue
c. Cartilage
d. Bone

298. The hormone primarily responsible for preventing hypercalcemia is:
a. T4
b. Parathyroid hormone
c. Calcitonin
d. Vitamin D

299. The mammary glands contain which type of connective tissue?
a. Tubular single
b. Alveolar single
c. Tubular multiple
d. Alveolar multiple

300. Which of the following bone tissues contain an internal meshwork of trabeculae with interconnected spaces that are filled with red bone marrow?
a. Cancellous bone
b. Compact bone
c. Spongy bone
d. Both a and c

301. Which substance covers the outer surface of all types of bone?
a. Cartilage
b. Bone marrow
c. Periosteum
d. Lamellae

302. The thorax is divided into right and left sides by a connective tissue septum known as the:
a. Mediastinum
b. Pericardium
c. Pulmonary pleura
d. Sternum

303. Which cavity lies immediately caudal to the thoracic cavity?
a. Pelvic cavity
b. Abdominal cavity
c. Pleural cavity
d. None of these

304. Which types of bones contain air-filled spaces known as sinuses that reduce the weight of the bone?
a. Sesamoid bones
b. Pneumatic bones
c. Splanchnic bone
d. Irregular bones

305. Cells that are responsible for laying down new bone are known as:
a. Osteoblasts
b. Osteoclasts
c. Ossification
d. Hemopoiesis

306. What is the formation called when one bone connects to another bone by articulation?
a. Hinge
b. Arthrosis
c. Cartilage
d. Ossification

307. Which of the following joints are immovable and connected by dense fibrous connective tissue?
a. Fibrous joints
b. Cartilaginous joints
c. Synovial joints
d. None, all joints are movable

308. The mandibular symphysis joins which of the following bones?
a. The two hip bones
b. Two vertebrae within the spinal column
c. Two halves of the mandible
d. The occipital and parietal bones

309. Which of the following is considered a range of movement that can occur in a synovial joint?
a. Abduction/adduction
b. Retraction
c. Protraction
d. All of the above

310. Which of the following correctly describes the joint movement of circumduction?
a. The moving body part twists on its own axis
b. The movement of an extremity of one end of a bone in a circular pattern
c. The animal moves the limb back toward the body
d. The animal moves the limb cranially

311. Which of the following is a type of synovial joint?
a. Plane/gliding
b. Condylar
c. Ball and socket
d. All of the above

312. Which of the following is an example of a hinge joint?
a. Hip
b. Shoulder
c. Stifle
d. Atlantoaxial joint

313. Which type of muscle contraction occurs when a muscle actually moves or shortens?
a. Isotonic contraction
b. Muscle tone
c. Isometric contraction
d. None of the above

314. Muscles that form a circular ring and serve to control the entrance or exit to a structure are known as:
a. Muscle tone
b. Sphincter muscles
c. Bursa
d. Extrinsic muscle

315. Which muscle type is responsible for moving the lips, cheeks, nostrils, eyelids, and external ears?
a. Sphincter muscle
b. Intrinsic muscle
c. Extrinsic muscle
d. Digastricus

316. Before birth, the testes begin to develop in the abdominal cavity near which organ?
a. Stomach
b. Kidneys
c. Bladder
d. Gallbladder

317. The scrotum is responsible for which of the following?
a. Regulation of temperature
b. Production of sperm
c. Housing of the testes
d. Both a and c

318. Which of the following male reproductive organs is a tube-like, connective tissue structure that contains blood vessels, nerves, lymphatic vessels, and the vas deferens?
a. Scrotum
b. Vaginal tunics
c. Spermatic cord
d. Pampiniform plexus

319. Which of the following is derived from the testicular veins, surrounds the testicular artery, and is described as multiple tiny veins?
a. Spermatic cord
b. Pampiniform plexus
c. Cremaster plexus
d. Vas deferens

320. What is the storage site for sperm after they detach from the Sertoli cells?
a. Epididymis
b. Vas deferens
c. Visceral vaginal tunic
d. Pampiniform plexus

321. The thick, outer layer that surrounds the testes in the scrotum and the spermatic cord is known as the:
a. Visceral vaginal tunic
b. Proper vaginal tunic
c. Parietal vaginal tunic
d. Both a and b

322. Below the tunics, a heavy, fibrous connective tissue capsule surrounds each testis. What is this known as?
a. Common vaginal tunic
b. Tunica albuginea
c. Pampiniform plexus
d. Septa

323. Where does spermatogenesis take place?
a. Seminiferous tubules
b. Epididymis
c. Spermatic cord
d. Pampiniform plexus

324. The vas deferens is responsible for which of the following actions?
a. To mature sperm
b. To store sperm before ejaculation
c. To propel spermatozoa and the fluid from the epididymis to the urethra during ejaculation
d. To produce spermatozoa

325. The accessory reproductive glands produce alkaline fluid that contains which of the following substances?
a. Electrolytes
b. Prostaglandins
c. Fructose
d. All of the above

326. Which of the following species does *not* contain seminal vesicles?
a. Bull
b. Cat
c. Dog
d. Both b and c

327. Which of the following animals does *not* have a prostate gland?
a. Dogs
b. Cats
c. Boar
d. Stallion
e. None of the above

328. The prostate gland completely surrounds which structure?
a. Testis
b. Epididymis
c. Urethra
d. Spermatic cord

329. Bulbourethral glands are also known as?
a. The prostate
b. Cowper's glands
c. Roots
d. Seminal glands

330. Which species contains short spines that cover the end of the glans of the penis?
a. Horses
b. Dogs
c. Ruminants
d. Cats

331. Which species contains a bone within the penis that is known as the os penis?
a. Dogs
b. Cats
c. Horses
d. Ruminants

332. Which structure can cause the male dog to become stuck or "tied" to the female during mating?
a. Testicles
b. Bulb of the glans
c. Os penis
d. None of the above

333. The anatomical plane that runs the length of the body and divides its right and left parts is known as the:
a. Median plane
b. Sagittal plane
c. Dorsal plane
d. Transverse plane

334. The thoracic cavity is considered to be in what anatomical direction from the abdomen?
a. Caudal
b. Cranial
c. Dorsal
d. Ventral

335. The duodenum exits the stomach on which side of the animal's abdomen?
a. Left
b. Right
c. Cranial
d. Caudal

336. A horse's shoulder is located in which anatomical direction to its hip?
a. Caudal
b. Cranial
c. Proximal
d. Ventral

337. The caudal end of the sternum is referred to as the:
a. Xiphoid process
b. Trochanter
c. Calcaneus
d. Cannon bone

338. The back of the hind leg distal to the tarsus is known as:
a. Plantar
b. Palmar
c. Lateral
d. Medial

339. An animal's body consists of how many main body cavities?
a. 1
b. 2
c. 5
d. 8

340. The dorsal body cavity contains which of the following structures?
a. Brain
b. Chest
c. Spinal cord
d. Both a and c

341. Which of the following body cavities is the largest?
a. Dorsal
b. Cranial
c. Spinal
d. Ventral

342. Which of the following is considered to be a major structure within the thoracic cavity?
a. Heart
b. Lungs
c. Esophagus
d. All of the above

343. All of the organs in the thoracic cavity are covered by a thin membrane known as:
a. Thorax
b. Pleura
c. Peritoneum
d. None of the above

344. The visceral layer of the peritoneum covers which organ?
a. Digestive
b. Urinary
c. Reproductive
d. All of the above

345. The animal body is made up of how many different tissues?
a. 1
b. 2
c. 4
d. 8

346. What is the main purpose of the epithelial tissue?
a. Provides support for the body
b. Covers body surfaces
c. Provides movement of structures
d. Controls the body function

347. Which types of cells carry oxygen throughout the body?
a. Red blood cells
b. White blood cells
c. Nerve cells
d. All cells carry oxygen

348. The secreting units of sweat glands, salivary glands, and mammary glands are all composed of what type of cellular tissue?
a. Connective tissue
b. Muscle tissue
c. Nervous tissue
d. Epithelial tissue

349. Which of the following is *not* a type of muscle tissue?
a. Cardiac
b. Skeletal
c. Striated
d. Smooth

350. Smooth muscle is found in which internal organ?
a. Urinary bladder
b. Heart
c. Digestive tract
d. All of the above
e. Both a and c

351. Which of the following is the first indication that the heart is starting to fail?
a. Decrease in blood pressure
b. Rise in blood pressure
c. Decrease in cardiac output
d. Drop in oxygen saturation

352. Which of the following elements is the component of all proteins and nucleic acids?
a. Hydrogen
b. Oxygen
c. Calcium
d. Nitrogen

353. Which element of the periodic table is required for muscle contraction, nerve impulse transmission, and blood clotting?
a. Nitrogen
b. Oxygen
c. Phosphorus
d. Calcium

354. Which of the following are considered major elements found in the body?
a. Nitrogen
b. Calcium
c. Magnesium
d. Potassium

355. Oxygen is an element that makes up approximately how much of the body mass?
a. 18.50%
b. 9.50%
c. 65%
d. 3.30%

356. Which of the following are considered as types of chemical bonds?
a. Covalent bonds
b. Ionic bonds
c. Hydrogen bonds
d. All of the choices are considered types of chemical bonds

357. A bond that is formed when electrons are transferred from one atom to another is known as what type of bond?
a. Covalent bond
b. Ionic bond
c. Hydrogen bond
d. Triple covalent bond

358. Which type of chemical reaction occurs in the body when the simple molecules absorbed during the digestive process are joined into larger molecules needed by cells for life processes?
a. Decomposition reaction
b. Synthesis reaction
c. Exchange reaction
d. None of the above

359. Which of the following are examples of inorganic compounds?
a. Water
b. Acids
c. Bases
d. All of the above

360. Which of the following is *not* an example of an organic compound?
a. Proteins
b. Bases
c. Lipids
d. Carbohydrates

361. What are chemicals that dissolve or mix well in water called?
a. Hydrophilic
b. Hydrophobic
c. Solute
d. Solvent

362. Which of the following are considered electrolytes?
a. Potassium
b. Sodium
c. Calcium
d. All of the above

363. Which of the following levels is considered the most acidic of the pH scale?
a. 2.5
b. 5
c. 7
d. 12

364. What does "buffering the solution" refer to?
a. Creating an acidic solution
b. Creating an alkaline solution
c. Creating a neutral solution with the pH close to 7
d. None of the above

365. Which of the following is an example of a buffer?
a. Lemons
b. Carbonic acid
c. Ammonia
d. Vinegar

366. What is the pH of distilled water?
a. 1
b. 5
c. 7
d. 11

367. Which of the following is an example of a carbohydrate?
a. Sugar
b. Starch
c. Cellulose
d. All of the above

368. Monosaccharides contain how many carbon atoms in a chain?
a. 2–5
b. 3–7
c. 5–10
d. 10–15

369. A sugar with five carbons is known as ______________ sugar.
a. Hexose
b. Pentose
c. Montose
d. Tritose

370. Which of the following molecules is *not* a lipid?
a. Ribose
b. Triglycerides
c. Prostaglandins
d. Steroids

371. What is the primary function of triglycerides?
a. Act as backbone of DNA and RNA
b. Regulate chemical reactions, enzymes
c. Synthesize hormones
d. Store energy

372. Which of the following molecules are nucleic acids?
a. DNA
b. RNA
c. Adenosine triphosphate
d. All of the above

373. Prostaglandins provide all of the following functions *except*:
a. Regulate hormone synthesis
b. Enhance immune system
c. Provide inflammatory response
d. Block the COX-2 pathway

374. When two monosaccharides join together, what type of reaction occurs?
a. Synthesis reaction
b. Hydrolysis reaction
c. Decomposition reaction
d. Exchange reaction

375. When water is extracted from saccharides, it is known as:
a. Hydrolysis
b. Dehydration synthesis
c. Decomposition reaction
d. Synthesis reaction

376. Lipids are made of all of the following components *except*:
a. Oxygen
b. Carbon
c. Hydrogen
d. Calcium

377. What are lipoproteins used for within the body?
a. Energy
b. To transport fats within the body
c. To regulate chemical reactions
d. To regulate hormone synthesis

378. Which type of lipids take the form of four interlocking hydrocarbon rings?
a. Steroids
b. Triglycerides
c. Prostaglandins
d. Phospholipids

379. Cholesterol is used by which of the following organs for the creation of steroid hormones?
a. Adrenal glands
b. Testes
c. Ovaries
d. All of the above

380. Which molecule is considered the most abundant organic molecule in the body?
a. Amino acids
b. Lipids
c. Proteins
d. Prostaglandins

381. Which characteristic of a protein molecule directly determines its function?
a. Size
b. Location
c. Shape
d. None, proteins all have the same function

382. All of the following are characteristics of structural proteins *except*:
a. Stability
b. Water-insoluble proteins
c. Rigidity
d. Steroid properties

383. Functional proteins are also known as:
a. Structural proteins
b. Globular proteins
c. Fibrous proteins
d. None of the above

384. Which of the following are considered the largest molecules in the body?
a. Lipids
b. Proteins
c. Nucleic acids
d. Carbohydrates

385. Nucleic acids consist of which of the following classes?
a. RNA
b. DNA
c. Ribose
d. Both a and b

386. The molecular building blocks of nucleic acids are known as:
a. Chromosomes
b. Nucleotides
c. Proteins
d. Carbohydrates

387. All of the following are nucleotides *except*:
a. Adenine
b. Guanine
c. Thiamine
d. Cystosine

388. Which nucleotide occurs in both DNA and RNA?
a. Thiamine
b. Guanine
c. Uracil
d. Thymine

389. Which nucleotide occurs only in RNA?
a. Adenine
b. Guanine
c. Cytosine
d. Uracil

390. The aorta originates from which structure?
a. Right ventricle
b. Left ventricle
c. Left atrium
d. Right atrium

391. Which type of blood vessel carries blood away from the heart?
a. Veins
b. Arteries
c. Capillaries
d. Vena cava

392. Which type of blood vessel contains one-way valves?
a. Arteries
b. Veins
c. Capillaries
d. Aorta

393. Which blood vessel carries CO_2-rich blood from the right ventricle of the heart to the lungs?
a. Aorta
b. Inferior vena cava
c. Pulmonary vein
d. Pulmonary artery

394. Which of the following is the first main branch of the aorta?
a. Left subclavian artery
b. Brachiocephalic trunk
c. The left common carotid artery
d. Superior mesenteric artery

395. Plasma is composed of what percentage of water?
a. 7%
b. 92%
c. 1%
d. Plasma does not contain water

396. Which blood cell is the most numerous blood cell in the body?
a. White blood cells
b. Plasma
c. Red blood cells
d. Leukocytes

397. Which protein gives erythrocytes their red color?
a. Granulocytes
b. Hemoglobin
c. Fibrinogen
d. Eosinophil

398. Blood makes up approximately what percentage of body weight?
a. 93%
b. 55%
c. 45%
d. 7%

399. All of the following are a type of white blood cell *except*:
a. Neutrophil
b. Reticulocyte
c. Lymphocyte
d. Eosinophil

400. Which structure is composed of several C-shaped incomplete rings of hyaline cartilage?
a. Esophagus
b. Trachea
c. Larynx
d. Pharynx

401. Where does gas exchange occur in the lungs?
a. Bronchi
b. Alveolus
c. Alveolar duct
d. Larynx

402. Which of the following is true about the thoracic cavity?
a. It contains positive pressure
b. It contains negative pressure
c. It does not contain any fluid
d. It is located below the diaphragm

403. What makes up the bulk of the tooth?
a. Enamel
b. Crown
c. Dentin
d. Root

404. Which of the following are the most rostral teeth in the mouth of small animals?
a. Canines
b. Premolars
c. Molars
d. Incisors

405. The hypoglossal cranial nerve is in charge of which of the following functions?
a. Eye movement
b. Tongue movement
c. Smell
d. Balance

406. What regulates the size of the opening of the esophagus into the stomach?
a. Duodenum
b. Pyloric sphincter
c. Cardiac sphincter
d. Epiglottis

407. After food leaves the stomach, it is referred to as which of the following terms?
a. Rugae
b. Chyme
c. Rumen
d. Bile

408. Which is the longest segment of the small intestines?
a. Duodenum
b. Ileum
c. Jejunum
d. Colon

409. Which is the longest segment of the large intestines?
a. Ileum
b. Colon
c. Cecum
d. Rectum

410. Which vein carries nutrient-rich blood from the intestines to the liver?
a. Inferior vena cava
b. Portal vein
c. Hepatic vein
d. Splenic vein

411. Which gland is located caudal to the diaphragm and is the largest gland in the body?
a. Spleen
b. Pancreas
c. Liver
d. Gallbladder

412. The diencephalon of the brain consists of which of the following structures?
a. Thalamus
b. Pons
c. Hypothalamus
d. Both a and b
e. Both a and c

413. What is the largest most rostral part of the brain?
a. Cerebellum
b. Cerebrum
c. Thalamus
d. Brainstem

414. Systems of folds located within the cerebrum are known as which of the following?
a. Gyri
b. Sulci
c. Meninges
d. Arachnoid villi

415. What is considered the most primitive part of the brain?
a. Cerebellum
b. Cerebrum
c. Brainstem
d. Gray matter

416. Which portion of the spinal cord is located at the cranial end?
a. Sacral
b. Cervical
c. Thoracic
d. Lumbar

417. Spinal nerves from the sacral region carry which type of nerve fiber?
a. Sympathetic nerve fibers
b. Parasympathetic nerve fibers
c. Both
d. Neither

418. How many types of cranial nerves exist?
a. 5
b. 8
c. 10
d. 12

419. Which cranial nerve is responsible for balance and hearing?
a. Trochlear
b. Vestibulocochlear
c. Accessory
d. Optic

420. The glossopharyngeal nerve is responsible for which of the following?
a. Sensations from the head and teeth, chewing
b. Eye movement
c. Facial and scalp movement
d. Tongue movement, swallowing, salivation, and taste

421. Which of the following cranial nerves is a sensory nerve?
a. Vestibulocochlear
b. Accessory
c. Trochlear
d. Hypoglossal

422. Which of the following cranial nerves is the longest cranial nerve that innervates many organs in the body?
a. Trigeminal
b. Vestibulocochlear
c. Vagus
d. Hypoglossal

423. Visceral sensations include which of the following?
a. Heat and cold
b. Hunger and thirst
c. Odors
d. Touch and pressure

424. Which of the following is *not* considered part of the special senses?
a. Taste
b. Hearing
c. Equilibrium
d. Proprioception

425. Which of the following is a cartilaginous funnel that collects sound waves and directs them medially into the external auditory canal?
a. Pinna
b. Eustachian tube
c. Cochlea
d. Tympanic membrane

426. Which of the following is part of the inner ear?
a. Cochlea
b. Malleus
c. Incus
d. Tympanic membrane

427. Which of the following contains receptor cells for hearing?
a. Tympanic membrane
b. Organ of Corti
c. Vestibule
d. Incus

428. The vestibular sense is responsible for:
a. Taste
b. Balance and head position
c. Vision
d. Hearing

429. The clear window on the rostral portion of the eye is known as:
a. Eyelids
b. Cornea
c. Iris
d. Sclera

430. Which structure is located immediately caudal to the cornea?
a. Lens
b. Iris
c. Anterior chamber
d. Vitreous humor

431. Where are visual images formed within the eye?
a. Lens
b. Cornea
c. Vitreous humor
d. Retina

432. In which layer of the eye are the rods and cones located?
a. Cornea
b. Retina
c. Iris
d. Vitreous humor

433. Which area is known as the blind spot of the eye?
a. Optic nerve
b. Optic disc
c. Rod
d. Cone

434. Which of the following is responsible for draining tears from the eye?
a. Lacrimal glands
b. Conjunctiva
c. Lacrimal puncta
d. Membrana nictitans

435. What happens to the iris of the eye in dim light?
a. The muscles relax, allowing the pupil to dilate
b. The muscles contract, allowing the pupil to constrict
c. The muscles constrict, closing the pupil
d. Nothing, light does not affect the iris of the eye

436. For what is the ciliary body within the eye responsible?
a. To change the diameter of the iris
b. To change the shape of the lens
c. To produce tears
d. To drain tears

437. Which hormones are produced by the corpus luteum and are necessary to maintain pregnancy?
a. FSH
b. LH
c. Progesterone
d. Estrogen

438. Which of the following hormones are the main hormones produced by the testicles?
a. Testosterone
b. Luteinizing hormone
c. Estrogen
d. Progesterone

439. Which of the following forms the tail of the horse?
a. The cervical vertebrae
b. The sacrum
c. The coccygeal vertebrae
d. The lumbar vertebrae

440. Which of the following bones is located immediately distal to the scapula of the horse?
a. Humerus
b. Metacarpus
c. Femur
d. Ulna

441. The carpus of the horse is located proximal to which of the following bones?
a. Humerus
b. Radius
c. Ulna
d. Metacarpus

442. Which of the following bones is located distal to the tarsal bone in the horse?
a. Femur
b. Patella
c. Metatarsal
d. Fibula

443. How many ribs does the horse have?
a. 5
b. 15
c. 18
d. 6

444. At what level of vertebrae are the withers of a horse located?
a. C1
b. C2
c. C3–C7
d. T4–T9

445. Which of the following bones is considered one of the strongest bones in the horse?
a. Humerus
b. Carpus
c. Scapula
d. Patella

446. Which of the following bones is also referred to as the cannon bone of the horse?
a. Phalanges
b. Carpus
c. Metacarpals
d. Femur

447. Which of the following joints lies between the cannon bone and the long pastern?
a. Stifle joint
b. Fetlock joint
c. Pastern joint
d. Carpal joint

448. Which of the following bones is encased in the hoof?
a. Navicular bone
b. Cannon bone
c. Pedal bone
d. Sesamoid bone

449. The glenoid cavity is located immediately proximal to which of the following bones of the horse?
a. Scapula
b. Humerus
c. Ulna
d. Cannon bone

450. The deltoid tuberosity is located on which of the following bones of the horse?
a. Radius
b. Ulna
c. Humerus
d. Scapula

451. Which bone forms the floor of the pelvis of the horse?
a. Pubis
b. Ischium
c. Ilium
d. Tuber coxae

452. Which of the following is the largest bone of the pelvis of the horse?
a. Ischium
b. Ilium
c. Pubis
d. Acetabulum

453. The interosseous space is located between which two bones on the limb of a horse?
a. Fibula/tibia
b. Radius/ulna
c. Cannon bone/split bone
d. Humerus/scapula

454. The femoral condyle is located _______________ to the head of the femur in a horse.
a. Proximal
b. Distal
c. Lateral
d. Medial

455. The coxal tuber is located on which of the following bones of the horse?
a. Talus
b. Metatarsal
c. Hip bone
d. Femur

456. The calcaneus bone in a horse forms which of the following?
a. Pastern
b. Fetlock
c. Point of the hock
d. The horse does not have a calcaneus bone, it is only found in small animals

457. The tarsus of the horse is composed of how many bones?
a. 1
b. 3
c. 4
d. 6

458. Metatarsal IV in the horse is also known as the:
a. Lateral splint bone
b. Cannon bone
c. Talus
d. Hock

459. Approximately how much of a horse's weight does its forelimbs carry?
a. 20%
b. 40%
c. 60%
d. 80%

460. Which muscle is responsible for movement of the head and neck of a horse?
a. Rhomboideus
b. Brachiocephalicus
c. Splenius
d. Deltoid

461. Where is the insertion of the sternocephalicus muscles of a horse?
a. Mandible
b. Humerus
c. Spine of the scapula
d. Proximal tibia

462. Which muscle of a horse supports the rider's weight?
a. Pectoral
b. Semitendinosus
c. Longissimus dorsi
d. Rhomboideus

463. Where is the point of origin of the pectoral muscle of horses?
a. Scapula
b. Pelvis
c. Thoracic vertebrae
d. Sternum

464. All of the following muscles of a horse extend the hock *except*?
a. Gastrocnemius
b. Semimembranosus
c. Semitendinosus
d. Biceps femoris

465. The point of origin of which muscle of the horse is at the tuber coxae of the pelvis?
a. Gastrocnemius
b. Infraspinatus
c. Latissimus dorsi
d. Superficial gluteals

466. Which of the following muscles of the horse is responsible for extending the elbow?
a. Infraspinatus
b. Gastrocnemius
c. Pectoral
d. Triceps

467. Which of the following muscles originates behind the poll (at the base of the skull) of a horse?
a. Trapezius
b. Splenius
c. Sternocephalicus
d. Brachiocephalicus

468. Which of the following muscles insert at the distal femur and tibia of a horse?
a. Gastrocnemius
b. Semitendinosus
c. Biceps femoris
d. Semimembranosus

469. Tendons attach __________ to bone.
a. Ligaments
b. Muscles
c. Blood vessels
d. Bone

470. Which of the following tendons flexes the toe in horses?
a. Suspensory ligament
b. Deep digital flexor tendon
c. Superficial digital flexor tendon
d. Lateral digital extensor tendon

471. What is the function of cheek ligaments in horses?
a. Support and suspend the fetlock and prevent overextension
b. Assist in the extension of the pastern joint
c. Prevent strain and overextension of the joint
d. Flexes the toe

472. Which of the following allows the horse to rest and sleep in a standing position?
a. The cheek ligaments
b. Stay apparatus
c. Deep digital flexor tendon
d. Superficial digital flexor tendon

473. A protective external capsule, called the __________, surrounds the internal structures of the foot on a horse.
a. Frog
b. Hoof
c. Horseshoe
d. Sole

474. Which of the following structures of a horse's hoof allows for expansion and provides strength?
a. Bars
b. Frog
c. Sole
d. Coronet

475. How long does it take for a horn to grown down from the coronet to the tip of the toe (on the ground surface) of a horse?
a. 1–2 months
b. 4–5 months
c. 9–12 months
d. 12–24 months

476. What forms the outer layer to protect the hoof and maintain moisture levels?
a. Hoof
b. Sole
c. Frog
d. Periople

477. What provides nourishment to the digital cushion and functions with the frog in a horse's foot?
a. Sole corium
b. Frog corium
c. Laminar corium
d. Perioplic corium

478. The sequence in which a horse lifts its feet from the ground is described as what?
a. Trot
b. Gait
c. Gallop
d. Canter

479. In which type of gait does the floating phase occur?
a. Walk
b. Trot
c. Gallop
d. Canter

480. During which gait are there never more than two legs on the ground at the same time?
a. Canter
b. Trot
c. Walk
d. Gallop

481. A horse's vision is primarily which type?
a. Binocular
b. Monocular
c. 3D
d. All of the above

482. Which area is the blind spot for a horse?
a. In front of the muzzle
b. Behind the ears
c. Right side of face
d. Left side of face

483. Which structure in horses provides additional shading for the retina to limit the entry of light?
a. Cornea
b. Iris
c. Ciliary muscle
d. Corpora nigra

484. What is the normal heart rate for a horse at rest?
a. 25–42 bpm
b. 40–140 bpm
c. 48–84 bpm
d. 260–600 bpm

485. Which of the following forms the ventral margin of each nostril of a horse?
a. External nares
b. False nostril
c. Alar fold
d. Ethmoturbinates

486. Which sinus lies in the dorsal part of the skull medial to the orbit?
a. Frontal sinus
b. Two maxillary sinuses
c. Oropharynx
d. Nasopharynx

487. Which of the following structures suspends the larynx from the skull?
a. Epiglottis
b. Arytenoid cartilages
c. Laryngopharynx
d. Hyoid apparatus

488. Which of the following is *not* part of the lower respiratory tract?
a. Trachea
b. Bronchi
c. Lungs
d. Pharynx

489. Which animal has a cotyledonary placenta?
a. Cat
b. Dog
c. Horse
d. Sheep

490. On an electrocardiogram, the P wave is most closely associated with:
a. Atrial depolarization
b. Atrial repolarization
c. Ventricular depolarization
d. Ventricular repolarization

491. Lymph nodes found on the caudal aspect of the leg at the level of the patella are the:
a. Popliteal nodes
b. Inguinal nodes
c. Mandibular nodes
d. Prescapular nodes

492. At what age do permanent teeth begin to erupt in a horse?
a. 1 year
b. 2½ years
c. 5 years
d. 6 years

493. How many permanent teeth does an adult male horse have (minus the wolf teeth)?
a. 24
b. 36
c. 40
d. 46

494. At what age do wolf teeth develop in a horse?
a. Less than 12 months
b. 18 months to 5 years
c. 5–10 years
d. Greater than 10 years

495. How much are the occlusal surfaces worn down every year in a horse?
a. 1–2 mm
b. 5–10 mm
c. 10–20 mm
d. None, they grow continuously and are never worn down

496. What does the term hypsodontic in a horse represent?
a. Thick layer of enamel
b. The lack of enamel over the occlusal surface
c. The crown reserve
d. Continuous growth of the teeth

497. The section between the canine teeth and the first premolar of a horse is termed:
a. Hypsodontic
b. Wolf teeth
c. Diastema
d. Infundibulum

498. What is the average length of the esophagus in an average sized horse?
a. 1.5 inches
b. 1.5 cm
c. 1.5 mm
d. 1.5 m

499. What volume can an adult horse's stomach hold?
a. 1–2 L
b. 2–3 L
c. 7–14 L
d. 20–25 L

500. Food passes from the esophagus into the stomach via what structure in a horse?
a. Pyloric sphincter
b. Epiglottis
c. Cardiac sphincter
d. Duodenum

501. At what level of "fullness" does a horse's stomach empty?
a. ¼ full
b. ½ full
c. ⅔ full
d. Completely full

502. Where does digestion and absorption of food take place in a horse?
a. Duodenum
b. Jejunum
c. Ileum
d. Ileocecal junction

503. Where does the microbial digestion of cellulose take place in a horse?
a. Ileocecal junction
b. Large intestine
c. Small intestine
d. Stomach

504. All of the following are part of the small intestine *except*:
a. Cecum
b. Duodenum
c. Jejunum
d. Ileum

505. In an average horse, how many liters of ingesta can the cecum hold?
a. 10 L
b. 20 L
c. 25 L
d. 35 L

506. In an average horse, how many liters of ingesta can the colon hold?
a. 10 L
b. 35 L
c. 65 L
d. 100 L

507. How long does food remain in the colon of a horse?
a. 1–2 hours
b. 5–15 hours
c. 25–35 hours
d. 36–65 hours

508. The left kidney of a horse lies __________ to the right kidney, is located ventral to the last rib, and is near the first two or three lumbar transverse processes.
a. Cranial
b. Caudal
c. Lateral
d. Medial

509. How many grams does an average equine kidney weigh?
a. 100–200 g
b. 400–600 g
c. 800–1000 g
d. 1000–1500 g

510. How many mL of urine does an equine patient produce per day of body weight?
a. 10 mL/kg/day
b. 20 mL/kg/day
c. 45 mL/kg/day
d. 60 mL/kg/day

511. What is the normal pH of equine urine?
a. Less than 3 pH
b. 3–6 pH
c. 7–8 pH
d. Greater than 9 pH

512. At what age do the male testicles of a horse reach their full adult size?
a. 6 months
b. 1 year
c. 2 years
d. 5 years

513. Which of the following glands is a pair of smooth-surfaced, pear-shaped glands located on either side of the male bladder and are also considered an accessory gland for the production of seminal fluid?
a. Bulbourethral gland
b. Seminal vesicles
c. Adrenal glands
d. Thyroid glands

514. The prostate gland is responsible for which of the following?
a. Cleans the urethra before the ejaculation of sperm
b. Neutralizes acidity of any remaining urine before ejaculation
c. Secretes a clear fluid
d. All of the above

515. Where does fertilization normally occur in a horse?
a. Testicles
b. Ovaries
c. Fallopian tubes
d. Infundibulum

516. What occurs to unfertilized ova?
a. They are expelled
b. They are reabsorbed
c. They remain in the fallopian tube until fertilization occurs
d. None of the above

517. The ovaries of a mare are largely inactive until sexual maturity, which occurs at what age?
a. 6 months
b. 1–2 years
c. 3–5 years
d. 7 years

518. Which of the following terms correctly describes a mare's parity?
a. Nulliparity
b. Uniparous
c. Multiparous
d. None of these

519. What is the typical breeding season of a mare?
a. Spring–summer
b. Summer–fall
c. Fall–winter
d. Winter–spring

520. A mare is considered a/an __________ ovulator, which means she will ovulate without the stimulus of mating.
a. Spontaneous
b. Polyestrous
c. Anestrous
d. Multiparous

521. How long does the typical estrous cycle last in a mare?
a. 5–7 days
b. 7–14 days
c. 17–21 days
d. 23–31 days

522. During the estrus phase of a mare, which of the following occurs?
a. Follicle development
b. Ovulation
c. Secretion of estrogen
d. Estrus does not occur in the mare

523. How long does the diestrus phase of a mare last?
a. 7–21 days
b. 3–5 days
c. 14–16 days
d. 35 days

524. The sternum of birds is extended into a laterally flattened ___________, which provides a large surface area for the attachment of the major flight muscles.
a. Coracoid
b. Keel
c. Beak
d. Quadrate

525. Many of the larger bones of the bird are filled with air contained in membranous sacs that connect with the respiratory system and are referred to as which type of bones?
a. Compact
b. Irregular
c. Long
d. Pneumatic

526. What division are birds missing that is normally seen between the thorax and abdomen of other animals?
a. Lungs
b. Diaphragm
c. Liver
d. Keel

527. Which of the following is responsible for the perching reflex in birds?
a. Tibiotarsus
b. Digital flexor tendon
c. Craniofacial hinge
d. Supracoracoid muscle

528. Most birds have how many toes pointing forward?
a. 1
b. 2
c. 3
d. None

529. The pygostyle found in birds is located distal to which of the following?
a. Sternum
b. Coccygeal vertebrae
c. Tibiotarsus
d. Hallux

530. Which of the following structures is the first digit in birds?
a. Alula
b. Major metacarpal
c. Tarsometatarsus
d. Hallux

531. Which digit of birds carries the primary feathers?
a. Digit 1
b. Alula
c. Digit 3
d. Metacarpal

532. The central shaft of a bird's feather is also referred to as:
a. Dentary
b. Talon
c. Hallux
d. Rachis

533. As feathers mature in birds, what happens to the rachis?
a. Fills with blood
b. Becomes hollow
c. Molts
d. Nothing, it stays the same throughout life

534. Secretions from which gland keeps feathers waterproof?
a. Alula
b. Preen
c. Gizzard
d. Coracoid

535. Secondary feathers are attached to which structure in birds?
a. Digit 1
b. Digit 3
c. Ulna
d. Hallux

536. Which types of feathers cover the outermost layer of the body?
a. Primary feathers
b. Secondary feathers
c. Contour feathers
d. Filoplume feathers

537. How often do birds go through a molting process?
a. Once a month
b. Every 3–6 months
c. Once a year
d. Once after 1 year of age

538. Which surface of the wing is longer and convex? And which surface is shorter and more concave?
a. Ventral/dorsal
b. Dorsal/ventral
c. Proximal/distal
d. Distal/proximal

539. Which side of the wing does air pass over more quickly?
a. Dorsal
b. Ventral
c. Proximal
d. Distal

540. The lift force must equal which of the following parameters for flight to occur in a bird?
a. Size of the bird
b. Shape of the wings
c. Weight of the bird
d. Gravity

541. Lift is reduced if the angle of tilt of a bird's wing is greater than how many degrees?
a. 5 degrees
b. 15 degrees
c. 25 degrees
d. 45 degrees

542. For a bird to land, the tail is used as a __________ and the wings are extended into a stall position.
a. Brake
b. Guide
c. Thrust
d. Perch

543. All of the following special senses of birds are well developed for survival *except*:
a. Sight
b. Hearing
c. Touch
d. All of the above are well developed in the bird

544. Which structure do birds move to view an image?
a. Eye muscles
b. Eyes
c. Head
d. Optic lobes

545. Predator birds have which type of vision?
a. Monocular
b. Binocular
c. 3D
d. None of the above

546. Which of the following structures reinforces the large circumference of the eye in birds?
a. Cornea
b. Sclerotic ring
c. Optic lobe
d. Optic nerve

547. Which muscle forms the iris of a bird's eye, enabling the bird to control the size of the pupil voluntarily?
a. Smooth
b. Striated
c. Cardiac
d. None of these

548. The vitreous humor in the posterior chamber of the eye contains a ribbon-like structure attached to the retina, which is known as what?
a. Nictitating membrane
b. Pecten
c. Third eyelid
d. Optic nerve

549. Which type of vision do photoreceptor cells, known as rods, provide in birds?
a. Color vision
b. Monocular vision
c. Binocular vision
d. Night vision

550. Which avian species contain ear pinnae?
a. Eagle
b. Parakeet
c. Parrot
d. None, there are no external ear pinnae in any avian species

551. Where is the columella bone located?
a. Caudal to the clavicle
b. Proximal to the ulna
c. Cranial to the sternum
d. In the ear

552. Where are the free spaces within the bird located?
a. Thorax
b. Abdomen
c. Major bones
d. Wings

553. The combined effect of air passing through the larynx and what other structure produces the characteristic sounds associated with the bird species?
a. Glottis
b. Syrinx
c. Bronchi
d. Choana

554. How many air sacs do most birds have?
a. 3
b. 5
c. 7
d. 9

555. The nine different air sacs within birds are responsible for all of the following *except*:
a. Lightening the weight of the skeleton
b. Gaseous exchange
c. As a reservoir for air
d. The bellows effect

556. During the respiration process of birds, air circulates continuously and passes through the lungs how many times?
a. 2
b. 3
c. 4
d. 5

557. The air in which air sac passes straight through the lungs and out?
a. Cranial
b. Thoracic
c. Abdominal
d. Humerus

558. How many chambers does the avian heart contain?
a. 1
b. 2
c. 3
d. 4

559. The pericardial sac covers which of the following structures in birds?
a. Bronchi
b. Keel
c. Heart
d. Syrinx

560. There is a large blood supply to the flight muscles and wings of birds via which artery?
a. Pectoral artery
b. Carotid artery
c. Brachial artery
d. All of the above
e. Both a and c

561. The pudendal artery in birds is located near what other structure?
a. Ulnar artery
b. Pectoral artery
c. Brachiocephalic artery
d. Rectum

562. Which of the following arteries runs parallel to the trachea in birds?
a. Brachial
b. Jugular
c. Subclavian
d. Carotid

563. Which of the following arteries runs parallel with the radial artery in birds?
a. Brachial
b. Ulnar
c. Femoral
d. Ischiatic

564. Which artery is distal to the femoral artery in birds?
a. Coeliac
b. Renal
c. Pectoral
d. External iliac

565. Food passes down the esophagus on the right side of the neck of birds and enters what structure?
a. Gizzard
b. Crop
c. Duodenum
d. Proventriculus

566. Which structure is located distal to the cecum of birds?
a. Gizzard
b. Cloaca
c. Proventriculus
d. Crop

567. Food leaves the gizzard and enters the duodenum by which of the following structures in birds?
a. Cloaca
b. Pylorus
c. Proventriculus
d. Ileum

568. How many lobes does the pancreas of birds have?
a. 1
b. 2
c. 3
d. None, birds do not have a pancreas

569. Via what structure do ureters carry urine to the outside of the body in birds?
a. Isthmus
b. Vagina
c. Cloaca
d. Proventriculus

570. Which of the following systems attach to the cloaca in birds?
a. Reproductive
b. Digestive
c. Urinary
d. All of the above

571. In female birds during the breeding season, how often is one ovum released until the clutch is complete?
a. Every 2 hours
b. Every 6 hours
c. Every 12 hours
d. Every 24 hours

572. Which of the following structures is the largest and most glandular structure of the oviduct in birds?
a. Infundibulum
b. Magnum
c. Isthmus
d. Cloaca

573. The majority of the albumen is added to the egg as it travels down which structure in birds?
a. Infundibulum
b. Cloaca
c. Magnum
d. Isthmus

574. How long does it take for calcification of the egg to occur in birds?
a. 1 hour
b. 5 hours
c. 10 hours
d. 15 hours

575. Which structure connects the testes of birds to the cloaca?
a. Vas deferens
b. Magnum
c. Infundibulum
d. Ureters

576. Where are the testes located compared with the kidneys in birds?
a. Lateral
b. Distal
c. Caudal
d. Cranial

577. In what location are spermatozoa stored in birds?
a. Vas deferens
b. Seminiferous tubules
c. Ductus deferens
d. Cloaca

578. During mating, the phallus of male birds becomes engorged with:
a. Blood
b. Air
c. Lymph
d. Water

579. Which type of vision do rabbits have?
a. Monocular
b. Binocular
c. 3D
d. Both a and b

580. Mature female rabbits develop a large fold of skin under the chin that is known as the:
a. Philtrum
b. Dewlap
c. Crepuscular
d. None of the above

581. Where are scent glands located on the rabbit?
a. Under the chin
b. On either side of the perineum
c. At the anus
d. All of the above

582. How many toes do the forelegs of rabbits have?
a. 2
b. 3
c. 4
d. 5

583. How many cervical vertebrae do rabbits have?
a. 7
b. 8
c. 13
d. 15

584. How many thoracic vertebrae do rabbits have?
a. 7
b. 12–13
c. 4
d. 8

585. Which characteristic is true about the fibula of rabbits?
a. It is twice the length of the tibia
b. It is half the length of the tibia
c. It is fused with the tibia
d. Both b and c

586. What is the average life span of rabbits?
a. 3–4 years
b. 2–3 years
c. 6–8 years
d. 10 years

587. What is the normal body temperature of rabbits?
a. 36.2–37.5°C
b. 38.3°C
c. 38.3–39.2°C
d. None of the above

588. What is the normal respiratory rate of rabbits?
a. 35–60 breaths/min
b. 40–80 breaths/min
c. 100–250 breaths/min
d. 90–150 breaths/min

589. What is the average heart rate of rabbits?
a. 250–500 bpm
b. 220 bpm
c. 130–190 bpm
d. 260–450 bpm

590. What is the average adult weight of rabbits?
a. 400–600 g
b. 50–60 g
c. 100 g
d. 1000–8000 g

591. What is the length of the estrous cycle in rabbits?
a. Every 4 days
b. Every 30–35 days
c. Every 15–16 days
d. Every 4–6 days

592. What is the gestational period of rabbits?
a. 28–32 days
b. 111 days
c. 63 days
d. 19–21 days

593. What is the average litter size of rabbits?
a. 1–2
b. 2–3
c. 2–7
d. 6–12

594. What is the weaning age of rabbits?
a. 6–8 weeks
b. 3–4 weeks
c. 4–6 weeks
d. 18 days

595. What is the age of sexual maturity for rabbits?
a. 3–4 weeks
b. 10–12 weeks
c. 12 months
d. 5–8 months

596. How many canine teeth does the rabbit have?
a. 2
b. 4
c. 6
d. None, they do not contain canine teeth

597. The premolars of rabbits are also known as:
a. Incisors
b. Canines
c. Cheek teeth
d. Diastema

598. Rabbits are unable to vomit because of the arrangement of the ____________ in relation to the stomach.
a. Esophagus
b. Pylorus
c. Duodenum
d. Cardia

599. The ileum in rabbits terminates at which of the following structures?
a. Ileocecal tonsil
b. Cecum
c. Rectum
d. Duodenum

600. What is the largest organ in the abdominal cavity of rabbits?
a. Liver
b. Spleen
c. Cecum
d. Colon

601. All of the following are true about rabbits *except*:
a. Rabbits are omnivores
b. Rabbits are hindgut fermenters
c. Rabbits are monogastric
d. Rabbits are herbivores

602. Hard fibrous pellets from the digestive system of rabbits are produced within how many hours of eating?
a. 3
b. 4
c. 6
d. 8

603. Food material of rabbits passes through the digestive system twice within how many hours?
a. 6
b. 8
c. 12
d. 24

604. What does it mean when rabbits breathe through their mouths?
a. Normal breathing
b. Good prognosis
c. Poor prognosis
d. Rabbits never breathe through their mouths

605. How often does the nose of a rabbit twitch during general anesthesia?
a. 10–20 times
b. 25–50 times
c. 50–100 times
d. 20–120 times

606. How many renal medullary pyramid(s) do rabbits have?
a. 1
b. 2
c. 6
d. 9

607. At what age do the testes descend in rabbits?
a. Less than 10 days
b. 8 weeks
c. 12 weeks
d. Rabbits' testes do not descend

608. The female rabbit has which type of uterus?
a. Bicornuate
b. Didelphys
c. Unicornuate
d. Septate

609. The term altricial refers to:
a. Born hairless
b. Born deaf
c. Born blind
d. All of the above

610. A male guinea pig is known as a:
a. Doe
b. Buck
c. Boar
d. Sow

611. How long is the gestational period of guinea pigs?
a. 28–32 days
b. 63 days
c. 111 days
d. 19–21 days

612. Ferrets have which type of vision?
a. Monocular
b. Binocular
c. 3D
d. Both a and b

613. What is the main source of a ferret's body odor?
a. Fur
b. Sebaceous glands
c. Anal glands
d. Mouth

614. How many thoracic vertebrae do ferrets have?
a. 7
b. 15
c. 5–6
d. 3

615. The coccygeal vertebra of a ferret is located in which part of the body?
a. Neck
b. Thorax
c. Pelvis
d. Tail

616. The spine of a ferret is flexible and allows the ferret to bend at an angle of at least:
a. 15 degrees
b. 45 degrees
c. 90 degrees
d. 180 degrees

617. The lumbar vertebra of the ferret is located distal to the:
a. Thoracic vertebrae
b. Sacrum
c. Coccygeal vertebrae
d. Pelvis

618. What is the average litter size of ferrets?
a. 3–4
b. 5–6
c. 8–10
d. More than 20

619. After mating occurs in ferrets, ovulation occurs within:
a. 30 minutes
b. 1–2 hours
c. 30–40 hours
d. 3 days

620. What is the average gestational period of a ferret?
a. 28–32 days
b. 42 days
c. 63 days
d. 111 days

621. A castrated male ferret is referred to as a:
a. Jill
b. Hobble
c. Hob
d. Gelding

622. Where are the lungs located in a tortoise?
a. The ventral surface above the carapace
b. The dorsal side below the carapace
c. Caudal to the stomach
d. Caudal to the heart

623. In a male tortoise, the testes are located adjacent to what other organ?
a. Stomach
b. Urinary bladder
c. Kidneys
d. Liver

624. All of the following are face bones in small animals *except*:
a. Zygomatic bones
b. Pterygoid bones
c. Vomer bone
d. Sphenoid bone

625. The incus, malleus, and stapes are all bones that create the ________ in small animals.
a. Ear
b. Face
c. Foot
d. Cranium

626. Which bone is the most caudal bone of the skull in small animals?
a. Parietal bone
b. Occipital bone
c. Interparietal bone
d. Temporal bone

627. The spinal cord exits the skull through which structure?
a. Temporal bone
b. Atlas
c. Foramen magnum
d. Occipital condyles

628. The calcaneus of dogs is also referred to as the:
a. Manubrium
b. Point of hock
c. Point of elbow
d. Olecranon

629. Which of the following animals have an os cordis?
a. Horses
b. Cattle
c. Sheep
d. All of the above
e. Both b and c

630. The tibia and fibula of dogs are located immediately proximal to which bones?
a. Metatarsal bones
b. Metacarpal bones
c. Tarsal bones
d. Olecranon

631. The sacrum of dogs is cranial to what structure?
a. Ligamentum nuchae
b. Coccygeal
c. Lumbar vertebrae
d. Atlas

632. The mental foramen of the cat is located on which bone?
a. Occipital bone
b. Mandible
c. Tympanic bulla
d. Nasal bone

633. Which skull bone is the most rostral bone?
a. Occipital
b. Interparietal
c. Incisive
d. Lacrimal

634. A space within the lacrimal bones houses which of the following structures?
a. Lacrimal sac
b. Maxillary sinuses
c. Hard palate
d. Nasal cavity

635. The zygomatic bones of dogs are also referred to as:
a. Premaxillary bones
b. Hard palate
c. Malar bones
d. Cochlea

636. The ____________ of the mandible is the horizontal portion that houses all the teeth.
a. Ramus
b. Shaft
c. Palate
d. Malar

637. Which of the following are the inner bones of the face of small animals?
a. Vomer bone
b. Palatine bone
c. Pterygoid bone
d. All of the above

638. The two small pterygoid bones support the lateral walls of what structure?
a. Pharynx
b. Mandibular symphysis
c. Nasal septum
d. Nasal conchae

639. Which animal contains the highest number of sacral vertebrae?
a. Horse
b. Dog
c. Cat
d. Pig

640. How many cervical vertebrae does a cat have?
a. 3
b. 7
c. 13
d. 18

641. The bodies of adjacent vertebrae are separated by what structure?
a. Spinal canal
b. Articular process
c. Intervertebral disks
d. Ligamentum nuchae

642. The junction between the bone and the cartilage of the ribs is referred to as the:
a. Costochondral junction
b. Xiphoid process
c. Asternal ribs
d. Manubrium

643. Which of the following is the most proximal bone of the thoracic limb?
a. Ulna
b. Humerus
c. Scapula
d. Brachium

644. Which of the following are considered to be organic molecules?
a. Lipids
b. Proteins
c. Nucleic acids
d. Carbohydrates
e. All of the above

645. All of the following are lipids *except*:
a. Steroids
b. Glycogen
c. Triglycerides
d. Prostaglandins

646. A sugar that contains five carbons is referred to as a:
a. Monosaccharide
b. Hexose sugar
c. Pentose sugar
d. Disaccharide

647. Which part of the cell contains and processes genetic information and controls cell metabolism?
a. Nucleus
b. Cell membrane
c. Cilia
d. Chromatin

648. The digestion of absorbed material is performed by which organelle?
a. Peroxisomes
b. Ribosomes
c. Lysosomes
d. Mitochondria

649. Which of the following move cells through fluid?
a. Flagella
b. Cilia
c. Basal bodies
d. Centrioles

650. What is the fluid of a cell called?
a. Cytoplasm
b. Cytosol
c. Cytoskeleton
d. Tubulins

651. Glucose that is *not* immediately used by cells is converted to glycogen and is stored in which organ?
a. Gallbladder
b. Pancreas
c. Spleen
d. Liver

652. Amphibians and reptiles are commonly referred to as ectothermic, which is correctly described by which of the following?
a. Warm-blooded
b. Cold-blooded
c. Endothermic
d. Behavioral thermoregulation

653. The term ecdysis refers to:
a. Cold-blooded
b. Shedding of skin
c. Hibernation
d. Active at night

654. When tension is generated in the muscle, muscle tone increases but the muscle does *not* shorten. Which of the following correctly names this action?
a. Isotonic contraction
b. Isometric contraction
c. Muscle tone
d. None of the above

655. Which of the following muscles opens the jaw and is located on the caudoventral surface of the mandible?
a. Temporalis
b. Dorsal rectus
c. Digastricus
d. Masseter

656. Which of the following muscles are responsible for side-to-side movements of the mouth?
a. Masseter
b. Temporalis
c. Medial and lateral pterygoids
d. Digastricus

657. The ___________ of the muscles of the jaw is responsible for closure and helps keep the mouth closed when it is *not* in use.
a. Shape
b. Length
c. Tone
d. Atrophy

658. Which of the following muscles originates at the zygomatic arch and inserts on the masseteric fossa on the lateral surface of the mandible?
a. Temporalis
b. Masseter
c. Digastricus
d. Medial and lateral pterygoids

659. How many extrinsic muscles of the eye are responsible for moving the eye up, down, and side to side within its socket?
a. 1
b. 2
c. 3
d. 4

660. Which muscle of the eye is responsible for rotating the eye about its visual axis?
a. Dorsal oblique
b. Dorsal rectus
c. Ventral oblique
d. Both a and c

661. What is the function of the retractor bulbi muscle?
a. To move the eye upward
b. To move the eye downward
c. To move the eye outward
d. To pull the eye deeper in the socket

662. Where do the epaxial muscles lie?
a. Dorsal to the transverse process of the vertebrae
b. Ventral to the transverse process of the vertebrae
c. Between the thoracic and abdominal cavity
d. Along each side of the linea alba

663. Which muscle originates from the caudal border of one rib and inserts on the cranial border of the rib behind it?
a. Internal intercostals
b. External intercostals
c. External abdominal oblique
d. Internal abdominal oblique

664. All of the following structures pass through the aortic hiatus *except*:
a. Aorta
b. Thoracic duct
c. Azygous vein
d. Vagal nerve

665. Which opening lies within the central tendon and transmits the caudal vena cava?
a. Aortic hiatus
b. Caval foramen
c. Esophageal hiatus
d. Foramen magnum

666. Which canine muscle originates from the dorsal midline from C2 to C7 and inserts on the spine of the scapula?
a. Pectoralis
b. Trapezius
c. Latissimus dorsi
d. Brachiocephalicus

667. Which muscle is responsible for retracting the forelimb of dogs?
a. Pectoralis
b. Trapezius
c. Latissimus dorsi
d. Supraspinatus

668. Which muscle is responsible for stabilizing and flexing the shoulder joint?
   a. Supraspinatus
   b. Infraspinatus
   c. Triceps brachii
   d. Biceps brachii
669. Which muscle group extends the hip joint and abducts the thigh?
   a. Sartorius
   b. Gluteals
   c. Quadriceps femoris
   d. Gastrocnemius
670. Which muscle is the most medial muscle of the hamstring?
   a. Semitendinosus
   b. Gastrocnemius
   c. Semimembranosus
   d. Quadriceps femoris
671. Which muscle flexes the hock and rotates the paw medially?
   a. Gastrocnemius
   b. Anterior tibialis
   c. Pectineus
   d. Gracilis
672. All of the following are muscles of the hind limb in dogs *except*:
   a. Biceps femoris
   b. Quadriceps femoris
   c. Semitendinosus
   d. Biceps brachii
673. The ________________ is a projection of bone on the lateral edge above its condyle.
   a. Foramen
   b. Epicondyle
   c. Head
   d. Periosteum
674. The protuberances on bones, which are used for the attachment of muscles, are referred to as which of the following?
   a. Fossa
   b. Tendon
   c. Tuberosity
   d. Shaft
675. Grooves on bones that allow tendons to act as pulleys are known as:
   a. Fossa
   b. Ligament
   c. Trochlea
   d. Epicondyle
676. Which of the following dogs has a mesaticephalic head?
   a. Boxer
   b. Greyhound
   c. Beagle
   d. Bulldog
677. Which artery carries deoxygenated blood to the lungs?
   a. Pulmonary
   b. Carotid
   c. Subclavian
   d. Renal
678. The azygous vein drains venous blood from what structure?
   a. Head
   b. Thoracic body wall
   c. Hind limbs
   d. Liver
679. The veins that drain the stomach, intestine, and pancreas drain into which of the following?
   a. Hepatic veins
   b. Hepatic arteries
   c. Portal veins
   d. Iliac veins
680. Which artery supplies the stomach, spleen, and liver with blood?
   a. Renal artery
   b. Portal vein
   c. Hepatic vein
   d. Celiac artery
681. Which artery supplies the small intestines with blood?
   a. Celiac artery
   b. Cranial mesenteric artery
   c. Caudal mesenteric artery
   d. Femoral artery
682. Which vein returns deoxygenated blood from the pelvic region, hind limbs, and abdominal viscera?
   a. Caudal vena cava
   b. Aorta
   c. Iliac veins
   d. Pulmonary vein
683. What are the smallest veins called?
   a. Capillaries
   b. Venules
   c. Iliacs
   d. Vessels
684. Which of the following are present in all organs/tissues and are the sites of exchange between blood and tissue fluid?
   a. Venules
   b. Capillaries
   c. Valves
   d. Lymph
685. A venous shunt within the liver that connects the umbilical vein to the caudal vena cava is known as what?
   a. Ductus venosus
   b. Ligamentum arteriosus
   c. Foramen ovale
   d. Ductus arteriosus
686. Blood leaves the right ventricle to enter what structure?
   a. Caudal vena cava
   b. Aorta
   c. Cranial vena cava
   d. Left atrium
687. Blood leaving the lungs enters which section of the heart?
   a. Right atrium
   b. Left atrium
   c. Right ventricle
   d. Left ventricle

688. Which is the largest lymphoid organ?
a. Liver
b. Cisterna chyli
c. Lymph node
d. Spleen

689. When an animal becomes severely dehydrated, it loses both tissue fluid and plasma fluid. What effect would this have on the hematocrit and the PCV?
a. Increase both values
b. Decrease both values
c. Increase the hematocrit but no effect on the PCV
d. No change in either value

690. Which of the following is a short irregular tube of cartilage and muscle that connects the pharynx with the trachea?
a. Larynx
b. Epiglottis
c. Bronchi
d. Esophagus

691. Which organelle is the site of protein synthesis?
a. Golgi apparatus
b. Ribosomes
c. Endoplasmic reticulum
d. Mitochondria

692. Which structure extends along the ventral midline from the xiphoid process of the sternum to the pubic symphysis?
a. Spinal cord
b. Linea alba
c. Diaphragm
d. Transversus abdominis

693. Which muscle forms the caudal half of the medial surface of the thigh?
a. Sartorius
b. Semitendinosus
c. Biceps femoris
d. Gracilis

694. Which type of cells make up bone?
a. Osteoblasts
b. Osteocytes
c. Osteoclasts
d. All of these

695. The bones of the head and trunk are referred to as the:
a. Axial skeleton
b. Appendicular skeleton
c. Visceral skeleton
d. Metacarpal bones

696. Which of the following is classified as an internal bone of the cranium?
a. Ethmoid bone
b. Temperal bone
c. Incisive bone
d. Parietal bone

697. The two small bones that form part of the orbit of the eye are which of the following:
a. Ossicles
b. Malleus
c. Incus
d. Lacrimal

698. Which of the following is located at the proximal end of the trochlear notch?
a. Antebrachium
b. Olecranon process
c. Styloid process
d. Anconeal process

699. Which of the following are four, thin, scroll-like bones that fill most of the space in the nasal cavity and are also called the nasal conchae?
a. Palatine bones
b. Pterygoid bones
c. Turbinates
d. Vomer bone

700. The ribs that make up the caudal part of the thorax are called:
a. The sternal ribs
b. The asternal ribs
c. The floating ribs
d. The costochondral junction

SECTION

2 Hospital Management

Brooke Lockridge

QUESTIONS

1. Credentialed veterinary technicians are allowed to perform certain duties under the direct supervision of whom?
   a. Office manager
   b. Lead veterinary technician
   c. Veterinarian
   d. Practice owner
2. Which of the following health care team members is allowed to diagnose, prescribe medication, and perform surgery?
   a. Veterinarian
   b. Office manager
   c. Credentialed veterinary technician
   d. Veterinary technologist
3. Which of the following tasks is the responsibility of a veterinary assistant?
   a. Perform dental prophylaxis
   b. Calculate drug dosages
   c. Perform surgical procedures
   d. Maintain legible and accurate medical records
4. The term "petty cash" refers to which of the following?
   a. Change owed back to an owner on a bill
   b. Cash set aside in the practice to purchase items needed for business when a check is not available
   c. The cash balance in the drawer at the start and end of every day
   d. Payment received from a third party
5. How many components does the human voice contain?
   a. 2
   b. 4
   c. 8
   d. 10
6. Which of the following is the correct definition of a mission statement in a hospital?
   a. The desired future of the practice
   b. The purpose of a hospital; the fundamental reason a hospital exists
   c. Guiding principles that are not to be compromised during change
   d. None of the above
7. Which of the following are characteristics of effective leaders?
   a. Team player
   b. Effective communicator
   c. Self-confident
   d. All of the above
8. Which of the following are methods that can be used to decrease loss of revenue in a hospital?
   a. Use travel sheets to decrease missed charges
   b. Implement internal controls to prevent employee theft
   c. Manage inventory appropriately
   d. All of the above
   e. Both a and b
9. To receive maximum value for time spent and to avoid loss of interest, what is the maximum time a staff meeting should last?
   a. 15 minutes
   b. 30 minutes
   c. 45 minutes
   d. 1 hour
10. How many branches of veterinary ethics exist?
    a. 2
    b. 4
    c. 6
    d. 8
11. Descriptive ethics refers to which of the following?
    a. The study of the ethical views of veterinarians and veterinary professionals regarding their behavior and attitudes.
    b. The creation of the official ethical standards adopted by organizations of professionals and imposed on their members.
    c. The search for correct principles of good and bad, right and wrong, justice or injustice.
    d. Actions by administrative government bodies that regulate veterinary practice and activities in which veterinarians engage.
12. Law is divided into how many categories?
    a. 1
    b. 2
    c. 4
    d. 5
13. A noncompete agreement falls under which division of the law?
    a. Civil
    b. Criminal
    c. Both criminal and civil
    d. Neither criminal nor civil
14. Animal abuse falls under which division of the law?
    a. Civil
    b. Criminal
    c. Both criminal and civil
    d. Neither criminal nor civil

15. Which of the following correctly defines negligence?
    a. A civil offense to an opposing party in which harm has occurred.
    b. An intentional action that has taken place in which harm has occurred to another member of society.
    c. The performance of an act that a reasonable person under the same circumstances would not perform.
    d. The unlawful activity against a member of the public that is prosecuted by a public official.
16. Lawsuits against veterinarians are almost always based on what?
    a. Defamation
    b. Breach of warranty
    c. Neglect
    d. Breach of contract
17. Which of the following is considered an act of malpractice?
    a. Abandonment
    b. Incorrect drug administration
    c. Disease transmission
    d. Failure to communicate
    e. All of the above
18. When a mistake is written in the medical record, what is the proper method to correct it?
    a. Erase the mistake and start over
    b. Use white-out to cover the written mistake, initial it, and rewrite it
    c. Draw a single line through the mistake, initial it, and write the correction
    d. Scratch out the mistake with ink and rewrite with initials
19. Which of the following acts was created to establish minimum wage and overtime pay standards, and to regulate the employment of minors?
    a. Family and Medical Leave Act
    b. Fair Labor and Standards Act
    c. Equal Employment Opportunity
    d. Occupational Safety and Health Administration
20. Which of the following laws/acts does *not* apply to veterinary facilities?
    a. Uniformed Services Employment and Reemployment Rights Act
    b. Immigration Reform and Control Act
    c. Employee Polygraph Protection Act
    d. None of the above
21. Which of the following are considered to be employee benefits?
    a. Sick leave
    b. Veterinary care
    c. Continuing education
    d. All of the above
22. Employee discounts on services greater than what percent must be reported to the IRS as pay?
    a. 10%
    b. 15%
    c. 20%
    d. 50%
23. Which of the following is an example of incorporeal property?
    a. Buildings
    b. Equipment
    c. Vehicles
    d. Practice goodwill
24. What is the correct procedure when a veterinary technician is pregnant?
    a. Have the employee placed on a temporary resignation status for the duration of the pregnancy
    b. Have the employee transferred to a receptionist position for the duration of the pregnancy
    c. Limit the employee on all safety issues such as lifting, anesthesia exposure, and radiation exposure
    d. Address the safety issues within the facility but allow the employee to decide their own safety level
25. Which of the following questions should *not* be asked during an interview?
    a. What is your salary requirement?
    b. Are you currently employed?
    c. Do you have any children?
    d. What are some areas you feel you need improvement on?
26. Which of the following is an example of a social symptom of compassion fatigue?
    a. Isolation
    b. Pain
    c. Depression
    d. Nightmares
27. All of the following are true about compassion fatigue *except*:
    a. Only occurs with caregivers
    b. Has a sudden onset of symptoms
    c. Occurs with any industry
    d. Can be resolved with time spent away from the caregiving role.
28. How many stages does a business life cycle have?
    a. 2
    b. 3
    c. 4
    d. 5
29. Which of the following descriptions are considered cognitive signs of compassion fatigue?
    a. Decreased concentration and/or ability to concentrate
    b. Questioning life's meaning
    c. Failure to develop non–work-related aspects of life
    d. Dread of working with certain co-workers
30. Which of the following correctly describes the term ergonomics?
    a. The organization of materials in a logical sequence
    b. The science that studies the relationship between people and their work environments.
    c. The positioning of objects as close to the point of use as possible
    d. The amount of time and degree of motion required to perform a given task
31. Which of the following is the correct acronym when referring to the proper use of a fire extinguisher?
    a. FIRE
    b. PASS
    c. CODE
    d. CARE

32. How often should the lead aprons, gloves, and thyroid collars be radiographed to ensure there is no damage or cracks in the lead?
a. Monthly
b. Yearly
c. Every 5 years
d. Never, lead cannot be damaged

33. Occupations Safety and Health Administration (OSHA) protects which of the following?
a. Employees and clients with disabilities
b. The sale and distribution of pharmaceuticals
c. Employee radiation exposure
d. Malpractice lawsuits

34. What device is used to measure an employee's exposure to radiation?
a. Dosimeter badge
b. Lead
c. Cathode unit
d. MPD badge

35. Which of the following abbreviations is used to indicate "both eyes"?
a. BID
b. OD
c. OU
d. AU

36. Which of the following imaging modalities uses a magnet to produce images?
a. Ultrasound
b. MRI
c. CT scan
d. Radiographs

37. What is ethylenediamine tetraacetic acid?
a. An anticoagulant added to blood collection tubes
b. A serum separator agent added to blood collection tubes
c. Rubbing alcohol added to the skin for aseptic purposes
d. None of the above

38. When submitting a tissue sample for pathology, what should the ratio of formalin to tissue volume be?
a. 1:01
b. 5:01
c. 10:01
d. 20:01

39. Serum separator tubes should *not* be used for which of the following therapeutic monitoring?
a. Phenobarbital levels
b. Theophylline levels
c. Digoxin levels
d. All of the above

40. All of the following are anticoagulants used in blood collection tubes *except*:
a. Potassium citrate
b. Lithium heparin
c. Sodium heparin
d. ETDA

41. An anaerobic culture should be kept at room temperature and processed within how many hours of collection?
a. 8 hours
b. 12 hours
c. 24 hours
d. 48 hours

42. What does a SWOT analysis evaluate within a marketing plan?
a. Weaknesses
b. Opportunities
c. Strengths
d. All of the above

43. Which of the following is an example of internal marketing?
a. Web page/social media
b. Yellow pages
c. Client education
d. Newspaper advertisement

44. Recalls should be performed for which of the following patient scenarios?
a. Yearly exams
b. Vaccines
c. Wound care/infection
d. Surgery
e. All of the above

45. Which of the following is *not* an example of external marketing?
a. Outdoor building sign
b. Lectures
c. Media advertising
d. Client education

46. Which message component contributes the most during communication?
a. Verbal
b. Nonverbal
c. Paraverbal
d. All components of a message are equal in contribution

47. Which of the following is an example of a nonverbal skill?
a. Folded arms
b. High-pitched tone
c. Slang word choice
d. Using "yeah" instead of "yes"

48. Which team members should present treatment plans to clients?
a. Receptionist
b. Office manager
c. Veterinary technician
d. Veterinarian

49. The percentage of clients who accept a recommendation is defined as:
a. Quantity
b. Turnover
c. Retention
d. Compliance

50. When should client grievances be addressed?
a. After a meeting with the office manager
b. Immediately, at the time of the grievance
c. A week later after the pet, client, and employee have recovered
d. Depends on the severity of the grievance

51. When a client is not present to sign a euthanasia form, to verify the euthanasia how many team members must the owner talk to?
a. 1
b. 2
c. 3
d. 4

52. Euthanasia comes from the Greek terms "eu" and "Thanatos". What does the term "eu" stand for?
  a. Right
  b. Death
  c. Good
  d. Both a and c
53. Which of the following characteristics would be examples of a barrier to communication?
  a. Cultures
  b. Exam room tables
  c. Reception desk
  d. Lack of eye contact
  e. All of the above
54. Which of the following correctly defines mass cremation?
  a. A cremation service held within a church
  b. A cremation of multiple animals without private ashes returned
  c. A cremation of a single animal with private ashes returned
  d. A cremation of a single animal without ashes returned
55. How should a pet be presented to an owner after it has been euthanized?
  a. In a box
  b. In a trash bag
  c. In a waterproof body bag
  d. Without any covering
56. What drug is commonly used for euthanasia?
  a. Barbiturate
  b. Morphine
  c. Acepromazine
  d. Telazol
57. When scheduling appointments, which of the following factors should be considered?
  a. Number of veterinarians seeing appointments
  b. Veterinary technician appointments
  c. Length of time for client education
  d. All of the above
58. Which of the following is an example of a nonsterile procedure?
  a. Spay procedures
  b. Orthopedic surgeries
  c. Abscess debridement
  d. Exploratory surgery
59. To help reduce client overload at the front desk, appointments should be:
  a. Set every 15 minutes
  b. Set every 30 minutes
  c. Staggered every 5 minutes
  d. None of the above
60. Appointment lengths may vary for all of the following *except*:
  a. Specific client
  b. Appointment type
  c. Veterinarian
  d. Patient
61. Which of the following people must be able to read medical records?
  a. Veterinarians
  b. Team members
  c. Legal personnel
  d. All of the above
62. What are computerized medical records filed under?
  a. Pet's name
  b. Client's last name
  c. Client number
  d. Both b and c
63. Which of the following is considered a disadvantage of computerized medical records?
  a. Legibility
  b. Client perceives progressive, higher-quality medicine
  c. Computer-generated records can lack medical details
  d. Can target specific clients quickly and efficiently when promoting specific services
64. Medical record entry should follow the standard SOAP format, which includes all of the following *except*:
  a. Plan
  b. Obsession
  c. Subjective
  d. Assessment
65. Which of the following correctly defines the term prognosis?
  a. The surgical procedure
  b. The medication prescribed
  c. The prediction of the outcome of a disease
  d. The treatment plan
66. Which of the following correctly defines the objective portion of the exam?
  a. The reason for the visit, history, and observations made by the client
  b. Information gathered directly from the patient, physical exam, diagnostic workup
  c. Conclusion reached along with a definitive diagnosis
  d. Treatment, surgery, medication, and diagnostics recommended
67. Surgical patients must be examined within what time frame before anesthesia is administered?
  a. 2 hours
  b. 12 hours
  c. 24 hours
  d. 48 hours
68. Which of the following is considered the correct entry for medication?
  a. Cefazolin 0.2 mL IV
  b. 0.5 mL Cefazolin
  c. 0.4 mL Cefazolin (100 mg/mL) IV
  d. Cefazolin .3 100 mg/mL
69. When a medication is being dispensed, all of the following must be included in the medical record *except*:
  a. Drug lot number
  b. Drug strength
  c. Drug administration route
  d. Drug duration of treatment
70. An inactive medical record is defined as a client who has not been seen by the practice in how long?
  a. 6 months
  b. 12 months
  c. 3 years
  d. 7 years

71. All of the following are rules for medical records *except*:
    a. Records can be written in any color ink desired
    b. The author of the entry must date and initial each time an entry is made
    c. Correction fluid may never be used
    d. Use standard and approved abbreviations only
72. Which of the following are considered losses associated with poor inventory management?
    a. Backorders
    b. Shrinkage
    c. Frequent ordering
    d. All of the above
73. Which of the following correctly defines "turnover rate" in reference to inventory?
    a. The most popular product used in the facility
    b. The number of times a specific product turns over in a practice
    c. How quickly the product will expire
    d. The time it takes to receive product after it has been purchased
74. Which of the following is the proper way to handle expired drugs?
    a. Prescribe them to owners to get them out the facility
    b. Flush them down the drain
    c. Dissolved in an appropriate pouch that inactivates the medication then disposed of in the trash
    d. Throw them in the trash
75. What does a dispensing fee cover?
    a. The label on the bottle
    b. The vial used to package the medication
    c. The wear and tear on the label machine
    d. All of the above
76. Missed charges account for approximately how much of gross revenue?
    a. 5%
    b. 10%
    c. 25%
    d. 45%
77. Any pharmaceutical that is a controlled substance will have what letter on the bottle?
    a. A
    b. C
    c. D
    d. S
78. Controlled substance prescriptions administered to clients for classes III, IV, and V can have five refills available for how long?
    a. 1 month
    b. 6 months
    c. 12 months
    d. None, they cannot have refills
79. Which class level of controlled drugs has the highest potential for abuse?
    a. I
    b. IV
    c. V
    d. VII
80. Class II controlled substances can be filled for 30 days with how many refills?
    a. 1
    b. 3
    c. 5
    d. None, this class is not allowed refills on the original script
81. Which controlled substance class level does not have DEA dispensing limits?
    a. Class I
    b. Class II
    c. Class IV
    d. Class V
82. Which controlled substance class must have separate logs and invoices from other classes?
    a. I
    b. II
    c. IV
    d. V
83. All of the following information is included in drug logs *except*:
    a. Amount of drug administered
    b. Balance of drug after use
    c. Client name
    d. Drug lot number
84. Which of the following will not be found on an inventory log?
    a. Date of purchase
    b. Date and time of inventory
    c. Client name, patient name
    d. Product name, strength, and count in a full bottle
85. When a drug loss or theft has been identified, who must be notified?
    a. DEA
    b. Police
    c. Both a and b
    d. No one; it just needs to be recorded
86. How many witnesses are required to sign off on the destruction of controlled substances?
    a. 1
    b. 2
    c. 3
    d. None, controlled substances must be disposed of by a reverse distributor and not through the practice
87. A loss equal to or greater than what amount must be reported to the DEA?
    a. 1%
    b. 2%
    c. 3%
    d. 5%
88. The law requires which of the following logs?
    a. Compliance logs
    b. Controlled substance logs
    c. Laboratory logs
    d. All of the above
89. Controlled substance logs should be kept for ______ year(s) beyond the last recorded entry.
    a. 1
    b. 2
    c. 3
    d. 4

90. Accounts receivable should not be greater than what percentage of gross revenue?
   a. 1.50%
   b. 5%
   c. 10%
   d. 12.50%

91. Which of the following best describes the Fair Debt Collection Practices Act of 1996?
   a. Any facility or collecting agency is allowed to call anytime in an effort to collect its debt
   b. Any collecting agency is allowed to state that it is a government agency attempting to collect its debt
   c. Protects the public from unethical collection procedures
   d. Protects the businesses on past-due accounts made by the patron

92. Which of the following is *not* allowed to be given to a collection agency?
   a. Client's full name, address, and telephone number
   b. Client's occupation
   c. Client's driver's license number
   d. None of the above

93. What does indemnity insurance provide?
   a. A contract for veterinarians to provide medical service at a set price
   b. A reimbursement the veterinarian collects directly from the insurance company for services rendered
   c. Compensation for treatment of injured or sick pets paid directly to the client, following the company policy
   d. None of the above

94. Which of the following correctly defines a per-incident limit?
   a. The maximum dollar amount a company will pay out on one policy for the lifetime of the pet
   b. The maximum dollar amount an insurance company will pay out per incident filed
   c. Injury or illness contracted, manifested, or incurred before the policy effective date
   d. An extension of coverage that can be purchased and added to a base medical policy

95. A team member must be able to walk to an eyewash station within what amount of time after being exposed to a chemical?
   a. 10 seconds
   b. 30 seconds
   c. 60 seconds
   d. 2 minutes

96. What is the minimum PPE that must be worn when performing x-rays?
   a. Lead gown only
   b. Lead gown and thyroid collar
   c. Lead gown, thyroid collar, and lead gloves
   d. Lead gown, thyroid collar, lead gloves, and goggles

97. Where should dosimeter badges be worn?
   a. Under the lead gown
   b. In the pocket of the team member
   c. On the outside of the PPE
   d. Dosimeter badges are not worn and should be kept outside of the x-ray room at all times

98. How long should dosimetry reports be kept in accordance with OSHA standards?
   a. 2 years
   b. 10 years
   c. 15 years
   d. 30 years

99. Noise protection should be provided for employees when noise levels reach which decibel level?
   a. 75 dB
   b. 85 dB
   c. 95 dB
   d. Ear protection is not required in the veterinary practice

100. All of the following are provided in SDS sheets *except*:
   a. Health hazards
   b. The nearest emergency facility
   c. Permissible exposure limits
   d. Emergency first aid procedures

101. Which of the following is *not* included in a spill kit?
   a. Cat litter
   b. Water
   c. Eye protection
   d. Nitrile gloves

102. Which of the following would be found under the HCS pictogram of the skull and crossbones?
   a. Explosives
   b. Skin irritant
   c. Flammables
   d. Acute toxicity (fatal or toxic)

103. A urine sediment evaluation checks for which of the following?
   a. White blood cells
   b. Crystals
   c. Epithelial cells
   d. All of the above

104. A urine dipstick analysis tests for all of the following *except*:
   a. Glucose
   b. pH
   c. Bacteria
   d. Leukocytes

105. Which of the following diagnostic imaging procedures uses sound waves?
   a. MRI
   b. x-ray
   c. Fluoroscopy
   d. Sonography

106. Which of the following abbreviations indicates "every other day"?
   a. QID
   b. QOD
   c. BID
   d. OD

107. Drugs that reduce inflammation are termed:
   a. Anthelmintics
   b. Antimicrobials
   c. Anti-inflammatories
   d. Antifungal

108. Insulin is an example of what type of drug?
   a. Anthelmintic
   b. Gastric
   c. Endocrine
   d. Nervous

109. A positive practice culture has all of the following characteristics *except*:
   a. Warm, welcoming environment
   b. Teamwork
   c. Gossip
   d. Team etiquette

110. When placing a caller on hold in the veterinary practice, how long is an acceptable wait time?
   a. 1 minute
   b. 2 minutes
   c. 5 minutes
   d. 10 minutes

111. What percentage of phone shoppers should become clients in each veterinary hospital?
   a. 20%
   b. 50%
   c. 70%
   d. 100%

112. Clients are expected to complete which forms?
   a. Rabies certificates
   b. Spay or neuter certificates
   c. Medical records
   d. Patient information sheet

113. When clients ask for their medical records to be released to anyone other than themselves, which act regulates how those records can be released?
   a. Privacy Act of 1974
   b. Family and Medical Leave Act
   c. Fair Credit and Reporting Act
   d. There is no act that regulates how to release medical records

114. The Red Flags Rule establishes that practices must:
   a. Give clients the option to purchase medication wherever they choose
   b. Verify identification when the client has presented credit cards to pay for services
   c. Give team members time off for jury duty
   d. Verify team member citizenship in advance of hiring

115. Which of the following are acceptable methods of payment in most veterinary practices?
   a. Credit cards
   b. Check
   c. Care Credit
   d. All of the above

116. Which of the following methods would the receptionist use to ensure the safety of both clients and patients in the reception area?
   a. Place every client and pet in an exam room when they arrive
   b. Make sure every dog is on a leash and every cat is in a carrier
   c. Provide signage advising of animal restraint policies
   d. Provide separate reception areas for well and ill pets

117. Clients and visitors observe a heated argument between two staff members regarding whose responsibility it is to clean up urine from a "doggie mishap" in the reception area. This type of staff interaction will have an effect on which of the following:
   a. Etiquette
   b. Job descriptions
   c. Cleaning product selection
   d. Team culture

SECTION

3 Calculations

Heather Prendergast

QUESTIONS

1. The doctor asks you to administer 5 g of 25% mannitol to a patient. How many mL do you give?
   a. 5 mL
   b. 20 mL
   c. 40 mL
   d. 25 mL
2. Many drugs do not have X mg/mL listed on their labels but instead have their concentrations listed as a percentage (e.g., X% solution). Which of the following most accurately reflects the conversion of a percentage of a solution to a weight per volume format?
   a. X% = X g/mL
   b. X% = X g/10 mL
   c. X% = X g/100 mL
   d. X% = X mg/10 mL
3. A 75-lb dog must be dewormed. If the daily dose of the dewormer is 1 tsp/25 lb of body weight for 3 days, approximately how much should be administered each day?
   a. 3 tbs
   b. 1 tbs
   c. 5 tsp
   d. 1 tsp
4. A cat on intravenous fluids must receive 30 mL/h of normal saline. If this cat has a drip set that provides 60 drops/mL, what should the drip rate be?
   a. 1 drop/2 s
   b. 1 drop/6 s
   c. 3 drops/s
   d. 16 drops/s
5. The concentration of furosemide is 5%. How many mg are in 0.5 mL?
   a. 150 mg
   b. 2.5 mg
   c. 25 mg
   d. 50 mg
6. How many mL of a drug with a concentration of 100 mg/mL should be administered to a 75-lb dog at a dose of 1 mg/lb?
   a. 75 mL
   b. 100 mL
   c. 0.75 mL
   d. 0.34 mL
7. How many mL are in a teaspoon?
   a. 1 mL
   b. 3 mL
   c. 5 mL
   d. 10 mL
8. A prescription in which 3 mL of lactulose is administered orally twice daily will require how many ounces to last at least 30 days?
   a. 3 oz
   b. 6 oz
   c. 90 oz
   d. 180 oz
9. A commercial dog food is 420 kcal/cup. A dog weighing 60 lb fed at a rate of 70 kcal/lb/day should be fed how many cups at each meal if he is fed twice daily?
   a. 5 cups
   b. 10 cups
   c. 2 cups
   d. 1 cup
10. A cockatiel needs 100 mg/kg piperacillin via intramuscular injection. If the bird weighs 80 g, and the concentration of piperacillin is 100 mg/mL, how many mL should be administered?
    a. 0.08 mL
    b. 0.8 mL
    c. 80 mL
    d. 1.6 mL
11. A rabbit needs 300 mg/kg of a 1% ivermectin solution. If the rabbit weighs 8 lb, how many mL of ivermectin should be administered?
    a. 8 mL
    b. 10 mL
    c. 0.1 mL
    d. 0.8 mL
12. How many mL of a 50% dextrose solution are needed to make 1000 mL of a 5% dextrose solution?
    a. 1 mL
    b. 10 mL
    c. 50 mL
    d. 100 mL
13. Six 12-oz puppies need deworming medication. If the dose is 1 mL/lb, how many mL do you dispense?
    a. 12 mL
    b. 4.5 mL
    c. 6 mL
    d. 3 mL
14. The doctor asks you to start a fentanyl constant rate infusion (CRI) at 3 μg/kg/h in a 50-kg dog. The fentanyl you have available in the hospital is 50 μg/mL. What will the rate per hour be?
    a. 1 mL/h
    b. 3 mL/h
    c. 5 mL/h
    d. 50 mL/h

15. To make a solution with a concentration of 15 mg/mL, how many mL of sterile water should be added to 30 g of powdered drug?
a. 5 mL
b. 200 mL
c. 150 mL
d. 2000 mL

16. A prescription reads "2 tab q4h po prn until gone." The translation of these instructions is:
a. Two tablets are to be taken four times per day for pain until all tablets are gone.
b. Two tablets are to be taken four times per day under supervision by the veterinarian until all tablets are gone.
c. Two tablets are to be taken every 4 hours with food and water until all tablets are gone.
d. Two tablets are to be taken every 4 hours by mouth as needed until all tablets are gone.

17. How many tablets would you dispense for a 30-day supply of a drug with a dose of 1.5 tablets three times daily?
a. 500 tablets
b. 45 tablets
c. 135 tablets
d. 90 tablets

18. One gram of powdered drug diluted with how many mL of sterile water will make a concentration of 20 mg/mL?
a. 0.05 mL
b. 0.2 mL
c. 100 mL
d. 50 mL

19. You regularly order six 10 mL vials per month of a drug that has a concentration of 50 mg/mL. This month that same drug is available only in 20 mL vials of 10 mg/mL. How many vials should you order this month to obtain the same total amount of drug?
a. 150
b. 60
c. 10
d. 15

20. If a dog that receives fluids at a rate of 120 mL/h has a rate reduction of 20%, what is the new rate in mL/h?
a. 1.6 mL/h
b. 0.4 mL/h
c. 24 mL/h
d. 96 mL/h

21. Generally 1 fluid ounce is equal to approximately how many mL of liquid?
a. 1 mL
b. 15 mL
c. 30 mL
d. 60 mL

22. A cat that weighs 5 kg is given 0.1 mL of a drug with a concentration of 10 mg/mL. What dose did this cat receive?
a. 0.05 mg/kg
b. 0.2 mg/kg
c. 2 mg/kg
d. 25 mg/kg

23. You give 5 mg of a drug to a 10-kg animal. What is the dose of the drug in mg/kg?
a. 2 mg/kg
b. 10 mg/kg
c. 0.5 mg/kg
d. 50 mg/kg

24. A bird that weighs 50 g requires a particular drug at 4 mg/kg divided twice daily. What is the morning dose?
a. 1 mg
b. 4 mg
c. 0.1 mg
d. 100 mg

25. A 1-mg/kg dose of diazepam is to be administered to a 50-lb dog. How many mg will he be given?
a. 50 mg
b. 22.7 mg
c. 500 mg
d. 2.27 mg

26. How long will it take to give a whole blood transfusion of 60 mL at a rate of 2 mL/min?
a. 30 h
b. 3 h
c. ½ hour
d. 1.8 h

27. If a prescription calls for one tablet to be administered for 3 days BID, then one tablet for 5 days sid, then ½ tablet administered every other day for 2 weeks, how many tablets should be dispensed?
a. 15 tablets
b. 18 tablets
c. 20 tablets
d. 11 tablets

28. Fifty mL of a solution of 50% dextrose is added to a liter of 0.45% NaCl with 2.5% dextrose to yield a solution with a final dextrose concentration of what percentage?
a. 3%
b. 4.80%
c. 5%
d. 10%

29. A dog consumes five bowls of water in a 24-hour period. Each bowl contained exactly 100 mL. If you collect 475 mL of urine over the same 24-hour period, approximately how many mL constitute insensible loss?
a. 475 mL
b. 500 mL
c. 25 mL
d. 5 mL

30. If you measure an animal and set the x-ray machine at 70 kVp and 1/60 second and the resulting radiograph is 20% too light, to what setting should the new kVp be increased?
a. 84
b. 87
c. 90
d. 114

31. Tidal volume for a dog is 15 mL/kg. If a 10-kg male dog is taking 10 breaths/min, what is his minute volume?
a. 150 mL/min
b. 1500 mL/min
c. 15 mL/min
d. 10 mL/min

32. A 10-kg dog has a diaphragmatic hernia and his tidal volume is only 10 mL/kg. If this dog were on a ventilator, what should his breathing rate be, when a normal tidal volume is 15 mL/kg and 10 breaths/min?
 a. 15 breaths/min
 b. 5 breaths/min
 c. 8 breaths/min
 d. 100 breaths/min
33. You are asked to administer a drug that is supplied as an enteric-coated tablet at 100 mg, 50 mg, and 25 mg; you require 25 mg but have available 50-mg tablets only. You should:
 a. Use a pill splitter to divide the 100-mg tablet into quarters to obtain the smallest piece
 b. Use a pill splitter to divide the 50-mg tablet into halves to obtain the most accurate dose
 c. Administer the 50-mg tablet but then skip the next scheduled dosing
 d. Order or purchase 25-mg tablets for the dosing schedule
34. An anesthesia machine is set to deliver 1 L/min oxygen and 3% isoflurane. Approximately how many mL of isoflurane will be used for a 1-hour procedure?
 a. 30 mL
 b. 180 mL
 c. 2400 mL
 d. 1800 mL
35. A 300-g bird must be tube fed 2 mL liquid formula/100 g body weight three times daily. One gram of powdered formula will yield 15 mL of liquid formula after reconstitution, which is good for 24 hours only. How many mL of reconstituted formula should you measure out for a 24-hour period, assuming no waste?
 a. 0.8 mL
 b. 0.4 mL
 c. 2.5 mL
 d. 1.2 mL
36. A cat with a gastrostomy tube must receive 300 kcal daily. A 15-oz can of the prescribed diet has 1500 kcal. The prescribed diet must be diluted 50:50 with water to flow through the tube, and a maximum of 45 mL can be administered at one feeding. Approximately how many feedings does this cat need daily?
 a. 10
 b. 8
 c. 4
 d. 2
37. If the cat in the previous question requires an additional 160 mL of water daily, how many additional 45-mL boluses of water must be given?
 a. 3.5 mL
 b. 2.5 mL
 c. 1.5 mL
 d. 5.5 mL
38. Five tonometer readings in millimeters of mercury are 14, 15, 19, 14, and 18. What is the average (mean) reading?
 a. 17
 b. 18
 c. 16
 d. 15
39. A patient requires 3 units of insulin every 12 hours. If the concentration of insulin is 100 U/mL, how many mL should be given at each administration?
 a. 0.3 mL
 b. 30 mL
 c. 0.03 mL
 d. 0.15 mL
40. If the concentration of the insulin in the previous question were 30 U/mL, what would be the volume of insulin given at each administration?
 a. 0.1 mL
 b. 10 mL
 c. 0.05 mL
 d. 0.01 mL
41. A diagnostic laboratory requires 1 mL of serum to run a chemistry panel. A bird with a PCV of 50% would need how many full HCT tubes collected to have enough serum for the panel? (Each HCT tube holds 0.1 mL of whole blood.)
 a. 100
 b. 20
 c. 10
 d. 5
42. A 20-kg dog with a PCV of 40% has 300 mL of blood collected. The red blood cells are separated from the serum. What volume of saline would you add to the red cells to make a PCV of 50%?
 a. 360 mL
 b. 240 mL
 c. 180 mL
 d. 120 mL
43. You are taking the heart rate of a cat. If you count 10 beats in 5 seconds, what is the rate in beats/min?
 a. 50
 b. 120
 c. 300
 d. 220
44. Six blood pressure readings are 115, 120, 123, 121, 121, and 112 mmHg. What is the average (mean) value?
 a. 123
 b. 120
 c. 121
 d. 119
45. A growth in the skin is 2 inches in diameter. What is the diameter of the growth in centimeters?
 a. 2.5 cm
 b. 30 cm
 c. 20 cm
 d. 5 cm
46. The veterinary dermatologist is asking you to prepare a dog for a patch test. Forty antigens need to be tested and each antigen must be 1 cm from the next. What size patch should you shave on the dog?
 a. 4 cm × 4 cm
 b. 20 cm × 20 cm
 c. 8 cm × 5 cm
 d. 16 cm × 10 cm
47. A 16-oz bottle contains how many mL?
 a. 480 mL
 b. 240 mL
 c. 40 mL
 d. 1.6 mL

48. Four hundred pounds is how many kilograms?
a. 880 kg
b. 182 kg
c. 600 kg
d. 18 kg

49. A commercial poultry diet contains 18 g of calcium per pound of feed on an as-fed basis. If calcium carbonate, the sole calcium source, is 60% elemental calcium, how much calcium carbonate is in 1 ton of feed?
a. 21.6 kg
b. 30 g
c. 6000 g
d. 18 kg

50. How many mg are in each mL of a 24% solution?
a. 24 mg
b. 2.4 mg
c. 240 mg
d. 0.24 mg

51. In a feed that includes 20 lb of corn, 5 lb of beet pulp, 1 lb of bone meal, and 2 lb of whey, approximately what percentage is corn?
a. 98%
b. 28%
c. 40%
d. 71%

52. Approximately how many ounces of bleach diluted with water make 1 gal of a 30% bleach solution (1 qt = 32 oz)?
a. 19 oz
b. 38 oz
c. 3 oz
d. 76 oz

53. A dose of 30 mEq KCl has been added to 1 L of normal saline. What drip rate would provide a patient with 2 mEq KCl/h?
a. 15 mL/h
b. 67 mL/h
c. 6.7 mL/h
d. 60 mL/h

54. Which of the following is a concentration of a drug solution?
a. 15 mg/kg
b. 1000 U/mL
c. 20 gr/mg
d. 250 g/lb

55. You have an injectable calcium solution that is 30 mg/mL. How much do you add to 1 L of lactated Ringer solution to deliver 4 mg/h of calcium at a fluid rate of 30 mL/h?
a. 133 mL
b. 13.3 mL
c. 4.4 mL
d. 0.67 mL

56. A 5% dextrose solution is diluted with 100 mL of sterile water. The volume of the sterile water added is 40% of the volume of the 5% dextrose solution. What approximately is the new dextrose concentration?
a. 1.40%
b. 2.30%
c. 3.60%
d. 6.50%

57. Most pharmaceutical agents that are measured in grains have how many mg/gr?
a. 32.4
b. 64.8
c. 100
d. 120

58. The volume of an injection for a small iguana is 0.005 mL. This amount is too small to measure accurately. What dilution would allow you to give a volume of 0.05 mL?
a. 1:10
b. 0.11111111111
c. 0.73611111111
d. 1:50

59. Ten cockatiels consume a total of approximately 60 mL/day of water. How many mg of tetracycline powder should you add to the daily measured drinking water so that each 100-g bird receives 10 mg/kg/day?
a. 100 mg
b. 10 mg
c. 60 mg
d. 36 mg

60. The veterinarian asks you to fill 250 mg po BID of metronidazole for 6 days. You have 500-mg tablets in stock. How many tablets will you fill?
a. 3 tablets
b. 6 tablets
c. 12 tablets
d. 24 tablets

61. You need to deworm 100 head of cattle with a pour-on product that is applied at a rate of 1 mL/100 lb and is sold in 250-mL bottles. The cattle weigh 825 to 1050 lb each. Approximately how many bottles of dewormer should you purchase?
a. 4 bottles
b. 8 bottles
c. 10 bottles
d. 16 bottles

62. The level of fluid in the 1-L IV bag reads halfway between the 4 and 5 marks. How much fluid remains in the bag?
a. 1000 mL
b. 550 mL
c. 450 mL
d. 0.5 L

63. The level of fluid in the 1-L IV bag reads at the 700 mark. How much fluid has been administered?
a. 700 mL
b. 300 mL
c. 0.3 L
d. 300 cc

64. How many pounds does a 10-kg animal weigh?
a. 2 lb
b. 15 lb
c. 18 lb
d. 22 lb

65. How many mg of dextrose does 1 mL of 50% dextrose solution contain?
a. 5 mg/mL
b. 50 mg/mL
c. 500 mg/mL
d. 5000 mg/mL

66. The doctor orders a patient to receive a CRI of fentanyl. How often will this drug be administered?
    a. Every 2 h
    b. Every 4 h
    c. Every 6 h
    d. At a constant rate
67. The "French" unit is commonly used to express the diameter of a urinary catheter. Each French unit is equivalent to ⅓ mm. What is the diameter of a 12-French catheter in millimeters?
    a. 3 mm
    b. 4 mm
    c. 18 mm
    d. 36 mm
68. What is the correct volume of epinephrine, in mL, to administer to a 28-lb dog, if the dose is 0.1 mg/kg and the concentration in the bottle is 1:1000 (1 mg/mL)?
    a. 2.8 mL
    b. 1.4 mL
    c. 1.3 mL
    d. 0.28 mL
69. How many mg of epinephrine are administered in the previous calculation?
    a. 0.13 mg
    b. 2.8 mg
    c. 0.41 mg
    d. 1.3 mg
70. How many mg of doxapram (Dopram) should be administered to a 7-lb cat, if the dose range is 1 to 5 mg/kg IV and the concentration in the bottle is 20 mg/mL?
    a. 9.5 mg
    b. 0.59 mg
    c. 21 mg
    d. 0.21 mg
71. How many mL will be administered in the previous calculation?
    a. 1.3 mL
    b. 2.1 mL
    c. 0.95 mL
    d. 0.48 mL
72. How many mL of a 50:50 mixture of diazepam and ketamine at a dose of 1 mL/20 lb should be administered to an 8-lb cat?
    a. 0.4 mL diazepam; 0.4 mL ketamine
    b. 0.2 mL diazepam; 0.2 mL ketamine
    c. 2 mL diazepam; 2 mL ketamine
    d. 1 mL diazepam; 1 mL ketamine
73. The suggested oxygen flow rate for a circle rebreathing system is 25 to 50 mL/kg/min and 130 to 300 mL/kg/min for a nonrebreathing system. What is the most appropriate flow setting for a 10-lb cat?
    a. 0.3 L/min
    b. 900 mL/min
    c. 3 L/min
    d. 0.9 mL/min
74. Using the same suggested oxygen flow rates as in the previous question, what is the most appropriate oxygen flow rate for a 32-lb spaniel?
    a. 8 L
    b. 1.6 L
    c. 435 mL
    d. 0.435 mL
75. You have just administered an injection of 0.02 mL of acepromazine (10 mg/mL). How many mg did you give?
    a. 2 mg
    b. 0.2 mg
    c. 20 mg
    d. 200 mg
76. You have just administered one tablet of 64.8 mg of phenobarbital. How many grains of drug did you deliver?
    a. 0.25 gr
    b. 0.5 gr
    c. 0.6 gr
    d. 1 gr
77. A 0.25 gr (grain) of phenobarbital is how many mg?
    a. 15.2 mg
    b. 14 mg
    c. 16.2 mg
    d. 32.4 mg
78. The doctor asks you to fill oral metronidazole, 10 mg/kg po BID for 7 days. The dog weighs 37.5 kg and you have 250 mg tablets available in the hospital. How many tablets do you fill?
    a. 7 tablets
    b. 14 tablets
    c. 21 tablets
    d. 42 tablets
79. 2% lidocaine is prescribed for a 13-lb beagle at a dose of 2 mg/kg IV. How many mL will you deliver?
    a. 1.6 mL
    b. 0.16 mL
    c. 0.6 mL
    d. 6 mL
80. You just administered 1.2 mL of penicillin (300,000 U/mL). How many units did you administer?
    a. 260,000 U
    b. 360,000 U
    c. 360 U
    d. 0.26 U
81. What unit of measure is most commonly used for serum potassium?
    a. French
    b. mEq
    c. International units (IU)
    d. German
82. Your patient is a 42-lb shepherd mix with a history of vomiting. The order reads: metoclopramide HCl (5 mg/mL); give 0.3 mg/kg IM q6h prn. How many mL will you deliver?
    a. 8 mL
    b. 1 mL
    c. 5 mL
    d. 2 mL
83. In the situation described in the previous question, how many mg will you deliver?
    a. 8 mg
    b. 1 mg
    c. 5.7 mg
    d. 2 mg

84. NPH insulin is labeled 100 U/mL. The order is for a 12-lb poodle and reads: NPH insulin 1 U/kg QD. How many units do you deliver?
a. 4 U
b. 3 U
c. 5.5 U
d. 6 U

85. How many mL will you draw up to deliver the number of units in the previous question?
a. 4 mL
b. 3 mL
c. 6 mL
d. 0.05 mL

86. You are preparing an insulin drip. If you add 1 U of insulin/100 mL of IV fluid, how many units will you add to the 1-L bag of fluids?
a. 100 U
b. 1 U
c. 10 U
d. 1000 U

87. The insulin drip prepared in the previous question is to be administered at 1 U/h. How many mL will this be per hour?
a. 1 mL
b. 10 mL
c. 0.01 mL
d. 100 mL

88. What would be the drip rate per second for 6 units of insulin (1 U/100 mL) administered during a 2-h period using a 60 gtt (drops)/mL administration set?
a. 1 gtt/s
b. 0.5 gtt/s
c. 1.5 gtt/s
d. 5 gtt/s

89. A cat in end-stage renal disease is receiving epoetin (2000 U/mL). The dose is 100 U/kg. Your patient weighs 5.5 lb. How many units will you deliver?
a. 250 U
b. 25 U
c. 0.25 U
d. 100 U

90. How many mL will you draw up to administer 25 units of epoetin (2000 U/mL)?
a. 2.5 mL
b. 0.25 mL
c. 0.01 mL
d. 0.1 mL

91. Potassium gluconate is administered ¼ tsp/4.5 kg po BID. How many mL will you deliver in 1 day to a 10-lb cat?
a. 4.5 mL
b. 2 mL
c. 0.15 mL
d. 2.5 mL

92. If the potassium is labeled 5 mEq/5 mL, how many milliequivalents of potassium are delivered in 2 mL?
a. 2 mEq
b. 0.2 mEq
c. 20 mEq
d. 5.5 mEq

93. Chemotherapy medications are dosed by:
a. mL/kg
b. cc/lb
c. Body surface area
d. mg/mL

94. What is the fluid deficit in mL for a 33-lb dog with 9% dehydration?
a. 297 mL
b. 1350 mL
c. 135 mL
d. 330 mL

95. To prepare 128 oz of a 1:7 dilution of iodine and alcohol, you would use:
a. 480 oz iodine, 3360 oz alcohol
b. 12.8 oz of iodine, 115.2 oz of alcohol
c. 128 mL of iodine, 896 mL alcohol
d. 480 mL iodine, 3360 mL alcohol

96. What is the fluid deficit for a 10-lb cat with 12% dehydration?
a. 120 mL
b. 60 mL
c. 545 mL
d. 1200 mL

97. To prepare 1 cup of instrument milk using the suggested 1:6 dilution ratio, you would use:
a. 1 oz milk, 6 oz water
b. 34.3 mL milk, 205.7 mL water
c. 30 mL milk, 210 mL water
d. 1 mL milk, 6 mL water

98. You need to deliver 450 mL of 5% glucose. You have a liter of sterile water and a 500-mL bottle of 50% glucose. Which of the following is the correct preparation?
a. 45 mL of 50% glucose in 405 mL sterile water
b. 0.45 mL of 50% glucose in 40.5 mL sterile water
c. 90 mL of 50% glucose in 360 mL of sterile water
d. 4.5 mL of 50% glucose in 445.5 mL sterile water

99. A 25% solution of sulfamethazine contains how many mg of sulfamethazine per mL?
a. 2500 mg/mL
b. 250 mg/mL
c. 25 mg/mL
d. 2.5 mg/mL

100. How much sodium chloride is required to produce 5 L of 0.85% saline solution?
a. 42.5 mg
b. 4.25 kg
c. 425 mg
d. 42.5 g

101. What volume of a 1.2% sodium hydroxide (NaOH) solution can be made from 600 mg of NaOH?
a. 50 mL
b. 5 mL
c. 250 mL
d. 500 mL

102. What volume of distilled water must be added to a 5-g vial of thiopental sodium to create a 2.5% solution?
a. 40 mL
b. 200 mL
c. 250 mL
d. 500 mL

103. A stock solution was diluted 1:5, then 1:3, then 1:2, and finally 1:6 to produce a final concentration of 0.4 mg/mL. The original concentration of the stock solution was:
a. 0.03%
b. 6.4 mg/mL
c. 7.20%
d. 7.2 mg/mL

104. What volume of water must be added to 12.5 mL of a 6% stock solution to produce a 0.5% solution?
a. 150 mL
b. 137.5 mL
c. 37.5 mL
d. 6.25 mL

105. A 30% stock solution of potassium permanganate ($KMnO_4$) was diluted four times as follows: 0.1 mL of stock was added to 0.4 mL of distilled water; 4.5 mL of distilled water was added; the resulting solution was diluted 1:3; the resulting solution was again diluted to 0.06 L. The final concentration of the solution was:
a. 1.36%
b. 50 mg/mL
c. 5 mg/mL
d. 0.05%

106. What volume of 4.5% potassium chloride (KCl) solution is needed to prepare 0.75 L of a 9-mg/mL KCl solution?
a. 15 mL
b. 375 mL
c. 1.5 mL
d. 150 mL

107. The concentration of a culture medium produced by dissolving 2.5 g in 0.4 L of distilled water is:
a. 0.15%
b. 0.63%
c. 0.16%
d. 6.25%

108. The amount of glucose to be weighed to produce 500 mL of a 4.5% solution is:
a. 22.5 g
b. 2.25 g
c. 0.225 kg
d. 22.5 mg

109. How many mg of a drug should be administered to a patient weighing 22 lb if the dose is 0.2 mg/kg?
a. 2 mg
b. 4.4 mg
c. 20 mg
d. 44 mg

110. A stock solution was diluted four times as follows: 18 mL of distilled water was added to 2 mL of stock; the resulting solution was diluted 1:3; 240 mL of distilled water was added; the resulting solution was diluted to 0.9 L. If the final concentration of the diluted solution was determined to be 100 mg/mL, the original concentration of the stock solution was:
a. 4.5 mg/mL
b. 4.50%
c. 60 mg/mL
d. 0.21%

111. What volume of sulfuric acid (H_2SO_4) is in 275 mL of a 12% v/v solution?
a. 33 mL
b. 22.9 mL
c. 3.3 mL
d. 4.36 mL

112. The concentration of a glucose solution produced when 4500 mg of glucose is dissolved in 3.6 L of water is:
a. 0.80%
b. 0.01%
c. 0.13%
d. 1.25%

113. How many cubic centimeters are in a tablespoon?
a. 5 cc
b. 15 cc
c. 25 cc
d. 30 cc

114. The basic unit of mass in the metric system is the:
a. Kilogram
b. Gram
c. Milligram
d. Microgram

115. The doctor ordered a patient to receive Unasyn, 1200 mg IV. Once reconstituted, the Unasyn has a concentration of 375 mg/mL. How many mL will you administer?
a. 0.31 mL
b. 1.2 mL
c. 3.2 mL
d. 6.4 mL

116. 50 g is equal to:
a. 0.005 kg
b. 0.05 kg
c. 500,000 mg
d. 5,000,000 µg

117. The mean cellular hemoglobin (MCH) for a particular blood sample is calculated to be 24.3 pg. This is equal to:
a. 24,300 mg
b. 2430 µg
c. 24.3 × 1012 g
d. 24.3 × 10–12 g

118. The mean corpuscular volume (MCV) for a particular blood sample is calculated to be 66.5 femtoliter (fl). This is equal to:
a. 66.5×10^{-15} L
b. 66.5×10^{15} mL
c. 66.5×10^{-3} µl
d. 66.5×10^{-9} L

119. The basic unit of length in the metric system is the:
a. Millimeter
b. Centimeter
c. Meter
d. Kilometer

120. 485 km is equal to:
a. 4.85 × 103 m
b. 485 × 104 mm
c. 4.85 × 108 mm
d. 48,500 cm

121. 250 cc is equal to:
a. 25 mL
b. 0.25 L
c. 25,000 µl
d. 2.5 L

122. One metric ton of livestock feed is equal to:
a. 1000 lb
b. 10,000 g
c. 2200 lb
d. 1,000,000 mg

123. One centimeter is:
a. Greater than 1 mm but shorter than 1 μ (1 micron)
b. Shorter than both 1 m and 1 mm
c. Greater than both 1 mm and 1 μ
d. Shorter than 1 km but greater than 1 m

124. A dog weighs 55 lb. Its weight can also be stated as:
a. 121 kg
b. 25 g
c. 121 mg
d. 25 kg

125. 8 oz is equal to approximately:
a. 227,200 mg
b. 454 g
c. 227 mg
d. 2.27 kg

126. 10 inches is equal to approximately:
a. 25 mm
b. 4 cm
c. 25 cm
d. 0.04 m

127. The volume of a stock solution required to prepare 3.5 L of a 1:40 dilution is:
a. 0.14 L
b. 87.5 mL
c. 630 mL
d. 0.875 L

128. A stock solution of atropine sulfate has a concentration of 2.2 mg/mL. It may also be used clinically as a 0.05% solution. The volume of the more concentrated atropine solution required to prepare 40 mL of the dilute solution is:
a. 17.6 mL
b. 9.1 mL
c. 4.4 mL
d. 0.91 mL

129. The doctor would like to place a patient on a metoclopramide CRI at 2 mg/kg/day. He would like this added to a 1-L bag of fluids that will last 24 hours. The patient weighs 20 kg. How many mL of 5 mg/mL metoclopramide should be added to the bag?
a. 2 mL
b. 8 mL
c. 20 mL
d. 40 mL

130. The volume of a 1:25 dilution that can be prepared from 150 mL of stock solution is:
a. 3750 mL
b. 6 L
c. 6000 mL
d. 75 mL

131. If a 0.75% solution results from the addition of 380 mL of water to 20 mL of stock solution, the concentration of the stock solution is:
a. 15%
b. 0.375 mg/mL
c. 14.25%
d. 300 mg/mL

132. If you are asked to administer 0.1 mg of epinephrine to an animal with threatened cardiac collapse, how much of a 1:10,000 solution should you inject?
a. 10 mL
b. 0.01 mL
c. 0.1 mL
d. 1 mL

133. When the doctor orders an intravenous infusion, you need three pieces of information to calculate the flow rate in drops per minute. Which of the following is *not* relevant to this calculation?
a. Total volume to be infused
b. Type of fluid to be delivered
c. Calibration of the administration set being used (in drops/mL)
d. Duration of the infusion

134. The doctor orders an intravenous infusion to run at 20 mL/h. Calculate the flow rate using an
a. 30 drops/min
b. 33 drops/min
c. 20 drops/min
d. More information is needed.

135. Calculate the flow rate for an intravenous infusion of 1 L of fluid to run over 8 hours with a set calibrated at 20 drops/mL.
a. 20 drops/min
b. 42 drops/min
c. 50 drops/min
d. 125 drops/min

136. Calculating drug doses involves routine conversion between units of measure within the metric system. Which of the following conversions is *not* correct?
a. 3 cc = 3 mL
b. 1 μg = 1000 mg
c. 1 kg = 1000 g
d. 1 L = 1000 mL

137. Which metric conversion is *not* correct?
a. 3500 mL = 3.5 L
b. 520 mg = 0.52 g
c. 950 μg = 9.5 mg
d. 750 cc = 0.75 L

138. Which common equivalent is *not* correct?
a. 1 tbs = 3 tsp = 15 mL
b. 1 oz = 30 mL = 2 tbs
c. ½ gr = 64 mg
d. 1 L of H_2O = 1000 g of H_2O

139. Which equivalent is *not* correct?
a. 1 tbs = 1 tablespoonful = 15 mL
b. 1 tsp = 1 teaspoonful = 5 mL
c. 1 gtt = 1 drop
d. 1 g = 1 gram = 30 mL

140. A doctor's order calls for prednisone at a dosage of 2 mg/kg to be delivered orally to a 7.5-kg cat. How many 5-mg tablets of prednisone would you administer to the cat?
a. ¼ tablet
b. 1 tablet
c. 2 tablets
d. 3 tablets

141. You are asked to give a patient phenobarbital po at 2.2 mg/kg. The medication is available in ½-gr tablets. How many tablets should you give a 35-lb dog?
 a. ¼ tablet
 b. ½ tablet
 c. 1 tablet
 d. 2 tablets

142. A prescription reads "amoxicillin, 750 mg, po BID, 10 days." The drug is available in 500-mg tablets. How many tablets must you count out to fill this prescription?
 a. 30 tablets
 b. 60 tablets
 c. 90 tablets
 d. 120 tablets

143. Diphenhydramine elixir, 25 mg po, is ordered for a 12-year-old, 12.5-kg beagle. The solution contains 12.5 mg/5 mL. What volume should you give to this patient?
 a. 0.5 mL
 b. 2 mL
 c. 10 mL
 d. 20 mL

144. You are asked to give a dog with head trauma 20% mannitol at 0.5 g/kg by slow intravenous injection. You check the record and see that the dog weighs 44 lb. What volume should you give?
 a. 10 mL
 b. 25 mL
 c. 50 mL
 d. 250 mL

145. How much drug does 100 mL of a 10% solution contain?
 a. 0.1 g
 b. 1 g
 c. 10 g
 d. More information is needed.

146. You are asked to draw up 2 mL of 50% dextrose in water to give to a hypoglycemic kitten. What volume should you draw into the syringe?
 a. 1 mL
 b. 2 mL
 c. 10 mL
 d. More information is needed.

147. To mix a 4% solution in a bottle that contains 5 g of drug powder, how much water should you add?
 a. 50 mL
 b. 125 mL
 c. 125 mL
 d. 500 mL

148. To prepare a dose of 0.2 mg of atropine using a solution that contains 400 μg/mL, how much do you draw into the syringe?
 a. 0.05 mL
 b. 0.2 mL
 c. 0.5 mL
 d. 2 mL

149. You are asked to administer intravenously 20 mg of furosemide. The solution contains 25 mg/mL. What volume should you draw into the syringe?
 a. 0.8 mL
 b. 1.25 mL
 c. 2.5 mL
 d. The weight of the patient must be known.

150. You are asked to prepare 20 mEq of KCl for addition to a 1-L bag of lactated Ringer solution. The solution contains 30 mEq/15 mL. How much should you draw into a syringe to add to the fluid bag?
 a. 10 mL
 b. 20 mL
 c. 30 mL
 d. 40 mL

151. You are asked to infuse fluids intravenously at 50 mL/h. The administration set is calibrated at 60 drops/mL. How fast should you set the drip rate?
 a. 1 drop/min
 b. 10 drops/min
 c. 50 drops/min
 d. 60 drops/min

152. You are asked to infuse intravenously 3 L of 0.9% saline over 24 hours. The administration set is calibrated at 15 drops/mL. How fast should you set the drip rate?
 a. 200 drops/min
 b. 125 drops/min
 c. 31 drops/min
 d. 15 drops/min

153. You are asked to infuse fluids intravenously at 60 drops/min. The drip rate is currently at 7 drops/15 s. What adjustment in the drip rate is necessary?
 a. No adjustment
 b. Double the flow rate
 c. Reduce the flow rate by 50%
 d. Increase the flow rate by 25%

154. You are asked to infuse intravenously 1 L of fluids at 25 drops/min over 10 hours. After 5 hours you observe that 650 mL have been administered. What adjustment in the drip rate is necessary?
 a. No action is necessary; the IV infusion will be completed on schedule.
 b. Rate must be slowed from 25 drops/min to 18 drops/min to complete the infusion as ordered.
 c. Rate must be increased from 25 drops/min to 32 drops/min to complete the infusion as ordered.
 d. Rate must be slowed from 100 mL/h to 60 mL/h to complete the infusion as ordered.

155. You are asked to infuse intravenously 750 mL of fluids over 6 hours. The administration set is calibrated at 20 drops/mL. After 2 hours you observe that 300 mL have been infused. What should the adjusted drip rate be?
 a. 8 drops/min
 b. 19 drops/min
 c. 27 drops/min
 d. 38 drops/min

156. You are asked to infuse intravenously 500 mL of fluids over 6 hours. The administration set is calibrated at 20 drops/mL. After 4 hours you observe that only 150 mL have been given. What should the adjusted drip rate be?
 a. 19 drops/min
 b. 25 drops/min
 c. 39 drops/min
 d. 58 drops/min

157. How much 50% dextrose must be added to 1 L of lactated Ringer solution to make a solution that contains 5% dextrose?
a. 5 mL
b. 50 mL
c. 55 mL
d. 110 mL

158. Diphenhydramine elixir is prescribed at 12.5 mg po q8h. The drug is available in 30-mL bottles that contain 25 mg/5 mL. How long will one bottle last?
a. 2 days
b. 4 days
c. 6 days
d. 1 week

159. You are asked to prepare a bottle of heparinized saline with a concentration of 4 IU heparin/mL to flush indwelling catheters. The stock sodium heparin solution contains 1000 IU/mL. How much heparin must be added to each 250-mL bottle of sterile physiologic saline (0.9% NaCl) to make the flushing solution?
a. 1 mL
b. 2 mL
c. 3 mL
d. 4 mL

160. A 1-L sample contains:
a. 1 mL
b. 10 mL
c. 100 mL
d. 1000 mL

161. A 10-cc syringe can hold:
a. 1 mL
b. 10 mL
c. 100 mL
d. 1000 mL

162. A 5-kg dog weighs approximately:
a. 2.5 lb
b. 5 lb
c. 7.5 lb
d. 11 lb

163. A 354-g rat weighs:
a. 0.0354 kg
b. 0.354 kg
c. 3.54 kg
d. 35.4 kg

164. A 450-μg sample contains:
a. 4.5 g
b. 0.45 g
c. 0.045 g
d. 0.00045 g

165. A 3700-cc sample contains:
a. 370 mL
b. 37 L
c. 0.37 L
d. 3.7 L

166. An 11-lb cat weighs approximately:
a. 22 kg
b. 5 kg
c. 500 g
d. 5000 g

167. A 6.2-g sample contains:
a. 3 kg
b. 3100 mg
c. 6,200,000 μg
d. 6200 μg

168. A 0.5 g/mL sample contains:
a. 5 mg/mL
b. 50 g/100 mL
c. 5 g/100 mL
d. 500 mg/100 mL

169. A 500-kg horse weighs approximately:
a. 250 lb
b. 750 lb
c. 1100 lb
d. 1000 lb

170. A 20-dram vial of digitalis contains approximately:
a. 1.5 oz
b. 2 oz
c. 2.5 oz
d. 4 oz

171. A 120-gr aspirin contains approximately:
a. 7.8 mg
b. 78 mg
c. 780 mg
d. 7800 mg

172. A solution of 45 gr/30 mL contains approximately:
a. 100 mg/mL
b. 450 mg/mL
c. 10 g/mL
d. 1 g/100 mL

173. A 12-fl dram bottle contains approximately:
a. 36 mL
b. 45 mL
c. 68 mL
d. 120 mL

174. A 1/120-gr tablet contains approximately:
a. 0.005 mg
b. 0.05 mg
c. 0.5 mg
d. 5 mg

175. A 2-qt container holds:
a. 12 oz
b. 18 oz
c. 32 oz
d. 64 oz

176. A 14-oz bottle contains approximately:
a. 420 mL
b. 210 mL
c. 105 mL
d. 56 mL

177. A 6-tbs dose administered BID requires:
a. 2 oz/day
b. 240 mL/day
c. 1.8 L for a 10-day supply
d. 2.6 L for a 2-week supply

178. A dosage of 1 tbs daily requires:
a. 2 oz for a 14-day supply
b. 5 oz for a 14-day supply
c. 7 oz for a 14-day supply
d. 10 oz for a 14-day supply

179. A dosage of 2 tbs BID requires approximately:
   a. 16 oz for a 16-day supply
   b. 1 qt for a 16-day supply
   c. 36 oz for a 16-day supply
   d. 2.5 pt for a 16-day supply
180. A dosage of 1.5 tsp BID requires:
   a. 8 tbs for a 2-week supply
   b. 1 oz for a 2-week supply
   c. 10 tbs for a 2-week supply
   d. 14 tbs for a 2-week supply
181. A dosage of 5 mL TID equals approximately:
   a. 1 tsp/day
   b. 2 tsp/day
   c. 3 tsp/day
   d. 5 tsp/day
182. A dosage of 1 tbs every other day requires approximately:
   a. 45 mL for a 2-week supply
   b. 90 mL for a 2-week supply
   c. 105 mL for a 2-week supply
   d. 210 mL for a 2-week supply
183. A 554-kg mare needs sulfadimethoxine at 10 mg/lb daily. It is available as a 40% solution. How much sulfadimethoxine should be administered daily?
   a. 13.85 mL
   b. 138.5 mL
   c. 45.32 mL
   d. 30.5 mL
184. Fenbendazole liquid is available as a 22.2% concentration and a 45-lb German shorthaired pointer needs 50 mg/lb. How many teaspoons does it require?
   a. 1 tsp
   b. 1.5 tsp
   c. 2 tsp
   d. 3 tsp
185. Procaine penicillin is available in a concentration of 300,000 IU/mL and is administered at 20,000 IU/kg. How much do you give a 900-lb Arabian gelding?
   a. 2.7 mL
   b. 27 mL
   c. 60 mL
   d. 132 mL
186. Altrenogest for horses is available as a 0.22% solution. The daily dosage is 0.044 mg/kg. If you treated a 990-lb Morgan mare for 15 days, how much would you dispense for the client?
   a. 9 mL
   b. 135 mL
   c. 165 mL
   d. 254 mL
187. A 9-month-old female Great Dane is admitted for a routine ovariohysterectomy. The animal weighs 65 lb and the veterinarian wants to use the following preanesthetic regimen: butorphanol (10 mg/mL) IM at 0.2 mg/kg; acepromazine (10 mg/mL) IM at 0.05 mg/kg; and atropine (0.02% solution) SC at 0.02 mg/kg. How much butorphanol should be administered?
   a. 0.6 mL
   b. 1.3 mL
   c. 2.9 mL
   d. 6 mL
188. A 9-month-old female Great Dane is admitted for a routine ovariohysterectomy. The animal weighs 65 lb and the veterinarian wants to use the following preanesthetic regimen: butorphanol (10 mg/mL) IM at 0.2 mg/kg; acepromazine (10 mg/mL) IM at 0.05 mg/kg; and atropine (0.02% solution) SC at 0.02 mg/kg. How much acepromazine should be administered?
   a. 0.15 mL
   b. 0.3 mL
   c. 0.7 mL
   d. 1.5 mL
189. A 9-month-old female Great Dane is admitted for a routine ovariohysterectomy. The animal weighs 6 lb and the veterinarian wants to use the following preanesthetic regimen: butorphanol (10 mg/mL) IM at 0.2 mg/kg; acepromazine (10 mg/mL) IM at 0.05 mg/kg; and atropine (0.02% solution) SC at 0.02 mg/kg. How much atropine should be administered?
   a. 1.43 mL
   b. 3.0 mL
   c. 6.5 mL
   d. 14.3 mL
190. A yearling paint colt is admitted for castration. The animal weighs 700 lb and the veterinarian wants to use the following regimen: butorphanol (10 mg/mL) IV at 0.02 mg/kg; xylazine (10 mg/mL) IV at 0.2 mg/kg; and ketamine (100 mg/mL) IV at 2.2 mg/kg. How much butorphanol should be administered?
   a. 0.6 mL
   b. 1.4 mL
   c. 3.1 mL
   d. 6 mL
191. A yearling paint colt is admitted for castration. The animal weighs 700 lb and the veterinarian wants to use the following regimen: butorphanol (10 mg/mL) IV at 0.02 mg/kg; xylazine (10 mg/mL) IV at 0.2 mg/kg; and ketamine (100 mg/mL) IV at 2.2 mg/kg. How much xylazine should be administered?
   a. 3.2 mL
   b. 6.4 mL
   c. 14 mL
   d. 31 mL
192. A yearling paint colt is admitted for castration. The animal weighs 700 lb and the veterinarian wants to use the following regimen: butorphanol (10 mg/mL) IV at 0.02 mg/kg; xylazine (10 mg/mL) IV at 0.2 mg/kg; and ketamine (100 mg/mL) IV at 2.2 mg/kg. How much ketamine should be administered?
   a. 2.8 mL
   b. 7.0 mL
   c. 15.4 mL
   d. 34 mL
193. A pet needs 100 mg of a medication, and the medication is available as a 50-mg tablet. How many tablets will be needed?
   a. 1 tablet
   b. 2 tablets
   c. 3 tablets
   d. 4 tablets

194. A pet needs 35 mg of a solution and the medication is available as a 100-mg/mL solution. How many mL will be needed?
a. 0.03 mL
b. 0.35 mL
c. 3.5 mL
d. 35 mL

195. A pet needs medication at a dose of 5 mg/kg and the medication is available in 25-mg tablets. The pet weighs 10 lb. How many tablets will be administered?
a. 1 tablet
b. 2 tablets
c. 5 tablets
d. 10 tablets

196. A pet needs a medication at a dose of 100 mg/kg and the medication is available in a 100-mg/mL solution. The pet weighs 25 lb. How many mL will be administered?
a. 1 mL
b. 11 mL
c. 12 mL
d. 114 mL

197. A pet needs 25 mg of a 2% solution. How many mL will be administered? 2% solution = 20 mg/mL
a. 25 mL
b. 20 mL
c. 1.25 mL
d. 0.1 mL

198. A pet needs butorphanol for pain at a dose of 0.04 mg/kg and the medication is available in a 10-mg/mL solution. The pet weighs 4 lb. How many mL will be administered?
a. 1.8 mL
b. 0.07 mL
c. 0.1 mL
d. 0.01 mL

199. A veterinarian writes a script for 25 mg of acepromazine to be administered every 8 hours for 5 days and the medication is available in 25-mg tablets. How many tablets will be dispensed?
a. 3 tablets
b. 5 tablets
c. 10 tablets
d. 15 tablets

200. A pet needs 5 mg/kg of Albon po sid on day 1, then 2.5 mg/kg po sid for 5 more days. The medication is available in 125-mg tablets and the pet weighs 25 lb. How many tablets will be dispensed for the owner?
a. 0.5 tablets
b. 1 tablet
c. 2 tablets
d. 5 tablets

201. A 22-lb dog needs IV fluids at a maintenance rate of 66 mL/kg/24 h. How many mL/h will the patient receive?
a. 660 mL/h
b. 60 mL/h
c. 27.5 mL/h
d. 2.7 mL/h

202. A 7-lb cat will have a dental procedure and needs IV fluids at the surgical rate of 11 mL/kg/h. How many mL/h will the patient receive?
a. 1.5 mL/h
b. 3 mL/h
c. 11 mL/h
d. 35 mL/h

203. A 120-lb dog is experiencing vomiting and diarrhea and must have IV fluids at two times maintenance (132 mL/kg/24 h). How many mL will he receive per hour?
a. 132 mL/h
b. 54 mL/h
c. 300 mL/h
d. 400 mL/h

204. A 32-lb dog needs IV fluids at a surgical rate (11 mL/kg/h). How many mL/h will the patient receive?
a. 32 mL/h
b. 15 mL/h
c. 100 mL/h
d. 160 mL/h

205. A 50-lb dog needs IV fluids at two times maintenance (132 mL/kg/24 h). How many fluids will the patient receive in a 24-hour period?
a. 125 mL
b. 132 mL
c. 2200 mL
d. 3000 mL

206. A 4.5-lb cat requires maintenance fluids (66 mL/kg/24 h). How many mL/h will be administered in a 24-hour period?
a. 5 mL
b. 28 mL
c. 132 mL
d. 300 mL

207. Lidocaine at 2% is prescribed for a 33-lb beagle at a dose of 2 mg/kg IV. How many mL will you deliver?
a. 1.5 mL
b. 0.15 mL
c. 0.5 mL
d. 5 mL

208. You just administered 3.2 mL of penicillin (300,000 U/mL). How many units did you administer?
a. 960,000 U
b. 96,000 U
c. 960 U
d. 0.96 U

209. Your patient is a 66-lb shepherd mix with a history of vomiting. The order reads: metoclopramide HCl (5 mg/mL); give 0.6 mg/kg IM q8h prn. How many mL will you deliver?
a. 5 mL
b. 1 mL
c. 0.36 mL
d. 3.6 mL

210. In the situation in the previous question, how many mg will you deliver?
a. 18 mg
b. 8 mg
c. 1 mg
d. 3.6 mg

211. Vetsulin insulin is labeled 40 U/mL. The order is for a 12-lb poodle and reads: Vetsulin 2 U/kg QD. How many units do you deliver?
   a. 1 U
   b. 2 U
   c. 8 U
   d. 11 U
212. How many mL will you draw up to deliver the number of units in the previous question?
   a. 0.27 mL
   b. 0.5 mL
   c. 1 mL
   d. 11 mL
213. A cat on intravenous fluids must receive 20 mL/h normal saline. If this cat has a drip set that provides 60 drops/mL, what should the drip rate be?
   a. 1 drop/2 s
   b. 1 drop/3 s
   c. 3 drops/s
   d. 16 drops/s
214. The concentration of furosemide is 10%. How many mg are in 1.2 mL?
   a. 100 mg
   b. 83 mg
   c. 25 mg
   d. 8.3 mg
215. How many mL of a drug with a concentration of 200 mg/mL should be administered to a 60-lb dog at a dose of 3 mg/lb?
   a. 90 mL
   b. 9 mL
   c. 3 mL
   d. 0.9 mL
216. A prescription in which 3 mL of cisapride is administered orally three times daily will require how many ounces to last at least 30 days?
   a. 3 oz
   b. 9 oz
   c. 90 oz
   d. 270 oz
217. A commercial cat food is 120 kcal/cup. A cat weighing 5 lb fed at a rate of 40 calories/lb/day should be fed how many cups at each meal if you feed him twice a day?
   a. 5 cups
   b. 10 cups
   c. 2 cups
   d. 1 cup
218. A cockatiel needs 80 mg/kg piperacillin via intramuscular injection. If the bird weighs 30 g and the concentration of piperacillin is 100 mg/mL, how many mL should be administered?
   a. 0.03 mL
   b. 0.3 mL
   c. 3 mL
   d. 30 mL
219. A dose of 40 mEq KCl has been added to 1 L of normal saline. What drip rate would provide a patient with 1 mEq KCl/h?
   a. 2.5 mL/h
   b. 20 mL/h
   c. 25 mL/h
   d. 40 mL/h
220. You have an injectable calcium solution that is 50 mg/mL. How much do you add to 1 L of lactated Ringer solution to deliver 5 mg/h of calcium at a fluid rate of 50 mL/h?
   a. 200 mL
   b. 20 mL
   c. 2 mL
   d. 0.2 mL
221. A 45-kg animal weighs how many pounds?
   a. 2.2
   b. 20
   c. 45
   d. 99
222. How many mg of dextrose does 6 mL of 50% dextrose solution contain?
   a. 3 mg/mL
   b. 30 mg/mL
   c. 300 mg/mL
   d. 3000 mg/mL

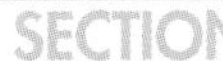

SECTION 4

Terminology

Brooke Lockridge

QUESTIONS

1. What is the correct term for an intact male cat?
   a. Sire
   b. Tom
   c. Dam
   d. Stud
2. Which of the following correctly defines the prefix *poly-*?
   a. Joint
   b. Many
   c. Disease
   d. Cartilage
3. A group of turkeys is referred to as which of the following?
   a. Poult
   b. Rafter
   c. Paddling
   d. Gaggle
4. The study of the cause of disease correctly corresponds to which term?
   a. Etiopathology
   b. Neogenic
   c. Pathology
   d. Idiopathic
5. Which of the following prefixes refers to bone?
   a. Myelo-
   b. Corpo-
   c. Osteo-
   d. Cerebro-
6. Which of the following correctly defines *kaliopenia*?
   a. Presence of an excess amount of sodium in the blood
   b. Presence of an excess amount of potassium
   c. Excretion of an abnormal amount of sodium in the urine
   d. Presence of a less than normal amount of potassium
7. A group of cats is also referred to as:
   a. Clowder
   b. Cluster
   c. Pounce
   d. All of the above
8. An atypical heart sound associated with a functional or structural valve abnormality is known as:
   a. Arrhythmia
   b. Fibrillation
   c. Murmur
   d. Infarct
9. A whelp refers to which of the following?
   a. An intact female dog
   b. A young feline
   c. A young canine
   d. The male parent of his offspring
10. The prefix *myring-* refers to which of the following?
    a. Ear
    b. Eardrum
    c. Embryo
    d. Empty
11. What is the correct term for an intact male horse older than 4 years?
    a. Gelding
    b. Mare
    c. Colt
    d. Stallion
12. An equine that is about to turn 1 year old is referred to as a:
    a. Yearling
    b. Foaling
    c. Weanling
    d. Filly
13. A male donkey that has not been castrated and is capable of breeding is referred to as a:
    a. Jenny
    b. Dam
    c. Jack
    d. Sire
14. A female calf (usually sterile) born twin to a bull calf is referred to as a:
    a. Freshening
    b. Freemartin
    c. Heifer
    d. Cow
15. Which of the following definitions correctly defines the term *wether*?
    a. An intact male sheep
    b. A young ovine
    c. The process of giving birth to lambs
    d. A castrated/neutered male ovine
16. The process of giving birth to pigs is referred to as:
    a. Stag
    b. Freshening
    c. Farrowing
    d. Kidding
17. A young female pig that has not yet given birth is referred to as:
    a. Dam
    b. Gilt
    c. Sow
    d. Stag

18. A young male chicken between 10 and 32 weeks of age is referred to as:
 a. Rooster
 b. Cockerel
 c. Capon
 d. Pullet

19. An egg-type chicken more than 32 weeks of age is referred to as a:
 a. Roaster
 b. Layer
 c. Hen
 d. Chick

20. Which of the following correctly defines the term *drake*?
 a. An intact male duck
 b. An intact female duck
 c. An immature duck of either sex
 d. A young turkey

21. An intact male ferret is known as a:
 a. Gib
 b. Jill
 c. Sprite
 d. Hob

22. The prefix *blephar-* refers to which of the following?
 a. Eye
 b. Eyelid
 c. False
 d. Fat

23. A disease that is transmitted from animals to humans is defined as:
 a. Zoology
 b. Zoonotic
 c. Enzootic
 d. Epizootic

24. The number of animals within a population that become sick can be defined as:
 a. Morbidity
 b. Mortality
 c. Chronic
 d. Acute

25. The suffix *-itis* refers to:
 a. Disease
 b. Inflammation
 c. False
 d. Bone

26. *Oste-* refers to what structure?
 a. Bone
 b. Many
 c. Cartilage
 d. Inflammation

27. The prefix *hyster-* refers to which of the following?
 a. Oviduct
 b. Uterus
 c. Ovary
 d. Surgical removal

28. The suffix *-ac* refers to which of the following?
 a. Pertaining to
 b. Condition
 c. Structure
 d. To act on

29. Which of the following terms means *within a living body*?
 a. Benign
 b. In vivo
 c. Infection
 d. In vitro

30. Which of the following means becoming progressively worse, recurring, and/or leading to death?
 a. Remission
 b. Malignant
 c. Exacerbation
 d. Idiopathic

31. Which is the correct definition of *chondrology*?
 a. The study of cartilage
 b. The study of malignancy
 c. The study of the cardiovascular system
 d. The study of bones

32. *Neoplasm* refers to which of the following?
 a. The process of abnormal or difficult growth
 b. A malignant growth of tissue
 c. Any new and abnormal growth
 d. Death of tissue

33. What is the correct term for the resting phase of a heartbeat that occurs between filling of the lower chamber of the heart and the start of contraction?
 a. Diastole
 b. Systole
 c. Arrhythmia
 d. Tachycardia

34. Which of the following terms means *toward the median plane*?
 a. Medial
 b. Lateral
 c. Anterior
 d. Posterior

35. The term *rostral* refers to which of the following definitions?
 a. Toward the head end of the body
 b. Toward the nose when referring to the head
 c. Toward the tail end of the body
 d. Posterior surface of the body

36. The transverse plane divides the body into which parts?
 a. Anterior/posterior
 b. Cranial/caudal
 c. Left/right
 d. Transverse refers to a position on a limb closer to the point of attachment

37. A collection of blood in the cranial portion of the ventral cavity is known as:
 a. Pneumothorax
 b. Pneumonia
 c. Hemothorax
 d. Hemostasis

38. An abnormal presence of tissue cells in the blood is known as:
 a. Histology
 b. Histiocytosis
 c. Karyogenic
 d. Homeostasis

39. The term *myelodysplasia* refers to which of the following?
    a. A specialized cell for the storage of fat
    b. An abnormal growth of tissue
    c. An abnormal development of muscles
    d. Slower than normal heartbeat
40. The term *abrasion* refers to which of the following descriptions?
    a. A localized collection of pus
    b. A group of furuncles in adjacent hairs
    c. Loss of hair, wool, or feathers
    d. A skin scrape
41. Blood leaking from a ruptured vessel into subcutaneous tissue is known as:
    a. Cicatrix
    b. Ecchymosis
    c. Eschar
    d. Fissure
42. The term *excoriate* means:
    a. Scratching the skin
    b. A boil or skin abscess
    c. Dried serum, blood, or pus
    d. A scar
43. An overgrowth of scar tissue at the site of injury is known as:
    a. Papule
    b. Petechia
    c. Laceration
    d. Keloid
44. A circumscribed craterlike lesion of the skin or mucous membrane is known as:
    a. Wheal
    b. Suppurate
    c. Ulcer
    d. Papule
45. Which of the following suffixes refers to a blood condition that is usually abnormal?
    a. -staxis
    b. -emia
    c. -clast
    d. -pnea
46. A bridge that forms as part of the healing process across the two halves of a bone fracture is known as a:
    a. Condyle
    b. Callus
    c. Crest
    d. Cull
47. What term is defined as a joint dislocation when the joint is displaced or goes out of alignment?
    a. Fracture
    b. Luxation
    c. Olecranon
    d. Subluxation
48. A rough projection on a bone is known as a:
    a. Suture
    b. Wing
    c. Tuberosity
    d. Trochanter
49. *Osteomalacia* refers to :
    a. Hardening of bones
    b. Softening of bones
    c. Collection of abnormal cells that accumulate within the bones
    d. Thickened skin
50. Which term is defined as the incomplete development or underdevelopment of an organ or tissue?
    a. Osteoporosis
    b. Hypoplasia
    c. Hyperplasia
    d. Ankylosis
51. Which of the following means a small opening or perforation?
    a. Fossa
    b. Foramen
    c. Exacerbation
    d. Process
52. What structure connects muscles to bones?
    a. Ligaments
    b. Tendons
    c. Foramen
    d. Process
53. Which of the following provides a smooth joint surface, allowing the bones to move freely over one another?
    a. Cartilage
    b. Ligaments
    c. Callus
    d. Fossa
54. The prefix *chondro-* refers to which of the following?
    a. Bone
    b. Muscle
    c. Cartilage
    d. Cheek
55. A rare benign tumor derived from striated muscle is known as:
    a. Cervicomuscular
    b. Rhabdomyoma
    c. Myopathology
    d. Rhabdomyosarcoma
56. *Myofibrosis* is defined as which of the following?
    a. Spasm of the muscle
    b. Abnormal condition of muscle fibers
    c. A disorder in which muscles are slow to relax
    d. A technique used for evaluating and recording the electrical activity produced by skeletal muscles
57. A connective tissue membrane that surrounds each muscle fiber is referred to as:
    a. Epimysium
    b. Endomysium
    c. Myopathy
    d. Sarcoma
58. The prefix *cephal-* means which of the following?
    a. Hard
    b. Head
    c. Hearing
    d. Heart
59. Skeletal muscle is also known as:
    a. Striated muscle
    b. Smooth muscle
    c. Cardiac muscle
    d. None of these

60. The term *ipsilateral* means which of the following?
a. Opposite side affected
b. Located on or affecting the same side of the body
c. Near or connected to the maxilla or jawbone
d. Movement away from the point of origin

61. Pain affecting half of the body is known as which of the following?
a. Semiconscious
b. Hemialgia
c. Analgesia
d. Bicaudal

62. The presence of four digits on one foot is known as:
a. Tetradactyly
b. Polydactyl
c. Multiarticular
d. Quadrilateral

63. Inflammation of all bones or inflammation of every part of one bone is known as:
a. Panosteitis
b. Polypathia
c. Pandemic
d. Osteoporosis

64. The word root *digitorum* refers to which of the following?
a. Rib
b. Wrist
c. Digit
d. Thigh

65. The word root *brachii* refers to which of the following?
a. Shin bone
b. Thigh
c. Upper foreleg
d. Shoulder blade

66. Which type of muscle attaches a limb to the body?
a. Intrinsic muscles
b. Extrinsic muscles
c. Adductor muscles
d. Abductor muscles

67. The term *amyoplasia* refers to the:
a. Lack of muscle formation or development
b. Paralysis of muscles
c. Muscular weakness or partial paralysis restricted to one side of the body
d. Any disease of a muscle

68. ____________________ is known as the destruction of the rod-shaped muscle cells?
a. Hypertrophy
b. Rhabdomyolysis
c. Hypoplasia
d. Necrosis

69. Which of the following is the definition of *aponeurosis*?
a. An acute tendon injury in which the tendon is forcibly torn away from its attachment side on the bone
b. Temporary muscular stiffening that follows death
c. Rapid involuntary muscle contractions that release waste heat
d. Sheet-like dense fibrous collagenous connective tissue that binds muscles together or connects muscle to bone

70. The prefix *onych-* refers to which of the following?
a. Claw, nail
b. Cell
c. Clotting process
d. Cornea

71. Clonic spasm refers to:
a. An acute involuntary muscle contraction
b. A continuous spasm
c. Alternating spasm and muscle relaxation
d. Painful, sustained muscle contractions caused by toxins

72. The term *atrophy* refers to:
a. All four limbs
b. Wasting away
c. Muscle stretch
d. Inflammation of muscles

73. The term *tetraparesis* refers to the:
a. Muscular weakness in all four limbs
b. Inflammation of nerves
c. Inflammation of many muscles
d. A continuous spasm

74. The suffix *-rrhage* refers to which of the following?
a. Expansion, dilation
b. Excessive flow
c. Sensation
d. Flow, flowing

75. The term *acardia* refers to which of the following?
a. Disease affecting the muscles of the heart
b. Excessive growth of the auricles
c. Absence of the heart
d. Pertaining to the heart and to the blood vessels

76. Which of the following terms pertains to the upper and lower chambers of the heart?
a. Atriotomy
b. Atrioventricular
c. Valvulosis
d. Avascular necrosis

77. *Hydremia* means which of the following?
a. Inadequate supply of blood to a part of the body
b. Disorder in which there is an excess of fluid in the blood
c. Low red blood cell count
d. The narrow pointed bottom of the heart

78. The prefix *eu-* refers to which of the following?
a. Glucose
b. Gland
c. Good
d. Hair

79. The demarcation line that separates the left and right ventricles of the heart is termed as an:
a. Interventricular septum
b. Atrium
c. Interventricular groove
d. Auricle

80. Which vessel carries blood to the lungs?
a. Aorta
b. Inferior vena cava
c. Pulmonary artery
d. Carotid artery

81. The inside surface of the chamber of the heart is lined by a thin membrane known as the:
   a. Pericardium
   b. Endocardium
   c. Atrium
   d. Epicardium
82. The bicuspid valve is also known as the __________ valve.
   a. Tricuspid
   b. Semilunar
   c. Mitral
   d. Atrioventricular
83. Which of the following suffixes means crushing or grinding?
   a. -tripsy
   b. -lytic
   c. -osis
   d. -pathy
84. A benign tumor that is composed of newly formed blood vessels is known as:
   a. Hemangioma
   b. Hamartoma
   c. Hepatoma
   d. Hepatocellular carcinoma
85. The rupture of an artery is known as:
   a. Hemorrhage
   b. Arteriorrhexis
   c. Arteriostasis
   d. Venostasis
86. Which of the following is the largest artery in an animal's body?
   a. Carotid artery
   b. Pulmonary artery
   c. Aorta
   d. Inferior vena cava
87. The prefix *ultra-* refers to which of the following definitions?
   a. Beyond, excess
   b. Below, decrease
   c. Black
   d. Back surface of rear limb
88. The term *bradycardia* refers to:
   a. A slower than normal heart rate
   b. An abnormally rapid heart rate
   c. An irregular heart rate
   d. Narrowing of the arteries
89. Enlargement of the heart is termed:
   a. Agnathia
   b. Cardiomegaly
   c. Dactyledema
   d. Pericarditis
90. An accumulation of fluid in the abdominal cavity is known as:
   a. Auscultate
   b. Infarct
   c. Ascites
   d. Edema
91. What is the term for the inflammation of a vein?
   a. Arteritis
   b. Stenosis
   c. Phlebitis
   d. Venostasis
92. An increase in arterial blood pressure is called:
   a. Hypertension
   b. Hypotension
   c. Edema
   d. Pleural effusion
93. *Pericardiocentesis* refers to which of the following definitions?
   a. Abnormal buildup of fluid within a space
   b. Buildup of fluid between the layer of the pericardial sac and the epicardium
   c. When the pericardial sac is full of fluid that the heart can no longer beat
   d. The removal of fluid via a needle inserted into the pericardial sac
94. The suffix *-ptosis* refers to which of the following?
   a. To act on
   b. Downward placement
   c. Enzyme
   d. Engage in a specific activity
95. ____________ is defined as the extensive loss of blood resulting from bleeding.
   a. Hematology
   b. Exsanguination
   c. Electrohemostasis
   d. Anemia
96. An abnormal new growth of plasma cells is known as:
   a. Plasmacytoma
   b. Plasmocyte
   c. Serosanguineous
   d. Polycythemia
97. Which of the following is the definition of *karyoclastic*?
   a. The rupture of a nucleus
   b. A cell that breaks down cartilage
   c. The breaking up of a cell nucleus
   d. The condition of many cells in the blood
98. ____________ refers to redness of the skin.
   a. Erythrocyte
   b. Erythematous
   c. Leukocyte
   d. Leukocytosis
99. Which of the following prefixes refers to the chest?
   a. Baso-
   b. Chyl-
   c. Col-
   d. Steth-
100. A blood cell that has both pale red and blue granules visible in the cytoplasm is known as a/an:
   a. Basophil
   b. Neutrophil
   c. Eosinophil
   d. Agranulocyte
101. Inflammation of the lymph vessels is known as:
   a. Leukocytosis
   b. Lymphangitis
   c. Lymphoma
   d. Immunocyte
102. Difficulty in eating or swallowing is termed:
   a. Dysphagia
   b. Dystocia
   c. Dysraphism
   d. Aphagia

103. _______________ is a primitive blood cell.
a. Hematopoiesis
b. Hematoblast
c. Hemoglobin
d. Hemolysis

104. An abnormally low white blood cell count is referred to as:
a. Normocytic
b. Leukocytosis
c. Leukopenia
d. Anemia

105. The term *idiopathic* means:
a. A general term for an abnormality
b. A disease that has an unknown cause
c. An uncoordinated and dehydrated patient
d. A blood clot that forms and adheres to the wall of a blood vessel

106. The prefix *cox-* refers to which of the following?
a. Heat
b. Hip
c. Hernia
d. Humerus

107. The increased destruction of RBCs within the vascular system is known as:
a. Macrocytic anemia
b. Hemolytic anemia
c. Polychromasia
d. Hypochromic anemia

108. Which of the following means an abnormally low number of neutrophils?
a. Pancytopenia
b. Neutropenia
c. Monocytosis
d. Eosinophilia

109. The measure of the percentage of red blood cells in a volume of blood is known as:
a. Hematocrit
b. Packed cell volume
c. Total protein
d. Both a and b

110. *Hematopoiesis* is defined as:
a. The formation of blood cells in the body
b. An abnormally low number of neutrophils in the blood
c. A high number of white blood cells
d. Resembling a white blood cell

111. The destruction of a blood clot is known as:
a. Exsanguination
b. Monocyte
c. Thrombolysis
d. Leukemia

112. Which of the following defines *neutropenia*?
a. An abnormal condition of too many white blood cells
b. The formation of blood cells in the body
c. An abnormally low number of neutrophils in the blood
d. An abnormal increase in the number of platelets

113. Which of the following means an increased amount of carbon dioxide in the blood?
a. Olfaction
b. Hypercapnia
c. Hyperemia
d. Hypoxia

114. The term *apnea* means which of the following?
a. Absence of breathing
b. A collection of air in the chest from a wound or tear in the lung
c. Surgical puncture of the lung
d. The abnormal development of the air sacs of the lung

115. The last breath taken near or at death is referred to as:
a. Emphysema
b. Agonal breathing
c. Asthma
d. Furcation

116. Which of the following is defined as a nosebleed?
a. Cardiectasis
b. Epistaxis
c. Atelectasis
d. Tussiculation

117. A lack of digestion is which of the following?
a. Bradypepsia
b. Apepsia
c. Monogastric
d. Anastomosis

118. A pathological softening of any of the structures of the mouth is known as:
a. Hyperphagia
b. Polydipsia
c. Cheilophagia
d. Stomatomalacia

119. The term *buccal* refers to which of the following?
a. Pertaining to toward the side of the mouth or cheek
b. Oriented toward the tongue
c. Toward the nose
d. Away from midline

120. The act of spitting up blood is known as:
a. Esophagoplegia
b. Hemoptysis
c. Xerostomia
d. Hypoptyalism

121. A surgical fixation of the stomach of a ruminant to the body wall is which of the following?
a. Gastropexy
b. Abomasopexy
c. Omasal stenosis
d. Laparosplenotomy

122. An infection of the common bile duct is known as:
a. Hepatitis
b. Pancreatitis
c. Cholangitis
d. Cholecystitis

123. A generalized wasting of the body as a result of disease is known as:
a. Eructation
b. Anemia
c. Necrosis
d. Cachexia

124. The term *melena* refers to which of the following?
a. Passing of dark, tarry feces containing blood that has been acted on by bacteria in the intestines.
b. A semifluid mass of partially digested food that enters the small intestine from the stomach.
c. A protein produced by living cells that initiates a chemical reaction but is not affected by the reaction.
d. To fall back into a disease state after an apparent recovery.

125. A progressive wave of contraction and relaxation of the smooth muscles in the wall of the digestive tract that moves food through the digestive tract is known as:
a. Ingesta
b. Rumination
c. Retrograde
d. Peristalsis

126. Which of the following describes incisor teeth?
a. Teeth that are used for tearing food
b. The most rostral teeth that are used for grasping food
c. The most caudal teeth in the mouth that are used for grinding food
d. Baby teeth or temporary teeth

127. A large amount of fat in the feces is known as which of the following?
a. Lipase
b. Steatorrhea
c. Lipolysis
d. Malodorous

128. The pathological condition that results from a stone is referred to as:
a. Enteroptosis
b. Lithiasis
c. Lipolysis
d. Lithogenesis

129. Tube feeding through a stomach tube is known as which of the following terms?
a. Emesis
b. Gavage
c. Emetic
d. Enema

130. Slipping or telescoping of one part of a tubular organ into a lower portion, causing the type of obstruction typically seen in the intestines, is known as what?
a. Impaction
b. Nosocomial
c. Intussusception
d. Ileus

131. Which of the following refers to an overdistention of the reticulorumen as a result of rumen gas being trapped in the rumen when the ruminant is unable to eructate?
a. Ruminal tympany
b. Retch
c. Volvulus
d. Torsion

132. Total parenteral nutrition is defined as which of the following?
a. No food or water given
b. Nutrition must be administered by means other than the mouth
c. Specialized diet for a certain disease process
d. Giving as much food as necessary for the desired result

133. Hair loss is referred to as which of the following?
a. Abrasion
b. Alopecia
c. Proud flesh
d. Aphagia

134. The destruction of skeletal muscle is which of the following?
a. Papule
b. Osteochondritis
c. Rhabdomyolysis
d. Pneumothorax

135. A disease of the nerves is known as:
a. Neuropathy
b. Enchondroma
c. Neuromyelitis
d. Poliomyelitis

136. The prefix *sarc-* refers to which of the following?
a. Flesh
b. Femur
c. Flank
d. First

137. The wasting away of brain tissue is referred to as which of the following?
a. Meningocele
b. Cerebroatrophy
c. Necrosis
d. Neuromyelitis

138. Which of the following means a head that is abnormally small or thin?
a. Ataxia
b. Arachnoid
c. Leptocephaly
d. Hydrocephalus

139. The term *aberrant* means which of the following?
a. To carry to or bring toward a place
b. Abnormal, deviating from the usual or ordinary
c. To carry out or take away from a place
d. An abnormal convex curvature of the spine

140. The __________ is the second largest portion of the brain?
a. Corpus callosum
b. Cortex
c. Cerebrum
d. Cerebellum

141. A *syrinx* is which of the following?
a. The part of the brain that relays sensory impulses to the cerebral cortex
b. A pathological tube-shaped lesion in the brain or spinal cord
c. The junction across which a nerve impulse passes from an axon to another neuron, to a muscle cell, or to a gland cell
d. The space or cavity that can exist between two adjacent body parts that are not tightly adjoined

142. ______________ are short, fine-branching fibers that extend from the cell body?
a. Dendrites
b. Perikarya
c. Axons
d. Microglial cells

143. Which of the following is a protein manufactured by the liver that maintains the osmotic fluid balance between capillaries and tissues?
a. Aldosterone
b. Albumin
c. Alkaline
d. Acetylcholine

144. The recognition by the nervous system of an injury or painful stimulus is known as:
a. Nociperception
b. Proprioception
c. Anesthesia
d. Visceral sensation

145. A painful response to a normally nonpainful stimulus is known as:
a. Allodynia
b. Proprioception
c. Nociperception
d. Tactile agnosia

146. Normal digestion is described by the term:
a. Rhinitis
b. Eupepsia
c. Malodorous
d. Anosmia

147. The surgical removal of the eardrum is:
a. Splenectomy
b. Cholecystectomy
c. Nephrectomy
d. Myringectomy

148. Which of the following means pertaining to the eyes and the skin?
a. Ophthalmology
b. Oculocutaneous
c. Audiology
d. Blepharospasm

149. *Palpebration* means:
a. An abnormal contraction of the eyelid
b. The method of feeling with fingers or hands during the physical examination
c. Inflammation of the cornea
d. Flow of tears mixed with pus

150. An abnormal dilation of the pupil of the eye is defined as:
a. Iridocele
b. Keratitis
c. Corneitis
d. Corectasis

151. An inflammation affecting both the optic nerve and the retina is known as:
a. Neuroretinitis
b. Conjunctivitis
c. Cholecystitis
d. Hepatitis

152. Which of the following means prolonged constriction of the pupil of the eye?
a. Mydriasis
b. Iridocele
c. Miosis
d. Canthus

153. Which of the following statements describes a pheromone?
a. A nerve ending that responds to a stimulus, found in the internal or external environment of an animal
b. An animal that is active at night
c. A surrounding substance in which something else is contained
d. A liquid substance released in small quantities by an animal, which causes a specific response if it is detected by another animal of the same species

154. An ear flap is also known as a:
a. Pinna
b. Papilla
c. Callus
d. Canthus

155. Which of the following is defined as pertaining to the study of cells?
a. Cytology
b. Morphology
c. Zoology
d. Oncology

156. Difficult or labored breathing is also known as:
a. Epistaxis
b. Lysis
c. Leukopenia
d. Dyspnea

157. Which blood cells carry oxygen to body cells?
a. White blood cells
b. Red blood cells
c. Neutrophils
d. Eosinophils

158. A stone found in the stomach is a:
a. Hepatolith
b. Cholelith
c. Coprolith
d. Gastrolith

159. Which of the following is a stone found within the artery?
a. Arteriolith
b. Cardiolith
c. Hysterolith
d. Broncholith

160. Which of the following is a surgical puncture of the vagina?
a. Vaginodynia
b. Colpocentesis
c. Paracentesis
d. Cystocentesis

161. Crushing of a stone into fragments that may pass through natural channels is known as:
a. Lithogenesis
b. Lithologist
c. Lithiasis
d. Lithoclasty

162. Which of the following terms describes a substance produced by one tissue or by one group of cells that is carried by the bloodstream to another tissue or organ to affect its physiological functions such as metabolism or growth?
a. Hormone
b. Endorphin
c. Protein
d. Enzyme

163. The disease of a gland is referred to as:
a. Amyotrophy
b. Adenopathy
c. Adrenomegaly
d. Cardiomyopathy

164. The surgical removal of the thyroid gland is a/an:
a. Splenectomy
b. Oophorectomy
c. Thyroidectomy
d. Cholecystectomy

165. Which of the following hormones is responsible for testosterone production in males and estrogen production and ovulation in females?
a. Prolactin
b. Thyroid-stimulating hormone
c. Follicle-stimulating hormone
d. Luteinizing hormone

166. Which of the following is a *nephroblastoma*?
a. A record made of the kidney, such as an x-ray
b. A rapidly developing tumor the of the kidney that is most often malignant
c. A tumor of the soft tissue usually found in the muscle
d. A tumor found within the liver

167. The term *uremia* is defined as:
a. Painful urination
b. Surgical repair of the kidney pelvis
c. Urine constituents that are found in the blood
d. Blood found in the urine

168. Pain felt in the ureter is termed:
a. Cystitis
b. Ureteralgia
c. Dysuria
d. Menorrhagia

169. Which of the following means crushing of a stone?
a. Lithogenesis
b. Lithotripsy
c. Lithiasis
d. Lithology

170. Which of the following terms means the downward displacement of the kidney?
a. Nephrectomy
b. Nephroptosis
c. Nephrostomy
d. Nephrology

171. A *concretion* is defined as:
a. A solid or calcified mass formed by disease found in a body cavity or tissue
b. A stone
c. A chemical element that carries an electrical charge when dissolved in water
d. The functional tissue of an organ

172. The act of urination is called:
a. Micturition
b. Concretion
c. Voiding
d. Both a and c

173. Which of the following is the definition of *denude*?
a. The process in the kidney whereby blood pressure forces material through a filter
b. A tube for injecting or removing fluids
c. The loss of epidermis, caused by exposure to urine, feces, body fluids, drainage, or friction
d. The end product of muscle metabolism; waste product excreted in urine

174. Painful urination as a result of muscle spasms in the urinary bladder and urethra is called:
a. Dysuria
b. Stranguria
c. Urea
d. Slough

175. The lack of voluntary urination or defecation is called:
a. Urolithiasis
b. Uremia
c. Incontinence
d. Anuria

176. The term *azotemia* means:
a. The presence of urinary calculi
b. The lack of voluntary urination
c. The increased production of urine
d. The buildup of nitrogenous waste material in the blood

177. The excess dilution of urine is called:
a. Oliguresis
b. Albuminuria
c. Hydruria
d. Hydrocephalus

178. A higher than normal blood level of nitrogen-containing compounds in the blood is called:
a. Bilirubinuria
b. Azotemia
c. Hydruria
d. Natriuresis

179. When the amount of glycogen in the liver is depleted, it is known as:
a. Hypoglycemia
b. Hyperglycemia
c. Ketosis
d. Sepsis

180. A diseased condition of pus within the ureter is defined as:
a. Ureteropyosis
b. Bacterium
c. Ketonuria
d. Pyometra

181. *Nephrolithotomy* refers to the:
a. Surgical removal of the gallbladder
b. Surgical incision into the kidney to remove a stone
c. Surgical removal of a kidney
d. Surgical removal of spleen

182. A *cystocentesis* refers to the:
a. Microscopic examination of a urine sample
b. Collection of urine directly from the bladder through a surgical puncture
c. Surgical incision into the bladder
d. Removal of free fluid from the abdominal cavity

183. *Hypokalemia* is defined as:
a. High sodium level
b. Low sodium level
c. High potassium level
d. Low potassium level

184. Which of the following means the surgical removal of testicles?
a. Orchectomy
b. Oophorectomy
c. Cryptorchidism
d. Hysterectomy

185. *Spermaturia* refers to which of the following?
a. Pertaining to sperm
b. The presence of sperm in the urine
c. Presence of blood in the urine
d. Painful urination

186. The surgical removal of the penis is:
a. Castration
b. Penectomy
c. Hysterectomy
d. Oophorectomy

187. Inflammation of the penis is called:
a. Priapitis
b. Megalopenis
c. Micropenis
d. Hypospadias

188. *Phimosis* is defined as a/an:
a. Persistent erection of the penis
b. Idiopathic protrusion of the nonerect penis with the inability to retract it
c. Inability to extend the penis
d. Hypertrophy of the penis

189. ________________ is defined as the release of an egg from the ovary.
a. Ovum
b. Ovulation
c. Oocyte
d. Paraphimosis

190. Which of the following terms correlates with bleeding from the ovary?
a. Ovariectomy
b. Oophorrhagia
c. Menorrhagia
d. Vaginodynia

191. Inflammation of the vulva is referred to as which of the following?
a. Vulvitis
b. Cystitis
c. Vaginitis
d. Pyometra

192. The term *corpus* refers to the:
a. Horn
b. Flared end of a funnel-shaped duct
c. Body
d. A sensitive female external organ homologous to the penis

193. The ________________ is a fringe-like structure found in the infundibulum.
a. Caruncle
b. Fimbria
c. Oviduct
d. Follicle

194. The prefix *hetero-* refers to which of the following?
a. Digestion
b. Digit
c. Different
d. Disease

195. The surgical removal of an animal in the early stages of development in the womb is known as:
a. Hysterectomy
b. Oophorectomy
c. Embryectomy
d. Penectomy

196. A false pregnancy is known as:
a. Primigravida
b. Pseudocyesis
c. Pseudoaneurysm
d. Uniparous

197. The term *bipara* refers to what?
a. The period of time just after the birth of offspring
b. A false pregnancy
c. A female that has given birth twice in two separate pregnancies
d. A female that has never given birth

198. Which term refers to the capability of producing offspring?
a. Fetus
b. Natal
c. Perineum
d. Fecund

199. A vascular membranous organ in the womb between a mother and her offspring is known as the:
a. Fecund
b. Perineum
c. Placenta
d. Umbilical cord

200. The injection of semen into the vagina or uterus by the use of syringe is termed:
a. Copulation
b. In vitro fertilization
c. In vivo fertilization
d. Artificial insemination

201. Which of the following refers to a species that has two estrous cycles per year?
a. Monestrous
b. Polyestrous
c. Diestrous
d. Anestrous

202. An abnormally slow or difficult birth is which of the following?
a. Dysuria
b. Dystocia
c. Ectopic
d. Pyometra

203. When an animal is not able to produce offspring it is:
a. Stillborn
b. Sterile
c. Pseudocyesis
d. Hermaphroditism

204. Which of the following terms pertains to the skin of animals?
a. Zoogenous
b. Zoogamous
c. Endozoic
d. Zoodermic

205. Which of the following terms refers to feeding on animals?
a. Zoophile
b. Zooplasty
c. Zooid
d. Zoophagy

206. Any human disease that may be transmitted from an animal is referred to as which of the following?
a. Zooscopy
b. Zootomy
c. Zoonosis
d. Zootrophic

207. An _______________ is a substance that prevents blood from clotting when it is added to the blood.
a. Anticodon
b. Anticoagulant
c. Antigen
d. Anticonvulsant

208. The bare area of the skin of birds where feathers do not originate is referred to as what?
a. Apteria
b. Aponeurosis
c. Anuria
d. Ataxia

209. The lack of normal muscle tone is known as:
a. Atrophy
b. Auricle
c. Atony
d. Ataxia

210. Which of the following is the definition of *avascular*?
a. Blood clot
b. Increased amount of blood supply
c. Decreased amount of blood supply
d. Without a blood supply

211. A lower respiratory tract infection affecting the lining of the larger air passageways in the lungs is:
a. Pneumonia
b. Bronchitis
c. Pleural effusion
d. Conjunctivitis

212. The dorsal shell of turtles and tortoises is the:
a. Canthus
b. Capsular space
c. Carapace
d. Cardia

213. Which of the following is defined as the movement of white blood cells into an area of inflammation in response to chemical mediators released by injured tissue or other white blood cells at the site?
a. Leukocytosis
b. Chemotaxis
c. Anemia
d. Leukopenia

214. The term *circumduction* refers to which of the following?
a. The removal of the male testicles
b. A joint motion whereby the distal end of an extremity moves in a circle
c. A reservoir that stores fluid
d. The movement of a joint where the distal end of the extremity moves away from the body

215. The initial secretion of the mammary gland before milk is produced is known as:
a. Colloidal
b. Columella
c. Colostrum
d. Cisterna

216. The process of shaping or trimming a bird's beak is referred to as:
a. Corium
b. Coping
c. Culling
d. Crop

217. The process by which white blood cells leave the blood vessel and enter tissue by squeezing through the tiny spaces between the cells' lining is:
a. Leukopenia
b. Diapedesis
c. Leukocytosis
d. Chemotaxis

218. A freely movable synovial joint is known as:
a. Diastole
b. Diestrous
c. Diarthrosis
d. Diaphysis

219. The prefix *dys-* refers to which of the following?
a. Before, anterior
b. Painful, defective
c. Below
d. Between

220. An immature goose of either sex is referred to as which of the following?
a. Poult
b. Rafter
c. Gosling
d. Gander

221. *Ovariohysterectomy* is defined as which of the following?
a. Surgical removal of the ovaries
b. Surgical removal of the uterus
c. Surgical removal of the testicles
d. Surgical removal of the uterus and oviducts/ovaries

222. *Pruritus* refers to:
a. Swelling of tissue
b. Itching
c. Containing or consisting of pus
d. An overgrowth of scar tissue

223. Red blood cells that remain pale after staining indicate which of the following?
a. Hypochromic
b. Hemoglobin
c. Agranulocytes
d. Anucleate

224. The auditory canal is also referred to as the:
a. Humerus
b. Cochlea
c. Eustachian tube
d. Pinna

225. A surgical incision into the windpipe is defined as:
a. Glottis
b. Epistaxis
c. Tracheotomy
d. Endoscope

226. Which of the following is an increase in urine production?
a. Dysuria
b. Diuresis
c. Polyuria
d. Anuria

227. The excretion of an abnormal amount of sodium in the urine is referred to as:
a. Hypernatremia
b. Natriuresis
c. Hydruria
d. Albuminuria

228. Pain within the testicle is termed:
a. Orchectomy
b. Orchialgia
c. Menorrhagia
d. Myalgia

229. Which of the following is known to be the thickest layer of the uterine wall?
a. Perimetrium
b. Endometrium
c. Myometrium
c. Caruncle

230. The prefix *atel-* refers to which of the following?
a. Injury
b. Intestines
c. Incomplete
d. Inward

SECTION 5

Pharmacology

Brandy Tabor

QUESTIONS

1. Neonatal animals are less tolerant of some drugs than older animals because in neonates the drugs are:
   a. Biotransformed more rapidly
   b. Absorbed more slowly from the gastrointestinal tract
   c. Not biotransformed
   d. Biotransformed more slowly
2. Which of the following is most responsible for biotransformation?
   a. Kidney
   b. Liver
   c. Pancreas
   d. Spleen
3. The generic name for a drug is also called the:
   a. Trade name
   b. Chemical name
   c. Proprietary name
   d. Nonproprietary name
4. You are asked to administer a drug that is supplied as an enteric-coated tablet at 100 mg, 50 mg, and 25 mg; you require 25 mg but only have 50-mg tablets. You should:
   a. Use a pill splitter to divide the 100-mg tablet into quarters to have the smallest piece.
   b. Use a pill splitter to divide the 50-mg tablet into halves to have the most accurate dose.
   c. Administer the 50-mg tablet but then skip the next scheduled dosing.
   d. Order or purchase 25-mg tablets for the dosing schedule.
5. A prescription reads "2 tab q4h po prn until gone." The translation of these instructions is:
   a. Two tablets are to be taken four times per day for pain until all tablets are gone.
   b. Two tablets are to be taken four times per day under supervision by the veterinarian until all tablets are gone.
   c. Two tablets are to be taken every 4 hours with food and water until all tablets are gone.
   d. Two tablets are to be taken every 4 hours by mouth as needed until all tablets are gone.
6. Ten mL of a 2.5% solution of thiopentone contains:
   a. 2.5 mg of thiopentone
   b. 25 mg of thiopentone
   c. 250 mg of thiopentone
   d. 2500 mg of thiopentone
7. The percentage of the total dose that ultimately reaches the bloodstream is determined by:
   a. Absorption
   b. Bioavailability
   c. Clearance
   d. Distribution
8. Cholinergic agents do all of the following *except*:
   a. Cause bradycardia
   b. Control vomiting
   c. Increase intraocular pressure
   d. Increase gastrointestinal motility
9. The nonsteroidal anti-inflammatory drug (NSAID) that is extremely toxic to cats is:
   a. Aspirin
   b. Acetaminophen
   c. Carprofen
   d. Flunixin
10. The most common adverse side effect(s) of aminoglycoside antimicrobials is/are:
    a. Nephrotoxicity
    b. Nephrotoxicity and ototoxicity
    c. Ototoxicity and neurotoxicity
    d. Nephrotoxicity, ototoxicity, and neurotoxicity
11. Which statement regarding tetracyclines is true?
    a. They are bactericidal
    b. They alter the permeability of the cell wall and cause lysis
    c. Currently many bacteria are resistant to tetracyclines
    d. They are unable to penetrate the bacterial cell wall
12. Cephalosporins are closely related to what other drug class?
    a. Tetracyclines
    b. Sulfas
    c. Penicillins
    d. Fluoroquinolones

13. Because of the manner in which they are excreted, sulfonamides are often effective against infections found in:
    a. Nervous tissue
    b. Urinary tract
    c. Skin
    d. Joint capsules
14. The Food and Drug Administration does not approve the use of fluoroquinolones in:
    a. Dogs
    b. Cats
    c. Poultry
    d. Birds
15. The antibiotic that should be avoided in all food-producing animals is:
    a. Lincosamides
    b. Cephalexin
    c. Enrofloxacin
    d. Chloramphenicol
16. Penicillins are primarily excreted by the:
    a. Small intestine
    b. Liver
    c. Kidney
    d. Stomach
17. Acepromazine must be used with caution or not at all in:
    a. Bitches
    b. Tomcats
    c. Heifers
    d. Stallions
18. The benzodiazepine derivative diazepam is often administered in combination with:
    a. Droperidol
    b. Morphine
    c. Ketamine
    d. Xylazine
19. If using a regular disposable-type syringe, which of the following drugs should not be preloaded and left for a time before use?
    a. Acepromazine
    b. Atropine
    c. Diazepam
    d. Ketamine
20. A 10-kg dog has inadvertently been administered a dose of xylazine hydrochloride intended for a 30-kg dog. The correct reversal agent for this overdose is:
    a. Atropine
    b. Flumazenil
    c. Naloxone
    d. Yohimbine
21. Griseofulvin acts on:
    a. Gram-positive bacteria
    b. Gram-negative bacteria
    c. Gram-negative and gram-positive bacteria
    d. Dermatophytes
22. Which of the following is not a side effect of sulfonamides?
    a. Crystalluria
    b. Keratoconjunctivitis sicca
    c. Seizures
    d. Thrombocytopenia
23. Which class of antibiotics, when administered to juvenile animals, can impair cartilage development?
    a. Cephalosporins
    b. Fluoroquinolones
    c. Macrolides
    d. Penicillins
24. Potentiated penicillins:
    a. Have a narrow spectrum of action relative to regular penicillins
    b. Include cephalosporins
    c. Are active against beta-lactamase–producing bacteria
    d. Are not used in treating mastitis
25. If you are instructed to give a medication IP, the medication should be injected into:
    a. The jugular vein
    b. The popliteal artery
    c. The abdominal cavity
    d. A major muscle mass
26. Which of the following statements is true when considering the use of xylazine?
    a. It is safe in all dog breeds
    b. It can be reversed with naloxone
    c. It provides some analgesia
    d. It can cause priapism in stallions
27. Which of the following statements is true when considering the use of propofol?
    a. It is a potent analgesic
    b. It can be given via the IM and IV routes
    c. It is best administered as a single bolus
    d. It can be given in incremental doses
28. Which of the following statements is true when considering the use of butorphanol?
    a. It is an antibiotic
    b. It is an antitussive
    c. It can be reversed using yohimbine
    d. It is contraindicated in the cat
29. Which of the following statements is true regarding an iodophor?
    a. It has a longer action than basic iodine compounds
    b. Organic materials do not inactivate it
    c. It is not an irritant at concentrations generally used
    d. It provides adequate disinfection with a single application
30. Heartgard contains ivermectin, which:
    a. Prevents dogs from developing congestive heart failure
    b. Is also effective in treating tapeworms
    c. Is used to prevent heartworm infection
    d. Is only administered orally
31. The active drug in ProHeart is moxidectin and it is a member of which drug class?
    a. Arsenical
    b. Organophosphate
    c. Milbemycin
    d. Pyrantel
32. A risk to veterinary technicians who administer prostaglandins is:
    a. Acne
    b. Liver failure
    c. Kidney damage
    d. Inducing an asthma attack

33. Loop diuretics such as furosemide:
   a. Cause dehydration in normal animals
   b. Cannot be used simultaneously with ACE inhibitors
   c. Are unsafe for use in animals with pulmonary edema
   d. May cause hypokalemia with chronic use
34. Pain receptors are known as:
   a. Nociceptors
   b. C fibers
   c. Proprioceptors
   d. Prostaglandins
35. If it is accidentally administered as an IV bolus, lidocaine may cause:
   a. Full body numbness
   b. Seizures
   c. Sinus arrest
   d. Polyuria
36. Which of these opioids is an agonist/antagonist?
   a. Oxymorphone
   b. Meperidine
   c. Butorphanol
   d. Fentanyl
37. Acepromazine maleate causes:
   a. Respiratory depression
   b. Tachycardia
   c. Hypotension
   d. Reduced salivation
38. What is the ratio between the toxic dose and therapeutic dose of a drug used as a measure of the relative safety of the drug for a particular treatment?
   a. Toxic index
   b. LD50
   c. ED50
   d. Therapeutic index
39. The biotransformation of aspirin takes much longer in cats than in dogs. The half-life of aspirin in cats is approximately:
   a. 10 hours
   b. 20 hours
   c. 30 hours
   d. 40 hours
40. Which statement is most accurate pertaining to insect growth regulators?
   a. They prevent the female from laying eggs
   b. They effectively kill all adult stages
   c. They interfere with development
   d. They are neurotoxic to mammals
41. What drug is approved for the treatment of old dog dementia?
   a. Clomipramine
   b. Meloxicam
   c. Diazepam
   d. Anipryl
42. What is *not* a short-term effect of corticosteroid therapy?
   a. Polyuria
   b. Polyphagia
   c. Delayed healing
   d. Osteoporosis
43. A common side effect of antihistamine drugs such as diphenhydramine is:
   a. Polyuria
   b. Sedation
   c. Pruritus
   d. Panting
44. The H2 receptors are found in the:
   a. Gastric mucosa
   b. Saliva
   c. Carotid arteries
   d. Aortic arch
45. Thiobarbiturates should be administered with great care, or not at all, to:
   a. Collies
   b. Greyhounds
   c. Rottweilers
   d. Spaniels
46. What drug is *not* used in the treatment of glaucoma?
   a. Chloramphenicol
   b. Carbachol
   c. Latanoprost
   d. Pilocarpine
47. A chronotropic agent affects the:
   a. Force of a contraction
   b. Rate of a contraction
   c. Rhythm of a contraction
   d. Rate of relaxation
48. Puppies born via cesarean section that are not breathing well may benefit from _____ drops administered sublingually.
   a. Diazepam
   b. Digitalis
   c. Dobutamine
   d. Doxapram
49. Parenteral administration of phenylbutazone should be only via:
   a. Subcutaneous injection
   b. Intramuscular injection
   c. Intradermal injection
   d. Intravenous injection
50. Intradermal injections are used primarily for:
   a. Allergy testing
   b. Antibiotics
   c. Insulin
   d. Vaccinations
51. Most biotransformation of drugs occurs in the:
   a. Liver
   b. Kidney
   c. Lungs
   d. Skin
52. The main reason that generic forms of drugs are less expensive than trademark drugs is because generic brands:
   a. Use less expensive ingredients
   b. Are not advertised heavily
   c. Do not incur the expense of developing a new drug
   d. Do not work as well as trademark name drugs

53. Repository forms of parenteral drugs:
  a. Contain a special coating that protects the drug from the harsh, acidic environment of the stomach
  b. Are formulated to prolong absorption of the drug from the site of administration
  c. Are composed of specially prepared plant or animal parts rather than being manufactured from chemicals
  d. Are extremely irritating to the tissues

54. All of the following organs may facilitate the elimination of drugs *except* the:
  a. Kidneys
  b. Liver
  c. Lungs
  d. Spleen

55. What liquid form of drug is administered intravenously?
  a. Syrup
  b. Solution
  c. Tincture
  d. Elixir

56. When a drug is said to have a narrow therapeutic range, it means that:
  a. The effective dosing range is small
  b. It may be used for treatment of a few disorders only
  c. It must be dosed frequently
  d. The concentration administered must be high in order to be effective

57. The regulatory agency that oversees the development and approval of animal topical pesticides is the:
  a. FDA
  b. EPA
  c. USDA
  d. DEA

58. A drug that has extreme potential for abuse and no approved medicinal purpose in the United States is classified as:
  a. C-I
  b. C-II
  c. C-IV
  d. C-V

59. A drug given by which of the following routes reaches its peak plasma concentration the fastest?
  a. Orally
  b. Intramuscularly
  c. Subcutaneously
  d. Intravenously

60. Which of these drugs is not an antifungal drug?
  a. Fluconazole
  b. Clotrimazole
  c. Ketoconazole
  d. Sulfadimethoxine

61. An example of an antibiotic that is considered to be a beta-lactamase inhibitor is:
  a. Amoxicillin
  b. Clavamox
  c. Tetracycline
  d. Penicillin

62. In what class of antibiotic drugs are nephrotoxicity and ototoxicity potential side effects?
  a. Aminoglycosides
  b. Barbiturates
  c. Dissociative anesthetics
  d. Phenothiazine tranquilizers

63. The best means of assuring that a particular antibiotic treatment will be successful is to:
  a. Treat for no less than a full 2-week course
  b. Collect a sample from the infected area for culture and sensitivity
  c. Use the highest dose that is considered nontoxic
  d. Use a broad-spectrum antibiotic

64. Dr. Blackman prescribed a particular antibiotic for a rabbit with a Pasteurella infection and asked you to educate the client regarding special instructions for administration of the drug. You told the client that she should wear gloves when handling this medication because it has been associated with a rare adverse reaction in humans: aplastic anemia. Based on this information, the drug that you dispensed was most likely:
  a. Gentamicin
  b. Tetracycline
  c. Erythromycin
  d. Chloramphenicol

65. A useful group of broad-spectrum drugs, whose popularity has recently declined because of numerous potential side effects, including keratoconjunctivitis sicca, polyarthritis (especially in Doberman pinschers), hematuria, allergic reactions, thrombocytopenia, and leukopenia, is the:
  a. Sulfonamides
  b. Macrolides
  c. Tetracyclines
  d. Fluoroquinolones

66. Which of the following statements about tetracyclines is true?
  a. Tetracyclines are bactericidal
  b. Oral absorption of tetracyclines is increased in the presence of food
  c. Tetracyclines are potentially nephrotoxic and ototoxic
  d. Tetracyclines may lead to bone or teeth problems if given to young animals

67. A 50-lb dog is to be given 1 mg/kg dose of diazepam. How many milligrams should he receive?
  a. 50 mg
  b. 22.7 mg
  c. 500 mg
  d. 500 mg

68. Amoxicillin (Amoxi-Drop) was prescribed for Tallulah, a 4-year-old female Chihuahua, who was being discharged after hospitalization. Dr. Segal asks you to provide her owner with discharge instructions. You advise the client of all of the following *except*:
  a. She should call if she notices any adverse side effects as a result of the medication.
  b. She should complete all the medication dispensed, even if Tallulah is feeling well and her symptoms have resolved.
  c. She must administer the medication on an empty stomach, even if Tallulah vomits.
  d. The medication should be refrigerated

69. Antimicrobial drugs such as enrofloxacin, marbofloxacin, and orbifloxacin all belong to which group of antibiotics?
    a. Fluoroquinolones
    b. Cephalosporins
    c. Penicillins
    d. Aminoglycosides
70. Which of the following drugs is least likely to kill the normal flora in the gut of a rabbit, thus avoiding severe diarrhea?
    a. Clavamox
    b. Clindamycin
    c. Cefotaxime
    d. Enrofloxacin
71. Guaifenesin is an example of a/an:
    a. Expectorant
    b. Antitussive
    c. Bronchodilator
    d. Decongestant
72. Which of the following drugs is available over the counter as an antitussive?
    a. Codeine
    b. Dextromethorphan
    c. Hydrocodone
    d. Butorphanol
73. Dr. Charles is performing a C-section on Sadie, a 3-year-old Dalmatian. The smallest pup was not breathing spontaneously, and the doctor asks you administer which of the following drugs as a respiratory stimulant?
    a. Theophylline
    b. Albuterol
    c. Doxapram HCl
    d. Terbutaline
74. Butorphanol tartrate is an example of a drug that functions on more than one body system. It is both an analgesic and a/an ________.
    a. Antitussive
    b. Expectorant
    c. Tranquilizer
    d. Emetic
75. The type of drug that would be most helpful for a patient with a productive cough is:
    a. Antitussive
    b. Antihistamine
    c. Expectorant
    d. Analgesic
76. The anticoagulant diluted in saline or sterile water for injection to form a flush solution for preventing blood clots in intravenous catheters is:
    a. Heparin
    b. EDTA
    c. Coumarin
    d. Acid citrate dextrose (ACD)
77. Sox, a 10-year-old M/C Siamese X, was brought to the emergency hospital, crying in pain and unable to walk. He was diagnosed with an aortic thromboembolism secondary to cardiomyopathy. The drug class used to treat this condition is:
    a. Anticoagulant
    b. Fibrinolytic
    c. Hematinic
    d. Hemostatic
78. The diuretic drug used most commonly in patients with congestive heart failure is:
    a. Mannitol
    b. Spironolactone
    c. Chlorothiazide
    d. Furosemide
79. The function of epinephrine is to:
    a. Increase the heart rate
    b. Decrease the heart rate
    c. Decrease the blood pressure
    d. Reverse the effects of acepromazine
80. The most common side effect(s) of drugs that cause vasodilation is/are:
    a. Anorexia, vomiting, and diarrhea
    b. Cardiac arrhythmias
    c. Bradycardia
    d. Hypotension
81. Cosmo, an 11-year-old M/C pug, has been diagnosed with mitral insufficiency and was referred to a veterinary cardiologist. The specialist decided to initiate treatment with digoxin, which is a positive inotrope and negative chronotrope. This means that it:
    a. Increases the force of contraction and decreases the heart rate
    b. Increases the peripheral vascular resistance and decreases the cardiac output
    c. Increases the blood pressure and decreases the cardiac output
    d. Increases the heart rate and decreases the blood pressure
82. Scooter, a 13-year-old miniature schnauzer, has arrested under anesthesia for routine dentistry. You run to the crash cart and grab what you know to be the drug of choice for cardiac arrest, which is:
    a. Epinephrine
    b. Lidocaine
    c. Sodium bicarbonate
    d. Dobutamine
83. A 3-month-old chow chow is presented to the pet emergency clinic because it has eaten a box of warfarin-based rat poison. Which of the following would be most useful to treat this toxicity?
    a. Protamine sulfate
    b. Coumarin
    c. Streptokinase
    d. Vitamin K
84. Which statement is true about the drugs used for cancer chemotherapy?
    a. They are usually given by mouth
    b. They usually have relatively low margins of safety
    c. They are available over the counter
    d. They are all nephrotoxic
85. Which of the following side effects is commonly seen with many cancer chemotherapeutic drugs?
    a. Hyperglycemia
    b. Immunosuppression
    c. Constipation
    d. Hyperphagia

86. Which of the following would be the least common side effect expected with common cancer chemotherapeutic drugs?
a. Myelosuppression
b. Vomiting and diarrhea
c. Pruritus
d. Alopecia

87. Common drugs of plant origin, such as digoxin and atropine, are ineffective in a cow when administered orally because of:
a. Eructation
b. The large size of the rumen
c. Methane gas
d. Digestive microorganisms

88. Which of these organs/tissues is not a normal site for drugs to accumulate to be released later, thereby prolonging the effect of the drug?
a. Pancreas
b. Fat
c. Bone
d. Liver

89. Chronic use of moderate-to-high doses of glucocorticoids may result in the development of:
a. Hypoadrenocorticism
b. Hyperadrenocorticism
c. Hypothyroidism
d. Hyperthyroidism

90. Glucocorticoids are often used in veterinary medicine for the treatment of all of the following conditions *except*:
a. Allergies
b. Musculoskeletal problems
c. Infections
d. Immune-mediated disease

91. Glucocorticoids have different durations of activity, a fact that plays an important role in their risk of side effects with long-term use. Which of the following glucocorticoids has the shortest duration of activity?
a. Hydrocortisone
b. Prednisone
c. Dexamethasone
d. Triamcinolone

92. Which of the following statements about glucocorticoids is true?
a. If adverse effects are seen after long-term administration, treatment should be discontinued immediately
b. They are generally considered safer to use than NSAIDs
c. They are a type of NSAID
d. They may cause immune-system suppression

93. What drug is *not* an NSAID?
a. Prednisone
b. Flunixin
c. Phenylbutazone
d. Aspirin

94. Flunixin meglumine (Banamine) is an NSAID most commonly used in:
a. Dogs for the treatment of chronic osteoarthritis
b. Horses for the treatment of colic
c. Horses for reducing fever
d. Dogs for its anticoagulant activity

95. The species that generally clears NSAIDs most slowly is:
a. Dog
b. Cat
c. Horse
d. Ruminant

96. What NSAID is administered to cats with a dosing interval of 2 days or more?
a. Aspirin
b. Ibuprofen
c. Carprofen
d. Naproxen

97. The most common side effect of NSAIDs is:
a. Polyuria
b. Gastrointestinal ulceration
c. Diarrhea
d. Constipation

98. What precautions should you take when applying DMSO to an animal's skin?
a. Wear a facial mask to avoid inhaling the fumes
b. Apply a bandage to cover the area of application
c. DMSO is irritating and should not be applied to skin
d. Wear latex gloves to avoid contact with the drug

99. The surgeon has completed Buffy's surgical procedure and asks you to discontinue the inhalant anesthesia. What is absolutely necessary to do when terminating anesthesia in a patient that has been receiving nitrous oxide?
a. Give an injection of the reversal agent
b. Observe carefully for signs of seizures
c. Allow the patient to recuperate in a quiet, dark area
d. Oxygenate for 5 to 10 minutes

100. Which of the following is not a controlled substance?
a. Apomorphine
b. Diazepam
c. Ketamine
d. Hydromorphone

101. Malignant hyperthermia is a phenomenon associated primarily with the use of what inhalant anesthetic?
a. Nitrous oxide
b. Sevoflurane
c. Halothane
d. Isoflurane

102. What drug is in the same class as thiopental?
a. Ketamine
b. Diazepam
c. Phenobarbital
d. Atropine

103. An opioid analgesic often used in transdermal patches to control postsurgical pain is:
a. Fentanyl
b. Pentazocine
c. Meperidine
d. Butorphanol

104. Mrs. Stillman's poodle Roxy has been diagnosed with idiopathic epilepsy. In the event of a seizure at home, which drug has the doctor decided to dispense, which Mrs. Stillman can administer per rectum?
a. Pentobarbital
b. Phenobarbital
c. Diazepam
d. Acepromazine

105. A recent graduate veterinary technician is concerned that a sedated patient has a heart rate of 50 beats/min when the heart rate in a dog is normally 60 to 120 beats/min. She also mentions that the blood pressure is normal. You ask her which sedative the veterinarian used and you were not surprised when she told you that the drug used was________________.
a. Dexmedetomidine
b. Diazepam
c. Ketamine
d. Acepromazine

106. All of the following drugs are antagonists and are used to reverse the effects of another drug *except*:
a. Yohimbine
b. Detomidine
c. Flumazenil
d. Naloxone

107. For which gas does anesthesia demand the greatest degree of patient monitoring, because the anesthetic depth changes occur most rapidly?
a. Desflurane
b. Sevoflurane
c. Halothane
d. Isoflurane

108. Norepinephrine, epinephrine, and dopamine are the primary neurotransmitters for the:
a. Parasympathetic nervous system
b. Sympathetic nervous system
c. Central nervous system
d. Peripheral nervous system

109. Beuthanasia solution is back-ordered at the distributor, so your employer asks you to order a different euthanasia solution. In researching the available drugs, you are reminded that the active ingredient in most euthanasia solutions is:
a. Phenobarbital
b. Pentobarbital
c. Methohexital
d. Thiopental

110. You are working with an equine veterinarian on a breeding farm. You will be sedating a young stallion for an oral examination. Which tranquilizer are you well aware that the veterinarian will probably *not* use for the procedure?
a. Xylazine
b. Diazepam
c. Detomidine
d. Acepromazine

111. The newly hired veterinary assistant is cleaning up after a procedure and returns an opened bottle of propofol to the refrigerator, stating that it can be used the next day on another patient. You explain to her that:
a. Propofol should be stored at room temperature rather than in the refrigerator.
b. The bottles are designed to contain only enough drug for one patient, and it is likely there will not be enough drug left to anesthetize another patient the next day.
c. Bacteria will readily grow in propofol and will produce endotoxins, so it is unwise to use the remains of an opened bottle.
d. The bottle has been contaminated from the first patient, and there is a possibility that contagious diseases can be transmitted in this way.

112. You are on an ambulatory call to Milkman's Dairy with Dr. Burrows. You are asked to bring the xylazine from the truck to sedate the patient. You are aware that when using this drug in a bovine, you must:
a. Use adequate doses, because cattle tend to be resistant to its effects
b. Always use it concurrently with a barbiturate to achieve adequate analgesia
c. Not use xylazine because it is contraindicated in this species
d. Use it at about 1/10 of the equine dose

113. You were assigned to work the front office at the hospital today. When you walk back to the treatment area, you notice a cat under anesthesia. The cat has eyes wide-open, lack of blinking, the limbs are stiffly distended, and is salivating profusely. Your highly educated guess is that this cat was anesthetized using which of the following drugs?
a. Xylazine
b. Medetomidine
c. Ketamine
d. Propofol

114. A cow is accidentally dosed with an equine dose of xylazine. What drug should be immediately administered?
a. None; the equine and bovine doses of xylazine are the same
b. Epinephrine
c. Naloxone
d. Yohimbine

115. Acepromazine should be avoided in:
a. Patients with a history of seizures
b. Aggressive patients
c. Geriatric patients
d. Doberman pinschers

116. The behavioral drug group that may be sent home to stimulate appetite in cats is:
a. Benzodiazepines
b. Tricyclic antidepressants
c. Selective serotonin reuptake inhibitors
d. Progestins

117. A progestin was often used in the past for the treatment of inappropriate elimination in cats and it has now fallen out of favor because of serious potential side effects, including mammary hyperplasia and adenocarcinoma. This drug is known as:
a. Megestrol acetate
b. Oxazepam
c. Amitriptyline
d. Fluoxetine

118. Which tricyclic antidepressant is now approved for use in dogs and cats to control separation anxiety?
a. Buspirone
b. Selegiline
c. Paroxetine
d. Clomipramine

119. A 12-year-old spayed female golden retriever is brought into your clinic with a history of waking up in her bed in a puddle of urine. A complete blood count (CBC), profile, and urinalysis show no sign of urinary tract disease. The doctor tells you to fill a prescription for phenylpropanolamine. The doctor is choosing this drug because it treats:
a. Bladder atony by increasing bladder tone
b. Urinary incontinence by decreasing urethral sphincter tone
c. Urinary incontinence by increasing urethral sphincter tone
d. Bladder atony by decreasing bladder tone

120. Erythropoietin is primarily used in the following feline patients:
a. Cats with anemia because of chronic renal failure
b. Cats with anemia resulting from rodenticide toxicity
c. Cats with aortic thromboembolism secondary to cardiomyopathy
d. Cats suffering from Tylenol toxicity

121. Which of the following drugs is used to decrease gastric acid production by blocking histamine receptors in the stomach?
a. Famotidine
b. Sucralfate
c. Omeprazole
d. Misoprostol

122. Amphojel and Basaljel are drugs in the general category of:
a. Potassium supplements
b. Antihypertensives
c. Urinary acidifiers
d. Phosphate binders

123. A heartworm preventative that is also approved for the treatment of ear mites and sarcoptic mange is:
a. Diethylcarbamazine
b. Milbemycin
c. Ivermectin
d. Selamectin

124. If a drug package insert states that the drug is a coccidiostat; what group of parasites will this drug be effective against?
a. Ascarids (Toxocara, Toxascaris)
b. Tapeworms (Taenia)
c. Protozoa (Eimeria, Isospora)
d. Flukes (liver fluke, lung fluke)

125. Which of the following drugs can cause severe tissue necrosis if administered perivascularly?
a. Phenylbutazone
b. Oxymorphone
c. Dexmedetomidine
d. Ketamine

126. Which statement about organophosphates is incorrect?
a. They are neurotoxic
b. They are used for control of endoparasites and ectoparasites
c. They have a narrow margin of safety
d. They have relatively few side effects

127. In cases of uncomplicated diabetes, by what route is insulin usually administered?
a. Intramuscular
b. Subcutaneous
c. Intravenous
d. Oral

128. Insulin concentration is measured in:
a. Milligrams
b. Milliequivalents
c. Units
d. Grams

129. Oral hypoglycemic drugs, such as glipizide (Glucotrol), are used to treat:
a. Diabetic ketoacidosis
b. Non–insulin-dependent diabetes
c. Hypoglycemia
d. Pancreatitis

130. The primary function of insulin is to:
a. Regulate the metabolic processes of the body
b. Regulate digestion through secretion of gastrointestinal hormones
c. Facilitate the entry of glucose into cells
d. Control reproductive function

131. Resuspension of NPH insulin is achieved by:
a. Gently rolling the bottle
b. Vigorously shaking the bottle
c. Gently heating the bottle in warm water
d. Refrigerating the bottle

132. Altrenogest, which is used for estrus synchronization in female animals, is a synthetic:
a. Estrogen
b. Androgen
c. Progestin
d. Follicle-stimulating hormone (FSH)

133. When diethylstilbestrol (DES), a synthetic estrogen, is used at higher doses, it can have the potentially dangerous side effect of:
a. Gastric ulceration
b. Cardiac arrhythmias
c. Bone marrow suppression
d. Hepatopathy

134. Kaolin, pectin, and bismuth subsalicylate are examples of:
a. Narcotic analgesics
b. Antispasmodics
c. Anticholinergics
d. Protectants

135. Psyllium and Metamucil are examples of:
a. Saline cathartics
b. Bulk laxatives
c. Lubricants
d. Irritant cathartics

136. What is *not* a potential side effect of the phenothiazine antiemetics?
a. CNS depression
b. Diarrhea
c. Lowering of the seizure threshold
d. Hypotension

137. A stool softener that often helps patients recovering from anal surgery is:
a. Docusate sodium succinate (DSS)
b. Magnesium hydroxide
c. Mineral oil
d. Bran

138. The most widely used type of antiemetic drug to prevent motion sickness in dogs and cats is:
a. Phenothiazine
b. Antihistamine
c. Anticholinergic
d. Antispasmodic

139. The emetic of choice in cats is:
a. Xylazine
b. Syrup of ipecac
c. Apomorphine
d. Hydrogen peroxide

140. The emetic of choice in dogs is:
a. Xylazine
b. Syrup of ipecac
c. Apomorphine
d. Hydrogen peroxide

141. Spike the dog ingested his owner's cardiac medication about a half-hour ago. The veterinarian instructs you to give him an emetic that may be administered into the conjunctival sac and then flush as necessary. The name of the drug is:
a. Xylazine
b. Syrup of ipecac
c. Apomorphine
d. Hydrogen peroxide

142. A coating agent that forms an ulcer-adherent complex at the ulcer site is:
a. Kaopectate
b. Sucralfate
c. Cimetidine
d. Misoprostol

143. In what species are Fleet (sodium phosphate) enemas contraindicated?
a. Horses
b. Ruminants
c. Cats
d. Pigs

144. The principal site of drug biotransformation is the:
a. Liver
b. Kidney
c. Stomach
d. Small intestine

145. What drug is most likely to be prescribed to prevent motion sickness in dogs and cats?
a. Apomorphine
b. Syrup of ipecac
c. Atropine
d. Maropitant Citrate

146. A veterinarian prescribes erythropoietin for use in a dog in terminal renal failure. Why was this drug prescribed?
a. For its fibrinolytic activity
b. For its immunosuppressive activity
c. For its ability to stimulate red blood cell production and release
d. For its ability to reduce hypertension

147. Which of the following drugs is considered a biologic response modifier?
a. Interferon
b. Streptokinase
c. Cephalosporin
d. EDTA

148. Atropine is often given as a preanesthetic agent. It is classified as an anticholinergic drug. That means that it will probably have the following effects on an animal receiving the drug:
a. Decreased heart rate, decreased salivation, and decreased GI motility
b. Increased heart rate, increased salivation, and increased GI motility
c. Increased heart rate, decreased salivation, and decreased GI motility
d. Decreased heart rate, increased salivation, and increased GI motility

149. A drug classified as an antagonist may exert its influence by:
a. Mimicking the activity of a neurotransmitter
b. Preventing the breakdown of a neurotransmitter
c. Blocking the binding of a neurotransmitter
d. Enhancing the release of a neurotransmitter

150. A client is advised to discontinue aspirin therapy in his dysplastic dog before the dog undergoes surgery to remove a mammary tumor. The client asks you why this request was made. You tell him:
a. Aspirin decreases platelet aggregation and may increase the likelihood of hemorrhage
b. Aspirin may result in gastrointestinal ulceration
c. Aspirin may adversely affect hepatic biotransformation
d. Aspirin has an anti-inflammatory effect

151. Duragesic (Fentanyl) transdermal patches are used most commonly in veterinary medicine to control:
a. Diarrhea
b. Vomiting
c. Seizures
d. Pain

152. Acetylcysteine (Mucomyst) is an antidote for what type of drug toxicity?
a. Opioid
b. Acetaminophen
c. Lidocaine
d. Digoxin

153. An expectorant is a drug that acts to:
a. Suppress a productive cough
b. Liquefy and dilute viscous secretions in the respiratory tract
c. Suppress inflammatory cells in the respiratory tract
d. Reduce the allergic component of respiratory disease

154. The therapeutic range of a drug refers to which of the following?
a. The plasma concentration at which therapeutic benefits should be observed
b. The relationship of a drug's ability to achieve a desired effect versus causing a toxic effect
c. The range of curative properties that a drug may exhibit
d. The frequency of idiosyncratic reactions

155. Which of the following drugs are contraindicated in a patient with a history of seizures?
   a. Diazepam
   b. Thiopental
   c. Acepromazine
   d. Fentanyl
156. Nutraceuticals is a category of drugs that includes which of the following characteristics?
   a. Genetically derived materials that enhance immune function
   b. Drugs that are derived from humans for use in animals
   c. Drugs that are undergoing clinical trials before FDA approval
   d. Nontoxic food components that have proven health benefits
157. What is the reversal agent for xylazine?
   a. Fentanyl
   b. Naloxone
   c. Acepromazine
   d. Yohimbine
158. The reversal agent used for opioid toxicity is:
   a. Naloxone (Narcan)
   b. Yohimbine
   c. Acetylcysteine
   d. Diazepam
159. One of the adverse side effects of opioid administration is:
   a. Increased seizure activity in epileptic animals
   b. Induction of cardiac arrhythmias
   c. Significant respiratory depression
   d. Systemic hypertension
160. In which of the following circumstances should a thiobarbiturate drug be avoided?
   a. In a patient with respiratory alkalosis
   b. In obese patients
   c. In sighthounds and very thin patients
   d. In hyperproteinemic animals
161. What is a potential electrolyte imbalance that can occur as a result of administering a loop diuretic to a small animal?
   a. Hypokalemia
   b. Hyperkalemia
   c. Hypercalcemia
   d. Hypocalcemia
162. Which of the following drugs is used to treat hypertension?
   a. Amlodipine
   b. Erythromycin
   c. Amitriptyline
   d. Atropine
163. A cat is given ketamine as an anesthetic induction agent. The veterinary technician monitoring this animal may observe which of the following side effects?
   a. Bradycardia
   b. Hypotension
   c. Apneustic breathing
   d. Flaccid muscle tone
164. The category of drugs classified as ACE inhibitors has which of the following effects on the body?
   a. Increases preload and afterload on the heart
   b. Decreases preload and afterload on the heart
   c. Enhances fluid retention in the body
   d. Enhances the production of angiotensin II
165. Nitroglycerin is administered primarily to:
   a. Cause vasodilation
   b. Cause vasoconstriction
   c. Treat arrhythmias
   d. Act as an ace inhibitor
166. For cats diagnosed with hypertrophic cardiomyopathy, a calcium channel blocker is often prescribed to relax the heart in an attempt to improve cardiac output. Which of the following drugs falls in this category?
   a. Procainamide
   b. Diltiazem
   c. Lidocaine
   d. Digoxin
167. Lidocaine is primarily used to control which of the following abnormalities?
   a. Supraventricular bradycardia
   b. Ventricular tachycardia
   c. Hypertension
   d. Supraventricular tachycardia
168. In dogs that have been receiving long-term glucocorticoid therapy (months to years), a sudden discontinuation of the drug may result in which of the following medical problems?
   a. Immunosuppression
   b. Hypoadrenocorticism
   c. Polyuria and polydipsia
   d. Iatrogenic thyroid disease
169. In dogs that have been receiving long-term glucocorticoid therapy (months to years), which of the following endocrinopathies can occur?
   a. Hypothyroidism
   b. Hyperthyroidism
   c. Iatrogenic Cushing's disease/hyperadrenocorticism
   d. Estrogen-responsive incontinence
170. Which of the following is/are *not* a side effect of oral steroid administration in dogs?
   a. Polyuria and polydipsia
   b. Polyphagia
   c. Hyperglycemia
   d. Vomiting
171. Glucocorticoids are often used to treat all of the following conditions *except*:
   a. Autoimmune skin disease
   b. Asthma
   c. Lymphocytic neoplasia
   d. Hyperadrenocorticism
172. An example of an anticholinergic drug is:
   a. Acetylcholine
   b. Pilocarpine
   c. Atropine
   d. Nicotine

173. The term "drug compounding" refers to which of the following activities?
   a. Diluting or combining drugs for ease of administration
   b. Delivering a drug via a different route than is directed on the label
   c. Delivering a drug at a different dose than is directed on the label
   d. Delivering the drug to a different species than is directed on the label

174. Which of the following drugs is most commonly used to treat urinary incontinence in dogs?
   a. Phenylpropanolamine
   b. Diethylcarbamazine
   c. Acepromazine
   d. Bethanechol

175. Which of the following drugs is classified as an osmotic diuretic and is often used to reduce intracranial pressure or treat oliguric renal failure?
   a. Furosemide
   b. Chlorothiazide
   c. Mannitol
   d. Spironolactone

176. Which of the following drugs does *not* have an antiemetic action?
   a. Chlorpromazine
   b. Metoclopramide
   c. Maropitant citrate
   d. Apomorphine

177. Which of the following antibiotics should *not* be given to an animal that demonstrates an allergic response to penicillin administration?
   a. Lincosamides
   b. Cephalosporins
   c. Sulfonamides
   d. Fluoroquinolones

178. Griseofulvin is used in cats, dogs, and horses to treat which of the following disorders?
   a. Dermatophytosis
   b. Staphylococcus pyoderma
   c. Rickettsial disease
   d. Nematode infection

179. Which of the following drugs provides analgesic relief to a patient who undergoes a painful procedure?
   a. Acepromazine
   b. Diazepam
   c. Thiopental
   d. Fentanyl

180. Which of the following drugs is used as an adulticide to treat a heartworm-positive dog?
   a. Melarsomine
   b. Ivermectin
   c. Milbemycin
   d. Moxidectin

181. The antidote for warfarin poisoning is:
   a. Vitamin C
   b. Naloxone
   c. Vitamin K
   d. 4-methylpyrazole

182. An example of an alpha-2 agonist is:
   a. Xylazine
   b. Propranolol
   c. Hydralazine
   d. Epinephrine

183. The number of species of bacteria that are affected by an antibiotic is known as the antibiotic's:
   a. Effectiveness
   b. Efficacy
   c. Spectrum
   d. Affinity

184. Which of the following drugs does *not* have an immunosuppressive effect?
   a. Cyclosporine
   b. Azathioprine
   c. Prednisone
   d. Ivermectin

185. An example of an aminoglycoside antibiotic is:
   a. Erythromycin
   b. Ampicillin
   c. Neomycin
   d. Doxycycline

186. A reported side effect of fluoroquinolone administration (Baytril) in cats given sid dosing at a higher dosing schedule is:
   a. Retinal damage
   b. Hypertension
   c. Renal failure
   d. Hepatic failure

187. Which of the following clinical signs may indicate that an animal is experiencing lidocaine toxicity?
   a. CNS signs: drowsiness, ataxia, muscle tremors
   b. Renal signs: oliguria
   c. Hepatic signs: jaundice, clotting problems
   d. Respiratory signs: labored respirations, bronchoconstriction

188. An asthmatic cat may receive which of the following drugs for its bronchodilatory effect?
   a. Histamine
   b. Digoxin
   c. Prednisone
   d. Theophylline

189. The class of antibiotics most commonly prescribed to treat rickettsial infections, such as Rocky Mountain spotted fever, is:
   a. Tetracyclines
   b. Penicillins
   c. Aminoglycosides
   d. Sulfonamides

190. What drug will not cause nephrotoxicity?
   a. Amikacin
   b. Banamine
   c. Cisplatin
   d. Oxymorphone

191. Why is it an accepted practice for cats receiving aspirin therapy to be dosed on a 2-day interval schedule only (i.e., a minimal dose every 2 days)?
a. Liver metabolism of salicylates occurs at a very slow rate in comparison to other species, thereby making cats extremely susceptible to overdose in comparison to dogs.
b. Salicylates cause severe respiratory depression in cats.
c. Salicylates often result in severe hypertension.
d. Salicylates may result in hypercoagulable states in cats.

192. A cat diagnosed with hyperthyroidism may be offered a number of treatment options, including all of the following, *except*:
a. Radioactive iodine-131 treatment
b. Methimazole medical management
c. Thyroidectomy surgery
d. Levothyroxine

193. Older sulfonamides were more likely to cause __________ than the newer sulfonamides.
a. Diarrhea
b. Crystalluria
c. Bronchospasms
d. Seizures

194. A dog diagnosed with a mast cell tumor is scheduled for surgery. The veterinarian chooses to pretreat the dog with an H1 blocker to prevent the negative effects of histamine release when the tumor is manipulated. Which of the following drugs may be chosen?
a. Diphenhydramine
b. Methimazole
c. Vincristine
d. Sulfasalazine

195. Which of the following drugs is used for its sedative, antiseizure, and appetite-stimulant effects?
a. Diazepam
b. Cyproheptadine
c. Ketamine
d. Potassium bromide

196. A cat is given methionine in an effort to dissolve his urinary struvite stones. The drug has which of the following intended effects?
a. Acidification of the urine
b. Alkalinization of the urine
c. Dilution of urine
d. Concentration of the urine

197. Which of the following types of insulin has the shortest duration of action?
a. NPH insulin
b. Regular insulin
c. Glargine insulin
d. Vetsulin

198. It is essential for veterinary technicians to educate clients expecting to treat their pets with insulin. Which of the following statements is true?
a. Insulin can be stored at room temperature between uses
b. The bottle of insulin should be shaken before use
c. The injection is given in the same site each time
d. Insulin should be given with a meal

199. Which type of antimicrobial drug would be effective against organisms such as Giardia or Eimeria?
a. Bactericidal
b. Virucidal
c. Antiprotozoal
d. Fungistatic

200. Many antibiotic drug inserts (information included in packages of drugs) make reference to the MIC at which the antibiotic is effective. What is the MIC?
a. Minimum inflammatory concentration
b. Maximum infusion concentration
c. Minimum inhibitory concentration
d. Maximum inhalation concentration

201. Antimicrobial drugs such as neomycin, gentamicin, and amikacin each belong to what group of antibiotics?
a. Penicillins
b. Cephalosporins
c. Quinolines
d. Aminoglycosides

202. Aminoglycosides, if given at high dosages or by continuous IV infusion, cause damage to the:
a. Lungs and liver
b. Liver and inner ear
c. Kidney and liver
d. Inner ear and kidney

203. Bacterial resistance to antibiotics is a significant problem in veterinary medicine. What factor is *not* considered to be a significant contributor to the development of bacterial resistance?
a. Prolonged levels of higher-than-recommended dosages of antibiotics
b. Normal dosages of antibiotics for half the recommended duration
c. Low dosages of antibiotics in the feed for prolonged periods
d. Antibiotics that do not reach the infection site in concentrations that exceed MIC

204. Which of the following drug groups is most likely to provoke an allergic reaction in treated animals?
a. Aminoglycosides
b. Quinolines
c. Penicillins
d. Tetracyclines

205. Antimicrobial drugs that work against bacterial deoxyribonucleic acid (DNA) have the potential for causing birth defects or other problems in the host animal if they also alter mammalian DNA. One group of antimicrobial agents known for this tendency is:
a. Antifungals
b. Antibacterials
c. Antivirals
d. Antiprotozoals

206. Unlike many other penicillins, penicillin G is not recommended for use by mouth. Why?
a. It upsets the stomach.
b. It is destroyed by gastric acid.
c. It causes severe diarrhea and intestinal cramping.
d. It is ineffectively absorbed from the gastrointestinal tract.

207. Which type of adverse reaction is most commonly observed when penicillins are administered to rabbits?
 a. Kidney damage and subsequent change in urine production
 b. Hives and swelling of the face from allergic reaction
 c. High fever and severe depression
 d. Severe diarrhea

208. Certain bacteria, especially staphylococcus, produce an enzyme (beta-lactamase) that destroys many penicillin drugs. Which is one of the penicillins *not* destroyed by beta-lactamase?
 a. Penicillin G
 b. Ampicillin/Sulbactum
 c. Amoxicillin
 d. Hetacillin

209. What is added to amoxicillin to make it resistant to the penicillin-destroying beta-lactamase enzymes produced by some bacteria?
 a. Trimethoprim
 b. Clavulanic acid
 c. Piperonyl butoxide
 d. Ormetoprim

210. Some penicillin G injectable products contain procaine or benzathine and some penicillin G products contain neither. What effects do procaine and benzathine have on penicillin G?
 a. They act as a local anesthetic to decrease the pain of injection.
 b. They prolong absorption of penicillin G from the injection site.
 c. They increase the rate at which penicillin G enters the bloodstream.
 d. They enhance the bacterial killing activity of the penicillin.

211. Ceftiofur is classified on the package insert as a third-generation cephalosporin antibiotic; cefadroxil is classified as a first-generation cephalosporin. How do third-generation cephalosporins differ from first-generation cephalosporins?
 a. Third-generation drugs are better absorbed when given orally.
 b. Third-generation drugs have better gram-negative activity.
 c. Third-generation drugs last longer in the body; they are given once daily only.
 d. Third-generation drugs have fewer side effects and adverse reactions.

212. Aminoglycoside antibiotics (e.g., amikacin and gentamicin) are powerful agents against bacteria. Unfortunately, they do not seem to work well in deep puncture wounds or in the lumen of the colon. Why?
 a. These are anaerobic sites and bacteria require oxygen to take up aminoglycosides.
 b. These sites often have enzymes that inactivate aminoglycosides.
 c. Gram-positive bacteria commonly infect these sites and aminoglycosides are ineffective against gram-positive bacteria.
 d. The DNA of bacteria at these sites is resistant to aminoglycosides.

213. How can a drug such as neomycin, which has severe risk of nephrotoxicity when administered by injection, have little risk when administered topically or orally?
 a. Some species are resistant to kidney damage.
 b. Little of the drug is absorbed through the skin.
 c. The absorbed drug is excreted so quickly that it does not have time to damage the kidneys.
 d. Subcutaneous enzymes inactivate the drug.

214. What antibiotic is most likely to cause damage to the ear?
 a. Amoxicillin
 b. Gentamicin
 c. Tetracycline
 d. Enrofloxacin

215. What route of administration of amikacin or gentamicin causes the highest risk for nephrotoxicity?
 a. Per os
 b. Intramuscular
 c. Continuous intravenous infusion
 d. Intravenous bolus

216. What can a technician do to recognize early signs of nephrotoxicity in an animal that receives aminoglycosides?
 a. Monitor blood urea nitrogen (BUN) and creatinine levels
 b. Monitor the CBC and total protein level
 c. Monitor feces for change in consistency
 d. Monitor urine for casts and protein

217. Why is it important that pus-filled wounds or ear canals with purulent debris be thoroughly cleaned before applying a topical aminoglycoside (e.g., gentamicin)?
 a. Purulent material shields bacteria from the antibiotic.
 b. The alkaline nature of the purulent material reduces bacterial uptake of the drug.
 c. Nucleic acids in the cellular debris bind the aminoglycoside.
 d. Irritation from the purulent material causes the tissue to produce enzymes against the aminoglycoside.

218. What drugs are considered fluoroquinolones?
 a. Oxytetracycline, doxycycline
 b. Danofloxacin, enrofloxacin
 c. Sulfadimethoxine, sulfamethazine
 d. Chloramphenicol, lincomycin

219. What organ blocks the entrance of many drugs because of a barrier similar to the blood–brain barrier?
 a. Prostate gland
 b. Thyroid gland
 c. Pancreas
 d. Spleen

220. In what animal is the use of enrofloxacin safest?
 a. 1-year-old Dutch rabbit
 b. 3-month-old Doberman puppy
 c. 6-month-old quarter horse colt
 d. 2-year-old Siamese cat

221. What is the drug group of choice for treating Lyme disease (borreliosis)?
   a. Antifungal
   b. Antiviral
   c. Antibiotic
   d. Antiprotozoal
222. With what type of diet should oral tetracyclines not be administered?
   a. High fat
   b. Low sodium
   c. High calcium
   d. Low potassium
223. Why should tetracycline use be avoided in pregnant bitches?
   a. It may cause changes in the joint cartilage that may result in arthritis at an older age in the pup.
   b. It may be deposited in dental enamel and give the pup's teeth a mottled yellow appearance.
   c. It may impair normal central nervous system development in the pups that may show up as behavioral changes later in life.
   d. It may damage the developing pups and may result in liver impairment later in life.
224. What is the effect of prostaglandin F2 alpha on the reproductive system?
   a. Ovulation
   b. Luteolysis
   c. Follicle stimulation
   d. Corpus luteum formation
225. What drug readily penetrates the blood–brain and corneal barriers and achieves therapeutic concentrations of antibiotic in the central nervous system?
   a. Amoxicillin
   b. Enrofloxacin
   c. Oxytetracycline
   d. Chloramphenicol
226. Which drug will have a prolonged half-life when used with chloramphenicol?
   a. Phenobarbital
   b. Penicillin
   c. Sulfadimethoxine
   d. Tetracycline
227. Why is chloramphenicol used with extreme caution in cats and neonates?
   a. It can bind with dietary calcium and become deactivated.
   b. The liver is unable to metabolize chloramphenicol effectively in these animals.
   c. It can alter developing bone, enamel, and cartilage.
   d. It may drastically alter gut bacterial flora, resulting in fatal diarrhea.
228. What fatal reaction to chloramphenicol has been reported in cats and people?
   a. Kidney failure
   b. Aplastic anemia
   c. Pulmonary edema
   d. Liver failure
229. When are drugs such as sulfadimethoxine, sulfadiazine, and other sulfa drugs most likely to cause kidney problems?
   a. When an animal is receiving intravenous fluids and it has a diuretic effect on the kidneys
   b. When an animal is dehydrated
   c. When an animal has only one functional kidney
   d. When an animal has a bladder infection
230. What are trimethoprim and ormetoprim?
   a. Agents that are growth regulators
   b. Agents that enhance bactericidal activity of sulfonamides
   c. Agents that enhance the spectrum of the activity of penicillins
   d. Agents that reduce the risk of liver damage from hepatotoxic drugs
231. Within the past few years there have been reports of dogs having adverse reactions to sulfadiazine, which is a commonly used sulfonamide. What reaction should clients and veterinary professionals watch for?
   a. Cardiac arrest
   b. Sudden liver failure
   c. Decreased tear production
   d. Increased urination
232. What antibacterial drug is also effective against protozoa such as Giardia?
   a. Clindamycin
   b. Griseofulvin
   c. Metronidazole
   d. Monensin
233. Ketoconazole, miconazole, and griseofulvin are effective against:
   a. Viruses
   b. Flukes
   c. Intestinal nematodes
   d. Fungi
234. What drug is used intravenously to treat status epilepticus?
   a. Potassium bromide
   b. Levetiracetam
   c. Diazepam
   d. Phenobarbital
235. What anticonvulsant drug is converted by the liver primarily to phenobarbital, which accounts for most of its anticonvulsant activity?
   a. Diazepam
   b. Primidone
   c. Phenytoin
   d. Clonazepam
236. What traditional anticonvulsant is now being used simultaneously with phenobarbital in dogs that are nonresponsive to phenobarbital alone?
   a. Diazepam
   b. Potassium bromide
   c. Phenytoin
   d. Strychnine
237. What drug is a respiratory stimulant?
   a. Oxytocin
   b. Dobutamine
   c. Propranolol
   d. Doxapram

238. Drugs that effectively block the cough reflex are called:
a. Mucolytics
b. Expectorants
c. Antitussives
d. Decongestants

239. Drugs that reduce the viscosity of secretions in the respiratory tract are called:
a. Anti-inflammatories
b. Expectorants
c. Antitussives
d. Antihistamines

240. Drugs used to increase airflow, through respiratory passageways narrowed by the relaxation of smooth muscle around them, are called:
a. Bronchodilators
b. Expectorants
c. Antitussives
d. Antihistamines

241. Butorphanol and hydrocodone are examples of:
a. Mucolytics
b. Expectorants
c. Antitussives
d. Antihistamines

242. What effect do beta-receptor agonists have on the respiratory tree?
a. Increase the volume of watery secretions
b. Increase the volume of sticky mucoid secretions
c. Cause bronchoconstriction
d. Cause bronchodilatation

243. Terbutaline, albuterol, and metaproterenol are used in veterinary medicine to:
a. Treat feline asthma or other bronchoconstrictive diseases
b. Treat low blood pressure caused by shock
c. Suppress a productive cough, such as in bronchopneumonia
d. Stimulate secretions within the respiratory tree to aid the mucociliary apparatus

244. Methylxanthines are often used to improve breathing in cardiac patients and patients with respiratory disease. Which of the following drugs are methylxanthines used for this purpose?
a. Theophylline and aminophylline
b. Codeine and dextromethorphan
c. Hydrocodone and butorphanol
d. Guaifenesin and propranolol

245. Most drugs that control arrhythmias of the heart are said to be "negative inotropes." What does this mean?
a. They increase the heart rate.
b. They decrease the heart rate.
c. They increase the force of contractions.
d. They decrease the force of contractions.

246. What drug reduces tachyarrhythmias by blocking sodium and decreasing automaticity of the cardiac cells?
a. Propranolol
b. Lidocaine
c. Procainamide
d. Digoxin

247. Hyperthyroid cats have heart rates of more than 200 beats per minute because of the large numbers of alpha-1 sympathetic receptors in their hearts, which make the heart more sensitive to epinephrine and norepinephrine. This high heart rate is an anesthetic risk. What drug is used to slow the heart rate and decrease arrhythmias associated with alpha-1 receptor stimulation?
a. Lidocaine
b. Propranolol
c. Quinidine
d. Digoxin

248. Digoxin has a narrow therapeutic index. What does this mean?
a. Plasma drug concentrations that produce toxicity are very low.
b. Plasma drug concentrations required to achieve a beneficial effect are very high.
c. Plasma drug concentrations that produce toxicity are very close to the concentration at which a beneficial effect occurs.
d. Plasma drug concentrations are extremely variable from animal to animal.

249. Because digoxin has a narrow therapeutic index, veterinary technicians and owners of animals that receive digoxin must be able to detect early signs of digoxin toxicity, such as:
a. Increased urination and increased water consumption
b. Increased coughing and difficulty breathing
c. Decreased appetite, anorexia, diarrhea, and vomiting
d. Ataxia, syncope, and disorientation

250. Some drugs commonly used to treat veterinary patients with cardiovascular disease alter the electrolyte levels (Na^+, K^+, Cl^-) within the body. Which electrolyte change greatly enhances the risk of digoxin toxicity?
a. Hypernatremia
b. Hyperkalemia
c. Hypochloremia
d. Hypokalemia

251. What drug would be most effective against dermatophytes?
a. Tylosin
b. Enrofloxacin
c. Sulfadimethoxine
d. Itraconazole

252. Drugs classified as ACE inhibitors have what effect on the body?
a. Increase the strength of heart contractions
b. Cause vasodilatation
c. Cause bronchodilatation
d. Increase the heart rate

253. Captopril is an example of a/an:
a. Positive inotrope
b. Antiarrhythmic
c. Bronchodilator
d. Vasodilator

254. Nitroglycerin is sometimes used as a paste applied to the pinna or to the abdominal skin in dogs with cardiovascular disease. Nitroglycerin has what therapeutic effect?
a. Increases strength of heart contractions
b. Causes vasodilation
c. Causes bronchodilation
d. Decreases the heart rate

255. Spironolactone, chlorothiazide, and furosemide are classified as:
a. Diuretics
b. Positive inotropes
c. Antiarrhythmics
d. Vasodilators

256. What controlled substance rating indicates a drug with the greatest potential for abuse?
a. C-III
b. C-II
c. C-V
d. C-IV

257. Why is apomorphine used in canine patients in emergency veterinary medicine?
a. To keep blood pressure elevated for animals in shock
b. To alleviate pain
c. To produce emesis after ingestion of a toxin
d. To maintain kidney function during periods of reduced blood flow to the kidneys

258. What drug is most likely to be prescribed to prevent motion sickness?
a. Apomorphine
b. Maropitant
c. Xylazine
d. Diphenhydramine

259. Why is syrup of ipecac used?
a. To stimulate defecation to flush out poisons from the distal bowel
b. To induce vomiting
c. To stimulate duodenal movement to overcome constipation
d. To increase blood supply to the gastrointestinal tract

260. Why should apomorphine and activated charcoal not be given simultaneously?
a. The resultant vomiting is too severe and too prolonged.
b. Each cancels the beneficial effects of the other.
c. The patient will vomit and may aspirate the charcoal.
d. Severe diarrhea and intestinal cramping result.

261. What effect are anticholinergic drugs expected to have on the gastrointestinal tract?
a. Increased secretions by the bowel
b. Increased movement of feces through the bowel
c. Decreased ability of compounds to irritate the bowel wall
d. Decreased bowel motility

262. Bismuth subsalicylate is the active ingredient in several common over-the-counter (OTC) preparations used for some types of gastrointestinal disease. Which of the following is it *not* used for?
a. Antiemetic
b. Anti-inflammatory
c. Antidiarrheic
d. To increase motility in the stomach

263. NSAIDs often produce side effects in the gastrointestinal tract with long-term use or high-dosage use, especially in dogs. What are the side effects?
a. Increased bowel motility, resulting in fluid diarrhea
b. Decreased ability to digest fat, resulting in fatty stool (steatorrhea)
c. Decreased mucus production, resulting in ulcers or gastritis
d. Decreased bowel motility, resulting in constipation

264. Cimetidine and ranitidine are used as:
a. Antidiarrheals
b. Laxatives
c. Rumen stimulants
d. Antacids

265. What type of medication is sucralfate (Carafate)?
a. Gastric protectant
b. Prostaglandin analogue
c. Proton pump inhibitor
d. H2 receptor antagonist

266. The drug most commonly used in treating animals with hypothyroidism is:
a. Thyroid-stimulating hormone (TSH)
b. Thyroid extract
c. Synthetic levothyroxine (T4)
d. Synthetic liothyronine (T3)

267. For what disease is methimazole used?
a. Hypothyroidism in dogs
b. Hyperadrenocorticism
c. Hyperthyroidism
d. Hypoadrenocorticism

268. What drug is used to return a mare to proestrus from diestrus through lysis of the corpus luteum?
a. Progesterone
b. Estrogen
c. Prostaglandin
d. Gonadotropin

269. What hormone is given to mares or cows for several days to mimic diestrus and then withdrawn to mimic natural lysis of the corpus luteum and a return to proestrus?
a. Estradiol cypionate
b. Prostaglandin F2 alpha
c. Human chorionic gonadotropin
d. Progestin

270. What drug is used as a contraceptive in dogs and sometimes for the correction of behavioral problems in cats (e.g., inappropriate urination)?
a. Altrenogest
b. Megestrol acetate
c. Estradiol cypionate
d. Dinoprost tromethamine

271. Which of the following is most likely to cause gastrointestinal ulcerations?
a. Aspirin
b. Deracoxib
c. Carprofen
d. Meloxicam

272. The glucocorticoid drug commonly used orally to treat immune-mediated diseases in dogs and cats is:
a. Hydrocortisone
b. Prednisone
c. Triamcinolone
d. Dexamethasone

273. Predictable, short-term side effects of glucocorticoid therapy of which every client should be aware include:
a. Polyuria and polydipsia
b. Cough and nasal discharge
c. Anorexia and diarrhea
d. Dry skin and skin irritations

274. Glucocorticoids may cause what changes to a CBC?
a. Neutrophils decreased, eosinophils increased, lymphocytes decreased
b. Neutrophils increased, eosinophils increased, lymphocytes increased
c. Neutrophils increased, eosinophils decreased, lymphocytes decreased
d. Neutrophils decreased, eosinophils decreased, lymphocytes increased

275. Chronic administration of high doses of glucocorticoids can cause iatrogenic:
a. Renal failure
b. Addison's disease
c. Cushing's disease
d. Johne's disease

276. In what species might dexamethasone administration lead to abortion during the last few weeks of gestation?
a. Horses and cattle
b. Pigs and dogs
c. Dogs and cats
d. Horses and cats

277. NSAIDs are most likely to cause side effects in what two organ systems?
a. Renal and pulmonary
b. Renal and gastrointestinal
c. Pulmonary and cardiac
d. Cardiac and hepatic

278. Which NSAID, when administered perivascularly in horses, can cause skin necrosis and sloughing?
a. Phenylbutazone
b. Etodolac
c. Carprofen
d. Meclofenamic acid

279. One of the following anti-inflammatory drugs is sometimes applied topically. Care must be taken to clean the area where it is applied because it readily penetrates the skin and can carry bacterial toxins or other chemicals with it into the body. What drug is it?
a. Dexamethasone
b. Dimethyl sulfoxide
c. Flunixin meglumine
d. Hydrocortisone

280. Which of these drugs most recently became controlled?
a. Butorphanol
b. Buprenorphine
c. Fentanyl
d. Tramadol

281. A drug's package insert states that the drug is an anticestodal. Against which type of parasite will this drug be effective?
a. Ascarids (Toxocara, Toxascaris)
b. Tapeworms (Taenia)
c. Protozoa (Eimeria, Giardia)
d. Flukes (liver fluke, lung fluke)

282. What breed of dog has a blood–brain barrier that allows ivermectin to reach toxic concentrations within the brain more readily than in other breeds?
a. German shepherd
b. Collie
c. Schnauzer
d. Cocker spaniel

283. Which drug is used most commonly as a microfilaricide in the treatment of heartworm disease?
a. Thiacetarsamide
b. Melarsomine
c. Ivermectin
d. Piperazine

284. If an animal receives an overdose of organophosphate insecticide (from dips, powders, sprays), what is the treatment of choice?
a. Diphenhydramine
b. Corticosteroids
c. Intravenous fluids
d. Atropine

285. Which insecticide is effective in treating demodectic mange?
a. Fenoxycarb
b. Amitraz
c. Pyrethrin
d. Allethrin

286. Methoprene and fenoxycarb are ingredients increasingly found in flea and other insect products. What are they?
a. Insecticides
b. Repellents
c. Insect growth regulators
d. Synergists

287. The following information was provided for a prescription written by a veterinarian: "Dr. Pete Bill, Veterinary Associates, Inc., 325 Sentry Highway, West Lafayette, IN 47907. Indiana License Number #4xxx. (317) 555-8636. For: Mr. R. K. Jones, 111, Melrose Place, Loomisville, IN 47905. Canine patient Ruby, Amoxicillin 100 mg tablets, Sig: 1 tab q8h po no refills. Date: 06/08/2019. Signature: Pete Bill." What vital information is missing from this prescription?
a. Veterinarian's Drug Enforcement Administration (DEA) license number
b. Pet's name
c. Owner's telephone number
d. Number of tablets

288. The following information was provided for a prescription written by a veterinarian: "Canine patient, Metoclopramide 10 mg tablets, Sig: 1 tab q8h po TID 2 refills. 07/09/2019." In the prescription what does po mean?
a. Administer with a meal
b. Administer by mouth
c. Administer as needed
d. Administer on an empty stomach

289. The following information was provided for a prescription written by a veterinarian: "Canine patient, Clavamox 375 mg tablets, Sig: 1 tab po BID no refills. Date: 11/12/2019." How many times a day is this medication to be given?
a. One
b. Two
c. Three
d. Four

290. The following information was provided for a prescription written by a veterinarian: "Canine patient, trazadone 100 mg tablets, Sig: 1 tab po TID prn 2 refills. Date: 8/12/2019." What does prn mean?
a. Administer every other day
b. Administer by mouth
c. Administer as needed
d. Administer on an empty stomach

291. The abbreviations od and os on a prescription refer to:
a. Administer by mouth and by rectum
b. Right eye and left eye
c. Administer every other day and every 3 days
d. Right ear and left ear

292. What do 15 gr and 10 g mean on a prescription?
a. 15 grains and 10 grams
b. 15 grains and 10 grains
c. 15 grams and 10 grams
d. 15 grams and 10 grains

293. Most pharmaceutical agents that are measured in grains have how many milligrams per grain?
a. 32.4
b. 64.8
c. 100
d. 120

294. Which of the following is a dose?
a. 100 mg po TID
b. One tablet
c. 100 mg
d. 10–20 mg/kg

295. How many milliliters are in a teaspoon?
a. 1
b. 3
c. 5
d. 10

296. How many cubic centimeters are in a tablespoon?
a. 5
b. 15
c. 25
d. 30

297. Which equivalent is correct?
a. q12h = QD
b. q6h = QID
c. q4h = TID
d. q8h = BID

298. A 10-kg animal weighs how many pounds?
a. 2
b. 15
c. 18
d. 22

299. Which of the following must be shaken before administration to an animal?
a. Solution
b. Ointment
c. Gel
d. Suspension

300. When a drug is used by an alternative route in a species, or for an indication other than what is specified by the manufacturer, this use is termed:
a. A felony offense
b. Extra-label use
c. Prohibited by the AVMA
d. Implied consent from the manufacturer

301. Each drug approved for use in food-producing animals has a time period given on the label between the last dose and when the animal can be slaughtered for food or when the milk can be sold. What is this period called?
a. Half-life period
b. Secretion period
c. Refractory period
d. Withdrawal period

302. Sometimes drugs are first administered in a large dose and then given as a series of smaller doses. What is the first dose called?
a. Initial dose
b. Loading dose
c. Distribution dose
d. Bolus dose

303. Many drugs do not have X mg/mL listed on their labels but instead have their concentrations listed as a percentage (e.g., X% solution). Which of the following most accurately reflects the conversion of a percentage of a solution to a weight per volume format?
a. X% = X g/mL
b. X% = X g/10 mL
c. X% = X g/100 mL
d. X% = X mg/10 mL

304. How many milligrams are in each milliliter of a 24% solution?
a. 24
b. 2.4
c. 240
d. 0.24

305. Which class of drugs generally poses the greatest potential health threat to those handling the medication?
a. Antibiotic
b. Antineoplastic
c. Antinematodal
d. Antiprotozoal

306. What effect does renal failure or compromised liver function have on the pharmacokinetics of many drugs?
a. Decreased absorption of drugs given orally
b. Increased elimination rate of drugs from the body
c. Decreased volume of distribution of drugs
d. Increased half-life of drugs

307. Controlled substances are drugs that:
  a. Cannot be used in any animal intended for use as human food
  b. Have a high potential for abuse
  c. Are very hazardous to anyone handling them
  d. Are environmentally hazardous

308. Drugs that are administered intra-articularly are injected into the:
  a. Bone marrow
  b. Subdural space
  c. Heart
  d. Joint

309. Extravasation of a chemotherapeutic agent should first be treated by:
  a. Applying a tourniquet to prevent movement of the drug up the leg
  b. Infiltrating the area with sterile saline or another sterile isotonic fluid
  c. Withdrawing as much drug as possible from the intravenous catheter
  d. Stopping the injection

310. Generally, 1 fluid ounce is equal to approximately how many milliliters of liquid?
  a. 1
  b. 15
  c. 30
  d. 60

311. Which of the following interferes with the development of an insect's chitin?
  a. Griseofulvin
  b. Lufenuron
  c. Methoprene
  d. Spinosad

312. The trade name for diphenhydramine is:
  a. Benadryl
  b. Prozac
  c. Dulcolax
  d. Panacur

313. Which of the following will *not* be used to decrease the potassium in a cat with a urethral obstruction?
  a. Calcium gluconate
  b. Dextrose
  c. Insulin
  d. Sodium bicarbonate

314. Which of the following medications was approved for use in the United States in 2014 and is being compared to propofol?
  a. Alfaxalone
  b. Etomidate
  c. Thiopental
  d. Telazol

315. Malignant hyperthermia is a possible side effect of which of the following?
  a. Etomidate
  b. Fentanyl
  c. Halothane
  d. Propofol

316. The specific treatment for malignant hyperthermia is:
  a. Dexmedetomidine
  b. Dantrolene
  c. Diazepam
  d. Acepromazine

317. Diffusion of drug molecules across the cell membrane that does not require energy and is a result of a difference in the concentration of that drug on the inside side of the cell versus the outside is called:
  a. Active transport
  b. Diffusive transport
  c. Passive transport
  d. Facilitated transport

318. Maropitant is the active ingredient in:
  a. Carafate
  b. Cerenia
  c. Flagyl
  d. Reglan

319. What can be done to decrease the risk of esophageal lesions in cats secondary to oral medications?
  a. Do not give oral medications
  b. Crush the medications
  c. Advise the owner to bring in the cat for medicating
  d. Follow the medication with water

320. Lidocaine is in which cardiac drug class?
  a. IA
  b. II
  c. IV
  d. IB

321. Which fibers in the central nervous system are responsible for sharp, localized pain?
  a. A
  b. A delta
  c. C
  d. C delta

322. Cyclooxygenase-1 (COX-1) is associated with:
  a. Blood flow to the kidney
  b. Healing
  c. Inflammation
  d. Pain

323. Which of the following will decrease the efficacy of lidocaine when used to address cardiac arrhythmias?
  a. Hypocalcemia
  b. Hypochloremia
  c. Hypokalemia
  d. Hyponatremia

324. A drug's tendency to bind to a receptor is called its:
  a. Affinity
  b. Efficacy
  c. Specificity
  d. Effective dose

325. Transport of a drug molecule that occurs when the majority of the cell surrounds the molecule, engulfs it, and brings it into the cell is referred to as:
  a. Facilitated
  b. Passive
  c. Phagocytosis
  d. Pinocytosis

326. Carprofen is the active ingredient in:
  a. Deramaxx
  b. Previcox
  c. Metacam
  d. Rimadyl

327. Cyclooxygenase-2 (COX-2) is associated with:
   a. Blood flow to the kidney
   b. Maintenance of the gastric mucosa
   c. Inflammation
   d. Normal physiological function
328. Furosemide is the active ingredient in:
   a. Lasix
   b. Osmitrol
   c. Aldactone
   d. HydroDIURIL
329. Which of the following is associated with central nervous signs if it is overdosed?
   a. Carprofen
   b. Chloramphenicol
   c. Furosemide
   d. Metronidazole
330. Levetiracetam is the active ingredient in:
   a. Keppra
   b. Valium
   c. Luminal
   d. Zonegran
331. Enrofloxacin works by:
   a. Inhibiting cell wall synthesis
   b. Inhibiting DNA
   c. Inhibiting protein synthesis
   d. Inhibiting the metabolic pathway
332. Diffusion of a drug molecule that involves a carrier protein but does not require energy is known as:
   a. Facilitated
   b. Passive
   c. Active
   d. Pinocytosis
333. The veterinarian asks you to fill metronidazole 250 mg po BID for 6 days. You have 500 mg tablets in stock. How many tablets will you fill?
   a. 3
   b. 6
   c. 12
   d. 24
334. Baytril is the trade name for:
   a. Acepromazine
   b. Cephalexin
   c. Enrofloxacin
   d. Gabapentin
335. With regard to the plasma concentration of a drug, what is the highest point in the concentration called?
   a. Peak
   b. Maximum
   c. Trough
   d. Minimum
336. What does it mean when a drug is at a steady state?
   a. The owner is giving the drug on a regular basis.
   b. The patient is responding as expected.
   c. The peak and trough are steady.
   d. The patient has been on the drug more than 6 months.
337. In a dog with a bite wound on the forelimb, which of the following will increase blood flow and thus delivery of a drug to the area of interest?
   a. Acute inflammation
   b. Shock
   c. Necrosis
   d. Hemorrhage
338. Metronidazole is the active ingredient in:
   a. Carafate
   b. Cerenia
   c. Flagyl
   d. Reglan
339. A patient is hospitalized for vomiting and diarrhea. The doctor orders metronidazole to be given BID. What is the most likely route the doctor will use?
   a. PO
   b. IV
   c. IM
   d. SQ
340. How long should a patient with pneumonia be on antibiotics?
   a. Two weeks past resolution of clinical signs
   b. Two weeks past resolution of radiographic signs
   c. Four weeks, no matter the clinical or radiographic signs
   d. Six weeks, no matter the clinical or radiographic signs
341. Why are prophylactic antibiotics given during surgery?
   a. To prevent contamination when the skin is entered
   b. To prevent contamination when a hollow viscous is entered
   c. To prevent contamination from the surgeon
   d. To prevent contamination from the instruments
342. Reglan is the trade name for:
   a. Metronidazole
   b. Dolasetron
   c. Maropitant
   d. Metoclopramide
343. After surgery has begun, how often should antibiotics be administered?
   a. Every 15–30 minutes
   b. Every 30–60 minutes
   c. Every 60–90 minutes
   d. Every 90–120 minutes
344. Of the following drugs, which must be in an anaerobic environment to be effective?
   a. Chloramphenicol
   b. Clindamycin
   c. Metronidazole
   d. Neomycin
345. Which of the following is generally used for infections not susceptible to other antibiotics?
   a. First-tier antibiotics
   b. Second-tier antibiotics
   c. Third-generation antibiotics
   d. Negative-tier antibiotics

346. An owner gives you a list of products and asks you which is most likely to prevent her dog from acquiring Rocky Mountain spotted fever. What would you advise her?
a. Advantix
b. Heartgard
c. Revolution
d. Interceptor

347. Which drug listed belongs in the drug class azole (imidazole derivatives)?
a. Amoxicillin
b. Cephalexin
c. Enrofloxacin
d. Ketoconazole

348. Which of the following is most likely to be used against Malassezia?
a. Griseofulvin
b. Itraconazole
c. Metronidazole
d. Tetracycline

349. Acylovir is an:
a. Antibacterial
b. Antifungal
c. Antiparasitic
d. Antiviral

350. Which of the following should be avoided or at least diluted 1:100 when cleaning an ear?
a. Chlorhexidine
b. Saline solution
c. Vinegar and water
d. Aural cleaning solution

351. In response to hyperkalemia, calcium gluconate will:
a. Cause potassium to move into the cell
b. Increase urination to excrete potassium
c. Protect the heart from the effects of the potassium
d. Cause potassium to move out of the cell

352. Of the following antibiotics, which is best suited to treat tetanus caused by Clostridium tetani?
a. Enrofloxacin
b. Metronidazole
c. Neomycin
d. Penicillin G

353. Cardiac drugs that belong in class IA act by:
a. Stabilizing myocardial cells
b. Blocking beta receptors
c. Decreasing myocardial automaticity
d. Blocking calcium channels

354. Propranolol is a:
a. Beta-1 blocker
b. Beta-2 blocker
c. A nonselective beta blocker
d. Not a beta blocker

355. Which drug class does diltiazem belong in?
a. Beta-1 blocker
b. Beta-2 blocker
c. Calcium channel blocker
d. Sodium channel blocker

356. Which of the following drugs can be used to increase platelet numbers?
a. Chlorambucil
b. Doxorubicin
c. Vinblastine
d. Vincristine

357. Which of the following products will provide oxygen-carrying capacity?
a. Cryoprecipitate
b. Fresh frozen plasma
c. Frozen plasma
d. Oxyglobin

358. The doctor ordered a patient to receive Unasyn, 1200 mg IV. After reconstitution, the Unasyn has a concentration of 375 mg/mL. How many mL will you administer?
a. 0.31 mL
b. 1.2 mL
c. 3.2 mL
d. 6.4 mL

359. How many half-lives does a drug go through before reaching a steady state?
a. 2
b. 3
c. 4
d. 5

360. The doctor asks you to fill oral metronidazole, 10 mg/kg po BID for 7 days. The dog weighs 37.5 kg and you have 250-mg tablets available in the hospital. How many tablets do you fill?
a. 7
b. 14
c. 21
d. 42

361. Cardiac drugs that belong in class IB act by:
a. Stabilizing myocardial cells
b. Blocking beta receptors
c. Decreasing myocardial automaticity
d. Blocking calcium channels

362. Of the fluids listed, which has the lowest sodium content?
a. 0.9% NaCl
b. D5W
c. 0.45% NaCl
d. Lactated ringers

363. The doctor orders a dose of calcium gluconate be administered to a patient. In addition to drawing up the medication, what other procedure should you prepare for?
a. To monitor an EKG
b. To monitor the BP
c. To monitor the SpO_2
d. To monitor the temperature

364. The transport mechanism requiring a carrier protein that also requires energy is called:
a. Facilitated
b. Passive
c. Active
d. Pinocytosis

365. What type of fluid is hetastarch considered to be?
a. Blood product
b. Crystalloid
c. Natural colloid
d. Synthetic colloid

366. Potassium-sparing diuretics, such as spirolactone, act on which part of the kidneys?
   a. Loop of Henle
   b. Collecting duct
   c. Proximal tubule
   d. Bowman capsule
367. Esmolol is:
   a. A nonselective beta blocker
   b. A beta-1 blocker
   c. A beta-2 blocker
   d. Not a beta blocker
368. The doctor expresses concern that a patient's cardiac output is poor and he is considering something to increase the contractility of the heart. You know he will want to use a:
   a. Positive inotrope
   b. Negative inotrope
   c. Positive chronotrope
   d. Negative chronotrope
369. The doctor asks you to fill acepromazine, 50 mg po TID for 7 days. You have 25-mg tablets available in the hospital. How many tablets do you fill?
   a. 14
   b. 21
   c. 28
   d. 42
370. Cardiac drugs that belong in class II act by:
   a. Stabilizing myocardial cells
   b. Blocking beta receptors
   c. Decreasing myocardial automaticity
   d. Blocking calcium channels
371. Which of the following processes will decrease the efficacy of an antibiotic in a dog with a bite wound on the forelimb?
   a. Acute inflammation
   b. Shock
   c. Necrosis
   d. Chronic inflammation
372. Cisapride is a/an:
   a. Antiemetic
   b. Prokinetic
   c. GI protectant
   d. Antidiarrheal
373. What condition does dirlotapide treat?
   a. Obesity in dogs
   b. Obesity in cats
   c. Anorexia in dogs
   d. Anorexia in cats
374. Ondansetron is an antiemetic that belongs in which drug class?
   a. Anticholinergic
   b. Barbiturate
   c. Phenothiazine
   d. Serotonin antagonist
375. Lactulose can be given to a patient with a portosystemic shunt to help:
   a. Decrease gastrointestinal transit time
   b. Convert ammonia to ammonium
   c. Prevent diarrhea
   d. Prevent water loss though the colon
376. The drug that treats autoimmune diseases and pruritus associated with atopic dermatitis is known as:
   a. Cyclosporine
   b. Interferon omega
   c. Ketoconazole
   d. Phytosphingosine
377. Atopica is the brand name for:
   a. Anzemet
   b. Cyclosporine
   c. Dolasetron
   d. Furosemide
378. Which of the following is a benzodiazepine tranquilizer?
   a. Fentanyl
   b. Ketamine
   c. Medetomidine
   d. Midazolam
379. Which type of diuretic is used to treat increased intracranial pressure?
   a. Loop
   b. Osmotic
   c. Potassium-sparing
   d. Thiazide
380. Which of the following medications is an opioid?
   a. Buprenorphine
   b. Carprofen
   c. Lidocaine
   d. Naloxone
381. The doctor orders a patient to receive a CRI of fentanyl. How often will this drug be administered?
   a. Every 2 hours
   b. Every 4 hours
   c. Every 6 hours
   d. At a constant rate
382. Which of the following drugs is a synthetic analog of codeine?
   a. Dextromethorphan
   b. Gabapentin
   c. Methocarbamol
   d. Tramadol
383. You are placing an intravenous catheter to administer chemotherapy. When placing the catheter you go through the vein, but you are able to reposition it and place it successfully. What should you do next?
   a. Use the catheter, but monitor it closely during the injection
   b. Pull the catheter and place it in a different vein
   c. Pull the catheter and place it higher up in the same vein
   d. Use it without concern
384. L-asparaginase, a chemotherapeutic, is used most commonly for:
   a. Hemangiosarcoma
   b. Mast cell tumors
   c. Lymphoma
   d. Osteosarcoma
385. A solution that contains so much solute that it cannot be dissolved is known as:
   a. Concentrated
   b. Dilute
   c. Saturated
   d. Supersaturated

386. Regarding the concentration of a solution, molality is known as:
a. The number of moles per liter of solution
b. The amount of solute per kilogram of solvent
c. The grams per liter of solution
d. The number of solute particles per liter

387. The doctor asks you to start a fentanyl constant rate infusion (CRI) at 3 mcg/kg/h in a 50-kg dog. The fentanyl you have available in the hospital is 50 mcg/mL. What will the rate per hour be?
a. 1 mL/h
b. 3 mL/h
c. 5 mL/h
d. 50 mL/h

388. Which injectable anesthetic is *not* recommended in patients with neurological disease?
a. Barbiturates
b. Etomidate
c. Ketamine
d. Propofol

389. Which of the following antiseizure medications should be avoided in a patient with existing liver disease?
a. Levetiracetam
b. Phenobarbital
c. Potassium bromide
d. Gabapentin

390. Which of the following anesthetics has the fewest cardiorespiratory effects?
a. Etomidate
b. Propofol
c. Ketamine
d. Thiopental

391. Methocarbamol is labeled as an adjunctive therapy for:
a. Seizures
b. Skeletal muscle trauma
c. Increased intracranial pressure
d. Joint pain

392. Which medication can be used to confirm a diagnosis of acquired myasthenia gravis?
a. Acepromazine
b. Metoclopramide
c. Tensilon
d. Theophylline

393. Bloat-Pac is indicated for frothy bloat in:
a. Cattle
b. Dogs
c. Pigs
d. Horses

394. Which of the following should never be used in cats?
a. Carboplatin
b. Hydroxyurea
c. 5-Fluorouracil
d. Procarbazine

395. Robaxin-V is the brand name for:
a. Gabapentin
b. Methocarbamol
c. Methimazole
d. Methionine (S-Adenosyl)

396. Cardiac drugs that belong in class IV act by:
a. Stabilizing myocardial cells
b. Blocking beta receptors
c. Decreasing myocardial automaticity
d. Blocking calcium channels

397. Antibiotics should be administered when abdominal surgery is longer than:
a. 30 minutes
b. 60 minutes
c. 90 minutes
d. 120 minutes

398. The doctor asks you to administer 5 g of 25% mannitol to a patient. How many mL do you give?
a. 5 mL
b. 20 mL
c. 40 mL
d. 25 mL

399. Which of the following drugs is most likely to require therapeutic drug monitoring?
a. Enrofloxacin
b. Metoclopramide
c. Metronidazole
d. Phenobarbital

400. An aerotolerant organism is one that:
a. Is not affected by the presence or absence of oxygen
b. Can tolerate elevated temperatures
c. Prefers and environment that is dehydrated
d. Is tolerant of environments lacking moisture

401. Some bacteria have an outer layer defined as a biopolymer matrix. This layer is called the:
a. Cell wall
b. Biofilm
c. Matrix layer
d. Bio layer

402. The mechanism of action of beta-lactams is interference with:
a. Cell wall synthesis
b. Protein synthesis
c. The uptake of nutrients
d. DNA synthesis

403. The doctor would like to start a patient on a drug that increases gastrointestinal motility. He would like to be able to add it to the intravenous fluids and also to send the dog home with an oral dose on discharge. Which drug fulfills these criteria?
a. Diphenhydramine
b. Dolasetron
c. Maropitant
d. Metoclopramide

404. One method of resistance to sulfonamides is through the bacteria's ability:
a. To survive without folic acid
b. To use the host's folic acid
c. To produce a substitute for folic acid
d. To turn the antibiotic into folic acid

405. Macrolides inhibit bacterial ribosomal action by binding which subunit?
a. 30s
b. 40s
c. 50s
d. 60s

406. A drug that requires biotransformation before it becomes active is called a:
a. Pretransformed drug
b. Nonactive drug
c. Predrug
d. Prodrug

407. When discharging a cat, you would explain to the owner that the buprenorphine should be given:
a. po
b. SQ
c. TM
d. IM

408. Which of the following drugs minimally crosses the placental barrier and is safe to use in pregnant dogs?
a. Acepromazine
b. Atropine
c. Fentanyl
d. Glycopyrrolate

409. In geriatric patients, drug doses are generally:
a. The same as in puppies
b. Decreased
c. Increased
d. The same as in adults

410. Which of the following can increase the risk of digoxin toxicity?
a. Hypokalemia
b. Hypochloremia
c. Hyponatremia
d. Hypocalcemia

411. While drawing up injectable Amikacin for a patient, you note that it has developed a pale yellow color. What should you do?
a. Discard the rest of the bottle
b. Don't be concerned because you know this can be normal
c. Dilute it with saline
d. Dilute it with sterile water

412. When applying nitroglycerin ointment, it is important to wear gloves and:
a. Wash it off after it has had contact with the patient for 5 minutes
b. Avoid placing it directly on the skin
c. Make a note where it was placed
d. Make sure it is placed thickly in a small area

413. Low-molecular-weight heparin is different from unfractionated heparin in that it:
a. Is less pure than unfractionated heparin
b. Does not block the activity of thrombin whereas unfractionated heparin does
c. Is less expensive than unfractionated heparin
d. Is more likely to cause hemorrhage than unfractionated heparin

414. Plavix is the brand name for:
a. Clopidogrel
b. Nitroprusside
c. Sildenafil
d. Tadalafil

415. An oral antiarrhythmic that includes an action similar to injectable propranolol is:
a. Hydralazine
b. Pimobendan
c. Prazosin
d. Sotalol

416. Which of the following drugs can be used for atrial fibrillation?
a. Digoxin
b. Hydralazine
c. Lidocaine
d. Pimobendan

417. What can be used in the hospital, given IV, to increase a patient's phosphorus?
a. Amphojel
b. Dexamethasone sodium phosphate
c. Potassium phosphate
d. Tums

418. Feline asthma can be treated with:
a. Amphotericin B
b. Digoxin
c. Hydralazine
d. Terbutaline

419. Aminophylline is known as a:
a. Bronchodilator
b. Decongestant
c. Expectorant
d. Mucolytic

420. Which of the following is not absorbed systemically?
a. Diphenhydramine
b. Dolasetron
c. Sucralfate
d. Tramadol

421. Tums can be administered to supplement:
a. Calcium
b. Vitamin B
c. Vitamin C
d. Vitamin E

422. Vitamin B1 is:
a. Ascorbic acid
b. Cyanocobalamin
c. Riboflavin
d. Thiamine

423. Which of the following is used to increase calcium uptake from the gastrointestinal tract, mobilize calcium from the bone, and conserve calcium from the kidneys?
a. Alendronate
b. Calcitonin
c. Calcitriol
d. Calcimimetics

424. Which species should receive prednisolone instead of prednisone?
a. Cats
b. Cows
c. Dogs
d. Swine

425. The doctor would like to place a patient on a metoclopramide CRI at 2 mg/kg/day. He would like this added to a 1-L bag of fluids that will last 24 hours. The patient weighs 20 kg. How many mL of 5-mg/mL metoclopramide should be added to the bag?
a. 2 mL
b. 8 mL
c. 20 mL
d. 40 mL

426. Which of the following can be used to decrease intraocular volume (via dehydration of the vitreous humor) as treatment for glaucoma?
a. Mannitol
b. Methazolamide
c. Pilocarpine
d. Timolol

427. Because administration of medications via this route has more potential for adverse effects, what type of injection should be given slowly?
a. IP
b. IV
c. IM
d. SQ

428. What is the maximum rate at which you can administer IV potassium?
a. 0.09 mEq/kg/h
b. 1.0 mEq/kg/h
c. 0.5 mEq/kg/h
d. 0.7 mEq/kg/h

429. When a patient has received a spinal epidural, which of the following must be monitored closely?
a. Appetite
b. Attitude
c. Urination
d. Walking

430. Which of the following is primarily used as a sedative that can also be used to increase the duration of an epidural?
a. Bupivacaine
b. Dexmedetomidine
c. Hydromorphone
d. Morphine

431. What can be used to decrease the damage caused by reperfusion injury?
a. Bupivacaine
b. Lidocaine
c. Marcaine
d. Procaine

432. Glucosamine/chondroitin is a nutraceutical that is used to treat:
a. Anemia
b. Arthritis
c. Pruritus
d. Urinary incontinence

433. Which antibiotic also has anti-inflammatory actions in the gastrointestinal tract?
a. Ciprofloxacin
b. Enrofloxacin
c. Metronidazole
d. Tetracycline

434. Because sucralfate is more effective in an acidic environment, it should be administered before:
a. Cisapride
b. Famotidine
c. Lactulose
d. Metoclopramide

435. The doctor asks you to perform a local block on a patient in preparation for a laceration repair. You know you should not exceed a dose of:
a. 2–4 mg/kg
b. 4–6 mg/kg
c. 6–8 mg/kg
d. 8–10 mg/kg

436. Which of the following *cannot* be phoned in to the pharmacy and will require a written prescription?
a. Buprenorphine
b. Diazepam
c. Morphine
d. Phenobarbital

437. Vetmedin is the brand name for:
a. Atenolol
b. Pimobendan
c. Procainamide
d. Quinidine

438. Lidocaine can be diluted with sodium bicarbonate to decrease pain associated with injection. What should this dilution be (sodium bicarbonate: lidocaine)?
a. 1:01
b. 1:04
c. 1:05
d. 1:09

439. Which of the following will have the longest duration of action when used as an epidural?
a. Bupivacaine
b. Butorphanol
c. Ketamine
d. Morphine

440. Alpha-tocopherol is the most active form of:
a. Vitamin E
b. Vitamin D2
c. Vitamin D3
d. Vitamin B2

441. DMSO should not be used in patients with:
a. Hemangiosarcoma
b. Lymphoma
c. Mast cell tumors
d. Osteosarcoma

442. A vaccine that produces immunity to a toxin is called a:
a. Live
b. Modified live
c. Recombinant
d. Toxoid

443. An example of a semisolid dosage form is:
a. Implant
b. Injectable
c. Ointment
d. Syrup

444. Which of the following can affect drug absorption, distribution, metabolism, and elimination?
a. Cardiac disease
b. Kidney disease
c. Liver disease
d. Pancreatic disease

445. Idiosyncratic drug reactions are those that are:
a. Predictable
b. Unpredictable
c. Synchronized with other reactions
d. Unsynchronized with other reactions

446. Regarding the storage of drugs, room temperature (in Fahrenheit) falls in the range of:
a. Less than 46°
b. 46°–59°
c. 60°–86°
d. 87°–104°

447. Which of the following drugs can become inactivated by shaking?
a. Amoxicillin
b. Clavamox
c. Insulin
d. Metronidazole

448. Which drug is preferred over Atropine for use in rabbits, because Atropine is less predictable in this species?
a. Acepromazine
b. Glycopyrolate
c. Diazepam
d. a and b

449. Midazolam can be administered to rabbits in all of the following methods *except*:
a. Intraperitoneal
b. Intramuscular
c. Intravenous
d. Subcutaneous

450. Yohimbine can be used to reverse all of the following alpha-2 adrenoreceptor agonists except:
a. Xylazine
b. Metetomadine
c. Midazolam
d. Dexmedetomadine

451. Atipamezole, when administered SC to rabbits, can reverse the effects of medetomadine within:
a. 2–5 minutes
b. 5–10 minutes
c. 10–25 minutes
d. 25–30 minutes

452. Anticholinergic drugs are used for:
a. Tachycardia
b. Tachypenia
c. Bradycardia
d. Bradypenia

SECTION 6

Surgical Nursing

Nicholas Raimondi

QUESTIONS

1. If you notice an item at the edge of a sterile field during surgery, you should:
   a. Ask others to find out whether it was contaminated
   b. Consider it unsterile if you are not absolutely certain
   c. Consider it sterile
   d. Move it further into the sterile field
2. What type of instrument is a Kelly?
   a. Needle holder
   b. Scissors
   c. Towel clamp
   d. Hemostatic forceps
3. Which of the following suffixes is used to describe the surgical alteration of a shape or form?
   a. -pexy
   b. -plasty
   c. -ostomy
   d. -rrhapy
4. What agent, method, or device is most appropriate for sterilizing a needle holder to be used in a surgical procedure?
   a. Autoclave
   b. Dry heat
   c. Ethylene oxide gas
   d. Liquid chemical disinfectant
5. What is the significance of an autoclave that will *not* properly seal but still has steam rising from it?
   a. Because it is the sterilizing agent, it will work fine, but you must be more cautious to prevent burns to personnel.
   b. The microbes are killed by the pressure and therefore the autoclave will not work.
   c. It will continue to sterilize but will require more water as the steam escapes.
   d. The pressure will not increase, which is required to meet the minimum temperature for sterilization.
6. When attaching an ECG, which leg should have the red lead attached to it?
   a. Right foreleg
   b. Left foreleg
   c. Right hind leg
   d. Left hind leg
7. Preparing a patient's skin for surgery:
   a. Renders the skin sterile
   b. Does nothing to affect the outcome of the surgery
   c. Reduces the bacterial flora to a level that can be controlled by the patient's immune system
   d. Is not necessary if antibiotics are administered
8. During a surgical procedure, which of the following does *not* have to be sterile to maintain aseptic conditions?
   a. Mask
   b. Drapes
   c. Instruments
   d. Gloves
9. The effectiveness of a surgical scrub on the hands and arms with an antibacterial soap depends on the:
   a. Combination of contact time and scrubbing action
   b. Amount of soap used throughout the scrub
   c. Scrubbing action of the brush
   d. Temperature of the water
10. Which statement regarding first-intention wound healing is false?
    a. It occurs without infection.
    b. It occurs when the skin edges are held together in apposition.
    c. It usually has some degree of suppuration.
    d. It occurs with minimal scar formation.
11. Which of the following statements about electrocautery is false?
    a. If the patient is not properly grounded, the surgeon may receive a shock.
    b. The intensity of the current passed through the unit is adjustable.
    c. Small bleeding blood vessels are sealed with a controlled electrical current that burns the bleeding end.
    d. All portions of the electrocautery unit can and should be sterilized.
12. Which size of scalpel blade should be used for making an abdominal skin incision in a dog?
    a. No. 10
    b. No. 11
    c. No. 12
    d. No. 20
13. Before starting the surgical procedure, the technician who has scrubbed in with the surgeon should do all of the following *except*:
    a. Count the gauze sponges in the pack
    b. Arrange the instruments to be located quickly and easily
    c. Place the scalpel blade on the handle
    d. Open the suture material
14. An ovariohysterectomy might be performed for all of the following reasons *except*:
    a. Prevention of prostate cancer
    b. Prevention of pyometra
    c. Sterilization of the animal
    d. Prevention of estrus

15. Place the following surgeries in the order in which they should be scheduled, from first to last:
    a. Cruciate repair, OHE, compound fracture repair, intestinal resection
    b. Intestinal resection, cruciate repair, compound fracture repair, OHE
    c. Compound fracture repair, cruciate repair, OHE, intestinal resection
    d. Cruciate repair, compound fracture repair, OHE, intestinal resection
16. If an animal goes home with a bandage, the client should observe the bandage daily and remove it if any of the following are observed *except*:
    a. Skin irritation at the edge of the bandage
    b. All bandages should be removed 24 hours after being applied
    c. The bandage is wet
    d. The position of the bandage has shifted
17. Which of the following is *not* true about dogs that are spayed before their first estrus cycle?
    a. The hair coat will change and become easier to manage with less shedding.
    b. The surgery is generally considered easier to perform if the bitch has not been through an estrus cycle.
    c. Mammary cancer is less likely to occur in a bitch that has been spayed before her first estrus cycle.
    d. The uterus and ovaries enlarge after the first estrus cycle. This necessitates a larger abdominal incision when the bitch is spayed.
18. Which of the following statements regarding pyometra is false?
    a. The bitch that goes to surgery will have the ovaries and uterus removed.
    b. The bitch that goes to surgery will have only her uterus removed.
    c. The uterus might have ruptured before surgery begins.
    d. The patient represents a high-risk anesthesia case, because other organs in the body might be compromised.
19. All of the following statements regarding cesarean sections are true *except*:
    a. After the newborns are removed, the mother is out of danger, and most of the technician's attention should be on the newborns.
    b. A cesarean section is also known as a hysterotomy.
    c. For some breeds of dogs, such as the English bulldog, it is expected that a cesarean section will need to be performed.
    d. Wait to place the mother with the newborns until after she has adequately recovered from anesthesia.
20. Which of the following statements regarding cesarean sections is false?
    a. Bloody vaginal discharge is expected following surgery.
    b. The newborns delivered by cesarean section are under the effects of anesthesia.
    c. The client should observe the surgical incision after 1 week, because the newborns do not start moving around the mammary area until then.
    d. The newborn should be immediately removed from the membranous sac that covers its body when it is removed from the uterus.
21. When a male dog is presented to the hospital for a castration procedure, the technician should do all of the following *except*:
    a. Ensure that the dog is a male
    b. Ensure that there are two testicles in the scrotum
    c. Ensure that the dog is not in heat
    d. Ensure that there is a telephone number to reach the client
22. All of the following are benefits to having a peripheral IV catheter placed in advance of surgery *except*:
    a. Administering anesthesia
    b. Administering emergency drugs in case of anesthetic complications
    c. Administering intravenous fluids
    d. Administering enteral nutrition
23. When a bitch is presented to the hospital for an ovariohysterectomy, the technician should do all of the following *except*:
    a. Ensure the dog is a female
    b. Obtain a telephone number where the client can be reached that day
    c. Ensure that the bitch does not have an abdominal scar
    d. Give the dog aspirin, because the surgical procedure will be painful
24. Clipper burn can cause all of the following adverse effects *except*:
    a. Excessive licking of the area
    b. Follicular damage preventing hair regrowth
    c. Inhibition of wound healing
    d. Promotion of bacteria growth
25. When a dog is presented for castration, and both testicles are descended, the veterinary technician will prepare the surgical site. In which area is the incision most commonly made?
    a. Flank
    b. Scrotum
    c. Prescrotal prepuce
    d. Mid-abdomen
26. Which of the following suffixes is used to describe the surgical creation of an artificial opening?
    a. -ectomy
    b. -otomy
    c. -ostomy
    d. -rrhapy
27. When a cat is presented for castration and both testicles are descended, the veterinary technician will prepare the surgical site. In which area is the incision most commonly made?
    a. Flank
    b. Scrotum
    c. Prescrotal prepuce
    d. Mid-abdomen
28. When a dog is presented to the hospital to be spayed, the veterinary technician should prepare the surgical site. In which area is the incision most commonly made?
    a. Inguinal
    b. Scrotum
    c. Prescrotal prepuce
    d. Abdominal ventral midline

29. What is the primary function of a Brown-Adson?
 a. Retractor
 b. Rongeur
 c. Periosteal elevator
 d. Thumb forceps

30. The hair coat can be most efficiently and gently removed when preparing a dog for spaying by which of the following methods?
 a. Plucking
 b. Clipping with sharp scissors
 c. Clipping against the grain of the hair with electrical clippers using a No. 40 blade
 d. Clipping against the grain of the hair with electrical clippers using a No. 10 blade

31. Which of the following statements is false after serious oral surgery, such as mandibular fracture repair or oral-nasal tumor resection?
 a. The patient might refuse to eat.
 b. The patient might need a gastrotomy tube.
 c. The patient might refuse to drink.
 d. The patient will no longer be in pain.

32. When feeding the patient through a gastrostomy tube, the technician should:
 a. Rapidly inject the fluids and food
 b. Flush the tube with water
 c. Flush the tube with air
 d. Feed a full day's caloric requirement immediately after placement

33. Postoperative physical therapy can help the patient in each of the following ways *except* in:
 a. Enhancing patient comfort
 b. Preventing complications from disuse
 c. Slowing the healing process
 d. Decreasing edema

34. A semi-permanent feeding tube may be placed in all of the following ways *except*:
 a. Through the nose
 b. Through a pharyngostomy site
 c. Through a gastrostomy site
 d. Through the mouth

35. All of the following statements are true regarding gastrointestinal (GI) surgery *except*:
 a. It is absolutely essential that all patients fast before GI surgery. The GI tract must be empty before surgery.
 b. At no point is the GI tract sterile; therefore, it is important to guard against contamination.
 c. Irrigation of the peritoneal cavity with a sterile isotonic solution after GI surgery helps reduce the number of microorganisms that remain free in the peritoneum following the procedure.
 d. The surgical assistant must be alert to the possibility of intestinal contents contaminating the abdominal cavity and must help the surgeon prevent this from happening.

36. It is important that the nursing care provided to paralyzed patients focuses on patient comfort. The prevention of decubital ulcers can be accomplished by all of the following procedures *except*:
 a. Frequent turning or repositioning of the patient
 b. Adequate padding in the cage or bed
 c. Appropriate analgesic therapy
 d. Massage

37. A proptosed globe:
 a. Can be caused by overzealous restraint of the animal
 b. Is not considered an emergency
 c. Can most easily occur in dolicocephalic breeds, such as collies
 d. Is commonly a consequence of conjunctivitis

38. An abscess is:
 a. Usually lanced, drained, flushed, and sutured closed
 b. A solid infiltration of inflammatory cells
 c. A rare consequence of bite wounds
 d. A "walled-off" or circumscribed accumulation of pus

39. All of the following are instructions provided to a client when the patient has had a Penrose drain placed *except*:
 a. An Elizabethan collar may be needed.
 b. Clean the skin around the drain with warm water or dilute chlorhexidine.
 c. The drain will fall out and there is no need to return for removal.
 d. Carefully watch the animal and prevent it from licking or chewing at the drain.

40. The client should be instructed to contact the veterinary hospital if any of the following occur with a splint or cast *except*:
 a. The animal chews at the splint or cast.
 b. The splint or cast is wet.
 c. The leg looks swollen above or below the cast.
 d. The animal is walking on or using the splinted or casted leg.

41. Proper splint and bandage care includes all of the following *except*:
 a. Washing the splint or bandage daily
 b. Preventing the bandage or splint from becoming wet
 c. Inspecting the bandage or splint daily for any change, such as swelling above or below the splint or bandage
 d. Inspecting the bandage or splint for any shifting or change in position on the limb

42. Which of the following is *not* true of an aural hematoma?
 a. An aural hematoma must be drained.
 b. Trimming back the pinna repairs it.
 c. It is painful and bothersome to the animal.
 d. An aural hematoma may be drained and bandaged by wrapping the head with the ear folded back across the top of the head.

43. Which of the following instruments should be available for use during abdominal exploratory surgery?
 a. Balfour retractor
 b. Weitlaner retractor
 c. Gelpi retractor
 d. Senn retractor

44. Suture materials are:
 a. Absorbable only
 b. Nonabsorbable only
 c. Braided or monofilament
 d. Only supplied with a needle attached

45. When passing surgical instruments to the surgeon, the technician should do all of the following *except*:
  a. Gently but firmly slap the palm of the surgeon with the instrument
  b. Pass the instrument in the open position
  c. Pass the instrument with the handle placed into the surgeon's hand
  d. Pass the curved instrument so that it is oriented in the surgeon's hand with the concave side up
46. When assisting the surgeon, the technician should:
  a. Always cut sutures on top of the knot
  b. Cut sutures with the middle tip part of the scissors blade
  c. Blot the surgical site with a gauze square to clear the site of blood
  d. Attach the scalpel blade to the handle using a pair of hemostats
47. Staples and other metal clips can:
  a. Resist infection
  b. Cause little scarring
  c. Be removed easily using scissors
  d. Be applied by hand without any special application device
48. Surgical instruments should be:
  a. Lubricated with oil between uses
  b. Cleaned without water to avoid the possibility of rusting
  c. Placed on surfaces and never dropped or thrown
  d. Cleaned with abrasive cleaners
49. External fixation devices include all of the following *except*:
  a. Cast
  b. Splint
  c. Bone plate
  d. Kirschner-Ehmer (K-E) apparatus
50. Overinflation or underinflation of the endotracheal tube cuff can result in all of the following *except*:
  a. Prevention of fluid aspiration into the lungs
  b. Pressure necrosis of the cells lining the trachea
  c. Inability to keep the patient under anesthesia with the expected concentration of gas anesthetic
  d. Increased levels of waste gas anesthesia in the surgical room
51. A chest tube is placed when an animal has:
  a. Subcutaneous emphysema
  b. Pulmonary edema
  c. Ascites
  d. Pneumothorax
52. There is more concern about pulling out the endotracheal tube too soon in the _______ than in an English mastiff:
  a. English bulldog
  b. German shepherd
  c. Jack Russell terrier
  d. Greyhound
53. *Dystocia* is:
  a. Difficulty in breathing
  b. A side effect of opioid drugs
  c. A difficult or abnormal birth
  d. Difficulty in urinating
54. Surgical procedures of the ear include all of the following *except*:
  a. Otoplasty
  b. Bulla osteotomy
  c. Aural hematoma drainage
  d. Enucleation
55. Surgical procedures of the eye and adnexal structures include all of the following *except*:
  a. Entropion repair
  b. Keratectomy
  c. Onychectomy
  d. Enucleation
56. A patient is to be prepared for a cystotomy. What part of the body is prepped?
  a. Ventral abdomen
  b. Lumbar spine
  c. Ventral cervical area
  d. Top of the head
57. A patient is to be prepared for an ovariohysterectomy. What part of the body is prepped?
  a. Paw
  b. Ventral chest wall
  c. Ventral abdomen
  d. Ear
58. A patient is to be prepared for a femoral head ostectomy. What part of the body is prepped?
  a. Top of the head
  b. Hip
  c. Shoulder
  d. Lumbar spine
59. A patient is to be prepared for an orchidectomy. What part of the body is prepped?
  a. Ventral abdomen
  b. Scrotal/prescrotal area
  c. Paw
  d. Ear
60. The patient is to be prepared for a popliteal lymph node biopsy. What part of the body is prepped?
  a. Caudal aspect of the stifle
  b. Cranial aspect of the elbow
  c. Medial aspect of the thigh
  d. Area cranial to the shoulder
61. A declaw is also known as an:
  a. Orchidectomy
  b. Onychectomy
  c. Ovariohysterectomy
  d. Onychotomy
62. Which structure is *not* part of the spermatic cord?
  a. Pampiniform plexus
  b. Vas deferens
  c. Testicular artery
  d. Epididymis
63. Which of the following is *not* completely removed in an ovariohysterectomy?
  a. Broad ligament
  b. Ovaries
  c. Uterine horns
  d. Oviducts

64. An enucleation may be required to correct a/an:
   a. Third eyelid prolapse
   b. Penile prolapse
   c. Proptosis of the eye
   d. Aural hematoma

65. Which of the following is a needle driver that is also able to cut suture material?
   a. Olsen-Hegar
   b. Mayo-Hegar
   c. Adson-Brown
   d. Rochester-Pean

66. Which of the following forceps has the best crushing action?
   a. Rochester-Carmalt
   b. Adson-Brown
   c. Ochsner
   d. Crile

67. Which of the following is a nondesirable characteristic of ethylene oxide?
   a. Carcinogenic
   b. Teratogenic
   c. Mutagenic
   d. Mitogenic

68. Which of the following suture materials remains in the body for the longest period?
   a. Polydioxanone
   b. Prolene
   c. Chromic catgut
   d. Vicryl

69. Scrotal swelling after orchidectomy is most likely caused by a:
   a. Hematoma
   b. Ascites
   c. Hemangioma
   d. Lipoma

70. Which of the following instruments is the only one appropriate for handling tissues during surgery?
   a. Dressing forceps
   b. Standard surgical scissors
   c. Sponge forceps
   d. Rat-tooth forceps

71. What suture pattern is commonly used to close the skin of cattle following a rumenotomy?
   a. Simple interrupted
   b. Simple continuous
   c. Continuous Ford interlocking pattern
   d. a and c

72. Which of the following suture materials is most appropriate to close the muscle layers of a cow following a left-displaced abomasum surgery?
   a. 3-0 nylon
   b. 3-0 polydioxanone
   c. 3 chromic nylon
   d. 3 polydioxanone

73. Which of the following statements regarding pyometra is incorrect?
   a. Onychectomy is usually curative.
   b. A purulent vaginal discharge is always present.
   c. Affected females usually have polyuria and polydipsia.
   d. It often occurs soon after a heat cycle.

74. Which of the following procedures is *not* considered elective?
   a. Orchidectomy
   b. Ovariohysterectomy
   c. Onychectomy
   d. Enucleation of a proptosed eye

75. *Nephrectomy* refers to:
   a. An incision into the kidney
   b. The removal of a kidney
   c. The removal of a tumor from the kidney
   d. The biopsy of a kidney

76. When preparing for an orthopedic surgery, shaving the surgical site should be performed:
   a. The previous night to shorten the anesthesia time
   b. First thing in the morning to help the procedures run more smoothly
   c. Immediately before the induction of anesthesia
   d. Just after the induction of anesthesia

77. Fracture apposition reduction refers to:
   a. Placing bones back in their normal positions
   b. Keeping bones still until healing has occurred
   c. Removing small fragments from around the fracture
   d. Placing pins through the marrow cavity

78. Which of the following suffixes is used to describe the removal of an organ?
   a. -ectomy
   b. -otomy
   c. -ostomy
   d. -rrhapy

79. A *Caslick* operation is performed in horses to:
   a. Stop roaring
   b. Prevent uterine infection
   c. Treat navicular disease
   d. Clean out the guttural pouches

80. Which of the following agents can be used as both an antiseptic and a disinfectant?
   a. Quaternary ammonium compounds
   b. Mercurial chloride compounds
   c. Isopropyl alcohol
   d. Formaldehyde

81. For which of the following surgeries are stay sutures *not* normally necessary?
   a. Cystotomy
   b. Gastrotomy
   c. Intestinal anastomosis
   d. Hepatic biopsy

82. What is the minimum number of throws required when making a surgical knot?
   a. One
   b. Two
   c. Three
   d. Four

83. When would it be considered an advantage to use a hand tie versus an instrument tie?
   a. When suturing very tough tissue
   b. When suturing the linea alba or areas that are difficult to reach
   c. When suturing the skin
   d. When suturing hollow organs

84. The chemical or mechanical destruction of pathogens is known as:
a. Disinfection
b. Decontamination
c. Barrier
d. Aseptic technique

85. Which of the following is an advantage of monofilament material over multifilament material?
a. Greater knot security
b. Greater suture strength
c. Less likely to cause suture reactions
d. Passes through tissue more easily

86. What type of instrument is a *Mayo-Hegar*?
a. Needle holder
b. Scissors
c. Towel clamp
d. Hemostatic forceps

87. Which of the following suture sizes is most appropriate for eye surgeries?
a. 0
b. 3-0
c. 6-0
d. 1

88. All of the following are important reasons to reduce the amount of dead space with drains in a wound *except*:
a. To decrease the chance of infection
b. To decrease the chance of seroma formation
c. To decrease hemostasis
d. To minimize necrosis

89. Which of the following is an absorbable suture material?
a. Polydioxanone
b. Prolene
c. Silk
d. Cotton

90. What factor will *not* influence how rapidly the body absorbs suture materials?
a. Age of the patient
b. Presence of infection
c. The location of the suture
d. The composition of the suture material

91. Which of the following is *not* considered a contaminated surgery and would be considered the cleanest?
a. Cruciate repair
b. Dental extractions
c. Intestinal anastomosis
d. Gastrotomy

92. Which of the following forceps should *not* be used to hold the edges of the incision open?
a. Rat-tooth
b. Brown-Adson
c. Crile
d. Allis tissue

93. Which of the following does *not* describe a type of surgical scissors?
a. Mayo
b. Metzenbaum
c. Iris
d. Lembert

94. A sponge count should be done:
a. At the beginning of the surgery and before closure
b. Several times during the surgery
c. Before surgery only
d. Before closure only

95. To maintain sterility throughout the surgical procedure, the method by which contamination with microorganisms is prevented is known as:
a. Sterile technique
b. Sterile field
c. Sterility
d. Terminal sterilization

96. Which of the following clinical signs would *not* normally be seen if a dog were suffering from hemorrhage after an ovariohysterectomy?
a. Decreased respiratory rate
b. Pale mucous membranes
c. Slow recovery from anesthesia
d. Slow capillary refill time

97. You are monitoring a cat during an exploratory surgery and notice the pupils are central and dilated. The cat is:
a. Too light
b. Too deep
c. Under the influence of atropine
d. In a state impossible to determine without more information

98. Which of the following does *not* cause an increase in respiratory rate (RR) in an anesthetized animal?
a. Increased blood CO_2
b. Anesthesia is too light
c. Increased PaO_2
d. Hyperthermia

99. What is the proper term for trimming the edges of a jagged tear before suturing?
a. Debridement
b. Decoupage
c. Curettage
d. Cauterization

100. Which of the following is *not* a factor influencing the formation of exuberant granulation tissue?
a. Presence of infection
b. Amount of missing tissue
c. Depth of the wound
d. Location of the wound

101. If a surgical incision is dehiscing, the discharge, if present, is probably:
a. Mucopurulent
b. Serosanguineous
c. Serous
d. Purulent

102. Which of the following techniques is considered an extracapsular repair of a torn cranial cruciate ligament?
a. Femoral head osteotomy (FHO)
b. Tibial plateau-leveling osteotomy (TPLO)
c. Tibial tuberosity advancement (TTA)
d. Placement of a nylon suture outside the joint

103. If a nonsterile person must move to the other side of a sterile person, the nonsterile person should pass:
a. Back to back
b. Front to front
c. Facing the back of the surgeon
d. With his or her side facing the back of the surgeon

104. When opening a double-wrapped gown pack, nonscrubbed surgical personnel may touch the:
a. Autoclave tape
b. Indicator
c. Towel
d. Gown

105. Which of the following suture materials is most likely to cause stitch granulomas if left in too long?
a. Silk
b. Cotton
c. Nylon
d. Prolene

106. When the surgeon and surgical technician are scrubbing for surgery, their hands should be held:
a. Below the elbows
b. Parallel to the elbows
c. Above the elbows
d. Above the head

107. When cleaning instruments, the instruments should first be soaked in a surgical soap solution (e.g., Asepti-Zyme) to:
a. Remove bacteria
b. Remove blood
c. Sterilize them
d. Enhance the effect of the ultrasonic cleaner

108. Which of the following patterns is *not* suitable for the closure of an intestinal biopsy incision?
a. Simple continuous
b. Simple interrupted
c. Everting
d. Inverting

109. Which of the following does *not* need to be included when labeling a surgical pack?
a. Contents of the pack
b. Date the pack was made up
c. Initials or name of the person making up the pack
d. Date by which the pack must be used

110. Which of the following hemostatic forceps has striations different from the others?
a. Halstead mosquitoes
b. Crile
c. Rochester-Pean
d. Rochester-Carmalt

111. Which of the following is *not* the formal name of a retractor?
a. Finochietto
b. Gelpi
c. Lembert
d. Balfour

112. Which of the following is *not* a requirement for fracture healing?
a. Apposition
b. Shearing
c. Fixation
d. Reduction

113. Using the dissection method, which parts of the distal forelimb are removed in an onychectomy?
a. Nail and proximal phalanx
b. Proximal and distal phalanges
c. Middle and distal phalanges
d. Distal phalanx and nail

114. What type of instrument is an *Adson*?
a. Retractor
b. Rongeur
c. Periosteal elevator
d. Thumb forceps

115. Anterior drawer movement detects a problem with the:
a. Elbow
b. Stifle
c. Hip
d. Hock

116. An incision into the bladder is known as a:
a. Cystotomy
b. Cystectomy
c. Cystocentesis
d. Cystostomy

117. Which of the following conditions does *not* require surgical repair?
a. Gastric dilatation and volvulus (GDV)
b. Intussusception
c. Mesenteric torsion
d. Ileus

118. A laminectomy is used to treat:
a. Intervertebral disk disease
b. Fractures of spinous processes
c. Hip dysplasia
d. Foot disorders in horses

119. If a fracture is found on the proximal part of the tibia, it is:
a. Distal to the femur
b. Proximal to the femur
c. In the middle of the bone
d. Distal to the metatarsals

120. If the testicles are *not* palpable and a cryptorchidectomy is performed, the incision would probably be:
a. Prescrotal
b. Scrotal
c. Ventral midline
d. Perineal

121. In dogs, the most common location for a thoracotomy incision is:
a. Through the sternum
b. Through the diaphragm
c. Along the linea alba
d. Between the ribs

122. What is the minimum number of air changes per hour required for adequate ventilation in a surgical suite?
a. 2
b. 5
c. 10
d. 15

123. Which of the following disinfectants includes the weakest virucidal activity?
a. Glutaraldehyde (2%)
b. Quaternary ammonium compounds at standard concentrations
c. Formalin (37%)
d. Isopropyl alcohol (70%)

124. Which of the following instruments is *not* considered surgical scissors?
- a. Iris
- b. Metzenbaum
- c. Wire-cutting
- d. Mayo-Hegar

125. Which of the following instruments is most suitable for the removal of bone to perform spinal surgery?
- a. Rongeur
- b. Curette
- c. Periosteal elevator
- d. Trephine

126. Clear fluid removed from thoracic cavity is known as:
- a. Pleural effusion
- b. Pulmonary edema
- c. Ascites
- d. Pyothorax

127. Where is the most likely place for a rumenotomy incision in a dairy cow?
- a. Right paralumbar fossa
- b. Left paralumbar fossa
- c. Linea alba
- d. Paramedian

128. What does a change in color in autoclave tape indicate to a surgical nurse?
- a. The surgical instruments in the pack have been adequately sterilized.
- b. During the autoclaving process, steam has reached the tape.
- c. Adequate temperature and pressures have been achieved.
- d. The pack has been exposed to adequate pressures.

129. A surgeon drops an instrument on the floor during a procedure and asks for it to be flash sterilized. How should the instrument be flash sterilized?
- a. instrument is wrapped and sterilized at 272° F for 15 minutes
- b. instrument is wrapped and sterilized at 272° F for 4 minutes
- c. instrument is unwrapped and sterilized at 272° F for 15 minutes
- d. instrument is unwrapped and sterilized at 272° F for 4 minutes

130. Which of the following is *not* a common concern when assisting a surgeon with canine cesarean section surgery?
- a. Minimizing anesthetic drugs that may pass on to the puppies
- b. Minimizing the time the bitch is in dorsal recumbency because of the weight of the uterus on the aorta
- c. Suctioning fluid from the puppies' nasal cavities and mouths to stimulate breathing
- d. Intubating the puppies

131. Which of the following is *not* a primary concern when assisting a surgeon performing a pyometra surgery?
- a. Providing preoperative and intraoperative antibiotics for the patient
- b. Gentle handling of the friable tissue to prevent rupture and drainage of the contents of the uterus into the abdominal cavity
- c. Fluid therapy to diurese the kidneys
- d. Lidocaine infusion to prevent ventricular arrhythmia

132. When assisting a surgeon in a gastric dilatation and volvulus surgery, which of the following is *not* your immediate concern?
- a. Establishing intravenous access to deliver shock doses of fluids
- b. Calculating lidocaine dose for constant rate infusion
- c. Monitoring for cardiac arrhythmia intraoperatively and postoperatively
- d. Preparing the ultrasound unit to confirm gastric dilatation and volvulus status of animal

133. What size scalpel blade fits on a No. 3 scalpel handle?
- a. No. 10
- b. No. 20
- c. No. 21
- d. No. 30

134. What size scalpel blade fits on a No. 4 scalpel handle?
- a. No. 10
- b. No. 12
- c. No. 15
- d. No. 20

135. Which of the following suffixes is used to describe the surgical repair by suturing?
- a. -ectomy
- b. -otomy
- c. -ostomy
- d. -rrhapy

136. Pathogenic bacteria is defined as bacteria that:
- a. Produce toxins
- b. Cause disease
- c. Live off and gain nutrients from the host
- d. Multiply in the host

137. Which of the following need *not* be considered in the timing of the autoclave cycle?
- a. Time required to heat up the interior of the chamber
- b. Time required to allow the steam to penetrate the interior of the packs
- c. Time required to seal the chamber
- d. Time required to sterilize those items in contact with the steam

138. The definition of sterile is:
- a. Without microbes or living spores
- b. Without pathogenic microbes
- c. With the presence of commensal organisms only
- d. Without bacteria or their byproducts

139. Which items should all personnel wear when entering the operating room?
- a. Cap and mask
- b. Cap, mask, and booties
- c. Cap, mask, booties, and clean scrubs or gown
- d. Cap, mask, and sterile gown

140. Which of the following surgical packs would *not* be considered contaminated and would *not* need to be reautoclaved?
- a. Single-wrapped crepe paper pack stored on an open shelf for 8 weeks
- b. Pack that was opened for a procedure but was not used and was needed for the next day's procedure
- c. Double-wrapped paper pack stored in a closed cabinet for 6 weeks
- d. Instrument in an autoclave pouch that has a very small tear near the top of the pack

141. Instruments are autoclaved:
a. With the ratchets closed to prevent tearing the wrap material
b. With the ratchets open to allow steam exposure to the entire surface
c. Always in a surgical tray to prevent the instruments from shifting
d. Without touching any other instruments to prevent corrosion

142. An advantage of using a Gelpi retractor over a Senn retractor is:
a. The Gelpi is much less expensive to purchase.
b. The Gelpi is smaller overall than the Senn.
c. The Senn must be molded to fit the position required.
d. The Gelpi is self-retaining.

143. Which of the following suffixes is used to describe the surgical fixation?
a. -pexy
b. -otomy
c. -ostomy
d. -rrhapy

144. All of the following are true regarding aseptic technique *except*?
a. It provides a clean surgical environment.
b. It prevents pathogenic microbes from entering the surgical suite.
c. It provides a sterile surgical environment.
d. It reduces the likelihood of fatal infections.

145. What specifically does the strip on the autoclave tape indicate when it turns dark?
a. The correct temperature has been reached.
b. The correct pressure has been reached.
c. The correct temperature for the proper amount of time has been reached.
d. The correct temperature, pressure, and time have been reached.

146. Metzenbaum scissors are used only for:
a. Cutting suture
b. Cutting paper drape
c. Ophthalmic surgery
d. Cutting tissue

147. Where is the sterile zone located on scrubbed personnel?
a. Front and sides, from the neck below the neckline to the bottom of the gown, including the arms
b. Front, from below the neckline to the bottom of the gown, including the arms
c. Front, sides, and back, from the neck to the waist
d. Front, from below the neckline to the waist, including the arms

148. Rank the following from greatest tensile strength to least:
a. 00 gut, 3-0 Vicryl, 1 chromic gut, 6-0 silk
b. 1 chromic gut, 0 chromic gut, 3-0 Vicryl, 6-0 silk
c. 6-0 silk, 3-0 Vicryl, 00 gut, 1 chromic gut
d. 6-0 silk, 3-0 Vicryl, 1 chromic gut, 00 gut

149. Why must instrument milk be used after ultrasonic cleaning?
a. To complete the sterilization process
b. To provide further cleaning and sanitizing of the instruments
c. To replace lubrication removed by the ultrasonic cleaner
d. To prevent rust spots from forming on the instruments

150. What type of needle is reusable?
a. Swaged-on
b. Taper point
c. Trocar tip
d. Eyed

151. Which of the following operating room personnel should face the sterile field during a procedure?
a. The surgeon only
b. The scrubbed-in technicians and surgeon only
c. All personnel, both scrubbed in and nonsterile
d. Only the surgeon and nonsterile personnel; the scrubbed-in technician should face the instrument field.

152. All of the following sutures have a degree of capillarity *except*?
a. Polyglycolic acid
b. Silk
c. Surgical gut
d. Polypropylene

153. An advantage of the braided suture over the monofilament is:
a. Knot security
b. Tensile strength
c. It does not hide bacteria in contaminated wounds.
d. Tissue reactivity

154. When attaching an animal to an ECG, which lead is hooked up to the right foreleg?
a. Red
b. Black
c. White
d. Green

155. A disinfectant labeled as a virucidal:
a. Prevents bacteria from growing
b. Kills all spores
c. Kills viruses
d. Prevents viruses from growing

156. What is the purpose of the surgical drape?
a. To keep the animal warm
b. To keep the surgeon focused on the surgical area
c. To establish a sterile field
d. To protect the table and mayo stand from contamination

157. When autoclaving, the minimum temperature and exposure times for the center of the surgical packs are:
a. 121.5° F for 10 minutes
b. 250° F for 15 minutes
c. 250° F for 20 minutes
d. 300° F for 30 minutes

158. In general, the difference between a disinfectant and an antiseptic is:
a. Disinfectants are agents used on inanimate objects and antiseptic agents are used on living tissue.
b. Disinfectants are used on living tissues and antiseptics are used on inanimate objects.
c. Disinfectants are bacteriostatic and antiseptics are bactericidal.
d. Disinfectants kill microbes whereas antiseptics inhibit their growth only.

159. How can you help prevent "strike through" during surgery?
a. Make sure sharp instruments are protected so that they do not puncture the wrap and cause contamination
b. Assist in keeping the surgical drapes and gown from becoming wet during surgery
c. Make sure the drape is properly placed and opened so that the fenestration is not over a contaminated area
d. Have reverse cutting needles available so that the suture does not pull through the tissue

160. The agent used in gas sterilization is:
a. Glutaraldehyde
b. Chlorhexidine
c. Ethylene oxide
d. Formaldehyde

161. Needle holders that do *not* have scissors, but have a needle-holding surface, are called:
a. Mayo-Hegar
b. Olsen-Hegar
c. Metzenbaum
d. Crile-Wood

162. Rochester-Carmalt Pean forceps:
a. Are generally smaller than a Kelly forceps
b. Have longitudinal serrations with interdigitating teeth at the tips
c. Have longitudinal serrations with a crosshatched pattern at the tips
d. Have transverse longitudinal serrations along the entire length

163. A Buhner needle is used in:
a. The repair of bovine vaginal and uterine prolapses
b. Eye enucleations in dogs
c. Intestinal anastomosis surgeries
d. Orthopedic surgeries

164. A Snook hook is typically used during:
a. A castration
b. An ovariohysterectomy
c. A diaphragmatic hernia repair
d. Declawing

165. What does the medical term ovariohysterectomy mean?
a. Removal of the ovaries only
b. Removal of the uterus only
c. Removal of the ovaries and uterus only
d. Removal of the entire reproductive tract, including ovaries, uterus, cervix, and vagina

166. An accumulation of purulent discharge within the uterus is called:
a. Pyometritis
b. Mastitis
c. Peritonitis
d. Vaginitis

167. A pack double wrapped in muslin and kept in a closed cabinet is good for how long?
a. 1 week
b. 3 to 4 weeks
c. 6 to 7 weeks
d. 6 months

168. Instruments suitable for cutting sutures include:
a. Scissors on Mayo-Hegar needle holders, operating scissors, and Mayo scissors
b. Operating scissors, scissors on Olsen-Hegar needle holders, and Metzenbaum scissors
c. Operating scissors, scissors on Olsen-Hegar needle holders, and Mayo scissors
d. Suture (stitch) scissors, Mayo scissors, and Metzenbaum scissors

169. What is a Steinmann IM pin?
a. An intramedullary pin used in orthopedics
b. An intramuscular pin used in orthopedics
c. A type of screw used in orthopedics
d. A staple used to hold muscle or bone fragments together

170. You are checking a recent surgical wound and find that the tissue is slightly warmer and redder than the surrounding tissue. What is the significance of this?
a. It is an indication that the wound is contaminated and requires an emergency intervention.
b. The wound will likely dehisce and should be checked immediately by the veterinarian.
c. It is normal because the first stage of wound healing is inflammation.
d. It is an indication that the sutures are interfering with blood flow and necrosis is likely.

171. What is the correct order of tasks when preparing an animal for routine surgery?
a. Premedicate, place IV catheter, clip and prep, move into surgery, final prep
b. Place IV catheter, premedicate, clip and prep, final prep move into surgery
c. Premedicate, IV catheter, move into surgery, clip and prep, final prep
d. Move into surgery Place IV catheter, premedicate, clip and prep, final prep

172. What should you wear when working as a nonsterile surgical assistant?
a. Mask and clean scrubs
b. Mask, cap, and clean scrubs
c. Mask, cap, shoe covers, and clean scrubs
d. Mask, cap, shoe covers, and sterile gown

173. While you are working as a sterile surgical assistant, your mask slips down below your nose. What should you do?
a. The nonsterile assistant may stand in front of you and secure the mask in its proper position.
b. The nonsterile assistant may secure the mask in position while standing behind you.
c. You may take a nonsterile piece of gauze and place it over the mask to allow you to adjust it into position.
d. You are completely contaminated and must leave surgery.

174. Which of the following is *not* a recommended agent for patient surgical preparation?
a. Chlorhexidine
b. Roccal
c. Alcohol
d. Povidone iodine

175. Abscesses are generally left open to allow continuous drainage. This type of wound healing is considered:
  a. Primary intention
  b. Second intention
  c. Third intention
  d. Fourth intention

176. Which of the following best describes the location of an incision through the skin and linea alba, extending from the xiphoid process to the umbilicus?
  a. Flank
  b. Paracostal
  c. Paramedian
  d. Ventral midline

177. Cesarean sections in cattle are most commonly performed via what surgical approach?
  a. Through a right paracostal incision
  b. Through a right paravertebral approach
  c. Through the left paralumbar fossa
  d. Through the ventral midline approach

178. Emasculators are used:
  a. In large-animal castrations
  b. During surgical ovariectomies in heifers and mares
  c. During enucleations in large-breed dogs
  d. To remove dewclaws in dogs

179. You are to assist with a rumenotomy. Where on the patient would you prep for the surgery?
  a. Ventral midline from xiphoid to pubic bone
  b. Left paralumbar fossa
  c. Right paralumbar fossa
  d. Right paramedian region

180. A disadvantage of tilting the surgical table so that the patient's head is lower than its tail is that:
  a. The increased pressure on the diaphragm can interfere with respiration.
  b. The tension on the large bowel may initiate defecation.
  c. It interferes with visualization of the caudal abdomen.
  d. It can cause a gastric volvulus.

181. A visiting relief veterinarian whom you are assisting in surgery asks you to provide a nonabsorbable suture that is less than 2-0 in size. Which of the following would meet the request?
  a. 3-0 chromic gut
  b. 4-0 silk
  c. 00 Dermalon nylon
  d. 0 polydioxanone

182. A surgical prep for feline castration:
  a. Involves clipping the prescrotal region from the umbilicus to the scrotum
  b. Involves clipping the scrotum with a No. 40 clipper blade
  c. Does not involve hair removal because the entire scrotal area is prepped with Nolvasan and alcohol
  d. Includes plucking or pulling the hair from the scrotum before the surgical scrub

183. Which of these is *not* a common surgical site for the correction of a left-displaced abomasum in cattle?
  a. Right paralumbar
  b. Left paralumbar
  c. Ventral midline
  d. Right paramedian

184. Postoperative care for horses following castration:
  a. Includes strict confinement to the stall for at least 1 week to prevent hemorrhage
  b. Includes suture removal at 10 to 14 days
  c. Involves antibiotic administration for 5 days following surgery
  d. Involves exercise twice daily to promote drainage

185. Which of the following terms means surgically opening the abdominal cavity?
  a. Laparotomy
  b. Pleurotomy
  c. Thoracotomy
  d. Cystotomy

186. What parameter(s) does the pulse oximeter measure?
  a. Pulse rate only
  b. Respiration rate and depth
  c. Oxygen saturation of hemoglobin and pulse rate
  d. Respiration rate and pulse rate

187. Which of the following is false regarding the ECG?
  a. It measures the electrical impulses of the heart.
  b. There can be a normal ECG tracing when there is no cardiac output.
  c. There is always a pulse beat with each QRS complex.
  d. Alcohol and sterile lubricant will enhance the connection of the skin leads.

188. What orthopedic fixation consists of pins that penetrate fractured bones and skin from the outside and are held in place externally by bolts attached to another cross pin?
  a. Rush pinning
  b. External fixators
  c. Steinmann fixation
  d. Bone plating

189. What is a nosocomial infection?
  a. Infection arising from bacteria in the gastrointestinal tract
  b. Infection originating from the respiratory tract, especially the nose
  c. Hospital-acquired infection
  d. Resistant infection

190. Which of the following should *not* be used to help prevent hypothermia in surgical patients?
  a. Electric heating pad set on low
  b. Warm-water circulating pad
  c. Warm air convection blankets
  d. Wrapping the patient's extremities with bubble wrap

191. In what type of surgical procedure would you make sure that the Jacobs bone chuck is sterilized and available?
  a. Onychectomy
  b. Celiotomy
  c. Thoracotomy
  d. Orthopedic

192. Which of the following is *not* an advantage of neutering a male dog?
  a. Decreased risk of perineal hernias
  b. Decreased roaming
  c. Prevention of it lifting its leg to urinate
  d. Decreased aggression toward other dogs

193. Which of the following can be used as a surgical scrub on a patient?
a. Povidone iodine solution
b. Chlorhexidine scrub
c. Alcohol
d. Nolvasan solution

194. Which of the following need *not* be done before moving a horse into surgery for a general anesthesia procedure?
a. Remove the shoes
b. Rinse the mouth
c. Clip as much of the surgical area as possible
d. Perform a complete tail wrap

195. What is an important measure that can help prevent myositis during equine surgery?
a. Providing proper padding
b. Ensuring that the horse does not experience hypothermia
c. Not overinflating the endotracheal tube cuff
d. Withholding food for 12 hours

196. If a single technician is responsible for setting the patient up in surgery, what task should be performed first?
a. Tying the animal to the table
b. Applying the final prep
c. Attaching the monitoring devices
d. Opening the surgery pack

197. Which of the following statements regarding compartment syndrome in the equine surgical patient is correct?
a. Compartment syndrome only affects the surgery compartment.
b. The "up" side of the patient can be affected.
c. Following all proper precautions can prevent compartment syndrome.
d. Compartment syndrome rarely results in euthanasia.

198. A gastrotomy refers to a surgical incision into the:
a. Gastrocnemius muscle
b. Peritoneal wall
c. Stomach
d. Small intestines

199. During a surgical scrub, you bump your hand on the faucet. What should you do?
a. Continue the scrub, giving the bumped area double the number of brush strokes to compensate
b. Start the entire scrub again because you have contaminated yourself
c. Rescrub the area immediately, rinse the brush, and then continue the scrub
d. Continue the scrub and add one more cycle on the bumped hand because you cannot make your hands truly sterile anyway

200. Why are such elaborate measures taken to maintain aseptic technique during surgery?
a. To protect personnel from pathogenic microbes encountered in the animals
b. To decrease the risk of nosocomial infections spread among patients
c. To decrease the risk of contamination into the surgical site and interference with wound healing
d. To decrease the virulence of the microbes in the hospital

201. A fenestrated drape:
a. Has a window opening in the middle through which the surgery is performed
b. Is folded in half in accordion style for ease of opening
c. Is folded such that the middle of the drape can easily be found
d. Is a cloth drape made of three doubled layers of muslin

202. What is the pressure that must be reached in a steam autoclave for the temperature to reach 121.5°C?
a. 1 psi
b. 10 psi
c. 15 psi
d. 45 psi

203. Healing of a properly sutured surgical wound is most appropriately termed:
a. First-intention healing
b. Granulation
c. Second-intention healing
d. Third-intention healing

204. Which of the following has the poorest potential for healing and return to normal function after damage and effective surgical repair?
a. Bone
b. Gastrointestinal tract
c. Liver
d. Nervous tissue

205. What is the correct location to administer a caudal epidural injection on a horse?
a. Between the last lumbar vertebrae and the sacrum
b. Between the sacrum and the first coccygeal vertebrae
c. Between the first and second coccygeal vertebrae
d. None because it is not safe to administer caudal epidural injections to horses.

206. What agent, method, or device is most appropriate for sterilizing an electric drill to be used in an orthopedic surgical procedure?
a. Autoclave
b. Dry heat
c. Ethylene oxide gas
d. Liquid chemical disinfectant

207. Which of the following is the most effective and timely indicator that sterilization conditions have been met in an autoclaved surgery pack?
a. Autoclave tape
b. Chemical indicator
c. Culture test
d. Melting pellet

208. What is the proper term for microorganisms that gain entrance into an incision during a surgical procedure?
a. Contamination
b. Debridement
c. Infection
d. Septicemia

209. Which of the following do/does *not* have to be sterile during a surgical procedure to maintain aseptic technique?
a. Drapes
b. Gloves
c. Gown
d. Mask

210. Which of the following is the agent for autoclave sterilization?
a. Chemical disinfectant solution
b. Dry heat
c. Ethylene oxide gas
d. Steam

211. What size of electrical clipper blade is most commonly used for removing the hair from a surgical site?
a. No. 10
b. No. 20
c. No. 30
d. No. 40

212. Which of the following is *not* an effective form of surgical hemostasis?
a. Crushing
b. Curettage
c. Ligation
d. Pressure

213. Which of the following is *not* a likely cause of dehiscence of an abdominal incision?
a. Excessive physical activity
b. Stormy recovery from anesthesia
c. Surgical wound infection
d. Suture material larger than needed

214. Which of the following is *not* an effective aseptic surgical technique?
a. Considering a sterile item to be nonsterile if it touches a nonsterile item
b. Considering an item sterile if its sterility is in doubt
c. Allowing nonscrubbed personnel to touch nonsterile items only
d. Allowing sterile items to touch only other sterile items

215. Which of the following does *not* enhance the healing of an open wound?
a. Debridement
b. Exuberant granulation tissue
c. Granulation tissue
d. Wound flushing

216. Which of the following is *not* a characteristic of first-intention wound healing?
a. Minimal contamination
b. Minimal tissue damage
c. No continuous movement of wound edges resulting from body movement
d. Wound edges not approximated

217. What incision is the most appropriate for exploratory surgery of the abdomen of a dog if the precise location of the problem is *not* known?
a. Flank
b. Paracostal
c. Paramedian
d. Ventral midline

218. Which of the following is *not* an early sign of wound dehiscence during the first 24 hours after abdominal surgery?
a. Increase in body temperature of between 1°C and 2°C
b. Serosanguineous discharge from the incision
c. Swollen incision
d. Very warm incision

219. The main goal of aseptic surgical technique is to prevent contamination of the:
a. Sterile fields
b. Sterile zones
c. Surgical instruments
d. Surgical wound

220. What factor relating to the infection of a surgical wound can an aseptic technique reasonably be expected to influence significantly?
a. Number of microorganisms entering the wound
b. Pathogenicity of microorganisms entering the wound
c. Route of exposure to infectious microorganisms
d. Susceptibility of the patient to infection

221. An animal waking up from surgery and general anesthesia exhibits signs of excitement with exaggerated and uncontrolled movements. The animal is probably displaying signs of:
a. Dysphoria
b. Emergence delirium
c. Euphoria
d. Pain

222. A veterinarian may elect to apply a bandage to an orthopedic patient for additional postoperative support. The type of bandage that would be applied to stabilize the hip after a hip luxation would be a/an:
a. Ehmer sling
b. Robert Jones bandage
c. Spica splint
d. Velpeau sling

223. Which of the following does *not* normally need to be sterilized as part of good aseptic surgical technique?
a. Cap
b. Drapes
c. Gown
d. Scrub brush

224. Liquid chemical sterilization is used primarily for:
a. Electrical equipment
b. Endoscopic equipment
c. Orthopedic equipment
d. Surgical drapes

225. The time necessary to disinfect surgical instruments with liquid chemicals can be shortened by:
a. Cooling the solution
b. Making the solution less concentrated than recommended
c. Making the solution more concentrated than recommended
d. Warming the solution

226. What surgical drape material prevents bacteria from penetrating the drape by capillary action when the top surface of the drape becomes wet?
a. Polyester
b. Muslin
c. Paper
d. Plastic

227. The best surgical monitoring device is:
a. An esophageal stethoscope
b. A pulse oximeter
c. A capnograph with ECG capability
d. A skilled veterinary technician

228. What is the most appropriate wound-flushing solution?
a. Hydrogen peroxide
b. Isotonic saline
c. Povidone-iodine solution
d. Tap water

229. How should a ventral midline surgical wound dehiscence of the muscle, subcutaneous tissue, and skin layers be dealt with?
a. As an emergency
b. As a candidate for cosmetic surgery
c. As of minor significance
d. As serious but not as an emergency

230. Why is a recent surgical wound usually slightly warmer than surrounding normal tissues?
a. Contamination
b. Debridement
c. Infection
d. Inflammation

231. When does a sutured surgical wound begin to gain significant strength from the production of collagen strands so that the wound edges are held together not only by the sutures?
a. Immediately
b. In 5 days
c. In 14 days
d. In 35 days

232. Wound contraction is produced by:
a. Reproduction of the dermis
b. Movement of the epidermis only
c. Movement of the whole thickness of skin
d. Reproduction of epidermal cells

233. As part of effective aseptic technique, surgical gowns:
a. Are commonly made of cloth, paper, or plastic
b. Are folded so that the inside of the gown faces outward
c. Are routinely sterilized by ethylene oxide gas
d. Do not need to be sterile, only clean

234. Which of the following is *not* a sign of hemorrhagic shock in a postsurgical patient?
a. Deep, slow breathing
b. Slow capillary refill
c. Tachycardia
d. Weakness

235. The usual significance of a small seroma beneath a suture line in the skin is:
a. Emergency
b. Cosmetic only
c. Major problem
d. Serious but not an emergency

236. The healing potential for a fractured bone that is properly aligned and kept immobile is:
a. Excellent
b. Fair
c. Good
d. Poor

237. All of the following can transmit microorganisms in the veterinary hospital *except*:
a. Team members
b. Contaminated instruments
c. Equipment contamination
d. Uterus

238. What abdominal incision is most appropriate for a standing cesarean section on a heifer?
a. Ventral midline
b. Flank
c. Paracostal
d. Ventral paramedian

239. Patients suffering from gastric dilation and volvulus (GDV) need to be stabilized prior to surgery. Which of the following is *not* a step in stabilizing a patient prior to surgery for a GDV?
a. Treating for shock with aggressive IV fluid therapy
b. Decompression of the stomach with an orogastric tube or trocharization
c. Administration of medications such as po simethicone to decrease gas production
d. Monitor the patient for potential cardiac arrhythmia

240. The first phase of the wound-healing process involves:
a. Endothelial cell proliferation
b. Fibroblast proliferation
c. Inflammation
d. Equilibrium of collagen synthesis

241. In the first 24 hours of primary union wound healing, most of the resistance to the opening of the wound is provided by:
a. Collagen strands
b. Fibrin strands
c. Granulation tissue
d. Sutures

242. In what type of abdominal incision can the muscle wall be most effectively closed with one layer of sutures?
a. Flank
b. Paracostal
c. Paramedian
d. Ventral midline

243. Scrubbed surgical personnel become contaminated if they touch:
a. Objects in sterile fields
b. Objects outside the sterile zone
c. Properly sterilized surgical instruments
d. Freshly exposed tissues of the patient

244. Nonscrubbed surgical personnel may properly touch anything that is:
a. Contaminated
b. Inside the patient's body
c. Inside the sterile zone
d. Part of a sterile field

245. When *not* otherwise occupied, scrubbed surgical personnel should stand with:
a. Arms folded
b. Hands above shoulder level
c. Hands clasped between waist and shoulder level
d. Hands down at their sides

246. When is it permissible for nonscrubbed surgical personnel to pass between scrubbed personnel and the patient during surgery?
a. Never
b. When opening suture material
c. When adjusting the anesthesia machine
d. When adjusting the intravenous drip

247. When aseptically opening a sterile surgical pack on an instrument stand, it is *not* proper for nonscrubbed surgical personnel to touch:
a. Autoclave tape
b. Contents of the pack
c. Corners of the wrap
d. Instrument stand

248. Which characteristic is true of ethylene oxide gas?
a. It is flammable.
b. Exposure to it is not considered a health hazard.
c. It is noncombustible.
d. It is nontoxic to tissues.

249. Which of the following is *not* a likely contributor to postoperative wound dehiscence?
a. Chronic postoperative vomiting
b. Internal suture ends cut too short
c. Infection
d. Skin sutures left in too long

250. Which type of dressing best helps debride a wound with extensive tissue damage?
a. Dry gauze
b. Gauze dressing with an oily antiseptic
c. Gauze dressing with a water-soluble antiseptic
d. Wet saline dressing

251. Most of the clinical signs seen in an animal in shock from excessive blood loss are attributable to:
a. Acidosis
b. Alkalosis
c. Cell death
d. Redistribution of blood flow

252. The main goal of surgery to remove a pus-filled uterus (pyometra) is:
a. A prophylactic measure
b. To make a diagnosis
c. To restore the animal to a normal reproductive state
d. To return the animal to health without restoring normal reproductive function

253. Which tissue must form in a wound that is healing by second intention before wound contraction or epithelial regeneration can occur?
a. Collagen fibers
b. Fibrin clot
c. Granulation tissue
d. Scar tissue

254. When gloving for surgery, which of the following is *not* permitted?
a. One gloved thumb touches the other gloved thumb
b. The scrubbed fingers touch the outside of the glove
c. The outside of the gown cuff is touched by inside of the glove cuff
d. The scrubbed fingers touch the inside of the glove cuff

255. How should a pack be placed in an autoclave for sterilization?
a. Diagonally
b. Horizontally
c. Upside down
d. Vertically

256. Metzenbaum scissors are used for:
a. Cutting sutures
b. Soft-tissue dissection
c. Cutting the linea alba
d. Cutting skin

257. What retractors are *not* handheld?
a. Deaver
b. Senn
c. Rake
d. Gelpi

258. What is the appropriate time to soak an instrument in a cold sterilization solution before adequate sterilization is achieved?
a. 30 minutes
b. 15 minutes
c. 45 minutes
d. 10 hours

259. How long does an instrument remain sterile if sterilized and wrapped in paper?
a. 6 months
b. 1 week
c. 1 month
d. 1 year

260. Instrument milk is used for all of the following *except*:
a. Lubrication
b. Rust inhibition
c. Extending the life of the instrument
d. Cleaning the instrument

261. What type of instrument is a Backhaus?
a. Needle holder
b. Scissors
c. Towel clamp
d. Hemostatic forceps

262. For which bovine surgical procedure are obstetric chains used?
a. Rumenotomy
b. Abomasopexy
c. Cesarean section
d. Uterine torsion correction

263. Which of the following does *not* have to be gas sterilized?
a. Arthroscope
b. Plastic pipette tips
c. Polyethylene tubing
d. Plastic spray bottles

264. Ultrasonic cleaners are used for:
a. Removing small particles of blood and tissue from instruments
b. Removing rust from instruments
c. Disinfecting instruments
d. Lubricating instruments

265. All of the following are causes of hypotension during surgery *except*:
a. Excessive vasodilation
b. Hypovolemia
c. Hyperthermia
d. Anesthetic depth

266. Which of the following is *not* a consideration when evaluating a surgical pack for sterility?
a. Sterilization date
b. Indicator color change
c. Holes or moisture damage
d. Incorrect labeling

267. Mayo-Hegar scissors are used in all of the following situations *except* for cutting:
a. Sutures
b. Delicate tissue
c. Paper drapes
d. Skin or muscle

268. All of the following are duties assigned to the sterile surgical assistant *except*?
a. Passing instruments
b. Draping the patient
c. Identifying suture patterns
d. Administering drugs intraoperatively

269. Which animal would have additional steps required in preparing the patient for abdominal surgery?
a. Female cat
b. Female dog
c. Male cat
d. Male dog

270. What size scalpel blade is generally used in an arthroscopy for making the stab incision into the joint because of its pointed, rather than rounded or hooked, end?
a. No. 10
b. No. 11
c. No. 12
d. No. 15

271. What type of sterilization technique is *not* acceptable for instruments used in canine castration?
a. Gas sterilization
b. Autoclaving
c. Chemical sterilization
d. Boiling

272. All of the following are objectives of the surgical hand scrub *except*:
a. To remove gross dirt and oil from the hands
b. To sterilize the hands
c. To reduce the microorganism count on the hands to as close to zero as possible
d. To produce a prolonged depressant effect on the number of microflora on the hands and forearms

273. What type of surgical scrub solution is most effective in reducing the number of bacteria on the skin and maintaining the longest residual activity?
a. Hexachlorophene alcohol
b. Povidone-iodine
c. Chlorhexidine gluconate
d. Polypropylene parachormeta-xylenol

274. When a surgeon encounters bleeding, all of the following can be used to control it *except*:
a. Electrocautery
b. A hemostat
c. Suction
d. Rat-tooth forceps

275. How long does a sealed item remain sterilized after being sterilized by gamma radiation?
a. 1 year
b. 6 months
c. Until it is opened
d. 1 month

276. Which retractor is *not* self-retaining?
a. Weitlaner
b. Alms
c. Senn
d. Balfour

277. Sterilization is the process of killing microorganisms by physical or chemical means. What is the quickest and most reliable form of sterilization?
a. Steam under pressure
b. Gas
c. Dry heat
d. Radiation

278. Instruments wrapped in a single linen wrap can become contaminated with microbes within 2 to 3 days. By how long does double wrapping an instrument extend the sterility period?
a. 6 months
b. 4 weeks
c. 4 to 6 days
d. 1 year

279. Which is the best type of cleaner to use when washing surgical instruments by hand?
a. Ordinary hand soap
b. Abrasive compounds
c. Low-sudsing detergents
d. Plain hot water

280. Which of the following is an absorbable suture?
a. Prolene
b. Vicryl
c. Mersilene
d. Silk

281. All of the following are considered benefits of using skin staples *except*:
a. Skin is more resistant to abscess formation than when sutures are used.
b. Staples provide excellent wound healing.
c. Staples are more cost effective.
d. Staples save time.

282. If skin edges are under extreme tension (e.g., in a large skin wound), which is the suture pattern of choice?
a. Simple continuous
b. Simple interrupted
c. Interrupted horizontal mattress
d. Continuous horizontal mattress

283. All of the following can contribute to a prolonged recovery *except*:
a. Breed predisposition
b. Poor perfusion
c. Hyperglycemia
d. Hypothermia

284. What suture is *not* recommended for skin closure?
a. Polydioxanone
b. Nylon
c. Chromic gut
d. Stainless steel

285. What is the purpose of using a subcuticular suture pattern for final closure?
a. To decrease the amount of suture material needed
b. To eliminate the need for skin sutures
c. To eliminate infection
d. To be more cost effective

286. What suture pattern would *not* be used to close skin?
a. Cushing
b. Horizontal mattress
c. Simple interrupted
d. Ford interlocking

287. Which of the following suture patterns is an inverting stitch?
a. Cruciate
b. Cushing
c. Horizontal mattress
d. Vertical mattress

288. How is a surgeon's knot different from a square knot?
a. A surgeon's knot has one throw on the first pass and two throws on the second pass; a square knot has two throws on each pass.
b. A surgeon's knot has two throws on the first pass and one throw on the second pass; a square knot has one pass on each throw.
c. A surgeon's knot has one throw on each pass; a square knot has two throws on each pass.
d. A surgeon's knot has two throws on the first pass and one throw on the second pass; a square knot has one throw on each pass.

289. Why is it better to ligate many small vessels rather than one mass ligation of tissues?
a. Mass ligation of tissues is unsightly.
b. Mass ligation of tissue might result in an infected area.
c. Mass ligation of tissue is more likely to fail.
d. Tissues included in a mass ligation may be too difficult for the body to resorb.

290. What is the purpose of a transfixation ligature?
a. To make the ligature stronger
b. To close a hollow organ
c. To prevent breakage of the suture
d. To prevent slippage of the suture

291. All of the following are good reasons for using an instrument tie (with the use of a needle holder) *except*:
a. It is economical; small pieces of suture can be used and therefore suture material is not wasted.
b. It saves time.
c. It is more accurate than a one- or two-handed tie.
d. It is readily adaptable to any type of wound closure.

292. Which of the following is *not* a consideration when choosing a needle for use in a surgical procedure?
a. Type of tissue to be sutured
b. Location of the tissue to be sutured
c. Size of suture material
d. Strength of suture material

293. When suturing skin, the needle of choice is:
a. Blunt
b. Reverse cutting
c. Cutting
d. Tapered

294. What is the most significant advantage of using a swaged-on needle as opposed to a closed-eye needle?
a. The needle never separates from the suture.
b. The suture diameter is smaller than the needle diameter.
c. The tissue is subjected to fewer traumas because a single strand is pulled through the tissue.
d. It saves time and money.

295. Suture patterns can be classified into three types: appositional, inverting, and tension. What tissue is most appropriately sutured in an appositional pattern?
a. Tendon
b. Hollow viscus
c. Skin
d. Nerve

296. Which of these sequences correctly lists suture material diameter, from largest to smallest?
a. 3-0, 2-0, 0, 1, 2, 3
b. 000, 00, 0, 1, 2, 3
c. 3, 2, 1, 1-0, 2-0, 3-0
d. 7-0, 5-0, 3-0, 1

297. Which of the following suffixes is used to describe the process of cutting into an organ?
a. -ectomy
b. -otomy
c. -ostomy
d. -rrhapy

298. All of the following are contributing factors of wound dehiscence *except*:
a. Suture failure
b. Infection
c. Tissue weakness
d. Optimal nutrition

299. Wound dehiscence is usually seen within the first:
a. 1–2 days
b. 3–4 days
c. 5–6 days
d. 10–14 days

300. When the term eviscerates is used, it can indicate that:
a. The wound has dehisced.
b. Abdominal contents protrude through the suture line.
c. The aseptic technique has been broken and contamination has occurred.
d. Infection has entered the body through the surgical wound.

301. All of the following are factors that determine whether infection occurs *except*:
a. Number of microorganisms
b. Virulence of microorganisms
c. Susceptibility of the patient
d. Length of exposure time

302. Increased risk of nosocomial infection may result from improper application of methods of:
a. Sanitation
b. Sterilization
c. Disinfection
d. All of the above

303. Sterile patient preparation generally consists of ______ round(s) of alternating antiseptic solution with saline rinse and every pass with gauze moves in a circular motion from the anticipated incision site radiating outward.
a. 1
b. 2
c. 3
d. 4

304. All of the following are clinical signs of pain that a patient may exhibit when recovering from an ovariohysterectomy *except*:
   a. Tachycardia
   b. Hyperpnea
   c. Muscle tension
   d. Hypotension

305. For suturing a uterine incision in a cow, the proper suture size is:
   a. 2-0
   b. 1
   c. 2
   d. 3-0

306. Which of the following is a disadvantage of multifilament suture material?
   a. Less knot security than monofilament suture material
   b. Tears tissue more easily than monofilament suture material
   c. Has a greater tendency for wicking bacteria than monofilament suture material
   d. Has less strength than monofilament suture material

307. Which of the following is a monofilament suture material?
   a. Polyglactin 910 (Vicryl)
   b. Polyester (Mersilene)
   c. Polyethylene (Dermalene)
   d. Cotton

308. Which of the following has the poorest handling ease?
   a. Silk
   b. Braided polyglycolic acid (Dexon-Plus)
   c. Chromic catgut
   d. Monofilament stainless steel wire

309. Characteristics of an ideal suture material include all of the following *except*:
   a. Minimal tissue reaction
   b. Favorability for bacterial growth
   c. Comfort in working with it
   d. Economical to use

310. An example of an inverting suture pattern is the:
   a. Purse-string
   b. Simple interrupted
   c. Interrupted horizontal mattress
   d. Simple continuous

311. After how long does a synthetic absorbable suture lose its tensile strength?
   a. 120 days
   b. 60 days
   c. 30 days
   d. 6 months

312. What suture material is absorbed most rapidly from an infected wound through increased local phagocytic activity?
   a. Vicryl (polyglactin 910)
   b. PDS (polydioxanone)
   c. Catgut
   d. Nylon

313. Which of the following is *not* a consideration when choosing a suture material?
   a. The surgeon's training and experience
   b. The part of the body where it will be used
   c. The size of the animal on which it will be used
   d. The age of the animal on which it will be used

314. Regarding wound healing, it is better to:
   a. Increase the size of the suture material rather than the number of sutures
   b. Increase the number of sutures rather than the size of the suture material
   c. Decrease both the size of the suture material and the number of the sutures
   d. Increase both the size of the suture material and the number of the sutures

315. Which of these statements concerning surgical catgut is false?
   a. It can be used for ligating superficial blood vessels.
   b. It is recommended for epidermal use.
   c. It is recommended for internal use.
   d. It absorbs quickly.

316. Chromic catgut is produced by exposure to basic chromium salts. How does this process affect it?
   a. Increases intermolecular bonding
   b. Decreases its strength
   c. Increases tissue reaction to it
   d. Decreases absorption time

317. Perioperative antibiotics:
   a. Should never be used
   b. Should always be used
   c. Are indicated in surgical procedures longer than 1.5 hours
   d. Are questionable in their effectiveness

318. What is the primary function of a Balfour?
   a. Retractor
   b. Rongeur
   c. Periosteal elevator
   d. Thumb forceps

319. What is the primary function of a Lempert?
   a. Retractor
   b. Rongeur
   c. Periosteal elevator
   d. Thumb forceps

320. All of the following statements regarding chlorhexidine gluconate surgical scrub are true *except*:
   a. Tends to stain the skin and hair coat
   b. Is effective against the Pseudomonas species
   c. Is marketed as Nolvasan
   d. Should be rinsed with alcohol

321. What if a gauze sponge that is being used for the surgical scrub inadvertently touches the patient's hair?
   a. It can continue to be used for the scrub, because the antimicrobial agents in the scrub will kill any bacteria picked up from the hair.
   b. It should be thrown out and replaced with a new sponge.
   c. It should now be used only for the edges of the clipped site.
   d. It should not be considered contaminated unless gross contamination is visible.

322. Surgical scrubs are applied to the surgically prepared site:
- a. In any pattern, as long as the area is covered thoroughly
- b. In target fashion, starting with the incision site and spiraling outward toward the edge of the clipped area
- c. Starting with the edges, because they are the dirtiest areas, and working in toward the incision site
- d. Without subsequent rinsing because dilution reduces the antimicrobial effect

323. Why is an anal purse-string suture placed before perianal surgery?
- a. To keep the tail out of the surgical field
- b. To prevent fecal contamination during surgery
- c. To close the urethra
- d. To tighten loose folds of perianal skin

324. In male dogs, the prepuce is:
- a. Sutured closed before an abdominal surgical procedure to prevent contamination
- b. Considered an uncontaminated area that is not given special consideration
- c. Flushed with alcohol while the dog is awake
- d. Flushed with a weak povidone-iodine and saline solution before abdominal surgery

325. What structure is commonly emptied before abdominal surgery?
- a. Stomach
- b. Anal sac
- c. Urinary bladder
- d. Gallbladder

326. What type of instrument is a Metzenbaum?
- a. Needle holder
- b. Scissors
- c. Towel clamp
- d. Hemostatic forceps

327. The most effective use for a Rongeur is to:
- a. Pinch off a bleeding vessel
- b. Elevate soft tissue off a bony surface
- c. Remove small pieces of bone
- d. Retract soft tissue away from bone

328. Talking in the surgery room should be kept to a minimum to:
- a. Prevent unnecessary injection of bacteria into the operating theater
- b. Prevent distractions
- c. Expedite the surgery
- d. Talking does not need to be kept to a minimum.

329. The instrument suitable for cutting a paper drape is:
- a. Operating scissors
- b. Metzenbaum scissors
- c. Scalpel blade
- d. Wire scissors

330. What instrument is *not* a self-retaining tissue retractor?
- a. Finochietto
- b. Army-Navy
- c. Balfour
- d. Gelpi

331. A surgical scrub with residual antibacterial activity is important because:
- a. Bacteria below the superficial dermal area are constantly rising to the surface.
- b. It makes it unnecessary to worry about touching a scrubbed area with an ungloved hand.
- c. It makes it unnecessary to be as fastidious in the scrubbing technique.
- d. It makes it unnecessary to worry about prepping the area with alcohol, in addition to the surgical scrub.

332. The most effective sterilizing method for an object that could be damaged by heat is:
- a. Autoclaving
- b. Gas sterilization
- c. Flash flaming
- d. Alcohol scrub

333. What term best describes freedom from infection as it applies to the surgical technique?
- a. Uncontaminated
- b. Asepsis
- c. Healthy
- d. Clean

334. What surgical materials are sterilized by filtration?
- a. Nutrient solutions
- b. Irrigation solutions
- c. Surgical solutions
- d. Pharmaceutical solutions

335. What piece of equipment delivers saturated steam under pressure?
- a. Oven
- b. Crematorium
- c. Autoclave
- d. Plasma sterilizer

336. A safeguard to ensure that a pack is sterilized adequately is:
- a. Sterilization tape
- b. Sterilization indicators
- c. Feeling how hot the instrument is after the sterilization process is complete
- d. Visually inspecting the pack for microorganisms

337. An autoclave:
- a. Is not a safe method to sterilize metal implants for orthopedic procedures
- b. Must not be overloaded because this decreases its effectiveness
- c. Can be used to sterilize syringes for future vaccination clinics
- d. Is expensive and is therefore not practical for most veterinary clinics

338. Electrocautery is:
- a. An effective way to sterilize skin
- b. Used to coagulate blood flow from a cut vessel
- c. Cannot be used for most surgical procedures
- d. Atraumatic and can be used liberally

339. All of the following should be performed to resuscitate puppies and kittens following a cesarean section delivery *except*:
  a. Warming the puppies or kittens
  b. Swinging the puppies or kittens to remove fluid from the airway
  c. Stimulating the puppies and kittens with gentle rubbing
  d. Suctioning the airway of the puppies or kittens with a bulb syringe to remove fluid from the airway

340. An abdominal surgery is finished and the surgical team realizes that they forgot to perform a sponge count. Upon completing the count it is noted that a radiopaque sponge is missing and cannot be located. The next step is to:
  a. Perform another surgical prep on the patient and re-explore the abdomen to look for the sponge
  b. Take a radiograph of the patient to look for the sponge
  c. Not worry about the missing sponge because they are absorbable
  d. Notify the owner of symptoms to watch for in case the sponge causes a problem

341. When preparing a feline patient for a routine spay, administration of antibiotics before surgery:
  a. Should be given only if the surgeon does not wear a cap or a mask
  b. Is not indicated for short, uncomplicated procedures
  c. Should always be given as a precaution to prevent infection
  d. Is never useful in conjunction with surgery

342. The main function of bactericidal disinfectants is to:
  a. Slow bacterial proliferation
  b. Kill bacteria
  c. Remove organic debris from the site
  d. Flush bacteria from the site

343. Keeping the environment (floors, walls, counters) clean throughout the hospital is:
  a. Not important if your surgery areas are separate from other areas of the clinic
  b. Advisable because it is good for public relations
  c. Mandated by the AVMA
  d. Mandatory to prevent cross-contamination into the surgery area

344. The sterile field in the surgery room:
  a. Is the entire surgical suite
  b. Consists of the shaved and prepared area on the animal's skin
  c. Consists of the draped field and instrument table
  d. All of the above

345. The surgical nurse circulating for the scrubbed-in surgeon(s):
  a. Has the task of keeping the animal anesthetized
  b. Does not need a cap and mask because he or she is not assisting with surgery
  c. Must constantly be concerned with maintaining an aseptic technique
  d. Need not wear sterile surgical gloves

346. Perineal urethrostomies are performed only on:
  a. Pregnant cats
  b. Male cats with urethral obstruction
  c. Large-breed dogs with gastric torsion
  d. Small dogs with pyometra

347. Assuming that good aseptic technique is being followed, the most common source of contamination in a surgical wound is:
  a. The patient's skin or internal organs
  b. Your own breath
  c. Dust falling from the ceiling
  d. Dust from the floor

348. The clothing worn in a surgical room:
  a. Can be clothes worn on the street
  b. Should be clothes worn while in the clinic only
  c. Should be a scrub suit dedicated to surgery use
  d. Is required to be clean only and not torn

349. Surgical masks:
  a. Prevent unpleasant odors from reaching the surgeon's nose
  b. Lose their effectiveness when saturated with moisture
  c. Are used for orthopedic procedures only
  d. Can be tied loosely so that they are not as confining

350. When folding surgical gowns for sterilization:
  a. Tie the arms together so they do not dangle when the surgeon is gowning
  b. Have the ends of the sleeves on top for easy grasping
  c. Make sure the ties are on top so they can be used to pick up the gown
  d. Place the inside of the shoulder seams on top and fold all outer areas of the gown to the inside

351. During surgery, the back outside aspect of a surgeon's gown should be considered:
  a. Sterile
  b. Sterile as long as someone has not touched it
  c. Unsterile
  d. Neither sterile nor unsterile because it is not likely to contact the patient

352. Excessive bleeding from the surface of a bone can be controlled with:
  a. Bipolar cautery
  b. Bone wax
  c. Monopolar cautery
  d. Gel foam

353. The counted brush stroke method for surgical scrubbing:
  a. Is not practical on a routine basis
  b. Is quicker than a timed scrub
  c. Refers to scrubbing the arms and hands in a methodical, consistent manner
  d. Is more thorough than a timed scrub

354. A timed scrub should last at least:
  a. 15 minutes
  b. 5 minutes
  c. 30 minutes
  d. 1 minute

355. The preferred method for gloving is:
   a. Open
   b. Closed
   c. Assisted
   d. Double
356. Which of the following statements about open gloving is false?
   a. Gloves should be picked up with a cuffed hand.
   b. Only the skin surface of the glove is to be touched.
   c. The gloved hand picks up the second glove under the folded cuff.
   d. The cuff of the first glove is not pulled up until the second glove is fully on.
357. Iodophors, such as povidone-iodine scrub:
   a. Are the ideal surgical preparation solutions
   b. Have been replaced by newer, more effective scrubbing agents
   c. Are effective when used with alcohol only
   d. Have better residual activity than chlorhexidine
358. The number of personnel in the operating theater:
   a. Has no bearing on the outcome of the surgery
   b. Cannot be controlled in most situations
   c. Must be high to keep the temperature in the room high
   d. Should be kept to a minimum to keep airborne bacteria levels low to reduce the likelihood of contamination
359. Cleaning instruments before sterilization:
   a. Must be performed carefully by hand
   b. Is done only if there is time
   c. Can be done exclusively with ultrasonic cleaners
   d. Is not necessary if proper sterilization practices are followed
360. Ethyl and isopropyl alcohols:
   a. Have characteristics that make them ideal for sterilizing instruments
   b. Have the ability to act both as disinfectants and as antiseptics
   c. Have excellent residual effects because of rapid evaporation
   d. Have no place in veterinary surgery
361. An effective disinfectant to clean a cage after an animal has had a pseudomonas-contaminated wound is:
   a. Chlorhexidine
   b. Isopropyl alcohol
   c. Quaternary ammonium
   d. Povidone-iodine
362. A good solution to instill in the conjunctival sac before surgery is:
   a. 10% chlorhexidine gluconate
   b. 10% povidone-iodine solution
   c. 5% isopropyl alcohol
   d. Dilute soapy water
363. Clean-contaminated surgery refers to:
   a. All surgeries
   b. Incisions in sterile areas that become contaminated during surgery
   c. A clean wound in which a drain is placed
   d. Incisions in a previously contaminated area that has been rendered sterile
364. In terms of surgical contamination, endogenous organisms are those that:
   a. Originate from the patient's own body
   b. Come from the external surgical environment
   c. Rarely cause any problem in surgical wounds
   d. Come from the surgeon
365. When a break in aseptic technique occurs:
   a. The surgery must be called off immediately.
   b. The break can be ignored and surgery can continue if the surgery is nearly finished.
   c. The patient is unlikely to recover from the surgery because of infection.
   d. Steps must be taken to remedy the situation immediately to the best of everyone's ability.
366. A good time to clean the surgery room is:
   a. On the night before surgery to allow airborne dust to settle before surgery
   b. Immediately before the surgery so things can be as clean as possible
   c. Once a week
   d. Once a month
367. Lavaging (flushing) a body cavity with warm, sterile saline after completing a surgical procedure and before closing the incision:
   a. Is of minimal value in abdominal surgeries
   b. Decreases the amount of bacteria left behind and warms the patient
   c. Serves as a medium in which bacteria can multiply and should therefore be avoided
   d. Is necessary only if a break in aseptic technique has occurred
368. An example of an elective procedure is:
   a. Ovariohysterectomy
   b. Nephrotomy
   c. Exploratory laparotomy
   d. Splenectomy
369. A tapered suture needle is:
   a. Best to use in skin
   b. The least traumatic and most often used in deep tissue layers
   c. Not used very often because of its relative inability to penetrate tissue
   d. Too expensive for routine surgical use
370. A thoracotomy is an incision into the:
   a. Abdomen
   b. Chest
   c. Skull
   d. Ear
371. The suffix *-ectomy* refers to:
   a. Surgical removal
   b. Reduction
   c. Drainage
   d. Incision into
372. Which orthopedic fixation consists of pins that penetrate fractured bones that are held in place externally by bolts?
   a. Rush pinning
   b. Steinmann fixation
   c. Stack pinning
   d. Kirschner-Ehmer fixation

373. The term *arthrotomy* refers to an incision into a/an:
  a. Artery
  b. Joint
  c. Muscle
  d. Long bone

374. Arresting the flow of blood from a vessel or to a part is called:
  a. Aspiration
  b. Fibrinolysis
  c. Hemostasis
  d. Hemolysis

375. Peritonitis refers to:
  a. Inflammation of the pericardial space
  b. Inflammation of the lining of the abdominal cavity
  c. Inflammation caused by parasite infection
  d. Inflammation of the perianal area

376. Cryptorchidectomy is performed on male dogs:
  a. When one or both testicles have not descended into the scrotal sac
  b. When no other treatment for cryptosporidiosis is available
  c. And is similar to the vasectomy procedure performed in people
  d. When complications from routine castration arise

377. Fenestration refers to:
  a. Cutting a part exactly in half
  b. Creating a window in tissue
  c. The draping procedure
  d. Folding back the top skin layer

378. Ovariohysterectomy is routinely performed:
  a. In excitable dogs that need immediate calming
  b. In young female dogs that the owners wish rendered sterile
  c. In male dogs with female characteristics
  d. Exclusively in female dogs who have already had litters of puppies

379. Hepatic refers to:
  a. Heparin preparations
  b. Liver
  c. Blood
  d. Stomach

380. Blood vessels are ligated:
  a. To remove them completely from the body
  b. When blood flow needs to be stopped
  c. With suture material only
  d. Rarely and in emergency situations only

381. Chemical cauterization:
  a. Releases toxic fumes, exposing team members to a potential hazard
  b. Is rarely used in veterinary medicine
  c. Is traumatic to adjacent tissues and therefore is not used in surgical cases
  d. Is a misnomer; chemicals cannot stop bleeding

382. Keeping tissues moist during a surgical procedure:
  a. Is important because dry tissues are less resistant to bacterial infection
  b. Is undesirable because wet tissue is an ideal medium for bacterial regeneration
  c. Is of little value
  d. Should be accomplished with 70% isopropyl alcohol

383. Plating a fractured bone:
  a. Refers to coating the bone with a rigid metallic solution to induce healing
  b. Is beyond the scope of most veterinary practices
  c. Is an internal method of fracture fixation involving stainless steel plates and screws
  d. Can be done without skin incision

384. The distal portion of a long bone is:
  a. The one closest to the trunk of the body
  b. The one farthest away from the trunk of the body
  c. The inner portion of the bone
  d. The outer layer of the bone

385. Torsion of an organ or part refers to:
  a. Swelling or expansion
  b. Inflation with fluid
  c. Inflation with gas
  d. Twisting or rotation

386. What surgical procedure is least likely to combat the debilitating complications of canine hip dysplasia?
  a. Triple pelvic osteotomy
  b. Total hip replacement
  c. Intramedullary pinning
  d. Pectineal myotomy

387. Ear canal ablation refers to:
  a. Irrigation of the ear canal
  b. Instilling antibiotics to correct otitis media
  c. Surgical removal and closure of the external ear canal
  d. The instrument used to examine the ear canal

388. Perioperative refers to:
  a. The day before surgery
  b. The day after surgery
  c. Immediately before and after surgery
  d. During surgery

389. Onychectomy:
  a. Is the procedure used to remove a cat's testicles and spermatic cord
  b. Is the procedure used to remove a cat's claws and associated phalanges
  c. Can be performed without anesthesia
  d. Can be performed on female cats only

390. Postoperative complications:
  a. Do not occur if the surgeon is skilled
  b. Should never be discussed with a client
  c. Can occur even if the surgery went well
  d. Are almost always attributable to poor assistance in surgery

391. Fracture reduction:
  a. Involves trimming the areas of bone adjacent to the fracture site
  b. Involves apposing (pulling together) the fractured bone ends
  c. Is rarely necessary for good healing
  d. Can usually be performed without anesthesia

392. A diaphragmatic hernia:
  a. Is a diaphragm that is in continuous spasm
  b. Is displacement of the heart and part of the lungs into the abdomen
  c. Cannot be corrected and is considered fatal
  d. Should be suspected if the animal is dyspneic following a traumatic experience

393. When an animal is sent home after surgery:
- a. The wound should already be completely healed.
- b. The client should be given written detailed home care instructions.
- c. The animal is no longer legally your patient and no longer your concern.
- d. The technician should make daily visits to ensure that the patient is given the same care as in the hospital.

394. Absorbable gelatin sponges:
- a. Are typically soaked or sutured into a bleeding site
- b. Should never be left in the body after surgery
- c. Are radiopaque
- d. Are not available for veterinary surgery

395. Exteriorizing a body part or organ during surgery:
- a. Is a routine practice when the part or organ contains contaminants
- b. Is very hazardous to the patient and is not routinely done
- c. Precludes the need for lavaging
- d. Is done only if that part or organ is to be resected (surgically removed)

396. A dog presents at your clinic with a suspected intestinal foreign body. During the laparotomy the doctor removes the object and notes that a section of the intestines is necrotic. What is the name of the procedure to remove the necrotic area and to rejoin the healthy intestines?
- a. Resection and intussusception
- b. Resection and enterotomy
- c. Resection and anastomosis
- d. Resection and celiotomy

397. During a cystotomy, the doctor requests a suture to close the bladder. Which suture is the most appropriate?
- a. Monofilament, absorbable with a taper point
- b. Monofilament, nonabsorbable with a taper point
- c. Multifilament, absorbable with cutting point
- d. Multifilament, nonabsorbable with a taper point

398. While monitoring a patient under anesthesia, you notice its blood pressure begins to drop. After notifying the veterinarian, what steps do you initially take to correct the situation?
- a. Decrease fluid rate and increase oxygen flow
- b. Increase fluid rate and increase oxygen flow
- c. Decrease fluid rate and increase anesthetic
- d. Increase fluid rate and decrease anesthetic

399. Which of the following situations can cause hypocarbia?
- a. Decreased respiratory rate
- b. Increased respiratory rate
- c. Exhausted soda lime
- d. Kinked endotracheal tube

400. What is considered the most painful portion of a routine spay procedure?
- a. The initial abdominal incision
- b. Applying the angiotribe
- c. The plucking/tearing of the suspensory ligament
- d. Ligation of the ovarian pedicle

401. How soon after surgery should animals be offered food?
- a. 8 hours after recovery
- b. 12 hours after recovery
- c. 24 hours after recovery
- d. As soon as possible after recovery

402. Which of the following is used primarily to determine patient safety as opposed to anesthetic depth?
- a. Respiratory rate
- b. Palpebral reflex
- c. Eye position
- d. Muscle tone

403. If a patient is at an adequate surgical plane of anesthesia, which of the following statements would be true?
- a. The pedal reflex would be present.
- b. The palpebral reflex would be present.
- c. The swallowing reflex would be present.
- d. The corneal reflex would be present.

404. How many phases of wound healing are present in animals?
- a. 1
- b. 2
- c. 3
- d. 4

405. During the debridement phase of wound healing, all of the following are components of exudate *except*:
- a. WBC
- b. RBC
- c. Dead tissue
- d. Wound fluid

406. Moist wound healing:
- a. Enhances wound healing
- b. Slows wound healing
- c. Has no effect on healing
- d. Increases the bacterial contamination of the wound

407. Which of the following external factors can delay wound healing?
- a. Steroids
- b. Radiation therapy
- c. Chemotherapeutic agents
- d. All of the above

408. All of the following items are removed when debriding a wound *except*?
- a. Dead or damaged tissue
- b. Foreign bodies
- c. Microorganisms
- d. WBCs

409. How often should the surgery room floor be cleaned?
- a. As needed
- b. Daily
- c. Morning and evening
- d. Weekly

410. Regarding disinfectants, to what does "contact time" refer?
   a. The time required for disinfectants to be in contact with microorganisms to achieve the intended effect
   b. The time of day when the manufacturer can be contacted for assistance
   c. The time required for a microorganism to develop resistance to a disinfectant
   d. The latent phase of microorganisms, providing the disinfectant "a window of opportunity" to kill the microorganism

411. The surgical preparation room is located:
   a. Within the surgical suite
   b. Adjacent to the surgical suite
   c. Separated from the surgical suite by a treatment room
   d. Upstairs, above the surgical suite

SECTION

7 Dentistry

Jeanne Perrone

QUESTIONS

1. Apical means "toward the __________."
   a. Root tip
   b. Crown
   c. Cheeks
   d. Tongue
2. When assessing and quantifying gingivitis, the modified Löe and Silness index is often referred to. According to this index, a gingival index 3 indicates:
   a. Clinically healthy gingiva
   b. Mild gingivitis with slight reddening and swelling of the gingival margins
   c. Moderate gingivitis, with gentle probing resulting in bleeding
   d. Severe gingivitis, in which there is spontaneous hemorrhage and/or ulceration of the gingival margin
3. Hypodontia is defined as:
   a. Congenital absence of many, but not all, teeth
   b. Total absence of teeth
   c. Absence of only a few teeth
   d. Inflammation of the mouth
4. Abbreviations are commonly used in veterinary practice and some abbreviations are exclusive to dental terminology. Which abbreviation best aligns with the complicated crown fracture?
   a. CCF
   b. UCF
   c. UCRF
   d. CCRF
5. When grading furcation involvement, which of the following descriptions is termed Grade 3?
   a. No furcation involvement
   b. The furcation can be felt with the probe/explorer, but horizontal tissue destruction is <⅓ of the horizontal width.
   c. The furcation can be explored, but the probe cannot pass through it.
   d. The probe can be passed through the furcation from buccal to palatal/lingual.
6. When grading tooth mobility, which of the following grades corresponds to a Grade 3?
   a. No mobility
   b. Horizontal movement <1 mm
   c. Horizontal movement >1 mm
   d. Vertical and horizontal movement
7. Which teeth on each side of the dog's mouth have three roots?
   a. Maxillary: third and fourth premolars and first molar
   b. Maxillary: fourth premolars and first and second molars
   c. Mandibular: fourth premolars and first and second molars
   d. Mandibular and maxillary: fourth premolars and first and second molars
8. At what age do the permanent canine and premolar teeth in dogs generally erupt?
   a. 3–5 months
   b. 4–6 months
   c. 5–7 months
   d. 6–8 months
9. Using the Triadan system, the proper way to describe a dog's first maxillary left permanent premolar is:
   a. 205
   b. 105
   c. 306
   d. 502
10. Using the Triadan system, the proper way to describe a cat's first mandibular right molar is:
    a. 407
    b. 409
    c. 109
    d. 909
11. The pulp canal of a tooth contains:
    a. Nerves
    b. Blood vessels
    c. Connective tissue and blood vessels
    d. Blood vessels, nerves, and connective tissues
12. As part of normal tooth development, what part of the tooth widens?
    a. Enamel
    b. Pulp
    c. Dentin
    d. Gingiva
13. Which of the following statements regarding enamel is true?
    a. Contains living tissue
    b. Covers the tooth crown and root
    c. Continues production by the ameloblasts after eruption
    d. Is relatively nonporous and impervious

14. Dentin is covered by:
    a. Enamel and bone
    b. Bone and pulp
    c. Cementum and enamel
    d. Pulp and cementum
15. Normal scissor occlusion occurs when the maxillary fourth premolars occlude:
    a. Level with the mandibular fourth premolar
    b. Buccally to the mandibular first molar
    c. Buccally to the mandibular fourth premolar
    d. Lingually to the mandibular first molar
16. Which of the following describes the adult feline dental formula?
    a. 2 × {I 2/1:C 0/0:P 3/2:M 3/3}
    b. 2 × {I 3/3:C 1/1:P 4/4:M 2/3}
    c. 2 × {I 3/3:C 1/1:P 3/2:M 1/1}
    d. 2 × {I 3/3:C 1/1:P 3/3}
17. The carnassial teeth in dogs are:
    a. $^{4}P4$ and $_{1}M_{1}$
    b. $4P^{4}$ and $^{4}P4$
    c. $^{1}M^{1}$ and $_{1}M_{1}$
    d. $^{1}C^{1}$ and $_{1}C_{1}$
18. The free or marginal gingiva:
    a. Occupies the space between the teeth
    b. Is the most apical portion of the gingiva
    c. Forms the gingival sulcus around the tooth
    d. Is tightly bound to the cementum
19. The periodontium includes the periodontal ligament and all of the following *except*:
    a. Gingiva
    b. Cementum
    c. Alveolar bone
    d. Enamel
20. A bulldog would be described as having what type of head shape?
    a. Brachycephalic
    b. Dolichocephalic
    c. Mesaticephalic/mesocephalic
    d. Prognacephalic
21. In veterinary dentistry, chlorhexidine solutions are used because they:
    a. Prevent cementoenamel erosion
    b. Have antibacterial properties
    c. Remove enamel stains and whiten teeth
    d. Are used to treat gingival hyperplasia in brachycephalic breeds
22. When using hand instruments to clean teeth, you should:
    a. Use a modified pen grasp with a back-and-forth scraping motion
    b. Use a modified pen grasp with overlapping pull strokes that are directed away from the gingival margin
    c. Use the sickle scaler for subgingival curettage
    d. Use a curette supragingivally
23. Pocket depth is measured from the:
    a. Cementoenamel junction to the bottom of the pocket
    b. Current free gingival margin to the bottom of the gingival sulcus
    c. Cementoenamel junction to the current free gingival margin and then adding 1–2 mm
    d. Cementoenamel junction to the apical extent of the defect
24. Between patients, it is best to maintain instruments in the following order:
    a. Use, sharpen, wash, and sterilize
    b. Use, wash, sterilize, and sharpen
    c. Use, wash, sharpen, and sterilize
    d. Wash, sterilize, use, and sharpen
25. When performing a dental prophylaxis, minimal safety equipment includes:
    a. Gloves only
    b. Gloves and mask only
    c. Safety glasses only
    d. Safety glasses, mask, and gloves
26. You have an instrument in your hand that has two sharp sides: a rounded back and a rounded point. Which instrument are you holding?
    a. Sickle scaler
    b. Morse scaler
    c. Universal curette
    d. Sickle curette
27. When polishing teeth using an air-driven unit, at what speed should the hand piece be set?
    a. High speed
    b. Low speed
    c. Either high or low is acceptable
    d. Finishing speed
28. The term that best describes a dog with an abnormally short mandible is:
    a. Prognathism
    b. Brachygnathism
    c. Mesaticephalic
    d. Dolichocephalic
29. A malocclusion, where one side of the mandible or maxilla is disproportionate to its other side, is known as:
    a. Posterior/caudal crossbite
    b. Base-narrow mandibular canines
    c. Wry mouth
    d. Rostral/anterior crossbite
30. A malocclusion in which the upper fourth premolar lies palatal to the first molars is known as:
    a. Posterior/caudal crossbite
    b. Base-narrow mandibular canines
    c. Wry mouth
    d. Rostral/anterior crossbite
31. A malocclusion that causes the canines to erupt lingually displaced as a result of an abnormally narrow mandible or the delayed exfoliation of the deciduous mandibular canine teeth is known as:
    a. Posterior/caudal crossbite
    b. Base-narrow mandibular canines
    c. Wry mouth
    d. Rostral/anterior crossbite
32. A malocclusion in which one or more of the upper incisor teeth are palatal to the lower incisors is known as:
    a. Posterior/caudal crossbite
    b. Base-narrow mandibular canines
    c. Wry mouth
    d. Rostral/anterior crossbite

33. To prep a patient for surgical tooth extraction, which of the following should occur?
   a. No prep is needed. It is best to extract, and then to clean the remaining teeth (this is a more efficient process, yielding a shorter anesthesia time).
   b. Rinse the mouth with chlorhexidine, then extract.
   c. Scale, polish, then extract.
   d. Scale, polish, rinse with chlorhexidine, then extract.

34. Dry socket is more likely to occur if:
   a. An increased blood supply to the area is ensured.
   b. Good surgical technique is practiced.
   c. A blood clot is allowed to form to encourage fibroblasts.
   d. The tooth socket is overirrigated so that no clot can form.

35. Gingivoplasty is the:
   a. Addition of more gingiva to the site
   b. Binding of the loose teeth together to stabilize them during a healing process
   c. Removal of hyperplastic gingival tissue
   d. Removal of a portion of the tooth structure

36. Which of the following should be done to protect the pulp tissue of teeth from thermal damage during ultrasonic scaling?
   a. Use constant irrigation
   b. Change tips frequently
   c. Use slow rotational speed
   d. Use appropriate amounts of paste

37. Another term for neck lesions often seen on feline teeth is:
   a. Peripheral odontogenic fibroma
   b. Stomatitis
   c. Feline odontoclastic resorptive lesions
   d. Enamel fracture

38. The most common dental procedure performed on a horse is:
   a. Quidding
   b. Curettage
   c. Scaling
   d. Floating

39. Stomatitis is defined as:
   a. Bad breath, malodor
   b. Inflammation of the lip
   c. Resorption of hard dental tissues by odontoclasts
   d. Inflammation and infection of some or all of the tooth's supportive tissues

40. A client would like to know what chew toy would be safest for her dog's teeth. You suggest that she is best to give "Fido" a:
   a. Dried cow hoof
   b. Nylon rope toy
   c. Dense rubber exerciser
   d. Large knucklebone

41. When taking radiographs of the canine tooth in a large breed dog, what size of dental film should be used to ensure that the whole tooth is included?
   a. 0
   b. 2
   c. 4
   d. 8" × 10" screen film

42. Dental film should be placed in the mouth with the dimple facing:
   a. Up and pointing rostrally
   b. Up and pointing caudally
   c. Down and pointing rostrally
   d. Down and pointing caudally

43. The flap side of the dental film should face:
   a. Any direction, because it does not matter
   b. Toward the tube head
   c. Away from the tube head
   d. The caudal side of the animal

44. The bisecting angle principle states that the plane of an x-ray beam should be 90 degrees to the:
   a. Long axis of the tooth
   b. Plane of the film
   c. Imaginary line that bisects the angle formed by the tooth's long axis and the film plane
   d. Imaginary line that bisects the angle formed by the animal's head and the film plane

45. You are looking at a dental radiograph and notice that the tooth is elongated. This happened because the beam was perpendicular to the:
   a. Film
   b. Tooth
   c. Bisecting angle
   d. Wrong tooth

46. Abbreviations are commonly used in veterinary practice and some abbreviations are exclusive to dental terminology. Which abbreviation best aligns with a complicated crown and root fracture?
   a. CCF
   b. UCF
   c. UCRF
   d. CCRF

47. A hand scaler is used to:
   a. Check the tooth's root surface for any irregularities
   b. Measure the depth of gingival recession
   c. Scale large amounts of calculus from the tooth surface
   d. Scale calculus from the tooth surface located in the gingival sulcus

48. What mineralized tissue covers the root of the tooth?
   a. Calculus
   b. Enamel
   c. Cementum
   d. Dentin

49. The nerves and blood vessels of a tooth are located in the:
   a. Sulcus
   b. Pulp cavity
   c. Marrow cavity
   d. Calculus

50. When scaling gross calculus from the teeth, you should:
   a. Hold the scaler using a modified pen grasp
   b. Hold the scaler using a modified screwdriver grasp
   c. Use long controlled strokes toward the gums
   d. Hold the curette using a modified pen grasp

51. Which of the following statements is true about ultrasonic scaling?
  a. Ultrasonic scaling is the only method to clean a tooth surface fully.
  b. Ultrasonic scaling causes thermal damage to the tooth if the tip is kept on a tooth for <5 seconds.
  c. The ultrasonic scaler works by spraying the tooth with water to wash the tooth clean.
  d. The purpose of the water spray on an ultrasonic scaler is to cool the tip of the instrument and cool the tooth to prevent pulp damage.

52. The following statements are all true *except*:
  a. Sulcus depth is measured using a periodontal probe.
  b. A sulcus depth ≤3 mm is normal in a cat.
  c. A sulcus depth >3 mm indicates periodontal disease.
  d. The probe is inserted gently into the gingival sulcus parallel to the root of the tooth.

53. All of the following are complications that may result from extraction *except*:
  a. Hemorrhage
  b. Jaw fracture
  c. Stomatitis
  d. Oronasal fistula

54. An older dog with dental disease is presented to the clinic with a draining tract below his right eye. What is the most likely cause?
  a. Right-sided maxillary carnassial tooth root abscess
  b. Left-sided maxillary carnassial tooth root abscess
  c. Right-sided mandibular carnassial tooth root abscess
  d. Maxillary incisor tooth root abscess

55. What members of the veterinary staff make up the oral health care team?
  a. The veterinarian
  b. The veterinary technician
  c. The receptionists
  d. All of the above

56. Why would thermal bone injury be a complication of tooth extraction?
  a. The bur will overheat and damage the soft tissue and bone.
  b. Thermal injury is not a concern, as you are removing the tooth anyway.
  c. Tooth elevators cause excessive heat, which could injure the soft tissue around the tooth that is being extracted.
  d. Tooth extractors cause excessive heat, which could injure the remaining teeth.

57. Mandibular Brachygnathism is a genetic defect best characterized as:
  a. A maxilla that is longer than the mandible
  b. A mandible that is longer than the maxilla
  c. A lack of incisors
  d. Polydontia

58. Prognathism is a normal condition in brachycephalic breeds but is considered a genetic defect in other breeds. It is best characterized as:
  a. A mandible that is longer than the maxilla
  b. A maxilla that is longer than the mandible
  c. One side of the head being longer than the other
  d. An overly long soft palate

59. Malocclusions can lead to dental disease for all of the following reasons *except*:
  a. Soft-tissue trauma from teeth that are abnormally positioned
  b. Accelerated development of periodontal disease resulting from the lack of normal wear and the normal flushing of teeth with saliva
  c. Abnormal wear of teeth resulting from malposition leading to fracture and pulp exposure
  d. Presence of resorptive lesions leading to the destruction of teeth

60. Which of the following teeth are *not* normally present in the adult cat?
  a. Maxillary P1 and Mandibular P1 and P2
  b. P1 and P1 and 2P
  c. I2 and I1
  d. PM3 and PM4

61. The furcation is best described as:
  a. The area between the cementum and the enamel
  b. The space between two roots where they meet the crown
  c. The space between the root and the alveolar bone
  d. The space between two teeth

62. What is the most common clinical sign of feline stomatitis?
  a. Fractured crowns and/or granulation tissue at the cementoenamel junction
  b. Thickening or bulging of the alveolar bone of the maxillary canine teeth
  c. Erythematous, ulcerative, proliferative lesions affecting the gingiva, glossopalatine arches, tongue, lips, buccal mucosa, and/or hard palate
  d. Granular, orange-colored ulcerations found on the upper lips adjacent to the philtrum

63. An oronasal fistula can often occur secondary to:
  a. Abscess of the mandibular canine tooth
  b. Incisor root abscess
  c. Abscess of the maxillary canine tooth
  d. Retained deciduous incisors

64. Which of the following statements about canine toy breeds is true?
  a. Chronic impaction of incisor teeth with hair and debris often results in a chronic osteomyelitis.
  b. Malocclusions are rare in toy breeds in comparison with giant-breed dogs.
  c. Enamel hypoplasia is a common finding in toy breeds.
  d. Prognathism is considered a genetic defect in brachycephalic breeds.

65. A biopsy report confirms that an oral mass is an acanthomatous ameloblastoma or an acanthomatous epulis. Which of the following statements is true regarding this growth?
  a. It is a nonmalignant tumor.
  b. It is a malignant tumor.
  c. It is very likely to metastasize.
  d. It is related to the presence of a malocclusion.

66. While performing a routine prophylactic dentistry, the veterinary technician notes a large, red raised lesion on the lip of her feline patient. The client noted that the lesion "comes and goes." What is a reasonable differential for this lesion?
   a. Feline resorptive lesion
   b. Trauma-related lesion
   c. Eosinophilic ulcer
   d. Tumor

67. Feline cervical line lesions/feline neck lesions/feline resorptive lesions are of great concern to veterinarians. Which of the following statements regarding these lesions is false?
   a. Feline resorptive lesions are aggressive dental caries that result in resorption of roots and subsequent tooth loss.
   b. Feline resorptive lesions often present with a raspberry seed-type sign at the base of the tooth where it meets the gingival margin.
   c. Feline resorptive lesions are effectively managed with steroid administration.
   d. It is common to find more than one feline cervical line lesion in the oral cavity.

68. Which of the following statements about the eruption of permanent teeth is false?
   a. The permanent upper canines erupt mesial to the deciduous canines.
   b. The permanent lower canines erupt buccal to the deciduous canines.
   c. The permanent incisors erupt distal to the deciduous incisors.
   d. The permanent canine teeth erupt at 5 to 6 months of age in the dog.

69. The pulp of the tooth has which of the following functions?
   a. Anchors the root to the alveolar bone with a fibrous ligament
   b. Provides the crown with a protective, hard surface
   c. Contains blood vessels and nerves that provide nutrition and sensation to the tooth
   d. Makes up the bulk of the tooth structure

70. When the pulp cavity of a tooth is exposed, what is/are the appropriate procedure(s) that should be performed if the patient is an adult and the time of fracture is unknown?
   a. Tooth extraction or root canal therapy
   b. No procedure required
   c. Crown amputation with intentional root retention
   d. Prophylactic dentistry to reduce tartar and plaque buildup on the tooth

71. In patients with severe, chronic periodontal disease, medication can be administered before a dental cleaning is performed. What is the most common type of medication chosen for these animals?
   a. Corticosteroids
   b. Antimicrobials
   c. Nonsteroidal antiinflammatories
   d. Immunostimulants

72. From birth to 9 months of age, what condition is *not* present in the oral cavity?
   a. Occurrence of oral masses
   b. Missing teeth
   c. Extra teeth
   d. Abnormal jaw length

73. Perioceutics refers to which of the following?
   a. Procedure to restore the periodontal ligament
   b. Application of time-released antibiotics directly within the oral cavity
   c. Use of antibiotics before dental procedure
   d. Procedure to cap the pulp cavity of the tooth

74. The bisecting angle technique is a method for radiographing the oral cavity. The description that adequately describes this technique is:
   a. The central radiation beam is directed perpendicular to the line that bisects the angle formed by the film and the long axis of the tooth.
   b. The central radiation beam is directed parallel to the line that bisects the angle formed by the film and the perpendicular axis of the tooth.
   c. The central radiation beam is directed perpendicular to the tooth root.
   d. The central radiation beam is directed perpendicular to the film or sensor.

75. A curette is used to:
   a. Check the tooth's surface for any irregularities
   b. Measure the depth of gingival recession
   c. Scale large amounts of calculus from the tooth supragingivally
   d. Scale calculus from the tooth surface subgingivally

76. Which of the following statements is false when performing an ultrasonic scaling during routine dental prophylaxis?
   a. The ultrasonic scaler should not be on the tooth for longer than 10–15 seconds at a time to prevent thermal damage to the pulp cavity.
   b. The ultrasonic scaler should be grasped like a pencil.
   c. The side of the instrument should be used against the tooth rather than the tip.
   d. The ultrasonic scaler can be used for supragingival scaling only.

77. Which of the following statements is false regarding patient safety during dentistry?
   a. Thermal support should be provided to the patient during the dental procedure because hypothermia can result, especially in cats and smaller dogs.
   b. The endotracheal tube should be uncuffed so that the tube can be easily manipulated when performing dentistry.
   c. Large-breed dogs should be rolled with their legs under them to prevent a gastric dilatation and volvulus crisis.
   d. The patient must be monitored to ensure that fluids and debris from the dentistry do not gain access to the trachea.

78. A dog exposed to distemper as a puppy may develop which of the following oral conditions?
   a. Anodontia
   b. Polydontia
   c. Enamel hypoplasia
   d. Enamel staining

79. Sometimes a 0.12%-chlorhexidine solution is sprayed in the patient's mouth before beginning dental prophylaxis. What is the benefit of this activity?
   a. Sterilizes the patient's mouth before the procedure
   b. Reduces the bacterial load in the mouth to reduce exposure to the technician who performs the procedure
   c. Substitutes for prophylactic antibiotic therapy
   d. Provides topical anesthetic activity

80. Which of the following statements is false with respect to polishing an animal's teeth following scaling?
   a. The polishing paste should be of medium or fine granularity.
   b. Polishing removes microscopic grooves left by the scaling process.
   c. The polishing instrument should be moved from tooth to tooth to prevent thermal damage to the pulp.
   d. Polishing is a means for removing stubborn plaque that occurs below the gumline.

81. The Triadan system is a:
   a. Tooth identification system designed to aid in dental charting
   b. Complete system that includes an ultrasonic scaler and polisher
   c. Method for performing radiographs of molars
   d. Complete home care dental system for use by clients

82. Oligodontia is defined as:
   a. Congenital absence of many, but not all, teeth
   b. Total absence of teeth
   c. Absence of only a few teeth
   d. Difficult eating

83. When considering the size of an upper canine tooth, how much of the tooth is exposed compared with that below the gumline?
   a. 1/3 of the tooth is exposed
   b. 1/2 of the tooth is exposed
   c. 2/3 of the tooth is exposed
   d. 3/4 of the tooth is exposed

84. The upper fourth premolar communicates with what sinus?
   a. Mandibular
   b. Occipital
   c. Maxillary
   d. Orbital

85. The crown of a tooth is defined as:
   a. The portion above the gumline and covered by enamel
   b. The most terminal portion of the root
   c. That portion below the gumline
   d. The layer of bony tissue that attaches to the alveolar bone

86. The range for acceptable gingival sulcus measurements in cats is:
   a. 1–3 mm
   b. 0.5–1 mm
   c. 1.5–4.5 mm
   d. 0.005–0.007 mm

87. How does tracheal rupture occur in feline dental patients?
   a. Packing the pharyngeal area too tightly
   b. Using a cuffed endotracheal tube
   c. Overinflation of the endotracheal tube cuff
   d. Disconnecting the breathing circuit before turning the patient

88. What stage of periodontal disease shows no change to the alveolar height but includes mild gingival inflammation?
   a. Stage I
   b. Stage II
   c. Stage III
   d. Stage IV

89. When assessing and quantifying gingivitis, the modified Löe and Silness index is often used. According to this index, a gingival index 0 indicates:
   a. Clinically healthy gingiva
   b. Mild gingivitis with slight reddening and swelling of the gingival margins
   c. Moderate gingivitis, with gentle probing resulting in bleeding
   d. Severe gingivitis, in which there is spontaneous hemorrhage and/or ulceration of the gingival margin

90. What drug should *not* be given to pregnant dogs because it may cause discoloration of the puppies' teeth?
   a. Amoxicillin
   b. Tetracycline
   c. Chloramphenicol
   d. Penicillin

91. The occlusal surface is defined as the:
   a. Surface facing the hard palate
   b. Surface nearer the cheek
   c. Chewing surface of the tooth
   d. Surface nearer the tongue

92. The normal adult canine mouth has how many permanent teeth?
   a. 40
   b. 42
   c. 48
   d. 52

93. When grading tooth mobility, which of the following grades corresponds to a Grade 2?
   a. No mobility
   b. Horizontal movement of <1 mm
   c. Horizontal movement >1 mm
   d. Vertical and horizontal movement

94. Which of the following is a complication that might develop if a curette is used improperly?
   a. Etched tooth enamel
   b. Torn epithelial attachment
   c. Overheated tooth
   d. Bitten technician

95. Which tooth has three roots?
   a. Upper canine
   b. Lower first premolar
   c. Lower first molar
   d. Upper fourth premolar

96. Which statement concerning the polishing aspect of dental prophylaxis is the least accurate?
   a. A slow speed should be used.
   b. Adequate prophy paste is needed for lubrication and polishing.
   c. The polisher should remain on the tooth for as long as is needed to polish the tooth.
   d. If teeth are not polished, the rough enamel will promote bacterial plaque formation.
97. What term means the wearing away of enamel by tooth-against-tooth contact during mastication?
   a. Plaque
   b. Attrition
   c. Calculus
   d. Abrasion
98. When grading furcation involvement, which of the following descriptions would be termed Grade 1?
   a. There is no furcation involvement.
   b. The furcation can be felt with the probe/explorer, but horizontal tissue destruction is <⅓ of the horizontal width.
   c. The furcation can be explored, but the probe cannot pass through it.
   d. The probe can be passed through the furcation from buccal to palatal/lingual.
99. What term identifies the loss of tooth structure by an outside cause?
   a. Plaque
   b. Attrition
   c. Calculus
   d. Abrasion
100. The thin film covering a tooth that is composed of bacteria, saliva, and food particles is:
   a. Plaque
   b. Attrition
   c. Calculus
   d. Abrasion
101. What is the minimum age for a cat to have all of its permanent teeth?
   a. 6 months
   b. 8 months
   c. 10 months
   d. 1 year
102. In general, most dental instruments should be held as you would hold a:
   a. Knife
   b. Pencil
   c. Hammer
   d. Toothbrush
103. What is the most common dental disease found in dogs and cats?
   a. Endodontic disease
   b. Oral tumors
   c. Jaw fractures
   d. Periodontal disease
104. Removal of calculus and necrotic cementum from the tooth roots is called:
   a. Curettage
   b. Splinting
   c. Gingivoplasty
   d. Scaling
105. Prevention of periodontal disease involves all of the following *except*:
   a. Daily teeth brushing or mouth rinsing
   b. Full mouth extractions
   c. Routine professional scaling and polishing
   d. Proper diet
106. Luxation of a tooth *cannot* be termed as:
   a. Attrition
   b. Intrusion
   c. Extrusion
   d. Avulsion
107. Ideally, the cutting edge of the scaler should be held at what angle to the tooth surface?
   a. 5–10 degrees
   b. 35–45 degrees
   c. 15–30 degrees
   d. 45–90 degrees
108. Which of the following correctly describes the puppy dental formula?
   a. 2 × {I 2/1:C 0/0:P 3/2:M 3/3}
   b. 2 × {I 3/3:C 1/1:P 4/4:M 2/3}
   c. 2 × {I 3/3:C 1/1:P 3/2:M 1/1}
   d. 2 × {I 3/3:C 1/1:P 3/3}
109. Mrs. Walker comes to collect her dog after a dental cleaning has been performed. Which of the following topics would be least helpful to discuss as a part of the discharge instructions?
   a. Postoperative complications
   b. Home care
   c. How to give injections
   d. Dietary concerns
110. After plaque bacteria have formed on the tooth, the bacteria will absorb calcium from the saliva to form what substance?
   a. Calculus
   b. Pellicle
   c. Biofilm
   d. Lipopolysaccharides
111. The most common dental problem found in rodents is:
   a. Tooth root abscess
   b. Malocclusion
   c. Scurvy
   d. Cheek pouch impaction
112. What tissue is *not* part of the periodontium?
   a. Periodontal ligament
   b. Alveolar bone
   c. Root
   d. Gingiva
113. Which of the following statements is false?
   a. Tooth brushing and avoiding treats containing sugars prevent caries in dogs.
   b. Abrasion and tooth fracture are prevented by monitoring play behaviors or changing the chewing object.
   c. There is no magic bullet that we can feed our pets to prevent periodontal disease; daily tooth brushing remains the single most effective method of restoring inflamed gingivae to health and then maintaining clinically healthy gingivae.
   d. After receiving instructions, clients will always perform dental home care program on a daily basis.

114. Which cells are responsible for destroying the hard surfaces of the root?
  a. Macrocytes
  b. Osteoclasts
  c. Chondrocytes
  d. Odontoclasts
115. What term identifies the space between the roots of the same tooth?
  a. Apical
  b. Rostral
  c. Furcation
  d. Buccal
116. What term identifies the tooth surface facing the cheeks?
  a. Apical
  b. Rostral
  c. Furcation
  d. Buccal
117. What is the directional term for "toward the root"?
  a. Apical
  b. Rostral
  c. Furcation
  d. Buccal
118. What is the directional term for "toward the front of the head"?
  a. Apical
  b. Rostral
  c. Furcation
  d. Buccal
119. Chlorhexidine contributes to dental prophylaxis by:
  a. Preventing plaque from mineralizing into calculus
  b. Bonding to the cell membrane and inhibiting bacterial growth
  c. Bleaching stained teeth
  d. Decreasing tooth sensitivity
120. The normal occlusion in a dog or cat can also be called a:
  a. Scissor bite
  b. Straight bite
  c. Occlusal bite
  d. Razor bite
121. What is the proper dilution of chlorhexidine solution for use in the mouth?
  a. 20%
  b. 2.00%
  c. 0.20%
  d. 10%
122. Topical fluoride:
  a. Will stain the remaining calculus red
  b. Helps to desensitize teeth and to strengthen enamel against cariogenic bacteria that cause cavities
  c. Should never be used on feline teeth
  d. Enhances odontoclastic activity and helps desensitize teeth
123. What instrument is used for root planing?
  a. Periodontal probe
  b. Explorer
  c. Scaler
  d. Curette
124. What instrument is used to detect subgingival calculus?
  a. Periodontal probe
  b. Explorer
  c. Scaler
  d. Curette
125. What instrument is used to remove supragingival calculus?
  a. Periodontal probe
  b. Explorer
  c. Scaler
  d. Curette
126. An elongation of one side of the animal's jaw results in:
  a. Anterior crossbite
  b. Wry mouth
  c. Brachygnathism
  d. Prognathism
127. The bulk of a tooth is composed of:
  a. Enamel
  b. Pulp
  c. Dentin
  d. Cementum
128. The most common mistake made in treating periodontal disease is:
  a. Inadequate removal of supragingival calculus
  b. Inadequate root planing
  c. Insufficient polishing
  d. Iatrogenic trauma to subgingival tissues
129. What is the purpose of a dentifrice when used in the dog and cat?
  a. Removes subgingival calculus
  b. Removes microetchants caused by scaling the teeth
  c. Removes supragingival calculus
  d. Provides a pleasant taste and improves the effectiveness of brushing
130. Applying fluoride and rinsing with diluted chlorhexidine at the same time:
  a. Is less effective, because the binding of one product may inactivate the other
  b. Results in temporary staining of the teeth
  c. Enhances the activity of both fluoride and chlorhexidine
  d. May be toxic to the patient
131. If the lower incisors seem excessively loose in a brachycephalic or miniature-breed dog:
  a. The teeth should be extracted
  b. The depth of the gingival sulcus should be tested
  c. The dog is calcium deficient
  d. The dog has advanced periodontal disease
132. Fractured deciduous teeth:
  a. Should be left in place until they are normally shed
  b. Should be repaired
  c. Are insignificant
  d. Should be extracted
133. The first dental examination should occur when:
  a. The patient is 2–3 years old.
  b. The client requests it.
  c. A problem such as drooling or bad breath is noticed.
  d. The patient is 6–8 weeks old.

134. What is true about deciduous incisors?
   a. They erupt at 4–12 weeks of age.
   b. They have roots that are long, thin, and fragile.
   c. They are the most frequently retained teeth.
   d. They are not usually replaced with permanent incisors until the dog is 6 months old.
135. Nerves and blood vessels enter the tooth through the:
   a. Apical delta
   b. Crown
   c. Pulp
   d. Sulcus
136. When one or more of the upper incisors rest caudally on the lower incisors and the rest of the occlusion is normal, the condition is known as:
   a. Level bite
   b. Wry mouth
   c. Rostral crossbite
   d. Anodontia
137. The term polydontia refers to:
   a. Retained deciduous teeth
   b. Supernumerary teeth
   c. Supernumerary teeth and retained deciduous teeth
   d. Tooth loss as a result of periodontal disease
138. The normal sulcus depth in the dog is:
   a. 3 mm
   b. 7 mm
   c. 10 mm
   d. 8 mm
139. Excessive growth of gingival tissue is termed:
   a. Gingivitis
   b. Gingival hyperplasia
   c. Gingival recession
   d. Gingivectomy
140. The shrinkage of free gingiva in the presence of bacteria, plaque, and/or dental calculus is termed:
   a. Gingival hyperplasia
   b. Periodontitis
   c. Gingivectomy
   d. Gingival recession
141. Two tooth buds that grow together to form one larger tooth is called:
   a. Gemini
   b. Fusion
   c. Polydontia
   d. Oligodontia
142. The space between two roots, where they meet the crown, is called:
   a. Crook
   b. Furcation
   c. Apex
   d. Fissure
143. The term for a tooth that has one root but two crowns is:
   a. Gemini
   b. Fusion
   c. Polydontia
   d. Oligodontia
144. The surface of the tooth toward the lips is known as the:
   a. Occlusal
   b. Labial
   c. Buccal
   d. Mesial
145. Fewer teeth than normal is known as:
   a. Polydontia
   b. Oligodontia
   c. Fusion
   d. Wry mouth
146. The surface of the tooth that is toward the cheek is known as:
   a. Occlusal
   b. Labial
   c. Buccal
   d. Mesial
147. Where do tooth resorption lesions first appear clinically in the cat?
   a. On the cementum
   b. On the alveolar mucosa
   c. At the cementoenamel junction
   d. At the tip of the crown
148. The purpose of fluoride treatment is to:
   a. Prevent thermal damage and lubrication
   b. Strengthen enamel and help desensitize teeth
   c. Remove plaque and strengthen the enamel
   d. Irrigate and lubricate
149. Sometimes referred to as distemper teeth, the name for a condition in which sections of the tooth enamel are pitted or discolored is:
   a. Prognathic
   b. Enamel hypoplasia
   c. Attrition
   d. Abrasion
150. Malocclusion in which the mandible is caudal to the maxilla is termed:
   a. Class 3 mandibular mesioclusion
   b. Class 2 mandibular distoclusion
   c. Class 1 neutroclusion
   d. Dental malocclusion
151. Malocclusion in which the mandibular is rostral to the maxilla is termed:
   a. Class 3 mandibular mesioclusion
   b. Class 2 mandibular distoclusion
   c. Class 1 neutroclusion
   d. Dental malocclusion
152. The maxillary carnassial tooth in the cat is also known as the:
   a. Upper first premolar
   b. Upper first molar
   c. Upper last premolar
   d. Upper canine
153. Using the modified Triadan system, the right maxillary teeth would be in the ___ series.
   a. 100
   b. 200
   c. 300
   d. 400
154. Which dental radiographic projection shows teeth 101, 102, 103, 201, 202, and 203?
   a. Rostral maxillary
   b. Parallel mandibular view
   c. Rostral mandibular view
   d. Lateral oblique view

155. Which dental radiographic projection shows teeth 301–304 and 401–404?
a. Rostral maxillary
b. Parallel mandibular view
c. Rostral mandibular view
d. Lateral oblique view

156. The only radiographic view that can be made with a true parallel technique is:
a. Rostral maxillary
b. Parallel mandibular view
c. Rostral mandibular view
d. Parallel oblique view

157. In dental radiographs, periapical disease appears as a:
a. Radiopaque area around the apex of the tooth
b. Radiolucent area around the apex of the tooth
c. Radiopaque area inside the tooth pulp
d. Radiolucent area inside the tooth pulp

158. Which discipline deals with dental conditions specific to puppies and kittens?
a. Exodontics
b. Orthodontics
c. Pedodontics
d. Prosthodontics

159. Which statement is incorrect regarding the importance of dental radiographs?
a. They are used to measure sulcus depth.
b. They help to reach a diagnosis.
c. They are used in the performance of certain procedures.
d. They are considered part of the creation of a treatment plan.

160. What is the general appearance of a Class 5 feline resorptive lesion?
a. The tooth will appear fractured with a red dot in the middle.
b. The tooth looks normal but the gums are inflamed.
c. The tooth is not visible, only gum tissue.
d. Only a little of the enamel is missing, exposing the dentin.

161. Internal resorption primarily affects the:
a. Enamel
b. Crown
c. Pulp
d. Dentin

162. Horizontal bone loss occurs in cases of:
a. Periodontal disease
b. Fractured teeth
c. Tooth resorption
d. Orthodontic disease

163. Vital pulp therapy refers to:
a. Operating outright on the pulp on a live tooth
b. Root canal therapy
c. Procedure to turn a live tooth into a dead tooth
d. Generally used when the tooth has been dead for a long time

164. If a tooth is fractured and there is a black spot in the center of the cut surface into which you can place a dental explorer, the best treatment would be:
a. An x-ray to see whether there are changes in the tooth or surrounding areas, with treatment provided according to findings
b. Either a root canal or an extraction
c. A discussion of fees with the client and a determination of whether or not the patient experiences pain before therapy
d. An extraction

165. Which nerve block will anesthetize all the maxillary teeth on the injected side?
a. Infraorbital
b. Middle mental
c. Maxillary
d. Mandibular

166. The goal of orthodontic care is to:
a. Allow a dog or cat to compete better in breed shows
b. Correct abnormalities so a puppy or kitten can sell for a better price
c. Provide a better-looking pet
d. Return the pet to a comfortable or functional bite

167. What is the best time to use the extraction forceps?
a. At the end of the procedure when the tooth is very mobile
b. In the middle of the procedure to help with the elevation process
c. At the beginning of the procedure to chip off calculus
d. An extraction forceps should not be used

168. The placement of an esophagostomy feeding tube benefits the dental patient after which procedure?
a. Routine cleaning and polishing
b. Extraction of a maxillary canine tooth
c. Mandibulectomy or maxillectomy
d. Excisional biopsy of a 3-mm epulis

169. What breed would be associated with a dolichocephalic head shape?
a. German shepherd
b. Seal point Siamese
c. Persian
d. Corgi

170. For what is crown reduction and restoration used?
a. Care for the tooth affected by near pulpal exposure
b. Care for the tooth affected by pulpal exposure
c. Tooth affected by Stage 3 periodontal disease
d. A palatal trauma caused by a lingually displaced mandibular canine

171. What breed is prone to lip fold dermatitis?
a. Bulldogs
b. Chihuahuas
c. Labradors
d. Miniature pinschers

172. Which of the following mm increments do periodontal probes with Williams markings have?
a. 1, 2, 3, 4, 5, 6, 7, 8, 9, 10, 11, 12, 13, 14, 15
b. 1, 2, 3, 4, 5, 7, 8, 9, 10
c. 3, 6, 8
d. 1, 2, 3, 5, 7, 8, 9, 10

173. When conducting a tooth-by-tooth evaluation with dental radiographs, when is the client given the total estimate for care?
 a. On the telephone when the appointment is made
 b. In the examination room
 c. When the animal is picked up after treatment
 d. After the evaluation is completed while the patient is still anesthetized
174. Local antibiotic therapy is provided:
 a. Intravenously
 b. Into a foramen
 c. Into the periodontal pocket
 d. Subcutaneously
175. What is epinephrine's role in local anesthesia in relation to a dental procedure?
 a. Prolongs the anesthetic through vasoconstriction
 b. Prolongs the anesthetic through vasodilation
 c. Helps the heart beat regularly
 d. Has no effect in local anesthesia
176. Which disease causes a cat to start spontaneously and aggressively pawing at its face and mouth and to cry out in pain?
 a. Tooth resorption
 b. Chronic ulcerative gingivostomatitis
 c. Squamous cell carcinoma
 d. Orofacial pain syndrome
177. Which material is used to fill the pulp chamber inside the tooth during root canal therapy?
 a. Gutta percha
 b. Dental cement
 c. Calcium hydroxide
 d. Acrylic resin
178. What is the least effective method of local anesthesia in dental patients?
 a. Rostral maxillary block
 b. Rostral mandibular block
 c. Infiltration or splash block
 d. Caudal mandibular block
179. What is the most common cause of dental malocclusions?
 a. Retained deciduous teeth
 b. Overbite
 c. Skeletal defects
 d. Bad breeding
180. What inheritable oral condition, causing a non-neoplastic bone formation, is primarily seen in West Highland white terriers?
 a. Mandibular periostitis ossificans
 b. Cranial mandibular osteodystrophy
 c. Odontoma
 d. Osteomyelitis
181. When referring to dental-related conditions, staging is a method of:
 a. Classifying tumors
 b. Planning periodontal care
 c. Planning surgical care for cancerous tumors
 d. Determining the size of a tumor
182. Equine cheek teeth are used primarily for:
 a. Grinding and mastication
 b. Prehension and cutting of food
 c. Defense and offense
 d. All of the above
183. In horses, the term coronal refers to which portion of the tooth?
 a. The area of the tooth farthest away from the occlusal surface
 b. The area closest to the tongue
 c. The crown
 d. The tooth closest to the incisors
184. Which of the following statements is true regarding the teeth of equine patients?
 a. Brachydont teeth fully erupt before maturity and are normally long and hard enough to survive for the life of the individual.
 b. Brachydont teeth do not fully erupt before maturity; however, they are hard enough to survive for the life of the individual.
 c. Brachydont teeth fully erupt before maturity; however, they are not hard enough to survive for the life of the individual.
 d. Hypsodont teeth do not have a limited time of growth.
185. Teeth that grow throughout an equine patient's life are termed:
 a. Brachydont
 b. Hypsodont
 c. Anelodont
 d. Elodont
186. How many deciduous teeth do horses have?
 a. 20
 b. 24
 c. 36
 d. 44
187. How many incisors are present in the adult equine patient?
 a. 6
 b. 12
 c. 24
 d. 36
188. Canine teeth are always present in which of the following patients?
 a. Donkeys
 b. Female horses
 c. Male horses
 d. All of the above
189. At what age do premolars erupt in foals?
 a. Foals are born with teeth
 b. 5–7 days after birth
 c. 3–4 weeks after birth
 d. 3–4 months after birth
190. An adult equine mouth normally contains ______ cheek teeth.
 a. 12
 b. 20
 c. 24
 d. 34
191. Which teeth are the most appropriate for determining the age of horses?
 a. Incisors
 b. Wolf teeth
 c. Premolars
 d. Molars

192. All of the following factors must be considered when aging a horse *except*:
a. Breed
b. Quantity of food
c. Environmental conditions
d. Injury

193. Parrot mouth in foals is also known as an:
a. Underbite
b. Overbite
c. Overjet
d. Underjet

194. Dental dysplasia is the abnormal development of teeth that involve which of the following?
a. Crown
b. Roots
c. The entire tooth
d. Pulp

195. All of the following are common soft-tissue neoplasms seen in horses *except*:
a. Squamous cell carcinoma
b. Sarcoid
c. Ossifying fibroma
d. Osteoma

196. All of the following are common non-neoplastic conditions seen in the oral cavity of horses *except*:
a. Cementoma
b. Polyps
c. Papilloma
d. Epulis

197. Which of the following antiseptics is considered choice oral rinses for horses?
a. Chlorhexidine gluconate
b. Chlorhexidine acetate
c. Dilute betadine
d. Glutaraldehyde

198. When using motorized equipment for an equine prophylaxis, which speed should be used to prevent thermal damage?
a. 100–200 rpm
b. 2000–3000 rpm
c. 3000–4000 rpm
d. 4000–5000 rpm

199. Which of the following safety items should be used when operating motorized dental instruments on the equine patient?
a. Protective eyewear
b. Air filter mask
c. Ear protection
d. All of the above

200. All of the following instruments may be used to remove deciduous cheek tooth remnants *except*:
a. Forceps
b. Elevators
c. Gelpi retractors
d. Dental picks

201. Which of the following instruments should be used to reduce the crown of sharp canine teeth?
a. Nippers
b. Cutters
c. Small files
d. Elevators

202. Which of the following patients would benefit from prophylactic antibiotics?
a. A 1-year-old Yorkshire terrier with Stage 2 periodontal disease
b. A 10-year-old King Charles spaniel with cardiomyopathy
c. A 5-year-old gelding
d. All of the listed patients would benefit from prophylactic antibiotics.

203. Which of the following options are best suited for rinsing a mouth before a dental prophy?
a. 10% dilute betadine solution
b. 0.12% Chlorhexidine gluconate
c. 50% dilute ampicillin solution
d. There is no need to rinse a mouth before a prophylaxis, but rinsing should be done after the procedure is completed.

204. What is a common cause of pain/discomfort and severe oral pathology in dental patients?
a. Malocclusion
b. Periodontal disease
c. Stomatitis
d. Gingival recession

205. All of the following would be considered part of an oral assessment *except*:
a. Facial bones and zygomatic arch
b. Temporomandibular joint
c. Popliteal lymph nodes
d. Salivary glands

206. When inspecting the mucous membranes during an oral assessment, which of the following should be looked at?
a. Vesicle formation and ulceration
b. Gingival recession
c. Tonsillary crypts
d. Fauces

207. When inspecting the pathology of a patient during an oral assessment, which of the following should be looked at?
a. Vesicle formation and ulceration
b. Gingival recession
c. Tonsillary crypts
d. Fauces

208. When assessing and quantifying gingivitis, the modified Löe and Silness index is often referred to. According to this index, a gingival index 2 indicates:
a. Clinically healthy gingiva
b. Mild gingivitis with slight reddening and swelling of the gingival margins
c. Moderate gingivitis with gentle probing resulting in bleeding
d. Severe gingivitis in which there is spontaneous hemorrhage and/or ulceration of the gingival margin

209. Which of the following is the correct dental term/definition describing a tooth surface?
a. Mesial: farthest from the midline
b. Mesial: nearest the front
c. Distal: nearest the midline
d. Distal: farthest from the midline

210. A curette:
a. Is used strictly as a supragingival instrument
b. Can be used either supragingivally or subgingivally
c. Is used to remove microetchants on the tooth surface after power scaling
d. Is used to irrigate the teeth with air or water

211. When grading furcation involvement, which of the following descriptions would be termed Grade 2?
a. There is no furcation involvement.
b. The furcation can be felt with the probe/explorer, but horizontal tissue destruction is <⅓ of the horizontal width.
c. The furcation can be explored, but the probe cannot pass through it.
d. The probe can be passed through the furcation from buccal to palatal/lingual.

212. The dental formula for the permanent teeth in dogs is 2 (I 3/3 and C 1/1) in addition to:
a. P 3/4 and M 3/2 = 40
b. P 3/4 and M 3/3 = 42
c. P 4/4 and M 2/3 = 42
d. P 4/4 and M 3/2 = 42

213. What term identifies the hard, mineralized substance on the tooth surface?
a. Plaque
b. Attrition
c. Calculus
d. Abrasion

214. When grading tooth mobility, which of the following corresponds to Grade 1?
a. No mobility
b. Horizontal movement <1 mm
c. Horizontal movement >1 mm
d. Vertical and horizontal movement

215. What is the main purpose of premolar teeth?
a. Holding and tearing
b. Cutting and breaking
c. Grinding
d. Gnawing and grooming

216. The instrument used to measure pocket depth is a periodontal ________________.
a. Explorer
b. Scaler
c. Curette
d. Probe

217. Abbreviations are commonly used in veterinary practice and some abbreviations are exclusive to dental terminology. Which abbreviation best aligns with the uncomplicated crown fracture?
a. CCF
b. UCF
c. UCRF
d. CCRF

218. Which of the following is an incorrect dental term/definition for describing a tooth surface?
a. Palatal
b. Labial
c. Buccal
d. Rostral

219. Fluoride accomplishes all of the following *except*?
a. Desensitizing the tooth
b. Providing antibacterial activity
c. Strengthening the enamel
d. Strengthening the periodontal ligament

220. Which statement is true?
a. Full oral examination is only possible without general anesthesia.
b. Oral examination should proceed in an orderly and structured fashion, using appropriate instrumentation.
c. Adequate recording should take place at the end of the prophy, preferably on published or adapted dental charting systems.
d. One radiograph should be obtained to complement visual assessments; for example, gingival index, periodontal probing depth, or periodontal/clinical attachment level.

221. Which of the following statements is false?
a. Radiography is mandatory for good dental practice.
b. Intraoral technique using parallel and bisecting angle views is essential for meaningful results to be obtained.
c. Dental x-ray machines and digital software and hardware are ideal and such equipment proves convenient and cost-effective.
d. Full mouth radiographs (1–2 views) are strongly advocated in cats to detect odontoclastic resorptive lesions.

222. Anodontia is defined as:
a. Congenital absence of many, but not all, teeth
b. Total absence of teeth
c. Absence of only a few teeth
d. Cleft palate

223. How many maxillary and mandibular premolars does the cat have in one half of the mouth?
a. 3 in the maxilla and 2 in the mandible
b. 3 in the maxilla and 3 in the mandible
c. 2 in the maxilla and 3 in the mandible
d. 2 in the maxilla and 2 in the mandible

224. Which of the following species does *not* have continually growing teeth?
a. Equine
b. Rabbit
c. Rat
d. Cat

225. The primary difference between primary and permanent teeth is:
a. There is no difference in size between primary and permanent teeth.
b. Primary teeth are smaller than permanent teeth, with short, stubby roots.
c. Primary teeth are larger than permanent teeth, with long slender roots.
d. Primary teeth are smaller than permanent teeth, with long, slender roots.

226. Enamel hypoplasia is also referred to as:
a. Dysplasia
b. Odontalgia
c. Anodontia
d. Oligodontia

227. Which of the following systemic factors may affect enamel development?
a. Nutritional deficiency
b. Febrile disorders
c. Hypocalcemia
d. All of the above

228. Local factors that could affect enamel development include all of the following *except*:
a. Trauma
b. Infection
c. Bite injury
d. Hypocalcemia

229. Medium- and large-breed dogs are most commonly affected by dental decay, which is also known as:
a. Trauma
b. Enamel hypoplasia
c. Caries
d. Furcation

230. Which of the following statements regarding common oral conditions is false?
a. Osteomyelitis requires differentiation from neoplasia.
b. The most common malignant oral tumors are malignant melanomas and squamous cell carcinomas.
c. Most epulides are neoplastic.
d. Odontogenic tumors are benign neoplasms arising from odontogenic tissues.

231. Periodontal disease is the result of the inflammatory process from:
a. Dental plaque
b. Systemic bacteria
c. Systemic lupus
d. Chronic stomatitis

232. The inflammatory reactions in periodontitis result in the destruction of which of the following structures?
a. Periodontal ligament
b. Alveolar bone
c. Tooth enamel
d. a and b

233. How long does it take plaque to accumulate on a clean tooth surface?
a. Minutes
b. Hours
c. Days
d. Weeks

234. What is the first sign that alerts owners to the fact that their pet may have dental disease?
a. Periodontal disease
b. Gingivitis
c. Halitosis
d. Visualization of plaque

235. A pseudopocket can be defined as:
a. Deep pocket
b. Shallow pocket
c. False pocket
d. Missing a pocket

236. The veterinary technician's role in treating periodontal disease includes all of the following *except*:
a. Supragingival scaling
b. Subgingival scaling
c. Subgingival lavage
d. Periodontal surgery

237. Which of the following statements is false?
a. Gingivitis is reversible.
b. If owners brush their pet's teeth with a toothbrush and pet toothpaste, gingivitis can be prevented/reduced.
c. Dental cleanings do not need to be performed under general anesthesia to reduce the incidence of gingivitis.
d. Untreated gingivitis may lead to periodontitis.

238. When scaling a tooth that has a large amount of calculus, the process should occur in which order?
a. Remove gross dental deposits with rongeurs or extraction forceps; remove residual supragingival deposits with hand instruments; use power scaler to remove remaining deposits.
b. Remove residual supragingival deposits with hand instruments; use power scaler to remove deposits; remove gross dental deposits with rongeurs or extraction forceps.
c. Use power scaler to remove calculus buildup and deposits; remove gross dental deposits with rongeurs or extraction forceps; remove residual supragingival deposits with hand instruments.
d. A three-step process is not needed, and a power scale will remove all calculi.

239. Which of the following statements regarding teeth polishing is false?
a. Scaling, even when performed correctly, will cause minor scratches of the tooth.
b. A rough surface will impede plaque retention.
c. Polishing smooths the roughness and helps remove any remaining plaque and stained pellicle.
d. Polishing is performed by applying a mildly abrasive prophylaxis paste to the tooth surface with a prophylaxis cup mounted in a slowly rotating low-speed handpiece.

240. Why would a veterinary technician lavage a pathological pocket with chlorhexidine?
a. To remove bacteria
b. To remove free-floating debris
c. To prevent the formation of an abscess
d. All of the above

241. All of the following dental conditions could be avoided with preventive care *except*:
a. Periodontal disease
b. Stomatitis
c. Excessive wear
d. Tooth fracture

242. An owner's goal when providing oral home care is:
a. Suprascaling
b. To remove or reduce the accumulation of plaque
c. Subgingival lavage
d. All of the above

243. Which of the following is the single most effective means of removing plaque?
a. Tooth brushing
b. Toothpaste
c. Dental diets
d. All of the above

244. Why is human toothpaste *not* recommended for pets?
a. Pets do not like the taste.
b. It foams and pets do not like that sensation in their mouths.
c. The fluoride content is too high.
d. The salt content is too high.

245. When brushing a pet-patient's teeth, which angle should the brush be held at?
a. 20 degrees
b. 35 degrees
c. 45 degrees
d. 65 degrees

246. A common cause of excessive wear and abrasion in teeth is:
a. Stone chewing
b. Playing ball
c. Loss of teeth
d. All of the above

247. All of the following are preventative measures that can be taken to prevent malocclusion *except*:
a. Extraction of persistent primary teeth
b. Interceptive orthodontics
c. Extraction of persistent permanent teeth
d. A removable orthodontic device

248. Which of the following correctly describes the lagomorph dental formula?
a. 2 × {I 2/1:C 0/0:P 3/2:M 3/3}
b. 2 × {I 3/3:C 1/1:P 4/4:M 2/3}
c. 2 × {I 3/3:C 1/1:P 3/2:M 1/1}
d. 2 × {I 3/3:C 1/1:P 3/3}

249. The heaviest calculus deposition in dogs and cats is typically located on the:
a. Lingual surfaces of the lower cheek teeth
b. Lower canine teeth
c. Incisor teeth
d. Buccal surfaces of the upper cheek teeth

250. The surface of the tooth toward the tongue is:
a. Lingual
b. Labial
c. Buccal
d. Mesial

251. Most abnormal dental conditions experienced by lagomorphs and rodents are a result of:
a. Diet
b. Environment
c. Husbandry
d. All of the above

252. The purpose of polishing during the dental prophy is to:
a. Massage the gums
b. Smooth out the rough areas and retard plaque formation
c. Apply fluoride
d. Disinfect the surface of the tooth

253. The most common benign soft-tissue tumor of the oral cavity is a/an:
a. Epulis
b. Fibrosarcoma
c. Malignant melanoma
d. Squamous cell carcinoma

254. The correct dental formula for an adult dog is:
a. 2(I 3/3 C 1/1 P 3/4 M 3/3) = 42
b. 2(I 3/3 C 1/1 P 4/4 M 3/2) = 42
c. 2(I 3/3 C 1/1 P 4/4 M 2/3) = 42
d. 2(I 4/4 C 1/1 P 3/4 M 3/3) = 46

255. The correct dental formula for an adult cat is:
a. 2(I 3/3 C 1/1 P 3/2 M 1/1) = 30
b. 2(I 4/4 C 1/1 P 2/3 M 1/1) = 34
c. 2(I 3/3 C 1/1 P 2/3 M 1/1) = 30
d. 2(I 3/3 C 1/1 P 3/2 M 2/1) = 32

SECTION 8

Laboratory Procedures

Rachel Poulin

QUESTIONS

1. What is the morphology of *Vibrio* spp. bacteria?
   a. Bacillus
   b. Coccus
   c. Spirochete
   d. Coccobacillus
2. All of the following are important functions of bacterial fimbriae *except*:
   a. Attachment
   b. Locomotion
   c. Ion transport
   d. Antibiotic resistance
3. Bacterial endospores are:
   a. Resistant to heat and desiccation
   b. A form of asexual reproduction
   c. A consequence of mating
   d. Highly susceptible to antiseptics
4. Blood levels of total bilirubin will *not* be a significant finding in:
   a. Hepatocellular damage
   b. Bile duct injury or obstruction
   c. Hemolytic disorders
   d. Acute pancreatitis
5. A bacterial genus can best be described as:
   a. Composed of one or more species
   b. Composed of classes
   c. Composed of families
   d. Belonging to a species
6. An iodine scrub on skin would result in:
   a. Antisepsis
   b. Disinfection
   c. Fumigation
   d. Sterilization
7. Which of the following would be a parenteral route of pathogen transmission?
   a. Transfusion
   b. Contaminated food
   c. Droplet infection
   d. Direct contact
8. Most bacteria grow best at a pH of:
   a. 1
   b. 3
   c. 9
   d. 7
9. Which of the following is an important function of bacterial flagella?
   a. Attachment
   b. Locomotion
   c. DNA replication
   d. Ion transport
10. Which parasite only uses the cat as its definitive host?
    a. *Toxoplasma gondii*
    b. *Giardia lamblia*
    c. *Isospora rivolta*
    d. *Balantidium coli*
11. _________ is the temperature that must be reached and maintained for 13 minutes in a steam autoclave to destroy microorganisms.
    a. 110°C
    b. 121°C
    c. 170°C
    d. 240°C
12. With which of the following is the humoral immune system involved?
    a. Monocytes
    b. B cells
    c. T cells
    d. Erythrocytes
13. Which of the following is a lentivirus?
    a. Coronavirus
    b. Feline immunodeficiency virus (FIV)
    c. Herpes virus
    d. Parvovirus
14. Which of the following is *not* a method of culturing animal viruses?
    a. Laboratory animal inoculation
    b. Cell culture
    c. Agar plate inoculation
    d. Embryonated egg inoculation
15. What immunoglobulin is usually present in the greatest quantity?
    a. IgA
    b. IgD
    c. IgE
    d. IgG
16. Blood levels of total bilirubin are used primarily to evaluate the function of the:
    a. Kidneys
    b. Liver
    c. Pancreas
    d. Bile ducts
17. Phagocytes are a type of:
    a. Red blood cell
    b. White blood cell
    c. Platelet
    d. Antibody

18. A hospital-acquired disease is known as:
 a. Endemic
 b. Nosocomial
 c. Ergasteric
 d. Iatrogenic
19. Leukopenia is defined as:
 a. A decrease in white blood cells
 b. An increase in white blood cells
 c. A bone marrow disease
 d. A type of blood cancer
20. What laboratory test evaluates kidney function and is a breakdown product of protein?
 a. Glucose
 b. SGTP (ALT)
 c. Creatinine
 d. BUN
21. The function of hemolysins is to:
 a. Coagulate blood
 b. Break down fibrin
 c. Destroy red blood cells
 d. Indicate a viral infection
22. Nonrenal causes of increased levels of urea might include:
 a. The amount of carbohydrate ingested
 b. The amount of protein ingested
 c. Insufficient insulin
 d. Insufficient ADH
23. A decrease in albumin may occur in cases experiencing:
 a. Chronic liver disease
 b. A carnivorous diet
 c. Gastroenteritis
 d. A vegetarian diet
24. To what color does "icteric serum" refer?
 a. Yellow
 b. Red
 c. Brown
 d. Green
25. What color are blood collection tubes that contain heparin?
 a. Purple
 b. Green
 c. Blue
 d. Gray
26. Which of the following substances is used to evaluate kidney filtration and function, is excreted, and is then reabsorbed?
 a. Urea
 b. Creatinine
 c. Glucose
 d. Sodium
27. With significant dehydration in an otherwise healthy patient, which of the following would probably appear on a urinalysis and CBC?
 a. Increased urine SG and increased PCV
 b. Increased urine SG and decreased PCV
 c. Decreased urine SG and decreased PCV
 d. Decreased urine SG and increased PCV
28. Water deprivation tests should never be performed on patients with:
 a. High MCV
 b. Suspected sufficient ADH
 c. Dehydration
 d. Suspected tubular malfunction
29. Glycosuria exists:
 a. When blood glucose levels exceed the renal threshold for absorption of glucose
 b. When blood glucose levels are lower than the renal threshold for absorption of glucose
 c. When urine glucose levels are lower than the renal threshold for absorption of glucose
 d. When urine glucose levels are higher than the serum threshold for absorption of glucose
30. Horses typically have higher __________ values than other species.
 a. AST
 b. ALP
 c. ALT
 d. GGT
31. What blood chemistry test should be used to measure cholangiocyte damage?
 a. ALKP
 b. AST
 c. ALT
 d. GGT
32. Which method is commonly used to measure electrolytes?
 a. Ion-specific electrodes
 b. Refractometry
 c. Adsorption
 d. Enzymatic digestion
33. A test that can be performed to help diagnose hyperthyroidism is:
 a. LH
 b. Cortisol
 c. Bile acids
 d. T4
34. When performing urinalysis testing, the sample should be analyzed within ___ minutes, otherwise refrigeration is required.
 a. 10
 b. 20
 c. 30
 d. 40
35. For cytological evaluation of urine, which of the following conditions should be observed?
 a. The specimen should be refrigerated as soon as possible.
 b. The specimen should be centrifuged as soon as possible.
 c. The specimen may sit at room temperature for ≤6 hours.
 d. The specimen may be frozen for later analysis.
36. The average urine specific gravity for a healthy adult dog is __________.
 a. 1.025
 b. 1.035
 c. 1.04
 d. 1.045
37. The average urine specific gravity for a healthy adult cat is ___________.
 a. 1.025
 b. 1.03
 c. 1.035
 d. 1.04

38. Which of the following tests is *not* included in a routine CBC?
   a. Total WBC count
   b. Differential WBC count
   c. Total protein
   d. Reticulocyte count

39. Ketonuria is most commonly associated with what condition?
   a. Liver disease
   b. Urinary tract infection
   c. Renal failure
   d. Diabetes mellitus

40. Hoover, a canine patient, was diagnosed with a urinary tract infection 2 weeks earlier and was placed on a course of amoxicillin. The veterinarian asked that he return for a recheck to ensure the infection has resolved. The collection method of choice is:
   a. Catheterization
   b. Free catch
   c. Cystocentesis
   d. Manual expression

41. Leukocytes in the urine sediment and a positive nitrite reaction on the urinary colorimetric strip provide presumptive evidence that the patient might have a:
   a. Neoplasm
   b. Diabetic condition
   c. Renal failure
   d. Bacterial infection

42. Aged urine samples left at room temperature and exposed to UV light may cause a false-negative result in which of the following biochemical tests?
   a. Ketones
   b. Protein
   c. Glucose
   d. Bilirubin

43. Which of the following is the best time to collect a urine sample to evaluate the specific gravity of a canine patient?
   a. First morning sample
   b. Midday sample
   c. Late afternoon sample
   d. Last sample of the day

44. Mr. Downing has brought in a urine sample from Cleo, his 6-year-old female spayed cocker spaniel. The color of the urine appears red. On centrifugation of the sample, you find that the supernatant is now clear. What was the most likely cause of the red color?
   a. Hemoglobinuria
   b. Hematuria
   c. Myoglobinuria
   d. Uroglobinuria

45. Urinary pH is *not* affected by the:
   a. Patient's diet
   b. Presence of bacteria in the urine
   c. Patient's acid-base status
   d. Presence of crystals in the urine

46. Squamous epithelial cells are *not* normally seen in urine samples obtained by:
   a. Catheterization
   b. Manual expression
   c. Free catch
   d. Cystocentesis

47. The two most common problems encountered in samples to be evaluated for clinical chemistry are:
   a. Coagulation and separation
   b. Dilution and concentration
   c. Hemolysis and lipemia
   d. EDTA and heparin

48. What biochemical tests are *not* considered part of a primary hepatic profile?
   a. BUN and creatinine
   b. Cholestatic enzymes
   c. Hepatocellular leakage enzymes
   d. Total protein and albumin

49. A fecal smear can be stained for fat. An increased amount of fat is indicative of:
   a. Dyschezia
   b. Dysentery
   c. Steatorrhea
   d. Tenesmus

50. Which is the correct method to use when performing a serum bile acids assay?
   a. Draw a blood sample on a fasting animal
   b. Draw a blood sample on an animal immediately after it eats a meal
   c. Draw a blood sample on a fasting animal and another sample 2 hours later
   d. Draw a blood sample on a fasting animal, feed the animal, and draw another sample 2 hours later

51. The current test of choice for evaluating liver function is:
   a. Ammonia assay
   b. Bile acids
   c. Bilirubin
   d. Alanine aminotransferase

52. Total protein levels are __________ in a dehydrated animal.
   a. Unaffected
   b. Decreased
   c. Increased
   d. Variable

53. Which of the following crystals is most likely to be found in the urine of an animal with ethylene glycol toxicity?
   a. Ammonium biurate
   b. Tyrosine
   c. Triple phosphate
   d. Calcium oxalate

54. What species has multiple forms of reticulocytes?
   a. Horse
   b. Cow
   c. Cat
   d. Dog

55. The etiologic agent of Lyme disease is:
   a. *Borrelia burgdorferi*
   b. Coronavirus
   c. Lentivirus
   d. *Pasteurella multocida*

56. Which of these tubes must never be placed on a blood rocker after being filled with blood?
   a. Blue top
   b. Green top
   c. Purple top
   d. Red top

57. Which of the following options is least likely to interfere with blood chemistry test results?
   a. Postprandial serum
   b. Icteric serum
   c. Fasting serum
   d. Hemolyzed serum

58. Where on the blood smear would you select to start your WBC differential count?
   a. Thickest area
   b. Feathered edge
   c. Monocellular layer
   d. Thinnest area

59. In which of the following species is rouleaux formation common?
   a. Rats
   b. Dogs
   c. Horses
   d. Pigs

60. Serum chemistry tests for acute pancreatitis include:
   a. Amylase and lipase
   b. Lipase and trypsin
   c. Amylase and trypsin
   d. Amylase, lipase, and trypsin

61. Pollakiuria is defined as:
   a. Frequent urination with small volume voided
   b. Complete lack of urine production
   c. Excessive drinking and urinating
   d. Excessive urination at night

62. Which of the following might be indicated by an elevated hematocrit?
   a. Hyperglycemia
   b. Anemia
   c. Dehydration
   d. Leukocytosis

63. Which of the following results may be found in a patient with a degenerative left shift?
   a. Leukocytosis
   b. No bands are present
   c. Lymphocytes outnumber neutrophils
   d. Bands outnumber mature neutrophils

64. Which of the following options is another term for icterus?
   a. Jaundice
   b. Xanthochromia
   c. Ketonemia
   d. Hemoglobinuria

65. Bile acids aid in the digestion of:
   a. Proteins
   b. Carbohydrates
   c. Fats
   d. Globulins

66. When considering hematology tests, clots in an EDTA sample are:
   a. Acceptable if they are microscopic
   b. Acceptable if they are detected on a wooden stick only
   c. Acceptable if they are run through an automatic analyzer
   d. Never acceptable

67. Which is least likely to be a clinical sign of a patient experiencing allergies?
   a. Face rubbing
   b. Ear problems
   c. Loss of appetite
   d. Skin rashes

68. On a complete blood count (CBC), all of the following findings could be expected in a patient with an infection *except*
   a. Neutrophilia
   b. Leukocytosis
   c. Narrow buffy coat
   d. A left shift

69. To make a smear with anemic blood,
   a. Increase the angle of the pusher slide
   b. Decrease the angle of the pusher slide
   c. Use a larger drop of blood
   d. Wait for the drop of blood to dry partially

70. Which of the red blood cell indices indicates cell size?
   a. MCH
   b. MCHC
   c. MCV
   d. MPV

71. A correction for nucleated red blood cells (nRBC) is done to avoid a falsely:
   a. Elevated PCV
   b. Elevated WBC count
   c. Decreased PCV
   d. Decreased WBC count

72. RBCs with multiple, irregularly spaced projections are known as:
   a. Crenated cells
   b. Schistocytes
   c. Acanthocytes
   d. Anisocytes

73. Reticulocytes on a modified Wright stain (e.g., Diff-Quik) appear:
   a. Polychromatic
   b. Hypochromic
   c. Hyperchromic
   d. Crenated

74. What is the most useful way to report WBC differential results?
   a. As percentages
   b. As relative numbers
   c. As absolute numbers
   d. As decimal numbers

75. Determination of which of the following is useful in the detection of inflammatory processes?
   a. Total protein
   b. Hematocrit
   c. RBC morphology
   d. Fibrinogen

76. The buffy coat in a spun hematocrit tube consists of:
   a. WBCs
   b. WBCs and platelets
   c. WBCs and NRBCs
   d. Platelets and NRBCs

77. Postrenal azotemia refers to:
   a. An increase in BUN resulting from severe liver disease
   b. An increase in BUN resulting from the inability to urinate
   c. A decrease in BUN resulting from severe renal disease
   d. An increase in BUN resulting from dehydration
78. What cells are phagocytic?
   a. Granulocytes
   b. Lymphocytes
   c. Neutrophils and macrophages
   d. Macrophages and lymphocytes
79. Monocytes typically have:
   a. Segmented nuclei
   b. Band-shaped nuclei
   c. Lobular nuclei
   d. No nuclei
80. Which of the following options would *not* affect a manual WBC count?
   a. Condenser in the farthest "up" position
   b. Length of time that the hemocytometer has been loaded
   c. Objective lens used
   d. Mini clots in the blood
81. Which of the following options is *not* a sign of RBC regeneration?
   a. Polychromasia
   b. Nuclear remnants
   c. Spherocytes
   d. Anisocytosis with macrocytosis
82. A left shift refers to increased numbers of:
   a. Immature neutrophils
   b. Immature RBCs
   c. Immature platelets
   d. Immature lymphocytes
83. What special stain would be used in assessing anemia?
   a. Lactophenol cotton blue
   b. New methylene blue
   c. Gram
   d. Acridine orange
84. Which of the following is the most immature erythrocyte?
   a. Rubricyte
   b. Metarubricyte
   c. Rubriblast
   d. Reticulocyte
85. The intermediate host for heartworms is the:
   a. Flea
   b. Rodent
   c. Mosquito
   d. Snail
86. Serology tests can detect heartworms in a dog's blood:
   a. Immediately after becoming infected
   b. Several days after becoming infected
   c. Several weeks after becoming infected
   d. Several months after becoming infected
87. What are the two diagnostic forms of Giardia?
   a. Cysts and trophozoites
   b. Merozoites and schizonts
   c. Oocysts and sporocysts
   d. Ova and L3 larvae
88. Compared with roundworm ova, coccidia appear:
   a. Smaller
   b. The same size
   c. Twice as large
   d. Three times as large
89. In a healthy animal, diminished water intake or loss of water would result in __________ urine specific gravity.
   a. Increased
   b. Decreased
   c. Isosthenuric
   d. Isotonic
90. What urine sediment component would be of the most significant concern?
   a. Sperm
   b. Fat droplets
   c. Squamous epithelial cells
   d. Blood cells
91. Struvite crystals are also known as:
   a. Calcium carbonate crystals
   b. Calcium oxalate crystals
   c. Triple phosphate crystals
   d. Amorphous phosphate crystals
92. Crystals in urine sediment often indicate:
   a. Uroliths
   b. Nothing
   c. Inflammation
   d. Urethral blockage
93. Which of the following test results are *not* determined by a urine dipstick?
   a. Glucose
   b. Blood
   c. Total protein
   d. BUN
94. Casts that are seen in urine sediment are:
   a. Mucous threads filled with amorphous sediment
   b. Always significant
   c. Formed in the renal tubules
   d. Artifacts
95. The presence of protein in the urine may indicate:
   a. Acid-base imbalance
   b. Hemolytic anemia
   c. Kidney disease
   d. Diabetes mellitus
96. Which of these would *not* be associated with ketones in the urine?
   a. Diabetes mellitus
   b. Lactating cows
   c. Starvation
   d. Hemolysis
97. Mucus is normally seen in __________ urine.
   a. Canine
   b. Equine
   c. Feline
   d. Bovine

98. The appearance of calcium oxalate crystals is described as:
   a. Hexagonal
   b. Dark, needle-like rods
   c. Brown spheres with long spicules
   d. Small squares that contain an X
99. A common laboratory test for chronic pancreatitis is a fecal test for:
   a. Amylase
   b. Lipase
   c. Trypsin
   d. Bilirubin
100. Fat droplets in urine samples are most commonly seen in:
   a. Dogs
   b. Cats
   c. Horses
   d. Cows
101. Gram-negative bacteria retain what component of the Gram stain?
   a. Crystal violet
   b. Iodine solution
   c. Decolorizer
   d. Safranin
102. What gram-negative bacteria may "swarm" a blood agar plate, leaving a film over the entire surface?
   a. *Pseudomonas* sp.
   b. *Staphylococcus* sp.
   c. *Proteus* sp.
   d. *Escherichia coli*
103. What microorganism is frequently recovered from the ears of dogs with chronic otitis externa?
   a. *Candida* sp.
   b. *Cryptococcus* sp.
   c. *Microsporum* sp.
   d. *Malassezia* sp.
104. What microorganism is an etiologic agent of ringworm?
   a. *Microsporum* sp.
   b. *Mycobacterium* sp.
   c. *Micrococcus* sp.
   d. *Moraxella* sp.
105. Which species includes common contaminants and is the causative agent of anthrax?
   a. *Escherichia*
   b. *Corynebacterium*
   c. *Bacillus*
   d. *Enterobacter*
106. What is a common pathogen in mastitis, skin wounds, and abscesses that is also found in the environment?
   a. *Proteus vulgaris*
   b. *Escherichia coli*
   c. *Streptococcus* spp.
   d. *Staphylococcus aureus*
107. Stress and epinephrine release in cats might cause an increase in:
   a. BUN
   b. Total protein
   c. ALT
   d. Glucose
108. A kidney function test that has been found useful in birds and Dalmatians is:
   a. BUN
   b. Creatinine
   c. Uric acid
   d. AST
109. What serum component can be used as a screening test for hypothyroidism?
   a. ALT
   b. Cholesterol
   c. Total protein
   d. Creatine kinase
110. During a glucose tolerance test, glucose levels in a diabetic animal will:
   a. Show an initial peak and then diminish to normal
   b. Remain high throughout the test
   c. Show a delayed peak at the end of the test period
   d. Show below normal levels throughout the test
111. What organ conserves nutrients, removes waste products, maintains blood pH, and controls blood pressure?
   a. Kidney
   b. Liver
   c. Pancreas
   d. Spleen
112. The small intestine receives digestive enzymes from the:
   a. Kidney
   b. Pancreas
   c. Liver
   d. Spleen
113. Bile acids aid in the absorption of:
   a. Proteins
   b. Carbohydrates
   c. Fats
   d. Globulins
114. Fibrinogen is produced in the:
   a. Pancreas
   b. Bone marrow
   c. Liver
   d. Spleen
115. Which of the following samples can be frozen and successfully thawed for performing an analytic test at a later time?
   a. Feces for a fecal float test
   b. Whole blood for chemistry testing
   c. Serum for chemistry testing
   d. Whole blood for a CBC
116. If there is only a small amount of serum separated after centrifuging a tube of whole blood (and you need more for testing), what should you do?
   a. Invert the tube several times and respin it
   b. Assume the patient is dehydrated and draw off all of the serum you can
   c. Spin the tube again at a faster speed and a longer time
   d. Rim/ring the clot and spin again at a normal speed and time
117. Arterial blood is most commonly used to analyze:
   a. Hematology
   b. Blood gases
   c. Blood chemistry
   d. Organ function tests

118. All of the following cells are produced in the bone marrow *except*:
a. Erythrocytes
b. Lymphocytes
c. Neutrophils
d. Eosinophils

119. Looking under a microscope at a blood smear, you see erythrocytes that are elliptical, not nucleated, and lacking central pallor. From which species was this sample most probably collected?
a. Bird
b. Horse
c. Llama
d. Snake

120. Under the microscope you observe a leukocyte that you identify as an eosinophil. The eosinophil cytoplasm contains numerous rod-shaped granules. From which species was this sample most probably collected?
a. Dog
b. Cat
c. Horse
d. Cow

121. Which of the following is a common finding on a blood smear from an animal with autoimmune hemolytic anemia?
a. Heinz bodies
b. Howell-Jolly bodies
c. Spherocytes
d. Target cells

122. Serum electrolyte levels should be determined when evaluating the function of the:
a. Liver
b. Pancreas
c. Kidneys
d. Heart

123. Kidney disease leads to the accumulation of metabolic waste in the blood, a condition known as:
a. Hypernaturia
b. Hypernatremia
c. Azotemia
d. Azoturia

124. For which of the following diagnostics is low-power magnification on the microscope *not* used?
a. To detect the presence of rouleaux
b. To detect RBC agglutination
c. To detect clumping of platelets
d. To estimate platelet numbers

125. What characteristic is *not* found in toxic neutrophils?
a. Howell-Jolly bodies
b. Vacuolated cytoplasm
c. Döhle bodies
d. Basophilic cytoplasm

126. What laboratory test evaluates primary hemostasis?
a. Activated clotting time
b. Activated partial thromboplastin time
c. Buccal mucosal bleeding time
d. One-step prothrombin time

127. Secondary hemostasis refers to:
a. The coagulation cascade
b. Vascular spasm
c. Clot lysis
d. Platelet plug formation

128. A good presurgical screening test for von Willebrand disease is a/an:
a. Total platelet count
b. Buccal mucosal bleeding time
c. Activated clotting time
d. Activated partial thromboplastin time

129. When collecting blood for a coagulation profile, it is especially important to:
a. Use a gray-top Vacutainer
b. Analyze the sample immediately
c. Use EDTA as the anticoagulant
d. Minimize vascular trauma during venipuncture

130. Physical signs of hypocoagulation include all of the following *except:*
a. Petechiae or ecchymoses
b. Epistaxis
c. Hematuria
d. Thromboembolism

131. An animal that tested positive for heartworm infection might also have an elevation of which of the following blood cells?
a. Leukocytes
b. Lymphocytes
c. Eosinophils
d. Monocytes

132. When using Diff-Quik to stain bone marrow smears, it is especially important to
a. Use freshly filtered stain
b. Dip the smear twice as long as blood smears
c. Rinse thoroughly with distilled water
d. Let the smear dry for 30 minutes before staining

133. The ability of the renal tubules to concentrate or dilute a urine sample is assessed by what component of the urinalysis?
a. pH
b. Volume
c. Specific gravity
d. Examination of the sediment

134. Which epithelial cell is the largest of the cells found in urine?
a. Squamous epithelial cells
b. Caudate epithelial cells
c. Transitional epithelial cells
d. Renal epithelial cells

135. The most common uroliths found in feline and canine urine are:
a. Struvite
b. Calcium oxalate
c. Urate
d. Cystine

136. The best urine collection method to assess the patency of the urethra is:
a. Catheterization
b. Manual expression
c. Free catch
d. Cystocentesis

137. Which of the following statements regarding casts is incorrect?
   a. A few hyaline or granular casts may be seen in normal urine.
   b. All casts are cylindric with parallel sides.
   c. Casts dissolve in acidic urine.
   d. Casts may be disrupted with high-speed centrifugation and rough sample handling.
138. Puddin, a 2-year-old castrated male domestic short-hair cat, was missing for 5 days before coming home. Because his owners were very concerned that he appeared weak and tired, they brought him to the clinic. On initial physical examination, you find that he is significantly dehydrated. You are not at all surprised when you find that his urine specific gravity is:
   a. 1.002
   b. 1.012
   c. 1.03
   d. 1.06
139. Bilirubinuria is considered a normal finding in what species?
   a. Dogs
   b. Cats
   c. Horses
   d. Sheep
140. Sadie, a 17-year-old spayed female domestic short-hair cat, is in the final stages of chronic renal failure. On presentation, you anticipate that her urine specific gravity will probably be:
   a. 1.012
   b. 1.03
   c. 1.04
   d. 1.06
141. What method of urine sample collection would *not* be associated with traumatic hematuria?
   a. Catheterization
   b. Manual expression
   c. Free catch
   d. Cystocentesis
142. Sasha, an 11-year-old spayed female domestic short-hair cat, was accidentally overhydrated with IV fluids. What would you expect her urine specific gravity to be?
   a. 1.002
   b. 1.012
   c. 1.03
   d. 1.06
143. In a diabetic animal, blood chemistry analysis is commonly performed to monitor insulin therapy by measuring blood levels of:
   a. Sodium
   b. Potassium
   c. Glucose
   d. Insulin
144. Leukocytes in the urine sediment and a positive nitrite reaction on the urinary colorimetric strip provide presumptive evidence that the patient may have a:
   a. Neoplasm
   b. Diabetic condition
   c. Renal failure
   d. Bacterial infection
145. What gland is the most active producer of corticosteroids?
   a. Thyroid gland
   b. Pancreas
   c. Pituitary gland
   d. Adrenal glands
146. In an animal with a history of bone resorption or convulsions, blood chemistry analysis is commonly performed to measure blood levels of:
   a. Calcium and phosphorus
   b. Urea nitrogen and creatinine
   c. Aspartate aminotransferase and alanine transaminase
   d. Sodium and potassium
147. The gland function that is evaluated by measuring blood cortisol levels before and after administration of adrenocorticotropic hormone (ACTH) is the:
   a. Thyroid gland
   b. Pancreas
   c. Liver
   d. Adrenal glands
148. Struvite crystals are composed of:
   a. Calcium potassium carbonates
   b. Magnesium ammonium phosphates
   c. Oxalates
   d. Urates
149. The gland that is evaluated by measuring blood levels of T3 and T4 is the:
   a. Thyroid gland
   b. Pancreas
   c. Pituitary gland
   d. Thymus
150. Measurement of blood levels of thyroid-stimulating hormone (TSH) and ACTH is used to evaluate the function of the:
   a. Thyroid gland
   b. Pancreas
   c. Pituitary gland
   d. Adrenal glands
151. Blood chemistry analysis is commonly performed to evaluate function of the _______ in an animal showing lethargy, obesity, mild anemia, infertility, and alopecia.
   a. Thyroid gland
   b. Pancreas
   c. Thymus
   d. Adrenal glands
152. Which of the following statements regarding creatinine is false?
   a. It is an indicator of the glomerular filtration rate.
   b. It is produced as a result of normal muscle metabolism.
   c. It is a less reliable indicator of renal function than BUN.
   d. It is usually evaluated in conjunction with the BUN and urine specific gravity.
153. A good initial urinary screening test for suspected Cushing's disease is:
   a. Endogenous ACTH
   b. Low-dose dexamethasone suppression test
   c. ACTH stimulation
   d. Cortisol/creatinine ratio

154. Chemistry evaluation of the kidney includes measurement of metabolic wastes in the blood in the form of:
a. Aspartate aminotransferase and alanine transaminase
b. Urea nitrogen and creatinine
c. Ammonia and pyruvic acid
d. Bilirubin and urobilinogen

155. Measurement of blood levels of amylase and lipase is used to evaluate the function of the:
a. Kidneys
b. Liver
c. Pancreas
d. Adrenal glands

156. Ammonia is metabolized by the liver and eliminated by the kidneys. Levels of which metabolic by-product of ammonia are measured to assess kidney function?
a. Phosphorus
b. Creatinine
c. Aspartate aminotransferase
d. Urea nitrogen

157. The main function of bicarbonate is to maintain which of the following?
a. The proper osmotic pressure of fluids in the body
b. Normal muscular function
c. Normal cardiac rhythm and contractility
d. Balanced body pH levels

158. Kidney disease results in accumulation of metabolic waste in the blood, a condition known as:
a. Azotemia
b. Bilirubinemia
c. Hypernatremia
d. Hyperkalemia

159. Prerenal azotemia refers to:
a. An increase in BUN resulting from severe liver disease
b. A decrease in BUN resulting from severe renal disease
c. An increase in BUN resulting from dehydration, shock, and/or decreased blood flow to the kidneys
d. An increase in BUN resulting from the inability to urinate

160. A glucose tolerance test is used to help diagnose:
a. Cushing's disease
b. Hypothyroidism
c. Addison's disease
d. Diabetes mellitus

161. Which white blood cell is known as "the first line of defense" after a microorganism has entered the body?
a. Eosinophil
b. Lymphocyte
c. Monocyte
d. Neutrophil

162. The red-top Vacutainer tube should sit at room temperature for ___ before centrifugation, allowing a clot to form.
a. 5 minutes
b. 30 minutes
c. 1 hour
d. 0 minutes (no clot will form)

163. *Dioctophyma renale* is often found in the ___ of dogs.
a. Right kidney
b. Left kidney
c. Urinary bladder
d. Ureters

164. Which of the following is the best method of preservation if you are unable to perform a CBC within 1 hour of blood collection?
a. Freeze the sample
b. Spin down the sample, refrigerate cells, and freeze serum
c. Add formalin to the sample
d. Refrigerate the sample

165. The mucin clot test is performed on:
a. Joint fluid
b. Plasma
c. Serum
d. Urine

166. Which of the following is associated with clotting disorders?
a. Anemia
b. Leukopenia
c. Thrombocytopenia
d. Reticulocytosis

167. When preparing cytology samples for microscopic evaluation, what is the best technique to use?
a. Wet prep
b. Squash prep
c. Modified Knott prep
d. Willis prep

168. Which of the following would be considered an abnormal finding on healthy canine external ear canal cytology?
a. Cerumen
b. Epithelial cells
c. Malassezia
d. Debris

169. The main function of neutrophils is:
a. Phagocytosis
b. Hypersensitivity reaction
c. Allergic reaction
d. Immune response

170. What is the primary function of eosinophils?
a. Phagocytosis
b. Respond to autoimmune reactions
c. Respond to allergic reaction
d. Initiate an immune reaction

171. How long must the typical microhematocrit tube be centrifuged for packed cell volume determination?
a. 1 minute
b. 5 minutes
c. 10 minutes
d. 15 minutes

172. What determines the average size of an erythrocyte?
a. Mean corpuscular volume
b. Packed cell volume (PCV)
c. Mean corpuscular hemoglobin concentration (MCHC)
d. Mean corpuscular hemoglobin

173. In what type of blood cell can Döhle bodies be found?
a. Erythrocytes
b. Neutrophils
c. Platelets
d. Nucleated RBCs

174. In what species are the platelets normally larger than the red blood cells?
a. Bovine
b. Canine
c. Equine
d. Feline

175. The term for red blood cell formation is:
a. Erythropoietin
b. Erythropoiesis
c. Hematopoietin
d. Leukopoiesis

176. Which sequence lists cells from most immature to most mature?
a. Rubricyte, reticulocyte, rubriblast, erythrocyte
b. Rubriblast, reticulocyte, rubricyte, erythrocyte
c. Rubriblast, rubricyte, reticulocyte, erythrocyte
d. Reticulocyte, rubriblast, rubricyte, erythrocyte

177. What test is used to diagnose autoimmune hemolytic anemia?
a. Red cell fragility test
b. Modified Knott
c. Coombs
d. Coggins

178. What term indicates an abnormally high lymphocyte count?
a. Lymphocytosis
b. Leukosis
c. Lymphocytopenia
d. Lymphosarcoma

179. It is important to keep cytology samples and unstained slides away from ______ so that the samples can be stained properly later.
a. Acetone
b. Ether
c. Formalin
d. Saline

180. Which of the following is considered a tick-borne organism found in dogs?
a. Toxoplasma
b. Isospora
c. Ehrlichia
d. Cryptosporidium

181. Which of the following terms refers to an infestation with lice?
a. Myiasis
b. Acariasis
c. Paraphimosis
d. Pediculosis

182. A skin scraping will diagnose which parasite?
a. *Bovicola*
b. *Notoedres*
c. *Otodectes*
d. *Ctenocephalides*

183. Which of the following is the largest intermediate form of a tapeworm?
a. Cysticercus
b. Hydatid cyst
c. Coenurus
d. Cysticercoid

184. What canine parasite causes nodules in the esophagus, which may then become neoplastic?
a. *Physaloptera*
b. *Filaroides*
c. *Spirocerca*
d. *Neosporum*

185. Which of the following options is *not* zoonotic?
a. *Toxoplasma*
b. *Echinococcus*
c. *Dipylidium*
d. *Giardia*

186. Observing a "zippy" motility in fresh feces is used to help diagnose the presence of what parasite?
a. *Toxoplasma*
b. *Mycoplasma (Haemobartonella)*
c. *Tritrichomonas*
d. *Ehrlichia canis*

187. Which parasite causes blood loss, especially in young animals?
a. Roundworm
b. Tapeworm
c. Heartworm
d. Hookworm

188. What parasite causes a very pruritic disease in dogs?
a. *Cheyletiella*
b. *Sarcoptes*
c. *Demodex*
d. *Dermacentor*

189. What causes the sensitivity of the occult heartworm test to decrease?
a. No microfilariae present
b. Female worms only
c. Male worms only
d. No clinical signs

190. Which statement is true about *Dirofilaria* infection in the cat?
a. The life span of heartworms in cats is shorter than in dogs.
b. Microfilariae are commonly seen in cat infections.
c. Adult worm burden in cats is similar in numbers to that in dogs.
d. *Dirofilaria* causes severe anemia in cats.

191. What is the function of a megakaryocyte?
a. Phagocytosis
b. Produces granulocytes
c. Produces thrombocytes
d. Produces plasma cells

192. Which of the following is *not* associated with a responsive anemia?
a. Poikilocytosis
b. Reticulocytosis
c. Anisocytosis
d. Polychromasia

193. What erythrocyte index provides an indication of the average size of a red blood cell?
a. MCHC
b. MCV
c. M/E ratio
d. Reticulocyte count

194. What is the most immature cell in the granulocyte series?
a. Megakaryoblast
b. Leukoblast
c. Myeloblast
d. Progranuloblast

195. What large cell with multiple separate nuclei is found in bone marrow?
a. Osteoclast
b. Megakaryocyte
c. Osteoblast
d. Monoblast

196. What marrow finding is consistent with a responsive anemia?
a. Myeloid hypoplasia
b. Erythroid hyperplasia
c. Erythroid hypoplasia
d. Myeloid metaplasia

197. Which test is used to confirm a diagnosis of warfarin (rodenticide) toxicity?
a. Thrombocyte count
b. Calcium level
c. One-step prothrombin time
d. Partial thromboplastin time (PTT)

198. Which of the following is *not* observed when a patient is in DIC?
a. Icterus
b. Hemorrhage
c. Thrombocytopenia
d. Prolonged activated clotting time

199. Which clotting disorder is stimulated by hypothyroidism?
a. Hemophilia A
b. von Willebrand's disease
c. Disseminated intravascular coagulation
d. Coumarin toxicity

200. In what species is ketonuria most commonly found?
a. Canine
b. Feline
c. Equine
d. Bovine

201. What is the smallest epithelial cell seen on a urine sediment examination?
a. Leukocyte
b. Transitional cell
c. Renal cell
d. Squamous cell

202. For glucosuria to occur, which of the following must also be present?
a. Uremia
b. Hyperglycemia
c. Ketonemia
d. Azoturia

203. Which urolith is becoming quite common in cats?
a. Oxalate
b. Silica
c. Urate
d. Urate

204. What test on the urine dipstick is the least useful in animals?
a. Glucose
b. Urobilinogen
c. Protein
d. Ketones

205. What substance increases in the urine during glomerular disease?
a. Glucose
b. Ketones
c. Bilirubin
d. Protein

206. Which breed of dog has the most problems with uric acid stones?
a. Basenji
b. German shepherd
c. Dalmatian
d. Shetland sheepdog

207. Keeping the urine ____________ will keep struvite crystals dissolved in solution.
a. Acidic
b. Basic
c. Isosthenuric
d. Dilute

208. Which of the following is a disadvantage of an enzyme-linked immunosorbent assay?
a. Sensitivity
b. Specificity
c. Rapid results
d. Titer detection

209. Which of the following clinical tests may be influenced when a toxic dose of acetaminophen has been ingested?
a. Alanine aminotransferase
b. Ammonia
c. Blood pH
d. Calcium

210. Chemical neutropenia may result from the ingestion of which drug in dogs?
a. Chloramphenicol
b. Estrogen
c. Phenylbutazone
d. All of the above

211. Xylitol ingestion may result in which of the following conditions?
a. Hypophosphatemia
b. Hyperphosphatemia
c. Hypoglycemia
d. Hyper and hypophosphatemia

212. Which type of fluid sample is the major vehicle for transporting toxicants within the body?
a. Blood/Plasma
b. Feces
c. Hair
d. Urine

213. All of the following samples should be submitted when acetaminophen is suspected to have been ingested *except*:
a. Plasma (EDTA or heparin preserved)
b. Liver biopsy
c. Urine
d. Blood smear

214. What is the main constituent of a struvite crystal?
a. Calcium carbonate
b. Calcium oxalate
c. Magnesium phosphate
d. Silica

215. Which of the following is *not* considered an electrolyte?
a. Calcium
b. Sodium
c. Potassium
d. Chloride

216. Hyperkalemia is commonly associated with which endocrine disorder?
a. Diabetes insipidus
b. Hyperthyroidism
c. Hyperparathyroidism
d. Hypoadrenocorticism

217. A false-positive test result is one in which the:
a. Animal is affected and the test is negative.
b. Animal is not affected and the test is positive.
c. Animal is not affected and the test is negative.
d. Animal is affected and the test is positive.

218. Polyuria and polydipsia are *not* commonly seen in what endocrine disorder?
a. Hyperadrenocorticism
b. Diabetes insipidus
c. Hyperparathyroidism
d. Diabetes mellitus

219. What cat blood type is considered the universal donor?
a. A
b. O
c. AB
d. None exists in the cat.

220. How do transfusion reactions in the cat differ from transfusion reactions in the dog?
a. Transfusions are more severe in cats.
b. Transfusions are more acute in dogs.
c. Cats suffer from severe pruritus.
d. Transfusions are more severe in dogs.

221. When the spun hematocrit test is completed, which of the following can be evaluated?
a. PCV
b. Plasma color and PCV
c. Total protein, buffy coat, plasma color, and PCV
d. Total protein, buffy coat, plasma color, fibrin, and PCV

222. A monolayer of cells on a blood smear is best described as:
a. A feathered edge
b. Cells with no overlapping or touching
c. Cells touching each other very closely with some overlapping
d. The body of the blood smear

223. An example of capillary action is:
a. The blood coursing through smaller veins
b. The perfusion of mucous membranes
c. The action of blood filling a hematocrit tube
d. Removing serum from a clot with a pipette

224. Which of these is *not* a random laboratory error?
a. Variation in glassware
b. Electronic or optical inconsistency
c. Anisocytosis
d. Contamination

225. Prolonged exposure of serum to the blood cells before the serum is removed from the clot can result in:
a. Increased serum glucose
b. Increased serum phosphorus
c. Increased serum enzyme activity
d. Increased serum sodium

226. Phagocytes include all of the following *except*:
a. Neutrophils
b. Lymphocytes
c. Monocytes
d. Macrophages

227. Before beginning other diagnostics of the urine, a ____ examination of urine is recommended.
a. Darkfield
b. Gross
c. Taste
d. Microscopic

228. *Paragonimus kellicotti* is a:
a. Tapeworm
b. Tick
c. Mite
d. Fluke

229. Which of these is *not* a function of the lymphatic system?
a. Transport of waste materials
b. Leukocyte production
c. Removal of excess tissue fluid
d. Protein transport

230. What organ has both lymphatic and hematologic functions?
a. Spleen
b. Pancreas
c. Tonsil
d. Liver

231. What organ has storage sinuses that hold blood and release it into circulation when the need for oxygen is increased?
a. Spleen
b. Pancreas
c. Parathyroid
d. Liver

232. What organ releases T cells?
a. Thyroid
b. Thymus
c. Splenic trabeculae
d. Tonsils

233. What tissue processes B cells before they are sent to peripheral lymphoid tissue?
a. GLNB
b. GALB
c. GALT
d. GLAN

234. What would *not* cause shifts or trends in quality-control data?
a. New lot numbers of reagents
b. Change in calibration of the instrument
c. Outdated reagents
d. Change in laboratory personnel

235. What error is *not* detectable through the use of a quality-control program?
a. Poor technique
b. Sample quality
c. Equipment malfunctions
d. Reagent contamination or degeneration

236. For proper calibration, what solution should be used to calibrate a refractometer?
a. Tap water
b. Distilled water
c. Plasma
d. Urine

237. To separate serum, whole blood should be spun down in a centrifuge at:
a. 4500 rpm for 30 minutes
b. 10,000 rpm for 10 minutes
c. 8500 rpm for 30 minutes
d. 2500 rpm for 10 minutes

238. When using a centrifuge, it is important to do all of the following each time it is used *except*:
a. Balance the tubes
b. Open the lid as the centrifuge is in the process of stopping
c. Set the timer
d. Check tube holders for leaked liquid

239. As a general rule, enough blood should be collected to run any test at least three times. This compensates for all of the following *except*:
a. Instrument error
b. Technician error
c. Transcription error
d. Improper dilution of a sample

240. False decreases in serum glucose levels can be caused by:
a. Prolonged contact with red blood cells before separating the serum
b. Refrigerating the serum sample before analysis
c. Freezing the serum sample before analysis
d. A lipemic sample

241. Drawing a blood sample from an animal that has recently eaten may result in a sample that is:
a. Hemolyzed
b. Lipemic
c. Icteric
d. Anemic

242. Centrifuging a blood sample at high speed for a prolonged period may result in:
a. Lipemia
b. Icterus
c. Hemolysis
d. Bacterial contamination

243. Improper handling of a blood sample after it has been collected may result in:
a. Lipemia
b. Icterus
c. Hemolysis
d. Leukocytosis

244. A serum sample that is extremely icteric generally derives its color from an increased level of:
a. Lipids
b. Total bilirubin
c. Electrolytes
d. Glucose

245. What color is icteric plasma?
a. Brown
b. Red
c. Green
d. Yellow

246. Which statement is false concerning the collection of a plasma sample for a blood chemistry analysis?
a. If a needle and syringe are used, hemolysis can be minimized by removing the needle from the syringe before discharging the blood into a sample tube.
b. Volume changes caused by evaporation can be minimized by keeping the cap on the blood collection tube as much as possible.
c. To separate, allow the sample to clot for approximately 30 minutes; gently remove the clot from the sides of the tube, centrifuge, and then remove the plasma.
d. Avoid lipemia by fasting the animal before collecting the sample.

247. What sample condition cannot be minimized by proper animal preparation or proper sample collection and handling?
a. Hemolysis
b. Icterus
c. Lipemia
d. Evaporation

248. An allergic response that is frequently life-threatening is the result of:
a. Agglutination
b. Hemolysis
c. DIC
d. Anaphylaxis

249. A total of 99% of the domestic short-hair cats in the United States have which blood type?
a. A
b. B
c. AB
d. O

250. Canine blood types are preceded by the letters "DEA." What do these letters stand for?
a. Detectable erythrocyte antibody
b. Detectable erythrocyte antigen
c. Dog erythrocyte antibody
d. Dog erythrocyte antigen

251. Coagulation tests would be useful for diagnosing:
a. Rodenticide poisoning
b. Thyroid function
c. Adrenal function
d. Ethylene glycol poisoning

252. The calibrated device used to deliver a specified volume of patient sample when performing a blood chemistry analysis is known as a:
a. Cuvette
b. Pipette
c. Graduated flask
d. Graduated cylinder

253. Laser-flow technology is used in:
   a. Hematology analyzers
   b. Chemistry analyzers
   c. Coagulation analyzers
   d. Electrolyte analyzers

254. In dogs and cats, the blood chemistry tests most commonly used to evaluate liver function are:
   a. Alanine transaminase and aspartate aminotransferase
   b. Electrolytes and blood urea nitrogen
   c. Gamma-glutamyl transferase and sorbitol dehydrogenase
   d. Amylase and lipase

255. In horses the blood chemistry tests most commonly used to evaluate liver function are:
   a. Alanine transaminase and aspartate aminotransferase
   b. Electrolytes and blood urea nitrogen
   c. Gamma-glutamyl transferase and sorbitol dehydrogenase
   d. Amylase and lipase

256. Blood chemistry assays, including dye excretion, ammonia tolerance, and bile acid concentrations, are used to evaluate the function of the:
   a. Pancreas
   b. Kidneys
   c. Heart
   d. Liver

257. Impedance is:
   a. Used in analytic instruments to stop a test
   b. Blockage of light or electric current in analytic instruments
   c. Lack of synchronicity between the jugular pulse and the heartbeat
   d. Inability to feel pedal pulses

258. Which of the following is *not* a disadvantage of using the PCR testing in equine medicine?
   a. False-positive reactions
   b. Lack of viable virus isolates
   c. Inability to detect new viruses
   d. Sensitivity of the test

259. The adult form of the parasite _________ is a fly, and the larval stage is an endoparasite.
   a. *Otobius*
   b. *Capillaria*
   c. *Thelazia*
   d. *Gasterophilus*

260. Bots are:
   a. Lice eggs
   b. Fly larvae
   c. Flea feces
   d. Seed ticks

261. Nits are considered:
   a. Lice eggs
   b. Fly larvae
   c. Flea feces
   d. Seed ticks

262. Which parasite could cause anemia in horses through blood sucking?
   a. *Strongylus vulgaris*
   b. *Parascaris equorum*
   c. *Anoplocephala perfoliata*
   d. *Dictyocaulus arnfieldi*

263. Which product stains fat?
   a. New methylene blue
   b. Sudan III or IV
   c. Diff-Quik
   d. Giemsa

264. Which stain is referred to as a supravital stain?
   a. New methylene blue
   b. Camco Quik
   c. Eosin
   d. Sudan III or IV

265. Eosinophilia is commonly seen with a:
   a. Bacterial infection
   b. Parasitic infection
   c. Viral infection
   d. Hormonal disorder

266. What is the underlying cause of icterus?
   a. Anemia
   b. Hyperbilirubinemia
   c. Ketonuria
   d. Hyperhemoglobinemia

267. Basophilic stippling is often associated with:
   a. Lead poisoning
   b. Autoimmune disease
   c. Anemia
   d. Neoplasia

268. A common finding on a stained blood smear from an animal with autoimmune hemolytic anemia is:
   a. Lymphocytosis
   b. Basophilic stippling
   c. Spherocytosis
   d. Leukemia

269. Denatured hemoglobin found in erythrocytes is referred to as a/an:
   a. Heinz body
   b. Howell-Jolly body
   c. Anaplasma body
   d. Spherocyte

270. Fresh frozen plasma can be stored up to _________ and still contain clotting factors.
   a. 1 month
   b. 12 months
   c. 36 months
   d. 60 months

271. What cell produces antibodies?
   a. Hepatocyte
   b. Plasma cell
   c. Thymocyte
   d. T cell

272. What appears as a blue spherical nuclear remnant seen in some Wright-stained erythrocytes?
   a. Reticulocyte
   b. Howell-Jolly body
   c. Heinz body
   d. Leptocyte

273. Frozen fresh plasma (FFP) must be separated and frozen within ____ hours to maintain all coagulation factors in normal concentrations.
a. 2
b. 8
c. 12
d. 6

274. Which of the following stimulates antibody production?
a. Immunoglobulin
b. Antigen
c. T cell
d. Plasma cell

275. A normal leukocyte count with an increase in immature neutrophils that outnumber mature neutrophils is:
a. Leukocytosis
b. Leukopenia
c. A regenerative left shift
d. A degenerative left shift

276. A variation in erythrocyte size is known as:
a. Polycytosis
b. Anisocytosis
c. Poikilocytosis
d. Erythrocytosis

277. What is the name for a nonnucleated, immature erythrocyte found in small numbers in the peripheral blood of dogs?
a. Reticulocyte
b. Metarubricyte
c. Rubriblast
d. Rubricyte

278. What sample is recommended for hemoglobin testing?
a. Serum
b. Plasma
c. Whole blood
d. Blood smear

279. What part of the CBC is the most accurate procedure?
a. Erythrocyte count
b. Hemoglobin determination
c. Leukocyte count
d. Hematocrit

280. What part of the CBC cannot be done manually with adequate accuracy?
a. Erythrocyte count
b. Leukocyte count
c. Packed cell volume
d. WBC differential

281. What would you expect to see on a Diff-Quik stained blood smear from an animal with regenerative anemia?
a. Schistocytosis
b. Reticulocytosis
c. Eosinophilia
d. Polychromasia

282. What cell is described as a central rounded area of hemoglobin surrounded by a clear zone, with a dense ring of hemoglobin around the periphery?
a. Plasma cell
b. Target cell
c. Spherocyte
d. Reticulocyte

283. Where is the buffy coat found on the refractometer?
a. Beneath the packed red cells
b. Above the packed red cells
c. Above the plasma
d. Buffy coats are not seen on refractometers

284. What is the major difference between serum and plasma?
a. Plasma has higher protein levels.
b. Serum has higher electrolyte levels.
c. Plasma has a darker color.
d. Serum will clot.

285. What is the term used to describe plasma that appears white or milky?
a. Leukemia
b. Lipemia
c. Chylemia
d. Lactemia

286. Which term is used to describe the situation in which many of the erythrocytes stain varying shades of lavender?
a. Anemia
b. Anisocytosis
c. Polychromasia
d. Poikilocytosis

287. Which of the following is a breakdown product of hemoglobin?
a. Bilirubin
b. Erythropoietin
c. Urea
d. Carotene

288. What type of anemia is associated with icterus?
a. Responsive
b. Nonresponsive
c. Hemolytic
d. Megaloblastic

289. What is the most immature erythrocyte that can be identified in bone marrow?
a. Prorubricyte
b. Rubriblast
c. Erythrocytoblast
d. Multipotent stem cell

290. Rouleaux formation is most commonly seen on blood smears from:
a. Horses
b. Goats
c. Dogs
d. Cats

291. An MCV value below the normal reference range suggests:
a. Hyperchromasia
b. Hypochromasia
c. Macrocytosis
d. Microcytosis

292. If you count 40 reticulocytes per 1000 erythrocytes, what is the observed reticulocyte count?
a. 2%
b. 4%
c. 20%
d. 40%

293. What is indicated by a neutrophil that includes a nucleus with six lobes?
a. Toxemia
b. Female animal
c. Old cell
d. Normal cell

294. What causes dark granules called Döhle bodies in the cytoplasm of canine neutrophils?
a. Leukemia
b. Parasitic infection
c. Immaturity
d. Toxemia

295. What is normally the largest mature blood cell in the peripheral blood of domestic species?
a. Monocyte
b. Neutrophil
c. Eosinophil
d. Lymphocyte

296. When preparing a direct smear from feces, all of the following liquids can be mixed with the feces *except*:
a. Tap water
b. Distilled water
c. Hydrogen peroxide
d. Saline

297. With the exception of cats, most animals have a total blood volume equivalent to ___ of their body weight.
a. 7%
b. 15%
c. 25%
d. 40%

298. What is tested in a minor crossmatch?
a. T-cell production
b. Recipient serum against donor erythrocytes
c. Recipient erythrocytes against donor serum
d. Recipient urine against donor erythrocytes

299. What anticoagulant is used most commonly in animal-blood collection for CBCs?
a. Sodium heparin
b. Potassium oxalate
c. Potassium ethylenediamine tetraacetic acid
d. Sodium citrate

300. What anticoagulant is used to determine activated partial thromboplastin time and one-stage prothrombin time?
a. Heparin
b. Citrate
c. Fluoride
d. EDTA

301. What structure is normally found in the nuclei of immature blood cells?
a. Nucleolus
b. Golgi apparatus
c. Heinz body
d. Döhle body

302. Certain oxidant drugs can denature hemoglobin and cause the production of round structures in erythrocytes that are called:
a. Howell-Jolly bodies
b. Russell bodies
c. Döhle bodies
d. Heinz bodies

303. What is the most common cause of hypochromia in erythrocytes?
a. Hypertonic drugs
b. Decreased hemoglobin
c. Iron toxicity
d. Increased erythrocyte production

304. What is the primary function of fibrinogen?
a. Antibody production
b. Phagocytosis
c. Hemostasis
d. Complement fixation

305. *Haemobartonella felis* is seen most commonly in the erythrocytes of:
a. Cats
b. Cattle
c. Dogs
d. Horses

306. An increased number of bands in the peripheral blood indicate:
a. Leukemia
b. Autoimmune hemolytic anemia
c. Left shift
d. Neutropenia

307. The first line of defense that the body has against foreign invaders is the:
a. Hair
b. Neutrophils
c. Primary lymphoid tissue
d. Skin

308. Which of these white blood cells migrate through tissue as macrophages and function to remove and destroy bacteria, damaged cells, and neoplastic cells?
a. Lymphocytes
b. Neutrophils
c. Monocytes
d. Eosinophils

309. Which immunoglobulin is most abundant in the serum and plays the major role in humoral immunity?
a. IgG
b. IgM
c. IgA
d. IgD

310. Immunity that is generated by an animal's immune system following exposure to a foreign antigen is referred to as:
a. Passive immunity
b. Active immunity
c. Responsive immunity
d. Colostral immunity

311. Which immunoglobulin is the only one that can cross the placenta?
a. IgG
b. IgM
c. IgA
d. IgD

312. Which of the following correctly lists the progressive stages of phagocytosis?
a. Adherence, chemotaxis, ingestion, digestion
b. Ingestion, adherence, chemotaxis, digestion
c. Chemotaxis, adherence, ingestion, digestion
d. Ingestion, digestion, chemotaxis, adherence

313. An attenuated vaccine is one in which:
a. Microorganisms are killed.
b. Microorganisms are weakened but are still alive.
c. Microorganisms are 100% virulent.
d. No microorganisms are found.

314. Which statement concerning passive immunity is least accurate?
a. It involves antibodies that have been produced in a donor animal.
b. It provides immediate but short-lived immunity.
c. It may be natural or artificial.
d. It develops after exposure to a pathogen.

315. Myasthenia gravis is commonly associated with:
a. Megaesophagus
b. Exercise intolerance
c. Aspiration pneumonia
d. All of the above

316. Anaphylactic shock is:
a. A mild reaction that causes destruction of erythrocytes
b. A moderate reaction that causes hives
c. A severe, life-threatening reaction that occurs seconds after an antigen enters the circulation
d. A severe reaction caused by rapid loss of large volumes of blood or other bodily fluid

317. Combined immunodeficiency is a condition in which animals fail to produce functioning:
a. Plasma cells
b. B cells
c. T cells
d. B and T cells

318. Which of the following is *not* a malfunction of the immune system?
a. Allergy
b. Immunodeficiency
c. Autoimmune disease
d. Immunity by vaccination

319. What cells are chiefly concerned with the production and secretion of antibodies?
a. B lymphocytes
b. T lymphocytes
c. Neutrophils
d. Monocytes

320. What cells respond more quickly to a second antigen exposure than to the initial exposure?
a. Thymocytes
b. Monocytes
c. Memory B cells
d. Neutrophils

321. Serology is the branch of science involved with detection of:
a. Bacteria or fungi
b. Viruses or prions
c. Antibodies or antigens
d. Endoparasites and ectoparasites

322. ELISA is an acronym for:
a. Electro-linked immunosorbent assay
b. Enzyme-linked immunosorbent assay
c. Enzyme-linked immunoassay
d. Electrolytic isoantibody assay

323. Which statement concerning ELISA testing is true?
a. The test specificity is very low
b. Washing is a critical step in the methodology
c. It may be used to detect only antibodies in the serum
d. It is not available in kit form

324. What serologic test is used for the diagnosis of autoimmune hemolytic anemia?
a. Coombs test
b. Coggins test
c. Intradermal testing
d. Latex agglutination test

325. Which of these parasites sucks blood from its host?
a. *Macracanthorhynchus hirudinaceus*
b. *Onchocerca cervicalis*
c. *Metastrongylus apri*
d. *Ctenocephalides felis*

326. Which of these pig parasites can be diagnosed by muscle biopsy?
a. *Trichinella spiralis*
b. *Oesophagostomum dentatum*
c. *Eimeria suis*
d. *Fasciola hepatica*

327. Vaccines may be administered by any of the following routes *except*:
a. Subcutaneously
b. Intramuscularly
c. Intranasally
d. Intraperitoneally

328. Which of the following is least likely to cause vaccine failure?
a. Improper storage
b. Administration during anesthesia
c. Interference by maternal antibodies
d. Improper route of administration

329. Which of these parasites is a tapeworm?
a. *Strongyloides westeri*
b. *Paranoplocephala mamillana*
c. *Parascaris equorum*
d. *Oxyuris equi*

330. Which of these parasites is classified as coccidia?
a. *Cryptosporidium parvum*
b. *Bunostomum phlebotomum*
c. *Moniezia expansa*
d. *Haemonchus contortus*

331. Pemphigus is a group of autoimmune disorders that affect the:
a. Blood and lymph systems
b. Skin and oral mucosa
c. Eyes
d. Hooves and claws

332. Signs of immune-mediated thrombocytopenia (ITP) include all of these conditions *except*
a. Petechiae
b. Ecchymoses
c. Thrombocytosis
d. Anemia

333. Which of these cells is the most immature?
a. Rubricyte
b. Metarubricyte
c. Prorubricyte
d. Reticulocyte

334. Which of the following is a possible site of extramedullary hematopoiesis in times of increased blood cell production?
a. Spleen
b. Kidney
c. Umbilicus
d. Bone cortex

335. *Baylisascaris procyonis* larvae have been shown to cause __________ in humans.
a. Pneumonia
b. Hemolytic anemia
c. Brain damage
d. Bloody diarrhea

336. Hemagglutination is:
a. Clumping of erythrocytes
b. Lysing of erythrocytes
c. Crenation of erythrocytes
d. Swelling of erythrocytes

337. What test is routinely used to diagnose equine infectious anemia?
a. Indirect fluorescent antibody test
b. Coggins test
c. Coombs test
d. Hemoglobin electrophoresis

338. When reviewing a blood smear, you come across an erythrocyte that does *not* contain its full amount of hemoglobin. What is this known as?
a. Polychromasia
b. Hypochromasia
c. Basophilia
d. Hyperchromasia

339. A neutrophil with a four-segmented nucleus would be classified as a:
a. Hypersegmented neutrophil
b. Immature neutrophil
c. Normal neutrophil
d. Aged neutrophil

340. During an allergic response, what do sensitized cells produce in abnormal quantities when an allergen reappears after an initial exposure?
a. Antihistamines
b. Histamine
c. Toxins
d. Lysins

341. Gram-positive microorganisms stain ____________ using a Gram stain.
a. Purple
b. Red
c. Orange
d. Lavender

342. Acid-fast stains are used to identify:
a. Coccidia
b. Yeast
c. Fungi
d. Mycobacteria

343. What cells are sensitized by IgE to produce large quantities of histamines?
a. Mast cells and basophils
b. Eosinophils and basophils
c. Monocytes and lymphocytes
d. Neutrophils and eosinophils

344. T killer cells:
a. Release histamine
b. Recognize cancer cells as abnormal cells and eliminate them
c. Coat cancer cells with antibody
d. Release endorphin

345. Cats exposed to feline leukemia virus typically respond in any of the following ways *except*:
a. Not becoming infected at all
b. Becoming temporarily infected, developing immunity, and overcoming the infection
c. Becoming infected and continuing to shed the virus indefinitely without becoming ill
d. Becoming infected, becoming ill within 3 days, and dying within a week

346. Acid-fast positive organisms stain __________ when using an acid-fast stain.
a. Yellow
b. Blue
c. Pink
d. Brown

347. What is the predominant method for the transmission of feline immunodeficiency virus in cats?
a. Grooming
b. Bite wounds
c. Urine
d. Feces

348. In assessing titers, how long after the first serum sample is collected should the second sample be collected?
a. 7 days
b. 3 days
c. 2 to 6 weeks
d. 14 weeks

349. What microorganisms are *not* free living?
a. Algae
b. Fungi
c. Bacteria
d. Viruses

350. What is the correct way to write the genus and species of bacteria?
a. *Streptococcus Pyogenes*
b. Streptococcus pyogenes
c. S. pyogenes
d. *Streptococcus pyogenes*

351. The acid-fast stain is used to identify the organism that causes:
a. Anaplasmosis
b. Colibacillosis
c. Ringworm
d. Tuberculosis

352. What color do gram-negative organisms appear when they are stained with Gram stain?
a. Purple
b. Pink
c. Green
d. Clear

353. Viruses are best described as:
a. Free-living organisms
b. Obligatory interstitial parasites
c. Obligatory intracellular parasites
d. Eukaryotic cells

354. A positive catalase test will be indicated by the presence of:
   a. A color change
   b. Gel formation
   c. Bubbles
   d. Fibrin
355. A nosocomial infection is always:
   a. Present but not apparent at the time of hospitalization
   b. Acquired during the course of hospitalization
   c. Caused by medical personnel
   d. Acquired during surgery
356. Generally, endotoxins are products of:
   a. Viruses
   b. Gram-negative bacteria
   c. Gram-positive bacteria
   d. Fungi
357. What organism is most likely to grow on mannitol salt agar?
   a. *Streptococcus pyogenes*
   b. *Bacillus subtilis*
   c. *Clostridium perfringens*
   d. *Staphylococcus aureus*
358. Which virus causes warts?
   a. Papilloma
   b. Variola
   c. Herpes
   d. Pox
359. What organism exhibits fluorescence under ultraviolet light?
   a. *Microsporum gypseum*
   b. *Trichophyton mentagrophytes*
   c. *Microsporum canis*
   d. *Epidermophyton floccosum*
360. Pinkeye or contagious conjunctivitis in cattle is caused by:
   a. *Hemophilus aegypti*
   b. *Moraxella bovis*
   c. *Streptococcus pyogenes*
   d. *Staphylococcus aureus*
361. On a blood agar plate, an area of complete hemolysis is classified as:
   a. Alpha
   b. Beta
   c. Gamma
   d. Delta
362. Dipylidium caninum is a:
   a. Trematode
   b. Nematode
   c. Arthropod
   d. Cestode
363. Fasciola hepatica is a:
   a. Nematode
   b. Cestode
   c. Trematode
   d. Protozoan
364. A puppy infected with *Dirofilaria immitis* the day it is born will *not* test positive for heartworm microfilariae until it is _______ old.
   a. 12 months
   b. 6 to 7 months
   c. 3 to 4 months
   d. 1 month
365. The ELISA heartworm test kit detects the antigens of:
   a. Heartworm microfilariae
   b. Female adult heartworms
   c. Adult heartworms and microfilariae
   d. Toxins produced by adult heartworms
366. *Dirofilaria immitis* is a:
   a. Cestode
   b. Arthropod
   c. Nematode
   d. Trematode
367. *Otodectes cynotis* is a:
   a. Cestode
   b. Arthropod
   c. Nematode
   d. Trematode
368. A dog becomes infected with *Dipylidium caninum* by ingestion of:
   a. Saliva from an infected dog
   b. Feces from an infected dog
   c. Tissues of an infected rabbit
   d. Infected fleas
369. The most common intermediate host of *Taenia pisiformis* is a:
   a. Ruminant
   b. Flea
   c. Fly
   d. Rabbit
370. The parasite whose adult resembles a whip and whose eggs have bipolar plugs is:
   a. *Strongyloides stercoralis*
   b. *Trichuris vulpis*
   c. *Toxocara canis*
   d. *Toxascaris leonina*
371. In most areas of the world, rats are the reservoir host of the plague organism. However, in the western United States, the most common species harboring this organism is:
   a. Dogs
   b. Cats
   c. Beavers
   d. Prairie dogs
372. The kennel cough syndrome in dogs is often caused by a combination of boarding at a kennel, a viral infection, and infection with:
   a. *Pasteurella multocida*
   b. *Staphylococcus aureus*
   c. *Corynebacterium diphtheriae*
   d. *Bordetella bronchiseptica*
373. What organism is a spirochete?
   a. *Corynebacterium pyogenes*
   b. *Streptococcus pyogenes*
   c. *Mycobacterium tuberculosis*
   d. *Leptospira grippotyphosa*
374. What organism causes strangles in horses?
   a. *Staphylococcus aureus*
   b. *Streptococcus equi*
   c. *Corynebacterium equi*
   d. *Strongylus vulgaris*

375. What characteristic is unique to *Mycobacterium*?
a. It is a spore former.
b. It is anaerobic.
c. It is easily killed by antibiotics.
d. It survives phagocytosis.

376. Which of the following is *not* a simple stain?
a. Methylene blue
b. Crystal violet
c. Safranin
d. Gram stain

377. Acquired active immunity results from:
a. Vaccination
b. Antitoxin administration
c. Ingestion of colostrum
d. Administration of gamma globulin

378. *Escherichia coli* is normally found:
a. On the skin
b. In the intestinal tract
c. In the respiratory tract
d. In the stomach

379. Pediculosis is an infestation of:
a. Ticks
b. Flies
c. Lice
d. Mites

380. In humans, *Toxocara canis* is the causative agent of:
a. Creeping eruption
b. Scabies
c. Hydatidosis
d. Visceral larva migrans

381. A large ciliate protozoa that may be found in swine feces is:
a. *Balantidium* species
b. *Trichomonas* species
c. *Giardia* species
d. *Histomonas* species

382. The parasite diagnosed by vaginal washing is:
a. *Tritrichomonas* species
b. *Dictyocaulus* species
c. *Dioctophyma* species
d. *Anaplasma* species

383. The parasite diagnosed by tracheal wash is:
a. *Tritrichomonas* species
b. *Dictyocaulus* species
c. *Dioctophyma* species
d. *Anaplasma* species

384. The parasite diagnosed by examining urine is:
a. *Tritrichomonas* species
b. *Dictyocaulus* species
c. *Dioctophyma* species
d. *Anaplasma* species

385. The parasite diagnosed by examining blood is:
a. *Tritrichomonas* species
b. *Dictyocaulus* species
c. *Dioctophyma* species
d. *Anaplasma* species

386. The parasite known as a brown dog tick is:
a. *Rhipicephalus sanguineus*
b. *Ixodes dammini*
c. *Dermacentor variabilis*
d. *Dermacentor albipictus*

387. The parasite known as a winter tick is:
a. *Rhipicephalus sanguineus*
b. *Ixodes dammini*
c. *Dermacentor variabilis*
d. *Dermacentor albipictus*

388. The parasite known as the American dog tick is:
a. *Rhipicephalus sanguineus*
b. *Ixodes dammini*
c. *Dermacentor variabilis*
d. *Dermacentor albipictus*

389. The parasite known as a deer tick is:
a. *Rhipicephalus sanguineus*
b. *Ixodes dammini*
c. *Dermacentor variabilis*
d. *Dermacentor albipictus*

390. The parasite that lives in ears is:
a. *Sarcoptes* species
b. *Demodex* species
c. *Chorioptes* species
d. *Otodectes* species

391. The parasite that lives on the skin's surface is:
a. *Sarcoptes* species
b. *Demodex* species
c. *Chorioptes* species
d. *Otodectes* species

392. The parasite that burrows into the skin is:
a. *Sarcoptes* species
b. *Demodex* species
c. *Chorioptes* species
d. *Otodectes* species

393. The parasite that lives in hair follicles is:
a. *Sarcoptes* species
b. *Demodex* species
c. *Chorioptes* species
d. *Otodectes* species

394. Which of the following ticks is considered a single host tick?
a. *Boophilus annulatus*
b. *Otobius megnini*
c. *Ixodid* sp.
d. *Argasidae* sp.

395. Cheyletiella mites use ___ as their hosts.
a. Dogs, cats, and rabbits
b. Dogs, rabbits, and birds
c. Cats, birds, and rodents
d. Cats, dogs, and rodents

396. Infection of which of these parasites is via skin penetration?
a. *Trichuris vulpis*
b. *Taenia pisiformis*
c. *Dipylidium caninum*
d. *Strongyloides stercoralis*

397. People may act as the intermediate hosts of:
a. *Echinococcus granulosus*
b. *Anoplocephala magna*
c. *Taenia pisiformis*
d. *Moniezia benedeni*

398. What parasite ova have three pairs of hooklets?
a. *Trichuris* species
b. *Taenia* species
c. *Alaria* species
d. *Moniezia* species

399. What parasite ova have bipolar plugs?
a. *Trichuris* species
b. *Taenia* species
c. *Alaria* species
d. *Moniezia* species

400. The double-pore tapeworm is:
a. *Paragonimus kellicotti*
b. *Moniezia expansa*
c. *Dipylidium caninum*
d. *Echinococcus granulosus*

401. The parasite that infects the liver of its host is:
a. *Diphyllobothrium* species
b. *Hymenolepis* species
c. *Paragonimus* species
d. *Fasciola* species

402. The parasite whose larvae encyst in the subcutaneous tissue of rabbits is:
a. *Gasterophilus* species
b. *Hypoderma* species
c. *Oestrus* species
d. *Cuterebra* species

403. The parasite whose eggs are cemented to the hair of horses is:
a. *Gasterophilus* species
b. *Hypoderma* species
c. *Oestrus* species
d. *Cuterebra* species

404. The parasite whose larvae form warbles in subcutaneous tissue along the backs of cattle is:
a. *Gasterophilus* species
b. *Hypoderma* species
c. *Oestrus* species
d. *Cuterebra* species

405. The parasite whose larvae enter the nasal cavity of sheep is:
a. *Gasterophilus* species
b. *Hypoderma* species
c. *Oestrus* species
d. *Cuterebra* species

406. What parasite completes its life cycle on or in its host?
a. *Ctenocephalides* species
b. *Otodectes* species
c. *Hypoderma* species
d. *Dermacentor* species

407. What species causes a disease known as walking dandruff?
a. *Trombicula* species
b. *Sarcoptes* species
c. *Demodex* species
d. *Cheyletiella* species

408. Scabies is caused by:
a. *Trombicula* species
b. *Otodectes* species
c. *Melophagus* species
d. *Sarcoptes* species

409. In which stage of the tick life cycle does it have six legs?
a. Nymphal
b. Larval
c. Adult female
d. Adult male

410. What is the definition of hematopoiesis?
a. The destruction of platelets
b. The production of blood cells and platelets
c. The creation of fibrinogen
d. The decrease of red blood cells

411. What urinary stone is most associated with a urinary tract infection?
a. Calcium oxalate crystal
b. Struvite crystal
c. Calcium carbonite crystal
d. Cystine crystal

412. A urine specimen collected by free catch at 8 a.m. and left at room temperature until the afternoon could be expected to have:
a. Decreased number of bacteria
b. Increased number of bacteria
c. Decreased number of epithelial cells
d. Increased number of epithelial cells

413. An intestinal fluke is of the:
a. *Alaria* species
b. *Fascioloides* species
c. *Stephanurus* species
d. *Metastrongylus* species

414. The parasite known as a lungworm is of the:
a. *Alaria* species
b. *Fascioloides* species
c. *Stephanurus* species
d. *Metastrongylus* species

415. The parasite known as a kidney worm is of the:
a. *Alaria* species
b. *Fascioloides* species
c. *Stephanurus* species
d. *Metastrongylus* species

416. The parasite known as the large American liver fluke is of the:
a. *Alaria* species
b. *Fascioloides* species
c. *Stephanurus* species
d. *Metastrongylus* species

417. Which statement concerning fleas is true?
a. "Flea dirt" is flea feces.
b. Fleas are host specific.
c. Adults cannot survive for long periods without feeding.
d. Flea eggs are not sticky and they fall off into the environment.

418. The parasite that causes generalized pruritus is of the:
a. *Ancylostoma* species
b. *Melophagus* species
c. *Notoedres* species
d. *Echinococcus* species

419. The urine of an animal with hematuria is likely to be:
a. Cloudy and red
b. Clear and brown
c. Red and clear
d. Brown and cloudy

420. Calcium carbonate crystals are often seen in ________ urine.
a. Dog
b. Horse
c. Cat
d. Cattle

421. What crystal is commonly described as having a coffin-lid appearance?
a. Bilirubin crystal
b. Calcium oxalate crystal
c. Cystine crystal
d. Triple phosphate crystal (struvite)

422. An ammonium biurate crystal is sometimes described as:
a. Shaped like an envelope
b. Shaped like a pyramid
c. Like a thorny apple in appearance
d. Like a bicycle wheel in appearance

423. The best urine sample from a housebroken dog is collected in:
a. Late evening
b. Afternoon
c. Midmorning
d. Early morning

424. Urine samples collected in the morning from housebroken dogs tend to be:
a. Unacceptable for sediment analysis
b. The most concentrated samples
c. Bright orange
d. The least concentrated samples

425. What are the two preferred methods of collecting a urine sample for culture?
a. Catheterization and voiding
b. Expressing the bladder and cystocentesis
c. Cystocentesis and catheterization
d. Cystocentesis and voiding

426. Polyuria is:
a. Lack of urine production
b. Production of excessive amounts of urine
c. Lack of water intake
d. Excessive protein in the urine

427. Oliguria is:
a. Excessive eating
b. Green urine
c. Excessive bilirubin in the urine
d. Decreased urine output

428. Anuria is:
a. Decreased urine output
b. Decreased drinking
c. Complete lack of urine production
d. Excessive drinking

429. An alkaline urine pH can be the result of:
a. Urinary tract obstruction
b. Uncontrolled diabetes
c. Prolonged diarrhea
d. Starvation

430. Blood in the urine is reported as:
a. Dysuria
b. Hematuria
c. Pyuria
d. Proteinuria

431. An excessive number of WBCs in the urine is reported as:
a. Dysuria
b. Hematuria
c. Pyuria
d. Proteinuria

432. Painful urination is recorded as:
a. Dysuria
b. Hematuria
c. Pyuria
d. Proteinuria

433. Pancytopenia is characterized by:
a. Decreased numbers of white blood cells
b. Decreased numbers of all blood cells
c. Decreased numbers of red blood cells
d. Decreased numbers of granulocytes and monocytes

434. Erythropoietin is produced in the:
a. Bone marrow
b. Kidney
c. Liver
d. Pituitary gland

435. What is the appropriate amount of time needed for antibiotics to dissolve struvite crystals?
a. 3–5 days
b. 10–14 days
c. 2–3 months
d. 6 months

436. Prerenal azotemia is:
a. Dehydration without true impaired kidney function
b. Stage 1 renal disease
c. Urinary tract infection that is affecting kidney function
d. Dehydration with true impaired kidney function

437. What is an example of enteral nutrition?
a. ITP given through an IV catheter
b. Fasting or NPO
c. Coaxing: warming the food, feeding by hand, etc.
d. Water only

438. What are two examples of anticholinergic drugs?
a. Propofol and ketamine
b. Atropine and glycopyrrolate
c. Cyclosporine and mycophenolate
d. Dexdomitor and antisedan

439. What does the term MAC stand for?
a. Maximum arterial concentration
b. A sandwich at McDonalds
c. Minimum alveolar concentration
d. Mild acid concentration

440. What does an iohexol clearance test determine?
a. Estimated GFR in dogs and cats
b. Liver function
c. Blood glucose values
d. Food sensitivity

441. What is fructosamine?
a. Another term for blood glucose
b. A type of insulin
c. A carbohydrate molecule to which glucose binds
d. A protein to which glucose binds

442. What is the half-life of fructosamine?
a. 3–5 days
b. 1–2 weeks
c. 3–5 months
d. More than 6 months

443. How quickly must slides evaluating bone marrow samples be made if EDTA is used?
a. 1 hour
b. Immediately
c. 15 minutes
d. EDTA cannot be used for bone marrow samples.

444. What does the buccal mucosa bleeding time test assess?
a. Platelet function
b. Prothrombin time (PT)
c. Partial thromboplastin time (PTT)
d. Fibrinogen

445. A canine patient experiencing high triglycerides may have serum that is:
a. Milky
b. Yellow
c. Red
d. Clear

446. Which of the following specific gravity concentrations would be expected in a healthy, hydrated, 4-year-old Labrador patient?
a. 1
b. 1.005
c. 1.01
d. 1.04

447. To avoid serum lipemia, animals should be fasted for:
a. 2 hours
b. 4 hours
c. 8 hours
d. 12 hours

SECTION

9 Animal Nursing

Nicholas Raimondi

QUESTIONS

1. Which of the following animals are strict omnivores?
   a. Dogs
   b. Ferrets
   c. Prairie dogs
   d. Rabbits
2. Which of the following is a true effect of pain?
   a. It prevents further patient harm by preventing movement.
   b. It places the animal in an anabolic state, leading to weight gain.
   c. It suppresses the immune system, leading to an increased chance of infection.
   d. It promotes inflammation and increases the healing rate.
3. Taking a complete and accurate patient history:
   a. Is an important task that may be performed by veterinary technicians
   b. Should only be performed by a veterinarian
   c. Is only necessary if the patient has never been to the hospital
   d. Is not necessary for wellness exams in healthy patients
4. Which of the following animals are herbivores?
   a. Dogs
   b. Ferrets
   c. Prairie dogs
   d. Iguanas
5. Serum centrifuged in a microhematocrit tube characterized by varying degrees of redness is probably a result of:
   a. Hemolysis
   b. Hyperproteinemia
   c. Icterus
   d. Lipemia
6. Which of the following agencies regulates pet food labels and research facilities?
   a. AAFCO: Association of American Feed Control Officials
   b. FDA: Food and Drug Administration
   c. FTC: Federal Trade Commission
   d. USDA: United States Department of Agriculture
7. To fill prescriptions or administer a medication, technicians must be familiar with medical abbreviations. Which of the following abbreviations indicates a medication that is to be applied to both eyes?
   a. AU
   b. OD
   c. OS
   d. OU
8. Which of the following is a characteristic commonly seen in rabbits, in which the stool is ingested for nutritional purposes?
   a. Coprophagy
   b. Dysbiosis
   c. Dytrophic calcification
   d. Vitamin A deficiency
9. Which of the following is an example of a standardized method in assessing the effectiveness of analgesia in a patient?
   a. ASA Score
   b. Glasgow Coma Scale
   c. Colorado Pain Score
   d. Shock Index
10. When obtaining a patient history it is important to:
    a. Ask leading questions to save time and keep on schedule
    b. Ask open-ended questions
    c. Always use medical terms
    d. Ask leading questions when you already know what the problem is
11. When performing a physical examination on a patient:
    a. It is only necessary to examine the body part that is of concern to the client.
    b. Always start at the rear of the patient
    c. Always start at the patient's head
    d. All aspects of the exam should be examined in the same order whenever possible.
12. Which of the following is commonly seen in rabbits, in which the intestinal flora is disrupted?
    a. Coprophagy
    b. Dysbiosis
    c. Dytrophic calcification
    d. Vitamin A deficiency
13. The proper pathway in which an animal perceives pain is:
    a. Transduction, transmission, modulation, perception
    b. Transmission, modulation, transduction, perception
    c. Perception, transmission, modulation, transduction
    d. Transduction, transmission, perception, modulation
14. Which of the following results in infertility and neonatal mortality in rabbits?
    a. Coprophagy
    b. Dysbiosis
    c. Dytrophic calcification
    d. Vitamin A deficiency

15. Which of the following is the most commonly seen cardiovascular disease in the dog?
a. Boxer right ventricular cardiomyopathy
b. Dilated cardiomyopathy
c. Hypertrophic cardiomyopathy
d. Ventricular septal defect

16. Which of the following endocrine diseases results in hyponatremia and hyperkalemia in a dog?
a. Hyperadrenocorticism
b. Hypoadrenocorticism
c. Hyperthyroidism
d. Hypothyroidism

17. Halitosis is an indication of a problem with which of the following body systems?
a. Cardiovascular
b. Digestive
c. Nervous
d. Hematologic

18. When performing a TPR on a patient, you should:
a. Always auscultate the heart while palpating the pulse
b. Palpate the patient's pulse while taking its temperature
c. Always auscultate the heart because the pulse rate may be lower than the heart rate
d. Auscultate the heart if the patient does not like you touching its legs

19. The pulse pressure or quality of the pulse:
a. Is not of clinical significance as it is a subjective measurement
b. Might be an indicator of possible heart or blood pressure issues
c. Often feels very strong in older animals
d. May feel weak if the patient is excited

20. Which of the following endocrine diseases results in weight loss and a ravenous appetite in cats?
a. Hyperadrenocorticism
b. Hypoadrenocorticism
c. Hyperthyroidism
d. Hypothyroidism

21. When restraining a cat to draw blood from the medial saphenous vein, the patient is restrained in:
a. Dorsal recumbency
b. Lateral recumbency
c. Medial recumbency
d. Sternal recumbency

22. Weak, moderate, strong, bounding, or tall are terms often used to describe the patient's:
a. Attitude
b. Respiration quality
c. Pulse quality
d. Blood pressure

23. The transparent covering of the front of the eye is called the:
a. Lens
b. Iris
c. Pupil
d. Cornea

24. Which of the following endocrine diseases results in weight gain, bradycardia, exercise intolerance, and lethargy in a dog?
a. Hyperadrenocorticism
b. Hypoadrenocorticism
c. Hyperthyroidism
d. Hypothyroidism

25. A canine patient is being held in right lateral recumbency for venipuncture. Which of the following veins are most accessible?
a. Left lateral saphenous
b. Left medial saphenous
c. Right jugular
d. Right lateral saphenous

26. Hypoxemia is defined as:
a. A decreased circulating blood volume
b. Low blood oxygen levels
c. Low tissue oxygen levels
d. An increase in circulating fluid in the body

27. Which of the following is the most important first step when a dyspneic patient presents to the veterinary hospital?
a. Obtain thoracic radiographs
b. Obtain an arterial blood gas
c. Stabilize the patient before performing any diagnostic testing
d. Perform a complete physical examination

28. The normal temperature for an equine patient ranges from:
a. 99–101.5°F
b. 96.8–99°F
c. 101.5–102.5°F
d. 96.8–102.5°F

29. Which of the following is an appropriate method for restraining an animal that does not respond well to gentle words and handling?
a. Force the patient down and proceed with the procedure without full control
b. Recruit help from the owner for physical restraint
c. Running the patient around until it is too tired to struggle
d. Use chemical agents for restraint

30. The normal temperature range for a canine patient is:
a. 99.0–101.5°F
b. 96.8–99°F
c. 100.0–102.2°F
d. 96.8–102.5°F

31. Which of the following individuals should not participate in the restraining of patients?
a. Patient owners
b. Veterinarians
c. Veterinary technicians
d. Veterinary assistants

32. The normal temperature range for a feline patient is:
a. 99.0–101.5°F
b. 96.8–99°F
c. 100.0–102.2°F
d. 96.8–102.5°F

33. Which of the following conditions is a common sign of heart failure?
a. Tachypnea
b. Bradypnea
c. Tachycardia
d. Bradycardia

34. The most common presenting sign in a patient with undiagnosed severe hypertension is:
a. Anoxia
b. Cardiomyopathy
c. Blindness
d. Hypothyroidism

35. Which of the following is a precaution that should be taken before restraining a cat?
a. Maximal restraint should be used from the start to prevent any chance of the cat resisting
b. Make sure all doors, windows, and cabinets are closed
c. Prepare to use loud sounds as distraction
d. Take the same restraining approach for every cat

36. The normal heart rate for a feline patient is:
a. 16–32 bpm
b. 20–42 bpm
c. 60–160 bpm
d. 140–220 bpm

37. Which of the following is the passive expulsion of material from the mouth, pharynx, or esophagus?
a. Regurgitation
b. Vomiting
c. Hematemesis
d. Hypersalivation

38. During the first few days of life, the normal body temperature of a newborn puppy is:
a. 94.5–97.3°F
b. 94.7–100.1°F
c. 97.0–99.0°F
d. 99.0–101.5°F

39. A nervous dog should be taken out of its cage by:
a. Throwing a slip lead onto the neck and pulling them out
b. Luring the animal out with quiet, gentle urging, standing clear of the door
c. Quickly adjusting your position, reacting to each movement of the patient and making sure the dog knows it cannot escape
d. Reaching into the cage with your bare hands to restrain the animal

40. The normal heart rate for a canine patient is:
a. 16–32 bpm
b. 20–42 bpm
c. 60–160 bpm
d. 140–220 bpm

41. An intravenously delivered solution that distributes evenly throughout the interstitial and intravascular space is considered:
a. Isotonic
b. Hypotonic
c. Hypertonic
d. 0.45% sodium chloride

42. When a female dog is bred, the amount of food (calories) she is fed should be increased:
a. Immediately after breeding
b. 1 week after breeding
c. 2 or 3 weeks after breeding
d. 5 or 6 weeks after breeding

43. A device used to help make the vein of the limb stand out is:
a. Capture pole
b. Elizabethan collar
c. Muzzle
d. Tourniquet

44. The normal pulse for an equine patient is:
a. 16–32 bpm
b. 28–44 bpm
c. 60–160 bpm
d. 140–220 bpm

45. The gastrointestinal tracts of newborn puppies and kittens are uniquely suited to digest and absorb the milk produced by their mothers. The primary sources of energy in this milk is:
a. Fat and lactose
b. Fat and protein
c. Lactose and protein
d. Protein and starch

46. The loss of body water that has a solute concentration equal to that which remains in the compartment is called:
a. Isotonic dehydration
b. Hypovolemia
c. Hypotonic dehydration
d. Hypertonic dehydration

47. When two people are lifting a dog that weighs more than 50 lb, the person handling the front of the patient should:
a. Hold the mouth closed with one hand and lift the patient by the head
b. Lift the patient with one arm around the chest behind the front legs and the other arm over the back to interlock the fingers of the two hands
c. Use one hand to restrain each of the thoracic limbs
d. Wrap one arm around the dog's neck and the other under and around the dog's chest, behind the front leg

48. The normal respiratory rate for an equine patient is:
a. 6–16 bpm
b. 28–44 bpm
c. 60–160 bpm
d. 140–220 bpm

49. A patient with an increased pack cell volume (PCV) and an elevated total solids (TS) is probably suffering from:
a. Protein loss
b. Dehydration
c. Anemia
d. Poor perfusion

50. Which of the following is the largest unit of measure?
a. Microgram
b. Milligram
c. Gram
d. Kilogram

51. Which of the following is the series of joint, segment, and whole-body movements used for locomotion?
    a. Gait
    b. Gallop
    c. Stance
    d. Stride
52. The normal respiratory rate for a feline patient is:
    a. 6–16 bpm
    b. 16–32 bpm
    c. 20–42 bpm
    d. 42–55 bpm
53. Liquid preparations for oral administration may be purchased in several different forms. Which of the following is generally mixed with water and requires shaking well before administration?
    a. Elixir
    b. Emulsion
    c. Suspension
    d. Syrup
54. When preparing to draw up a drug into a syringe from a multidose vial, it is important to:
    a. Wipe the rubber diaphragm of the vial with 70% isopropyl alcohol before inserting the needle into the vial
    b. Wipe the rubber diaphragm of the vial with 70% isopropyl alcohol after inserting the needle into the vial
    c. Inspect the rubber diaphragm for foreign material
    d. Remove the rubber diaphragm
55. Which of the following is the correct progression of wound healing?
    a. Inflammatory phase, proliferative phase, maturation phase
    b. Inflammatory phase, proliferative phase, granulation phase, maturation phase
    c. Proliferative phase, inflammatory phase, maturation phase
    d. Proliferative phase, granulation phase, inflammatory phase, maturation phase
56. The normal respiratory rate for a canine patient is:
    a. 6–16 bpm
    b. 16–32 bpm
    c. 20–42 bpm
    d. 42–55 bpm
57. Which of the following needle sizes has the largest inside diameter?
    a. 16 gauge
    b. 18 gauge
    c. 20 gauge
    d. 22 gauge
58. When filling a prescription or administering medication to a patient, the technician must be familiar with medical abbreviations. Which of the following abbreviations indicates that a medication is to be applied to the right ear?
    a. AD
    b. AS
    c. AU
    d. OD
59. Which of the following is the act of manually providing movement of joints without muscle contraction in a repetitive manner?
    a. Active range of motion
    b. Passive range of motion
    c. Proprioception
    d. Stretching
60. The normal systolic blood pressure for a feline patient is:
    a. 120–160 mmHg
    b. 130–160 mmHg
    c. 140–180 mmHg
    d. 160–190 mmHg
61. When filling a prescription or administering medication to a patient, the technician must be familiar with medical abbreviations. Which of the following abbreviations indicates a medication is to be given once per 24 hours?
    a. s.i.d.
    b. t.i.d.
    c. q.i.d.
    d. q.o.d.
62. When filling a prescription or administering medication to a patient, the technician must be familiar with medical abbreviations. Which of the following abbreviations indicates milliequivalent?
    a. mcg
    b. mEq
    c. mg
    d. mm
63. Which of the following is a nursing intervention to allow a neurologic patient to void urine?
    a. Atonic bladder
    b. Bladder expression
    c. Bladder palpation
    d. Distension urination
64. The normal systolic blood pressure for a canine patient is:
    a. 120–160 mmHg
    b. 130–160 mmHg
    c. 140–180 mmHg
    d. 160–190 mmHg
65. Understanding common conversions from the metric system, used in veterinary medicine, to the common household systems of measurement can be helpful when instructing clients about dosage. Which of the following is equal to 30 mL?
    a. 1 tbsp
    b. 1 tsp
    c. 1 oz
    d. 1 cup
66. Which area of the brain is responsible for higher functions such as learning, memory, and interpretation of sensory input (e.g., vision and pain recognition)?
    a. Cerebrum
    b. Thalamus
    c. Hypothalamus
    d. Reticular formation

67. Which of the following statements is true of urinary catheterization?
   a. Disinfecting of the prepuce is not required.
   b. The catheter must be disinfected periodically.
   c. After the catheter is properly placed, there is no concern for dislodgment.
   d. Aseptic technique is not required when handling the collection bag.
68. At what age do the permanent canine and premolar teeth in dogs generally erupt?
   a. 3–5 months
   b. 4–6 months
   c. 5–7 months
   d. 6–8 months
69. The work of the respiratory system can be divided into the following four parts. The movement of gases across the alveolar membrane is called:
   a. Diffusion
   b. Distribution
   c. Perfusion
   d. Ventilation
70. Which of the following is a type of pain that can be beneficial in that it can allow the animal to avoid damaging stimuli?
   a. Neuropathic pain
   b. Physiologic pain
   c. Somatic pain
   d. Visceral pain
71. What is the name of the cycle of collecting subjective and objective data, identifying and prioritizing patient problems to be addressed, developing a nursing plan, implementing interventions, and assessing the treatment's effectiveness?
   a. Nursing process
   b. Physical exam
   c. Patient treatment
   d. Diagnosis
72. A bulldog would be described as having which type of head shape?
   a. Brachycephalic
   b. Dolichocephalic
   c. Mesaticephalic/mesocephalic
   d. Prognacephalic
73. Colloid solutions are used for expansion of the patient's plasma volume. Which of these fluid types is a colloid?
   a. Dextrose 5% in water
   b. Hetastarch
   c. Lactated Ringer solution
   d. Normosol R
74. Which of the following is an alkalizing agent that may be added to intravenous fluids to correct metabolic acidosis?
   a. Calcium chloride
   b. Calcium gluconate
   c. Potassium chloride
   d. Sodium bicarbonate
75. Which of the following is defined as an increase in serum creatinine and blood urea nitrogen level?
   a. Anemia
   b. Azotemia
   c. Hypoproteinemia
   d. Isosthenuria
76. The term that best describes a dog with an abnormally short mandible is:
   a. Prognathism
   b. Brachygnathism
   c. Mesaticephalic
   d. Dolichocephalic
77. When performing an electrocardiography (ECG) with a dog in right lateral recumbency, the green electrode is attached to the:
   a. Right forelimb
   b. Left forelimb
   c. Right hind limb
   d. Left hind limb
78. A common clinical sign of saddle thrombus in the cat is:
   a. Acute onset of front leg pain and paresis
   b. Acute onset of rear leg pain and paresis
   c. Bright red footpads
   d. Bounding pulses in the rear limbs
79. Consumption of colostrum after being born is important to a neonate's health because:
   a. The neonate immediately requires calories to start growing.
   b. Colostrum strengthens the bond between mother and neonate.
   c. Passive acquirement of immunoglobulins strengthens the immune system.
   d. Colostrum has a palatable taste that encourages neonates to continue suckling.
80. Stomatitis is defined as:
   a. Bad breath that is evident when dental work must be completed
   b. Inflammation of the mouth's soft tissue
   c. Resorption of hard dental tissues by odontoclasts
   d. Inflammation and infection of some or all of the tooth's supportive tissues
81. The stomach is located in the left cranial abdomen. When food is ingested, it mixes with gastric juices and is then propelled to which part of the small intestine?
   a. Cecum
   b. Duodenum
   c. Pylorus
   d. Serosa
82. Jaundice might develop as a disease progresses in which of the following organs?
   a. Heart
   b. Intestinal
   c. Kidney
   d. Liver
83. How soon should a kitten receive colostrum to obtain passive immunity?
   a. 8 hours
   b. 16 hours
   c. 24 hours
   d. 48 hours
84. Which of the following is least useful when resuscitating a dog in shock?
   a. D5W
   b. Hetastarch
   c. Hypertonic saline
   d. Plasma-Lyte 48

85. Which of the following is considered a zoonotic disease?
    a. Cholangiohepatitis
    b. Infectious canine hepatitis
    c. Leptospirosis
    d. Toxin-induced liver disease
86. Clients may not want to ask the veterinarian to repeat what he or she has said, especially if the client does not understand a lot of specialized terminology that the vet has used. The veterinary technician should:
    a. Repeat what the veterinarian said using the same terminology to be consistent
    b. Offer a dictionary of medical terms to the client so he or she can look up terms that are not understood
    c. Explain the veterinarian's words using laymen's terms
    d. Suggest the client use the Internet to obtain additional information
87. Which of the following are reasons for cautious drug dosing in neonates?
    a. Neonates have reduced liver function.
    b. The left and right ventricles are of approximately equal size.
    c. Appropriate immunoglobulin production is lacking.
    d. Neonates are susceptible to hypothermia.
88. The first drug of choice for a cat that experiences status epilepticus is:
    a. Diazepam
    b. Pentobarbital
    c. Potassium bromide
    d. Propofol
89. Which of these common radiology terms refers to a negatively charged electrode that produces electrons in the x-ray tube?
    a. Anode
    b. Artifact
    c. Cathode
    d. Collimator
90. Which of these abbreviations commonly used in radiology causes the electrons to move faster, increasing the force of the collision with the target?
    a. kVp
    b. mAs
    c. SID
    d. OID
91. Which of the following is a true feline blood type?
    a. AB
    b. DEA 1
    c. Q
    d. Tr
92. Which of the following is defined as the assessment of the patient through the tactile senses of hands and fingers?
    a. Auscultation
    b. Centrifugation
    c. Mentation
    d. Palpation
93. Tension pneumothorax occurs when pressure in the thoracic cavity is:
    a. Less than atmospheric pressure
    b. Equal to atmospheric pressure
    c. Greater than atmospheric pressure
    d. Constant as animal breathes in and out
94. Emesis should not be induced in patients that have ingested:
    a. Anticholinergics
    b. Hydrocarbons
    c. Organophosphates
    d. Salicylates
95. The mucous membranes of a dog in septic shock are:
    a. Cyanotic
    b. Hyperemic
    c. Icteric
    d. Pale
96. Diarrhea is a common clinical sign of a variety of diseases. Which of the following diseases is zoonotic?
    a. Canine parvovirus
    b. Campylobacteriosis
    c. Feline infectious enteritis
    d. Inflammatory bowel disease
97. When administering oral liquid medications the patient's neck should be:
    a. Hyperextended
    b. Flexed in a downward angle
    c. Flexed in an upward angle
    d. Held at a neutral angle
98. The most desirable induction agent for an emergency cesarean section in a dog is:
    a. Etomidate
    b. Diazepam
    c. Propofol
    d. Thiopental
99. The underlying disease for most cases of feline aortic thromboembolism is __________ in origin.
    a. Cardiac
    b. Hepatic
    c. Renal
    d. Respiratory
100. Which of the following points are true in gathering patient data during the nursing process?
    a. Past medical history should be ignored because the presenting problem might not be related.
    b. Consulting the veterinarian is unnecessary for a veterinary technician to assess a patient.
    c. The physical examination should be focused on the area of concern for efficiency.
    d. The owner's description of complaint and history should be taken.
101. To reduce intracranial pressure that results from trauma, __________ may be administered every 4 to 8 hours.
    a. Atropine
    b. Dexamethasone
    c. Diazepam
    d. Mannitol
102. Orogastric intubation is sometimes necessary for a variety of reasons. The length of the tube is measured from the nose to which of the following?
    a. Thoracic inlet
    b. 8th rib
    c. 13th rib
    d. Medial canthus

103. Certain medications applied topically to the skin have systemic and local effects. Many drugs commonly administered by the oral route, such as prednisone or methimazole, can be formulated into an ointment for this type of application. Other medications, such as nitroglycerin, are manufactured as a cream to be applied directly to the skin. Which of the following terms indicates this route of medication application?
   a. Diuretic
   b. Emetics
   c. Transdermal
   d. Viscus
104. Four patients present at the same time with emergency conditions. In which order should the patients be triaged?
   a. Dyspnea, dystocia, proptosis, laceration
   b. Proptosis, dyspnea, dystocia, laceration
   c. Laceration, dystocia, dyspnea, proptosis
   d. Dystocia, proptosis, laceration, dyspnea
105. Which of the following conditions will heal best through first intention?
   a. Abscess
   b. Degloving
   c. Simple laceration
   d. Puncture wound
106. A patient is experiencing cardiopulmonary arrest. The most desirable route of drug administration is:
   a. Intratracheal
   b. Intracardiac
   c. Intravenous
   d. Intraosseous
107. Which of the following routes of injectable drug administration is not recommended in dehydrated patients, especially in an emergency situation?
   a. Intramuscular
   b. Intraosseous
   c. Intravenous
   d. Subcutaneous
108. A patient that has been hit by a car and has no palpable pulse or detectable heartbeat requires chest compressions. These compressions should be performed at a rate of:
   a. 60–80 compressions per minute
   b. 80–100 compressions per minute
   c. 100–120 compressions per minute
   d. 120–140 compressions per minute
109. Serum centrifuged in a microhematocrit tube characterized as turbid and white in color is called:
   a. Hemolysis
   b. Hyperproteinemia
   c. Icterus
   d. Lipemia
110. In a patient, what does an elevated total protein measurement accompanied by elevated packed cell volume probably indicate?
   a. Anemia
   b. Dehydration
   c. Hemorrhage
   d. Red blood cell transfusion
111. Where should pressure be applied to minimize hemorrhage to the head of a canine trauma patient?
   a. At the thoracic inlet in both jugular grooves
   b. At the thoracic inlet of the left jugular groove
   c. To the area adjacent and ventral to the mandible
   d. To the lateral points of the temporomandibular joint
112. Which of the following is not included in the veterinary technician practice model?
   a. Technician assessment
   b. Technician evaluation
   c. Technician intervention
   d. Technician prescription
113. A calorie is a very small unit that is not of practical use in the science of animal nutrition. The commonly used unit of measure is the kilocalorie (kcal). One kcal is equal to how many calories?
   a. 10
   b. 100
   c. 1000
   d. 10,000
114. In emergency care cases in which it is not possible to administer large volumes of desired fluids, it may be beneficial to administer:
   a. D5W
   b. Hypertonic saline
   c. Hypotonic saline
   d. Isotonic saline
115. What does the presence of petechiae and ecchymoses indicate in a patient?
   a. Anemia
   b. Coagulation disorder
   c. Dehydration
   d. Hypertension
116. During emergency intubation, the cranial nerve ______ may be stimulated, resulting in ______.
   a. I; bradycardia
   b. IV; tachycardia
   c. X; bradycardia
   d. XII; tachycardia
117. Which of the following is an essential amino acid?
   a. Arginine
   b. Alanine
   c. Asparagine
   d. Aspartate
118. Which of the following is a nonessential amino acid?
   a. Histidine
   b. Isoleucine
   c. Methionine
   d. Tyrosine
119. A man phones the veterinary practice to say that he has just hit a dog with his car and the animal is now lying on the side of the road. It appears to be breathing with minimal distress; however, there is blood coming from both nostrils and there is a small river of dark blood coming from a laceration on the lateral side of its hind leg. The dog can raise its head and is attempting to stand. In advising the man, your recommendation is to do all of the following *except*:
   a. Be aware for any signs of aggression
   b. Tie the mouth securely closed with your shoelace
   c. Transport the dog on a board lying on its side
   d. Apply direct pressure to the wound

120. What does the presence of peripheral edema indicate?
   a. Coagulation disorder
   b. Hypoproteinemia
   c. Hypotension
   d. Hypoxia
121. A normal central venous pressure (CVP) range is:
   a. 0–5 cm H_2O
   b. 5–10 cm H_2O
   c. 10–15 cm H_2O
   d. 15–20 cm H_2O
122. Which of the following is a water-soluble vitamin?
   a. Vitamin A
   b. Vitamin C
   c. Vitamin E
   d. Vitamin K
123. Rickets is caused by a deficiency of which vitamin?
   a. Vitamin A
   b. Vitamin D
   c. Vitamin E
   d. Vitamin K
124. When monitoring patients on fluids and/or patients that undergo diuresis, urine output is an important consideration. The normal urine production for a healthy dog or cat is approximately:
   a. 0–1 mL/kg/h
   b. 1–2 mL/kg/h
   c. 2–3 mL/kg/h
   d. 3–4 mL/kg/h
125. On auscultation of the ventral side of the abdomen, which of the following is a normal finding?
   a. Borborygmus
   b. Crackles
   c. No audible sound
   d. Stertor
126. Multiple parameters are measured to determine a category of shock that an animal may be experiencing. In which of the following types of shock is the central venous pressure high?
   a. Cardiogenic
   b. Distributive
   c. Hypovolemic
   d. Septic
127. Most vitamins cannot be synthesized by the body and must be supplied in food. Well-balanced pet foods are formulated to provide the necessary supplementation. What is the one vitamin that can be synthesized from glucose by dogs and cats?
   a. Vitamin A
   b. Vitamin B6
   c. Vitamin C
   d. Vitamin K
128. Which of the following vitamins is a form of vitamin D?
   a. Cobalamin
   b. Ergocalciferol
   c. Pyridoxine
   d. Thiamin
129. Hypoglycemia is most common in patients that experience:
   a. Anaphylactic shock
   b. Cardiogenic shock
   c. Neurogenic shock
   d. Septic shock
130. For what purpose is an esophageal stethoscope most useful?
   a. Assessing megaesophagus
   b. Detecting ileus
   c. Monitoring anesthetized patients
   d. Routine physical exam
131. Blood levels of total bilirubin are used primarily to evaluate function of the:
   a. Kidneys
   b. Liver
   c. Pancreas
   d. Bile ducts
132. Deficiencies in iron may result in anemia. Which of these minerals may also cause anemia if it is deficient in a dog's or a cat's diet?
   a. Calcium
   b. Phosphorus
   c. Copper
   d. Zinc
133. Macrominerals are minerals that occur in appreciable amounts in the body and account for most of the body's mineral content. Microminerals, often referred to as trace minerals, include a larger number of minerals that are present in the body in very small amounts. Which of these minerals is a trace mineral?
   a. Phosphorus
   b. Nosocomial
   c. Sulfur
   d. Zinc
134. A hospital-acquired disease is known as:
   a. Endemic
   b. Magnesium
   c. Ergasteric
   d. Iatrogenic
135. Taste receptor cells are located at the tip of each taste bud. Taste receptors in dogs and cats are similar; however, there are also interesting differences. For which of the following do dogs show a preference that cats do not?
   a. Sweet
   b. Sour
   c. Salty
   d. Bitter
136. A decrease in albumin may occur in cases experiencing:
   a. Chronic liver disease
   b. Carnivorous diet
   c. Gastroenteritis
   d. Vegetarian diet
137. Which of the following describes a canine patient experiencing a fever?
   a. 97.8°F when presenting with pyometra
   b. 100.2°F after being left in a warm car for 30 minutes
   c. 103.9°F when presenting with septic peritonitis
   d. 105.7°F after exercising in heat
138. When palpating pulses, what do bounding pulses indicate?
   a. Adequate cardiovascular function
   b. Elevated diastolic blood pressure
   c. Elevated pulse pressure
   d. Elevated mean arterial pressure

139. With significant dehydration in an otherwise healthy patient, which of the following is likely to be seen on a urinalysis and CBC?
a. Increased urine UG and increased PCV
b. Increased urine SG and decreased PCV
c. Decreased urine SG and decreased PCV
d. Decreased urine SG and increased PCV

140. The majority of water and certain electrolytes, especially sodium, are absorbed in the:
a. Esophagus
b. Stomach
c. Small intestine
d. Large intestine

141. A domestic cat has a high dietary protein requirement. A diet containing animal tissue is required to meet this need. In addition, this species requires all of the following *except*:
a. Ascorbic acid
b. Arachidonic acid
c. Preformed vitamin A
d. Taurine

142. Ketonuria is most commonly associated with what condition?
a. Liver disease
b. Urinary tract infection
c. Renal failure
d. Diabetes mellitus

143. Which blood pressure measuring device obtains automated readings through sensing pressure oscillations on a cuff?
a. Doppler ultrasound
b. Direct blood pressure
c. Oscillometric device
d. Stethoscope

144. What does redness, swelling, and purulent discharges from an IV catheter site indicate?
a. Catheter site infection
b. Catheter leakage
c. Catheter occlusion
d. Normal insertion site

145. Total protein levels are ________ in a dehydrated animal.
a. Unaffected
b. Decreased
c. Increased
d. Variable

146. Which is least likely to be a clinical sign of a patient experiencing allergies?
a. Face rubbing
b. Ear problems
c. Loss of appetite
d. Skin rashes

147. Current recommendations for feeding critically ill patients are to begin feeding equal to the patient's estimated:
a. Resting energy requirement (RER)
b. Resting energy requirement (RER) × 2
c. Resting energy requirement (RER) × 4
d. Daily energy requirement (DER) × 4

148. The presence of protein in the urine may indicate:
a. Acid-base imbalance
b. Hemolytic anemia
c. Kidney disease
d. Diabetes mellitus

149. Arterial blood is most commonly used to analyze:
a. Hematology
b. Blood gases
c. Blood chemistry
d. Organ function tests

150. Various factors influence a pet's total daily energy expenditure. Which of the following is affected by gender, reproductive status, and age?
a. Basal metabolic rate
b. Voluntary muscular activity
c. Meal-induced thermogenesis
d. Adaptive thermogenesis

151. Which of the following agencies has no regulatory authority regarding pet food, however is made up of government employees?
a. AAFCO: Association of American Feed Control Officials
b. FDA: Food and Drug Administration
c. FTC: Federal Trade Commission
d. USDA: United States Department of Agriculture

152. Which clotting disorder is stimulated by hypothyroidism?
a. Hemophilia A
b. Von Willebrand disease
c. Disseminated intravascular coagulation
d. Coumarin toxicity

153. What is the most appropriate action when a catheter infection is detected?
a. Disinfect the catheter site and continue use.
b. Measure patient temperature and remove only if there is a fever.
c. Remove the catheter.
d. There is no need for intervention.

154. What is the most appropriate action when a catheter is determined to be leaking subcutaneously?
a. Leave as is and check the site 3 to 4 hours later.
b. Reduce the fluid rate and continue use.
c. Remove the catheter.
d. There is no need for intervention.

155. Hyperkalemia is commonly associated with which endocrine disorder?
a. Diabetes insipidus
b. Hyperthyroidism
c. Hyperparathyroidism
d. Hypoadrenocorticism

156. The forceful expulsion of stomach contents that requires abdominal contractions is:
a. Cachexia
b. Cathartics
c. Regurgitation
d. Vomiting

157. If the patient is vomiting fresh or digested blood, this is termed:
a. Hematemesis
b. Hematochezia
c. Hematuria
d. Hemoabdomen

158. In what endocrine disorder is polyuria and polydipsia not commonly seen?
a. Hyperadrenocorticism
b. Diabetes insipidus
c. Hyperparathyroidism
d. Diabetes mellitus

159. How do transfusion reactions in cats differ from transfusion reactions in dogs?
a. Transfusions are more acute in cats.
b. Transfusions are more acute in dogs.
c. Cats suffer from severe pruritus.
d. Transfusions are more severe in dogs.

160. Which of the following is the least effective method for delivering fluids to a 12% dehydrated patient?
a. Central intravenous
b. Intraosseous
c. Peripheral intravenous
d. Subcutaneous

161. How does marked dehydration affect an animal's eye?
a. Lateral nystagmus
b. Pinpoint pupils
c. Rotated ventrally
d. Sunken in the socket

162. An allergic response that is frequently life-threatening is the result of:
a. Agglutination
b. Hemolysis
c. DIC
d. Anaphylaxis

163. The letters "DEA" precede canine blood types. What do these letters stand for?
a. Detectable erythrocyte antibody
b. Detectable erythrocyte antigen
c. Dog erythrocyte antibody
d. Dog erythrocyte antigen

164. Which of the following describes a patient suffering from dystocia?
a. Hard, painful nipple, and galactostasis
b. Hypocalcemia, muscle spasms, fever, tachycardia, and seizures
c. In hard labor for 30 to 60 minutes with no new young produced
d. Vaginal discharge, vomiting, diarrhea, dehydration, anorexia, polyuria, and polydipsia

165. Which of the following is a technique to keep joints from becoming stiff?
a. Cold compress
b. Coupage
c. Passive range of motion
d. Warm compress

166. Coagulation tests are useful for diagnosing:
a. Rodenticide poisoning
b. Thyroid function
c. Adrenal function
d. Ethylene glycol poisoning

167. When the medical history of a patient with diarrhea is obtained, it is important to question the owner regarding the duration, severity, frequency, amount, and quality. This information can assist in localizing diarrhea as involving the small or large bowel. Which of these is a common indication of small bowel diarrhea?
a. Decreased volume of feces
b. Mucus in feces
c. Normal frequency of bowel movements
d. Tenesmus

168. Painful straining at urination or defecation is:
a. Hematochezia
b. Hematuria
c. Melena
d. Tenesmus

169. What is the underlying cause of icterus?
a. Anemia
b. Hyperbilirubinemia
c. Ketonuria
d. Hyperhemoglobinemia

170. Fresh frozen plasma can be stored up to __________ and still contain clotting factors.
a. 1 month
b. 12 months
c. 36 months
d. 60 months

171. Pancreatitis occurs in both dogs and cats. Which of the following statements is false?
a. Acute pancreatitis is seen more commonly in dogs.
b. Chronic pancreatitis is more common in cats.
c. Chronic pancreatitis is often caused by dietary indiscretion.
d. Acute pancreatitis is often caused by dietary indiscretion.

172. Treatment of acute pancreatitis includes administration of intravenous fluid therapy, analgesics, antiemetics, mucosal protectants, and antibiotics to prevent secondary sepsis. Treatment also includes which of the following?
a. Feeding a low-protein, high-fat diet
b. Feeding a bland, low-fat diet
c. Feeding a low-carbohydrate, high-fat diet
d. Feeding a diet high in fat and calories

173. Frozen fresh plasma (FFP) must be separated and frozen within __________ hours to maintain all coagulation factors in normal concentrations.
a. 2
b. 8
c. 12
d. 6

174. Which of the following choices characterizes skin turgor in a dehydrated dog or cat?
a. Prolonged
b. Normal
c. Shortened
d. Skin turgor is not a reliable indicator of hydration status.

175. Which type of anemia is associated with icterus?
a. Responsive
b. Nonresponsive
c. Hemolytic
d. Megaloblastic

176. With the exception of cats, most animals have a total blood volume equivalent to _________ of their body weight.
a. 7%
b. 15%
c. 25%
d. 40%

177. Which of the following choices characterizes the pulse rate and quality in a moderately dehydrated dog?
a. Pulse rate increased
b. Pulse rate decreased
c. Pulse rate inconsistent
d. Pulses not palpable

178. Which of the following choices characterizes the mucous membrane color and capillary refill time in a patient in hypovolemic shock?
a. Pale, prolonged
b. Pink, normal
c. Red, rapid
d. Yellow, normal

179. Myasthenia gravis is commonly associated with:
a. Megaesophagus
b. Exercise intolerance
c. Aspiration pneumonia
d. All of the above

180. Goals for the medical management of chronic kidney disease include all of the following *except*:
a. Slowing progression of the disease
b. Treating concurrent disease
c. Correcting electrolyte imbalances
d. Restoring loss of kidney function

181. Which of the following is a postpartum complication caused by hypocalcemia?
a. Eclampsia
b. Galactostasis
c. Mastitis
d. Metritis

182. Vaccines may be given by any of the following routes *except*:
a. Subcutaneously
b. Intramuscularly
c. Intranasally
d. Intraperitoneal

183. Pemphigus is a group of autoimmune disorders that affects the:
a. Blood and lymph systems
b. Skin and oral mucosa
c. Eyes
d. Hooves and claws

184. Signs of immune-mediated thrombocytopenia (ITP) include all of the following conditions *except*:
a. Petechiae
b. Ecchymoses
c. Thrombocytosis
d. Anemia

185. When the medical history of a patient with diarrhea is obtained, it is important to question the owner regarding the duration, severity, frequency, amount, and quality. This information can assist in localizing diarrhea as involving the small or large bowel. Which of these is a common indication of large bowel diarrhea?
a. Increased volume of feces
b. Mucus in feces
c. Normal frequency of bowel movements
d. Weight loss

186. Nasoesophageal (NE) feeding tubes may be used to provide short-term enteral nutrition to dogs and cats. Which of the following statements regarding NE feeding tubes is false?
a. Can be used for the continuous delivery of liquid food and/or water
b. Can be used for boluses of liquid food and/or water
c. Can often be placed without sedation
d. Can be used in unconscious patients

187. Which of the following is defined as the assessment of the patient through listening to sounds through a stethoscope?
a. Auscultation
b. Centrifugation
c. Mentation
d. Palpation

188. When setting up an IV fluid line to be used without an infusion pump, the drip chamber should be:
a. Filled completely to the top
b. Filled to the halfway line on the chamber
c. Left empty
d. Allowed to fill by gravity

189. Many hospitalized veterinary patients receive fluid therapy. The veterinary technician is responsible for many aspects of fluid therapy. Which of the following is the responsibility of the veterinarian and not the technician?
a. Calculating fluid rate
b. Ordering the fluid type
c. Initiating fluid therapy
d. Monitoring the infusion

190. Cats exposed to feline leukemia virus typically respond in any of the following ways *except*:
a. Not becoming infected at all
b. Becoming temporarily infected, developing immunity, and overcoming the infection
c. Becoming infected and continuing to shed the virus indefinitely without becoming ill
d. Becoming infected, becoming ill within 3 days, and dying within a week

191. Which of the following types of fluids is used primarily to replace intravascular volume?
a. Hypertonic crystalloid
b. Isotonic crystalloid
c. Synthetic colloid
d. Whole blood

192. What is the predominant method for transmission of feline immunodeficiency virus in cats?
a. Grooming
b. Bite wounds
c. Urine
d. Feces

193. Pinkeye or contagious conjunctivitis in cattle is caused by:
  a. *Hemophilus aegypti*
  b. *Moraxella bovis*
  c. *Streptococcus pyogenes*
  d. *Staphylococcus aureus*

194. How many drops per minute is equivalent to 20 mL/h using a 60 drops/mL drip set?
  a. 10
  b. 20
  c. 60
  d. 120

195. Which of the following allows oxygen supplementation with minimal stress and handling of the patient?
  a. Mask oxygen
  b. Nasal cannula
  c. Oxygen cage
  d. Transtracheal catheter

196. Inflammation, infection, sepsis, neoplasia, and reaction to transfusion of blood products are common causes of:
  a. Hyperthermia
  b. Hypothermia
  c. Pyrexia
  d. Pyridoxine

197. Which of the following is a common cause of bradycardia?
  a. Hypovolemia
  b. Hypoxia
  c. Hypokalemia
  d. Hyperkalemia

198. Polyuria is:
  a. A lack of urine production
  b. The production of excessive amounts of urine
  c. A lack of water intake
  d. Excessive protein in the urine

199. A urolith is a pathologic stone formed from mineral salts found in the urinary tract. Which of the following is not a factor in the formation of uroliths?
  a. Urine pH
  b. Urine concentration
  c. Urine saturation
  d. Urine protein

200. Lower urinary tract infections (UTIs) can be caused by a variety of bacteria. The most common pathogen in small animals is *Escherichia coli*. Which of the following statements is true?
  a. Bacterial infections of the bladder are common in dogs and rare in healthy cats.
  b. Bacterial infections of the bladder are common in cats and rare in healthy dogs.
  c. Male dogs are more prone to infection than female dogs.
  d. Treatment for bacterial infections consists of appropriate antimicrobial therapy for 2 to 4 days.

201. Oliguria is:
  a. Excessive eating
  b. Green urine
  c. Excessive bilirubin in the urine
  d. Decreased urine output

202. Urinary tract infection is a common secondary complication in cats and dogs with:
  a. Congestive heart failure
  b. Diabetes mellitus
  c. Hepatic lipidosis
  d. Hyperthyroidism

203. Common signs of bacterial infections of the urinary tract include hematuria, pollakiuria, urinating in inappropriate places, and which of the following?
  a. Azotemia
  b. Dehydration
  c. Dysuria
  d. Elevated BUN

204. Anuria is:
  a. Decreased urine output
  b. Decreased drinking
  c. Complete lack of urine production
  d. Excessive drinking

205. Painful urination is recorded as:
  a. Dysuria
  b. Hematuria
  c. Pyuria
  d. Proteinuria

206. Which of the following is false regarding nonpharmacologic interventions to provide pain relief?
  a. Stress from boredom, thirst, anxiety, and the need to urinate and defecate can mimic pain.
  b. The need for physical comfort of the patient is alleviated when adequate pain medication is administered.
  c. The patient may need to be placed in a position to reduce pain, to allow for easier breathing, and to promote sleep.
  d. Each patient has unique emotional needs.

207. How might anesthesia affect an animal's eye?
  a. Lateral nystagmus
  b. Pinpoint pupils
  c. Rotated ventrally
  d. Sunken in the socket

208. Hemolytic anemia is characterized by the destruction of:
  a. Erythrocytes
  b. Leukocytes
  c. Lymphocytes
  d. Monocytes

209. Which of the following laboratory tests would *not* be used to diagnose immune-mediated hemolytic anemia (IMHA)?
  a. Autoagglutination test
  b. CBC
  c. Coombs test
  d. Fructosamine

210. The veterinary technician can play an important role in pain management by:
  a. Monitoring urine and fecal output
  b. Changing the medication when it is ineffective
  c. Communicating directly with the clinician about particular concerns
  d. Directing the veterinary assistant to provide medications

211. Which of the following signs would a regurgitating patient show?
   a. Forceful contraction of the abdomen and diaphragm
   b. Restlessness
   c. Salivation
   d. Undigested food in the expelled substance
212. What does the presence of green fluid in the vomitus indicate?
   a. Gastric or esophageal disorder
   b. Gastrointestinal ulceration
   c. Involvement of bile in the duodenum
   d. Pyloric outflow obstruction
213. Which of the following characteristics do cats exhibit when they experience pain?
   a. Sleeping continuously, overeating, and attention-seeking behaviors
   b. Resentment of being handled, aggression, and abnormal posture
   c. Hyperactivity, pupillary enlargement, and tail swishing
   d. Hypotension, hypocapnia, hypopnea, bradycardia
214. During hospitalization, how often should pain assessment be performed?
   a. Every 4–6 hours
   b. Every 30 minutes to 1 hour
   c. Every 12–24 hours
   d. Every 8 hours
215. Which of the following drugs is a commonly used antiemetic?
   a. Apomorphine
   b. Chlorpromazine
   c. Hydrogen peroxide
   d. Xylazine
216. Patients with myasthenia gravis may also suffer from megaesophagus and regurgitation. These patients are at increased risk of:
   a. Acephalus
   b. Aspiration
   c. Asteatosis
   d. Astrocytoma
217. Which of the following choices characterizes the mucous membrane color and capillary refill time in a patient with liver disease?
   a. Pale, prolonged
   b. Pink, normal
   c. Red, rapid
   d. Yellow, normal
218. What do black "coffee grounds" in the vomitus indicate?
   a. Gastric or esophageal disorder
   b. Gastrointestinal ulceration
   c. Involvement of bile in the duodenum
   d. Pyloric outflow obstruction
219. When a veterinary technician is trying to distinguish pain from dysphoria, which of the following would the technician do?
   a. Place the patient on comfortable blankets
   b. Speak in low tones and interact with the animal, which makes the patient feel better, but behavior resumes when the interactions stop
   c. Move the animal to a different ward
   d. Reverse the analgesic medication
220. Which of the following is a zoonotic disease spread by fleas?
   a. *Borrelia burgdorferi*
   b. *Rickettsia rickettsii*
   c. *Ehrlichia*
   d. *Yersinia pestis*
221. Which of the following types of cancer commonly arises from cartilage or bone?
   a. Adenocarcinoma
   b. Sarcoma
   c. Lymphoma
   d. Carcinoma
222. Massage is an example of which type of rehabilitation technique?
   a. Manual therapy
   b. Effleurage techniques
   c. Physical modalities
   d. Therapeutic exercise
223. What does high-frequency diarrhea with straining and mucus indicate?
   a. Involvement of the stomach
   b. Involvement of the jejunum or ileum
   c. Involvement of the large intestine
   d. Colitis
224. Which of the following describes a patient suffering from pyometra?
   a. Hard, painful nipple, and galactostasis
   b. Hypocalcemia, muscle spasms, fever, tachycardia, and seizures
   c. In hard labor for 30 to 60 minutes with no new young produced
   d. Vaginal discharge, vomiting, diarrhea, dehydration, anorexia, polyuria, and polydipsia
225. Visceral pain is common among companion animals. Which of the following is not an example of visceral pain?
   a. Pancreatitis
   b. Gastroenteritis
   c. Bowel ischemia
   d. Osteosarcoma
226. Which of the following might a dysphoric or delirious animal experience because of opioid overdose?
   a. Thrashing and yowling continuously
   b. Claustrophobia
   c. Only rare response to soothing interaction
   d. Chewing on cage doors
227. Technicians administering IV chemotherapy drugs via an IV catheter must be vigilant. If you suspect some of the drug may have leaked out of the vessel into the surrounding tissue, you should:
   a. Immediately remove the IV catheter
   b. Leave the IV catheter in place
   c. Continue to administer the drug
   d. No action required
228. A blood sample from neonatal puppies and kittens is generally most easily obtained using the:
   a. Cephalic vein
   b. Jugular vein
   c. Lateral saphenous vein
   d. Medial saphenous vein

229. Which of the following is the shortest portion of the small intestine?
   a. Cecum
   b. Duodenum
   c. Ileum
   d. Jejunum
230. Which of the following behaviors is commonly associated with clinical signs of pain in dogs?
   a. Vocalization and increased appetite
   b. Playful actions and excessive licking of the owners
   c. Panting, anorexia, and depression
   d. Increased attention to the environment
231. Which device for measuring blood pressure is used to obtain manual blood pressure measurements, turning blood flow into an audible signal?
   a. Doppler ultrasound
   b. Direct blood pressure
   c. Oscillometric device
   d. Stethoscope
232. What does frank blood in the diarrhea indicate?
   a. Involvement of the stomach
   b. Involvement of the jejunum or ileum
   c. Involvement of the large intestine
   d. Colitis
233. The large intestine begins at the:
   a. Ascending colon
   b. Ileocolic valve
   c. Cecum
   d. Transverse colon
234. The energy required for a normal animal in a fasting state in a thermoneutral environment, awake but resting, is the:
   a. Basel energy requirement
   b. Resting energy requirement
   c. Maintenance energy requirement
   d. Daily energy requirement
235. It is sometimes difficult to distinguish normal from pain-associated behaviors in cats and dogs. Which of the following behaviors are most likely to be normal, nonpainful behaviors?
   a. Decreased appetite
   b. Unusual aggression
   c. Stretching all four legs when the abdomen is touched
   d. Decreased social interaction
236. Which of the following is most beneficial in preventing gastrointestinal ulceration?
   a. Antibiotic administration
   b. Enteral feeding
   c. Famotidine
   d. Withholding food (NPO)
237. Which of the following is true of artificial warming devices?
   a. Warm water blankets are the most effective in preventing hypothermia.
   b. Commercial warming devices do not require insulation because they are tested to be safe.
   c. They can solely provide sufficient heat support to prevent hypothermia.
   d. They should be directed at warming the core as opposed to the periphery.
238. Treatment for joint mobility includes:
   a. ROM
   b. Stretching exercises
   c. a and b
   d. None of the above
239. The US Food and Drug Administration regulates pet food labels and labels are required to contain the name of the product. Using chicken as an example, a label that includes “Chicken Dinner” in the product name, must contain:
   a. At least 70% chicken
   b. At least 10% chicken
   c. At least 3% chicken
   d. Less than 3% chicken
240. The principal display panel (PDP) is required to contain all of the following *except*:
   a. Manufacturer’s name
   b. Brand name
   c. Net weight
   d. Nutritional claim
241. The most common types of pain experienced by horses are:
   a. Ocular and head pain
   b. Spine and pelvic pain
   c. Orthopedic and abdominal/colic pain
   d. Foot and dental pain
242. Which of the following is optional (not required) on the information panel of all pet foods?
   a. Feeding guidelines
   b. Freshness date
   c. Manufacturer or distributor
   d. Nutritional adequacy statement
243. The guaranteed analysis panel on a cat food label is required to include all of the following *except*:
   a. Minimum percentage of crude protein
   b. Minimum percentage of crude fat
   c. Maximum percentage of moisture
   d. Minimum percentage of taurine
244. Which of the following are effects of hypothermia?
   a. Increased metabolic rate
   b. Decreased clotting time
   c. Cardiac dysfunction
   d. Increased peripheral blood flow
245. Which of the following clinical signs might a cow in pain exhibit?
   a. Dullness and depression
   b. Inappetence and grinding teeth
   c. A stance with one foot behind the other
   d. All of the above
246. What is the definition of obesity?
   a. 10% heavier than the optimal weight for the breed in question
   b. 20% heavier than the optimal weight for the breed in question
   c. An increase in fat tissue mass sufficient to contribute to disease
   d. None of the above
247. Which of the following drugs is a commonly used emetic?
   a. Acepromazine
   b. Apomorphine
   c. Chlorpromazine
   d. Prochlorperazine

248. Which of these drugs is a laxative used most commonly in small animals with chronic constipation?
a. Diphenoxylate
b. Lactulose
c. Loperamide
d. Paregoric

249. A traumatic cause of OA in dogs indicates obesity as a risk factor. What is the most common traumatic cause of OA in dogs?
a. Ruptured cruciate ligaments
b. Torn Achilles group
c. Hip dysplasia
d. Phalangeal fracture

250. Which of the following is detrimental to a patient with limited mobility?
a. Passive range of motion exercises
b. Sling walking
c. Adjusting position as little as possible to prevent pain
d. Neck and head being slightly elevated

251. What is "porphyrin staining" in rodents?
a. Hair standing on end
b. Color of cage litter from urine
c. Red tears that may encircle the eye
d. None of the above

252. How is pain typically characterized in rabbits?
a. Reduction in food and water intake
b. Bruxism
c. Closed eyes
d. Lateral recumbency

253. Which of these is an antiulcer drug used to treat ulcers of the stomach and upper small intestine?
a. Cimetidine
b. Famotidine
c. Ranitidine
d. Sucralfate

254. When attaching an ECG, which leg should have the red lead attached to it?
a. Right foreleg
b. Left foreleg
c. Right hind leg
d. Left hind leg

255. Which of the following is a sign of insulin overdose in treated diabetic patients?
a. Muscle wasting
b. Polyuria
c. Severe lethargy and seizures
d. Vomiting and halitosis

256. Which statement regarding first-intention wound healing is false?
a. It occurs without infection.
b. It occurs when the skin edges are held together in apposition.
c. It usually has some degree of suppuration.
d. It occurs with minimal scar formation.

257. Which of the following agencies is responsible for approving new pet food ingredients?
a. AAFCO: Association of American Feed Control Officials
b. FDA: Food and Drug Administration
c. FTC: Federal Trade Commission
d. USDA: United States Department of Agriculture

258. Which of the following is a common cause of tachycardia:
a. If skin irritation appears at the edge of the bandage
b. Hyperkalemia
c. Hypocalcemia
d. Toxin ingestion

259. If an animal goes home with a bandage, the client should check the bandage daily and remove it if any of the following are observed *except*:
a. Hypoxia.
b. All bandages should be removed 24 hours after application.
c. The bandage is wet.
d. The position of the bandage has shifted.

260. Which of the following describes a patient suffering from eclampsia?
a. Hard, painful nipple, and galactostasis
b. Hypocalcemia, muscle spasms, fever, tachycardia, and seizures
c. In hard labor for 30 to 60 minutes with no new young produced
d. Vaginal discharge, vomiting, diarrhea, dehydration, anorexia, polyuria, and polydipsia

261. When feeding the patient through a gastrostomy tube, the technician should:
a. Rapidly inject the fluids and food
b. Flush the tube with water
c. Flush the tube with air
d. Feed a full day's caloric requirement immediately after placement

262. Which of these drugs is an antacid used to reduce acidity of the stomach?
a. Amphojel
b. Misoprostol
c. Omeprazole
d. Sucralfate

263. A semipermanent feeding tube may be placed in all of the following ways *except*:
a. Through the nose
b. Through a pharyngostomy site
c. Through a gastrostomy site
d. Through the mouth

264. Which of the following are small bones that support part of the lateral walls of the throat?
a. Palatine bones
b. Pterygoid bones
c. Turbinates
d. Vomer bone

265. It is important that the nursing care provided to paralyzed patients focuses on patient comfort. The prevention of decubital ulcers can be accomplished by all of the following procedures *except*:
a. Frequent turning or repositioning the patient
b. Adequate padding in the cage or bed
c. Appropriate analgesic therapy
d. Massage

266. Which of the following is a technique used to increase blood flow to improve drainage and healing to an area?
a. Cold compress
b. Coupage
c. Passive range of motion
d. Warm compress

267. A proptosed globe:
    a. Can be caused by overzealous restraint of the animal
    b. Is not considered an emergency
    c. Can most easily occur in dolicocephalic breeds, such as collies
    d. Is commonly a consequence of conjunctivitis
268. The metabolic alterations that occur after nutritional support is started in a severely malnourished, underweight, and/or starved patient is known as:
    a. Refeeding syndrome
    b. Starvation
    c. Simple starvation
    d. None of the above
269. Proper splint and bandage care includes all of the following *except*:
    a. Washing the splint or bandage daily
    b. Preventing the bandage or splint from becoming wet
    c. Inspecting the bandage or splint daily for any change, such as swelling above or below the splint or bandage
    d. Inspecting the bandage or splint for any shifting or change in position on the limb
270. Serum centrifuged in a microhematocrit tube characterized as transparent and yellow or orange in color is called:
    a. Hemolysis
    b. Hyperproteinemia
    c. Icterus
    d. Lipemia
271. A chest tube is placed when an animal has:
    a. Subcutaneous emphysema
    b. Pulmonary edema
    c. Ascites
    d. Pneumothorax
272. Refeeding syndrome occurs in disease conditions such as:
    a. Starvation from feline hepatic lipidosis
    b. Overall malnutrition
    c. Prolonged diuresis
    d. All of the above
273. Which of the following are the bones in the tail of a dog?
    a. The cervical vertebrae
    b. The coccygeal vertebrae
    c. The lumbar vertebrae
    d. The sacral vertebrae
274. Which of the following agents has been associated with causing neurologic disorders in cats?
    a. Chlorhexidine
    b. Povidone iodine
    c. Quaternary ammonium compounds
    d. Hexachlorophene
275. Which blood pressure measuring technique requires an arterial catheter?
    a. Doppler ultrasound
    b. Direct blood pressure
    c. Oscillometric device
    d. Stethoscope
276. Anterior drawer movement detects a problem with the:
    a. Elbow
    b. Stifle
    c. Hip
    d. Hock
277. Nutrients given in excess of the patient's needs ____________ in a critically ill patient, as they would in a healthy patient.
    a. Will be used
    b. Will not be used
    c. Occasionally will be used
    d. Will be stored as fat for later use
278. What does the presence of subcutaneous fluid around an IV catheter site indicate?
    a. Catheter site infection
    b. Catheter leakage
    c. Catheter occlusion
    d. Normal insertion site
279. Clear fluid removed from thoracic cavity is known as:
    a. Pleural effusion
    b. Pulmonary edema
    c. Ascites
    d. Pyothorax
280. Which of the following choices characterizes skin turgor in an overhydrated dog or cat?
    a. Prolonged
    b. Normal
    c. Shortened
    d. Skin turgor is not a reliable indicator of hydration status.
281. Abscesses are generally allowed to heal open to provide continuous drainage. This type of wound healing is considered:
    a. Primary intention
    b. Second intention
    c. Third intention
    d. Fourth intention
282. Chronic mitral valvular disease (endocardiosis) affects more than one-third of patients older than:
    a. 2 years
    b. 5 years
    c. 8 years
    d. 10 years
283. The prevalence of dilated (congestive) cardiomyopathy in cats has decreased markedly since 1987, following the discovery that __________ deficiency was the principal cause.
    a. Glutamine
    b. Taurine
    c. Arginine
    d. Copper
284. What is the most appropriate wound-flushing solution?
    a. Hydrogen peroxide
    b. Isotonic saline
    c. Povidone-iodine solution
    d. Tap water
285. How might a neurologic issue affect an animal's eye?
    a. Lateral nystagmus
    b. Pinpoint pupils
    c. Rotated ventrally
    d. Sunken in the socket

286. Which of the following choices characterizes the mucous membrane color and capillary refill time in a patient with systemic inflammation?
a. Pale, prolonged
b. Pink, normal
c. Red, rapid
d. Yellow, normal

287. Most of the clinical signs seen in an animal in shock from excessive blood loss are attributable to:
a. Acidosis
b. Alkalosis
c. Cell death
d. Redistribution of blood flow

288. Within a few _________ of ingesting high levels of sodium, normal dogs and cats easily excrete the excess in their urine.
a. Hours
b. Days
c. Months
d. Weeks

289. Abnormalities in potassium or magnesium homeostasis may cause all of the following *except*:
a. Cardiac dysrhythmia
b. An increase in myocardial contractility
c. Profound muscle weakness
d. A potentiation of the effects of drugs

290. Which fatty acids have been shown to have a significant effect on survival times when used in dogs diagnosed with dilated cardiomyopathy (DCM) or chronic valvular disease (CVD)?
a. Omega-3
b. Omega-6
c. Omega-9
d. None of the above

291. All of the following are clinical signs a horse may show when experiencing respiratory disease *except*:
a. Stertor
b. Bilateral nasal discharge
c. Bradycardia
d. Cough

292. Which of the following are abnormal lung sounds heard in an equine patient on auscultation of the lower respiratory system?
a. Stridor
b. Wheezes
c. Stertor
d. Increased airflow

293. Projectile vomiting is most associated with:
a. Gastric or esophageal disorder
b. Gastrointestinal ulceration
c. Involvement of bile in the duodenum
d. Pyloric outflow obstruction

294. Which tests may be recommended for an equine patient experiencing upper airway complications?
a. BAL
b. TTW
c. MRI
d. Pulmonary function testing

295. All of these are typical clinical signs of advanced arthritis in dogs *except*:
a. Reduced appetite
b. Stiffness
c. Lameness
d. Difficulty in getting up

296. A respiratory disease that produces swelling of abscesses of the submandibular and retropharyngeal lymph nodes is known as:
a. Strangles
b. Equine influenza
c. Herpes
d. Viral arteritis

297. Which part of the gastrointestinal system is associated with melena?
a. Involvement of the stomach
b. Involvement of the jejunum or ileum
c. Involvement of the large intestine
d. Colitis

298. A causative agent of rhinopneumonitis is:
a. *Streptococcus equi*
b. Equine herpes virus
c. *Aspergillus* spp
d. None of the above

299. All of the following are risk factors for developing osteoarthritis in dogs *except*:
a. Trauma
b. Obesity
c. Large/giant breeds
d. Spaying or neutering

300. Which of the following is commonly seen in cats older than 10 years but is very rare in dogs?
a. Hyperadrenocorticalism
b. Hypoadrenocorticism
c. Hypothyroidism
d. Hyperthyroidism

301. Which of the following is not generally a symptom of osteoarthritis in cats?
a. Changes in mobility
b. Changes in activity level
c. Changes in grooming
d. Changes in eating habits

302. Which of the following is described as seizures involving loss of consciousness with tonic–clonic whole body movements, possibly with salivation, urination, and defecation?
a. Absence seizures
b. Focal seizures
c. Generalized seizures
d. Myoclonus

303. Which equine respiratory condition can cause abortion?
a. Strangles
b. Equine influenza
c. Herpes
d. Equine infectious anemia

304. Nutritional deficiencies and excesses in avian patients might result in:
a. Immune dysfunction
b. Increased susceptibility to infectious diseases
c. Metabolic and biochemical derangements
d. All of the above

305. Which of the following is described as seizures involving specific parts of the body, many times without a loss of consciousness?
a. Absence seizures
b. Focal seizures
c. Generalized seizures
d. Myoclonus

306. Which of the following is described as a transient alteration in consciousness, with or without external signs?
a. Absence seizures
b. Focal seizures
c. Generalized seizures
d. Myoclonus

307. Which of the following conditions is an allergic airway disease experienced by equine patients?
a. Heaves
b. Viral arteritis
c. Inflammatory airway disease
d. Exercise-induced pulmonary hemorrhage

308. Which of the following conditions matches a patient exhibiting a head tilt, facial paresis, nystagmus, positional strabismus, and ataxia?
a. Brachycephalic syndrome
b. Horner's syndrome
c. Wobbler's syndrome
d. Vestibular syndrome

309. Ferrets are which of the following?
a. Carnivores
b. Herbivores
c. Omnivores
d. Granivores

310. Pleuropneumonia in horses occurs when:
a. Viral infections spread from lung tissue to the pleural space.
b. Viral infections spread from the plural space to lung tissue.
c. Bacterial infections spread from the plural space to lung tissue.
d. Bacterial infections spread from lung tissue to the pleural space.

311. Which of the following is characterized as droopy eyelids, protruding nictitans, and miosis?
a. Brachycephalic syndrome
b. Horner's syndrome
c. Wobbler's syndrome
d. Vestibular syndrome

312. A contagious viral disease that produces limb swelling in horses is:
a. Equine infectious anemia
b. Equine viral arteritis
c. Heaves
d. Herpes

313. Lagomorphs have a rapid gut transit time resulting in starch and simple sugars not being completely digested in the:
a. Large intestine
b. Stomach
c. Small intestine
d. Colon

314. It is difficult to determine accurately how much food is being ingested by the following small mammal(s) that hoard food items:
a. Hamsters
b. Rabbits
c. Guinea pigs
d. Ferrets

315. Which of the following is described as ataxia and paresis resulting from spondylosis of the vertebrae?
a. Brachycephalic syndrome
b. Horner's syndrome
c. Wobbler's syndrome
d. Vestibular syndrome

316. Equine anaplasmosis exhibits all of the following clinical signs *except*:
a. Anemia
b. Icterus
c. Excitement
d. Stiffness

317. Clinical signs of gastric ulcers include:
a. Bruxism
b. Pyrexia
c. Hyposalivation
d. All of the above

318. Because guinea pigs lack the enzyme involved in synthesizing glucose to ascorbic acid, they require a dietary source of which of the following?
a. Vitamin K
b. Vitamin B
c. Vitamin C
d. All of these

319. Nutritional protein for ferrets should come from:
a. Carbohydrates
b. Animal-based ingredients
c. Plant-based ingredients
d. Fiber

320. Which of the following is the recommended method to prevent further exposure to chemicals spilled on an animal's fur (not caustic on touch)?
a. Applying chemical solvents
b. Bathed with mild dishwashing detergent
c. Induce emesis
d. Wipe it off with a dry towel

321. Phenylbutazone toxicosis in horses can produce:
a. Liver insufficiency
b. Oral, gastric, and colonic ulcerations
c. Icterus
d. Limb edema

322. A prescription for a controlled substance must be signed and dated when issued. The prescription must include the patient's (owner's) full name and address, the practitioner's full name and address, and the practitioner's DEA number. Which of the following is *not* required on the prescription?
a. Drug name and strength
b. Quantity prescribed and number of refills authorized
c. Directions for use
d. Drug manufacturer's name and address

323. All of the following can result from colitis in horses *except*:
a. Endotoxemia
b. Electrolyte loss
c. Hypervolemia
d. Hypovolemia

324. Which of the following is typically the largest vein to collect blood from a bird?
a. Cutaneous ulnar vein
b. Left jugular vein
c. Medial metatarsal vein
d. Right jugular vein

325. You must give a dog 250 mg of a medication that comes in tablets labeled 100 mg each. How many tablets will you give?
a. 1½
b. 2
c. 2¼
d. 2½

326. Complications of colitis in an equine patient could include:
a. Founder
b. Stertor
c. Stridor
d. Bruxism

327. What is the most common neoplasia seen in horses?
a. Lymphosarcoma
b. Osteosarcoma
c. Lymphoma
d. All of the neoplasia listed occur equally among the equine species

328. It is safe to draw ≅1% of a bird's body weight of blood. For a 450 g bird, how much blood can be taken safely?
a. 0.45 mL
b. 4.5 mL
c. 45 mL
d. 450 mL

329. All of the following are examples of viral equine encephalitis *except*:
a. Eastern
b. Western
c. Pacific
d. West Nile

330. A dog weighs 88 lb. What is this dog's weight in kilograms?
a. 20 kg
b. 24 kg
c. 40 kg
d. 44 kg

331. Clinical signs of West Nile encephalitis include:
a. Hypoesthesia
b. Bilateral nasal discharge
c. Ataxia
d. Mandibular lymph node swelling

332. When hemorrhaging from a broken blood feather occurs, what is the appropriate course of action?
a. Apply pressure to the broken edge
b. Apply styptic powder to the feather
c. Cut the feather at the base
d. Pull the feather out along the follicle

333. When should horses receive vaccines for encephalomyelitis viruses?
a. Autumn, before the first freeze
b. Before breeding
c. Spring, before mosquito season
d. At 3 months of age

334. A cat requires 60 mg of a liquid medication of strength 120 mg/mL. What quantity of the medication should be administered?
a. 2.0 mL
b. 0.5 mL
c. 0. 2 mL
d. 5.0 mL

335. __________ is a highly fatal neurologic disease in horses, characterized by a stiff, stilted gait, hyperexcitability, seizure, and coma.
a. West Nile
b. Tetanus
c. Equine degenerative myelopathy
d. Herpes

336. Which of the following is a common venipuncture site for a reptile?
a. Basilic vein
b. Caudal tail vein
c. Cephalic vein
d. Jugular vein

337. A symptom of botulism is:
a. Dysphagia
b. Bruxism
c. Pyrexia
d. Tachycardia

338. A dog on intravenous fluids has initially received 25% of the 1000 mL in the IV bag. How many mL has it received?
a. 100 mL
b. 250 mL
c. 350 mL
d. 500 mL

339. If a dog that weighs 25 kg has received 250 mL of IV fluids, how many mL/kg of body weight has it received?
a. 5
b. 10
c. 15
d. 25

340. Acute renal failure in horses is most often a result of:
a. Colic
b. Toxicity
c. Age
d. Hereditary factors

341. Which of the following is defined as an irreversible, progressive loss of functioning renal tissue?
a. Acute kidney injury
b. Chronic kidney disease
c. Acute liver failure
d. Chronic liver disease

342. Which of the following is the appropriate treatment when a patient experiences severe heartworm infestation and caval syndrome?
a. Adulticide therapy
b. Microfilaricide therapy
c. Surgical removal
d. No treatment is needed because it is transient.

343. What is an average amount of water intake per day for a full-sized horse?
a. 20–30 mL/day
b. 5–15 L/day
c. 20–30 L/day
d. 20–30 gal/day

344. A cat is to receive 90 kcal of canned food at each meal. The food has a caloric density of 360 kcal per can. How much of this food should the cat be fed at each meal?
a. 0.25 can
b. 0.20 can
c. 0.50 can
d. 1 can

345. The cell is the basic unit of the body. Cells contain all of the following *except*:
a. Cell membrane
b. Cytoplasm
c. Neuron
d. Nucleus

346. What is an average amount of urine output per day for a full-sized horse?
a. 20–30 mL/day
b. 1–3 L/day
c. 5–15 L/day
d. 5–15 gal/day

347. Which of the following is a sign of common complications to heartworm adulticide therapy?
a. Ecchymoses, anemia
b. Hemoptysis, dyspnea
c. Hematuria, stranguria
d. Melena, lethargy

348. Which of the following is the most common clinical sign of severe hypertension?
a. Acute blindness
b. Syncope
c. Tachycardia
d. Weakness

349. Which of the following is a common contributor to pancreatitis specific to dogs?
a. Blunt force trauma
b. Dietary indiscretion
c. Pancreatic hypoperfusion
d. Pancreotoxic drugs

350. Which of the following is another term for red blood cells?
a. Epithelial cells
b. Glandular cells
c. Osteoblasts
d. Erythrocytes

351. The highly convoluted ________________ extends from the glomerular capsule to the connection with the collecting duct.
a. Nephron
b. Renal tubule
c. Ureter
d. Urethra

352. The veterinary technician can use both subjective and objective observations to determine the patient's state. All of the following are examples of objective observations *except*:
a. Body temperature
b. Capillary refill time
c. Demeanor
d. Heart rate

353. All of the following may contribute to PU/PD in a horse *except*:
a. Lactation
b. Psychogenic water drinking
c. Glucocorticoid administration
d. All of the above

354. Which of the following is a technique used to help loosen purulent material within the pulmonary parenchyma?
a. Cold compress
b. Coupage
c. Passive range of motion
d. Warm compress

355. When monitoring a condition, the SOAP method may be used to ensure completeness. SOAP stands for:
a. Subjective, objective, assessment, and planning
b. Study, objective, assessment, and planning
c. See, objective, assessment, and planning
d. Subjective, objective, appraisal, and planning

356. Dermatophilosis in horses is also known as:
a. Ringworm
b. Rain rot
c. Culicoides hypersensitivity
d. Arcoid

357. Which of the following is an endocrine disease most commonly seen in cats?
a. Chronic kidney disease
b. Diabetes mellitus
c. Hyperthyroidism
d. Hypothyroidism

358. Production of fresh, bright red blood in the feces, indicating blood loss in the lower gastrointestinal tract, is:
a. Dyschezia
b. Hematochezia
c. Melaena
d. Tenesmus

359. Moon blindness in horses is also known as:
a. Ringworm
b. Rain rot
c. Corneal ulceration
d. Equine recurrent uveitis

360. Which of the following endocrine diseases results in weight gain, muscle weakness, polyuria, polydipsia, skin and hair coat abnormalities, and a pot-bellied appearance in a dog?
a. Hyperadrenocorticism
b. Hypoadrenocorticism
c. Hyperthyroidism
d. Hypothyroidism

361. Which of the following is an appropriate element for an isolation ward?
a. Sharing all equipment available to nonisolated patients
b. Positive-pressure air-ventilation system
c. Double-door entryway with an anteroom
d. Two walls of cage banks facing each other

362. Passage of large volumes of pale, fatty feces, usually associated with exocrine pancreatic insufficiency, is referred to as:
a. Anuria
b. Coprophagia
c. Steatorrhea
d. Oliguria

363. When passing urine is painful and uncomfortable, it is known as which of the following?
a. Dysuria
b. Poikuria
c. Polyuria
d. Stranguria

364. Equine recurrent uveitis results from:
a. An immune mediated condition
b. Ocular trauma
c. Antibiotic toxicity
d. Corticosteroid therapy

365. Which of the following is not part of a standard set of personal protective gear in an isolation ward?
a. Filtered respirator mask
b. Gloves
c. Gown
d. Shoe cover

366. Nauseous patients often:
a. Are unable to urinate
b. Vomit every time they eat
c. Appear unusually depressed and may intermittently lick their lips
d. All of the above

367. Conditions that may induce a coughing reflex include all of the following *except*:
a. Bronchitis
b. Infectious rhinotracheitis
c. Intestinal foreign body
d. Left-sided congestive heart failure

368. To perform coupage, cupped hands should be used to tap firmly on the chest wall, starting:
a. Caudally and working forward
b. Cranially and working upward
c. Caudally and working backward
d. Cranially and working backward

369. Pica is a term used to describe:
a. A partial reduction in appetite
b. Ingestion of an animal's own feces
c. Cravings for eating unusual food or objects
d. Loss of desire to eat

370. All of the following are common locations for decubital ulcers in recumbent horses *except*:
a. Pelvis
b. Elbow
c. Head
d. Hock

371. Why do tortoises require ultraviolet light in their habitat?
a. To prevent vitamin A deficiency
b. To promote cholecalciferol synthesis
c. To reduce vitamin D level
d. To regulate body temperature

372. Which of the following is not used to determine a patient's dehydration status?
a. Capillary refill time (CRT)
b. Eye position
c. Discharge in the pinna
d. Packed cell volume (PCV)

373. Which of the following methods of delivering fluids should not be used in severely dehydrated patients?
a. Intraosseous fluid administration
b. Intravenous fluid administration
c. Subcutaneous fluid administration
d. Intraperitoneal fluid administration

374. Recumbent equine patients should be rotated every:
a. 2–3 hours
b. 4–6 hours
c. 8–10 hours
d. 12–14 hours

375. Which of the following animals are strict carnivores?
a. Dogs
b. Ferrets
c. Prairie dogs
d. Rabbits

376. Which of the following are dorsal to the abdominal region?
a. The cervical vertebrae
b. The thoracic vertebrae
c. The lumbar vertebrae
d. The sacral vertebrae

377. Clinical signs associated with endotoxemia include:
a. Fever
b. Bradycardia
c. Cyanotic mucous membranes
d. Leukocytosis

378. Which of the following is seen as chalky-white or cream-colored urine in rabbits?
a. Coprophagy
b. Dysbiosis
c. Dytrophic calcification
d. Vitamin A deficiency

379. Which of the following complications associated with intravenous catheters is the term used to describe the formation of a blood clot resulting from an impeded blood flow?
a. Thrombophlebitis
b. Thrombus
c. Air embolism
d. Septicemia

380. After the medical resolution of colic, horses should be fed:
a. Twice daily
b. Three times daily
c. Frequent, small meals
d. A calorically dense food

381. Which of the following is true of hamsters?
   a. Male hamsters often attack newly introduced female hamsters
   b. Hamsters live 4–5 years
   c. Female hamsters may hide their young in their cheek pouches, leading to death
   d. The best method of restraint is to pick them up by the tail
382. Inappetent horses should be fed:
   a. Twice daily
   b. A calorically dense food
   c. Fresh grass
   d. High-fat food
383. Hypostatic pneumonia in hospitalized patients may be prevented by:
   a. Starting a course of antibiotics when the patient is admitted to the hospital
   b. Turning the patient every 4 hours
   c. Ensuring that the patient is fully awake and able to protect its own airway in advance of extubation
   d. All of the above
384. Which of the following might be useful in the prevention of muscle atrophy?
   a. Passive limb movement
   b. Hydrotherapy
   c. Massage
   d. All of the above
385. Physical therapy for companion animals presents multiple therapeutic benefits, improves the quality of life, and speeds functional recovery. Which of the following may be helped by physical therapy?
   a. Pain management
   b. Combating acute and chronic inflammatory processes
   c. Reducing edema
   d. All of the above
386. Septic thrombophlebitis is more likely to occur in which of the following equine patients?
   a. Patients experiencing endotoxemia
   b. Patients receiving enteral nutrition
   c. Patients that are recumbent
   d. Septic thrombophlebitis does not occur in horses.
387. Which of the following describes a patient suffering from mastitis?
   a. Hard, painful nipple, and galactostasis
   b. Hypocalcemia, muscle spasms, fever, tachycardia, and seizures
   c. In hard labor for 30 to 60 minutes with no new young produced
   d. Vaginal discharge, vomiting, diarrhea, dehydration, anorexia, polyuria, and polydipsia
388. Which of the following increases the supply of oxygen and nutrients to the tissues, while encouraging muscle relaxation? It is used to encourage the breakdown and mobilization of adhesions in damaged tissues, soften fascia, and prevent injury.
   a. Effleurage
   b. Petrissage
   c. Percussion
   d. Vibration
389. Life-threatening anaphylactic reactions are reported in equine patients that receive IV doses of:
   a. Aminoglycosides
   b. Procaine penicillin
   c. Trimethoprim-sulfa
   d. Metronidazole
390. Which of the following is one of the most important components of the successful rearing of lambs?
   a. The establishment of a strong ram–lamb bond
   b. The establishment of a strong ewe–lamb bond
   c. The establishment of a strong lamb–lamb bond
   d. The establishment of a strong ram–ewe bond
391. Which type of visit is not considered an outpatient service?
   a. Examination
   b. Vaccination
   c. Laboratory work
   d. Surgery
392. Which of the following qualifies an individual as a credentialed veterinary technologist?
   a. A 4-year Bachelor of Science degree in veterinary technology accredited by the AVMA
   b. A diploma from an accredited high school
   c. A 4-year Bachelor of Science degree in Animal Science
   d. An Associate of Science degree in veterinary technology
393. Which of the following team members is considered the face of the veterinary practice?
   a. Veterinary assistants
   b. Veterinarians
   c. Receptionists
   d. Veterinary technicians
394. What is the purpose of a safety program?
   a. To reduce or eliminate the possibility of injury or illness for everyone on the premises
   b. To reduce or eliminate the possibility of injury or illness for employees only
   c. To make OSHA happy
   d. To reduce or eliminate the possibility of injury or illness for clients only
395. Which potent chemical is used for "cold sterilization" of hard instruments?
   a. Ethylene oxide
   b. Glutaraldehyde
   c. Glutaraldehyde
   d. Formaldehyde
396. Which of the following can result from long-term work in an indoor kennel with barking dogs?
   a. Ear ablation
   b. Hearing loss
   c. Ear infections
   d. Hyphema
397. How high can noise levels in veterinary dog wards reach?
   a. 220 dB
   b. 440 dB
   c. 110 dB
   d. 880 dB

398. Which of the following describes the transmission path of a zoonotic disease?
a. From animals to humans
b. From animals to animals
c. From humans to humans
d. From humans to zoos

399. Which of the following routes may expose veterinary technicians to organisms that cause disease?
a. Inhalation
b. Ingestion
c. Needle sticks
d. All of the above

400. All of the following are adverse side effects with the use of corticosteroids in horses *except*:
a. Laminitis
b. Anuria
c. Progression of joint disease
d. Poor wound healing

401. Coupage is contraindicated in patients that have:
a. Proptosed eye
b. Fractured ribs
c. Pulmonary disease
d. Fractured femur

402. Orally administered drugs travel through the gastrointestinal tract and most are absorbed in the small intestine. After absorption across the intestinal wall, orally administered drugs:
a. Enter the stomach where the remainder of the drug is absorbed
b. Enter the hepatic portal circulation and are routed directly to the liver
c. Enter the kidney and are eliminated in the urine
d. Enter the colon and are eliminated in the feces

403. How long after birth does colostrum ingestion terminate?
a. 8 hours
b. 12 hours
c. 24 hours
d. 48 hours

404. Calf scours is common among young dairy and beef calves and is characterized by:
a. Muscle weakness
b. Diarrhea
c. Hyperglycemia
d. Hyperthermia

405. The movement of drug from the systemic circulation into the body tissues is known as which of the following?
a. Therapeutic effect
b. Protein binding
c. Distribution
d. Redistribution

406. A disease that is not caused by microorganisms but is usually a result of a disturbance in the normal metabolism of the animal is:
a. A contagious disease
b. An infectious disease
c. A noninfectious disease
d. A vector

407. Glomerulonephritis and pyelonephritis are two causes of:
a. Cardiac disease
b. Hepatic disease
c. Renal disease
d. Thyroid disease

408. Which of the following types of uroliths are found in alkaline urine?
a. Struvite uroliths
b. Ammonium urate uroliths
c. Calcium oxalate uroliths
d. Cystine uroliths

409. Nutritional myodegeneration is also known as:
a. Scours
b. Bacterial enteritis
c. Bovine viral diarrhea
d. White muscle disease

410. White muscle disease can be treated with:
a. Selenium
b. Vitamin E
c. First cut of alfalfa with higher levels of protein
d. Both a and b

411. Which of the following may be caused by right-sided heart failure?
a. Aortic stenosis
b. Mitral valve dysplasia
c. Dysrhythmias
d. Tricuspid dysplasia

412. Addison's disease is also known as which of the following:
a. Hyperadrenocorticalism
b. Hypoadrenocorticism
c. Hypothyroidism
d. Hyperthyroidism

413. Small ruminants are considered highly susceptible to enterotoxemia and should be vaccinated every ________ months.
a. 3
b. 6
c. 10
d. 12

414. Rumen fluid with a pH less than ________ suggests grain overload.
a. 3.5
b. 5.5
c. 7.5
d. 9

415. A vascular abnormality in which the hepatic portal vein empties directly into the caudal vena cava is:
a. Hepatic lipidosis
b. Portosystemic shunt
c. Cardiomyopathy
d. Aortic stenosis

416. Which of the following terms is used to describe a high-pitched, discontinuous inspiratory sound associated with the reopening of airways that closed during expiration?
a. Crackle
b. Stertor
c. Stridor
d. Wheeze

417. Rumen indigestion may result from:
a. Undercooked feeds
b. Vaccination
c. Slow transition within the rumen environment
d. Rapid feed change

418. Mucous membranes that appear deep brick red in color and appear injected are:
a. Pale
b. Icteric
c. Hyperemic
d. Cyanotic

419. Sites for intraosseous catheter placement include:
a. The cranial aspect of the greater tubercle of the humerus
b. The trochanteric fossa of the proximal femur
c. The flat medial aspect of the proximal tibia
d. All of these

420. Clinical signs of rumen indigestion include all of the following *except*:
a. Anorexia
b. Malodorous diarrhea
c. Reduced rumen motility
d. Increased rumen motility

421. Which of the following terms is used to describe passing larger volumes of urine than normal?
a. Fomite
b. Poikuria
c. Polyuria
d. Vector

422. Which of the following terms refers to excessive salivation?
a. Borborygmus
b. Dyschezia
c. Polyphagia
d. Ptyalism

423. The medical treatment for lactic acidosis in ruminants is:
a. Rapid removal of rumen contents
b. Intravenous administration of calcium
c. Intramuscular injection of sodium bicarbonate
d. Lactic acidosis cannot be treated.

424. Which of the following terms refers to the passive, retrograde movement of ingested material to a level above the upper esophageal sphincter?
a. Expectoration
b. Hematemesis
c. Regurgitation
d. Vomiting

425. Which plane across the body divides it into cranial (head end) and caudal (tail end) parts that are not necessarily equal?
a. Sagittal plane
b. Transverse plane
c. Median plane
d. Dorsal plane

426. Rumen tympany is also referred to as:
a. Lactic acidosis
b. Tetany
c. Bloat
d. Rumenitis

427. Which is a special term used only to describe positions or directions on the head?
a. Cranial
b. Caudal
c. Rostral
d. Ventral

428. Which surface of an animal's leg is closest to its body?
a. Medial
b. Lateral
c. Proximal
d. Distal

429. The technician who is involved in performing a professional dental cleaning should be capable of:
a. Performing assessment
b. Periodontal debridement
c. Polishing
d. All of the above

430. The American Veterinary Dental College (AVDC) position statement indicates it is appropriate for veterinary technicians to perform:
a. Dental cleanings
b. Root canals
c. Surgical extractions
d. All of the above

431. Dogs have all of the following types of teeth *except*:
a. Canines
b. Elodont teeth
c. Molars
d. Premolars

432. Which of the following terms is used to describe the tooth surface facing the lips?
a. Rostral
b. Caudal
c. Lingual
d. Vestibular

433. Which of the following may be caused by left-sided heart failure?
a. Mitral valve dysplasia
b. Pulmonic stenosis
c. Neoplasia
d. Myocarditis

434. Which of the following terms refers to a structure with a location that is closer to the crown of the tooth in relation to another structure?
a. Palatal
b. Mesial
c. Coronal
d. Apical

435. Treatment of free gas bloat in ruminant patients includes all of the following *except*:
a. Passing an orogastric tube
b. Administration of calcium
c. Exercise restriction
d. Rumen trocarization

436. Treatment of frothy gas bloat in ruminant patients includes the administration of all of the following products *except*:
a. Dioctyl sodium sulfosuccinate (DSS)
b. Poloxalene
c. Household detergent
d. Calcium

437. Most mammals have a first set of teeth, which are replaced with permanent or adult teeth. This first set of teeth is called:
a. Malocclusions
b. Occlusion
c. Deciduous
d. Cingulum

438. How many adult teeth does a normal cat have?
a. 30
b. 32
c. 40
d. 42

439. The heart is an organ that is commonly affected by age. Chronic valvular disease (CVD) results from thickening of the heart valves and affects many:
a. Young dogs
b. Older dogs, especially smaller dogs
c. Large breed dogs
d. Cats

440. Hardware disease in ruminants is also known as:
a. Grain overload
b. Rumen tympany
c. Traumatic reticuloperitonitis
d. Polioencephalomalacia

441. Bovine viral diarrhea can manifest with all of the following clinical symptoms *except*:
a. Oral ulcers
b. Pyrexia
c. Bloat
d. Lethargy

442. Chronic renal disease is one of the diseases seen most commonly in geriatric patients, especially cats. In addition to causing increased polyuria and polydipsia, renal disease may also cause:
a. Anemia
b. Anorexia
c. Gastric upset
d. All of the above

443. Which of the following treatments used to treat heartworm disease in dogs is a common microfilaricide treatment?
a. Thiacetarsamide
b. Melarsomine dihydrochloride
c. Ivermectin
d. All of the above

444. Increased intraocular pressure (IOP), caused by more aqueous fluid being produced than leaving the eye, might result in:
a. Pannus
b. Keratoconjunctivitis sicca
c. Glaucoma
d. Chronic superficial keratitis

445. The cornea is composed of four layers. Which of the following is not one of the four layers of the cornea?
a. Epithelium
b. Stroma
c. Endothelium
d. Sclera

446. Treatment for bovine viral diarrhea is:
a. IV fluid administration
b. Anti-inflammatory administration
c. Anthelmintic therapy
d. There is no treatment for BVD.

447. Overproduction of tears may be caused by:
a. Ocular pain or irritation
b. Sad or frightened patients
c. Ingesting too much protein in the patient's diet
d. All of the above

448. The term used to describe a group of hereditary eye diseases seen in many breeds of dogs, which causes loss of night vision or low-light vision, is:
a. Pannus
b. Keratoconjunctivitis sicca
c. Progressive retina atrophy
d. Chronic superficial keratitis

449. Pyrexic cows experiencing bovine respiratory disease syndrome commonly have a temperature of:
a. 99.0–101.5°F
b. 96.8–99.0°F
c. 100.0–102.2°F
d. 104.0–107.0°F

450. The mass treatment of animal populations before the onset of disease is termed:
a. Metaphylaxis
b. Preconditioning
c. Megascript
d. All of the above

451. External parasites are responsible for many skin problems seen in small-animal medicine. All of the following may be treated with shampoos and dips *except*:
a. Fleas
b. Ticks
c. Ear mites
d. Mange mites

452. The current recommended location for administering a rabies vaccine to a cat is:
a. Between the shoulder blades
b. The right shoulder
c. The right rear leg
d. The left rear leg

453. In the veterinary hospital, barrier nursing should be practiced:
a. To keep the staff's uniforms free of pet hair
b. To prevent the staining of staff uniforms
c. To avoid transmitting infection among patients
d. All of the above

454. Which of these endocrine disorders can result from the failure of the pituitary gland to produce antidiuretic hormone (ADH)?
a. Diabetes insipidus
b. Cushing's disease
c. Hypothyroidism
d. Insulinoma

455. BRDS, which affects primarily feedlot calves and dairy calves younger than 6 months of age, is caused by:
a. Respiratory viruses
b. Bacteria
c. Stress
d. All of the above

456. Ovine progressive pneumonia (OPP) causes all of the following *except*:
a. Mastitis
b. Arthritis
c. Neurologic signs
d. Pyometra

457. Which of the following types of cells makes up bone?
a. Osteoblasts
b. Osteocytes
c. Osteoclasts
d. All of the above

458. The bones of the head and trunk are referred to as the:
a. Axial skeleton
b. Appendicular skeleton
c. Visceral skeleton
d. Metacarpal bones

459. Which of the following bones is located where the spinal cord exits the skull?
a. Interparietal bones
b. Occipital bone
c. Parietal bones
d. Temporal bones

460. Which of the following are the two small bones that form part of the orbit of the eye?
a. Ossicles
b. Malleus
c. Incus
d. Lacrimal

461. Retained placentas in dairy cattle may result from all of the following *except*:
a. Delivery of twins
b. Abortion
c. Vitamin D deficiency
d. Dystocia

462. Postpartum uterine infections are known as:
a. Fetal membranes
b. Metritis
c. Pseudopregnancy
d. Milk fever

463. The two zygomatic bones are also known as the:
a. Malar bones
b. Maxillary bones
c. Lacrimal bones
d. Nasal bones

464. Which of the following are four thin, scroll-like bones that fill most of the space in the nasal cavity and are also called the nasal conchae?
a. Palatine bones
b. Pterygoid bones
c. Turbinates
d. Vomer bone

465. A condition that is characterized by the accumulation of fluid in the uterus and one or more corpus lutea in the ovaries is known as:
a. Fetal membranes
b. Metritis
c. Pseudopregnancy
d. Milk fever

466. Which of the following types of vertebrae are unique in that they form a single solid structure?
a. The cervical vertebrae
b. The thoracic vertebrae
c. The lumbar vertebrae
d. The sacral vertebrae

467. In accordance with the Association of American Feed Control Officials (AAFCO) guidelines ingredients on food labels are listed:
a. In descending order by volume
b. In ascending order by volume
c. In descending order by weight
d. In ascending order by weight

468. A metabolic disorder in which there is a severe decline in the serum calcium, usually occurring within 48 hours of calving, is known as:
a. Fetal membranes
b. Metritis
c. Pseudopregnancy
d. Milk fever

469. The most caudal sternebra is called the:
a. Sternebra
b. Manubrium
c. Xiphoid
d. Anticlinal

470. The most proximal bone of the thoracic limb is the:
a. Humerus
b. Scapula
c. Tubercle
d. Greater tubercle

471. The antebrachium is made up of which two bones?
a. Humerus and radius
b. Humerus and scapula
c. Ulna and radius
d. Radius and scapula

472. The anatomical term synarthroses refers to:
a. Fibrous joints
b. Palatine bones
c. Vomer bone
d. Pterygoid bones

473. Uterine infections in ruminants are associated with all of the following *except*:
a. Unbalanced prepartum diets
b. Viruses
c. Delivery of twins
d. Bacterium

474. Clinical symptoms of milk fever include:
a. Staggering gate
b. Bilateral nasal discharge
c. Polyuria
d. Lacrimation

475. The effect of the omega-3 fatty acids on cardiac patients may be attributed to:
a. Anti-inflammatory effects
b. Improved appetite
c. Antiarrhythmic effects
d. All of the above

476. The American Veterinary Dental College (AVDC) supports veterinary technicians with advanced training who are performing which of the following procedures?
a. Charting dental lesions
b. Taking dental radiographs
c. Performing nonsurgical subgingival root planing
d. All of the above

477. Milk fever can be prevented by:
a. Feeding a high-calcium diet during the dry period
b. Feeding a low-calcium diet during the dry period
c. The slow administration of calcium intravenously
d. The oral administration of 50% dextrose

478. Spheroidal joints are also called:
a. Trochoid joints
b. Pivot joints
c. Gliding joints
d. Ball-and-socket joints

479. Which of the following is commonly seen in dogs but is rare in cats?
a. Hyperadrenocorticalism
b. Hypoadrenocorticism
c. Hypothyroidism
d. Hyperthyroidism

480. Ketosis in dairy cows may result from all of the following *except*:
a. Deficient energy intake
b. Abomasal displacement
c. Metritis
d. Milk fever

481. Caseous lymphadenitis is:
a. The most common cause of lymph node abscess in small ruminants
b. A major cause of carcass condemnation in sheep
c. Endemic
d. All of the above

482. Which of the following is *not* a common risk factor for obesity in dogs?
a. Age
b. Feeding semi-moist food
c. Feeding homemade diets
d. Feeding dry dog food

483. Which of the following allows the body to withdraw calcium from the bone when blood calcium levels are low?
a. Osteoblasts
b. Osteocytes
c. Osteoclasts
d. Hematopoiesis

484. Copper toxicity results from the accumulation of copper in the:
a. Liver
b. Kidneys
c. Gallbladder
d. Lymph nodes

485. Keratoconjunctivitis in sheep or goats can be treated with:
a. Penicillin
b. Tetracycline
c. Aminoglycoside
d. Phenylbutazone

486. Which of the following bones are usually clearly visible in young animals but may become indistinguishable in older animals?
a. Interparietal bones
b. Occipital bone
c. Parietal bones
d. Temporal bones

487. In general, how many days should be allowed for diet changes in dogs and cats?
a. 5 to 7 days
b. 1 to 3 days
c. 48 to 72 hours
d. 28 days

488. As a dog or cat transitions from immature to mature, the recommended diet change is for the:
a. Increase in calories
b. Decrease in fat and increase in fiber
c. Addition of table scraps
d. Decrease in fiber

489. Which of the following is/are antioxidants?
a. Vitamin A, vitamin E, vitamin C
b. L-Carnitine
c. Vitamin
d. Krebs cycles

490. Which of the following has the least influence on the acceptability of food to dogs and cats?
a. Salt content
b. Size
c. Shape
d. Color

491. Interdigital necrobacillosis is also known as:
a. Polioencephalomalacia
b. Foot rot
c. Hardware disease
d. Hairy heel wart

492. Laminitis in cattle is a diffuse, aseptic inflammation of the:
a. Coronary band
b. Wall
c. Coffin bone
d. Corium

493. Horses are which of the following?
a. Ruminants
b. Omnivores
c. Hindgut fermenters
d. Carnivores

494. Puppies, kittens, and nursing mothers require:
a. Higher levels of protein in their diet than adult maintenance requirements
b. Vitamin supplementation
c. Higher levels of fiber than are required in adult maintenance diets
d. Fewer calories than adult maintenance requirements

495. Which of the following is/are examples of preservatives?
a. Omega-3 oils
b. Sucrose, dextrose
c. Lactated Ringer
d. Vitamin E

496. Which of the following organisms is responsible for ringworm in cattle?
   a. *Trichophyton verrucosum*
   b. *Microsporum gypseum*
   c. *Epidermophyton floccosum*
   d. *Microsporum canis*
497. Contagious ecthyma is a common viral disease of small ruminants that is zoonotic. What is this disease also known as?
   a. Orf
   b. Sore mouth
   c. Sorf
   d. Both a and b
498. Corticosteroids are used for which of the following?
   a. Decreasing appetite
   b. Stimulating tear production
   c. Increasing appetite
   d. Improving hair coat
499. Chondroitin sulfates are an example of:
   a. Flavor enhancement
   b. Nutraceuticals
   c. Dentifrices
   d. Parenteral medications
500. All of the following processes should be completed for piglets raised in confinement *except*:
   a. Iron injections at 3 days of age
   b. Clipping needle teeth
   c. Tail docking
   d. Removing dewclaws
501. The typical gestation period for pigs is:
   a. 42 days
   b. 63 days
   c. 114 days
   d. 147 days
502. Another term for exertional rhabdomyolysis is:
   a. Polydipsia
   b. Azoturia
   c. Anorexia
   d. Pyrexia
503. Which of the following vitamins is/are water soluble?
   a. Vitamins A and D
   b. Vitamins E and K
   c. Vitamins B12 and C
   d. Vitamins A and E
504. Patients with pancreatitis or hyperlipidemia should avoid foods that are:
   a. High in protein
   b. Low in protein
   c. High in fats
   d. Low in fats
505. Taurine and L-carnitine have been found to aid in:
   a. Inappetence
   b. Dysphagia
   c. Cardiac muscle function
   d. Temperament
506. Potassium deficiency results in:
   a. Neurologic disease
   b. Weight gain
   c. Increased palatability
   d. Improved growth
507. The typical gestation period for dogs is:
   a. 42 days
   b. 63 days
   c. 114 days
   d. 147 days
508. In the equine large intestine, the optimum pH for microbial activity that promotes volatile fatty acid (VFA) absorption is:
   a. 6.5
   b. 6.7
   c. 7.1
   d. 6.1
509. AAFCO feeding trials are used to evaluate pet foods in all of the following life stages *except*:
   a. Senior
   b. Gestation and lactation
   c. Adult maintenance
   d. Growth
510. Porcine stress syndrome is also known as:
   a. Malignant hypothermia
   b. Malignant hyperthermia
   c. Sodium ion toxicosis
   d. Porcine parvovirus
511. According to AAFCO rules, a pet food indicating "beef" on the label must have how much beef in the food?
   a. 70%
   b. 50%
   c. 40%
   d. 25%
512. If the client wants to feed a preservative-free food to a pet, which food should you recommend?
   a. Canned food
   b. Dry food
   c. Semi-moist food
   d. A combination of dry and semi-moist foods
513. Porcine stress syndrome results in all of the following *except*:
   a. Muscle tremors
   b. Death
   c. Hypothermia
   d. Dyspnea
514. Which of the following statements about cats is true?
   a. Cats need more protein in their diets than dogs.
   b. It is important to provide plenty of variety by buying different brands of foods.
   c. Hairballs are a sign of illness in a cat.
   d. Giving liver as a treat can result in vitamin A deficiency.
515. Which of the following diets is intended to be dispensed under the supervision of veterinarians in the context of a valid veterinarian–client–patient relationship (VCPR)?
   a. Veterinary therapeutic
   b. Holistic
   c. Raw
   d. Over-the-counter
516. Swine wallow in mud to:
   a. Forage for food
   b. Thermoregulate
   c. Remove parasites
   d. Prevent sunburn

517. Kittens are generally fed a growth formula food until they are approximately how old?
a. 10–12 months
b. 18 months
c. 2 years
d. 6 months

518. Most clients offer treats to their pets. How many treats can safely be given each day?
a. Not more than 20% of the pet's diet in treats
b. As long as the pet is not overweight, there is no limit on the number of treats that may be offered.
c. If the treats are low in calories, it should not matter.
d. Not more than 10% of the pet's diet in treats

519. What is the average weight of an adult pot-bellied pig?
a. 50 lb
b. 120 lb
c. 220 lb
d. 450 lb

520. Which amino acid must be present in cat food but not in dog food?
a. L-Carnitine
b. Glutamine
c. Taurine
d. Lysine

521. The list of ingredients appears on a pet food label in order of:
a. Dietary importance
b. Nutrient bioavailability
c. Caloric percentage
d. Weight

522. What is the most common nutritional disease of pot-bellied pigs?
a. Calcium deficiency
b. Vitamin E deficiency
c. Obesity
d. Malnourishment

523. Which government agency is responsible for inspecting the ingredients used in pet foods?
a. USDA
b. FDA
c. AAFCO
d. FTC

524. A bitch's food caloric needs are highest:
a. During the first trimester
b. During the fourth week of lactation
c. During the third trimester
d. Just before weaning

525. An atypical heart sound associated with a functional or structural valve abnormality is known as:
a. Arrhythmia
b. Fibrillation
c. Murmur
d. Infarct

526. Semi-moist food is not recommended for an animal that is:
a. Diabetic
b. Geriatric
c. Growing
d. Lactating

527. If "fish flavor" is stated on the pet food label, how much fish must be in the food?
a. 5%
b. 8%
c. 15%
d. An amount that is detectable by the pet

528. Which of the following is an example of a product designator from a pet-food label?
a. Beef entrée
b. Cat food
c. Nine Lives
d. Complete and balanced for adult dogs

529. An equine that is about to turn 1 year old is referred to as a:
a. Yearling
b. Foaling
c. Weanling
d. Filly

530. What does the guaranteed analysis on the pet-food label mean?
a. It states the exact measurements of the nutrients and moisture levels in the food.
b. It is a combination of maximum and minimum nutrient and moisture levels in the food.
c. It states the maximum levels of each nutrient in the food.
d. It states the minimum levels of each nutrient in the food.

531. The difference between the amount of a nutrient consumed and the amount absorbed by the body is described as:
a. Dry-matter basis
b. Energy density
c. Digestibility
d. Hydrolyzation

532. Which of the following is an acceptable method of making food more palatable to the pet?
a. Warming the food
b. Adding onion salt to the food
c. Heating the food above body temperature
d. Adding warm milk to the food

533. Fats are composed of triglycerides, which include:
a. Two fatty acids to a glycerol chain
b. Three fatty acids attached to three glycerol chains
c. Three fatty acids attached to a glycerol chain
d. One fatty acid attached to one glycerol chain

534. A male donkey that has not been castrated and is capable of breeding is referred to as a:
a. Jenny
b. Dam
c. Jack
d. Sire

535. The process of giving birth to pigs is referred to as:
a. Stag
b. Freshening
c. Farrowing
d. Kidding

536. What diet should be prescribed and monitored by animal health professionals and describes most veterinary therapeutic diets?
a. All purpose
b. Premium
c. Specific purpose
d. Value

537. Pet foods that use food ingredients that have not been exposed to insecticides, pesticides, or medications such as antibiotics or growth promotants, are known as:
a. Organic
b. Raw
c. Natural
d. Holistic

538. Pet food recipes found in books and on the Internet are almost always:
a. Perfectly balanced for dogs and cats
b. Complete and healthy
c. Highly palatable
d. Incomplete and unbalanced

539. The number of animals within a population that becomes sick can be defined as:
a. Morbidity
b. Mortality
c. Chronic
d. Acute

540. A collection of blood in the cranial portion of the ventral cavity is known as:
a. Pneumothorax
b. Pneumonia
c. Hemothorax
d. Hemostasis

541. The most common error in feeding growing puppies is providing:
a. Too much food
b. Too little food
c. The right amount of food
d. Too much milk

542. Cats that act hungry and tend to overeat should be:
a. Free fed
b. Meal fed twice a day
c. Fed once a day
d. Fed once a week

543. The most common form of malnutrition in hospitalized animals is ___________ because of the reluctance or inability to eat voluntarily.
a. Lack of energy and protein intake
b. Lack of sugar
c. Lack of carbohydrates
d. Lack of minerals

544. Which type of feeding is the most physiologic and often the safest route?
a. Intravenous
b. Intraosseous
c. Oral
d. Subcutaneous

545. Which of the following is *not* true of nasoesophageal (NE) or nasogastric (NG) tubes?
a. Inexpensive
b. Easy to place
c. Useful for short-term feeding support
d. Costly and inefficient

546. An overgrowth of scar tissue at the site of injury is known as:
a. Papule
b. Petechia
c. Laceration
d. Keloid

547. Osteomalacia is known as the:
a. Hardening of bones
b. Softening of bones
c. Collection of abnormal cells that accumulate within the bones
d. Thickened skin

548. Inadequate intake of protein and energy may result in:
a. A dry, dull hair coat and excessive pigmentation
b. Pyoderma
c. Skin depigmentation and crusting around the eyes
d. Hair loss and dry, dull hair coat

549. Which factor influences the success of a dietary elimination trial?
a. Type of protein contained in the elimination diet
b. Use of a homemade diet
c. Concurrent allergic skin disease
d. All of the above

550. Foods effective in the management of an adverse food reaction include:
a. Novel protein diets
b. Foods that contain high levels of proteins
c. Foods that contain a single carbohydrate source
d. Foods that use only natural preservatives

551. What is the name of the third party that evaluates veterinary dental foods and approves an oral care seal on its veterinary products?
a. Veterinary Oral Health Council
b. American Veterinary Dental Association
c. Academy of Veterinary Oral Health
d. Veterinary Dental Society

552. What structure connects muscles to bones?
a. Ligaments
b. Tendons
c. Foramen
d. Process

553. Acute diarrhea is usually caused by:
a. Malignancy
b. Diet or dietary indiscretion
c. Histoplasmosis
d. Pythiosis

554. Which of the following is not a typical sign of inflammatory bowel disease (IBD) in cats?
a. Vomiting
b. Diarrhea
c. Weight gain
d. Weight loss

555. Increased frequency of defecation and loose and watery stools are common when the ___________ is involved.
a. Small intestine
b. Large intestine
c. Colon
d. Stomach

556. A comprehensive nutritional history for patients presenting with acute diarrhea should include:
a. Ingestion of trash or any unusual foods
b. The diet fed
c. The household member responsible for feeding the pet
d. All of the above

557. Inflammation of all bones or inflammation of every part of one bone is known as:
a. Panosteitis
b. Polypathia
c. Pandemic
d. Osteoporosis

558. The term amyoplasia refers to the:
a. Lack of muscle formation or development
b. Paralysis of muscles
c. Muscular weakness or partial paralysis restricted to one side of the body
d. Any disease of a muscle

559. Patients suffering with short-bowel syndrome (SBS) should be fed the following type of diet in the long term:
a. High-protein, high-fat diets
b. Low-fat, highly digestible diets
c. High-fat, highly digestible diets
d. High-protein, moderately digestible diets

560. Dehydration is frequently encountered in patients suffering from GI disorders. Which of the following factors causes this?
a. Reduced oral water consumption
b. Vomiting
c. Diarrhea
d. All of the above

561. If vomiting patients lose hydrogen and chloride ions in excess of sodium and bicarbonate, which of the following should be expected?
a. Acidemia
b. Neutrality
c. Alkalemia
d. None of the above

562. Hydremia refers to which of the following?
a. Inadequate supply of blood to a part of the body
b. Disorder in which there is excess fluid in the blood
c. Low red blood cell count
d. The narrow, pointed bottom of the heart

563. The accumulation of fluid in the abdominal cavity is defined as:
a. Auscultate
b. Infarct
c. Ascites
d. Edema

564. Enteral feeding tubes of all types should be flushed:
a. Before and after use
b. After use only
c. Before use only
d. Never

565. Which type of nutrition is defined as providing nutrients intravenously?
a. Parenteral
b. Enteral
c. Oral
d. Emergency

566. Feeding dog food to a cat is ____________ advised.
a. Never
b. Sometimes
c. Seldom
d. Frequently

567. An abnormally low white blood cell count is referred to as:
a. Normocytic
b. Leukocytosis
c. Leukopenia
d. Anemia

568. A lack of digestion is referred to as which of the following?
a. Bradypeptic
b. Apepsia
c. Monogastric
d. Anastomosis

569. All but one of the following make up the five vital assessments:
a. Temperature
b. Pain
c. Weight
d. Nutrition

570. Which nutrient is the most important for patients with acute or chronic vomiting?
a. Protein
b. Vitamins
c. Minerals
d. Water

571. Acute diarrhea is typically the result of which of the following?
a. Diet
b. Parasites
c. Infectious disease
d. All of the above

572. The goals of the nutritional management of hepatic disease include:
a. Providing substrates to support hepatocellular repair and regeneration
b. Maintaining normal metabolic processes
c. Avoiding toxic byproduct accumulation
d. All of the above

573. Melena refers to which of the following?
a. Passing of dark, tarry feces containing blood that has been acted on by bacteria in the intestines
b. A semi-fluid mass of partially digested food that enters the small intestine from the stomach
c. A protein produced by living cells that initiates a chemical reaction but is not affected by the reaction
d. To fall back into a disease state after an apparent recovery

574. Which of the following is a technique used to decrease blood flow and minimize inflammation?
a. Cold compress
b. Coupage
c. Passive range of motion
d. Warm compress

575. What percentage in excess of the optimal weight for their breed classifies dogs and cats as obese?
a. ≥20%
b. 10%–19%
c. 35%
d. 50%

576. When reintroducing exercise into the pet's daily regimen to promote weight loss, the following recommendation should be made:
a. Start with a moderate exercise plan
b. Exercise should include running
c. Exercise as much as possible on the first day
d. Exercise is not necessary

577. Sebaceous glands that deposit cat scent are located in all of the following areas *except*:
a. Around the lips and chin
b. Between the toes
c. The tip of the tail
d. The perianal area

578. What amino acid does a cat require in its diet to avoid dilated cardiomyopathy?
a. Cysteine
b. Taurine
c. Guanine
d. Isoleucine

579. The most accurate formula to determine the pet's resting energy requirement is:
a. RER kcal/day = 50 (ideal body weight in kg) 0.75
b. RER kcal/day = 70 (ideal body weight in kg) 0.50
c. RER kcal/day = 70 (ideal body weight in kg) 0.75
d. RER kcal/day = 75 (ideal body weight in kg) 0.75

580. Specific recommendations that support a successful weight-loss program include:
a. Using an 8 oz measuring cup to measure food
b. Appropriate exercise for the pet
c. Emphasizing feeding consistency including feeding the pet from its designated dish only
d. All of the above

581. The most common cause of FLUTD in cats less than 10 years of age is:
a. Struvite uroliths
b. Feline idiopathic cystitis (FIC)
c. Calcium oxalate crystals
d. Urethral plugs

582. Which of the following is a clinical symptom of thromboemboli in cats?
a. Chronic onset or rear leg pain
b. Acute onset of rear leg pain
c. Palpable pulses in rear limbs
d. Warm foot pads

583. Causes of congenital heart disease include all of the following *except*:
a. Genetics
b. Viruses
c. Nutrients
d. Drugs

584. Litter box management for cats with FLUTD includes:
a. Using only covered litter boxes
b. Using highly scented litter so the unappealing urine odor is masked
c. Having one litter box per cat—plus one additional
d. Always using scoopable litter

585. Diagnostic evaluation of felines with recurrent or persistent lower urinary tract signs should include:
a. Urinalysis
b. Diagnostic imaging
c. Thyroid testing
d. Both a and b

586. To evaluate urine for crystalluria:
a. Urinalysis should be performed within 30 minutes of sample collection.
b. Evaluation is best performed after urine has been refrigerated for 12 hours.
c. Sample should always be sent out for evaluation.
d. Ultrasound is the most reliable means of evaluation.

587. Which of the following clinical symptoms is seen in a cat with heartworm disease?
a. Diarrhea
b. Left-sided chronic heart failure
c. Weight gain
d. Vomiting

588. The FDA's Center for Veterinary Medicine (CVM) regulates pet foods in cooperation with the individual states. Which of the following is *not* a responsibility of the FDA?
a. Establishing certain animal food-labeling regulations
b. Specifying certain permitted ingredients such as drugs and additives
c. Enforcing regulations about chemical and microbiologic contamination
d. Enforcing manufacturing procedures

589. Adverse reaction to food is an abnormal response to which of the following?
a. Ingested toxin
b. Ingested food
c. Inhaled food
d. Inhaled toxin

590. Protein malnutrition in patients with hepatic disease manifests clinically as:
a. Hypoalbuminemia, weight gain, and muscle atrophy
b. Weight loss, muscle atrophy, and hypoalbuminemia
c. Muscle atrophy, hyperalbuminemia, zinc accumulation
d. Vitamin K accumulation, weight loss, and muscle atrophy

591. Small frequent meals help the patient with hepatic disease by:
a. Optimizing blood flow through the liver
b. Managing fasting glucose
c. Minimizing hepatic encephalopathy
d. All of these

592. In cats, hepatic lipidosis often occurs as a result of which of the following?
a. Thyroid disease
b. Anorexia and weight loss
c. Lower urinary tract disease
d. Cardiac disease

593. Chronic hepatitis may be a result of:
a. Copper accumulation, infectious diseases, drugs
b. Breed-associated hepatitis, autoimmune disease, copper deficiency
c. Infectious diseases, unknown etiology, zinc accumulation
d. Autoimmune disease, Vitamin K deficiency, drugs

594. When administrating oral medications to cats, which of the following techniques should be practiced?
a. Placing medication inside a piece of cheese
b. Flushing water with a syringe into the mouth after the tablet has been given
c. Placing the tablet or capsule on the back of the tongue and holding the mouth shut
d. Cats cannot take oral medications

595. Clinical signs of acute gastritis may include:
a. Anorexia
b. Polyuria
c. Polydipsia
d. Anuria

596. The accumulation of inflammatory cells within the lining of the small intestine, stomach, or large bowel is known as:
a. Acute gastritis
b. Chronic gastritis
c. Inflammatory bowel disease
d. Colitis

597. Hematuria can be determined to exist:
a. When there is any positive reading for blood on the dipstick
b. If intact erythrocytes are present in the microscopic examination of the urine sediment
c. Only if there is a red tint to the urine sample
d. Whenever there is a case of feline idiopathic cystitis

598. Methods for increasing water intake in cats include:
a. Placing ice cubes in water
b. Adding broth to foods
c. Providing water fountains
d. All of the above

599. A key nutritional component to managing the inflammation seen in FIC is:
a. Adding salt to the cat's food
b. Adding omega-3 fatty acids to the diet
c. Feeding only once daily
d. Feeding various types of food

600. Currently the recommended treatment(s) for cats with FIC include:
a. Nutritional management
b. Environmental enrichment
c. Stress reduction
d. All of the above

601. The most common sign in dogs and cats with allergic disease is:
a. Reluctance to eat
b. Lethargy
c. Pruritus
d. Hyperpigmentation

602. All of the following information should be provided to clients when their pet has been diagnosed with inflammatory bowel disease *except*:
a. A definitive diagnosis requires a biopsy.
b. Therapy will only be required until the clinical signs resolve.
c. A special diet will be required for the remainder of the animal's life.
d. Pets cannot eat table food.

603. Which of the following medications is most commonly implicated in cases of gastric ulcers in horses, dogs, and cats?
a. NSAIDs
b. Antibiotics
c. Parasiticides
d. Immunotherapy

604. All of the following are among the most commonly diagnosed skin disorders in cats *except*:
a. Miliary dermatitis
b. Eosinophilic granuloma complex
c. Adverse reaction to food
d. Hyperthyroidism

605. Adverse reaction to food is an:
a. Abnormal response to an ingested toxin
b. Abnormal response to an ingested food
c. Abnormal response to an inhaled food
d. Abnormal response to an inhaled toxin

606. Feline eosinophilic granuloma complex involves which three conditions?
a. Indolent ulcers, eosinophilic plaques, and linear granulomas
b. Indolent ulcers, eosinophilic granulomas, and linear plaques
c. Linear ulcers, eosinophilic plaques, and linear granulomas
d. Eosinophilic ulcers, indolent granulomas, and linear plaques

607. Intestinal lymphangiectasia is defined as:
a. A protein-losing stomach disease
b. A fat-losing stomach disease
c. A fat-losing intestinal disease
d. A protein-losing intestinal disease

608. Which of the following factors is most important in the nutritional management of inflammatory skin disorders?
a. Assessment of current foods being fed and identification of an appropriate feeding plan
b. Assessment of the feeding method and elimination of corn from the diet
c. Determination of an appropriate feeding plan including the elimination of gluten from the diet
d. Assessment of the feeding plan and elimination of carbohydrates from the diet

609. Which of the following factors influences the success of a dietary elimination trial for pets suffering from adverse food reactions?
a. Type of protein contained in the elimination diet
b. Complete elimination of all other foods and treats
c. Concurrent allergic skin disease
d. All of the above

610. Feline obstipation is also known as:
a. IBD
b. Megacolon
c. Constipation
d. All of the above

611. Acute onset of hepatic disease may result from all of the following drugs *except*:
a. Acetaminophen
b. Phenobarbital
c. Antifungals
d. Vitamin K

612. Dogs and cats with diabetes mellitus (DM) typically present to the veterinary hospital with which of the following signs?
a. Polydipsia and lethargy
b. Weight gain and lethargy
c. Lethargy and chronic kidney disease (CKD)
d. All of the above

613. What is a relatively new option for managing hyperthyroidism in cats?
a. Thyroidectomy
b. Nutritional management
c. Anti-thyroid medications
d. Radioactive iodine

614. What percentage of hyperthyroid cats remained euthyroid when fed ≅0.32 ppm iodine DMB as the sole source of nutrition?
a. 60%
b. 80%
c. 90%
d. 75%

615. Clinical signs associated with liver disease could include:
a. Melena
b. Anuria
c. Weight gain
d. Hyposalivation

616. Which of the following hormones is produced by the thyroid gland?
a. Triiodothyronine
b. Tetraiodothyronine
c. Calcitonin
d. All of the above

617. If a patient is 12%–15% dehydrated, which characteristics would you expect to see?
a. Death
b. Slightly dry mucous membranes
c. Prolonged capillary refill time
d. Eyes are sunken in orbits

618. Which of the following is intended to provide long-term solutions for feline hyperthyroidism?
a. Surgery and oral anti-thyroid drugs
b. Radioactive iodine therapy and oral anti-thyroid drugs
c. Surgery and radioactive iodine therapy
d. Radioactive iodine therapy only

619. Feline hyperthyroidism is a result of:
a. Malnutrition
b. Excessive production of thyroid hormone
c. Excessive production of the pituitary glands
d. Diets containing excessive protein

620. Poorly controlled diabetic patients may experience muscle wasting because of:
a. Fat being catabolized to meet energy needs
b. Protein being catabolized to meet energy needs
c. Carbohydrates being catabolized to meet energy needs
d. All of the above

621. All of the following are symptoms of hyperthyroid disease *except*:
a. Weight gain
b. Polyphagia
c. Vomiting
d. Increased appetite

622. Which of the following hormones does the pancreas produce?
a. Oxytocin
b. Glucagon
c. Glycogen
d. Calcitonin

623. Key nutritional factors in the management of skin disorders include:
a. Carbohydrates, essential fatty acids, and calcium
b. Proteins, essential fatty acids, and calcium
c. Proteins, essential fatty acids, copper, and zinc
d. Proteins, carbohydrates, essential fatty acids, copper, and zinc

624. A paraneoplastic syndrome manifested by weight loss and a decrease in body condition, despite adequate nutritional intake, is known as:
a. Cancer anorexia
b. Cancer cachexia
c. Inappetence
d. None of the above

625. Key nutritional factors in animals with cancer include which of the following?
a. Soluble carbohydrate, protein, and omega-3 fatty acids
b. Soluble carbohydrate, polyphenols, and cysteine
c. Insoluble carbohydrate, polyphenols, and arginine
d. Insoluble carbohydrate, protein, and calcium

626. Which of the following types of diabetes are more common in dogs?
a. Insulin dependent diabetes
b. Type 1 diabetes
c. Non–insulin-dependent diabetes
d. Both a and b

627. Copper storage disease is an inherited autosomal recessive trait that is prevalent in:
a. Afghan hounds
b. Bedlington terriers
c. Pekinese dogs
d. Cats

628. The liver's main responsibility is:
a. Maintaining homeostasis
b. Removing waste products from the body
c. Both a and b
d. None of the above

629. The most common electrolyte disturbance in vomiting cats and dogs is:
a. Hypokalemia
b. Hypochloremia
c. Hypernatremia
d. All of the above

630. In clinical trials of dogs with spontaneous cancer, high levels of omega-3 fatty acids and arginine in food were shown to benefit dogs with:
a. Lymphoma
b. Nasal carcinomas
c. Hemangiosarcomas
d. All of the above

631. Which of the following types of diabetes is more common in cats?
a. Non–insulin-dependent diabetes
b. Type 2 diabetes
c. Insulin-dependent diabetes
d. All of the above

632. Which statement(s) regarding vitamin supplementation in dogs is/are true?
a. The vitamin E level should be appropriate to the levels of polyunsaturated fatty acids in the food.
b. Vitamin E can reverse cancer cachexia.
c. Mega doses of vitamins are recommended for dogs receiving commercial dry food diets.
d. All of the above.

633. Which of the following is considered to be the most commonly detected electrolyte disturbance when providing nutritional support to a patient suffering from refeeding syndrome?
a. Hyponatremia
b. Hypochloremia
c. Hypokalemia
d. Hypomagnesemia

634. Common symptoms of diabetes in both dogs and cats include:
a. Bradypnea/bradycardic
b. Polyuria/polydipsia
c. Weight gain/pitting edema
d. All of the above

635. Which of the following conditions can be life-threatening?
a. Hyperglycemia
b. Hypoglycemia
c. Polyuria
d. Polyphagia

636. Which disease involves the adrenal glands?
a. Diabetes
b. Addison's
c. IBD
d. Eclampsia

637. Which clinical signs would indicate small intestine diarrhea?
a. Mucus
b. Hematochezia
c. Increased stool volume
d. Dyschezia

638. Which clinical signs would indicate large intestinal diarrhea?
a. Halitosis
b. Borborygmus
c. Tenesmus
d. Steatorrhea

639. Which of the following toxic plants would have an effect on the cardiovascular system?
a. Oleander
b. Marijuana
c. Morning glory
d. Tobacco

640. Which of the following toxic plants would have an effect on the kidneys of cats?
a. Apricot seeds
b. Easter lily
c. Onion
d. Mistletoe

641. Which heart condition is most common in Pomeranians?
a. Patent ductus arteriosus
b. Aortic stenosis
c. Atrial septal defect
d. Ventricular septal defect

642. If a patient is 5%–6% dehydrated, which characteristics would you expect to see?
a. 5%–6% is not clinically detectable.
b. Subtle loss of skin elasticity
c. Prolonged capillary refill time
d. Eyes are sunken in orbits.

643. Which of the following symptoms would be common in dogs experiencing anemia?
a. Anorexia
b. Weakness
c. Tachypnea
d. All of the above

644. Which of the following diseases would cause a patient to become anemic?
a. Iron deficiency
b. Lethargy
c. Alopecia
d. Viral infection of the upper respiratory tract

645. Opaque pupillary opening and progressive vision loss may be seen in patients with:
a. Calcivirus
b. Parvovirus
c. Cataracts
d. Distemper

646. Which of the following may contribute to ringworm in companion animals?
a. *Microsporum canis*
b. *M. gypseum*
c. *Trichophyton mentagrophytes*
d. All of the above

647. What is a cause of flea allergy dermatitis?
a. Environmental allergens, including trees, grasses and pollens
b. Ctenocephalides infestation
c. Blastomyces infestation
d. Mite infestation

648. Which of the following would contribute to geriatric vestibular syndrome?
a. Increased intraocular fluid production
b. Otitis media
c. *Coccidioides immitis*
d. *Histoplasma capsulatum*

649. The accumulation of triglycerides in the liver is known as:
a. Renal lipidosis
b. Hepatic lipidosis
c. Hyperthyroidism
d. Hypothyroidism

650. Which of the following diseases exhibit coughing, fever, and mucopurulent discharge?
a. Kennel cough
b. Canine parvovirus
c. Canine distemper
d. Infectious canine tracheobronchitis

651. Which of the following contribute to Lyme disease?
a. *Rickettsia rickettsii*
b. *Scabies scabiei*
c. *Staphylococcus*
d. *Borrelia burgdorferi*

652. Viral rhinotracheitis is caused by:
a. Canine distemper
b. Canine parvovirus
c. Herpes virus
d. von Willebrand's disease

653. Which of the following may be a viral enteritis?
a. Parvovirus
b. Coronavirus
c. Rotavirus feline
d. All of the above
e. None of the above

654. Petechial hemorrhage, ecchymosis, epistaxis, and lethargy might be seen with:
a. Thrombocytopenia
b. Urolithiasis
c. Renal failure
d. Pyometra

655. The over-ingestion of fats may contribute to:
a. Patella luxation
b. Cushing's disease
c. Pancreatitis
d. Panosteitis

656. All of the following diseases are of orthopedic decent *except*:
a. *Osteochondrosis dissecans*
b. von Willebrand's disease
c. Panosteitis
d. Arthritis

657. All of the following would be considered a core vaccine *except*:
a. Distemper
b. Rabies
c. Canine adenovirus
d. Leptospira

658. All of the following would be considered a core vaccine *except*:
a. Modified live panleukopenia
b. Herpes-calicivirus
c. Leukemia
d. Rabies

659. What is the known duration of immunity for *Bordetella bronchiseptica*?
a. 6 months
b. 1 year
c. 3 years
d. 5 years

660. When charting a medical record, in which portion of the record is the TPR logged?
a. Subjective
b. Objective
c. Assessment
d. Plan

661. If a patient presents with a heart murmur that can be heard with the stethoscope bell slightly off of the thoracic wall, which grade would the heart murmur receive?
a. 1/6
b. 4/6
c. 6/6
d. Murmurs are not graded.

662. When choosing a specific restraint mechanism for a patient, which of the following should be taken into consideration before restraining?
a. Available equipment
b. The individual patient's behavior
c. Whether the client is watching
d. There are no considerations in advance of restraint

663. Which of the following devices is used to immobilize a patient with chemical restraint?
a. Muzzle
b. Towel
c. Drugs
d. Sandbags

664. Which of the following knots is used to secure the ends of two ropes together or to form a nonslipping noose?
a. Square knot
b. Nonslip knot
c. Surgeon's knot
d. Reefer's knot

665. Which of the following is a false statement?
a. Use minimal restraint with a cat to start the procedure
b. Treat all cats the same when it comes to handling
c. Use distraction techniques when retraining cats
d. Use towels to restrain cats rather than muzzles

666. All of the following procedures can be completed with a feline patient in sternal recumbency *except*:
a. Administration of ophthalmic medications
b. SQ injections
c. Cystocentesis
d. Cleaning ears

667. All of the following are signs of anxiety in a dog *except*:
a. Ears stand tall
b. An averted gaze
c. Raised hair along the back
d. Tail straight out

668. __________ feet is known as the "kill zone" in cattle, when considering restraint.
   a. 2–4 feet
   b. 4–6 feet
   c. 6–8 feet
   d. 8–10 feet

669. What device is used to restrain cattle?
   a. Nose ring
   b. Nose lead
   c. Chute
   d. Halter

670. The "blind spot" for horses is:
   a. Between their eyes
   b. Below their noses
   c. To the left of their heads
   d. To the right of their heads

671. In which direction can a horse kick?
   a. Directly behind itself
   b. To the front of itself
   c. To its side
   d. All of the above

672. A horse's tail can indicate its attitude. What does a horse do with its tail when it is afraid?
   a. Wringing or circling
   b. Held straight down
   c. Tightly clamped
   d. Held with an arch

673. What are the main tools of equine restraint?
   a. Halter
   b. Lead rope
   c. Nose twitch
   d. Only a and b

674. All of the following are distraction techniques for an equine patient *except*:
   a. Rocking an ear
   b. Skin roll
   c. Hand twitch
   d. Tail jacking

675. A hurdle is used to capture:
   a. Sheep
   b. Cows
   c. Pigs
   d. Horses

SECTION 10

Diagnostic Imaging

Brooke Lockridge

QUESTIONS

1. Which one of the following imaging modalities produces images without the use of radiation?
   a. X-ray
   b. Ultrasound
   c. Fluoroscopy
   d. CT
2. To obtain a radiographic image of both temporomandibular joints of a small animal, which of the following is the best position?
   a. Dorsal recumbency
   b. Ventral recumbency
   c. Right lateral recumbency
   d. Sternal recumbency
3. When obtaining a lateral projection of the skull of small animals, where should the centering of the image occur?
   a. Midway between the tip of the nose to just caudal to the occipital protuberance at the base
   b. Lateral canthus of the eye socket
   c. Between the eyes
   d. Above the base of the tongue and just below the palate, approximately at the commissure of the mouth
4. Which grade level on the ossification index for newborn foals does a closed metacarpal and metatarsal physes describe?
   a. Grade 1
   b. Grade 2
   c. Grade 3
   d. Grade 4
5. What element is found within the transducer of an ultrasound machine?
   a. Bucky
   b. Piezoelectric ceramics
   c. Magnets
   d. All of the above
6. To obtain a dorsoventral view of the abdomen of a rabbit, where should the center of the beam be focused?
   a. Center over the heart
   b. Center over the liver
   c. Center of the body cranial to caudal
   d. Center over the thoracolumbar area
7. What happens to crystals within the ultrasound transducer when strong, short electrical pulses strike them?
   a. They harden
   b. They melt
   c. They vibrate
   d. They break apart
8. Radioisotopes used in nuclear medicine studies are administered by which route?
   a. Orally
   b. Injection
   c. Inhalation
   d. All of the above
9. At what age in foals does the closure of the proximal growth plate of P2 occur?
   a. 4–22 weeks
   b. 18–30 weeks
   c. 22–38 weeks
   d. 18–38 weeks
10. A deformity, in which the interior angle of the joint, viewed frontally, is <180 degrees is known as what?
    a. Axial rotation
    b. Windswept
    c. Valgus deformity
    d. Varus deformity
11. Where should the cassette be held when obtaining a dorsomedial-palmarolateral oblique view of the carpus of a horse?
    a. Against the palmarolateral aspect of the leg
    b. Against the medial aspect of the leg
    c. Against the palmaromedial aspect of the leg
    d. Against the palmar aspect of the carpus
12. Which of the following effects is a result of radiation overdose to lymphoid tissue?
    a. Cataract
    b. Ulcers
    c. Atrophy
    d. Necrosis
13. Which of the following radiographic terms describes the caudal surface of the hind limb distal to the carpus?
    a. Plantar
    b. Dorsopalmar
    c. Palmar
    d. Caudocranial
14. Approximately how many shades of gray are incorporated into the display of an image obtained through ultrasound?
    a. 50 shades of gray
    b. 100 shades of gray
    c. 226 shades of gray
    d. 256 shades of gray

15. What is the correct definition of the abbreviation *B-mode* in ultrasound?
   a. Brightness
   b. Bits
   c. Binary
   d. Power mode

16. Which of the following best describes the use for Doppler ultrasound?
   a. Doppler uses a motion mode that simultaneously creates a B-mode image while displaying the motion of the tissues over a two-dimensional scale.
   b. Doppler is used to image the flow of blood and other liquids as well as to measure their velocity.
   c. Doppler units display the different shades of gray.
   d. None of the above

17. When using color-flow Doppler in ultrasound, what do the displayed red and blue colors mean?
   a. Blue colors are veins and red colors are arteries.
   b. Blue colors are arteries and red colors are veins.
   c. The colors show blood flow; blue indicates flow away and red indicates flow toward.
   d. The colors show different velocities of blood.

18. Which radiographic view provides the best accuracy for evaluating major fracture dislocation and conformational abnormalities in horses?
   a. Lateral view
   b. Medial oblique view
   c. The flexed lateral view
   d. Dorsopalmar view

19. What is the difference between color Doppler and power Doppler ultrasound?
   a. Color Doppler indicates velocity and power Doppler indicates direction of flow.
   b. Power Doppler is sensitive to slow flow and color Doppler indicates direction of flow.
   c. Power Doppler indicates direction of flow and color Doppler indicates slow flow.
   d. Color Doppler indicates arteries and power Doppler indicates veins.

20. Pulse wave imaging can detect velocities up to a maximum of __________ m/s.
   a. 0.5
   b. 1
   c. 1.4
   d. 2.2

21. Which of the following best describes the Nyquist point in ultrasound?
   a. The point at which the maximum blood velocity is reached
   b. The point of deepest penetration
   c. The point at which a drop-out signal is reached and an image is no longer produced
   d. The Nyquist point is not an ultrasound concern

22. Dental film should be placed in the mouth with the dimple facing:
   a. Up and pointing rostrally
   b. Up and pointing caudally
   c. Down and pointing rostrally
   d. Down and pointing caudally

23. Which of the following allows measurements of very high blood flow velocities in ultrasound?
   a. Color Doppler
   b. PW Doppler
   c. CW Doppler
   d. Harmonics

24. What does the gain control knob adjust on the ultrasound machine?
   a. The power output
   b. The brightness of the image
   c. The PRF scale used in PW Doppler
   d. The depth of the image

25. What does the TGC or time gain compensation allow on the ultrasound machine?
   a. It allows the amount of time it takes sound to travel through a medium to be changed.
   b. It provides a faster time frame for clearer images with motion.
   c. It allows adjustment of the gain at various depths.
   d. None of the above.

26. Carpal hematomas usually result from the rupture of which vessel in the horse?
   a. Buccal vein
   b. Accessory cephalic vein
   c. Medial saphenous vein
   d. Superficial thoracic vein

27. What is the maximum number of focal points that are recommended for use in ultrasound?
   a. 2
   b. 3
   c. 4
   d. 5

28. Which of the following frequencies will allow the deepest level of penetration in ultrasound?
   a. 4 MHz
   b. 5 MHz
   c. 9 MHz
   d. 12 MHz

29. The ability to distinguish between two objects that are adjacent to each other, yet perpendicular to the sound wave in ultrasound, is described as:
   a. Axial resolution
   b. Lateral resolution
   c. Longitudinal resolution
   d. Azimuthal resolution

30. To obtain a lateromedial view of the femorotibial joint of the horse, the cassette should be placed against which surface?
   a. Cranial aspect
   b. Caudal aspect
   c. Lateral aspect
   d. Medial aspect

31. Which of the following is the proper way to disinfect an ultrasound probe?
   a. Autoclave
   b. Gas sterilization
   c. Wipe with a glutaraldehyde-based disinfectant
   d. Immerse in an alcohol-based cleaner

32. Which of the following ultrasound artifacts is likely to be produced when the sound wave strikes a metal object or a pocket of air?
    a. Edge shadowing
    b. Comet tail
    c. Mirror image
    d. Acoustic enhancement
33. Which of the following is the correct abbreviation to perform a *caudalocranial* radiograph?
    a. CdCr
    b. Dpa
    c. CrCd
    d. Cr
34. Which of the following is the correct definition for the ultrasound term *hypoechoic*?
    a. Bright gray
    b. Dark gray
    c. White
    d. Black
35. Which of the following can the piezoelectric crystal within an ultrasound probe do?
    a. Convert electrical energy into mechanical energy
    b. Convert mechanical energy into electrical energy
    c. Change shape in the presence of an electrical current
    d. All of the above
36. For a dorsolateral-palmaromedial oblique of the metacarpus of a horse, on which surface should the cassette be placed?
    a. The medial aspect
    b. The palmar aspect
    c. The palmaromedial aspect
    d. The palmarolateral aspect
37. Which of the following radiographic terms describes the view when the primary x-ray beam enters the dorsal surface and exits the ventral surface of the patient?
    a. Dorsoventral
    b. Ventrodorsal
    c. Craniocaudal
    d. Caudocranial
38. To obtain a craniocaudal view of the tibia of a small animal, the patient should be in which of the following positions?
    a. Sternal recumbency
    b. Dorsal recumbency
    c. Right lateral recumbency
    d. Left lateral recumbency
39. To perform an ultrasound in the intercostal region, which transducer would be ideal?
    a. Linear probe
    b. Microconvex probe
    c. Phase array probe
    d. All of the above produce the same images.
40. When scanning in the sagittal plane, where is the cranial aspect of the patient's body displayed on the ultrasound monitor?
    a. Left side of the monitor
    b. Right side of the monitor
    c. Top of the monitor
    d. Bottom of the monitor
41. The M in M-mode of ultrasound represents which of the following?
    a. Brightness
    b. Motion
    c. Harmonics
    d. Multiplanar reconstruction
42. Which of the following transducer frequencies allows the deepest imaging depth?
    a. 7.5 MHz
    b. 10 MHz
    c. 5 MHz
    d. 3 MHz
43. The radiation unit REM (radiation equivalent man/mammal), the unit measured by radiation monitoring dosimeters, has been changed to which international naming code?
    a. Sievert (Sv)
    b. Coulomb/kg (C/kg)
    c. Becquerel (Bq)
    d. Gray (Gy1)
44. Which of the following image receptors is used in dental imaging?
    a. Film
    b. Phosphor plates
    c. Neither
    d. Both
45. A biarticular fracture is also known as a:
    a. Corner fracture
    b. Slab fracture
    c. Chip fracture
    d. Biarticular fractures do not exist.
46. What size power outlet is required to run a digital dental unit?
    a. 70 kV
    b. 110 V
    c. 110 kV
    d. 8 mA
47. What is the purpose of the foil backing found on dental x-ray film?
    a. To absorb exiting remnant radiation
    b. To be able to mold to the shape of the tooth
    c. To create a waterproof barrier around the film
    d. None of the above
48. Which of the following is the correct order to process dental film?
    a. Passed through the developer, then the fixer, then the wash.
    b. Passed through the fixer, wash, developer, then the wash again.
    c. Passed through the developer, wash, fixer, then the wash again.
    d. Passed through the wash, developer, fixer, and wash again.
49. Which of the following radiographic terms describes the radiographic views distal to the carpus obtained by passing the primary x-ray beam from the dorsal direction to the palmar surface of the forelimb?
    a. Plantar
    b. Dorsopalmar
    c. Palmar
    d. Caudocranial

50. What is the typical kilovoltage preset on a dental unit?
   a. 110 kV
   b. 25 kV
   c. 50 kV
   d. 70 kV
51. Which of the following correctly describes a CT image?
   a. A two-dimensional image
   b. A matrix of pixel or picture elements
   c. A three-dimensional image
   d. A matrix of voxels
   e. Both c and d
   f. Both a and b
52. A computer tomography x-ray tube can rotate how many degrees?
   a. 270 degrees
   b. 180 degrees
   c. 360 degrees
   d. None, it does not rotate
53. When using computed tomography, what Hounsfield unit does blood have?
   a. –50 HU
   b. 160 HU
   c. 80 HU
   d. None of these
54. The number of detectors that are covered by the x-ray beam in CT scanning is known as which type of field of view?
   a. Display field of view
   b. Scan field of view
   c. Raw data
   d. Image data
55. Anything below what Hounsfield unit is displayed as black on CT imaging?
   a. –750 HU
   b. 0 HU
   c. 250 HU
   d. None; black is not displayed on CT
56. Which of the following Hounsfield units on CT imaging appears as white?
   a. –755 HU
   b. 120 HU
   c. 1200 HU
   d. 1260 HU
57. Modern CT scanners use multislice technology and are able to acquire image slices thinner than which of the following sizes?
   a. 10 mm
   b. 1 cm
   c. 10 cm
   d. 1 mm
58. What does the term *pitch* refer to in CT imaging?
   a. The calculation of an unknown value based on two known values on either side
   b. A ratio between the table movement in mm and the CT slice thickness
   c. A type of helical scanning
   d. None of the above
59. IV contrast used with CT imaging will help to view all of the following *except*:
   a. Veins
   b. Arteries
   c. Bone marrow
   d. Infection of the extremities
60. When using the shaded-surface display process with CT, which Hounsfield units should be selected to view bone?
   a. –750 HU
   b. 160 HU
   c. –200 HU
   d. –800 HU
61. Which of the following best describes the term *fulcrum*?
   a. The point of interest
   b. The distortion of the resolution of anatomy above and below the region of interest
   c. A series of boxes or individual shades of information
   d. None of the above
62. Which of the following best describes the word *tomography*?
   a. Cut or section
   b. Whole
   c. Point of interest
   d. A series of boxes or individual shades of information
63. Which of the following imaging modalities can cause radiation burns if the unit is too close to the skin and remains in exposure mode for too long?
   a. CT
   b. MRI
   c. Fluoroscopy
   d. Ultrasound
64. What does the acronym ALARA stand for?
   a. As low as reasonably achievable
   b. Animal limited anatomical radiation assessment
   c. As large as radiation accepts
   d. None of the above
65. Atoms that emit particles and energy to become stable are known as:
   a. Photons
   b. Radionuclides
   c. Radioactive decay
   d. Isotopes
66. What is an isotope termed when it is radioactive?
   a. Photon
   b. Radionuclide
   c. Radioisotope
   d. None of the above; isotopes do not become radioactive
67. Which particles have high linear energy transfer (LET) with low penetrability?
   a. Alpha particles
   b. Beta particles
   c. Gamma particles
   d. Both a and b
68. Which of the following types of tissue absorb the most radiation?
   a. Bone
   b. Soft tissue
   c. Fat
   d. Bone, fat, and soft tissue absorb the same amount of radiation

69. For a mediolateral view of the tarsal joint of a horse, the cassette should be placed in which position?
 a. On the lateral surface
 b. On the medial surface
 c. On the plantar surface
 d. On the plantaromedial surface
70. Which of the following kV will produce more scatter and secondary radiation?
 a. 40 kV
 b. 60 kV
 c. 70 kV
 d. 110 kV
71. Which of the following is considered to be a cardinal rule for radiation protection?
 a. Distance
 b. Time
 c. Shielding
 d. All of the above
72. When obtaining a dorsopalmar view of the carpus of a horse, where should the cassette be held?
 a. Against the palmarolateral aspect of the leg
 b. Against the medial aspect of the leg
 c. Against the palmaromedial aspect of the leg
 d. Against the palmar aspect of the carpus
73. Which time frame is the most critical for limiting radiation exposure to an unborn fetus of an employee?
 a. 2nd trimester
 b. 3rd trimester
 c. Between 2 and 10 weeks' gestation
 d. After 35 weeks
74. Which radiographic view provides the best option for detecting slab fractures in horses?
 a. Lateral view
 b. Medial oblique view
 c. Flexed lateral view
 d. Dorsopalmar view
75. *Meters to measure the rate of exposure* is also known as:
 a. Dosimeter
 b. Fluoroscopy
 c. Collimation
 d. Shielding
76. Which of the following is the best method for storing lead x-ray gowns?
 a. Folded and kept in a drawer to prevent overexposure
 b. Hung up by the shoulders when not in use
 c. Draped across the table with the tail end hanging off the side
 d. None of the above
77. Which of the following locations is best for storing a dosimeter badge?
 a. In the x-ray room
 b. At home with the employee
 c. In a box on a windowsill to receive natural light
 d. In a dry, cool place away from the x-ray room
78. How often should x-ray equipment in a veterinarian's office be tested?
 a. Every 6 months
 b. Every year
 c. Every 2 years
 d. Only once when the equipment is installed
79. To what level of kV radiation are most lead aprons effective?
 a. 50 kV
 b. 70 kV
 c. 90 kV
 d. 125 kV
80. All of the following people are allowed to view individual dosimetry reports *except*:
 a. OSHA inspector
 b. Owner of the practice
 c. The employee exposed
 d. All team members
81. Which of the following can occur if DNA is affected by radiation?
 a. Cell death.
 b. Cell damage may be obvious, with portions of the DNA compromised.
 c. Cell may display no immediate effects but damage may have occurred internally that will affect the individual later, when mitosis occurs.
 d. All of the above.
82. Which imaging modality is superior for demonstrating the brain and spinal cord?
 a. Ultrasound
 b. MRI
 c. X-ray
 d. Fluoroscopy
83. What is a major safety concern with MRI machines?
 a. The amount of radiation emitted
 b. The intensity of the magnet on the patient
 c. The potential projectile effect with metallic objects within the vicinity of the machine
 d. MRI machines are extremely safe and contain no safety concerns.
84. What is the term used to describe a medical magnet's field strength?
 a. Gauss
 b. Tesla
 c. Polarity
 d. Precession
85. Which type of magnet consists of two slabs of magnetic material facing each other?
 a. Permanent magnets
 b. Electromagnets
 c. Resistive magnets
 d. Superconducting magnets
86. Which of the following is the most common medical magnet?
 a. Resistive magnets
 b. Superconducting magnets
 c. Permanent magnets
 d. Electromagnets
87. Which of the following correctly defines the term *shims* in reference to MRI?
 a. Pieces or plates of metal used to correct the magnetic field within the magnet
 b. Coils or assemblies within the magnetic bore that enable the machine to create images in any plane
 c. Devices that receive radio-wave signals from a body part that is covered or contained by them
 d. None of the above

88. Which repetition time shows the T1 decay response of tissues when using MRI?
a. 899 ms
b. 1500 ms
c. 546 ms
d. 1680 ms

89. What does the MRI unit use to manipulate hydrogen atoms in and out of an excited energy state?
a. Helium
b. Water
c. Radio waves
d. Oxygen

90. In MRI what are the various shades of gray referred to as?
a. Densities
b. Signal intensities
c. Hypoechoic
d. Hyperechoic

91. How does cerebrospinal fluid appear on a true T1-weighted image of MRI?
a. White
b. Black
c. Different shades of gray
d. None of the above

92. What does MRI require to highlight injections, tumors, or vascular disease?
a. Gadolinium
b. Iodine contrast
c. Barium
d. None of the above

93. How is gadolinium that is used in MRI excreted from the body?
a. Liver
b. Kidneys
c. Lungs
d. GI tract

94. Which of the following radiographic terms describes the radiographic projection obtained by passing the primary x-ray beam from the caudal surface to the cranial surface of a structure?
a. Plantar
b. Dorsopalmar
c. Palmar
d. Caudocranial

95. MRI machines produce noise in which of the following ranges?
a. 20–30 dB
b. 40–50 dB
c. 60–90 dB
d. 100–110 dB

96. Which of the following factors should all personnel understand about MRI machines?
a. No loose metallic objects can be near the machine.
b. It consists of a strong magnetic field.
c. The magnet is always on.
d. Every patient/employee should be screened for safety purposes.
e. All of the above.

97. For a dorsopalmar view of the metacarpus of a horse, which surface should the cassette be on?
a. The medial aspect
b. The palmar aspect
c. The palmaromedial aspect
d. The palmarolateral aspect

98. In which imaging modality is Technetium-99m used?
a. MRI
b. Ultrasound
c. Nuclear medicine
d. Fluoroscopy

99. Which of the following is the best view for detecting distal corner fractures?
a. Lateral view
b. Flexed lateral view
c. Medial oblique
d. Dorsopalmar view

100. The amount of radioisotope used for each examination in a nuclear medicine study is measured in which of the following units?
a. kV
b. mAS
c. mCi
d. MHz

101. What is the term used to describe an area that indicates higher radiation has been emitted in nuclear medicine?
a. Cold spot
b. Hot spot
c. Gamma photon burst
d. None of the above

102. In dental radiographs, periapical disease appears as a:
a. Radiopaque area around the apex of the tooth
b. Radiolucent area around the apex of the tooth
c. Radiopaque area inside the tooth pulp
d. Radiolucent area inside the tooth pulp

103. When does the soft tissue phase occur in nuclear medicine?
a. 5–10 minutes after injection
b. Immediately during injection
c. 2–3 hours after injection
d. 48 hours after injection

104. What does the color blue indicate on a nuclear medicine study?
a. High activity
b. Low activity
c. No activity
d. Normal anatomy

105. Which of the following is the correct abbreviation to perform a *dorsopalmar* radiograph?
a. CdCr
b. Dpa
c. CrCd
d. Cr

106. What is the half-life of the radioisotope Technetium-99m, used in nuclear medicine studies?
a. 1 hour
b. 6 hours
c. 24 hours
d. 48 hours

107. Which parts of a patient's body are considered radioactive after they have received the radioisotope?
a. Skin
b. Hair
c. Waste products
d. All of the above

108. Which of the following PPE must the handler wear when a patient is considered radioactive?
a. Lab coat only
b. Lab coat and gloves
c. Lab coat, gloves, and disposable boots
d. Lab coat, gloves, disposable boots, and a dosimeter badge

109. Radiographic projections are named according to which of the following?
a. The direction in which the central beam anatomically enters the body parts, followed by the area of exit of the x-ray beam
b. The direction in which the central beam anatomically leaves the body parts, followed by the area of entrance of the x-ray beam
c. The side of the patient to which the film is closest, followed by the exposed side
d. Radiation that bounces off objects

110. The term *ventral recumbency* refers to the patient lying on the __________.
a. Back
b. Abdomen
c. Right side
d. Left side

111. The abbreviation *Cd* in x-ray positioning refers to which of the following?
a. Cranial
b. Caudal
c. Ventral
d. Palmar

112. The term *proximal* refers to which of the following abbreviations?
a. Pa
b. Pr
c. Pl
d. Di

113. The abbreviation *CrCd* refers to which of the following?
a. Craniocaudal
b. Mediolateral
c. Dorsopalmar
d. Dorsoplantar

114. Which of the following radiographic terms describes the view when the primary x-ray beam enters the cranial surface and exits the caudal surface of the patient?
a. Dorsoventral
b. Ventrodorsal
c. Craniocaudal
d. Caudocranial

115. The term *oblique* is generally used in reference to which of the following?
a. Abdomen
b. Spine
c. Limbs
d. Head

116. The term *rostral* refers to "toward the __________."
a. Head
b. Nose
c. Tail
d. Middle

117. The median plane divides the body into which of the following?
a. Left/right portions
b. Anterior/posterior portions
c. Cranial/caudal portions
d. None of the above

118. When a patient is receiving an x-ray and is in the right lateral recumbent position, which marker should be used to denote the correct side?
a. Left
b. Right
c. Front
d. Hind

119. When viewing a lateral radiograph, the cranial part of the animal is in which direction in relation to the illuminator?
a. To the left
b. To the right
c. To the top
d. To the bottom

120. The area of interest when obtaining an x-ray should be closest to what?
a. The end of the table
b. The back of the table
c. The image receptor
d. The restrainer

121. For a lateromedial view of the metacarpus of a horse, which surface should the cassette be on?
a. The medial aspect
b. The palmar aspect
c. The palmaromedial aspect
d. The palmarolateral aspect

122. What does it mean to collimate the x-ray beam?
a. To use the highest kV possible
b. To limit the beam exposure to the area of interest within the film
c. To allow for full exposure of the entire film
d. None of the above

123. Which of the following will help prevent motion artifacts?
a. Low milliamperage
b. High milliamperage
c. Higher kVp
d. Lower kVp

124. For a dorsoplantar view of the tarsal joint of a horse, the cassette should be placed in which position?
a. On the lateral surface
b. On the medial surface
c. On the plantar surface
d. On the plantaromedial surface

125. When obtaining an x-ray of a vomiting patient, which position is ideal?
a. Right lateral recumbency
b. Left lateral recumbency
c. Dorsal/ventral
d. Ventral/dorsal

126. Which of the following are ways to determine if the animal is properly positioned in the lateral view?
a. Coxofemoral joints are superimposed.
b. Intervertebral foramina are different sizes.
c. Rib heads are perpendicular.
d. Transverse processes are perpendicular at the origin from the vertebral bodies.

127. Which of the following are ways to determine whether the animal is properly positioned in the ventrodorsal view?
a. Rib and abdominal symmetry.
b. Wings of the ilium are symmetrical.
c. Coxofemoral joints are superimposed.
d. Rib heads are superimposed.
e. Both a and b.
f. Both c and d.

128. When obtaining a foramen magnum projection of the skulls of small animals, where should the centering of the image occur?
a. Midway between the tip of the nose to just caudal to the occipital protuberance at the base
b. Lateral canthus of the eye socket
c. Between the eyes
d. Above the base of the tongue and just below the palate, approximately at the commissure of the mouth

129. All of the following organs are normally seen on a radiograph *except*:
a. Liver
b. Kidney
c. Pancreas
d. Bladder

130. All of the following organs are seen on ultrasound *except*:
a. Lungs
b. Adrenal glands
c. Pancreas
d. Gallbladder

131. In a dorsoventral view on a small animal x-ray, which organ appears in the shape of a question mark?
a. Colon
b. Spleen
c. Right kidney
d. Diaphragm

132. When viewing a radiograph, which organ lies in the cranial abdomen between the diaphragm and stomach in small animals?
a. Adrenal glands
b. Pancreas
c. Liver
d. Spleen

133. In which radiographic view is the right kidney visualized cranial to the left kidney?
a. Left lateral view
b. Ventrodorsal view
c. Dorsoventral view
d. Right lateral view
e. All of the above

134. If pneumonia is suspected in small animals, which of the following radiographic views should be performed?
a. Both lateral views
b. Dorsoventral view
c. Both lateral views and ventrodorsal view
d. Right lateral and dorsoventral views

135. Which of the following could cause a false diagnosis of a pneumothorax on a radiograph?
a. Underexposure of film
b. Overexposure of film
c. Panting
d. Motion artifacts

136. Which radiographic view is best suggested for imaging the lungs?
a. Right lateral
b. Left lateral
c. VD
d. DV

137. What is the maximum permissible dose of radiation a person can receive per year?
a. 1000 mrems/y
b. 2000 mrems/y
c. 2500 mrems/y
d. 5000 mrems/y

138. How long should veterinary facilities maintain dosimetry reports?
a. 5 years
b. 20 years
c. 30 years
d. 1 year following separation of an employee

139. What is the best exposure time for a thoracic radiograph?
a. At any point during the respiratory cycle
b. At maximum inspiration
c. At maximum expiration
d. While the patient is panting

140. Before taking a radiograph of a patient, what is the proper way to obtain a measurement of the area of interest?
a. With the patient standing
b. When the patient is in the position in which it is to be x-rayed
c. When the thinnest part is targeted
d. With the patient lying in the dorsal recumbent position

141. When obtaining a caudocranial view of the scapula of a small animal, where should the central ray be located?
a. Center of the scapula
b. Center of the humerus
c. At the level of the eighth rib
d. At the first thoracic vertebral body

142. The only dental radiographic view that can be made with a true parallel technique is:
a. Rostral maxillary
b. Parallel mandibular view
c. Rostral mandibular view
d. Parallel oblique view

143. When obtaining a caudocranial view of the humerus of a small animal, in which position should the animal be?
   a. Ventral recumbency
   b. Left lateral recumbency
   c. Dorsal recumbency
   d. Right lateral recumbency
144. If the mA or exposure time is doubled, what happens to the film density?
   a. It is halved.
   b. It is doubled.
   c. It stays the same.
   d. It is unrelated to the mA or exposure time.
145. What does the milliamperage control on the x-ray machine affect?
   a. The amount of radiation that is produced
   b. The amount of incoming voltage
   c. The current to the cathode
   d. Both a and c
146. The degree of blackness on a radiograph is described as:
   a. Radiographic density
   b. Radiographic contrast
   c. Focal-film distance
   d. Radiographic fogging
147. What occurs when the object is *not* parallel to the recording surface of an x-ray?
   a. Distortion
   b. Penumbra
   c. Foreshortening
   d. Fogging
148. When an x-ray photon strikes an object, which of the following can occur?
   a. The object rejects the photon.
   b. The photon penetrates the object.
   c. The photon reduces scatter radiation.
   d. X-ray photons do not leave the housing unit.
149. Scatter radiation has a __________ wavelength than the primary beam used in an x-ray.
   a. Shorter
   b. Longer
   c. Wider
   d. Thinner
150. What is the typical wavelength of a medical x-ray?
   a. 0.05–0.01 mm
   b. 0.05–0.01 m
   c. 0.05–0.01 nm
   d. 0.05–0.01 dm
151. Lead shutters installed in the tube head of the x-ray machine are referred to as:
   a. Filters
   b. Diaphragms
   c. Cones
   d. Collimators
152. When obtaining a view of the tympanic bullae of small animals, where should the centering of the image occur?
   a. Midway between the tip of the nose to just caudal to the occipital protuberance at the base
   b. Lateral canthus of the eye socket
   c. Between the eyes
   d. Above the base of the tongue and just below the palate, approximately at the commissure of the mouth
153. For what are grids used on an x-ray machine?
   a. To decrease scatter radiation and to increase the contrast on the radiograph
   b. To absorb the less penetrating x-rays as they leave the tube head
   c. To restrict the primary beam to the size of the cone used
   d. To limit the size of the primary beam to the size of the diaphragm used
154. When obtaining a dorsolateral-palmaromedial oblique view of the carpus of a horse, where should the cassette be held?
   a. Against the palmarolateral aspect of the leg
   b. Against the medial aspect of the leg
   c. Against the palmaromedial aspect of the leg
   d. Against the palmar aspect of the carpus
155. A grid is a series of thin, linear strips made of alternating radiodense and radiolucent material. Of what are the radiodense strips made?
   a. Aluminum
   b. Fiber
   c. Lead
   d. Plastic
156. Where is the grid located in reference to an x-ray machine?
   a. Below the cassette
   b. Between the patient and the cassette
   c. On top of the patient
   d. Within the housing unit
157. Which of the following causes a black irregular border on one end of the film?
   a. Rough handling of the film before exposure
   b. Expired film
   c. Light exposure while still in the box in advance of exposure
   d. Exposure to radiation while still in storage
158. Which of the following will cause a fogged film?
   a. Chemical spills on the screen
   b. Exposure resulting from static electricity
   c. Exposure to excessive scatter radiation
   d. Foreign materials between the film and the screen
159. What causes grid lines on the entire film?
   a. Patient motion
   b. Poor film-screen contact
   c. Grid not being centered with the primary beam
   d. Focal-film distance not being in the range of the grid's focus
160. What is the correct temperature for an automatic processor tank that is used to develop x-ray film?
   a. 35°C
   b. 95°F
   c. 68°F
   d. Both a and b
   e. Both a and c
161. Decreased radiographic density with poor contrast results from which of the following?
   a. The film was overdeveloped.
   b. The film was overexposed.
   c. The film was underexposed.
   d. The film was developed in chemicals that were too hot.

162. To obtain a whole body view of the abdomen of a rabbit, where should the center of the beam be focused?
a. Center over the heart
b. Center over the liver
c. Center of the body cranial to caudal
d. Center over the thoracolumbar area

163. To obtain a mediolateral view of the brachio-antebrachial joint of a horse, how should the leg be positioned?
a. Adducted
b. Abducted
c. Extended cranially
d. Extended caudally

164. To obtain a lateral view of the tibia of a small animal, the patient should be in which of the following positions?
a. Sternal recumbency
b. Right lateral recumbency
c. Left lateral recumbency
d. Both b and c

165. Closure of the distal growth plate of MC3 occurs at what age of the foal?
a. 4–38 weeks
b. 4–22 weeks
c. 18–38 weeks
d. 22–38 weeks

166. Which of the following conditions results from uneven development of film?
a. Uneven chemical levels
b. Low-grade light leak in the darkroom
c. Film developed in chemicals that are too cold
d. Underexposed film

167. Which of the following causes the entire film to be clear?
a. Final wash was conducted improperly.
b. There was no exposure.
c. The film was placed in the fixer before the developer.
d. Both b and c.

168. When obtaining a lateral view of the cervical vertebrae of a small animal, which of the following techniques should *not* be performed?
a. Overextend the limbs caudally.
b. Place a pad beneath the mandible to superimpose the wings of the atlas.
c. Place a pad under the neck to prevent sagging of the spine.
d. Place the wings of the atlas and center of the spine of the scapula in the longitudinal center of the primary beam.

169. What is the topographic radiographic landmark for the caudal cervical vertebrae?
a. Base of the skull
b. Center of the spine of the scapula
c. At the C4 level
d. At the T4 level

170. What is the cranial landmark for an x-ray of the thoracic vertebrae in the lateral position?
a. The base of the skull
b. Halfway between the xiphoid process and the last rib
c. Spine of the scapula
d. Wings of the ilium

171. When obtaining a radiograph of the thoracic vertebrae, what level should be measured for the kVp setting?
a. The cranial end of the thoracic vertebrae
b. The caudal end of the thoracic vertebrae
c. The lowest point of the thorax
d. The highest point of the thorax

172. Which of the following is the correct abbreviation for a cranial radiograph?
a. CdCr
b. Dpa
c. CrCd
d. Cr

173. When imaging the lumbosacral vertebrae in the lateral position, which of the following should be done to ensure proper exposure?
a. Decrease the kVp
b. Increase the kVp
c. Increase the mAs
d. Decrease the mAs

174. To obtain a dorsopalmar x-ray of the metacarpus and digits, in which position should the patient be?
a. Right lateral recumbency
b. Left lateral recumbency
c. Sternal recumbency
d. Dorsal recumbency

175. When obtaining a ventrodorsal x-ray of the thorax, what is the cranial landmark?
a. The base of the skull
b. The manubrium
c. Halfway between the xiphoid and the last rib
d. The ilium wings

176. What is the caudal landmark for obtaining an abdominal x-ray in the lateral position?
a. Three rib spaces cranial to the xiphoid
b. Greater trochanter of the femur
c. The ilium wings
d. The manubrium

177. Which of the following is the best technique to consider for an abdominal x-ray?
a. Peak inspiration
b. Peak expiration
c. Panting
d. Consideration of breathing techniques is not necessary for abdominal x-rays

178. What caudal landmark is used when obtaining a lateral x-ray of the pelvis?
a. Border of the ischium
b. Wings of the ilium
c. The xiphoid process
d. The greater trochanter of the femur

179. Which of the following radiographic terms describes the view when the primary x-ray beam enters the caudal surface and exits the cranial surface of the patient?
  a. Dorsoventral
  b. Ventrodorsal
  c. Craniocaudal
  d. Caudocranial
180. When obtaining a caudocranial x-ray of the stifle joint, what should be palpated to determine the amount of rotation necessary for an exact caudocranial projection?
  a. The greater trochanter of the femur
  b. The tibial tuberosity
  c. The patella
  d. The manubrium
181. Which of the following terms is used to describe the white appearance on an x-ray?
  a. Radiolucent
  b. Radiopaque
  c. Hyperechoic
  d. Hypoechoic
182. You are looking at your dental radiograph and notice that the tooth is elongated. This happened because the beam was perpendicular to the:
  a. Film
  b. Tooth
  c. Bisecting angle
  d. Wrong tooth
183. Which contrast is commonly used for GI studies when perforation is *not* suspected?
  a. Barium sulfate
  b. Meglumine diatrizoate
  c. Sodium diatrizoate
  d. Betadine
184. How long does it take for barium sulfate to travel from the stomach to the colon?
  a. 30 minutes
  b. 1 hour
  c. 2 hours
  d. 3 hours
185. Which of the following is *not* a form of barium sulfate that can be administered to patients?
  a. Powder
  b. Colloid suspension
  c. Pastes
  d. Injectable
186. Which of the following could be considered as negative-contrast agents used in radiography?
  a. Oxygen
  b. Air
  c. Carbon dioxide
  d. All of the above
  e. b and c only
187. In which of the following circumstances should water-soluble organic iodides be avoided?
  a. Suspected bowel perforation
  b. Dehydrated patients
  c. Overhydrated patients
  d. Kidney failure
188. Which of the following will be caused by exposing a reptile to cool conditions, such as a cool metal surface?
  a. Temporary lethargy and immobility
  b. Temporary excitement
  c. Rapid breathing
  d. Aggressiveness
189. For a dorsolateral-plantaromedial oblique view of the tarsal joint of a horse, the cassette should be placed in which position?
  a. On the lateral surface
  b. On the medial surface
  c. On the plantar surface
  d. On the plantaromedial surface
190. When positioning a lizard in right lateral recumbency before taking an x-ray, the left limbs are always __________ to the right limbs.
  a. Cranial
  b. Caudal
  c. Lateral
  d. Medial
191. During an x-ray, a tabletop technique is most commonly used for exotic companion animals *except* when the species' girth exceeds which diameter?
  a. 2–5 cm
  b. 5–10 cm
  c. 10–12 cm
  d. 12–15 cm
192. When using a Plexiglas tube to obtain an x-ray, which of the following should be adjusted?
  a. The mAs should be increased.
  b. The mAs should be decreased.
  c. The kVp should be increased.
  d. The kVp should be decreased.
193. Which of the following is *not* considered a physical restraint?
  a. Tape
  b. Radiolucent Plexiglas
  c. Gloved hands
  d. Foam pads
194. Which of the following contains a filament consisting of a tightly coiled tungsten wire and is the site of electron generation in the x-ray tube?
  a. Anode
  b. Cathode
  c. B-mode
  d. Transducer
195. What is the amount used to express the dose equivalent that results from exposure to ionizing radiation known as?
  a. REM
  b. ALARA
  c. MPD
  d. Sv
196. The protective lead equipment required for wear during x-ray exposure can decrease the primary beam exposure by how much?
  a. 15%
  b. 25%
  c. 50%
  d. 100%

197. Film badges, TLDs, and OSL badges contain three or four elements for filtration. Which element monitors the highest level of exposure to radiation?
a. Open window
b. Plastic
c. Aluminum
d. Copper

198. Which type of monitoring badge is the most common method of monitoring ionizing radiation?
a. Thermoluminescent dosimeters
b. Film badges
c. Optically stimulated luminescence badges
d. Ion chambers

199. Digital radiography, CT, MRI, and ultrasound are stored using a universally accepted format known as which of the following?
a. CCD
b. DICOM
c. MOD
d. PACS

200. When obtaining a lateromedial view of the carpus of a horse, where should the cassette be held?
a. Against the palmarolateral aspect of the leg
b. Against the medial aspect of the leg
c. Against the palmaromedial aspect of the leg
d. Against the palmar aspect of the carpus

201. To obtain a flexed lateromedial view of the carpus of a horse, the limb should be flexed approximately how many degrees?
a. 15 degrees
b. 30 degrees
c. 60 degrees
d. 90 degrees

202. For standard radiographs of the tarsus of a horse, which of the following is the correct weight distribution?
a. The affected limb should be suspended with no weight on it for the duration of the x-ray.
b. There should be 25% weight bearing on the affected limb.
c. There should be 50% weight bearing on the affected limb.
d. The weight should be evenly distributed on all four legs.

203. For a lateromedial view of the tarsal joint of a horse, the cassette should be placed in which position?
a. On the lateral surface
b. On the medial surface
c. On the plantar surface
d. On the plantaromedial surface

204. To obtain a flexed dorsoplantar radiographic view of the tarsal joint of a horse, at what angle should the primary beam direction be?
a. 15 degrees
b. 45 degrees
c. 60 degrees
d. 90 degrees

205. For a standard radiograph of the metacarpus of a horse, the limb of interest should be in which position compared with the ground?
a. Parallel
b. Perpendicular
c. At 45 degrees
d. At 60 degrees

206. All of the following statements are true *except*:
a. Only personnel necessary to complete the procedure should be in the x-ray room at the time of exposure.
b. Persons younger than 18 years and pregnant women must not be in the x-ray room during the examination.
c. Personnel who assist with radiographic examinations should have a rotating duty roster to minimize exposure to any one person.
d. Sandbags, sponges, tape, or other restraining devices should not be used for positioning the patient rather than manual restraint.

207. To obtain a dorsopalmar view of the fetlock joint of a horse, the primary beam needs to be angled at __________ degrees proximal to distal.
a. 10
b. 20
c. 45
d. 60

208. To obtain a dorsopalmar view of the interphalangeal joint, what should the primary beam angle be proximal to distal?
a. 15–20 degrees
b. 30–45 degrees
c. 45–60 degrees
d. 90 degrees

209. Before imaging the coffin bone in horses, which of the following tasks should be performed in preparation?
a. Hoof should be trimmed to the new sole level.
b. The horseshoes need to be removed.
c. The sulcus should be packed with radiolucent material.
d. All of the above.

210. To obtain a caudocranial view of the femorotibial joint of the horse, the cassette should be placed against which surface?
a. Cranial aspect
b. Caudal aspect
c. Lateral aspect
d. Medial aspect

211. To obtain a craniocaudal view of the brachio-antebrachial joint of a horse, how should the leg be positioned?
a. Adducted
b. Abducted
c. Extended cranially
d. Extended caudally

212. To obtain a caudocranial view of the tibia of a small animal, the patient should be in which of the following positions?
a. Sternal recumbency
b. Dorsal recumbency
c. Right lateral recumbency
d. Left lateral recumbency

213. To obtain a dorsoventral view of the thorax of a rabbit, where should the center of the beam be focused?
a. Centered over the heart
b. Centered over the liver
c. Center of the body cranial to caudal
d. Centered over the thoracolumbar area

214. Which of the following is the best restraint to use in avian radiography?
a. Manual restraint
b. Physical restraint
c. Chemical restraint
d. None; birds should not be restrained for x-rays

215. Which should be avoided when manually restraining a bird?
a. Grasping the patient around the neck
b. Grasped by the mandibular articulation
c. Grasping the feet and gently stretching the bird
d. All of the above should be avoided

216. For a lateral avian view, where would the left wings and limbs be positioned?
a. Cranially to the right wings and limbs
b. Caudally to the right wings and limbs
c. Lateral to the right wings and limbs
d. Superimposed to the right wings and limbs

217. For a ventrodorsal avian radiographic view, the keel should be in which position related to the spine?
a. Superimposed
b. Lateral
c. Caudal
d. Cranial

218. For larger species of birds, which technique can be used to obtain a craniocaudal appendicular skeletal radiograph?
a. Tape the limb to a Plexiglas plate.
b. Tape the limb directly on the cassette.
c. Use a gloved hand placed behind the hock to restrain the limb for exposure.
d. Both a and c.

219. When restraining a sedated bird for a lateral x-ray, where should the wings be properly taped?
a. On the most distal end
b. Across the humerus
c. Across the radius-ulna
d. The wings should not be taped

220. For an avian lateral view, where should the dependent limb be placed compared with the contralateral limb?
a. Lateral
b. Medial
c. Superimposed
d. Cranial

221. For smaller-sized patients, which radiographic technique is preferred?
a. Grid technique
b. Lower mA
c. Tabletop technique
d. Higher kVp

222. When obtaining a dorsoventral view of the whole body of a rodent, how should the front legs be positioned?
a. Extended caudally
b. Extended cranially
c. Superimposed
d. Abducted from the body

223. What is an essential factor when using a nonscreen film to x-ray a snake?
a. The snake needs to move continuously across the film.
b. Movement needs to be minimal.
c. The snake needs to be short and thin.
d. Nonscreen films should never be used to x-ray a snake.

224. For digital radiography, what does the postprocessing step of image manipulation allow?
a. Magnification
b. Rotation
c. Contrast adjustment
d. All of the above
e. a and b only

225. Which of the following is *not* an advantage of digital x-ray versus analog x-ray?
a. Elimination of the darkroom
b. Image postprocessing
c. Elimination of damaging radiation
d. Exposure latitude and contrast optimization

226. A feature of digital radiography that is related to the bit depth of each pixel and the software that accompanies the digital-imaging system is referred to as which of the following?
a. Spatial resolution
b. Contrast optimization
c. Dynamic range
d. Exposure latitude

227. What is a concern of *exposure creep* with the use of digital x-rays?
a. Underexposed x-ray
b. Unnecessary patient and personnel exposure because of ionizing radiation
c. Excessive film blackening
d. Exposure creep is only an issue in analog x-rays

228. Horses have approximately how many carpal bones?
a. 4
b. 5
c. 6
d. 7

229. Which radiographic view of the carpal joint of a horse provides the best view to judge the width of the cartilage spaces?
a. Lateral
b. Dorsopalmar
c. Medial oblique
d. Flexed lateral

230. Which of the following is the best view for assessing the distal radial growth plate for closure in horses?
a. Lateral view
b. Flexed lateral view
c. Medial oblique
d. Dorsopalmar view

231. How does the adjacent bone density appear in fresh carpal chips in horses?
a. Decreased
b. Increased
c. Normal

232. Which of the following does *not* describe an old carpal chip seen on x-ray in horses?
  a. Sharp fragment margination
  b. Decreased adjacent bone density
  c. Presence of osteoarthritis
  d. Normal or cool surrounding tissue

233. Which of the following is the most serious of all carpal fractures seen in horses?
  a. Corner fracture
  b. Slab fracture
  c. Chip fracture
  d. All chip fractures are equal in severity

234. Which radiographic view provides the best accuracy for detecting carpal fractures in horses?
  a. Lateral view
  b. Medial oblique view
  c. Flexed lateral view
  d. Dorsopalmar view

235. Which of the following is *not* a radiographic characteristic of the bones of a newborn foal?
  a. Smooth
  b. Fused
  c. Round
  d. Wider joint spaces

236. At what age does the first radiographic appearance of the crena seen in foals occur?
  a. 18–38 weeks
  b. 22–38 weeks
  c. 4–22 weeks
  d. 0–4 weeks

237. Which of the following is *not* considered a key radiographic feature of carpal or tarsal bone immaturity?
  a. Increased calcification
  b. Increased number of visible vascular canals causing increased porosity
  c. Abnormally tapered profile
  d. One or more fringed margins

238. A deformity in the interior angle of the joint greater than 180 degrees when viewed frontally is known as what?
  a. Axial rotation
  b. Windswept
  c. Valgus deformity
  d. Varus deformity

239. An unossified carpal or tarsal bone describes which grade level on the ossification index for newborn foals?
  a. Grade 1
  b. Grade 2
  c. Grade 3
  d. Grade 4

240. Which of the following is the correct abbreviation for a *craniocaudal* radiograph?
  a. CdCr
  b. Dpa
  c. CrCd
  d. Cr

241. Which of the following radiographic terms describes the caudal surface of the forelimb distal to the carpus?
  a. Plantar
  b. Dorsopalmar
  c. Palmar
  d. Caudocranial

242. Which of the following radiographic terms describes the view when the primary x-ray beam enters the ventral surface and exits the dorsal surface of the patient?
  a. Dorsoventral
  b. Ventrodorsal
  c. Craniocaudal
  d. Caudocranial

243. Radiographs of long bones must include which of the following?
  a. The joint proximal to the long bone
  b. The joint distal to the long bone
  c. Both the joint proximal and the joint distal to the long bone
  d. The long bone only, excluding joints proximal and distal

244. Radiographs of joints must include which of the following?
  a. The bones proximal to the joint
  b. The bones distal to the joint
  c. Only the joint needs to be imaged, excluding any surrounding bones
  d. One-third of the bones proximal and distal to the joint

245. Films that are properly collimated will have which of the following appearances?
  a. Black, fully exposed edges of the film of a finished radiograph
  b. Clear, unexposed areas on all four edges of the film of a finished radiograph
  c. Clear, unexposed areas of the two long edges of a finished radiograph
  d. Clear, unexposed areas of the two short edges of a finished radiograph

246. When using a V-trough to aid in obtaining a radiograph, what needs to be measured before taking the x-ray?
  a. The thinnest portion of the body to be radiographed
  b. The thickest portion of the body to be radiographed
  c. The V-trough only
  d. The V-trough and the thickest portion of the body to be measured

247. When obtaining a radiograph, the thickest part of the area of interest is placed toward what?
  a. The anode end of the x-ray tube
  b. The cathode end of the x-ray tube
  c. The center of the x-ray beam
  d. Closest to the radiographer

248. To decrease magnification of an x-ray, which of the following would help?
a. Patients are positioned as close to the x-ray cassette as possible.
b. Patients are positioned are far away from the x-ray cassette as possible.
c. There should be as much collimation as possible.
d. There should be as little collimation as possible.

249. When capturing analog radiographs, which of the following descriptions refers to "splitting the plate"?
a. Creating a smaller x-ray cassette to use for small patients
b. Using a lead shield on half of the film to prevent exposure and to allow for two views to be obtained on the same film
c. Collimating the beam to accommodate small patients on a large cassette
d. Combining two small cassettes to accommodate a larger patient

250. What view is required for the evaluation of the nasal passages of small animals?
a. Dorsoventral view
b. Lateral view
c. Rostrocaudal view
d. Open-mouth view
e. All of the above
f. a and b only

251. What is the correct place of measurement for radiographs of the nasal passages of small animals?
a. The most rostral end of the cranium
b. The most caudal end of the cranium
c. Slightly rostral to the widest area of the cranium
d. At the widest portion of the cranium

252. When obtaining a VD projection of the skull of small animals, where should the centering of the image occur?
a. Midway between the tip of the nose and just caudal to the occipital protuberance at the base
b. Lateral canthus of the eye socket
c. Between the eyes
d. Above the base of the tongue and just below the palate, approximately at the commissure of the mouth

253. To obtain a radiographic image of the right temporomandibular joint of a small animal, which of the following is the best position?
a. Dorsal recumbency
b. Ventral recumbency
c. Right lateral recumbency
d. Left lateral recumbency

254. To obtain a radiograph of the VD extended hip projection, where is the center of the beam focused?
a. Greater trochanter of femur
b. Midline between the left and right ischial tuberosity
c. At the level of the 7th vertebrae
d. At the midfemur

255. To obtain a lateral projection of the pelvis, which area should be used for measurement?
a. At the highest level of the trochanter
b. The thickest part of the pelvis
c. The thinnest part of the pelvis
d. The level of the 7th vertebrae

256. To obtain a radiograph of the CdCr projection of the scapula of a small animal, which of the following is the correct position for the patient?
a. Sternal recumbency
b. Lateral recumbency
c. Dorsal recumbency
d. Standing

257. To obtain a CdCr projection of the humerus of small animals, where should the measurement be taken?
a. Measure from the table to the midshaft humerus.
b. Measure the thickest part of the humerus.
c. Measure on the dorsal side from the table to the height of the scapula.
d. Measure the midshaft humerus.

258. To obtain a flexed lateral projection of the carpus of small animals, where should the measurement be taken?
a. Caudal to the carpal joint
b. The thickest part of the flexed joint
c. Thickest part of the nonflexed joint
d. Cranial to the carpal joint

259. The bisecting angle principle states that the plane of an x-ray beam should be 90 degrees to the:
a. Long axis of the tooth
b. Plane of the film
c. Imaginary line that bisects the angle formed by the tooth's long axis and the film plane
d. Imaginary line that bisects the angle formed by the animal's head and the film plane

260. All of the following are components of an x-ray tube *except*:
a. Cathode
b. Anode
c. Grid
d. Tungsten filament

261. With film-based imaging, which of the following are receptor components?
a. Intensifying screen
b. Cassette
c. Film
d. All of the above

SECTION

11

Anesthesia

Mary Ellen Goldberg and Jody Nugent-Deal

QUESTIONS

1. Which of the following statements defines regional anesthesia?
   a. Loss of sensation in a limited area of the body produced by administration of a local anesthetic or other agent in proximity to sensory nerves
   b. Loss of sensation in a small area of the body produced by administration of a local anesthetic agent in proximity to the area of interest
   c. Loss of sensation in a localized area produced by administration of a local anesthetic directly to a body surface or to a surgical or traumatic wound
   d. A drug-induced sleep-like state that impairs the ability of the patient to respond appropriately to stimuli
2. If an oxygen flowmeter uses a ball for oxygen readings, where is the reading taken from to determine flow of oxygen in the system?
   a. The top of the ball
   b. The center of the ball
   c. The bottom of the ball
   d. None of the above
3. Which of the following statements defines balanced anesthesia?
   a. The administration of two or more agents in equal volume
   b. Administration of multiple drugs concurrently in smaller quantities than would be required if each were administered alone
   c. General anesthesia in which the patient's physiological status remains stable
   d. The administration of a local and general anesthetic concurrently
4. Which of the following terms refers to a loss of sensation in a small area of the body produced by administration of a local anesthetic?
   a. Sedation
   b. General anesthesia
   c. Surgical anesthesia
   d. Local anesthesia
5. Which of these statements regarding anesthesia is incorrect?
   a. Anesthetic agents have wide therapeutic indices.
   b. There is always a risk to patient safety when anesthetics are administered.
   c. Most anesthetics cause significant changes in cardiopulmonary function.
   d. All statements are false.
6. Which of the following opioids is preferable in a patient undergoing a painful ophthalmic procedure?
   a. Morphine
   b. Methadone
   c. Diazepam
   d. Midazolam
7. Which of the following drugs is classified as an opioid?
   a. Amantadine
   b. Carprofen
   c. Ketamine
   d. Butorphanol
8. Physical examinations are an important step when assessing the patient's risk factor. Which of the following statements is incorrect because it refers to PE findings?
   a. Dehydration increases the risk for hypotension.
   b. Anemia predisposes the patient to hypoxemia.
   c. Patients with bruising may be at higher risk of potentially life-threatening intraoperative and postoperative bleeding.
   d. A dog with a body condition score of 8/9 will require more anesthetic per unit body weight than a dog of the same breed with a body condition score of 5/9.
9. When a capnometer is combined with a continuous graphical display, the monitoring device is referred to as a:
   a. Capnometer
   b. Capnograph
   c. Pulse oximeter
   d. Capillary refill time
10. Using a Doppler for blood pressure measurement will yield which of the following readings?
    a. Systolic
    b. Mean
    c. Diastolic
    d. All of the above
11. When using the emergency oxygen flush valve, what must the technician also do simultaneously?
    a. Disconnect the patient from the breathing circuit to avoid barotrauma
    b. Disconnect the oxygen supply
    c. Close the pop-off valve
    d. Turn off the isoflurane
12. You have a patient that looks asleep, will not respond to voice, but will respond to pain. Which of the following would describe the animal's level of consciousness?
    a. Lethargic
    b. Obtunded
    c. Stuporous
    d. Comatose

13. Which of the following is used for direct blood pressure monitoring?
    a. Cardell
    b. Dinamap
    c. Arterial catheter
    d. Doppler
14. Which of the following products is considered a colloid solution?
    a. Lactated Ringer's solution
    b. Normal saline solution
    c. Hetastarch
    d. 5% dextrose
15. What is the function of a vaporizer?
    a. To regulate flow of oxygen into the anesthetic system
    b. To deliver safe and effective levels of anesthetic gas
    c. To measure the pressure of gas in the system
    d. All of the above
16. What is the American Society of Anesthesiologists (ASA) Physical Status Classification system rating for a patient that is anemic or moderately dehydrated?
    a. Class P1
    b. Class P2
    c. Class P3
    d. Class P4
17. Which of the following fluids is an example of a colloid?
    a. Lactated Ringer's solution
    b. Normosol-R
    c. Whole blood
    d. Hypertonic saline
18. You have a calm canine patient that must be anesthetized. Which of the following conditions could present the greatest risk to anesthesia?
    a. Wheezing while breathing
    b. Lethargy
    c. Temperature of 104.1°F
    d. Sinus arrhythmia
19. Which of the following inhaled anesthetics has a very low boiling point and therefore has to be contained within an electrically heated chamber?
    a. Halothane
    b. Desflurane
    c. Isoflurane
    d. Sevoflurane
20. Which of the following patients would be of greatest concern regarding the patent airway when anesthesia is being considered?
    a. Brachycephalic breeds
    b. Exotic breeds
    c. Cats and horses
    d. Sight hounds
21. Which of the following is often used to calculate a patient's tidal volume?
    a. 100 mL/kg
    b. 200 mL/kg
    c. 1–2 mL/kg
    d. 10–20 mL/kg
22. The width of the blood pressure cuff in a dog should be what percentage of the circumference of the leg?
    a. 40%
    b. 50%
    c. 25%
    d. 30%
23. What does the term *minute volume* mean?
    a. The volume of anesthetic agent used in 1 minute
    b. The flow of oxygen through the system in 1 minute
    c. The sum of all gas volumes exhaled in 1 minute
    d. The volume of gas exhaled in one breath
24. Placement of IV catheters is just as critical as the techniques used to administer medications. Which of the following actions should *not* be done?
    a. Choose an administration set with an injection port
    b. Provide all IV drugs slowly unless told otherwise
    c. Always follow IV injections through a catheter with sterile saline flush
    d. Choose a catheter that is small in diameter to minimize the risk of bleeding
25. What is the main component of soda lime (a substance used to absorb carbon dioxide from the breathing system)?
    a. Carbon dioxide
    b. Potassium hydroxide
    c. Calcium hydroxide
    d. Baking soda
26. Blood pressure cuff placement is common in all of the following areas *except* the:
    a. Tail
    b. Forelimb
    c. Hind limb
    d. Foot
27. What is the name given to the opening opposite the bevel of the endotracheal tube?
    a. Pilot hole
    b. Accessory opening
    c. Murphy eye
    d. Miller opening
28. The body of an adult animal contains a large amount of fluid. Which statement about body fluids is incorrect?
    a. About 40% of the body weight is water.
    b. About two thirds of the total body water resides inside the cells.
    c. Blood plasma makes up about 5% of the total body weight.
    d. Dogs have a larger total blood volume than cats.
29. A patient is admitted to the hospital with moderate dehydration. The veterinarian has asked that the patient be rehydrated. Which of the following solutions would be considered ideal for rehydration?
    a. Colloids
    b. Hypertonic saline
    c. Isotonic crystalloids
    d. 50% dextrose
30. Which of the following is a main disadvantage for using a chamber to induce anesthesia?
    a. Patient struggling causes increased catecholamines.
    b. Increased risk of cardiac arrhythmias
    c. Staff exposure to harmful waste anesthetic gases
    d. All of the above
31. All of the following factors would be indicators for placing a patient on a controlled ventilator *except*:
    a. An open thorax thoracotomy or chest wall trauma
    b. Neuromuscular blockade
    c. Pneumothorax
    d. Intestinal foreign body

32. Which of the following administration rates describes that of a microdrip set?
   a. 10 gtt/mL
   b. 10 - 15 gtt/mL
   c. 20 - 60 gtt/mL
   d. 60 gtt/mL
33. All of the following are clinical signs used to evaluate the depth of anesthesia *except*:
   a. Eye position
   b. Ear pinch
   c. Jaw tone
   d. Palpebral reflex
34. All of the following statements regarding fluid infusion rates are false *except*:
   a. Standard shock doses of fluids are about the same as doses used during routine surgery.
   b. Surgery patients with blood loss may require colloids instead of crystalloids.
   c. Crystalloids are generally given at lower administration rates than colloids.
   d. Hypertonic saline is administered in large volumes to patients in shock.
35. What is the function of an esophageal stethoscope?
   a. Cardiac and lung auscultation via the esophagus
   b. Temperature readings via the esophagus
   c. Measuring exhaled end tidal carbon dioxide
   d. Measuring central venous pressure
36. Which of the following monitoring parameters is used for the measurement and numerical display of the carbon dioxide concentration in the respiratory gas?
   a. Electrocardiogram
   b. Capnometry
   c. Pulse oximeter
   d. Capillary refill time
37. Fluid overload can carry serious consequences. All of the following clinical signs are consistent with that of fluid overload *except*:
   a. Ocular and nasal discharge
   b. Hypotension
   c. Increased lung sounds and respiratory rate
   d. Dyspnea
38. Which of the following describes capnometers where the measuring chambers are placed directly in the airway and the measurement signal is generated?
   a. Sidestream capnometer
   b. Invasive capnometer
   c. Mainstream capnometer
   d. Endstream capnometer
39. Which of the following locations would be acceptable for placement of a pulse oximeter probe?
   a. Tongue
   b. Prepuce
   c. Nonpigmented toe
   d. All of the above
40. In the equine patient, which heart rhythm is *not* normal?
   a. Normal sinus rhythm
   b. Sinus arrhythmia
   c. Second-degree AV block
   d. Third-degree AV block
41. Which of the following blood pressure measuring techniques is considered "gold standard" in terms of accurate measurements?
   a. Invasive blood pressure measurements
   b. Doppler blood pressure measurements
   c. Oscillometric blood pressure measurements
   d. All of the above
42. Which of the following terms describes the volume of gas exhaled in one breath?
   a. Tidal volume
   b. Minute volume
   c. Dead space volume
   d. Oxygen flow rate
43. What combination of drugs is in a neuroleptanalgesic cocktail?
   a. An opioid and an anticholinergic
   b. An anticholinergic and a tranquilizer
   c. An opioid and a tranquilizer
   d. An anticholinergic and a benzodiazepine
44. Where is the intravenous catheter placed for measurement of central venous pressures?
   a. Vena cava
   b. Right atrium
   c. Left ventricle
   d. Cephalic vein
45. Which of the following drugs is a phenothiazine tranquilizer most commonly used as a premedication in small animal practice?
   a. Acepromazine
   b. Midazolam
   c. Diazepam
   d. Morphine
46. Where does atropine block the release of acetylcholine?
   a. Muscarinic receptors of the parasympathetic system
   b. Nicotinic receptors of the parasympathetic system
   c. Muscarinic receptors of the sympathetic system
   d. Nicotinic receptors of the sympathetic system
47. All of the following are common side effects of acepromazine *except*:
   a. Peripheral vasodilation
   b. Decrease in body temperature
   c. Increase in body temperature
   d. Decrease in overall blood pressure
48. Which of the following is an example of an alpha-2 adrenoreceptor agonist?
   a. Dexmedetomidine
   b. Xylazine
   c. Medetomidine
   d. All of the above
49. How is it best to treat bradycardia induced by dexmedetomidine?
   a. Atropine
   b. Naloxone
   c. Epinephrine
   d. Atipamezole
50. Which of the following medications will reverse the effects of mu opioids?
   a. Atipamezole
   b. Naloxone
   c. Atropine
   d. Yohimbine

51. What class of drugs is not only used as a premedicant, but also as a first-line intervention for animals presenting in status epilepticus?
  a. Opioids
  b. Benzodiazepines
  c. Alpha-2 adrenoreceptor agonist
  d. Antibiotics
52. Of the following drugs listed, which one does *not* have analgesic properties?
  a. Dexmedetomidine
  b. Morphine
  c. Methadone
  d. Diazepam
53. What is the indication for induction with etomidate in dogs?
  a. Severe cardiac disease
  b. Renal failure
  c. Orthopedic disease
  d. Pediatric (younger than 4 weeks)
54. Which of the following represents how a drug can be eliminated from the body?
  a. Urine excretion
  b. Digestion
  c. Biotransformation
  d. Metabolized
55. Which of the following opioids would be the best choice as premedication in a patient with moderate to severe pain?
  a. Butorphanol
  b. Diazepam
  c. Methadone
  d. Naloxone
56. Which of the following is a dissociative anesthetic?
  a. Thiopental sodium
  b. Pentobarbital sodium
  c. Ketamine hydrochloride
  d. Propofol
57. What should the vaporizer be set at to maintain a surgical plane of anesthesia?
  a. 0.5 × MAC
  b. 1 × MAC
  c. 1.5 × MAC
  d. 2 × MAC
58. Which of the following is considered a reversal drug for opioid agonist effects at all receptors?
  a. Butorphanol
  b. Naloxone hydrochloride
  c. Morphine
  d. Hydromorphone
59. How do local anesthetic drugs function as analgesics?
  a. By reducing inflammation
  b. By blocking impulse conduction in nerve fibers
  c. By facilitating the breakdown of arachidonic acid
  d. By acting as an antipyretic
60. What can be done to avoid transient apnea from the drug propofol?
  a. Administer by infusion only
  b. Premedicate with opioids
  c. Administer intravenously only
  d. Titrate this drug in several boluses
61. Which problem can be caused by tiletamine-zolazepam in dogs on recovery?
  a. Excitement
  b. Bradycardia
  c. Hypotension
  d. Laryngospasm
62. An injection of a local anesthetic into the area around a peripheral nerve to block sensory and/or motor function such as a ring block before declaw procedure is an example of what?
  a. Spinal anesthesia
  b. Regional anesthesia
  c. Topical anesthesia
  d. Subcutaneous injection
63. Which of the following drugs is *not* considered an NMDA receptor antagonist?
  a. Ketamine
  b. Methadone
  c. Morphine
  d. Amantadine
64. Which of the following is a common adverse effect of isoflurane?
  a. Hepatic toxicity
  b. Accumulation in body fat stores
  c. Depression of respiration
  d. Seizures during recovery
65. Which of the following opioids has been shown to have the lowest likelihood of causing vomiting in cats?
  a. Morphine
  b. Methadone
  c. Fentanyl
  d. Hydromorphone
66. Which of the following drugs has been shown to be useful at reducing opioid-related nausea and vomiting that occur after administration of opioids when given preoperatively?
  a. Maropitant
  b. Carprofen
  c. Morphine
  d. Hydromorphone
67. What components of pain are involved in an ovariohysterectomy?
  a. Somatic pain only
  b. Visceral pain only
  c. Both somatic and visceral pain
  d. Neither somatic nor visceral pain
68. Which of the following opioids is most commonly used for epidural analgesia?
  a. Morphine
  b. Buprenorphine
  c. Bupivacaine
  d. Lidocaine
69. Rapid administration of morphine intravenously can cause release of what hormone?
  a. Testosterone
  b. Histamine
  c. Endogenous opioids
  d. Estrogen

70. Electrical signals (action potentials) are converted by thermal, mechanical, or chemical noxious stimuli during which process?
   a. Perception
   b. Modulation
   c. Transduction
   d. Transmission
71. Which of the following opioids would be best to use in cases where you want to avoid vomiting such as cases with increased intracranial pressure?
   a. Morphine
   b. Methadone
   c. Fentanyl
   d. Hydromorphone
72. Young puppies and kittens have limited glucose reserves and are at a greater risk of what condition because of the fasting required before anesthesia?
   a. Hypothermia
   b. Hypotension
   c. Hypoglycemia
   d. Hyperglycemia
73. Pain impulses can be altered by neurons that either suppress or amplify nerve impulses in the spinal cord during which process?
   a. Perception
   b. Modulation
   c. Transduction
   d. Transmission
74. Where does "wind-up" occur?
   a. Brain
   b. Spinal cord
   c. Visceral pain receptors
   d. Peripheral pain receptors
75. Which of the following is a common side effect when opioids such as morphine and hydromorphone are used preoperatively?
   a. Vomiting
   b. Decreased mucous membrane secretions
   c. Tachycardia
   d. Hypertension
76. Which of the following is *not* a barbiturate anesthetic drug?
   a. Pentobarbital
   b. Methohexital
   c. Propofol
   d. Thiopental
77. During multimodal analgesic therapy, which of the following statements is true?
   a. The dose of each drug is decreased when several drugs are used.
   b. Multiple pain receptor mechanisms are targeted by one drug.
   c. Several drugs target one pain receptor mechanism.
   d. Using several drugs increases side effects.
78. Which of the following drugs is *not* considered a benzodiazepine?
   a. Midazolam
   b. Methadone
   c. Zolazepam
   d. Diazepam
79. The drug Telazol is a combination of which two drugs?
   a. Ketamine and diazepam
   b. Ketamine and midazolam
   c. Tiletamine and zolazepam
   d. Methadone and midazolam
80. Choose an analgesic plan that targets three different pain receptor mechanisms:
   a. Morphine IM, fentanyl CRI, lidocaine nerve block
   b. Morphine IM, fentanyl CRI, bupivacaine nerve block
   c. Morphine IM, ketamine CRI, lidocaine nerve block
   d. Ketamine CRI, lidocaine and bupivacaine nerve block
81. Which of the following is a neuroactive steroid anesthetic?
   a. Alfaxalone
   b. Telazol
   c. Propofol
   d. Etomidate
82. In which organ are most inhalant anesthetic drugs metabolized (biotransformed)?
   a. Skin
   b. Lungs
   c. Eye
   d. Liver
83. Giving analgesics before tissue injury is known as:
   a. Premedication
   b. Local analgesia
   c. Multimodal analgesia
   d. Preemptive analgesia
84. Which of the following opioids would be the best choice for a surgery that is anticipated to be moderately to severely painful?
   a. Butorphanol
   b. Propofol
   c. Hydromorphone
   d. Naloxone
85. Which of the following opioid analgesics is often used as a continuous rate infusion because of its short duration of action (approximately 30 minutes)?
   a. Morphine
   b. Ketamine
   c. Buprenorphine
   d. Fentanyl
86. Opioid administration in cats and dogs can have side effects. Which one is *not* a side effect from opioid administration in cats and dogs?
   a. Vomiting
   b. Dysphoria
   c. Renal failure
   d. Respiratory depression
87. Which of the following terms refers to a specific stage in general anesthesia in which there is a sufficient degree of analgesia and muscle relaxation to allow surgery to be performed without patient pain or movement?
   a. Sedation
   b. General anesthesia
   c. Surgical anesthesia
   d. Local anesthesia

88. Which of the following preoperative tests should be performed on a patient with a suspected clotting disorder?
   a. Blood glucose measurement
   b. Urine specific gravity
   c. Buccal mucosal bleeding time
   d. Schirmer tear test
89. Nonsteroidal anti-inflammatory drugs have what mechanism of action (MOA)?
   a. They block sodium channels.
   b. They are alpha-2 receptor agonists.
   c. They inhibit prostaglandin synthesis.
   d. They are mu-opioid receptor agonists.
90. Which term describes the drugs given before general anesthesia?
   a. Induction agents
   b. Maintenance agents
   c. Preanesthetic medications
   d. Postanesthetic medications
91. Which of the following is the most commonly used alpha-2 agonist in dogs and cats?
   a. Dexmedetomidine
   b. Xylazine
   c. Morphine
   d. Detomidine
92. Which of the following options is *not* a side effect of NSAID administration?
   a. Liver damage
   b. Kidney damage
   c. Gastrointestinal ulcers
   d. Respiratory depression
93. Which of the following induction agents can cause muscle tremors, muscle twitching, nystagmus, and paddling?
   a. Thiopental
   b. Propofol
   c. Alfaxalone
   d. None of the above
94. What will the tank pressure gauge read when the oxygen tank is half full?
   a. 1100 psi
   b. 2000 psi
   c. 500 psi
   d. 2200 psi
95. Which of the following statements is true of isoflurane?
   a. A precision vaporizer is used to administer isoflurane.
   b. Isoflurane has no analgesic properties.
   c. Isoflurane is stable at room temperature.
   d. All of the above.
96. A tank of nitrous oxide is present in what state(s)?
   a. Liquid
   b. Gas
   c. Liquid and a gas
   d. Solid and liquid
97. All of the following sites can be used for placement of an arterial catheter used to measure arterial pressures during anesthesia *except*:
   a. Brachial artery
   b. Medial pedal artery
   c. Auricular artery
   d. Coccygeal artery
98. Which condition causes a decrease in the requirements for general anesthesia?
   a. Hypoventilation
   b. Hyperthermia
   c. Hypothermia
   d. Hypotension
99. What shows the amount of oxygen the patient is receiving?
   a. Oxygen tank pressure gauge
   b. Flowmeter
   c. Pressure manometer
   d. Vaporizer
100. Which of the following is *not* a recommended method of actively warming a patient while under anesthesia?
   a. Circulating warm water blankets
   b. Convective warm air devices
   c. Commercial bubble wrap
   d. Radiant heat via heat lamp
101. Which of the following is an example of a monitoring parameter that would be useful during the recovery process?
   a. Continuous ECG monitoring
   b. Temperature monitoring
   c. Postoperative pain scoring
   d. All of the above
102. The reservoir bag's minimum size can be calculated as:
   a. 20 mL/kg
   b. 60 mL/kg
   c. 80 mL/kg
   d. 100 mL/kg
103. If a patient regurgitates while waking up from anesthesia, what is the best course of action?
   a. Remove the regurgitation and lavage the esophagus with saline
   b. Feed the patient a meal as quickly as possible
   c. Place the patient back on gas anesthetic
   d. No treatment is needed
104. What is the function of the pop-off valve?
   a. To vaporize the liquid anesthetic
   b. To prevent excess gas pressure from building up within the breathing circuit
   c. To keep the oxygen flowing in one direction only
   d. To prevent waste gases from reentering the vaporizer
105. Which term describes the drugs given after general anesthesia and after the surgical stimulus is finished?
   a. Induction agents
   b. Maintenance agents
   c. Preanesthetic medications
   d. Postanesthetic medications
106. Which of the following drugs is a phenothiazine tranquilizer commonly used to calm patients in the recovery period?
   a. Acepromazine
   b. Midazolam
   c. Diazepam
   d. Morphine
107. The pressure manometer reading should *not* exceed __________ when a small animal patient is bagged.
   a. 5 cm H_2O
   b. 10 cm H_2O
   c. 15 cm H_2O
   d. 20 cm H_2O

108. Which of the following medications would be a good choice for providing sedation and analgesia in the recovery period?
 a. Midazolam
 b. Diazepam
 c. Acepromazine
 d. Dexmedetomidine
109. Of the following drugs listed, which would not be the best choice to use for a patient recovering from surgery because it *does not* have analgesic properties?
 a. Dexmedetomidine
 b. Morphine
 c. Methadone
 d. Diazepam
110. What is the maintenance flow rate of non-rebreathing systems?
 a. Very low (5–10 mL/kg/min)
 b. Low (20–40 mL/kg/min)
 c. Moderate (50–100 mL/kg/min)
 d. Very high (≥200 mL/kg/min)
111. Which of the following terms describes a diminished volume or a lack of air in part or all of a lung lobe?
 a. Atelectasis
 b. Hypoxia
 c. Tidal volume
 d. Functional residual capacity
112. All of the following techniques can be used to prevent laryngospasm in cats *except*:
 a. Spraying the endotracheal tube with lidocaine
 b. Spraying the larynx with local anesthetic
 c. Ensuring adequate depth before intubation
 d. Using a gentle intubation technique
113. When is the negative pressure relief valve important?
 a. When nitrous oxide is being used
 b. If there is no scavenging system present
 c. If there is a failure of oxygen flow through the system
 d. When the carbon dioxide absorber is no longer functioning
114. Which of the following is a reason why red rubber endotracheal tubes should no longer be used?
 a. The solid color of the tube makes it impossible to detect occlusions from mucus.
 b. Over time the tube can soften, making it more prone to cracking.
 c. Red rubber endotracheal tubes are less likely to cause cross contamination between patients.
 d. Red rubber endotracheal tubes are shorter and cannot provide adequate anesthesia delivery to the patient.
115. What is the tidal volume of an anesthetized animal in mL/kg of body weight?
 a. 5
 b. 10
 c. 19
 d. 20
116. What should the pressure be between the flowmeters and breathing circuit?
 a. 5 psi
 b. 15 psi
 c. 25 psi
 d. 45 psi
117. For which of the following patients would it be advantageous to use a laryngeal mask airway?
 a. Brachycephalic dogs
 b. Rabbits
 c. Pigs
 d. All of the above
118. What is the function of a laryngoscope?
 a. To obtain tissue samples from the trachea
 b. To facilitate endotracheal intubation by allowing direct visualization of the opening to the trachea
 c. To cover the esophagus and prevent regurgitation during surgery
 d. To provide a way for anesthetic gases to be delivered
119. Which anesthetic used in today's practice is associated with neurologic and adverse reproductive effects?
 a. Isoflurane
 b. Halothane
 c. Methoxyflurane
 d. Nitrous oxide
120. What is the function of an endotracheal tube?
 a. To obtain tissue samples from the trachea
 b. To facilitate endotracheal intubation by allowing direct visualization of the opening to the trachea
 c. To cover the esophagus and prevent regurgitation after surgery
 d. To provide a way for oxygen and anesthetic gases to be delivered to the lungs
121. Which type of laryngoscope is composed of a straight blade with a light source on a handle?
 a. Murphy
 b. Cole
 c. Miller
 d. Magill
122. Which of the following endotracheal tubes can be heat-sterilized with steam from an autoclave?
 a. Silicone tubes
 b. PVC tubes
 c. Red rubber tubes
 d. All of the above
123. In the United States, the National Institute for Occupational Safety and Health (NIOSH) recommends that the levels of waste anesthetic gases for anesthetics such as isoflurane, halothane, or methoxyflurane should *not* exceed _____ ppm.
 a. 0.2
 b. 2
 c. 20
 d. 200
124. Anesthesia machines do all of the following *except*:
 a. Deliver oxygen
 b. Deliver anesthetic gas
 c. Remove oxygen
 d. Remove carbon dioxide and waste gases
125. The minimum alveolar concentration (MAC) of isoflurane in horses is:
 a. 1.31%
 b. 1.55%
 c. 2.10%
 d. 1.80%

126. What is the function of a flush valve within the anesthetic circuit?
  a. To deliver oxygen to the system at a specific rate in L/min
  b. To deliver a burst of pure oxygen into the breathing system
  c. To flush more anesthetic gas into the system if the patient is in a light anesthetic plane
  d. To shut off the oxygen supply

127. Which of the following is used to effectively monitor waste anesthetic gases?
  a. Odor of waste gas
  b. Passive dosimeter badge
  c. Radiation monitor
  d. Regular preventive maintenance by qualified personnel

128. The numbers on the vaporizer dial indicate the:
  a. Concentration (in percent) delivered at the output of the vaporizer
  b. Depth of anesthesia
  c. Flow of oxygen through the system
  d. Amount of anesthetic gas left in the reservoir

129. How often is a low-pressure leak test conducted on an anesthesia machine?
  a. Each day that the machine is used
  b. At least once/week
  c. At least once/month
  d. When the anesthetist smells anesthetic gases

130. Which of the following breathing systems is made of an inspiratory tube running within an expiratory tube for the purpose of aiding in the warming and humidification of inspired gases?
  a. Mapleson
  b. Bain coaxial
  c. Modified Jackson Rees
  d. Universal F

131. What is the normal capillary refill time in veterinary patients?
  a. 1–2 seconds
  b. 3–4 seconds
  c. <1 second
  d. 10 seconds

132. If you want to transport a high-pressure O_2 tank, what is the safest way?
  a. Carrying it
  b. Rolling it along the floor
  c. Using a handcart
  d. Dragging it by the neck

133. What can pale mucous membranes indicate in a veterinary patient?
  a. Vasoconstriction because of drugs
  b. Vasodilation because of drugs
  c. Increased cardiac output
  d. Hypertension

134. If anesthetic waste gases are present in a room, how many air changes per hour should occur?
  a. 5
  b. 10
  c. 15
  d. 30

135. All of the following sites are acceptable for palpating peripheral pulses in patients under anesthesia *except*:
  a. Femoral artery
  b. Articular artery
  c. Dorsal pedal artery
  d. Lingual artery

136. How can a technician reduce the amount of waste anesthetic gases?
  a. Use uncuffed endotracheal tubes
  b. Ensure that the anesthetic machine has been tested for leaks
  c. Use a mask or chamber
  d. Use high fresh gas flows

137. What is a Doppler device used to measure?
  a. Patient oxygenation
  b. Temperature
  c. Blood pressure
  d. End-tidal carbon dioxide

138. How would a low-pressure test be conducted on a circle system?
  a. Open the pop-off valve and occlude the end of the circuit
  b. Turn off the oxygen tank
  c. Inflate the reservoir bag
  d. Pressurize the circuit with a volume of gas

139. What should be used to clean most monitoring devices?
  a. Bleach
  b. Mild soap and water
  c. Alcohol
  d. No cleaning is needed

140. Which side effects are common with injectable and inhalant anesthetics?
  a. A period of apnea
  b. Progressive depression of the cardiovascular and respiratory function as the depth of anesthesia increases
  c. Tachycardia followed by bradycardia
  d. Hypothermia-related event

141. Which of the following terms describes the amount of air left in the lungs after normal ventilation?
  a. Functional residual capacity
  b. Atelectasis
  c. Hypoxia
  d. Tidal volume

142. Which of the following would be a cause of spontaneous ventilations not being active enough, therefore requiring controlled ventilation?
  a. Deep level of anesthesia
  b. Use of neuromuscular blockers
  c. During intrathoracic surgery
  d. All of the above

143. What is the desired anesthetic plane for surgical procedures?
  a. Stage III, plane 1
  b. Stage III, plane 2
  c. Stage III, plane 3
  d. Stage III, plane 4

144. What is the term used to express when an animal is trying to breathe against the set respiratory rhythm and volume being delivered by the mechanical ventilator?
a. Checking
b. Pulling
c. Pushing
d. Bucking

145. Which of the following drugs provides sedation but *no* analgesia?
a. Butorphanol
b. Dexmedetomidine
c. Midazolam
d. Morphine

146. What is the stage of anesthesia when you see breath holding, vocalization, and involuntary movement of the limbs?
a. Stage I
b. Stage II
c. Stage III, plane 1
d. Stage III, plane 2

147. Which of the following terms describes a state in which patients are in a trance-like state and unaware of their surroundings?
a. Catalepsy
b. Sedation
c. Sleeping
d. Nystagmus

148. What is considered anatomic dead space?
a. Room air within the breathing circuit
b. Air within the digestive tract
c. Air within the trachea, pharynx, larynx, bronchi, and nasal passages
d. Air within the alveoli

149. Which of the following techniques helps to minimize the occurrence of respiratory depression when using propofol as an induction agent?
a. Administrating the entire dose as a fast IV bolus
b. Slow IV administration
c. Administrating subcutaneously
d. Administrating intramuscularly

150. All of the following patients would be a good candidate for etomidate as the induction drug *except* for patients that are experiencing:
a. Cesarean section
b. Known cardiac disease
c. Cardiovascular instability resulting from trauma
d. All of the above

151. What is the minimum acceptable heart rate for a large breed dog that is anesthetized?
a. 60 bpm
b. 70 bpm
c. 80 bpm
d. 100 bpm

152. Which of the following is *not* a characteristic of alpha-2 agonists?
a. Sedation
b. Increased heart rate
c. Analgesia
d. Muscle relaxation

153. An anesthetized dog that has a respiratory rate less than __________ should be reported to the veterinarian.
a. 4 bpm
b. 6 bpm
c. 10 bpm
d. 15 bpm

154. Patients given alpha-2 agonists often have pale mucous membranes and cold extremities in the initial phase because of what side effect of the drug?
a. Peripheral vasoconstriction
b. Hypothermia
c. Hypoglycemia
d. Decreased hepatic blood flow

155. Ketamine administration would be contraindicated in which of the following disease processes?
a. Hypotrophic cardiomyopathy
b. Congestive heart failure
c. Healthy patients
d. Panosteitis

156. Tachypnea is:
a. An increase in respiratory depth (tidal volume)
b. An increase in respiratory rate
c. A decrease in respiratory depth (tidal volume)
d. A decrease in respiratory rate

157. Which of the following opioids has been shown to have the highest likelihood of causing vomiting in cats?
a. Hydromorphone
b. Morphine
c. Fentanyl
d. Methadone

158. Your patient has a pulse oximetry reading of 89%. What does this indicate?
a. Normal value
b. Need for supportive therapy
c. State of hypoxemia, but no need for therapy
d. Medical emergency

159. Which anesthetic monitoring tool is important for patients on a ventilator to verify the efficiency of gas exchange and adequate ventilation?
a. Capnography
b. Pulse oximeter
c. ECG
d. Blood pressure

160. Which of the following could be a cause of an increase in intraocular pressure (IOP) in an ophthalmology patient?
a. Struggling and excitement in a poorly sedated pet
b. Vomiting or gagging
c. Pressure on the jugular vein from neck leads
d. All of the above

161. Which of the following statements regarding body temperature is true?
a. Body temperatures of 36°C to 38°C (96.8°F to 100.4°F) cause prolonged anesthetic recovery.
b. Dangerous central nervous system depression and changes in cardiac function may be seen at body temperatures <32°C (89.6°F).
c. There is no need to warm IV fluids before administration to surgery patients.
d. Circulating warm water blankets should be set at 45°C (approximately 111°F).

162. Which of the following induction methods should be avoided in patients undergoing an ophthalmic procedure?
a. Alfaxalone
b. Propofol
c. Etomidate
d. Mask or box inductions

163. When monitoring anesthesia and nystagmus is present, which statement is correct?
a. Nystagmus is commonly seen in horses in very light plane of anesthesia.
b. Nystagmus is a useful indicator of anesthetic depth in small animals.
c. In a cat, a "divergent eye sign" is typically associated with an adequate plane of anesthesia for surgery.
d. Ruminants often show nystagmus under anesthesia.

164. Which of the following inhalant anesthetics should be avoided in the ophthalmology patient?
a. Isoflurane
b. Sevoflurane
c. Nitrous oxide
d. Desflurane

165. Pale mucous membranes are indicative of:
a. Acidosis
b. Hypotension
c. Decreased perfusion
d. Hypertension

166. Which drug class is commonly used in ophthalmology procedures to prevent movement of the eye during the procedure and to keep the eye in a central position?
a. Inhalant anesthetics
b. Opioids
c. Neuromuscular blocking agents
d. Alpha-2 agonists

167. What nerve block is commonly used to desensitize nerves and add additional analgesia to an ocular procedure?
a. Retrobulbar block
b. Epidural
c. Circumferential nerve block
d. Sacrococcygeal block

168. Which sign would a patient under stage III, plane 2 anesthesia exhibit?
a. Very brisk palpebral reflex
b. Irregular respiration
c. Relaxed skeletal muscle tone
d. Very dilated pupils

169. Use of ophthalmic local anesthetic drops in the eye before an ophthalmic examination would be an example of ___________ anesthesia.
a. Topical
b. Surgical
c. General
d. Epidural

170. What is the main stimulus to breathe in healthy awake animals?
a. Excess oxygen concentration in the blood
b. Excess carbon dioxide concentration in the blood
c. Insufficient oxygen in the blood
d. Insufficient carbon dioxide in the blood

171. Which of the following is the most common form of heart disease seen in cats?
a. Dilated cardiomyopathy
b. Hypertrophic cardiomyopathy
c. Mitral valve insufficiency
d. Low blood pressure

172. Which of the following drugs should be avoided when premedicating the cat with hypertrophic cardiomyopathy because of its likelihood of causing tachycardia and tachyarrhythmia?
a. Hydromorphone
b. Midazolam
c. Atropine
d. Dexmedetomidine

173. What is the normal tidal volume in an awake animal?
a. 5–10 mL/kg
b. 10–15 mL/kg
c. 16–20 mL/kg
d. 20–25 mL/kg

174. Which of the following factors can cause an increase in intracranial pressure?
a. Hypercapnia
b. Ketamine administration
c. Pressure on the jugular vein
d. All of the above

175. Where is nerve impulse transmission blocked with local anesthetics?
a. Sensory neurons only
b. Motor neurons only
c. Sensory and motor neurons only
d. Sensory, motor, and autonomic neurons

176. Which of the following techniques is useful for reducing intracranial pressure and therefore reducing brain size during neurosurgery?
a. Controlled hyperventilation
b. Controlled hypoventilation
c. Starting a ketamine CRI
d. Placing the patient in a head down position

177. What effect do inhalant anesthetics such as isoflurane and sevoflurane have on intracranial pressure?
a. No change
b. Increased intracranial pressure
c. Decreased intracranial pressure
d. Isoflurane decreases intracranial pressure and sevoflurane decreases intracranial pressure.

178. Which of the following is the mechanism of action for local anesthetics?
a. Local anesthetics do not have a mechanism of action.
b. They interfere with the movement of sodium ions.
c. They block all impulses at the spinal cord level.
d. They affect neurotransmission within the brain.

179. Which of the following opioids would be the *best* choice for emergency department patients who have experienced some sort of head trauma and may need serial neurological exams?
a. Morphine
b. Methadone
c. Fentanyl
d. Remifentanil

180. Which of the following opioids would be the *best* choice of analgesic for a patient with suspected head trauma for whom vomiting and/or abdominal contractions are contraindicated?
a. Methadone
b. Midazolam
c. Morphine
d. Hydromorphone

181. If a cat was receiving an epidural, what is the most caudal aspect that the epidural could be administered?
a. T13
b. L6
c. L7
d. S1

182. Which drug is often used in patients with intracranial disease because of its effect of reducing brain edema and intracranial pressure?
a. Ketamine
b. Isoflurane
c. Glycopyrrolate
d. Mannitol

183. What is the maximum subcutaneous dose of lidocaine in a dog?
a. 1 mg/kg
b. 4 mg/kg
c. 10 mg/kg
d. 15 mg/kg

184. Which inhalant anesthetic causes the most dramatic increase in cerebral blood flow and intracranial pressure?
a. Desflurane
b. Isoflurane
c. Nitrous oxide
d. Halothane

185. Which of the following terms is used to describe a tumor of the pancreas that results in excessive insulin production, leading to hypoglycemia?
a. Pancreatitis
b. Insulinoma
c. Diabetes
d. Hyperglycemia

186. To what does *atelectasis* refer?
a. Excess fluid in the respiratory system
b. The absence of breathing
c. Collapse of the alveoli
d. Bronchial constriction

187. If a specific neuromuscular blocking drug is given and you see an initial surge of muscle activity before paralysis, what drug has most likely been used?
a. Succinylcholine
b. Gallamine
c. Pancuronium
d. Cisatracurium

188. What is the treatment of choice for an insulinoma?
a. Antibiotics
b. Start insulin therapy
c. Surgical removal
d. Antifungal medications

189. Which of the following drugs may *not* be the best choice in a diabetic patient undergoing surgery because of its effect of increasing glucose and then causing a decrease in insulin that can last several hours?
a. Dexmedetomidine
b. Isoflurane
c. Morphine
d. Fentanyl

190. When using neuromuscular blocking agents, which is the most affected type of muscle?
a. Cardiac
b. Smooth muscle
c. Skeletal muscle
d. All types are equally affected.

191. In preparation for an anesthetic procedure, you have drawn up a syringe of ketamine and midazolam and an identical syringe of saline. You are then called to the examination room to assist the veterinarian. About 10 minutes later you return to prepare the animal for induction. With the IV catheter in place, you are just about to inject some saline into the animal when you realize that you are not sure whether the syringe contains saline. The best thing to do is:
a. Inject a small amount of the solution and see what effect it has
b. Discard both syringes and begin again
c. Ask the person who was holding the animal which syringe had saline in it
d. Discard both syringes, label some new syringes, and begin again

192. Which of the following drug classes should be avoided in patients with renal disease?
a. Opioids
b. Nonsteroidal anti-inflammatory drugs
c. Inhalant anesthetics
d. Anticholinergics

193. Which of the following serum enzyme values are commonly used to directly evaluate liver function before an anesthetic event?
a. Glucose and fructosamine
b. PCV and total protein
c. Creatinine and blood urea nitrogen
d. Alanine aminotransferase (ALT) and alkaline phosphatase

194. What should you do if you are monitoring an anesthetic patient and you notice that the O_2 tank is empty?
a. Disconnect the patient from the circuit, put on a new oxygen tank, and then reconnect the patient to the circuit
b. Remove the circuit from the patient to allow it to breathe room air for the remainder of the procedure
c. Resuscitate the patient with an Ambu bag
d. Switch to an injectable anesthetic

195. Which of the following drug classes is not commonly used in pediatric patients because of its side effect of bradycardia?
a. Alpha-2 agonists
b. Anticholinergics
c. Opioids
d. Benzodiazepines

196. Which of the following methods is considered the least suitable choice for anesthetic induction in the pediatric canine and feline patient?
a. IV injection of propofol
b. IV injection of ketamine/diazepam mixture
c. IM injection of alfaxalone
d. Chamber induction with isoflurane

197. Inadequate oxygenation of the tissues for longer than_________ minutes could result in brain damage.
a. 2
b. 4
c. 6
d. 8

198. Which type of breathing system is commonly used in the pediatric patient because of lower resistance to breathing and minimal apparatus dead space?
a. Non-rebreathing system
b. Flow by oxygen via facemask
c. Rebreathing system
d. Ventilator

199. Which of the following fluids is an example of a crystalloid?
a. Dextran
b. Hetastarch
c. Plasma-Lyte 148
d. Plasma

200. What is a reason to suspect that the pop-off valve has been closed or that it is malfunctioning?
a. The anesthetist smells isoflurane
b. Patient has difficulty exhaling
c. Patient wakes up
d. Flow rate starts to drop

201. Which fluid type should be used with caution in patients with blood clotting abnormalities?
a. Plasma-Lyte
b. Normosol-R
c. Hetastarch
d. Lactated Ringer's solution

202. Which of the following procedures can be completed to reduce the risk of anesthesia for a brachycephalic dog?
a. Use dexmedetomidine as part of the anesthetic protocol
b. Preoxygenate the animal before administering any anesthetic
c. Chamber induce the dog
d. Use a laryngeal mask airway

203. Crystalloid solutions are considered balanced when they have a fluid composition that closely resembles the patient's extracellular fluid. Which of the following crystalloids is *not* considered a balanced solution?
a. Normal 0.9% saline
b. Lactated Ringer's solution
c. Normosol-R
d. Plasma-Lyte 148

204. What would the approximate tidal volume be for a 40-kg canine patient?
a. 40–80 mL
b. 400–800 mL
c. 4–8 mL
d. 10 mL

205. If a patient has cardiovascular disease, what anesthetic agents or drugs might you want to avoid?
a. Lidocaine
b. Isoflurane
c. Xylazine
d. Opioids

206. What is the formula to calculate minute volume?
a. Tidal volume multiplied by respiration rate
b. % of inhaled anesthetic multiplied by respiration rate
c. Tidal volume multiplied by % of inhaled anesthetic
d. There is no formula to calculate minute volume.

207. Which of the following patients would *not* be a good candidate for premedication with acepromazine?
a. A 2-year-old mixed breed canine presenting for ovariohysterectomy
b. A 6-year-old German shepherd presenting after being hit by a car
c. A 1-year-old male cat presenting for castration
d. All of the above are good candidates for premedication with acepromazine

208. What might cause tachypnea?
a. Increased levels of arterial oxygen
b. Increased levels of arterial CO_2
c. The use of ketamine
d. Too deep a plane of anesthesia

209. Consider the following scenario: You are performing a procedure on a canine patient that you feel is at an appropriate anesthetic depth. Which of the following settings would be most appropriate if using sevoflurane in this patient?
a. 2%
b. 2 L/min
c. 3%
d. 8 mL/min

210. Which of the following drugs is *not* considered an alpha-2 adrenoreceptor agonist?
a. Dexmedetomidine
b. Xylazine
c. Medetomidine
d. Yohimbine

211. When inducing anesthesia in a young healthy patient by using an IV agent such as propofol, which statement is false?
a. If the patient is not adequately anesthetized to allow intubation after giving the initial amount, give the rest of the calculated dose
b. Draw up the calculated dose, give about quater to half first, and give the rest to effect anesthetization
c. You must be sure the drug gets in the vein
d. Old, sick, or debilitated patients often require less

212. In what organ are most drugs metabolized (biotransformed) in the patient?
a. Skin
b. Liver
c. Eye
d. Intestines

213. Which of the following terms refers to a drug-induced central nervous system depression and drowsiness that varies in intensity from light to deep?
   a. Sedation
   b. General anesthesia
   c. Surgical anesthesia
   d. Local anesthesia

214. When giving IV induction agents, which statement is false?
   a. Ketamine-diazepam takes slightly longer to act and lasts somewhat longer than propofol.
   b. When using propofol, about 25%–50% of the calculated dose should be given every 30 seconds to have an effect.
   c. Significantly lower doses of thiopental sodium must be used in sick, old, or debilitated patients.
   d. Propofol is generally given intravenously but can be given intramuscularly in uncooperative patients.

215. Which of the following is *not* a recommended method of actively warming a patient during the recovery period?
   a. Circulating warm water blankets
   b. Convective warm air devices
   c. Commercial bubble wrap
   d. Electric heating blankets

216. Which of the following terms describes impaired oxygen delivery as a result of systemic delivery issues?
   a. Atelectasis
   b. Hypoxia
   c. Tidal volume
   d. Functional residual capacity

217. Which of the following is a short-acting neuroactive steroid induction agent?
   a. Pentobarbital
   b. Alfaxalone
   c. Propofol
   d. Midazolam

218. Which of the following is experienced by veterinary personnel who are exposed to waste anesthetic agents on a short-term basis?
   a. Headache
   b. Excitement
   c. Increased energy
   d. Happiness

219. Which of the following statements is false?
   a. Choosing a tube that is too short may cause increased mechanical dead space.
   b. Choosing a tube that is too small may result in increased resistance to breathing.
   c. Choosing a tube that is too long may result in hypoxemia.
   d. Failure to cuff the tube may result in aspiration of foreign material.

220. All of the following conditions are known health issues that result from long-term exposure to waste anesthetic gases *except*:
   a. Reproductive disorders
   b. Liver damage
   c. Hyperexcitability
   d. Kidney damage

221. How can you tell whether the endotracheal tube has been placed in the esophagus?
   a. The patient coughs when the tube is placed.
   b. The unidirectional valves do not move.
   c. The pressure manometer indicates 0–2 cm H_2O while the patient is spontaneously breathing.
   d. Only one firm structure in the neck is palpated.

222. All of the following are mechanisms to decrease the amount of waste anesthetic gases in the veterinary facility except:
   a. Anesthetic machine maintenance
   b. Scavenger system(s)
   c. Anesthetic technique used
   d. Using only inhalant gases

223. When should a dog be extubated after anesthesia?
   a. Right after you turn off the vaporizer
   b. About 10 minutes after turning off the vaporizer
   c. When the animal begins to swallow
   d. Any time that is convenient

224. Which of the following best describes a passive scavenger system?
   a. Uses suction created by a vacuum pump or fan to draw gas into the scavenger
   b. Uses positive pressure of the gas in the anesthetic machine to push gas into the scavenger
   c. Uses positive pressure created by a vacuum to draw gas out of the anesthetic machine
   d. Uses negative pressure of the gas in the anesthetic machine to push gas into the scavenger

225. What does the term *hypostatic congestion* mean?
   a. Accumulation of mucus in the trachea
   b. Pooling of blood in the dependent lung
   c. Leakage of fluid into the chest
   d. Pooling of ingesta in one area of the gastrointestinal tract

226. The advantages of a non-rebreathing system compared with a circle breathing system include all of the following *except*:
   a. Reduced resistance to breathing
   b. Greater potential for hypothermia caused by high flows needed
   c. Reduced mechanical dead space
   d. No soda lime required

227. Which anesthetic plan will give the fastest induction time and the best control over anesthetic depth?
   a. IM induction and maintenance
   b. IV induction with an ultra–short-acting agent and maintenance with bolus injections of the same
   c. Inhalant induction and maintenance
   d. IV induction with an ultra–short-acting agent and maintenance with an inhalant

228. An intravenous catheter should be:
   a. Large enough to allow adequate fluid delivery in the event of an emergency
   b. As small as possible to avoid pain
   c. Placed in critically ill patients only
   d. Left in place for at least 3 days after surgery

229. Pulse oximetry monitoring devices give an estimate of:
   a. Respiratory rate
   b. Cardiac output
   c. Percentage of hemoglobin saturation with oxygen in arterial blood
   d. Oxygen content of arterial blood

230. Which of the following techniques is used most often in general small animal practices?
 a. General anesthesia and sedation
 b. Sedatives and local techniques
 c. Neuromuscular blockade and neuroleptanalgesia
 d. Local and general anesthesia

231. Nitrous oxide cylinders are painted what color in the United States?
 a. Green
 b. Gray
 c. Blue
 d. Yellow

232. Activated charcoal devices absorb all inhalation agents *except*:
 a. Isoflurane
 b. Halothane
 c. Sevoflurane
 d. Nitrous oxide

233. What size endotracheal tube would an adult 18-kg non-brachycephalic dog require?
 a. 7–7.5 mm
 b. 8–8.5 mm
 c. 9–9.5 mm
 d. 11 mm

234. Which animal is most likely to experience laryngospasm during endotracheal intubation?
 a. Thoroughbred mare
 b. Hereford cow
 c. Persian cat
 d. Dalmatian dog

235. The best method for determining the proper inflation of an endotracheal tube cuff is:
 a. Use 1 mL of air for each mm of internal diameter of the tube
 b. Inject air while applying pressure from the reservoir bag until no air escapes around the tube
 c. Inject air until the bulb on the cuff tubing is too hard to collapse
 d. Use a 12-mL syringe and inject 12 mL of air into the cuff

236. What is the purpose of an endotracheal tube?
 a. To increase dead space
 b. To maintain a patent airway
 c. To protect the patient from reflex tachycardia
 d. To allow the anesthetist to monitor the patient

237. The preferred method for treating a cat with laryngospasm is to:
 a. Use a sharp stylet to insert the endotracheal tube between the vocal cords
 b. Return the animal to its cage and wait 20 minutes before trying again
 c. Place a drop of a topical anesthetic onto each arytenoid, wait several seconds, and then intubate the animal
 d. Use a stiffer endotracheal tube that can force the vocal cords open

238. In a pug, the endotracheal tube should be removed:
 a. As soon as the surgery or diagnostic technique is completed
 b. Only after the animal is fully conscious and able to maintain a free airway
 c. When the animal is taken off of the anesthesia machine
 d. As soon as the animal begins to swallow and cough

239. When monitoring the vital signs of an anesthetized patient, you must observe and record all of the following *except*:
 a. Mucous membrane color and capillary refill time
 b. Heart rate and respiratory rate and depth
 c. Reflexes
 d. Pulse quality and strength

240. What could be a complication from improper intubation?
 a. Increased dead space
 b. Pressure necrosis of the tracheal mucosa
 c. Intubation of alveoli
 d. Atelectasis

241. The responsibilities of the anesthetist during a surgical procedure include continuous monitoring of the patient's vital signs and recording observations at approximately:
 a. 10-minute intervals
 b. 5-minute intervals
 c. 2-minute intervals
 d. 15-minute intervals

242. It is recommended to wait longer before extubation because of the likelihood of an airway obstruction in patients with which of the following characteristics?
 a. Dolichocephalic
 b. Prognathism
 c. Brachycephalic
 d. Cleft palate

243. When performing maintenance anesthesia:
 a. The patient should be monitored every 30 minutes.
 b. The patient should be placed on an electric heating pad to prevent hypothermia.
 c. If a patient has one diseased lung, it should be positioned with the diseased side down.
 d. The anesthetist should avoid any more than a 5-degree elevation of the rear quarters.

244. Use of an indwelling catheter in an artery to monitor blood pressure is termed:
 a. Direct monitoring
 b. Central venous pressure
 c. Indirect monitoring
 d. Peripheral venous pressure

245. What can influence the anesthetic recovery period?
 a. Body temperature
 b. Patient condition
 c. The length of time the patient was under
 d. The breed of the patient
 e. All of the above

246. The most accurate way to evaluate the effectiveness of respiration is by:
  a. Observing abdominal and chest movements during respiration
  b. Counting the respiratory rate
  c. Feeling air move through the endotracheal tube or nostrils
  d. Measuring the arterial blood oxygen and carbon dioxide partial pressures
247. What is not a normal sign during recovery?
  a. Head bobbing
  b. Mydriasis
  c. Seizures
  d. Rapid limb paddling
248. Kidney function can be assessed by all of the following preanesthetic screening tests *except*:
  a. Blood urea nitrogen
  b. ALT
  c. Urinalysis
  d. Creatinine
249. A preanesthetic check of the anesthesia machine should include all of the following *except*:
  a. Leak testing
  b. Weighing the charcoal canister
  c. Calibrating the vaporizer
  d. Filling the vaporizer with anesthetic gas agent
250. Please choose the appropriate action for anesthetic recovery.
  a. Administer oxygen at a high flow rate for 5 minutes after discontinuation of the anesthetic or until extubation
  b. Leave the cage door open so you can monitor the patient from across the room
  c. Turn the patient about every 45 minutes
  d. Use cooling methods to prevent hyperthermia
251. A patient in ASA class I physical status is:
  a. A normal patient with no organic disease
  b. A moribund patient
  c. An adult animal with no signs of evident disease on physical examination
  d. In absolutely no danger while under anesthesia
252. Treatment for hypotension during anesthesia includes:
  a. Turning up the anesthetic gas
  b. Increasing the drip rate of the IV fluids
  c. Increasing the flow of oxygen
  d. Giving ventilating breaths
253. When performing surgery on a horse and administrating a standing chemical restraint, which statement is true?
  a. Horses must be intubated for standing chemical restraint.
  b. Risk of myopathy or neuropathy is higher with standing chemical restraint.
  c. The head must be supported in a normal position to avoid nasal congestion.
  d. Hypoxemia is a common complication of standing chemical restraint.
254. It is generally safe to extubate a canine or a feline when the patient:
  a. Vocalizes
  b. Swallows
  c. Stands
  d. Can rest in a sternal position
255. An epidural agent is most commonly administered where in a dog?
  a. Between L7 and the sacrum
  b. Just cranial to C1
  c. Immediately caudal to T13
  d. Directly into the spinal cord at T1
256. What is the next step for the anesthetist if a horse becomes excited after it has been premedicated with xylazine intravenously before general anesthesia?
  a. Allow the horse time to calm down before proceeding
  b. Physically restrain the horse using ropes
  c. Induce anesthesia with acepromazine
  d. Induce anesthesia with ketamine
257. Epidural anesthesia could be appropriately used for all of the following procedures *except*:
  a. Tail amputation
  b. Cesarean section
  c. Eye enucleation
  d. Femur fracture repair
258. What is prevented by appropriate positioning and padding of the horse on the surgery table?
  a. Hypoxemia and hypotension positions
  b. Myopathies and neuropathies
  c. Hypoventilation and hypertension positions
  d. Regurgitation and aspiration padding
259. Propofol is a/an:
  a. Neuroactive steroid
  b. Ultra–short-acting barbiturate
  c. Ketamine-like dissociative
  d. Short-acting hypnotic agent
260. Some anesthesiologists suggest that acepromazine be avoided in:
  a. Patients with a history of seizures
  b. Aggressive patients
  c. All senior dogs
  d. All Dobermans
261. In dogs, normal doses of opioids generally produce all of the following *except*:
  a. Respiratory depression
  b. Decreased heart rate
  c. Analgesia
  d. Excitement
262. What is the function of guaifenesin when added to an induction protocol in horses?
  a. Muscle relaxation
  b. Analgesia
  c. Sedation
  d. All of the above
263. The oxygen flush valve:
  a. Allows oxygen to flow into the breathing system without going through the vaporizer
  b. Increases the anesthetic concentration within the circuit
  c. Causes the patient to breathe deeper
  d. Is used primarily to keep the reservoir bag deflated

264. The minimum fresh gas flow in a semi-closed circle system is correctly determined by:
a. Patient's metabolic rate
b. Patient's respiratory rate
c. Drugs used for premedication
d. Size of the soda lime canister

265. When would an inhalant induction via nasotracheal tube be appropriate?
a. A 2-year-old Arabian stallion undergoing arthroscopy
b. A 25-year-old thoroughbred mare undergoing sinus surgery
c. A 3-week-old foal undergoing colic surgery
d. A 6-month-old foal undergoing umbilical hernia repair

266. All inhalant anesthetic machines should have:
a. A nitrous oxide flowmeter
b. Blood pressure monitors
c. Respiratory monitors
d. An anesthetic waste gas scavenging system

267. In a Siamese cat, the endotracheal tube should be removed:
a. As soon as the surgery or diagnostic procedure is completed
b. Only after the animal is fully conscious and able to maintain a free airway
c. When the animal is taken off of the anesthesia machine
d. As soon as the animal begins to swallow and cough

268. Which of the following best describes endotracheal intubation in the horse?
a. Intubation is performed blindly with the head and neck extended.
b. It is not advisable to rinse the horse's mouth out before intubation.
c. A laryngoscope is useful for visualization of the larynx.
d. An endoscope is commonly used to facilitate intubation.

269. What is the best technique for securing an endotracheal tube to an animal?
a. It is best not to secure the tube to the animal so that it can move freely if the animal starts to wake up.
b. It should be secured by a gauze tie or IV tubing around the maxilla, mandible, or behind the ears.
c. It can be secured with several wraps of cloth and tape around the animal's nose and the tube.
d. A rubber band can be looped tightly around the tube and the animal's nose.

270. Hypoventilation that occurs in the anesthetized patient is characterized by:
a. Reduced tidal volume and respiratory rate followed by increased carbon dioxide levels
b. Decreased carbon dioxide levels and decreased oxygen levels
c. Increased tidal volume and oxygen levels followed by decreased carbon dioxide levels
d. Increased respiratory rate and hypocarbia followed by hypotension

271. During maintenance of anesthesia in horses with inhalant anesthetics, what are the most common complications?
a. Hypoxemia, hypertension, and bradycardia
b. Hypoxemia, hypotension, and bradycardia
c. Hypoxemia, hypertension, and hypoventilation
d. Hypoxemia, hypotension, and hypoventilation

272. For which patients should mask induction with isoflurane be avoided?
a. Patients with impaired liver function
b. Patients with impaired cardiac function
c. Patients with impaired respiratory function
d. Patients with impaired gastrointestinal function

273. What anesthetic agent does the cat kidney excrete largely intact?
a. Atropine
b. Ketamine
c. Sevoflurane
d. Acepromazine

274. When treating hypotension in the anesthetized horse, what drug is commonly used?
a. Dextrose
b. Digoxin
c. Dobutamine
d. Doxycycline

275. Ideally, in a patient under anesthesia:
a. The PaO_2 should be high, and the $PaCO_2$ should be low
b. The PaO_2 should be high, and the $PaCO_2$ should be high
c. The PaO_2 should be low, and the $PaCO_2$ should be low
d. The PaO_2 should be low, and the $PaCO_2$ should be high

276. The approximate volume of oxygen in an E cylinder is:
a. 65 L
b. 650 L
c. 6500 L
d. 2000 L

277. The approximate volume of oxygen in an H cylinder is:
a. 69 L
b. 690 L
c. 6900 L
d. 2200 L

278. Which phase of anesthesia is the greatest risk for horses?
a. Pre-anesthesia
b. Induction
c. Maintenance
d. Recovery

279. In cattle, an epidural block is most commonly performed by inserting a spinal needle between which vertebrae?
a. T13 and L1
b. L7 and the sacrum
c. The sacrum and C1
d. Cy1 and Cy2

280. What is the most likely diagnosis in a horse that has recovered from anesthesia for arthroscopy and shows the following symptoms: hard, swollen gluteal muscles, stiff gait, and reluctance to walk?
a. Colic
b. Myopathy
c. Neuropathy
d. Nephropathy

281. You have been asked to perform low-flow anesthesia on a 40-kg canine patient needing repair of a fractured femur. Which of the following flow rates would be appropriate for this patient?
a. 80–280 mL/kg/min
b. 500–1000 mL/kg/min
c. 10–20 mL/kg/min
d. 600–800 mL/kg/min

282. Which of the following offers a continuous, noninvasive way to estimate the partial pressure of carbon dioxide in arterial blood?
a. Pulse oximetry
b. Direct arterial blood pressure
c. Central venous pressure
d. Capnometry

283. What is the best choice when comparing cattle, horses, and swine with xylazine usage?
a. Cattle are more sensitive than horses, which are more sensitive than swine.
b. Cattle are more sensitive than swine, which are more sensitive than horses.
c. Horses are more sensitive than cattle, which are more sensitive than swine.
d. Swine are more sensitive than cattle, which are more sensitive than horses.

284. A blood pH of 7.2 is referred to as:
a. Alkalemia
b. Acidemia
c. Hypoxemia
d. Hyponatremia

285. Blood flow to the major organs is jeopardized when mean arterial blood pressure drops below:
a. 60 mmHg
b. 100 mmHg
c. 80 mmHg
d. 90 mmHg

286. Which drug is normally used in premedication in cattle?
a. Anticholinergic
b. Local anesthetic
c. Alpha-2 adrenoceptor agonist
d. Inhalation agent

287. An increased or rising central venous pressure (CVP) is caused by:
a. Hypovolemia
b. Increased cardiac output
c. Hypertension
d. Fluid overload

288. What are the two main components of "double drip"?
a. Guaifenesin and dobutamine
b. Guaifenesin and ketamine
c. Xylazine and ketamine
d. Acepromazine and ketamine

289. Which of the following drugs may cause histamine release if given intravenously too quickly?
a. Butorphanol
b. Morphine
c. Methadone
d. Hydromorphone

290. Which of the following drugs is classified as a full mu opioid?
a. Butorphanol
b. Buprenorphine
c. Dexmedetomidine
d. Hydromorphone

291. You have been asked to anesthetize a 1000-kg bull and maintain anesthesia by using an inhalant technique. Which is the correct statement regarding intubation of this patient?
a. The inhalant can be safely delivered via a facemask.
b. The tube does not need to be lubricated before intubation.
c. You will have to intubate the bull manually.
d. All of the above.

292. Which of the following drugs produces the most profound analgesia in dogs and cats?
a. Methadone
b. Midazolam
c. Ketamine
d. Butorphanol

293. Mu opioid agonists cause which of the following?
a. Miosis in both dogs and cats
b. Miosis in cats and mydriasis in dogs
c. Mydriasis in cats and miosis in dogs
d. Mydriasis in both dogs and cats

294. Which of the following inhalants cannot be used safely in ruminants?
a. Nitrous oxide
b. Isoflurane
c. Halothane
d. Sevoflurane

295. Which of the following drugs is used to reverse the effects of mu-opioid agonists?
a. Flumazenil
b. Remifentanil
c. Atipamezole
d. Naloxone

296. Which of the following is *not* a contraindication for the use of NSAIDs?
a. Pulmonary disease
b. Impaired renal or hepatic function
c. Coagulopathies
d. Dehydration and hypovolemia

297. If you position the head of an anesthetized ruminant with the pharynx higher than the mouth, what can this help to prevent?
a. Hyperventilation
b. Hypotension
c. Aspiration
d. Hypoxemia

298. An infraorbital dental nerve block is used to block the sensation of pain to which of the following areas?
a. The lower dental arcade and hard palate
b. The rostral maxilla
c. The rostral mandible
d. The upper dental arcade and tongue

299. Why should ruminants be placed in sternal recumbency during recovery?
a. Eructation
b. Regurgitation
c. Salivation
d. Hyperventilation

300. You have been asked to perform an epidural in a canine patient that requires repair of a fractured ilium. This procedure is estimated to take at least 3 to 4 hours. The veterinarian would like you to use a combination of a local anesthetic and an opioid. Which of the following will you use?
a. Lidocaine and morphine
b. Bupivacaine and morphine
c. Lidocaine only
d. Bupivacaine only

301. All of the following items make it easier to intubate swine *except*:
a. Speculum
b. Laryngoscope
c. Stylet
d. Epiglotoscope

302. Unlike other domestic species, the spinal cord in the dog ends at which of the following vertebra?
a. S1
b. L6
c. L7
d. T13

303. In the feline patient, the spinal cord ends at the level of which of the following vertebra?
a. S1
b. L6
c. L7
d. T13

304. Which statement regarding swine anesthesia is true?
a. Oscillometric blood pressure monitors work well in pigs.
b. All pigs should have complete blood work before anesthesia.
c. Pigs are very sensitive to alpha-2 agonists.
d. Intravenous sedation is virtually impossible in healthy pigs.

305. Which of the following is *not* a contraindication for epidural administration?
a. Pyoderma
b. Coagulopathy
c. Breed
d. Septicemia

306. Which of the following drug combinations is considered neuroleptanalgesia?
a. Atropine and morphine
b. Midazolam and etomidate
c. Hydromorphone and acepromazine
d. Butorphanol and methadone

307. Which of the following conditions does *not* occur in porcine stress syndrome?
a. Hypothermia
b. Hyperthermia
c. Hyperkalemia
d. Hypercapnia

308. Which of the following fluids is considered a synthetic colloid?
a. Lactated Ringer's solution
b. Hetastarch
c. Fresh frozen plasma
d. 0.9% saline

309. Why should glycopyrrolate be used in rabbits instead of atropine?
a. Atropine is highly toxic in rabbits
b. Many rabbits have high levels of atropinase, so atropine is relatively ineffective
c. Rabbits are unable to metabolize atropine
d. Atropine causes marked bradycardia in rabbits

310. Which of the following is *not* a consideration for blood administration during surgery?
a. Type of procedure and blood loss anticipated
b. Age and breed of patient
c. Hemoglobin content of the patient's blood
d. Hematocrit of the patient's blood

311. Why might you *not* get an accurate reading from a pulse oximeter in small mammals?
a. The heart rate of the animal may exceed the upper range of the instrument.
b. The hemoglobin absorption characteristics are different in rodents and dogs and cats.
c. Pulse oximeters do not function on animals that have dark fur.
d. Small rodents have a rapid respiratory rate.

312. Which of the following drugs should probably be avoided in patients requiring ocular surgery because it causes an increase in intraocular pressure?
a. Propofol
b. Isoflurane
c. Fentanyl
d. Ketamine

313. Why can the position of the eyes *not* be used to assess depth of anesthesia in rodents?
a. The eye is too small to assess its position accurately.
b. The position of the eye does not change during anesthesia.
c. The eye rotates downward in very light planes of anesthesia.
d. The eyelids remain closed throughout anesthesia.

314. You have been asked to anesthetize a patient with a suspected brain tumor. This patient is at risk of increased intracranial pressure. Which of the following drugs does not contribute in any way to increasing intracranial pressure and is thus "safe" for this patient?
a. Propofol
b. Ketamine
c. Morphine
d. Hydromorphone

315. What is an advantage of using dexmedetomidine combined with ketamine for anesthesia of rodents and rabbits?
a. It is readily absorbed from body fat.
b. It can be given by mouth to produce anesthesia.
c. It promotes gut motility and therefore reduces the occurrence of postoperative inappetence.
d. It can be partially reversed by using atipamezole, allowing faster recovery.

316. Because of the enlarged fleshy tongue and a narrowed upper airway, which of the following statements is correct when dealing with neonatal and pediatric patients undergoing general anesthesia?
a. Neonatal and pediatric patients should be induced and maintained via an anesthetic mask and inhalant.
b. Neonatal and pediatric patients should not be preoxygenated because it increases the risk of obstruction.
c. Neonatal and pediatric patients should be intubated for all procedures requiring general anesthesia because they are at risk of upper airway obstruction.
d. Neonatal and pediatric patients are at no more risk of airway obstruction than adult patients.

317. What will the approximate blood volume of a 40-g adult mouse be?
a. 10 mL
b. 3 mL
c. 50 mL
d. 0.2 mL

318. Which of the following drugs is most likely the safest to give as part of an anesthetic protocol for a healthy, 1-year-old Labrador cesarean section?
a. Dexmedetomidine
b. Propofol
c. Midazolam
d. Acepromazine

319. Which of the following statements is correct?
a. Arteries carry blood to the heart
b. Veins carry blood to the heart
c. Both veins and arteries carry blood away from the heart
d. Both veins and arteries carry blood to the heart

320. What should be done to fluids such as lactated Ringer's solution when they are given to small mammals?
a. Used at about 4°C so that they are rapidly absorbed
b. Administered orally because it is not possible to use any other route
c. Warmed to body temperature before administration to avoid causing hypothermia
d. Given only postoperatively to avoid overloading the circulation

321. The P wave in the electrocardiograph represents which of the following?
a. Ventricular depolarization
b. Ventricular repolarization
c. Atrial depolarization
d. Atrial repolarization

322. The T wave in the electrocardiograph represents which of the following?
a. Ventricular depolarization
b. Ventricular repolarization
c. Atrial depolarization
d. Atrial repolarization

323. Which of the following is the most accurate description of an anesthetic breathing circuit used in a small rabbit?
a. Is constructed of only plastic components because rabbits are allergic to latex
b. Has low equipment dead space
c. Has high equipment dead space
d. Always includes soda lime to prevent rebreathing

324. The QRS complex in the electrocardiograph represents which of the following?
a. Ventricular depolarization
b. Ventricular repolarization
c. Atrial depolarization
d. Atrial repolarization

325. When giving postoperative analgesics to rodents and rabbits to alleviate pain, which of the following statements is true?
a. NSAIDs cannot be used because they cause gastric ulceration at normal therapeutic doses in these species.
b. Opioids (narcotics) cause severe respiratory depression and therefore must never be used.
c. Opioids must be given with care if a neuroleptanalgesic mixture has been used for anesthesia.
d. Local anesthetics cannot be used because they produce cardiac arrest even at low doses in these species.

326. Which of the following best represents systolic blood pressure?
a. The pressure measured when the left ventricle relaxes
b. The pressure measured when the right ventricle relaxes
c. The pressure measured when the left ventricle contracts
d. The pressure measured when the right ventricle contracts

327. What is the tidal volume range for a 20-kg beagle mix?
a. 200–400 mL
b. 20–40 mL
c. 2000–4000 mL
d. 2–4 mL

328. What will happen if postoperative pain is not alleviated in rabbits?
a. They will not eat or drink normally
b. They will recover much faster from anesthesia
c. They will spend a great deal of time grooming themselves
d. Porphyrin staining will appear around their eyes

329. Which of the following patients should have coagulation profile submitted before anesthetizing for an elective hernia repair?
a. Doberman
b. Labrador
c. Domestic short-hair
d. Chihuahua

330. Common locations for pulse palpation in the dog include all of the following *except*:
a. Femoral
b. Dorsopedal
c. Auricular
d. Palmar digital

331. What will pulse oximetry often allow you to estimate?
a. Arterial blood pressure
b. Pulse pressure
c. PaO_2
d. Percentage saturation of hemoglobin with oxygen

332. In relation to anesthesia, a patient with moderate risk that has systemic changes and some clinical alterations would be classified in which of the following categories?
a. ASA I
b. ASA II
c. ASA III
d. ASA IV

333. How many milligrams are in one microgram?
a. 100
b. 1000
c. 10
d. 1

334. A 2% solution of lidocaine has a mg/mL concentration of:
a. 2 mg/mL
b. 0.2 mg/mL
c. 200 mg/mL
d. 20 mg/mL

335. The drug xylazine is best described as an:
a. Anti-inflammatory
b. Analgesic and sedative
c. Antiemetic
d. Anesthetic

336. When pressure checking a rebreathing circuit, why is it important to keep your thumb over the end of the hose until the pressure is fully released from the system?
a. Releasing your thumb before releasing the pressure in the circuit can create a vacuum effect causing some of the carbon dioxide absorbent to be sucked into the circuit.
b. Releasing your thumb before releasing the pressure in the circuit can cause the pop-off valve to become stuck in the closed position.
c. Releasing your thumb before releasing the pressure in the circuit can cause the scavenge system to malfunction.
d. Releasing your thumb before releasing the pressure in the circuit can lead to a malfunction of the one-way valves.

337. The carbon dioxide absorbent should be changed when how much of the canister has changed to violet?
a. ½ of the canister
b. ¼ of the canister
c. ⅔ of the canister
d. ⅛ of the canister

338. An endotracheal tube should be checked and left inflated for about how many minutes before use?
a. 2–4 min
b. 1–2 min
c. 1–15 min
d. 5–10 min

339. Detomidine is approved for use in:
a. Dogs
b. Cats
c. Horses
d. Cattle

340. The benefits of placing an arterial catheter include all of the following *except*:
a. Ability to obtain central venous pressure
b. Ability to obtain direct blood pressure
c. Provides access to quick blood sample collection
d. Ability to obtain and monitor blood gas samples

341. Hypothermia in the anesthetized patient can cause all of the following complications *except*:
a. MAC reduction
b. Decreased tissue perfusion
c. Bradycardia
d. Hypertension

342. Butorphanol is best described as a/an:
a. Anti-inflammatory
b. Analgesic
c. Anesthetic
d. Diuretic

343. Which of the following is *not* an advantage to endotracheal intubation in an anesthetized patient?
a. It allows for complete control of the airway.
b. Oxygen and inhalant are delivered close to the lungs.
c. It increases anatomic dead space compared with a facemask.
d. It helps prevent aspiration of foreign material into the lungs.

344. One disadvantage of an endotracheal tube that has a low-volume high-pressure cuff is:
a. The endotracheal tube is hard to clean and sanitize.
b. A tight seal cannot be obtained without a large volume of air placed into the cuff.
c. A stylet must be used to advance these endotracheal tubes.
d. The high pressure in the cuff can cause tracheal necrosis over time.

345. Diazepam is considered a good choice in patients when which body system is compromised?
a. Hepatic
b. Renal
c. Cardiovascular
d. All body systems

346. Placing an endotracheal tube that is too small compared with the diameter of the trachea can cause:
a. Increase in airway resistance
b. Decrease in tidal volume
c. Increase in dead space
d. Decrease in peak inspiratory pressure

347. Before anesthetic induction, it is ideal to preoxygenate the patient for:
a. 1–2 min
b. 10 min
c. 3–5 min
d. Preoxygenation is not necessary.

348. In the United States, xylazine is *not* approved for use in:
a. Dogs
b. Cats
c. Horses
d. Cattle

349. You have just induced and intubated a canine patient. The patient has normal chest excursions, but the capnograph is reading zero. What has probably happened?
   a. The patient is not completely anesthetized.
   b. The endotracheal tube has been inserted too deeply.
   c. The oxygen flow rate is too high, thus flushing the system.
   d. The endotracheal tube is probably in the esophagus.
350. The small oxygen tank that attaches to the anesthesia machine is labeled as what type of tank?
   a. "E"
   b. "H"
   c. "J"
   d. "G"
351. Guaifenesin is most often used in horses and cattle to provide:
   a. Analgesia
   b. Muscle relaxation
   c. Anesthesia
   d. Diuresis
352. You have been asked to provide inhalant anesthesia to a patient by using low-flow anesthetic rates. Which of the following rates would you use to calculate low-flow anesthesia?
   a. 4–7 mL/kg/min
   b. 1–3 mL/kg/min
   c. 10–15 mL/kg/min
   d. 15–25 mL/kg/min
353. What is the purpose for higher flow rates when using a non-rebreathing system?
   a. To eliminate rebreathing of carbon dioxide
   b. To ensure the patient receives the proper percentage of inhalant
   c. To help keep the patient warm
   d. To provide humidity to the respiratory system
354. Which of the following ECG leads is most commonly used to monitor patients under general anesthesia?
   a. Lead I
   b. Lead II
   c. Lead III
   d. Lead IV
355. Your patient's ECG strip is showing a fast, regular rhythm with normal morphology. Which of the following do you suspect?
   a. First-degree AV block
   b. Atrial fibrillation
   c. Premature ventricular contractions
   d. Sinus tachycardia
356. The combination of xylazine and butorphanol is used to:
   a. Provide greater analgesia and muscle relaxation than either drug can alone
   b. Cause central nervous system (CNS) excitement
   c. Increase the dose of butorphanol
   d. Increase the dose of xylazine
357. Which of the following drugs is used to treat bradycardia in the anesthetized patient?
   a. Doxapram
   b. Glycopyrrolate
   c. Alfaxalone
   d. Ketamine
358. Which of the following arrhythmias is characterized by a prolonged P-R interval?
   a. First-degree AV block
   b. Second-degree AV block
   c. Third-degree AV block
   d. AV dissociation
359. Which drug is the most potent sedative?
   a. Xylazine
   b. Detomidine
   c. Acepromazine
   d. Diazepam
360. Which of the following arrhythmias is characterized by a P wave that lacks a QRS complex to follow?
   a. First-degree AV block
   b. Second-degree AV block
   c. Third-degree AV block
   d. AV dissociation
361. Which drug is most likely to cause hypotension in normal doses?
   a. Diazepam
   b. Butorphanol
   c. Acepromazine
   d. Flunixin meglumine
362. Which of the following arrhythmias is characterized by a fast, irregular rhythm with wide and bizarre QRS complexes?
   a. Third-degree AV block
   b. Atrial premature complexes
   c. Ventricular tachycardia
   d. Sinus bradycardia
363. You are monitoring a 12-year-old dog for a humeral fracture repair. You notice that the complexes on the ECG are intermittently wide and bizarre; otherwise, the rhythm is normal. Which arrhythmia is most probably occurring?
   a. Atrial fibrillation
   b. Ventricular fibrillation
   c. Atrial premature complexes
   d. Ventricular premature complexes
364. The combination drug Telazol contains:
   a. Diazepam and ketamine
   b. Diazepam and xylazine
   c. Zolazepam and tiletamine
   d. Xylazine and tiletamine
365. Which of the following drugs would most likely be the cause of atrioventricular block in a patient under anesthesia?
   a. Propofol
   b. Ketamine
   c. Dexmedetomidine
   d. Alfaxalone
366. All of the following cross the placental barrier in significant amounts *except*:
   a. Acepromazine
   b. Diazepam
   c. Isoflurane
   d. Neuromuscular blocking agents

367. Which of the following drugs is used to treat ventricular premature contractions (VPCs)?
a. Lidocaine
b. Doxapram
c. Dopamine
d. Phenylephrine

368. Which drug is *not* classified as a barbiturate?
a. Phenobarbital
b. Thiopental
c. Pentobarbital
d. Propofol

369. Common causes of ventricular premature contractions include all of the following *except*:
a. Hypoxia
b. Pain
c. Gastric dilation and volvulus
d. Anemia

370. Glycopyrrolate is an anticholinergic with all of the following advantages over atropine *except*:
a. It has a longer duration of action
b. It crosses the placental barrier
c. It is less likely to cause cardiac arrhythmias
d. It has a smaller dose volume

371. A patient breathing 100% oxygen should have a pulse oximetry reading of what percentage?
a. 95%–100%
b. 90%–100%
c. 93%–100%
d. 90%–95%

372. Which of the following drugs is most likely to affect a pulse oximetry reading?
a. Ketamine
b. Fentanyl
c. Hydromorphone
d. Dexmedetomidine

373. Which of the following is *not* a side effect of hypothermia under anesthesia?
a. Impaired platelet function
b. Death
c. Anemia
d. Coagulopathy

374. Which of the following reflexes should *always* be present in patients under anesthesia?
a. Palpebral reflex
b. Corneal reflex
c. Withdrawal reflex
d. Swallowing reflex

375. Normal capillary refill time in mammals is how long?
a. 1 second
b. 1–3 seconds
c. Less than 1–2 seconds
d. Greater than 2 seconds

376. At normal doses, what effect does atropine have on the heart rate?
a. Decreases
b. No effect
c. Increases
d. Depends on the species

377. Anesthetic drugs that cause vasoconstriction often cause the mucous membranes to become:
a. Pink
b. Red
c. Blue
d. Pale

378. Opioid drugs are used in anesthetic protocols primarily as:
a. Anesthetics
b. Analgesics
c. Anti-inflammatories
d. Antihistamines

379. The advantage of xylazine over acepromazine is that it:
a. Does not cause cardiac arrhythmias
b. Produces a short period of analgesia
c. Has antiemetic properties
d. Is an anti-inflammatory

380. Routine use of atropine in horses should be avoided because it may:
a. Cause colic
b. Slow the heart rate
c. Cause excitement
d. Increase salivation

381. Which drug should be avoided in the stallion because it may cause permanent prolapse of the penis?
a. Glycopyrrolate
b. Acepromazine
c. Xylazine
d. Diazepam

382. Anesthetic drugs that cause vasodilation often cause the mucous membranes to become:
a. Pink
b. Red
c. Blue
d. Pale

383. Which drug is a narcotic antagonist?
a. Naloxone
b. Atropine
c. Pancuronium
d. Droperidol

384. The width of the blood pressure cuff in a cat should be what percentage of the circumference of the leg?
a. 40%
b. 50%
c. 25%
d. 30%

385. The audible sound coming from the Doppler probe is produced by red blood cells circulating through the:
a. Vein
b. Artery
c. Capillaries
d. Mucous membranes

386. Depressant preanesthetic medication may have what effect on the anesthesia procedure?
a. Shorten the recovery time
b. Prolong the recovery time
c. Leave the recovery time unaltered
d. Necessitate increasing the dose of induction agent

387. The use of oscillometric blood pressure monitoring should be reserved for patients weighing more than how many kilos because of inaccuracies in smaller patients?
a. 2 kg
b. 3 kg
c. 4 kg
d. 5 kg

388. Which of the following provides a noninvasive method for assessing ventilation, cardiac output, pulmonary perfusion, and systemic metabolism?
a. Electrocardiograph
b. Capnograph
c. Central venous pressure
d. Arterial blood gas

389. Which drug is an antagonist of xylazine?
a. Butorphanol
b. Detomidine
c. Yohimbine
d. Pentazocine

390. Which of the following is considered mechanical dead space?
a. Excessively long endotracheal tube
b. Air in the nasal passages
c. Air in the trachea
d. Air in the mouth

391. Which of the following fluids is considered a colloid?
a. Lactated Ringer's solution
b. Plasma-Lyte
c. 0.9% saline
d. Hetastarch

392. Diazepam is used to produce:
a. Analgesia
b. Hypnosis
c. Muscle relaxation
d. Vomiting

393. Epinephrine:
a. Increases the heart rate
b. Decreases the heart rate
c. Decreases the blood pressure
d. Should be used to reverse the effects of acepromazine

394. The use of nitrous oxide in anesthesia:
a. Increases the amount of inhalation anesthetic required
b. Decreases the amount of inhalation anesthetic required
c. Slows the induction process
d. Has no effect on the time or amount of anesthetic required

395. Which of the following have a similar sodium and chloride concentration to that of the extracellular fluid as well as a similar osmolarity?
a. Hypertonic fluids
b. Hypotonic fluids
c. Isotonic fluids
d. None of the above

396. Which of the following fluids is considered an unbalanced solution?
a. Lactated Ringer's solution
b. Normosol-R
c. Plasma-Lyte 148
d. 0.9% saline

397. A disadvantage of breathing 50% nitrous oxide is that it:
a. Decreases the arterial oxygenation
b. Increases the arterial oxygenation
c. Slows the induction time
d. Prolongs the recovery time

398. Which of the following fluids is *not* a colloid?
a. Whole blood
b. Plasma-Lyte 148
c. Hetastarch
d. Hextend

399. Which of the following is considered a sensible loss?
a. Urine output
b. Fecal waste
c. Loss of fluid through the skin
d. Loss of fluid through the respiratory tract

400. How many milligrams per milliliter (mg/mL) does a 2% lidocaine solution contain?
a. 2
b. 0.2
c. 20
d. 200

401. You must anesthetize a patient that will require a whole blood transfusion. To avoid contamination, blood products should be given within how many hours after collection?
a. 2 hours
b. 4 hours
c. 8 hours
d. 12 hours

402. Apneustic breathing patterns are frequently seen in cats when high doses of ________ are used.
a. Pentobarbital
b. Thiamylal
c. Ketamine
d. Guaifenesin

403. If 180 mL of a 5% solution of guaifenesin is administered to a 150-kg foal, how many mg/kg would be administered?
a. 30
b. 60
c. 90
d. 15

404. Which of the following are tranquilizers that cause muscle relaxation and might also cause excitation in some young healthy animals?
a. Alpha-2 agonists
b. Opioids
c. Dissociates
d. Benzodiazepines

405. Which of the following premedication drugs would be contraindicated in patients that are tachycardic?
a. Morphine
b. Atropine
c. Methadone
d. Midazolam

406. Caudal epidural administration of lidocaine in the dog is:
a. Useful to prevent movement
b. Not to be used for cesarean section
c. An excellent caudal analgesic
d. An old procedure with little value in veterinary anesthesia today

407. Because diazepam is not water soluble, it should only be administered via which routes:
a. Intravenously and orally
b. Subcutaneously and intramuscularly
c. Intramuscularly and intravenously
d. Intramuscularly only

408. Which of the following opioids is *not* appropriate for a fracture repair in a dog or cat?
a. Methadone
b. Morphine
c. Hydromorphone
d. Butorphanol

409. Mask inductions are:
a. Best used in dogs and cats with airway obstruction
b. Best used in aggressive dogs and cats
c. Absolutely the best way to induce anesthesia in all dogs and cats
d. More appropriately used in calm dogs and cats

410. Which of the following drugs reverses the effects of a full μ-opioid?
a. Flumazenil
b. Atipamezole
c. Alfaxalone
d. Naloxone

411. Which of the following drugs is a partial agonist?
a. Butorphanol
b. Buprenorphine
c. Morphine
d. Naloxone

412. Which of the following is *not* an effect associated with atropine administration?
a. Tachycardia
b. Excessive salivation
c. Mydriasis
d. Decreased gastrointestinal motility

413. Which of the following drugs can cause the release of histamine when administered intravenously?
a. Buprenorphine
b. Hydromorphone
c. Butorphanol
d. Morphine

414. Which of the following induction drugs causes the palpebral reflex to be retained, increases the heart rate and blood pressure, causes the eyes to stay centrally located, and maintains a fair amount of jaw tone?
a. Propofol
b. Alfaxalone
c. Fentanyl
d. Ketamine

415. The dosage of acepromazine is 0.1 mg/kg and the maximum dose is 4 mg. How many milligrams would you administer to a 60-kg dog?
a. 2 mg
b. 4 mg
c. 6 mg
d. 8 mg

416. Which drug is a dissociative anesthetic?
a. Propofol
b. Ketamine
c. Alfaxalone
d. Etomidate

417. The adverse effects of anesthetic compounds are:
a. Nothing to worry about
b. Never present with smaller doses
c. Dose dependent
d. Not dose dependent

418. Heinz body formation, lethargy, vomiting, diarrhea, and anorexia can occur in cats given which of the following drugs repeatedly over a short period?
a. Propofol
b. Midazolam
c. Ketamine
d. Alfaxalone

419. Which of the following drugs should be avoided in cats with renal failure?
a. Propofol
b. Ketamine
c. Alfaxalone
d. Fentanyl

420. Which of the following factors do *not* influence MAC?
a. Age
b. Temperature
c. Sex
d. Stress

421. The definition for the rate at which a liquid will turn into a gas at a given temperature is:
a. Sublimation
b. Vapor pressure
c. Evaporation
d. Deposition

422. Which of the following statements is correct?
a. The higher the solubility of the anesthetic, the more rapid gas anesthetics will go from the alveoli into the blood.
b. The higher the solubility of the anesthetic, the slower the gas anesthetics will go from the alveoli into the blood.
c. The lower the solubility of the anesthetic, the less rapid gas anesthetics will go from the alveoli into the blood.
d. The lower the solubility of the anesthetic, the more rapid gas anesthetics will go from the alveoli into the blood.

423. Which of the following statements about inhalant anesthetics is incorrect?
a. Inhalant anesthetics affect the CNS.
b. The primary method of excretion of inhalant anesthesia is via hepatic metabolism.
c. Inhalants cause dose-dependent vasodilation.
d. Most inhalants decrease the rate and depth of respiration.

424. What is the MAC value of isoflurane in dogs?
a. 1.28
b. 1.65
c. 1.77
d. 1.17

425. What is the MAC value of isoflurane in cats?
a. 1.35
b. 1.63
c. 2.6
d. 2.1

426. What is the MAC value of sevoflurane in dogs?
a. 2.7
b. 1.82
c. 2.1
d. 1.61

427. What is the MAC value of sevoflurane in cats?
a. 2.6
b. 1.81
c. 2.25
d. 1.69

428. Which of the following affects the solubility coefficient of an inhalant anesthetic?
a. Patient weight
b. Age
c. Body temperature
d. Anesthetic drug protocol

429. Which of the following inhalants is twice as soluble as sevoflurane?
a. Isoflurane
b. Halothane
c. Desflurane
d. Nitrous oxide

430. Which of the following inhalant anesthetics does not need to be vaporized for administration?
a. Halothane
b. Isoflurane
c. Sevoflurane
d. Nitrous oxide

431. Which of the following drugs causes a dose-dependent vasodilation?
a. Fentanyl
b. Thiopental
c. Isoflurane
d. Midazolam

432. Which of the following contributes to a prolonged recovery?
a. Hypothermia
b. Reproductive status
c. Sex of patient
d. Hyperthermia

433. Ideally, vital signs should be monitored in all patients recovering from anesthesia how often?
a. Every 45 minutes
b. Every hour
c. Every 15 minutes
d. Every 1–2 hours

434. Respiratory acidosis is most often caused by:
a. Hyperventilation
b. Hypoventilation
c. Hypercarbia
d. Eupnea

435. A complete blockage of the endotracheal tube will cause which of the following?
a. Eupnea
b. Hypercarbia
c. Aspiration
d. Respiratory acidosis

436. Which of the following drugs can cause excitation in healthy patients when used as a premedication or induction agent?
a. Midazolam
b. Fentanyl
c. Morphine
d. Alfaxalone

437. Which of the following is a potential side effect of administering propofol too quickly?
a. Tachycardia
b. Apnea
c. Hypertension
d. Hypothermia

438. When is airway obstruction most likely to occur in a surgical patient?
a. During the surgical procedure
b. During the preanesthetic and recovery period
c. During surgery and postoperatively
d. During recovery as the patient is awakening

439. Using which of the following drugs can prevent laryngospasm?
a. Isoflurane
b. Methadone
c. Lidocaine
d. Diazepam

440. Which term best describes the following definition: “Reduced minute volume due to a reduction in tidal volume and/or respiratory rate”?
a. Hypoventilation
b. Dyspnea
c. Tachypnea
d. Hyperventilation

441. All of the following contribute to hypoventilation *except*:
a. Hyperthermia
b. Pulmonary disease
c. Accidental endobronchial intubation
d. Restrictive chest bandage

442. All of the following contribute to hyperventilation *except*:
a. Inadequate anesthetic depth
b. Pain
c. Hypoxia
d. Hypothermia

443. You have anesthetized a 9-year-old male, castrated mixed-breed dog for a right hind limb amputation. What would be the lowest acceptable mean arterial blood pressure for this patient?
a. 40 mmHg
b. 60 mmHg
c. 80 mmHg
d. 100 mmHg

444. Which of the following terms best describes the following definition: “Sudden cessation of functional ventilation and systemic perfusion”?
a. Bradycardia
b. Cardiopulmonary arrest
c. Ventricular tachycardia
d. Hypercapnia

445. How long does it take after cardiopulmonary arrest before irreversible neurological damage can occur?
   a. 5 minutes
   b. 10 minutes
   c. 7 minutes
   d. 3 minutes
446. During CPR what is the preferred order of routes for drug administration?
   a. Central venous, intraosseous, peripheral venous, intratracheal
   b. Peripheral venous, central venous, intraosseous, intratracheal
   c. Peripheral venous, central venous, intratracheal, intraosseous
   d. Central venous, peripheral venous, intraosseous, intratracheal
447. Which of the following is a direct response of epinephrine administration?
   a. Vasoconstriction
   b. Vasodilation
   c. Hypoventilation
   d. Hyperventilation
448. Which of the following drugs is used to treat ventricular tachycardia?
   a. Thiopental
   b. Lidocaine
   c. Alfaxalone
   d. Dopamine
449. Which of the following drugs is most commonly used to treat bradycardia?
   a. Lidocaine
   b. Dobutamine
   c. Alfaxalone
   d. Atropine
450. Which of the following devices is essential to monitor heart rate and rhythm?
   a. Capnograph
   b. Doppler
   c. Electrocardiogram
   d. Pulse oximeter
451. Why is placing alcohol onto ECG leads contraindicated in patients requiring CPR?
   a. Alcohol can cause skin irritation.
   b. Alcohol can cool the patient.
   c. Alcohol can cause a fire if defibrillation is performed.
   d. Alcohol is actually not contraindicated in these patients.
452. Which of the following best describes the term *multimodal anesthesia*?
   a. The use of one single drug to achieve analgesia.
   b. The use of multiple drugs to help reduce the doses of each agent, thus decreasing negative side effects.
   c. An anesthetic protocol that does not use a premedication in an attempt to decrease the negative side effects of anesthetic drugs.
   d. The use of opioids only to decrease anesthetic requirements.
453. Which of the following is the best technique for providing effective preoxygenation in a dog or cat before anesthetic induction?
   a. Using flow-by oxygen via the breathing circuit
   b. Using a mask without the diaphragm
   c. Using a mask with a fitted diaphragm
   d. Oxygen is not necessary before anesthetic induction
454. Which of the following best describes the inability to move blood forward effectively enough to meet metabolic needs?
   a. Liver failure
   b. Heart failure
   c. Renal failure
   d. Pulmonary failure
455. The normal peak inspiratory pressure delivered during mechanical ventilation should range between:
   a. 10–15 cm H_2O
   b. 10–20 cm H_2O
   c. 20–25 cm H_2O
   d. 15–20 cm H_2O
456. The normal respiratory rate in anesthetized dogs and cats is between:
   a. 4–6 breaths/min
   b. 8–12 breaths/min
   c. 6–10 breaths/min
   d. 10–15 breaths/min
457. An intact thoracic cavity is under ______________.
   a. Negative pressure
   b. Positive pressure
   c. Both negative and positive pressure
   d. Neutral pressure
458. What percentage decrease in renal function must be present before seeing any abnormalities on a blood chemistry panel?
   a. 40%–50%
   b. 25%–40%
   c. 60%–65%
   d. 70%–75%
459. Which of the following drugs is contraindicated in cats presenting with renal failure?
   a. Ketamine
   b. Propofol
   c. Hydromorphone
   d. Isoflurane
460. Which of the following organs plays a crucial role in the metabolism and clearance of most anesthetic drugs?
   a. Lungs
   b. Kidneys
   c. Pancreas
   d. Liver
461. Which of the following can result in decreased drug binding, prolonged recoveries, and relative overdose from highly protein-bound drugs?
   a. Low total protein and low albumin
   b. Low total protein and low blood urea nitrogen
   c. Low total protein and high creatinine
   d. Low total protein and high packed cell volume

462. Of the following drug protocols, which is most commonly used in ruminant patients undergoing minor surgical procedures?
a. Premedicate with butorphanol and mask down with isoflurane
b. Premedicate with atropine and morphine and induce with alfaxalone
c. Premedicate with acepromazine and induce with propofol
d. Premedicate with butorphanol and use a standing position with local blocks

463. To decrease regurgitation in ruminants undergoing anesthesia, food should be withheld for how many hours before induction?
a. 12 hours
b. 6 hours
c. 48 hours
d. 24 hours

464. Why is the neck of ruminants elevated with the head placed in a downward position during general anesthesia?
a. This position helps decrease intracranial pressure.
b. This position helps keep the endotracheal tube in place.
c. This position helps facilitate drainage of saliva and regurgitation.
d. This position is not necessary in ruminants.

465. Which of the following nerve blocks is used for dehorning ruminants?
a. Auriculopalpebral nerve block
b. Cornual nerve block
c. Peroneal nerve block
d. Digital nerve block

466. Which of the following local blocks would provide additional anesthesia/analgesia to a sheep undergoing a large abdominal surgery?
a. Epidural block
b. Caudal block
c. Peroneal block
d. Cornual block

467. Improper administration or an overdose of a local anesthetic into the epidural space can lead to all of the following *except*:
a. Seizures
b. Hypertension
c. Paralysis of the respiratory system
d. Unconsciousness

468. Which of the following is safe to use in animals that will be slaughtered?
a. Xylazine
b. Ketamine
c. Romifidine
d. None of the above

469. Which of the following drugs is *not* generally suggested for use in sheep?
a. Ketamine
b. Butorphanol
c. Propofol
d. Atropine

470. Which of the following vessels is most commonly used for intravenous catheter placement in cattle undergoing anesthesia?
a. Jugular
b. Cephalic
c. Lateral saphenous
d. Auricular

471. You have been asked to anesthetize a horse for a laceration repair. You just administered xylazine to the patient and realized it has been overdosed by 10 times. Which of the following drugs is used to reverse the effects of xylazine?
a. Flumazenil
b. Naloxone
c. Dexmedetomidine
d. Yohimbine

472. The MAC of isoflurane in equine patients is:
a. 1.7%–2.1%
b. 1.31%–1.64%
c. 2.11%–2.34%
d. 1.12%–1.54%

473. In horses, which of the following is considered unreliable when assessing anesthetic depth?
a. Respiratory rate
b. Swallow reflex
c. Heart rate
d. Lateral nystagmus

474. Which of the following is the ideal way to assess ventilation in horses?
a. Assessing mucous membrane color
b. Blood gas analysis
c. $ETCO_2$
d. Pulse oximetry

475. The average oxygen flow rate used for inhalant anesthetic induction in horses is:
a. 5–10 mL/kg/min
b. 10–15 mL/kg/min
c. 15–20 mL/kg/min
d. 20–25 mL/kg/min

476. The average oxygen flow rate used for maintenance anesthesia in the horse is:
a. 2–4 mL/kg/min
b. 5–10 mL/kg/min
c. 4–8 mL/kg/min
d. 1–2 mL/kg/min

477. Which of the following is a potential problem with maintaining a patient on room air during an anesthetic procedure?
a. Hypertension
b. Hyperthermia
c. Apnea
d. Hypoxemia

478. NSAIDs should *not* be administered in conjunction with corticosteroids because of:
a. Increased risk of liver failure
b. Increased risk of renal failure
c. Effects of the two drugs cancel each other
d. Increased risk of GI ulceration

479. Which of the following drugs used for postoperative analgesia is not a true opioid?
a. Hydromorphone
b. Meperidine
c. Tramadol
d. Deracoxib

480. Which of the following opioids is an NMDA antagonist?
a. Morphine
b. Methadone
c. Butorphanol
d. Fentanyl

481. Which of the following is an example of chronic pain?
a. Osteoarthritis
b. Fractured leg after being hit by a car 12 hours earlier
c. Fresh laceration
d. Bite wound from a dogfight earlier the same day

482. Which of the following is *not* an example of maladaptive pain?
a. Cancer
b. Fresh laceration
c. Osteoarthritis
d. Profound gingivitis

483. Which of the following types of pain dissipates as the initial source of pain resolves?
a. Chronic pain
b. Acute pain
c. Maladaptive pain
d. Wind-up pain

484. Which of the following types of pain is most associated with trauma or surgery?
a. Adaptive pain
b. Maladaptive pain
c. Chronic pain
d. Neuropathic pain

485. Which of the following drugs drastically reduces cardiac output?
a. Morphine
b. Meloxicam
c. Dexmedetomidine
d. Ketamine

486. You have been asked to anesthetize a 1-year-old Labrador for removal of a foreign body in the GI tract. This is a painful procedure, and you want to provide an opioid that will not induce vomiting. Which of the following would be the best choice for this?
a. Morphine
b. Fentanyl
c. Hydromorphone
d. Methadone

487. Which of the following drugs acts by preventing painful signals from reaching the spinal cord?
a. Morphine
b. Alfaxalone
c. Propofol
d. Bupivacaine

488. To avoid the risk of GI ulceration, NSAIDs should be stopped for how many days before starting a different NSAID?
a. 30 days
b. 15–30 days
c. 1–3 days
d. 4–10 days

489. Which of the following is considered an adjunct for pain management?
a. Weight loss
b. Laser therapy
c. Physical rehabilitation
d. All of the above

490. Which of the following is not a normal sign of pain in the dog?
a. Dilated pupils
b. Increased grooming
c. Lack of appetite
d. Licking wound or surgery site

491. Which of the following terms best describes: "An unpleasant sensory and emotional experience individuals have when they perceive actual or potential tissue damage to their body"?
a. Dysphoria
b. Pain
c. Anxiety
d. Aggression

492. Which of the following is best characterized by visceral pain?
a. Dull, diffuse pain in the kidneys
b. Chronic, deep, burning sensation in the bone
c. Superficial pain originating in the dermis
d. A throbbing pain originating in the mucous membranes

493. Which of the following types of pain is considered a protective pain?
a. Chronic pain
b. Acute pain
c. Neuropathic pain
d. Wind-up pain

494. Which of the following is best described as somatic pain?
a. Dull, diffuse pain in the liver
b. Achy pain in the bladder
c. Spasm-like pain in the intestines
d. Superficial pain originating in the skin

495. It is believed that the viscera may contain more kappa receptors than mu receptors. If this is correct, which of the following drugs would provide better analgesia for visceral pain?
a. Morphine
b. Fentanyl
c. Hydromorphone
d. Butorphanol

496. You have been asked to anesthetize a ferret for a small mass removal on the flank. How long should this patient be fasted before induction?
a. No fasting time is required
b. 1–2 hours
c. 2–4 hours
d. 4–6 hours

497. Premedication in ferrets is most often administered into which of the following sites?
a. Caudal thigh
b. Forelimbs
c. Caudal lumbar
d. Cephalic vein

498. Which of the following drugs is used to help prevent laryngospasm in ferrets before endotracheal intubation?
a. Ketamine
b. Lidocaine
c. Alfaxalone
d. Propofol

499. What is the most common site for an IO catheter in a rat?
a. Femur
b. Tibia
c. Fibula
d. Radius

500. You have anesthetized a patient that presented with a gastric dilatation-volvulus (GDV). After induction, you notice tachycardia, hypotension, prolonged capillary refill time, and pale mucous membranes. What is the likely cause of this?
a. Hyperthermia
b. Hypovolemic shock
c. Light plane of anesthesia
d. Hypocapnia

501. Which of the following crystalloid fluids would be the best choice for a patient with hyperkalemia currently undergoing a surgical procedure?
a. Lactated Ringer's solution
b. Normosol-R
c. 0.9% sodium chloride
d. D5W

502. An anesthetic patient has metabolic acidosis and a blood pH of 7.122. Which of the following drugs can be administered to help increase pH?
a. Dopamine
b. Sodium bicarbonate
c. Etomidate
d. Doxapram

503. You are preparing for a German shepherd patient presenting with a suspected GDV. It will probably require emergency surgery soon after arrival. In preparing for the procedure, where are you going to place the IV catheter?
a. Large-bore catheter in the jugular vein
b. Large-bore catheter in the lateral saphenous vein
c. Large-bore catheter in the auricular vein
d. Large-bore catheter in the medial saphenous vein

504. Which of the following preanesthetic drugs should be avoided in GDV patients?
a. Hydromorphone
b. Methadone
c. Fentanyl
d. Morphine

505. Which of the following is *not* an anticipated problem of a patient undergoing anesthesia for the repair of a GDV?
a. Arrhythmia
b. Electrolyte imbalance
c. Pain
d. Severe blood loss

506. Which of the following would be considered a complication of recovery for a patient that had a foreign body removed from the trachea?
a. Severe pain
b. Airway obstruction resulting from swelling
c. Aspiration
d. Hypovolemic shock

507. Which of the following is a potential complication for a patient anesthetized for a myelogram?
a. Hyperthermia
b. Seizures
c. Pain
d. Bleeding

508. A cat with a urethral obstruction presents to the hospital as an emergency. This patient needs to be anesthetized for a urethrotomy. Before induction you decide to place an ECG on the patient. You immediately notice wide QRS complexes with a lack of P waves. What does this indicate?
a. Hypernatremia
b. Hyperchloremia
c. Hypophosphatemia
d. Hyperkalemia

509. A 10-year-old mixed-breed intact male dog presents to the clinic after being rescued from a house fire. He is tachycardiac, dyspneic, and has a large wound on his left hind limb. This patient is compromised. Which of the following would be the best premedication protocol?
a. Midazolam and butorphanol
b. Hydromorphone and dexmedetomidine
c. Midazolam and methadone
d. Buprenorphine only

510. A 10-year-old mixed-breed intact male dog presents to the clinic after being rescued from a house fire. He is tachycardiac, dyspneic, and has a large wound on his left hind limb. This patient is compromised. Which of the following would be the best anesthetic induction protocol?
a. Etomidate and midazolam
b. Propofol
c. Mask induction
d. Any of the above would be acceptable for this patient

511. Which of the following drugs best fits this description: "Class IV controlled substance that acts as an anxiolytic, muscle relaxant, hypnotic, and anticonvulsant"?
a. Propofol
b. Midazolam
c. Fentanyl
d. Thiopental

512. How many hours after thoracic trauma does it take to show the full extent of pulmonary lesions via radiographs?
a. 12–16 hours
b. 12–24 hours
c. 20–25 hours
d. 24–36 hours

513. Which of the following statements about anesthesia for a cesarean section is true?
   a. Mask induction is the safest means of anesthetic induction.
   b. GI transit time and lower esophageal sphincter tone are decreased, leading to increased risk of regurgitation and aspiration.
   c. PCV and plasma protein levels are often increased in these patients.
   d. Urine specific gravity is decreased in these patients.

514. Because of the increase in cerebral oxygen demand, which of the following drugs is no longer recommended to stimulate respiration in newborns after cesarean section?
   a. Dobutamine
   b. Dopamine
   c. Doxapram
   d. Naloxone

515. Which of the following techniques can be considered for use in a cesarean section to help reduce the need for larger doses of other more detrimental drugs?
   a. Epidural
   b. Constant rate infusion of morphine
   c. Bier block
   d. Constant rate infusion of ketamine

516. Why are uncuffed endotracheal tubes suggested for use in birds undergoing anesthesia?
   a. The trachea in birds is too small for a cuffed endotracheal tube.
   b. The trachea is made up of a mixture of complete and incomplete tracheal rings.
   c. The trachea is made up of complete tracheal rings that lack elasticity.
   d. The trachea is made up of incomplete tracheal rings only.

517. Which of the following structures makes it possible for birds to vocalize even after they have been properly intubated?
   a. Choana
   b. Syrinx
   c. Larynx
   d. Operculum

518. Which of the following bones are pneumatic in birds and should therefore *not* be used for intraosseous catheter placement?
   a. Ulna and radius
   b. Femur and radius
   c. Humerus and tibiotarsus
   d. Femur and humerus

519. Guinea pigs are difficult to intubate because of which of the following anatomic structures?
   a. Enlarged nasopharynx
   b. Hyperplastic oropharynx
   c. Palatal ostium
   d. Nasopharyngeal diverticula

520. Nasotracheal intubation is possible in which of the following species?
   a. Chinchilla
   b. Ferret
   c. Rabbit
   d. Guinea pig

521. A sidestream capnograph samples approximately how much gas from the attachment site?
   a. 200–300 mL/min
   b. 100–400 mL/min
   c. 50–150 mL/min
   d. Sidestream capnography does not sample gas.

522. Intramuscular injections are most commonly administered into which of the following muscles in avian patients?
   a. Quadriceps muscle
   b. Biceps muscle
   c. Pectoral muscle
   d. Gastrocnemius muscle

523. Which of the following is the most commonly used drug for maintenance anesthesia in the fish and amphibian patient?
   a. MS-222
   b. Propofol
   c. Isoflurane
   d. Ketamine

524. A blood sample is needed to run a PCV and total solids before anesthetic induction in a small frog. What site is most commonly used for blood collection in amphibians?
   a. Cephalic vein
   b. Ventral abdominal vein
   c. Lingual venous plexus
   d. Lateral saphenous

525. Which of the following drugs might decrease the heart rate of a neonatal patient?
   a. Midazolam
   b. Glycopyrrolate
   c. Morphine
   d. Lidocaine

526. Reptiles have a three-chambered heart consisting of the following:
   a. One atrium and two ventricles
   b. One atrium, one ventricle, and a cavum venosum
   c. Two atria and one ventricle
   d. Reptiles actually have a four-chambered heart similar to birds.

527. Which of the following can profoundly affect cardiac output and blood pressure in neonates?
   a. Tachycardia
   b. Bradycardia
   c. Apnea
   d. Hyperthermia

528. Because pediatric patients have less functional contractile tissue, limited cardiac reserve, low ventricular compliance, and a reduced ability to increase stroke volume, they are highly dependent on heart rate to maintain which of the following?
   a. Cardiac output and blood pressure
   b. Body temperature and systemic vascular resistance
   c. Myocardial oxygen consumption and pulmonary reserve
   d. Glycogen storage and hepatic blood flow

529. Which of the following statements is correct regarding sedation and anesthesia in the pediatric patient?
   a. Because of an increased metabolic rate, drug doses need to be higher compared with that in adults.
   b. Pediatric patients are prone to hyperglycemia; therefore they should be monitored throughout the anesthetic period.
   c. Drug doses often need to be reduced because of slow metabolism, biotransformation, and excretion of drugs.
   d. Oxygen consumption is 10 times that in an adult because of a high metabolic rate.
530. The pliable rib cage of pediatric patients can lead to which of the following for efficient ventilation?
   a. More
   b. Less
   c. The pliable rib cage does not affect ventilation under anesthesia.
   d. The rib cage is actually less pliable compared with adult dogs.
531. You have been asked to induce and monitor anesthesia in an unweaned kitten presenting for wound care after being stepped on by a child. How long should you fast this patient before anesthetic induction?
   a. 1–2 hours
   b. 2–4 hours
   c. 4–6 hours
   d. Fasting is not recommended in these patients.
532. You have been asked to induce and monitor anesthesia in a 7-week-old puppy for a GI foreign-body removal from the stomach. How long should this patient be fasted before anesthetic induction?
   a. 1–3 hours
   b. 3–6 hours
   c. 6–9 hours
   d. Fasting is not recommended in these patients.
533. Water should be withheld from neonatal and pediatric patients for how long before anesthetic induction?
   a. Water is never withheld from these patients.
   b. 1–2 hours
   c. 2–4 hours
   d. 4–6 hours
534. Minimum laboratory tests that should be evaluated before induction of a pediatric patient includes which of the following?
   a. BUN, creatinine, PCV, TP
   b. PCV, TP, BUN, blood glucose
   c. PCV, TP, blood glucose
   d. BUN, PCV, TP, WBC count
535. Which of the following drugs is generally avoided in pediatric patients because of negative side effects such as severe bradycardia, respiratory depression, and extensive hepatic metabolism?
   a. Midazolam
   b. Morphine
   c. Glycopyrrolate
   d. Dexmedetomidine
536. Shivering during anesthetic recovery leads to which of the following?
   a. Increase in metabolic oxygen demand
   b. Decrease in metabolic oxygen demand
   c. Increase in glyconeogenesis
   d. Decrease in glyconeogenesis
537. Peak airway pressure in pediatric patients should be:
   a. 10–20 cm H_2O
   b. 5–10 cm H_2O
   c. 15–20 cm H_2O
   d. 5–15 cm H_2O
538. Which of the following methods is the most accurate way to assess blood pressure in pediatric patients?
   a. Oscillometric
   b. Doppler
   c. Palpation of pulse
   d. Direct
539. Fasting time in geriatric patients should be limited to how many hours before anesthetic induction?
   a. 8 hours
   b. 12 hours
   c. 24 hours
   d. 1–2 hours
540. Which of the following anesthetic drugs is not reversible?
   a. Acepromazine
   b. Diazepam
   c. Methadone
   d. Dexmedetomidine
541. You have been asked to induce and maintain a geriatric poodle with Addison's disease. Which of the following anesthetic drugs should be avoided?
   a. Fentanyl
   b. Midazolam
   c. Etomidate
   d. Alfaxalone
542. Which of the following is defined as the delivery of specific drugs for analgesia, sedation, amnesia, and muscle relaxation?
   a. Regional anesthesia
   b. Epidural anesthesia
   c. Balanced anesthesia
   d. Premedication
543. To help prevent artificially low or high blood pressure readings, the blood pressure cuff width should be approximately what percentage of the circumference of the limb where it will be placed?
   a. 25%
   b. 30%
   c. 40%
   d. 50%
544. Basic anesthetic patient parameters should be monitored and recorded in a permanent record every ______________ minutes.
   a. 5
   b. 10
   c. 15
   d. 20
545. All of the following are signs of hypotension *except*:
   a. Vasoconstriction
   b. Poor pulses
   c. Increasing heart rate
   d. Increasing $ETCO_2$

546. Hypotension is most often caused by which of the following?
 a. Hypovolemia and anesthetic drugs
 b. Hyperthermia and toxemia
 c. Cardiac arrhythmias and opioid administration
 d. Hypercarbia and increased central venous pressure

547. All of the following are potential signs of pain *except*:
 a. Vocalization
 b. Decreased heart rate
 c. Inappetence
 d. Increased temperature

548. Which of the following opioids can be used effectively in feline patients when administered via the transmucosal route?
 a. Butorphanol
 b. Morphine
 c. Methadone
 d. Buprenorphine

549. You have been asked to anesthetize a 5-year-old mixed breed, female spayed dog for a severe degloving injury of the left forelimb. Which of the following drugs might be beneficial in dealing with the acute neuropathic pain this patient may be experiencing?
 a. Ketamine
 b. Propofol
 c. Alfaxalone
 d. Hydromorphone

550. Which of the following drugs should be used with caution in cats because of its potential severe cardiotoxic effects?
 a. Ketamine
 b. Dexmedetomidine
 c. Lidocaine
 d. Morphine

551. A canine patient is recovering from a surgical procedure. On extubation, it is howling, paddling, and swaying from side to side. After a quick assessment, it is determined that it is dysphoric and not in pain. What can be done to help a patient that is experiencing opioid-induced dysphoria?
 a. Administer an additional dose of opioids to help calm the patient
 b. Hold the patient tightly until it calms down
 c. Induce anesthesia and try waking it up again
 d. Slowly titrate a dose of naloxone

552. During anesthesia, why is administering a constant rate infusion advantageous over providing intermittent boluses of a drug(s)?
 a. You can administer higher doses when using a CRI
 b. You can use multiple different drugs in a CRI
 c. A CRI allows continuous low doses of various analgesics
 d. It is not advantageous. Intermittent boluses are safer and more effective

553. A patient undergoing which of the following procedures would probably benefit from an epidural?
 a. Femoral head osteotomy
 b. Humeral fracture repair
 c. Total ear canal ablation
 d. Glossectomy

554. Which of the following blocks a particular opioid receptor?
 a. An agonist
 b. An antagonist
 c. COX-2 inhibition
 d. COX-1 inhibition

555. All of the following are primary goals of anesthesia *except*:
 a. Provide immobilization
 b. Ensure amnesia
 c. Eliminate pain
 d. Having a standard anesthetic protocol

556. Which of the following drugs causes Heinz body formation with repeated dosing in cats?
 a. Ketamine
 b. Propofol
 c. Alfaxalone
 d. Etomidate

557. Which of the following is the best indicator of anesthetic depth?
 a. Palpebral reflex
 b. Toe pinch
 c. Jaw tone
 d. Blood pressure

558. Which of the following is not an advantage of low-flow anesthesia?
 a. Less moisture is lost from the airways
 b. Less heat is lost because of low oxygen flow rates
 c. Low-flow is more economical
 d. Low-flow anesthesia can be used on any anesthetic circuit

559. Overventilation of a patient can lead to all of the following *except*:
 a. Decreased preload
 b. Decreased blood pressure
 c. Decreased cardiac output
 d. Decreased core body temperature

560. Which of the following statements is true regarding carbon dioxide absorbents?
 a. Storage of absorbent should consist of a sealable pail, canister, carton, or bag.
 b. High temperatures greatly affect absorbent, even when properly sealed.
 c. Freezing temperatures aid in the longevity of the absorbent.
 d. Absorbents are respiratory irritants but are not caustic to the skin.

561. Why are unidirectional valves an important part of an anesthesia machine?
 a. They are directly involved with scavenging waste gases.
 b. They play a large role in helping warm the anesthetic gases before they are delivered to patients.
 c. They ensure that gases flow toward the patient in one breathing tube and away from the patient in the other breathing tube.
 d. They act as a safety mechanism, ensuring the patient does not receive a tidal volume larger than 20 cm H_2O.

562. A respirometer is used for which of the following purposes?
a. To measure respiratory rate
b. To measure ventilatory volume
c. To measure $ETCO_2$
d. To measure the amount of moisture in the breathing circuit

563. Which of the following is false regarding a Mapleson breathing system?
a. Unidirectional valves are present.
b. Fresh gas flow must remain high to flush out carbon dioxide.
c. There is no device for absorbing carbon dioxide.
d. Mapleson systems are less economical compared with circle systems.

564. Why is the pin index safety system (PISS) an important feature for anesthetic cylinders?
a. The PISS ensures that the cylinders are properly identified by specific colors (i.e., green/oxygen, yellow/medical air, etc.).
b. The PISS ensures that waste gas is properly collected and removed from the surgical area.
c. The PISS aids in the delivery of oxygen from the house gas supply.
d. The PISS ensures that the correct cylinder is mounted into the correct yoke for delivery of the proper anesthetic gas.

565. What is the purpose for the vaporizer interlock device?
a. It prevents the vaporizer from becoming detached from the anesthesia machine during transport.
b. It reduces the amount of waste gases from entering the environment.
c. It prevents two vaporizers on the same machine from being turned on at the same time.
d. This device sounds an alarm when the vaporizer becomes dangerously low on inhalant gases.

566. You are examining the capnography waveform of the patient under anesthesia. You notice that the baseline is elevated (not going back to zero), but the waveform otherwise looks normal. Why might this be happening?
a. The patient is hyperventilating.
b. The patient is hypoventilating.
c. The patient has been intubated into the esophagus.
d. The patient is rebreathing carbon dioxide.

567. Monitoring carbon dioxide allows analysis of all of the following *except*:
a. Ventilation
b. Circulation
c. Equipment malfunction
d. Core body temperature

568. What is the purpose of the common gas outlet?
a. The common gas outlet is the area where the APL valve connects to the machine.
b. The common gas outlet connects anesthetic machine to the breathing systems, ventilator or oxygen supply device.
c. The common gas outlet connects the fresh gas to the scavenge system.
d. The common gas outlet connects the oxygen flowmeter to the vaporizer.

569. Which of the following receives oxygen directly from the cylinder, or pipeline, and bypasses the vaporizer?
a. Oxygen flush
b. Oxygen flowmeter
c. Rebreathing circuit
d. Non-rebreathing circuit

570. Which of the following is the volume of the breathing system occupied by gases that are rebreathed without any change in composition?
a. Tidal volume
b. Apparatus dead space
c. Peak inspiratory pressure
d. Minute volume

571. You have been asked to help prepare an anesthetic protocol for a glaucoma patient that needs multiple dental extractions. The patient is otherwise systemically healthy. Which of the following induction agents should be avoided in this patient?
a. Ketamine
b. Propofol
c. Diazepam
d. Alfaxalone

572. All of the following drugs have the potential to raise both intraocular and intracranial pressure *except*:
a. Morphine
b. Dexmedetomidine
c. Hydromorphone
d. Methadone

573. You are monitoring anesthesia on a patient undergoing an enucleation. The patient suddenly becomes severely bradycardiac during manipulation of the globe. What is probably occurring?
a. The patient is in a light anesthetic plane and can feel the surgical stimulation.
b. The patient has an underlying heart condition that went unrecognized until now.
c. This is probably a result of the oculocardiac reflex.
d. The patient is in an anesthetic plane that is too deep and it should be reduced.

574. Which of the following is a common side effect of opioid administration in cats?
a. Miosis
b. Mydriasis
c. Meiosis
d. Mitosis

575. A dog you are monitoring under anesthesia has lost a significant amount of blood during the surgical procedure. You must estimate current blood loss by assessing the sponges and suction canister volume. Before estimating volume deficit, you must first know what is normal for a dog. What is the normal blood volume in dogs?
a. 50–60 mL/kg
b. 10–20 mL/kg
c. 80–90 mL/kg
d. 30–50 mL/kg

576. Which solution has the same proportion of particles and water as that found in plasma?
a. A hypertonic solution
b. An isotonic solution
c. A hypotonic solution
d. A buffered solution

577. You must extract multiple molars and premolars on the lower left and right dental arcade. Which of the following local blocks can be used to provide pain relief both during and after the procedure?
   a. Infraorbital block
   b. Inferior alveolar block
   c. RUMM block
   d. Auriculotemporal block
578. Which of the following block the generation and conduction of nerve impulses by inhibiting voltage-gated sodium channels within neuronal membranes?
   a. Local anesthetics
   b. Full mu opioids
   c. Alpha-2 agonists
   d. Kappa agonists
579. Which of the following local blocks could be used to help manage pain in patients undergoing a lateral thoracotomy or in those that have rib fractures?
   a. RUMM block
   b. Paravertebral block
   c. Intercostal block
   d. Epidural block
580. Common side effects of acepromazine include all of the following *except*:
   a. Decreasing body temperature
   b. Antiemetic properties
   c. Antiarrhythmic
   d. Respiratory depressant
581. Which of the following drugs when administered alone produces minimal sedation in healthy dogs and cats?
   a. Acepromazine
   b. Midazolam
   c. Dexmedetomidine
   d. Morphine
582. A cat you are monitoring under anesthesia has lost a significant amount of blood during the surgical procedure. You must estimate current blood loss by assessing the sponges and suction canister volume. Before estimating volume deficit, you must first know what is normal for a cat. What is the normal blood volume in cats?
   a. 60–70 mL/kg
   b. 10–20 mL/kg
   c. 80–90 mL/kg
   d. 30–50 mL/kg
583. You must anesthetize a patient that was hit by a car and has suspected head trauma. This patient may have increased intracranial pressure as a result of the trauma. All of the following are techniques that can help reduce intracranial pressure *except*:
   a. Keeping head at a 30-degree angle
   b. Administering mannitol to decrease blood viscosity and increase blood volume
   c. Ventilate patient to provide normocapnia
   d. Only draw blood from the jugular vein
584. During CPR, adequate cardiac massage is present when:
   a. The electrocardiogram (ECG) is normal
   b. The heart rate is 60 beats/min
   c. A peripheral pulse can be palpated
   d. The end-tidal CO_2 is normal
585. No more than what percentage of nitrous oxide should be delivered to an anesthetized patient?
   a. 45%
   b. 30%
   c. 65%
   d. 75%
586. Which of the following is a concern when a patient is recovering from anesthesia when nitrous oxide has been used?
   a. Solubility
   b. Diffusion hypoxia
   c. Biotransformation
   d. Inflammation
587. Local anesthetics:
   a. Cause increased release of inhibitory neurotransmitters
   b. Block transmission of the impulse along the nerve fiber
   c. Work by acting on GABA receptors
   d. Block catecholamine release
588. In nonbrachycephalic breeds of dogs recovering from anesthesia, the endotracheal tube should be removed when:
   a. Palpebral reflex returns.
   b. Swallowing reflex returns.
   c. The eyes resume a central position.
   d. Animal shows voluntary movement of the limbs.
589. What agent should be avoided in geriatric patients with compromised liver function?
   a. Atropine
   b. Dexmedetomidine
   c. Isoflurane
   d. Midazolam
590. A capillary refill time that is over 3 seconds is indicative of:
   a. Renal failure
   b. Poor tissue perfusion
   c. Increased ventilation
   d. Hypertension
591. Normal urinary output in canine and feline patients is 1–2 mL/kg/h. Why is normal urinary output important in patients under general anesthesia?
   a. Normal urinary output is directly related to liver function.
   b. Normal urinary output is directly related to pulmonary function.
   c. Normal urinary output reflects cardiovascular status and normal renal perfusion.
   d. Normal urinary output reflects appropriate central venous pressure and ventilation status.
592. Cardiac output in the pediatric patient is primarily dependent on which of the following?
   a. Respiratory rate
   b. Heart rate
   c. Pulse quality
   d. Fluid rate

593. Which of the following is *not* a cause of barotrauma in patients undergoing anesthesia?
   a. Closed pop-off valve
   b. Excessive peak inspiratory pressure with positive pressure ventilation
   c. Repetitive collapse and re-expansion of normal or diseased lung during positive pressure ventilation
   d. Providing a ventilatory rate in excess of 25 breaths/min

594. Which of the following is the intrinsic pacemaker of the heart?
   a. Sinoatrial node
   b. Atrioventricular node
   c. Purkinje fibers
   d. Bundle of His

595. Spirometers are used to measure which of the following?
   a. Central venous pressure and respiratory rate
   b. Minute volume and tidal volume
   c. Respiratory rate and effort
   d. Pulmonary ventilation and mechanical dead space

596. The normal pH range of blood is 7.35–7.45. If a patient has a blood pH of 7.25, this patient is considered to have:
   a. Acidosis
   b. Alkalosis
   c. Ketoacidosis
   d. Ketoalkalosis

597. Which of the following drugs is *not* generally suggested for use in ruminants?
   a. Ketamine
   b. Butorphanol
   c. Propofol
   d. Atropine

SECTION

12 Emergency and Critical Care

Brandy Tabor

QUESTIONS

1. Which of the following is least useful when resuscitating a dog in shock?
   a. D5W
   b. Hetastarch
   c. Hypertonic saline
   d. Plasma-Lyte 48
2. The first drug of choice for a cat that experiences status epilepticus is:
   a. Diazepam
   b. Pentobarbital
   c. Levetiracetam
   d. Phenobarbitol
3. Tension pneumothorax occurs when pressure in the thoracic cavity is:
   a. Less than atmospheric pressure
   b. Equal to atmospheric pressure
   c. Greater than atmospheric pressure
   d. Constant as animal breathes in and out
4. Emesis should not be induced in patients that have ingested:
   a. Anticholinergics
   b. Hydrocarbons
   c. Organophosphates
   d. Salicylates
5. The mucous membranes of a dog in septic shock are:
   a. Cyanotic
   b. Hyperemic
   c. Icteric
   d. Pale
6. The most desirable induction agent for an emergency cesarean section in a dog is:
   a. Etomidate
   b. Diazepam
   c. Propofol
   d. Thiopental
7. Feline aortic thromboembolism is most commonly associated with __________ disease.
   a. Cardiac
   b. Hepatic
   c. Renal
   d. Respiratory
8. To reduce intracranial pressure that results from trauma, ___________ may be administered every 4 to 8 hours.
   a. Atropine
   b. Dexamethasone
   c. Diazepam
   d. Mannitol
9. Four patients present at the same time with emergency conditions. In which order should the patients be triaged?
   a. Dyspnea, dystocia, proptosis, laceration
   b. Proptosis, dyspnea, dystocia, laceration
   c. Laceration, dystocia, dyspnea, proptosis
   d. Dystocia, proptosis, laceration, dyspnea
10. Which of the following conditions heals best through first intention?
    a. Abscess
    b. Degloving
    c. Simple laceration
    d. Puncture wound
11. A patient is experiencing cardiopulmonary arrest. The most desirable route of drug administration is:
    a. Intratracheal
    b. Intracardiac
    c. Intravenous
    d. Intraosseous
12. A patient that has been hit by a car and has no palpable pulse or detectable heartbeat requires chest compressions. These compressions should be performed at a rate of:
    a. 60–80 compressions per minute
    b. 80–100 compressions per minute
    c. 100–120 compressions per minute
    d. 120–140 compressions per minute
13. To minimize hemorrhage from the head of a canine trauma patient, where should pressure be applied?
    a. At the thoracic inlet in both jugular grooves
    b. At the thoracic inlet of the left jugular groove
    c. To the area adjacent and ventral to the mandible
    d. To the lateral points of the temporomandibular joint
14. In emergency care cases in which it is not possible to administer large volumes of desired fluids, it may be beneficial to administer:
    a. D5W
    b. Hypertonic saline
    c. Hypotonic saline
    d. Isotonic saline
15. During emergency intubation, the cranial nerve _________________ may be stimulated, resulting in _________________.
    a. I; bradycardia
    b. IV; tachycardia
    c. X; bradycardia
    d. XII; tachycardia

16. A man phones the veterinary practice to say that he has just hit a dog with his car and it is now lying on the side of the road. It appears to be breathing with minimal distress; however, there is blood coming from both nostrils and there is a small river of dark blood coming from a laceration on the lateral side of its hind leg. The dog can raise its head and is attempting to stand. In advising the man, your recommendation is to do all of the following *except*:
   a. Be aware for any signs of aggression
   b. Tie the dog's mouth securely closed with your shoelace
   c. Transport the dog on a board lying on its side
   d. Apply direct pressure to the wound
17. A normal central venous pressure (CVP) range is:
   a. 0–5 cm H_2O
   b. 5–10 cm H_2O
   c. 10–15 cm H_2O
   d. 15–20 cm H_2O
18. When monitoring patients on fluids and/or patients that undergo diuresis, urine output is an important consideration. The normal urine production for a healthy dog or cat is approximately:
   a. 0–1 mL/kg/h
   b. 1–2 mL/kg/h
   c. 2–3 mL/kg/h
   d. 3–4 mL/kg/h
19. Multiple parameters are measured to determine a category of shock that an animal might be experiencing. The central venous pressure is high in which of the following types of shock?
   a. Cardiogenic
   b. Distributive
   c. Hypovolemic
   d. Septic
20. Hypoglycemia is most common in patients that experience:
   a. Anaphylactic shock
   b. Cardiogenic shock
   c. Neurogenic shock
   d. Septic shock
21. A patient has increased muscular tone in the thoracic limbs and flaccid paralysis in the pelvic limbs when lying on its side. He is able to ambulate when placed on its feet and has a normal mentation. What posture do these clinical signs indicate?
   a. Decerebellate
   b. Decerebrate
   c. Opisthotonus
   d. Schiff-Sherrington
22. The Schiff-Sherrington posture is indicative of injury to which part of the spine?
   a. Cranial-C6
   b. C6-T2
   c. T1-T3
   d. T3-L3
23. NSAIDs are also referred to as:
   a. Anti-prostaglandins
   b. Neoprostaglandins
   c. Pro-prostaglandins
   d. Prostaglandoids
24. Which of the following is a colloid solution?
   a. Hetastarch
   b. Lactated Ringer's
   c. Normosol-R
   d. Plasma-Lyte 148
25. Defibrillation is the passing of an electrical current through the heart to:
   a. Cause the already depolarized cardiac cells to repolarize in a uniform manner
   b. Cause the cardiac cells to depolarize and then repolarize in a uniform manner
   c. Prevent the cardiac cells from depolarizing, thus maintaining rhythm
   d. Prevent any contractile activity of the cardiac cells temporarily
26. Which of the following is least likely to be seen in a patient suffering from shock?
   a. Hyperthermia
   b. Hypotension
   c. Tachycardia
   d. Tachypnea
27. Gastric dilatation/volvulus (GDV) is a life-threatening emergency. Which of the following veins becomes obstructed as a result of GDV?
   a. Femoral vein
   b. Gastroduodenal vein
   c. Portal vein
   d. Renal vein
28. The unit of measurement for insulin is:
   a. Milliliters
   b. Microliters
   c. Milligrams
   d. International units
29. Dystocia in dogs or cats may be defined as active straining without delivery of a fetus for more than __________ minutes.
   a. 20
   b. 30
   c. 40
   d. 60
30. Which direction should you approach an animal that requires emergency treatment?
   a. Caudal
   b. Lateral
   c. Rostral
   d. Let the animal try to come to you.
31. Ocular exposure to a toxin has occurred in a dog. On examination, it is discovered that there is possible damage to the corneal epithelium. Which of the following procedures is contraindicated?
   a. Continuous flushing with physiologic saline
   b. Provision of mild sedative, analgesic, or both
   c. Corticosteroid administration to prevent inflammation
   d. Use of antibiotic cream after flushing

32. A client calls the veterinary practice indicating that their cat drank ethylene glycol 6 hours earlier. Everyone is at lunch and you immediately page the veterinarian; however, the client wants to make the cat vomit to rid it of the toxin. What should you advise?
    a. To use 3% hydrogen peroxide at 1 tbsp/20 lb
    b. To use salt on the back of the cat's tongue
    c. To use syrup of ipecac
    d. Not to induce vomiting and to bring in the cat immediately
33. Eclampsia produces elevated body temperatures as a result of:
    a. Increased levels of endotoxins that are present
    b. A large fetal mass that is present
    c. Heat produced through muscle movement
    d. Eclampsia does not result in elevated body temperature.
34. To place a nasal oxygenation catheter in a dog, a veterinary technician would measure to the:
    a. Beginning of the thoracic inlet
    b. Medial canthus of the eye
    c. Pharynx
    d. No measurement is needed; a standard catheter 1.5 inches in length is used.
35. A client calls to say they has come home to find their cat lying with the lamp cord in its mouth. The cat is breathing but is unresponsive. The first thing you should advise is:
    a. To place the cat in a carrier and bring it to clinic immediately
    b. To perform CPR and explain how to do it
    c. To disconnect the plug of the lamp cord from the wall socket immediately
    d. To take note of the amperage of the lamp
36. The most common artery to use when assessing the pulse of a dog or cat is the:
    a. Jugular
    b. Femoral
    c. Carpal
    d. Tarsal
37. A healthy, adult, small-breed dog is presented to the veterinary practice for a wellness examination. At what point should you become concerned about an elevated heart rate?
    a. 175 beats/min
    b. 250 beats/min
    c. 300 beats/min
    d. 350 beats/min
38. A pulse deficit occurs when the pulse:
    a. Occurs before the heartbeat
    b. Occurs with the heartbeat
    c. Occurs after the heartbeat
    d. Does not occur
39. A normal sinus arrhythmia occurs when heart rate:
    a. Increases with expiration
    b. Decreases with expiration
    c. May increase or decrease with expiration
    d. Does not increase or decrease with expiration
40. An abnormal increase in the depth and rate of respirations is called:
    a. Dyspnea
    b. Hyperpnea
    c. Orthopnea
    d. Tachypnea
41. An 18-gauge needle would be most appropriate for administering SQ fluids to which patient?
    a. Cockatiel
    b. Labrador retriever
    c. Kitten
    d. Rat
42. The proper site for an intraperitoneal injection is:
    a. On the lateral abdominal wall just caudal to the rib cage
    b. 2 to 3 inches caudal to the umbilicus on the midline
    c. At the level of the umbilicus to the right or left of the midline
    d. 2 to 3 inches cranial to the umbilicus on the midline
43. Which of the following statements is true regarding the administration of liquids via the oral cavity in a dog?
    a. Flush a large bolus of fluid directly into the mouth
    b. Flush a very small bolus of fluid directly into pharyngeal area
    c. Place fluid between the teeth and the cheek, and allow the patient to swallow on its own accord
    d. Place the fluid between the teeth and the cheek in large enough amounts so that the patient will be forced to swallow
44. Which area of the body is best to assess skin turgor in a canine patient?
    a. Lateral aspect of the neck
    b. Caudal abdomen
    c. Base of the tail
    d. Axillary region
45. Knuckling is an abnormality of which system?
    a. Cardiac
    b. Neurologic
    c. Respiratory
    d. Urinary
46. The rapid intravenous administration of large amounts of potassium can result in:
    a. Respiratory arrest
    b. Cardiac arrest
    c. Polyuria
    d. Polydipsia
47. Which of the following route(s) can potassium solutions be administered to dogs and cats without causing severe pain?
    a. Intravenous only
    b. Subcutaneous only
    c. Intramuscular only
    d. Intravenous and subcutaneous
48. Which of the following is *not* a contraindication for crystalloid fluid therapy?
    a. Pulmonary edema
    b. Cerebral edema
    c. Pitting of the soft tissues
    d. Swollen soft tissue from bruising caused by trauma

49. Which of the following is the *easiest* method for monitoring fluid therapy?
   a. Central venous pressure (CVP)
   b. Packed-cell volume/total protein (PCV/TP)
   c. Urine output (UOP)
   d. Weight
50. What part of the eye can be used to indicate fluid overload?
   a. Conjunctiva
   b. Lens
   c. Pupil
   d. Nictitating membrane
51. Rapid fluid replacement with crystalloids is contraindicated in conditions of:
   a. Severe dehydration
   b. Shock
   c. Cerebral edema
   d. Renal failure
52. Which of the following is a common colloid preparation that is administered intravenously?
   a. Lactated Ringer's solution
   b. Normosol-R solution
   c. Sodium chloride 9%
   d. VetStarch
53. Fluid-therapy solutions administered subcutaneously are:
   a. Colloids
   b. Hypertonic
   c. Hypotonic
   d. Isotonic
54. The best route for rapid fluid administration of large amounts of fluids to patients with poor venous access is:
   a. Intraosseous
   b. Intraperitoneal
   c. Oral
   d. Subcutaneous
55. Fluid therapy should be used with caution in which of the following scenarios?
   a. Hypovolemic shock
   b. Distributive shock
   c. Cardiogenic shock
   d. Obstructive shock
56. When a critical patient arrives at the veterinary practice, which body system should be evaluated first?
   a. Cardiac
   b. Neurologic
   c. Respiratory
   d. Urinary
57. Which of the following is the safest and most effective first aid for frostbite?
   a. Apply warm towels and massage the area
   b. Immerse the affected area in hot water
   c. Immerse the affected area in lukewarm water
   d. Rub the affected area with snow
58. Which of the following methods for controlling hemorrhage from a traumatic wound is least likely to cause further damage to the animal?
   a. Clamping the wound with a hemostat
   b. Direct pressure
   c. Tourniquet
   d. Applying silver nitrate
59. Which would be considered the least important physical measure evaluated during triage of a patient?
   a. Heart rate
   b. Respiratory rate
   c. Capillary refill time
   d. Weight
60. Which of the following statements is true regarding a patient in shock?
   a. An initial decrease in heart rate that then increases as the patient nears death
   b. A decreased heart rate
   c. An initial increase in heart rate that then decreases as the patient nears death
   d. An increased heart rate
61. The mucous membranes of patients in hemorrhagic shock are:
   a. Cyanotic
   b. Hyperemic
   c. Icteric
   d. Pale or white
62. What is the minimum concentration of hemoglobin required to detect cyanosis?
   a. 3 g/dL
   b. 4 g/dL
   c. 5 g/dL
   d. 6 g/dL
63. According to the principles of triage, which patient should the veterinarian see first?
   a. Cat with a closed fracture
   b. Dog in respiratory distress
   c. Dog with otitis externa
   d. Cat with a small laceration on a paw pad
64. Which of the following would petechiation on the mucous membranes indicate?
   a. Hemoglobinemia
   b. Methemoglobinemia
   c. Myoglobinemia
   d. Thrombocytopenia
65. Which of the following is not a characteristic of compensatory shock?
   a. Normal blood pressure
   b. Cool extremities
   c. Capillary refill time <1 second
   d. Tachycardia
66. According to the principles of triage, which patient should a veterinarian see first?
   a. Dog with a small laceration on a pinna
   b. Dog with acute gastric dilatation/volvulus
   c. Cat with dystocia, not in shock, no kitten in birth canal
   d. Cat with possible linear foreign body in the bowel
67. Which of these signs is not an indication of dystocia?
   a. Abnormal vulvar discharge
   b. Profuse vulvar hemorrhage
   c. Pup or kitten in the birth canal for 5 minutes
   d. More than 1 hour of vigorous contractions with no pup or kitten produced
68. What is not usually a sign of acute gastric dilatation/volvulus?
   a. Unproductive vomiting
   b. Hypersalivation
   c. Abdominal distention
   d. Profuse diarrhea

69. Crackles on thoracic auscultation indicate:
   a. Asthma
   b. Pleural effusion
   c. Pneumothorax
   d. Pulmonary edema

70. A client describes their male cat as lethargic and constipated; they has observed the cat straining in the litter box. You suspect that the cat is actually suffering from:
   a. Peritonitis
   b. Urethral obstruction
   c. Intestinal obstruction
   d. An upper respiratory viral infection

71. If the hindquarters were elevated in a dog with a severe diaphragmatic hernia, what effect would this have on respiration?
   a. There is no change in respiratory rate or labor of respirations.
   b. Respiratory rate decreases and respiration becomes less labored.
   c. Respiratory rate increases and respiration becomes more labored.
   d. A cough is induced.

72. A veterinarian is assessing a cat with a spinal injury. When the doctor pinches the cat's toe, a positive response to deep pain would be indicated by:
   a. Kicking of the foot without vocalizing
   b. Kicking of the foot while vocalizing
   c. Withdrawal of the foot without vocalizing
   d. Withdrawal of the foot while vocalizing

73. Signs of cardiopulmonary arrest include all of the following *except*:
   a. Alertness
   b. Dilated pupils
   c. Agonal breathing
   d. No femoral pulse

74. A patient that was hit by a car and has multiple pelvic fractures has not urinated in more than 24 hours. One may suspect the cause of anuria to be:
   a. A ruptured urinary bladder
   b. Severe dehydration
   c. Renal failure
   d. Urethral calculi

75. A free-roaming dog is brought to the hospital for listlessness and dyspnea. While performing venipuncture, you notice that the animal seems to have a prolonged clotting time. A possible cause of prolonged clotting times would be the ingestion of __________
   a. Anticoagulant rodenticide
   b. Ethylene glycol
   c. Organophosphate insecticide
   d. Strychnine

76. Which statement concerning status epilepticus is accurate?
   a. It occurs in geriatric animals only.
   b. It is a life-threatening medical emergency.
   c. It is treated by the administration of acepromazine.
   d. It will resolve spontaneously.

77. Signs of organophosphate toxicity include all of the following *except*:
   a. Bradycardia
   b. Lacrimation
   c. Mydriasis
   d. Salivation

78. Normal capillary refill time in dogs is:
   a. <1 second
   b. 1 to 2 seconds
   c. 2 to 4 seconds
   d. 4 to 6 seconds

79. A client calls the hospital and indicates that a car has just hit their cat. The recommendations that should be made include:
   a. Immediately bring the cat in to be examined by a veterinarian
   b. Observe the cat at home for an hour and call back if problems occur
   c. Bring the cat in for an examination by a veterinarian the following day
   d. Bring the cat to you for initial examination so that you can determine whether the animal needs to be seen by a veterinarian

80. A client calls the hospital and says that their puppy has walked through motor oil and is licking its paws. What should be recommended?
   a. Do not induce emesis and immediately bring the pet to the clinic for examination and treatment
   b. Induce emesis and then immediately bring the pet to the clinic for examination and treatment
   c. Induce emesis and no further treatment is required.
   d. Induce emesis and then bring the pet to the clinic only if it shows signs of toxicity

81. A client calls the practice and states that their dog has just ingested sugar-free gum. They are 90 minutes from the practice. What should be recommended?
   a. Do not induce emesis and immediately bring the pet to the clinic for examination and treatment
   b. Induce emesis then immediately bring the pet to the clinic for examination and treatment
   c. Induce emesis and no further treatment is required.
   d. Induce emesis then bring the pet to the clinic only if it shows signs of toxicity

82. A client owning a diabetic cat calls the practice and says that their cat has just had a seizure and collapsed. They gave the cat its usual dose of insulin that morning, but the animal has not eaten anything during the day. What should the next recommendation entail?
   a. Another dose of insulin, then bring the cat to the clinic for medical attention
   b. Some corn syrup or sugar solution on the gums, then observe the cat at home
   c. Some corn syrup or sugar solution on the gums, then bring the cat to the clinic for medical attention
   d. Another dose of insulin, then observe the cat at home

83. A client has just treated their 5-week-old kitten with a flea dip that contains lindane. The cat is slightly lethargic and the client notices that the label on the dip reads "for dogs only." The client calls the practice. What advice should be given?
   a. Observe the kitten at home
   b. Wash the kitten with mild dish soap, rinse well, and then bring the animal to the clinic for examination
   c. Wash the kitten with mild dish soap, rinse well, and then administer acetaminophen for discomfort
   d. Induce emesis and observe the kitten at home

84. A client calls the hospital because they have noticed that their cat has a string protruding from under the tongue. The client should be advised to:
   a. Gently attempt to pull out the string
   b. Induce emesis
   c. Cut the string and administer laxatives at home
   d. Bring the cat to the clinic for examination

85. A client calls the hospital because they have noticed a barbed fishhook embedded in their dog's lower lip. The client should be advised to:
   a. Gently attempt to pull out the fishhook
   b. Observe the dog at home; most fishhooks fall out spontaneously within 24 hours
   c. Bring the animal to see the veterinarian as soon as possible
   d. Administer aspirin for discomfort and see the veterinarian right away

86. A dog has a lacerated paw pad. The client has placed a small bandage over the wound, but blood is soaking through. The appropriate treatment is to:
   a. Remove the bandage and apply digital pressure to the wound
   b. Apply another bandage over the client's original bandage
   c. Remove the bandage and apply a tourniquet to the limb
   d. Do nothing; no further treatment is required if the bleeding is not excessive.

87. An extremely upset client calls the hospital. Their small poodle has stopped breathing and they cannot feel a heartbeat. What should the recommendation be?
   a. Attempt no treatment; immediately transport the pet to the hospital
   b. Start chest compressions; immediately transport the pet to the hospital
   c. Close the dog's mouth and attempt mouth-to-snout resuscitation; immediately transport the pet to the hospital
   d. Attempt resuscitation; transport the pet to the hospital if attempts at resuscitation are unsuccessful

88. How should a patient with a potential spinal injury be transported to the hospital?
   a. Sitting
   b. Standing
   c. Lying on a flat board
   d. Moving as it wishes

89. A patient with a possible herniated intervertebral disk should be:
   a. Allowed to move freely and if no improvement is evident after 24 hours, see the veterinarian
   b. Allowed to move freely; immediately see the veterinarian
   c. Kept strictly quiet and confined; if no improvement is evident in 24 hours, see the veterinarian
   d. Kept strictly quiet and confined; see the veterinarian immediately

90. Which of these items would be least useful on a crash cart used for emergency situations?
   a. Laryngoscope
   b. Intravenous catheter
   c. Otoscope
   d. Ambu bag

91. A patient who is apneic and cyanotic enters the practice. A quick oral examination shows a hard ball lodged in the glottal opening. Which of the following options should be performed next?
   a. Place the patient in an oxygen cage
   b. Attempt to pass a nasal oxygen catheter
   c. Attempt to pass an endotracheal tube
   d. Perform the Heimlich maneuver; if unsuccessful, prepare the patient for tracheotomy

92. A 16-year-old, 3-kg poodle is brought to the hospital with cyanosis, agonal respirations, and frothy fluid coming from the nose and mouth. Knowing the treatments that the doctor is likely to order, you prepare to:
   a. Administer intravenous fluids at 90 mL/kg/h
   b. Administer furosemide intramuscularly and place the patient in an oxygen cage
   c. Suction the airway and initiate cardiopulmonary resuscitation
   d. Assist with an immediate tracheostomy

93. The veterinarian has authorized you to start infusing intravenous fluids in a 0.25-kg Yorkshire terrier puppy that is critically ill. You are unable to insert a catheter into a jugular or cephalic vein. An alternative site that can be used to administer large volumes of fluids is the:
   a. Medullary cavity of the femur
   b. Carotid artery
   c. Lingual vein
   d. Ear vein

94. The veterinarian has directed you to give a whole blood transfusion to a 0.3-kg kitten with severe anemia from flea infestation. You are unable to insert an intravenous or intraosseous catheter. Which of the following would be the most effective alternative route to administer the blood effectively?
   a. Subcutaneous injection
   b. Intramuscular injection
   c. Intraperitoneal injection
   d. Per os

95. You are instructing a client to apply an emergency muzzle to their injured dog. Which of these is the least appropriate material for the muzzle?
   a. Rope
   b. Metal chain dog leash
   c. Pantyhose
   d. Necktie

96. Which of the following is least likely to be available for at-home induction of emesis?
a. Apomorphine
b. Syrup of ipecac
c. Hydrogen peroxide
d. Salt

97. Which of the following is not performed when treating acute gastric dilatation/volvulus?
a. Induction of emesis
b. Placement of an intravenous catheter
c. Passing of a gastric tube
d. Trocharization of the stomach

98. All of the following might be included in emergency treatment for epistaxis *except*:
a. Placing dilute epinephrine into the nares
b. Fresh frozen plasma transfusion
c. Applying a warm compress to the nose
d. Keep the patient quiet

99. Which statement concerning the administration of activated charcoal via stomach tube is least accurate?
a. Check tube placement by administering a small amount of water; listen for coughing or gagging
b. Measure the tube from the tip of the nose to the 13th rib
c. Measure the tube from the tip of the nose to the thoracic inlet
d. Use a roll of tape as a speculum to keep the mouth open and to prevent the animal from biting the tube

100. Oxygen can be administered to a patient via any of the following routes *except*:
a. Chest tube
b. Endotracheal tube
c. Nasal oxygen catheter
d. Tracheotomy tube

101. Which of the following is the most important goal when treating a patient with heat stroke?
a. Cooling
b. Infection control
c. Oxygen therapy
d. Pain control

102. All of the following are recommended treatments for a dog experiencing paraphimosis *except*?
a. Lubricating the penis
b. Cleaning the penis
c. Applying hypertonic solutions to the penis
d. Applying a warm compress to the penis

103. Initial treatment for a dog with an open fracture includes all of the following *except*:
a. Copiously cleaning and flushing the wound
b. Covering the wound
c. Applying a temporary splint to the limb
d. Taking radiographs of the fracture

104. Which is the most correct action when treating a dog having a seizure?
a. Grasp the dog's tongue and pull it forward to prevent airway obstruction
b. Administer oral anticonvulsants
c. Prevent the dog from injuring itself
d. Immediately start infusion of intravenous fluids

105. A client calls the hospital to say that their Pekingese has suffered an eye proptosis. Your advice to the client should include all of the following *except*:
a. Apply pressure to the globe to replace it in the socket
b. Protect the globe from further trauma
c. Keep the globe moist
d. Immediately bring the dog to the veterinarian

106. A client calls and says that their Rottweiler has been shot in the abdomen with a BB gun but appears perfectly fine. What should be recommended?
a. Observe the animal at home for vomiting or abdominal pain
b. See the veterinarian immediately
c. See the veterinarian at your earliest convenience
d. Observe the animal for hemorrhage

107. Initial treatment for a cat with an open pneumothorax may include all of the following *except*:
a. Thoracocentesis
b. Oxygen administration
c. Covering the wound
d. Radiographic examination

108. Which statement is least accurate concerning the emergency treatment of cats with urethral obstruction?
a. Cats must always be sedated to have a urinary catheter passed.
b. Massaging the tip of the penis can relieve the obstruction.
c. Cats with a slow, irregular heart rate probably have a high serum potassium level.
d. If the obstruction is not relieved, the cat will die.

109. Which procedure is not routinely performed to resuscitate neonates following cesarean section?
a. Cleaning the nose and mouth of secretions
b. Rubbing the neonate with a towel to stimulate breathing
c. Administering a drop of oxytocin under the tongue
d. Ligating the umbilical cord

110. Inducing emesis after ingestion of a solid toxin is imperative. However, emesis has little value if induced more than ________ after ingestion.
a. 0.5 hours
b. 1.5 hours
c. 4 hours
d. 8 hours

111. Which is not an immediate consideration in cardiopulmonary resuscitation?
a. Airway
b. Analgesia
c. Breathing
d. Circulation

112. At what rate (breaths per minute) should respirations be administered to a patient in cardiopulmonary arrest?
a. 4–8 breaths per minute
b. 8–12 breaths per minute
c. 12–26 breaths per minute
d. 16–20 breaths per minute

113. All of the following are signs of end-stage decompensatory shock *except*:
a. Hypothermia
b. Vasodilation
c. Prolonged capillary refill time
d. Tachycardia

114. Central venous pressure is used to guide:
a. Rewarming measures
b. Oxygen therapy
c. Fluid therapy
d. Pain management

115. Each of the following can be used to check mucous membrane color *except* the:
a. Sclera
b. Gingiva
c. Lining of vulva
d. Lining of prepuce

116. Dehydration is assessed by all of the following *except*:
a. Moistness of mucous membranes
b. Skin turgor
c. Packed-cell volume and total plasma protein
d. Nasal discharge

117. A 20-kg Springer spaniel is brought to the hospital because of anorexia and lethargy. Dehydration is estimated at 8%. The maintenance requirement of fluids is 66 mL/kg/day. To correct this dog's dehydration, how much fluid should it receive during the first 24 hours?
a. 2920 mL
b. 1600 mL
c. 1320 mL
d. 1336 mL

118. A 32-kg golden retriever is brought to the hospital because of anorexia and lethargy. Dehydration is estimated at 8%. The maintenance requirement of fluids is 66 mL/kg/day. To provide two times the daily maintenance requirements, what is the hourly rate of fluid infusion?
a. 55 mL
b. 176 mL
c. 235 mL
d. 1320 mL

119. Placement of a jugular catheter is contraindicated in which of the following situations?
a. Vomiting
b. Pancreatitis
c. Thrombocytopenia
d. Renal failure

120. Which of the following is *not* included in basic life support of CPR?
a. Chest compressions
b. Intubation
c. Ventilation
d. Medications

121. Tissue perfusion can be assessed by all of the following *except*:
a. Capillary refill time
b. Rectal temperature
c. Mucous membrane color
d. Mentation

122. During triage, which patient should be attended to first?
a. Dog with a penetrating wound of the abdomen
b. Cat in respiratory arrest
c. Cat with an intestinal foreign body
d. Dog with gastric dilatation/volvulus

123. What is the main determinant of the treatment of a hyperthermic patient?
a. Age of patient
b. Duration of hyperthermia
c. Cause of hyperthermia
d. Breed of patient

124. What is the recommended dosage for intratracheal drug administration during cardiac arrest?
a. Half the intravenous dosage
b. Same as the intravenous dosage
c. Up to five times the intravenous dosage
d. Up to ten times the intravenous dose

125. A client calls the practice and is worried about their Irish wolfhound. The dog ran loose in the neighborhood and it is now retching without bringing anything up and pacing the floor. The abdomen looks a little distended. What advice should be given?
a. Record the client's phone number and tell them the doctor will call them back
b. Tell the client to bring the dog in for examination immediately
c. Advise the client to give 3% hydrogen peroxide to induce vomiting
d. Tell the client that the dog may have eaten garbage and to call the hospital in the morning if the animal is not feeling better

126. A 6-year-old mongrel is brought to the hospital with ataxia and mydriasis. On presentation, you notice the dog is dribbling urine and seems overly sensitive to movement and sound. Which toxin is the most likely cause of these signs?
a. Chocolate
b. Grapes
c. Marijuana
d. Xylitol

127. When advising a client to move an injured animal, all of the following scenarios are appropriate *except*:
a. If a back injury is suspected, place the animal on a board to move it
b. Muzzle the injured animal because it may bite when being moved
c. Call the veterinary hospital to notify of your expected arrival time
d. Give a baby aspirin to reduce pain before moving the animal

128. Intraosseous catheters can be used in all of the following cases *except*:
a. In septic animals
b. When epinephrine and atropine must be administered during an arrest
c. In young and/or debilitated animals
d. When rapid access to the circulatory system is needed in hypovolemic animals

129. What is the preferred route of fluid administration in a critically ill animal?
a. Intravenous
b. Subcutaneous
c. Oral
d. Intramuscular

130. Which of the following products is a crystalloid?
a. Packed red blood cells
b. Lactated Ringer's solution
c. Hetastarch
d. Oxyglobin

131. In which of the following cases is whole blood indicated over packed red blood cells?
a. Hemorrhage during surgery
b. Hemorrhage secondary to an anticoagulant rodenticide
c. Autoimmune hemolytic anemia
d. Hemorrhage caused by trauma

132. Nutritional support can be administered in several ways. What is the preferred method?
a. Enteral nutrition
b. Partial parenteral nutrition
c. Total parenteral nutrition
d. Per rectum

133. Which of the following is the most common sign of a blood transfusion reaction?
a. Fever
b. Vomiting
c. Tachycardia
d. Seizure

134. The normal blood pH for a dog is:
a. 6.4
b. 7
c. 7.4
d. 8

135. What electrolyte imbalance is most likely to be found in a cat with total urethral obstruction?
a. Hyperkalemia
b. Hyperchloremia
c. Hypernatremia
d. Hypercalcemia

136. The heart rate of an unanesthetized patient can be determined (and monitored) using all of the following options *except*:
a. Stethoscope
b. Electrocardiographic monitor
c. Pulse rate
d. Esophageal stethoscope

137. All of the following are noninvasive ways of monitoring a critically ill patient *except*:
a. Respiratory rate using a stethoscope
b. Temperature using a tympanic thermometer
c. Blood pressure using an arterial catheter
d. Heart rate using an ECG

138. Which of the following options takes the lowest priority when preparing to treat a critical patient?
a. Oxygen source
b. Endotracheal tubes
c. Heating pad
d. Intravenous catheters

139. A dog presents with irregular movements over the surface of the muscle near its shoulder. This type of muscle movement is called:
a. Dyskinesia
b. Fasciculation
c. Myoclonus
d. Tremors

140. A dehydrated patient presents. Which of the following solutions would be the most appropriate fluid choice?
a. Fresh frozen plasma
b. Hetastarch
c. Packed red blood cells
d. Plasma-Lyte 48

141. A fellow veterinary technician is triaging a patient and notes the mucous membranes look brown in color. What might be the cause?
a. Anemia
b. Bilirubinemia
c. Hyperthermia
d. Methemoglobinemia

142. Which toxicity will cause salivation, lacrimation, urination, and defecation?
a. Acetaminophen
b. Grapes
c. Lilies
d. Organophosphates

143. The bandage layer that comes in contact with the wound is the:
a. Primary layer
b. Secondary layer
c. Tertiary layer
d. Quaternary layer

144. At what temperature will organ damage occur in a hyperthermic patient?
a. 105°F
b. 106°F
c. 107°F
d. 108°F

145. A dog presents to the practice with a history of waxing and waning vomiting, lethargy, and decreased appetite for several months. Bloodwork shows 122 mmoL/L sodium and 7.8 mmoL/L potassium. What disease can cause these symptoms and electrolyte changes?
a. Diabetic insipidus
b. Diabetic ketoacidosis
c. Hypoadrenocorticism
d. Thyroid storm

146. Which of the following bacteria is responsible for kennel cough?
a. *Bordetella bronchiseptica*
b. *Clostridium tetani*
c. *Neospora caninum*
d. *Toxoplasmosis gondii*

147. Which of the following medications should not be used to control seizures in a patient with liver disease?
a. Levetiracetam
b. Phenobarbital
c. Potassium bromide
d. Propofol

148. A dog presents 30 minutes after the owner saw him lacerate himself on a dirty nail. How would this wound be classified?
a. Clean
b. Clean-contaminated
c. Contaminated
d. Dirty-infected

149. Which insulin is quick-acting and short-lasting, making it appropriate for use as a CRI?
a. NPH
b. Regular
c. Glargine
d. PZI

150. A hospitalized patient is receiving intravenous fluids with a potassium supplementation; however, the potassium blood value continues to drop. What other blood value should be discussed with the veterinarian?
a. Calcium
b. Magnesium
c. Sodium
d. Chloride

151. Which of the following conditions can cause ventroflexion in cats?
a. Hypokalemia
b. Hyponatremia
c. Hypocalcemia
d. Hypomagnesemia

152. Which of the following options controls breathing in dogs and cats?
a. The level of carbon dioxide in the blood
b. The level of oxygen in the blood
c. The level of oxygen in the airway
d. The level of humidity in the airway

153. Which of the following blood tests can be diagnostic for anticoagulant rodenticide ingestion?
a. Activated clotting time (ACT)
b. Activated partial thromboplastin time (aPTT)
c. Buccal mucosal bleeding time (BMBT)
d. Prothrombin time (PT)

154. Which blood value will be elevated when a patient experiences decreased perfusion?
a. Creatinine
b. Glucose
c. Lactate
d. Sodium

155. The veterinarian has requested bloodwork on a patient. When reviewing the results, you notice that the patient has an elevated blood lactate level. What change would you expect to see on a blood gas analysis?
a. Normal pH
b. Elevated pH
c. Decreased pH
d. No change in pH

156. Which of the following options is not a ketone?
a. Acetone
b. Acetoacetate
c. Beta-hydroxybutyrate
d. Ketoacetone

157. Which of the following options is not a goal of oxygen therapy?
a. To decrease the work of breathing
b. To decrease myocardial work
c. To improve mentation
d. To treat hypoxemia

158. The stretch (or load) placed on the myocardial fibers right before the heart contracts is known as:
a. Afterload
b. Contractility
c. Preload
d. Resistance

159. A patient presents with a history of collapse. While obtaining vitals, you notice the pulses become weaker with inspiration and stronger with expiration. The heart sounds are muffled and the height of the QRS complex on the patient's ECG changes with each beat. Which of the following conditions may be the cause of these clinical signs?
a. Heart failure
b. Hypovolemia
c. Pericardial effusion
d. Pneumothorax

160. What coagulation factors are tested by a prothrombin time?
a. I, II, V, VII, X
b. I, II, III, IV
c. V, VII, X, XII
d. V, XI, XII, XIII

161. At what point should a veterinary technician become concerned that the mean arterial pressure of a patient is becoming too low and that perfusion to the brain, heart, and kidneys will be compromised if it continues to fall?
a. 40 mmHg
b. 50 mmHg
c. 60 mmHg
d. 70 mmHg

162. Which of the following rodenticides will cause neurological signs when ingested?
a. Bromethalin
b. Bromadiolone
c. Brodifacoum
d. Warfarin

163. A patient presents with a respiratory pattern consisting of periods of apnea alternating with periods of hyperpnea. What is this respiratory pattern known as?
a. Cheyne-Stokes
b. Kussmaul's
c. Paradoxical
d. Orthopnea

164. How many days after a tick attaches itself to a dog can the neurological signs associated with tick paralysis be seen?
a. 1
b. 3
c. 7
d. 11

165. Which of the following is not a cause of hypoglycemia in a septic patient?
a. Decreased dietary intake
b. Increase release of insulin
c. Increased consumption of glucose by the body
d. Decreased production of glucose by the body

166. Which of the following medications can cause abortions?
a. Clavamox
b. Misoprostol
c. Metronidazole
d. Metoclopramide

167. A Doppler is used to measure:
a. Blood pressure
b. Central venous pressure
c. SpO_2
d. End-tidal CO_2

168. ___________ is a disease that causes damage to the optic nerve resulting in blindness and it can be diagnosed by testing for an increase in intraocular pressure.
a. Blepharitis
b. Glaucoma
c. Uveitis
d. Ulcerative keratitis

169. What is the initial cause of blepharospasm?
a. Ocular discharge
b. Increased intraocular pressure
c. Lacrimation
d. Irritation to the eye

170. What is the most common cause of hypercalcemia in dogs?
a. Cancer
b. Pregnancy
c. Vomiting
d. Diarrhea

171. Which is the correct order of changes in mentation from best to worst?
a. Obtunded, comatose, quiet, stuporous
b. Quiet, obtunded, stuporous, comatose
c. Comatose, stuporous, quiet, obtunded
d. Quiet stuporous, obtunded, comatose

172. When falling from a building, at what height (story) will a cat's injuries be less likely to be life threatening?
a. 3 stories
b. 5 stories
c. 7 stories
d. 9 stories

173. What is the expected difference between a patient's end-tidal CO_2 ($ETCO_2$) and the actual $PaCO_2$ (carbon dioxide in the arterial blood)?
a. $ETCO_2$ 2–5 mmHg less than the $PaCO_2$
b. $ETCO_2$ 5–7 mmHg less than the $PaCO_2$
c. $PaCO_2$ 2–5 mmHg less than the $ETCO_2$
d. $PaCO_2$ 5–7 mmHg less than the $ETCO_2$

174. A young, healthy patient is on intravenous fluids before a routine spay. Immediately after the fluids are started, the patient goes into cardiorespiratory arrest. What might be the cause?
a. Fluid rate too high
b. The intravenous catheter was not patent
c. There was air in the fluid line
d. Unknown underlying disease

175. Which of the following tests can be used to diagnosis panleukopenia in a cat?
a. Complete blood count
b. Blood gas
c. Electrolytes
d. Canine Parvovirus snap test

176. What coagulation factors are tested with an activated partial thromboplastin time (aPTT)?
a. I, II, V, VII, X
b. I, II, V, VIII, IX, X, XI, XII
c. V, VII, IX
d. VIII, IX, X, XI

177. What is the correct formula when discussing cerebral perfusion pressure (CPP)?
a. CPP = ICP (intracranial pressure) – MAP (mean arterial pressure)
b. CPP = ICP + MAP
c. CPP = MAP – ICP
d. CPP = MAP + ICP

178. Which type of hypersensitivity occurs when antibodies destroy the body's own, normal cells?
a. Type I
b. Type II
c. Type III
d. Type IV

179. Which patient will experience more damage from an electrical shock?
a. A dry dog
b. A wet dog
c. A dog with its hair shaved
d. A dog wearing metal tags

180. Which of these metabolites contributes more to ketoacidosis but is least detectable on a urine ketone strip?
a. Acetone
b. Acetoacetate
c. Beta-hydroxybutyrate
d. Ketoacetone

181. A dog presents to the practice after being hit by a car and it has numerous injuries including a flail chest. How should the patient be positioned on the treatment table to minimize pain and maximize respiratory function?
a. Affected side up
b. Affected side down
c. Sternal
d. Dorsal

182. Metoclopramide is contraindicated in which of the following conditions?
a. Postoperative gastrotomy
b. Postoperative GDV
c. Pancreatitis
d. Gastrointestinal obstruction

183. A dog presents with pericardial effusion. Where should a you shave the patient for a pericardiocentesis?
a. Left side from the 3rd to the 7th ribs
b. Left side from the 8th to the 12th ribs
c. Right side from the 3rd to the 7th ribs
d. Right side from the 8th to the 12 ribs

184. At what temperature (related to hypothermia) will a patient become comatose and develop muscular rigidity as well as cardiac arrhythmia?
a. <83°F
b. 83–86°F
c. 86–93°F
d. 93–98°F

185. A patient receives chemotherapy for lymphoma, and 6 hours later you notice the patient is vomiting, has diarrhea, and seems depressed. When you examine the patient more closely, you note pale mucous membranes, a prolonged CRT, and bradycardia. What do you suspect is happening?
a. Extravasation of the chemotherapeutic agent
b. Heart failure
c. Tumor lysis syndrome
d. Sterile hemorrhagic cystitis

186. The oncology department brings a dog to the emergency department after vincristine (a vinca alkaloid) extravasation. Which of the following procedures is not recommended?
a. Administer the remainder of the medication
b. Inject saline, dexamethasone sodium phosphate, and sodium bicarbonate around the site
c. Withdraw as much of the medication as possible
d. Apply a warm compress

187. Which of the following is not a determinant of stroke volume?
a. Afterload
b. Contractility
c. Heart rate
d. Preload

188. A dog presents the emergency department with vomiting and diarrhea. The animal had received chemotherapy a week earlier and was doing well until today. When obtaining the patient's vital signs, you note a temperature of 104.0°F. The veterinarian asks you to draw blood and run a complete blood count. What do you expect the results to show?
a. Anemia
b. Monocytosis
c. Neutropenia
d. Thrombocytopenia

189. A 3-year-old boxer comes into the veterinary practice, and the owner states they were on a walk when the dog suddenly appeared weak, then fell over. It was unresponsive for 10–15 seconds and then recovered and seemed normal. The owner states that the dog did not thrash or lose control of its bladder or bowels. What condition may have occurred?
a. Anaphylaxis
b. Cardiac arrest
c. Seizure
d. Syncope

190. An owner calls the veterinary practice and states their dog cut its paw at the barn several days previously. The dog seemed to be fine and the cut was healing, but it started acting strangely yesterday. This morning they found the dog lying on its side with its head and neck extended backward. It was salivating heavily, and when the owner tried to open its mouth, they were unable to because the dog's jaw was so stiff. Which of the following conditions might the history and clinical signs indicate?
a. Botulism
b. Bromethalin toxicity
c. Seizure activity
d. Tetanus

191. A patient with a history of megaesophagus presents to the veterinary clinic with weakness associated with exercise. The owner says the dog seems fine for a short period and then is unable to walk. If he rests, he recovers and is normal for a few minutes, but then it happens again. What do you suspect is the cause?
a. Myasthenia gravis
b. Myopathy
c. Polyradiculoneuritis
d. Tick paralysis

192. While triaging a patient, you notice an increased respiratory effort on inspiration. What disease might this indicate?
a. Upper airway disease
b. Lower airway disease
c. Lung disease
d. Pleural space disease

193. A cat presents after being hit by a car. The veterinarian notes abdominal effusion, performs an abdominocentesis to obtain a sample, and asks you to run electrolytes on the abdominal fluid and compare it with serum electrolytes. Which of the following conditions is he trying to eliminate?
a. Hemoabdomen
b. Uroabdomen
c. Peritonitis
d. Septic abdomen

194. What is the cause of polyuria/polydipsia in dogs with a pyometra?
a. Increased thirst resulting from fever
b. Release of prostaglandin
c. Dehydration
d. Release of endotoxin

195. Which of the following drugs is the preferred antidote for ethylene glycol toxicity?
a. Acetylcysteine
b. Calcium EDTA
c. Deferoxamine
d. 4-methylprazole

196. When obtaining an ECG, how should the patient be positioned?
a. Standing
b. Right lateral
c. Left lateral
d. Sternal

197. With what is the P wave associated on an ECG?
a. Depolarization of the ventricles
b. Depolarization of the atria
c. Repolarization of the ventricles
d. Repolarization of the atria

198. While monitoring a patient you note the ECG suddenly flatlines. You immediately:
a. Start CPR
b. Auscultate the heart with your stethoscope
c. Do nothing; it is probably incorrect.
d. Check the ECG leads

199. When setting up direct arterial blood pressure monitoring, where should the transducer be placed?
a. At the level of the heart
b. At the level of the arterial catheter
c. At the level of the fluid bag
d. At the level of the monitor

200. The difference between the systolic and diastolic blood pressures is called:
a. Mean arterial pressure
b. Pulse pressure
c. Blood pressure
d. Central venous pressure

201. When measuring central venous pressure, where should the zero on the manometer be positioned?
a. At the level of the jugular catheter
b. At the level of the dorsal pedal artery
c. At the level of the left atrium
d. At the level of the right atrium

202. What is a patient's expected PaO_2 when breathing room air?
a. 21 mmHg
b. 40 mmHg
c. 75 mmHg
d. 100 mmHg

203. When preparing a patient for a temporary tracheostomy, where should the patient be shaved and scrubbed?
a. Mandible to manubrium
b. Between the cricoid and thyroid cartilages
c. The thyroid cartilage to the thoracic inlet
d. Caudal to the manubrium

204. How should a patient be positioned for a temporary tracheostomy?
a. Laterally with the legs pulled caudally
b. Laterally with the legs pulled cranially
c. Dorsally with the legs pulled caudally
d. Dorsally with the legs pulled cranially

205. When performing a thoracentesis, the needle should be placed:
a. Cranial to the rib with the bevel up
b. Caudal to the rib with the bevel down
c. Caudal to the rib with the bevel up
d. Cranial to the rib with the bevel down

206. When performing a diagnostic peritoneal lavage, how much fluid is infused into the abdomen?
a. 10 mL/kg
b. 15 mL/kg
c. 20 mL/kg
d. 25 mL/kg

207. When passing a nasogastric tube, where should the tube be measured?
a. From the nares to the thoracic inlet
b. From the nares to the last rib
c. From the nares inlet to the 10th rib
d. From the nares to the 5th rib

208. Which is the most important measure that can be taken to control nosocomial infections?
a. Antibiotics
b. Barrier nursing
c. Cleaning
d. Handwashing

209. Which of the following medications requires a filter when being administered?
a. Cerenia
b. Enrofloxacin
c. Mannitol
d. Propofol

210. A 10-kg dog requires a metoclopramide CRI at a rate of 2 mg/kg/day. The veterinarian asks that it be added to a new 1-L bag of Normosol-R. The fluid rate is 100 mL/h and the metoclopramide is 5 mg/mL. How many mL of metoclopramide should be added to the bag?
a. 0.8 mL
b. 1.7 mL
c. 3.2 mL
d. 4.1 mL

211. A dog presents to the hospital after being saved from a house fire. Its skin shows areas that are yellow/black in color, dry, and only mildly painful. How would this burn be classified?
a. Superficial
b. Superficial partial-thickness
c. Deep partial-thickness
d. Full-thickness

212. Which of the following procedures should *not* be used to cool a heatstroke patient?
a. Tepid water
b. A fan
c. Ice
d. Intravenous fluids

213. While writing in a patient's medical record you make a mistake. What should you do?
a. Scratch it out
b. Erase it
c. Draw a line through it
d. Black it out

214. What is the most likely cause of respiratory distress in a dog that has suffered from a choking episode?
a. Noncardiogenic pulmonary edema
b. Pneumothorax
c. Heart failure
d. Upper airway obstruction

215. Which of the following conditions is not a cause of central vestibular disease?
a. Neoplasia
b. Otitis interna
c. Infection
d. Inflammation

216. Which of the following techniques is appropriate for a radius fracture?
a. Robert Jones
b. Elmer sling
c. Spica splint
d. Velpeau sling

217. Where would a veterinary technician shave and surgically prep a patient that requires placement of an esophagostomy tube?
a. Left side of the neck
b. Right side of the neck
c. Left side of the abdomen
d. Right side of the abdomen

218. A patient with von Willebrand's disease requires surgery. Which product can be administered to prevent hemorrhage?
a. Cryoprecipitate
b. Fresh whole blood
c. Fresh frozen plasma
d. Packed red blood cells

219. A patient receives a packed red blood cell transfusion. How many days can pass before he will require a crossmatch for a second transfusion?
a. 2
b. 5
c. 8
d. 12

220. How many square meters of surface area are contained in one gram of activated charcoal?
a. 10
b. 100
c. 1000
d. 10,000

221. A patient will develop idiogenic osmoles in response to which condition?
a. Hypernatremia
b. Hyperkalemia
c. Hyperchloremia
d. Hyponatremia

222. What changes will be seen on the pulse oximeter of a patient with carbon dioxide poisoning?
a. It will be high
b. It will be low
c. No change
d. Normal

223. The veterinarian is concerned that a patient's platelets are not functioning properly. Which test will the doctor request?
a. Activated clotting time
b. Activated partial thromboplastin time
c. Buccal mucosal bleeding time
d. Prothrombin time

224. Which of the following bacteria is responsible for tetanus?
a. *Bordetella bronchiseptica*
b. *Clostridium tetani*
c. *Neospora caninum*
d. *Toxoplasmosis gondii*

225. Which of the following drugs would be used to treat organophosphate poisoning?
a. Atropine
b. Diazepam
c. Dexamethasone
d. Mannitol

SECTION

13 Pain Management and Analgesia

Mary Ellen Goldberg

QUESTIONS

1. The veterinary technician can play an important role in pain management by:
   a. Monitoring urine and fecal output
   b. Changing the medication when it is ineffective
   c. Communicating directly with the clinician about particular concerns
   d. Directing the veterinary assistant to provide medications
2. Which of the following characteristics do cats exhibit when they are experiencing pain?
   a. Sleeping continuously, overeating, and attention-seeking behavior
   b. Resentment of being handled, aggression, and abnormal posture
   c. Hyperactivity, pupillary enlargement, and tail swishing
   d. Hypotension, hypocapnia, hypopnea, and bradycardia
3. During hospitalization, how often should a pain assessment be performed?
   a. Every 4–6 hours
   b. Every 30 minutes to 1 hour
   c. Every 12–24 hours
   d. Every 8 hours
4. When a veterinary technician is trying to distinguish pain from dysphoria, which of the following would the technician do?
   a. Place the patient on comfortable blankets
   b. Speak in low tones and interact with the animal to make the patient feel better, but behavior resumes when interaction stops
   c. Move the animal to a different ward
   d. Reverse the analgesic medication
5. Which guidelines have elevated pain to the fourth vital sign?
   a. American College of Veterinary Anesthesiologist's Pain Management Guidelines
   b. The International Veterinary Academy of Pain Management's Guidelines
   c. AAHA/AAFP Pain Management Guidelines for Dogs and Cats
   d. The AVMA Pain Management Guidelines
6. Nociception is defined as:
   a. The activity in the peripheral pathway that transmits and processes information about the stimulus to the brain
   b. A normal response to tissue damage
   c. Pain without apparent biological origin that has persisted beyond the normal tissue healing time
   d. Any stimuli to the affected area that would normally be innocuous that become noxious
7. What is the correct sequence of steps to the pain pathway?
   a. Transduction, transmission, modulation, perception
   b. Modulation, transduction, perception, transmission
   c. Transduction, modulation, transmission, perception
   d. Transmission, transduction, modulation, perception
8. Which of the following describes "wind-up"?
   a. An increase in the excitability of spinal neurons, mediated in part by the activation of NMDA receptors in dorsal horn neurons.
   b. It occurs when tissue inflammation leads to the release of a complex array of chemical mediators, resulting in reduced nociceptor thresholds.
   c. When brief trauma or noxious stimulus result in physiological pain.
   d. The perceived increase in pain intensity with time when a given painful stimulus is delivered repeatedly in excess of a critical rate.
9. Which of the following is an example of an opioid agonist?
   a. Butorphanol
   b. Naloxone
   c. Morphine
   d. Buprenorphine
10. Prostaglandins play an important role in:
    a. Production of endorphins
    b. Mammalian cardiovascular physiology
    c. Production of leukotrienes
    d. Mammalian renal physiology
11. Which of the following is an NMDA antagonist medication?
    a. Ketamine
    b. Lidocaine
    c. Meperidine
    d. Dexmedetomidine

12. Which of the following classes of drugs would include gabapentin?
    a. Corticosteroids
    b. Sodium channel blockers
    c. Antiepileptics
    d. Nutraceuticals
13. An example of an agent that is only administered topically and provides analgesia is:
    a. Buprenorphine
    b. EMLA cream
    c. Bupivacaine
    d. Fentanyl
14. Which of the following statements can apply to an intratesticular block?
    a. Intratesticular blocks can only be used in large animal patients.
    b. Intratesticular blocks can be used in canine and feline orchiectomies.
    c. Intratesticular blocks require the use of a vaporizer.
    d. Intratesticular blocks should never been performed on veterinary patients.
15. Many veterinary technicians are asked to calculate and administer constant rate infusions because patients can benefit immensely. Which of the following statements is *not* a benefit of a CRI?
    a. CRIs provide a more stable plane of analgesia with less incidence of breakthrough pain.
    b. CRIs provide greater control over drug administration.
    c. CRIs allow a lower dose of drug to be delivered at any given time, resulting in a lower incidence of dose-related side effects.
    d. CRIs allow the veterinary technician to leave the practice for the evening while administering medication continuously.
16. Massage is an example of which type of rehabilitation technique?
    a. Manual therapy
    b. Effleurage techniques
    c. Physical modalities
    d. Therapeutic exercise
17. Which of the following is a benefit of cryotherapy?
    a. Decreased metabolism therefore patient is less hungry
    b. Decreased production of pain mediators, leading to analgesia
    c. Prevention of hyperthermia
    d. Useful 2–3 weeks postinjury
18. Which of the following describes a myofascial trigger point?
    a. A point in the muscle at which a reflex can be elicited
    b. A transcutaneous electrical nerve stimulation
    c. A painful area of sustained muscle contraction that cannot easily self-release
    d. A technique where needles are used to pierce the skin at certain points to bring about a physiologic change to treat or to prevent disease
19. Visceral pain is quite common among companion animals. Which of the following is *not* an example of visceral pain?
    a. Pancreatitis
    b. Gastroenteritis
    c. Bowel ischemia
    d. Osteosarcoma
20. Which of the following are three examples that are *all* considered chronic pain diseases?
    a. Lymphoma, diabetes, GDV
    b. Osteoarthritis, IVDD, cancer
    c. Respiratory infection, cardiac disease, blocked cat
    d. Broken leg, bronchitis, hypertension
21. Veterinary technicians that advocate pain management are most closely compared with which group of nurses?
    a. Orthopedic nurses
    b. Psychiatric nurses
    c. Human neonatal and pediatric nurses
    d. Emergency and critical care nurses
22. Which of the following is essential for good communication between veterinarians and veterinary technicians who are working in pain management?
    a. Knowing each other's routine and what is regularly done for patients.
    b. Knowledge of the physiology of pain and the pharmacology of analgesics.
    c. Veterinarians *and* veterinary technicians should have attained the Certified Veterinary Pain Practitioner status from IVAPM.
    d. Communication is not an essential skill and veterinary technicians should just do as the attending veterinarian tells them.
23. Why are the differences in expression among dogs and cats of all ages, and variations among certain breeds, important for pain assessment?
    a. Certain breeds vocalize and appear more sensitive to pain whereas others seem to remain stoic in the face of pain.
    b. Only cats exhibit facial expressions; dogs do not.
    c. No comprehensive pain scale has been developed for companion animals.
    d. Expressions are insignificant; physiological parameters are what should be used to determine pain.
24. The role of the veterinary technician in pain management includes:
    a. Patient assessment
    b. Differentiating pain from other stress
    c. Monitoring and treating drug effects
    d. All of the above
25. Which of the following might a dysphoric or delirious animal experience because of opioid overdose?
    a. Thrashing and yowling continuously
    b. Claustrophobia
    c. Only rare response to soothing interaction
    d. Chewing on cage doors
26. Which of the following behaviors is commonly associated with clinical signs of pain in dogs?
    a. Vocalization and increased appetite
    b. Playful actions and excessive licking of the owners
    c. Panting, anorexia, and depression
    d. Increased attention to the environment

27. It is sometimes difficult to distinguish normal from pain-associated behavior in cats and dogs. Which of the following is most likely to be a normal, nonpainful behavior?
    a. Decreased appetite
    b. Unusual aggression
    c. Stretching all four legs when the abdomen is touched
    d. Decreased social interaction
28. Which of the following statements regarding pain assessment in dogs is true?
    a. Physiological parameters, such as heart rate and blood pressure, are sensitive tools for assessing pain in dogs.
    b. A visual analog scale is a type of multidimensional pain scale and is useful for assessing pain in dogs.
    c. Multidimensional pain scales yield better interobserver agreement than unidimensional pain scales.
    d. Multidimensional pain scales correlate closely with vocalization and serum cortisol levels in chronically painful dogs.
29. Which of the following is the most common sign of osteoarthritic pain in cats?
    a. Hiding from company
    b. Eating fewer meals
    c. Reduced frequency of jumping up to high places
    d. Sleeping all day
30. The observer's subjective interpretation of behavior and assessment of physiologic pain can be described using a pain-rating instrument such as:
    a. Visual analog scale
    b. Force plate gait analysis
    c. Health-related quality-of-life instrument
    d. Serum cortisol levels
31. Regarding the use of pain scales in hospitalized animals, which of the following statements is *false*?
    a. Pain scales may encourage routine evaluation of hospitalized animals.
    b. Pain scales can be used to determine whether analgesic therapy should be discontinued.
    c. Effective analgesic therapy should result in an animal with a low pain score.
    d. A low pain score indicates that analgesic therapy is sufficient, even if an animal is exhibiting some questionable behaviors.
32. In cats, some diseases cause behavioral changes that are often ascribed to "old age" rather than pain. Examples include all of the following *except*:
    a. Facet pain of spondylosis
    b. Intervertebral disc disease
    c. Osteoarthritis
    d. Basal cell tumor
33. Frequency of pain assessment depends on the situation. Which of the following is the most appropriate guideline for frequency of chronic pain assessment?
    a. Every 8 hours during the postoperative period
    b. A minimum of every 3 months for an animal with chronic pain
    c. Every 12 hours for animals with traumatic injuries
    d. Yearly for an animal with chronic pain
34. The purpose of any pain scale is to:
    a. Help guide analgesic, medical, or surgical treatment
    b. Provide "concrete" diagnostic evidence
    c. Provide legal documentation
    d. Provide "happy faces" for the patient's chart
35. The preemptive scoring system is a:
    a. Visual analog scale
    b. Subjective scoring system
    c. Simple descriptive scale
    d. Numerical rating scale
36. The University of Melbourne Pain Scale is based on:
    a. Hematologic values
    b. Australian regulations
    c. Behavioral and physiologic responses
    d. Physiologic responses
37. The Colorado State University Veterinary Medical Center Acute Pain Scale uses which of the following options as an indication of pain?
    a. Number scale
    b. Recorded sounds
    c. Numeric and categoric convenient pain scales
    d. Happy and sad face drawings
38. A mental nerve block provides analgesia to the:
    a. Maxilla
    b. Lower lip and incisors on the ipsilateral side
    c. Upper lip and nose
    d. Premolars and molars
39. For which of the following can the lidocaine patch be used to provide analgesia?
    a. Skin abrasions
    b. Lacerations
    c. Hot spots
    d. All of the above
40. In a diffusion catheter, the MILA Soaker Catheter delivers the local anesthetic how?
    a. Elastomeric reservoir pump
    b. CRI
    c. Syringe pump
    d. All of the above
41. For which kind of pain would an interpleural block be recommended?
    a. Heart pain
    b. Pancreatic pain
    c. Colon pain
    d. Kidney pain
42. For which of the following would a brachial plexus block provide analgesia?
    a. Thorax
    b. Forefeet
    c. Distal to the elbow
    d. Proximal to the elbow
43. The sciatic nerve block provides analgesia to the:
    a. Medial portion of the thigh, tibia, and tarsus and akinesia of the quadriceps femoris muscle
    b. The stifle (partial) and the structures distal to it
    c. Portions distal to the elbow
    d. Lumbosacral space and the first or second intercoccygeal space

44. If a tourniquet is used when injecting a local anesthetic intravenously, the block is referred to as the:
   a. Baer's block
   b. Bayer's block
   c. Byer's block
   d. Bier's block
45. An epidural injection in a dog is injected between:
   a. L7 and S1
   b. L4 and L5
   c. L5 and L6
   d. S1 and S2
46. Which of the following statements is *not* true regarding acupuncture?
   a. The points and channels of acupuncture follow neurovascular pathways.
   b. Acupuncture treats pain by inducing neuromodulation along peripheral, central, and autonomic pathways.
   c. Acupuncture treatments can involve needling, electroacupuncture, low-level laser, and manual pressure.
   d. Acupuncture relies on nonspecific identification of the structures responsible for generating pain.
47. Which of the following examples does acupuncture usually involve?
   a. Veterinary manual therapy
   b. The use of herbs for analgesia
   c. The insertion of thin, sterile needles into specific anatomic sites richly supplied with nerve endings
   d. Diluted substances in homeopathic remedies
48. Which of the following is a contraindication for acupuncture?
   a. Pregnancy
   b. Sepsis
   c. Severe bleeding abnormalities
   d. All of the above
49. Myofascial pain syndrome entails the palpation of:
   a. Taut bands and trigger points
   b. Swollen segments of muscle
   c. Nodules of infection
   d. Nerve bundles
50. What is a substance that is naturally derived from chili peppers?
   a. Ginger
   b. Devils claw
   c. Capsaicin
   d. White willow bark
51. Examples of complementary therapy for pain management include:
   a. Acupuncture
   b. Massage
   c. Homeopathy
   d. All of the above
52. During cryotherapy, the cold temperature raises the activation threshold of:
   a. Reflex muscles
   b. Blood vessels
   c. Tissue nociceptors
   d. Painful nerves
53. When should cryotherapy be applied for best response?
   a. During the acute inflammatory phase of tissue healing
   b. After exercise to lessen inflammatory response
   c. Immediately following surgery
   d. All of the above
54. Caution should be used with cryotherapy if a patient has:
   a. A large percentage of fat
   b. Localized vascular compromise
   c. Areas of previous frostbite
   d. b and c
55. The primary benefit of cryokinetics is to:
   a. Aid the patient's ability to perform pain-free, low-level exercise
   b. Cool down a body that is overheating
   c. Allow an athlete to compete at the highest levels with no pain
   d. Take the place of local anesthetic injections in advance of athletic stress
56. Cold or white skin after a 20-minute cryotherapy session may indicate:
   a. Circulation is restored and normal
   b. Possible cold-induced tissue damage
   c. The need for external heat creams or rubs
   d. The need for more melanin in the diet
57. Cryotherapy can include:
   a. Ice packs
   b. Cold immersion baths
   c. Ice massage
   d. All of the above
58. Which of the following scenarios is thermotherapy *not* useful for?
   a. Chronic pain
   b. Muscle spasm
   c. Acute inflammation
   d. Stretching to enhance collagen extensibility
59. Treatment for joint mobility includes:
   a. ROM
   b. Stretching exercises
   c. a and b
   d. None of the above
60. Which of the following is *not* true for passive range of motion?
   a. Treatment should be in a quiet, comfortable area.
   b. A muzzle should be applied for initial treatments.
   c. The patient's limb (of interest) is fully supported.
   d. The patient's position is unimportant.
61. Which of the following is the target tissue for lengthening a muscle that is contracted?
   a. Joint capsule
   b. Muscle belly
   c. Tendon
   d. Ligament
62. Which of the following is an example of an active range of motion exercise?
   a. Aquatic therapy
   b. Walking in snow or sand
   c. Climbing stairs
   d. All of the above

63. Therapeutic exercises do not include:
- a. Pulling or carrying weights
- b. Cavaletti rails
- c. Treadmill walking
- d. Wheelbarrowing

64. Transcutaneous electrical nerve stimulation is a form of:
- a. LLLT
- b. NMES
- c. EEG
- d. EMG

65. A contraindication for transcutaneous electrical nerve stimulation (TENS) includes:
- a. Cruciate ligament reconstruction
- b. Rehab after orthopedic injury
- c. Animals with pacemakers
- d. Chronic OA

66. When should low-level laser therapy *not* be used?
- a. Over muscle trigger points
- b. Over acupuncture points
- c. With osteoarthritis and muscle spasms
- d. Over areas of malignancy or cancer

67. Massage techniques may include:
- a. Effleurage
- b. Petrissage
- c. Trigger point therapy
- d. All of the above

68. Extracorporeal shock wave treatment (ESWT) could be indicated for:
- a. Pregnancy
- b. Osteoarthritis
- c. Neoplasms
- d. Heart disease

69. Which tool is used to measure passive range of motion in companion animals?
- a. Calipers
- b. Slide rule
- c. Goniometer
- d. Oliometer

70. When should therapeutic ultrasound *not* be used?
- a. When the patient's area of interest has plastic or metal implants
- b. When the ultimate result is to decrease pain
- c. When the goal is to accelerate wound healing
- d. When the patient's ROM should be increased

71. Phototherapy can be used for:
- a. Soft-tissue injuries
- b. Wound healing
- c. Chronic pain
- d. All of the above

72. In cats, aquatic therapy is contraindicated for:
- a. Muscle weakness
- b. OA
- c. Cardiac dysfunction
- d. Geriatric care

73. An example of a proprioception exercise used for cats is:
- a. Jump rope
- b. Swimming
- c. Balance board
- d. Massage

74. Which organization requires pain to be included in every veterinary patient assessment regardless of a presenting complaint?
- a. North American Veterinary Technician Association
- b. American College of Veterinary Anesthesia and Analgesia
- c. American Animal Hospital Association
- d. American Veterinary Medical Association

75. How can pain negatively impact the patient?
- a. Treatment costs money therefore the client will refuse it.
- b. Pain promotes inflammation, which delays wound healing.
- c. Pain can induce viral diseases.
- d. Pain can cause cataracts to form.

76. Which pain scale should be used?
- a. It does not matter as long as you like it and it makes you happy.
- b. The longest and most complex is always the best.
- c. The shortest and simplest is always the best.
- d. It is important to choose one system to be used by the entire veterinary team.

77. How painful is abscess drainage?
- a. Mild
- b. Moderate
- c. Severe
- d. Extremely severe

78. How painful is an ovariohysterectomy?
- a. Mild
- b. Moderate
- c. Severe
- d. Extremely severe

79. How painful is a thoracotomy?
- a. Mild
- b. Moderate
- c. Severe
- d. Extremely severe

80. What kind of scale is a visual analog scale (VAS)?
- a. Subjective
- b. Objective
- c. a and b
- d. None of the above

81. The Colorado State Canine and Feline Pain Scales fall under which category?
- a. Objective
- b. Subjective
- c. a and b
- d. None of the above

82. Which pain scale is considered "state of the art"?
- a. Colorado State Canine and Feline Pain Scales
- b. A scale that you make for yourself
- c. Glasgow Pain Scoring System
- d. Client-specific outcome measures scale

83. How often should a pain score be given to the client?
- a. Never
- b. Every 6 months
- c. Yearly
- d. Every time the pain score is assessed

84. Which of the following parameters do horses most commonly exhibit for various states of pain?
  a. Behavior parameters
  b. Emotional parameters
  c. Physiologic parameters
  d. All of the above
85. Pain that is abnormal and *not* beneficial for the patient is called:
  a. Adaptive pain
  b. Maladaptive pain
  c. Physiologic pain
  d. Peripheral pain
86. Where can inflammatory pain occur?
  a. Muscles, joints, skin, and periosteum
  b. Thorax
  c. Abdomen
  d. All of the above
87. The most common types of pain experienced by horses are:
  a. Ocular and head pain
  b. Spine and pelvic pain
  c. Orthopedic pain and abdominal/colic pain
  d. Foot and dental pain
88. What pain scoring system is available for horses?
  a. Obel Laminitis Pain Scale
  b. AAEP lameness grade definition
  c. Horse Grimace Scale
  d. All of the above
89. Which of the following clinical signs might a cow in pain exhibit?
  a. Dull and depressed
  b. Inappetent and grinding teeth
  c. A stance with one foot behind the other
  d. All of the above
90. Goats are intolerant of painful procedures. How do sheep react to a painful procedure?
  a. They refuse to eat.
  b. They show subtle signs of pain.
  c. They always vocalize when in pain.
  d. They develop a fever from pain.
91. Squealing is a normal behavior in pigs. When could squealing be considered a result of pain?
  a. When a painful area is palpated
  b. When squealing becomes excessive
  c. When squealing involves a lack of social behavior
  d. All of the above
92. What is a benefit of using local anesthetics?
  a. Local anesthetics produce true analgesia resulting in the complete absence of pain for the duration of the block.
  b. Long-term (chronic) pain states may be diminished or eliminated.
  c. These drugs are nonscheduled agents.
  d. All of the above
93. Side effects of local anesthetics can include:
  a. Cardiovascular effects
  b. CNS effects
  c. Allergic reactions
  d. All of the above
94. Which of the following is a local block used for onychectomy procedures?
  a. Leg block
  b. Brachial plexus block
  c. Circumferential ring block
  d. Foot block
95. Of the following listed blocks, which is *not* a dental nerve block?
  a. Mandibular nerve block
  b. Mental nerve block
  c. Infraorbital nerve block
  d. Retrobulbar nerve block
96. Which block can be performed before surgery of the abdominal cavity?
  a. Sacrococcygeal block
  b. Incisional block
  c. Mental nerve block
  d. Bier's block
97. Which bones serve as a landmark for an intercostal block?
  a. Sternum
  b. Thoracic vertebrae
  c. Humerus
  d. Ribs
98. What are the advantages of an interpleural block over the intercostal block?
  a. Ability to redose easily
  b. Ease of administration
  c. Ability to provide analgesia following median sternotomy
  d. All of the above
99. Which block can be used in a castration procedure for companion animals, large animals, and exotic animals?
  a. Intratesticular block
  b. Epidural block
  c. Intra-articular block
  d. Intrapleural block
100. Which of the following is considered an excellent block that can be used for male cats with a urinary blockage?
  a. Epidural
  b. Sacrococcygeal block
  c. Pelvic block
  d. Penile block
101. Which of the following procedures is *not* an indication for an epidural block?
  a. Cesarean section
  b. Tibial–femoral fractures
  c. TECA procedure
  d. Cruciate ligament repair
102. What type of needle is recommended for an epidural catheter?
  a. Tuohy-type
  b. Butterfly catheter needle
  c. 16-gauge IV catheter needle
  d. Auto-vac needle
103. Which of the following is an indication for an epidural in a horse?
  a. Difficult parturition
  b. Caslick's closure
  c. Urethrostomy
  d. All of the above

104. What can happen to goats if they experience unrelieved pain?
  a. Faint
  b. Death
  c. Goats will roll and vocalize.
  d. Goats can suddenly become lame.

105. What type of nerve block is used to dehorn cattle?
  a. Cornual nerve block
  b. Epidural nerve block
  c. Facial nerve block
  d. Disbudding nerve block

106. In which ruminant species can an epidural nerve block be performed?
  a. Cattle
  b. Sheep and goats
  c. Camelids
  d. All of the above

107. Which of the following are goals of physical rehabilitation therapy?
  a. Decreased pain and inflammation
  b. Maintained or increased joint ROM and flexibility
  c. Maintained or increased strength
  d. All of the above

108. Benefits of massage include which of the following?
  a. Decreased muscle spasms and increased local blood and lymphatic flow
  b. Help for the patient to reach "nirvana"
  c. No physiological benefits
  d. Cannot be performed on canine species

109. What modalities does thermotherapy encompass?
  a. Heat therapy only
  b. Cold therapy only
  c. Laser therapy
  d. Heat and cold therapy

110. When starting a patient on aquatic swimming therapy, which of the following would be a main recommendation?
  a. Start the patient on a long, difficult program to increase tolerance
  b. Swim several times a day, building in 30-minute increments
  c. Slowly introduce aquatic therapy depending on patient's level
  d. Aquatic therapy swimming is recommended for all patients regardless of incisions

111. Traditional Chinese veterinary medicine (TCVM) includes what five branches?
  a. Diet and food, exercise Qigong, Tui Na, acupuncture, and herbal medicine
  b. Yin-yang, eight principles, zang-fu organs, four levels, and six stages
  c. Wood, fire, earth, metal, and water
  d. Heart, blood, spleen, lung, and kidney

112. Why is electrical stimulation used at select acupuncture points?
  a. To warm acupuncture points
  b. To release endorphins at high frequency
  c. To increase the duration of effect
  d. To cause a permanent effect

113. What is a myofascial trigger point (MTrP)?
  a. An area where muscle is excessively smooth
  b. A hyperirritable spot in skeletal muscle that is associated with a hypersensitive palpable nodule in a taut band
  c. A muscle spasm that causes intense pain
  d. None of the above

114. What is a "jump sign"?
  a. A reaction to pain from MTrP palpation
  b. When the patient has recovered and can jump high
  c. A behavior exhibited when a patient is startled
  d. A behavior exhibited when the patient receives an injection

115. In chiropractic practice, what is the role of the veterinary technician?
  a. Takes the preliminary history
  b. Conducts the initial examination
  c. Pain assessment
  d. All of the above

116. What is the definition of obesity?
  a. 10% heavier than the optimal weight for the breed in question
  b. 20% heavier than the optimal weight for the breed in question
  c. An increase in fat tissue mass sufficient to contribute to disease
  d. None of the above

117. Negative effects of obesity include:
  a. Specific disease conditions
  b. Reduced life span
  c. Abnormally high body condition scores
  d. All of the above

118. A traumatic cause of OA in dogs includes obesity as a risk factor. What is the most common traumatic cause of OA in dogs?
  a. Ruptured cruciate ligaments
  b. Torn Achilles group
  c. Hip dysplasia
  d. Phalangeal fracture

119. Which of the following statements is false regarding the negative effects of pain?
  a. Pain produces a catabolic state.
  b. Pain enhances immune response.
  c. Pain promotes inflammation.
  d. Pain increases the anesthetic risk.

120. What inhibits the aggrecanase enzymes responsible for cartilage degradation in cats?
  a. Docosahexaenoic acid (DHA)
  b. Eicosapentaenoic acid (EPA)
  c. Arachidonic acid (AA)
  d. Methionine

121. What is "porphyrin staining" in rodents?
  a. Hair standing on end
  b. Color of cage litter from urine
  c. Red tears that may encircle the eye
  d. None of the above

122. How is pain typically characterized in rabbits?
  a. Reduction in food and water intake
  b. Bruxism
  c. Closed eyes
  d. Lateral recumbency

123. What is a common cause of pain in ferrets?
   a. Arthritis
   b. Dystocia
   c. Ear mites
   d. Albinism
124. Signs of pain in birds can include:
   a. Weaving in cage
   b. Eating fecal droppings
   c. Self-isolation
   d. Aggressiveness
125. A sign of chronic pain in a reptile includes:
   a. Increased respiratory rate
   b. Restlessness
   c. Immobility
   d. Florid displays
126. Abnormal behavioral signs that could indicate pain in fish could include:
   a. Anorexia, rapid opercular movements, clamped fins
   b. Attempting to attack, eating tank mates, breathing air at surface
   c. Listing, "shimmies," curling
   d. Gasping, hurdling, drifting
127. During the initial onset of pain, all of the following physiologic changes occur *except*:
   a. Sympathetic tone increases
   b. Vasoconstriction
   c. Increased myocardial work
   d. Decreased oxygen consumption
128. What is meant by the term *noxious stimulus*?
   a. A toxic overdose of a drug
   b. A damaging or potentially damaging tissue stimulus
   c. An nitrous oxide reaction
   d. The changing of the nervous system based on the environment
129. If a painful stimulus is traveling in an afferent direction, what does this mean?
   a. Toward the area of inflammation
   b. Toward the central nervous system
   c. Away from the central nervous system
   d. Not moving at all
130. What is the minimal stimulus required to elicit a transmittable electrical signal from a peripheral sensory receptor?
   a. The action potential
   b. Polymodal nociceptors
   c. Threshold
   d. Secondary modulation
131. What are the two main nerve fiber types associated with transmitting pain sensation information to the central nervous system?
   a. A-delta and C fibers
   b. A-beta and C fibers
   c. A-nociceptors and C nociceptors
   d. Interleukins and substance P
132. Pain known as *first pain*, because it is often the first pain felt after injury, is often described as sharp and short lived. This pain signal is transmitted by which nociceptor?
   a. A-Beta
   b. C fibers
   c. Histamine
   d. A-delta
133. Which of the following correctly lists (in order) the four events involved in the pain pathway?
   a. Transduction, transmission, modulation, perception
   b. Perception, modulation, transmission, transduction
   c. Perception, inhibition, conduction, inflammation
   d. Transduction, modulation, transmission, perception
134. Which of the following terms describes the changing, inhibiting, or amplifying of an impulse within the spinal cord?
   a. Transmission
   b. Perception
   c. Modulation
   d. Inflammation
135. What is the function of the dorsal horn of the spinal cord?
   a. To sense an awareness of pain
   b. To regulate blood pressure
   c. To receive and manage sensory information from the peripheral nerves
   d. To excrete excitatory neurotransmitters.
136. Which type of fibers does the "gate control theory" state are responsible for increasing the inhibitory effects of interneurons, thereby reducing transmission of painful stimuli?
   a. C fibers
   b. A-beta
   c. Myelin
   d. A-delta
137. Pain originating from injury to the skin, muscles, joints, and deep tissues is termed:
   a. Somatic pain
   b. Visceral Pain
   c. Deep pain
   d. Referred pain
138. Where do the peripheral nerve fibers A-delta and C fibers terminate?
   a. The brain
   b. The hypothalamus
   c. The skin
   d. The dorsal horn of the spinal cord
139. What type of nociceptors respond to the release of endogenous chemicals from damaged cells?
   a. Chemoreceptors
   b. Thermoreceptors
   c. Mechanoreceptors
   d. Beta receptors
140. Which of the following chemicals is *not* considered a major inflammatory mediator of pain?
   a. Histamine
   b. Substance P
   c. Bradykinin
   d. Estrogen
141. Which type of nerve fiber is responsible for a diffuse, burning type of pain accompanying tissue damage and inflammation?
   a. A-beta fibers
   b. C fibers
   c. A-delta fibers
   d. Myelinated fibers

142. Which of the following answers represents the three zones of gray matter in the spinal cord?
   a. Dorsal horn, ventral horn, intermediate zone
   b. Dorsal horn, ventral horn, lateral horn
   c. Dorsal horn, intermediate zone, central zone
   d. Ventral horn, lateral horn, white matter
143. What area of the cerebrum is responsible for the higher processing and awareness of pain?
   a. Medulla oblongata
   b. Intermediate zone of the spinal cord
   c. Adrenal glands
   d. Somatosensory cortex
144. What type of pain can develop from damage to the peripheral nervous system?
   a. Visceral pain
   b. Somatic pain
   c. Neuropathic pain
   d. Referred pain
145. Pain arising from the skin and muscles is known as ________________.
   a. Referred pain
   b. Central sensitization
   c. Visceral pain
   d. Neuropathic pain
146. What type of pain can be felt as a result of damage to internal organs?
   a. Visceral pain
   b. Neuropathic pain
   c. Referred pain
   d. Somatic pain
147. What type of nerve fibers are responsible for carrying pain signals from the internal organs?
   a. A-delta fibers
   b. C fibers
   c. A-beta fibers
   d. Myelinated fibers
148. What nerve fibers are responsible for conducting harmless signals that provide information such as touch, pressure, vibration, and movement?
   a. A-beta fibers
   b. C fibers
   c. A-delta fibers
   d. None of the above
149. Which of the following painful conditions is *not* an example of chronic pain?
   a. Osteoarthritis
   b. Chronic otitis externa
   c. Incisional pain following castration
   d. Prolonged cancer treatment
150. Which of the following time frames describes chronic pain?
   a. Pain that lasts only 24 hours
   b. Pain that lasts minutes to hours
   c. Pain that is prolonged (days, weeks, months)
   d. The sharp pain that accompanies IV catheter placement
151. Which substance normally blocks the NMDA receptor so that it cannot allow ions to pass freely and generate an impulse?
   a. Sodium
   b. Magnesium
   c. Potassium
   d. Calcium
152. Which term describes the ability of neurons to change their structure and function in response to different environmental stimuli?
   a. Central sensitization
   b. Wind-up
   c. Peripheral sensitization
   d. Neuroplasticity
153. Which strategy can the veterinary clinic use to help decrease a patient's likelihood of developing central sensitization and all of the negative aspects associated with it?
   a. Provide comfortable bedding
   b. Discontinue vaccines
   c. Start IV fluids
   d. Provide preemptive analgesia
154. The high threshold A-delta nerve fiber is covered in an electrically insulating substance called:
   a. Synapse
   b. Neurotransmitter
   c. Myelin
   d. Substance-P
155. What is the function of myelin?
   a. To act as an inflammatory neurotransmitter
   b. To suppress central sensitization
   c. To decrease the rate of nerve impulse transmission
   d. To increase the rate of nerve impulse transmission
156. Where does the inflammatory mediator histamine originate?
   a. Mast cells
   b. Damaged tissue
   c. C fibers
   d. A-delta fibers
157. What is an area innervated by a sensory nerve fiber called?
   a. Dermatome
   b. Receptive field
   c. C fibers
   d. A-delta fibers
158. What term describes the series of events that occur within the body after a drug has been administered to a patient?
   a. Pharmacodynamics
   b. Pharmacokinetics
   c. Bioavailability
   d. Efficacy
159. Which of the following terms describes the phenomenon of drug metabolism in which the concentration of a drug is greatly reduced before it reaches the systemic circulation?
   a. First-pass effect
   b. Pass-fail effect
   c. Pharmacokinetics
   d. Pharmacodynamics

160. Which of the following does *not* play a role in a drug's rate of absorption?
   a. Route of administration
   b. Solubility of the drug
   c. Temperature of the patient
   d. Brand of syringe used
161. Which of the following terms means the amount of a drug that is absorbed and reaches systemic circulation?
   a. Pharmacodynamics
   b. Pharmacokinetics
   c. Bioavailability
   d. Efficacy
162. Which of the following is a representation of how a drug can be *eliminated* from the body?
   a. Urine excretion
   b. Digestion
   c. Biotransformation
   d. Metabolization
163. In what organ are most drugs metabolized (biotransformed)?
   a. Skin
   b. Liver
   c. Kidney
   d. Intestines
164. Which of the following words correctly identifies the tendency of a drug to combine with its intended receptor?
   a. Bioavailability
   b. Efficacy
   c. Affinity
   d. Adherence
165. A drug termed an *antagonist* has which characteristics?
   a. Affinity and efficacy are both present
   b. Affinity is present but poor efficacy
   c. No affinity and no efficacy present
   d. Affinity present but no efficacy
166. Which of the following is an example of an opioid agonist?
   a. Morphine
   b. Naloxone
   c. Butorphanol
   d. Nalbuphine
167. Which of the following opioids would be the best choice for moderate to severe pain?
   a. Butorphanol
   b. Propofol
   c. Hydromorphone
   d. Naloxone
168. Which of the following correctly lists the opioid receptor types?
   a. Kappa, beta, gamma
   b. Kappa, mu, gamma
   c. Kappa, mu, delta
   d. Delta, mu, gamma
169. Which of the following routes of administration in *not* commonly used for opioids in canine patients?
   a. Intravenous (IV)
   b. Intramuscular (IM)
   c. Subcutaneous (SQ)
   d. Oral administration (PO)
170. Opioids that are considered the most clinically useful analgesics act as agonists at which of the following receptors?
   a. Beta
   b. Mu
   c. Delta
   d. Kappa
171. Which of the following opioid analgesics is often used as a continuous rate infusion because of its short duration of action (approximately 30 minutes)?
   a. Morphine
   b. Ketamine
   c. Buprenorphine
   d. Fentanyl
172. Which of the following mu agonist opioids also has additional affinity for the NMDA receptor making it potentially useful for neuropathic pain?
   a. Morphine
   b. Methadone
   c. Ketamine
   d. Propofol
173. Which of the following opioids has been shown to cause hyperthermia in felines?
   a. Hydromorphone
   b. Butorphanol
   c. Morphine
   d. Methadone
174. Which of the following drugs is classified as an opioid?
   a. Amantadine
   b. Carprofen
   c. Ketamine
   d. Oxymorphone
175. Which of the following can be used to reverse all opioid agonist effects at all receptors?
   a. Butorphanol
   b. Naloxone hydrochloride
   c. Morphine
   d. Hydromorphone
176. Opioid agonist–antagonist drugs such as butorphanol and nalbuphine exert mild analgesic activity by stimulating which receptor?
   a. Mu
   b. Delta
   c. Kappa
   d. Somatic
177. How do nonsteroidal anti-inflammatory drugs (NSAIDs) exert their analgesic activity?
   a. Blocking sodium channels
   b. Slowing or stopping the conduction of nerve impulses
   c. Inhibition of the enzyme cyclooxygenase (COX).
   d. Nerve cell depolarization.
178. Newer NSAIDs that are COX selective have fewer side effects because they only block which isoenzyme?
   a. COX-1
   b. COX-2
   c. Kappa receptors
   d. Arachidonic acid

179. Many NSAIDs have been used for their role in fever reduction. If a drug is shown to be effective in reducing fever, we say it has ______________________.
   a. Gastrointestinal effects
   b. Antipyretic effects
   c. Renal effects
   d. Cowbell effects

180. Which of the following is *not* a technique the veterinary technician can use to prevent side effects of NSAID use?
   a. Refill the medication as soon as the owner requests
   b. Discuss adverse effects of the medication with the owner.
   c. Create a client information sheet for owners that describes the possible side effects
   d. Call owner to follow up on efficacy of the drug and any side effects the pet may be experiencing

181. Side effects of NSAIDs most commonly affect what major organ system?
   a. The gastrointestinal tract
   b. The eye
   c. The dermis
   d. The urinary bladder

182. If a client calls to report that their dog has started vomiting while taking the NSAID carprofen, what is the best course of action?
   a. Tell the client to give hydrogen peroxide to stimulate more vomiting to ensure all of the carprofen is out of the dog's system.
   b. Tell the client to give an antacid to help the pet feel better.
   c. Do nothing but monitor for further GI problems such as diarrhea.
   d. Tell the client to stop using the carprofen and have a veterinarian see the pet.

183. What drug class should be avoided when a patient is on NSAIDs because of the likelihood of adverse GI effects occurring from concurrent administration?
   a. Opioids
   b. Corticosteroids
   c. Local anesthetics
   d. Topical flea and tick treatments

184. Which of the following drugs is classified as a nonsteroidal anti-inflammatory drug?
   a. Amantadine
   b. Carprofen
   c. Ketamine
   d. Oxymorphone

185. When a patient is switching from one NSAID to another, what is the best course of action?
   a. The patient should experience a "washout" period of 3–5 days to minimize the risk of concurrent side effects.
   b. The patient should experience a "washout" period of 30 days to minimize the risk of concurrent side effects.
   c. The patient should start both drugs concurrently to minimize the likelihood of breakthrough pain.
   d. The patient should never switch NSAIDs.

186. Using which of the following COX-3–inhibiting NSAIDs is contraindicated in cats?
   a. Meloxicam
   b. Carprofen
   c. Acetaminophen
   d. Robenacoxib

187. Which NSAID is labeled for use in horses and cattle, but has extra label uses in other species?
   a. Acetaminophen
   b. Flunixin meglumine
   c. Carprofen
   d. Meloxicam

188. Which of the following NSAIDs has been proven effective in felines as an analgesic on the lower urinary tract associated with cystitis and urethritis?
   a. Aspirin
   b. Acetaminophen
   c. Flunixin meglumine
   d. Piroxicam

189. How do local anesthetic drugs function?
   a. By reducing inflammation
   b. By blocking impulse conduction in nerve fibers
   c. By facilitating the breakdown of arachidonic acid
   d. By acting as an antipyretic

190. Local anesthetics that are applied *topically* provide desensitization and analgesia to which body system?
   a. The internal organs
   b. The skin and mucous membrane surfaces
   c. The muscles
   d. The brain and spinal cord

191. Which of the following drugs is *not* considered a local anesthetic?
   a. Bupivacaine
   b. Lidocaine
   c. Meperidine
   d. Mepivacaine

192. Which of the following determines the potency and speed of onset of local anesthetics?
   a. The volume of local anesthetic infused into an area
   b. The lipid solubility of the drug
   c. The temperature of the local anesthetic
   d. The brand of local anesthetic used

193. Which of the following can be an early sign of toxicity associated with local anesthetics in dogs and cats?
   a. Hematuria
   b. Diarrhea
   c. Vomiting
   d. Muscle twitching and convulsing

194. What nerve block is commonly used to desensitize nerves and add additional analgesia to an onychectomy procedure?
   a. Retrobulbar block
   b. Epidural
   c. Circumferential nerve block
   d. Sacrococcygeal block

195. Which of the following terms is used to describe the injection of a local anesthetic into the area around a peripheral nerve to block sensory and/or motor function?
a. Spinal anesthesia
b. Regional anesthesia
c. Topical anesthesia
d. Subcutaneous injection

196. Which of the following terms describes the technique when a local anesthetic is injected into the cerebrospinal fluid?
a. Spinal anesthesia
b. Regional anesthesia
c. Topical anesthesia
d. Epidural anesthesia

197. In what types of procedures would a wound diffusion catheter with local anesthetic be useful?
a. Limb amputations
b. Radical mastectomies
c. Tooth extractions
d. Both a and b

198. To prolong the duration of action because of vasoconstriction, lidocaine is often available in combination with what other drug?
a. Bupivacaine
b. Epinephrine
c. Atropine
d. Dexmedetomidine

199. For what is EMLA cream most commonly used in veterinary medicine?
a. As a topical anesthetic to facilitate IV catheter placement
b. To desensitize the eye before ocular surgery
c. To desensitize the trachea before intubation
d. None of the above

200. Which type of nerve block is useful to provide analgesia before or after surgery of the thoracic cavity?
a. Infraorbital nerve blocks
b. Retrobulbar nerve blocks
c. Intercostal nerve blocks
d. Mental nerve blocks

201. Which of the following is *not* a property associated with the local anesthetic mepivacaine?
a. Approved for use in dogs and horses
b. Moderate duration of action
c. Metabolized by the lungs
d. Does not sting on injection

202. Which of the following drugs is *not* considered an alpha-2 agonist?
a. Dexmedetomidine
b. Medetomidine
c. Xylazine
d. Acepromazine

203. What is the name of the drug used to reverse the alpha-2 agonist dexmedetomidine?
a. Medetomidine
b. Levomedetomidine
c. Xylazine
d. Atipamezole

204. Which of the following is *not* a characteristic of alpha-2 agonists?
a. Sedation
b. Increased heart rate
c. Analgesia
d. Muscle relaxation

205. Patients given alpha-2 agonists often have pale mucous membranes and cold extremities in the initial phase because of what side effect of the drug?
a. Peripheral vasoconstriction
b. Hypothermia
c. Hypoglycemia
d. Decreased hepatic blood flow

206. In contrast to alpha-2 receptors, alpha-1 receptors produce which of the following physiological effects?
a. Sedation and muscle relaxation
b. Arousal and excitement
c. Analgesic and antianxiety effects
d. None of the above

207. Of the veterinary approved alpha-2 agonists, which one produces the most side effects because of its affinity for the alpha-1 receptor as well as the alpha-2 receptor?
a. Xylazine
b. Medetomidine
c. Dexmedetomidine
d. Atipamezole

208. Which of the following is *not* a route of administration commonly used for alpha-2 agonists?
a. Transmucosal
b. Subcutaneous
c. Transdermal
d. Intramuscular

209. What arrhythmias can be seen after administration of an alpha-2 agonist?
a. Ventricular bradycardia
b. Sinus bradycardia
c. First- and second-degree AV block
d. All of the above

210. What side effect of alpha-2 agonists would warrant their cautious use in diabetic patients?
a. Hyperglycemia
b. Initial vasoconstriction
c. Bradycardia
d. Decreased hepatic blood flow

211. Which drug is commonly used to reverse the effects of the alpha-2 agonist xylazine?
a. Dexmedetomidine
b. Levomedetomidine
c. Yohimbine
d. Detomidine

212. Which of the following does *not* function as an NMDA receptor antagonist?
a. Ketamine
b. Methadone
c. Hydromorphone
d. Amantadine

213. Which of the following is *not* an example of how *ketamine* can be administered as part of a multimodal pain therapy plan?
   a. As a continuous infusion during general anesthesia
   b. As an epidural injection
   c. When mixed with an opioid in the premedication
   d. By mouth in pill form after surgery
214. Ketamine administration would be contraindicated in which of the following disease processes?
   a. Hypertrophic cardiomyopathy
   b. Congestive heart failure
   c. Unstable shock patients
   d. All of the above
215. Which of the following drugs is an antiviral agent in human patients but was recently shown to function as an NMDA receptor antagonist similar to ketamine?
   a. Hydromorphone
   b. Methadone
   c. Amantadine
   d. Oxymorphone
216. Which of the following drugs classes has been shown to be the most efficacious in the management of neuropathic pain?
   a. Opioids
   b. NMDA receptor antagonists
   c. Nonsteroidal anti-inflammatory drugs
   d. Antibiotics
217. Serotonin syndrome can occur after patients are administered tramadol concurrently with which drug class?
   a. Antibiotics
   b. Antidepressants (SSRIs)
   c. Opioids
   d. Anticholinergics
218. Gabapentin is used to help alleviate the symptoms of neuropathic pain. Which of the following characteristics best describes the sensation associated with neuropathic pain?
   a. Burning or lancing pain
   b. Dull pain
   c. Aching pain
   d. Visceral pain
219. Gabapentin has proven useful for patients experiencing osteoarthritis pain, especially when used in combination with what other drug class?
   a. NSAIDs
   b. Anticholinergics
   c. Antibiotics
   d. Inhalant anesthetics
220. Cats with chronic cystitis are often in pain. Which of the following drugs has been shown to provide relief of pain associated with chronic cystitis?
   a. Amoxicillin
   b. Enrofloxacin
   c. Cefazolin
   d. Amitriptyline
221. Which drug is often administered to cats before undergoing limb amputation or declaw surgery to help prevent neuropathic pain and to lessen the chance of chronic pain developing?
   a. Glucose
   b. Osteoarthritis patients
   c. Cefazolin
   d. Carprofen
222. Tricyclic antidepressants are contraindicated in which of the following patients?
   a. Senior patients
   b. Gabapentin
   c. Diabetic patients
   d. Seizure patients
223. Which of the following drugs has been useful in not only reducing opioid-related nausea and vomiting, but also in reducing the MAC of anesthetic gases needed when given preoperatively?
   a. Maropitant
   b. Carprofen
   c. Morphine
   d. Hydromorphone
224. What is another term for an analgesic plan that involves combining different drug classes acting on different pain pathways?
   a. Multimodal analgesia
   b. Constant rate infusion
   c. Soaker catheter
   d. Take-home medications
225. Morphine has a strong tendency to cause physical dependency or addiction in humans. What is the classification of morphine in the United States and Canada?
   a. Schedule I
   b. Schedule II
   c. Schedule III
   d. Not a scheduled drug
226. Which of the following opioids is least likely to cause vomiting in cats?
   a. Morphine
   b. Methadone
   c. Oxymorphone
   d. Hydromorphone
227. Which of the following opioid drugs is commonly administered via a transdermal patch?
   a. Carprofen
   b. Lidocaine
   c. Morphine
   d. Fentanyl
228. What is a common problem with Fentanyl patches if they become overheated?
   a. They become ineffective.
   b. They release excessive amounts of fentanyl.
   c. They cause excessive sedation.
   d. Both b and c
229. Which of the following opioids is most commonly used for epidural analgesia?
   a. Morphine
   b. Buprenorphine
   c. Bupivacaine
   d. Lidocaine

230. Which of the following take-home medications should be reserved for canine patients only?
   a. Acepromazine
   b. Tramadol
   c. Tylenol with codeine
   d. Fentanyl patch
231. What term describes the administration of anesthetic and analgesic agents and adjuncts to calm and prepare the patient for anesthetic induction?
   a. Maintenance
   b. Recovery
   c. Premedication
   d. Induction
232. Which of the following methods is considered the least suitable choice for anesthetic induction in the canine and feline patient?
   a. IV injection of propofol
   b. IV injection of ketamine/diazepam mixture
   c. IM injection of alfaxalone
   d. Chamber induction with isoflurane
233. What term describes the type of pain that will be experienced from any surgery of the reproductive tract that involves manipulations of organs such as the uterus and ovaries?
   a. Somatic pain
   b. Visceral pain
   c. Preemptive pain
   d. Wind-up pain
234. What would be the most appropriate opioid for preemptive analgesia for a patient undergoing surgery for OVH as a treatment for pyometra?
   a. Hydromorphone
   b. Butorphanol
   c. Buprenorphine
   d. Midazolam
235. Which of the following local blocks is considered part of a multimodal analgesic plan for a castration?
   a. Ovarian ligament blocks
   b. Intratesticular blocks
   c. Infraorbital nerve block
   d. Maxillary nerve blocks
236. If your patient begins responding to surgical stimulation under anesthesia, what should the technician's next step optimally be?
   a. Turn down the % inhalant anesthetic
   b. Turn up the % of inhalant anesthetic
   c. Administer IV analgesics
   d. Administer more induction agent
237. If your patient begins responding to surgical stimulation under anesthesia and you choose to turn up the inhalant %, what next step also needs to be done to ensure your patient receives the % dialed on the vaporizer in a timely manner?
   a. Increase your fresh gas flow rate
   b. Decrease your fresh gas flow rate
   c. Start a constant rate infusion
   d. Preform local blocks
238. Which of the following surgeries would probably involve using a neuromuscular blocking agent?
   a. Ovariohysterectomy
   b. Castration
   c. Cataract removal surgery
   d. Digit amputation
239. What is the standard dose of lidocaine that should be administered as a "loading" dose before starting a lidocaine CRI?
   a. 1 mg/kg IV
   b. 2 mg/kg IV
   c. 0.2 mg/kg IV
   d. No loading dose is needed
240. What analgesic tool can be used to provide ≤72 hours of continuous analgesia for large incisions such as radical mastectomies?
   a. Wound diffusion catheter
   b. Infraorbital nerve block
   c. Intra-articular nerve block
   d. Intercostal nerve block
241. In patients with fractured ribs, what is the benefit of treating pain in advance of thoracotomy?
   a. Improved ventilation
   b. Decreased anxiety
   c. More consistent breathing pattern
   d. All of the above
242. What is the name of the regional anesthesia technique preferred for analgesia in thoracotomy patients?
   a. Intercostal nerve block
   b. Infraorbital nerve block
   c. Maxillary nerve block
   d. Intratesticular block
243. Which of the following is a risk associated with improperly placed retrobulbar nerve blocks?
   a. Hemorrhage
   b. Perforation of the globe
   c. Damage to the optic nerve
   d. All of the above are risks
244. Which of the following drugs is commonly used in the postoperative period for its combined effects of analgesia and sedation?
   a. Dexmedetomidine
   b. Propofol
   c. Diazepam
   d. Midazolam
245. Which nonpharmacologic analgesic technique can be used in the immediate postoperative period?
   a. Low-level laser therapy
   b. Icing
   c. Massage therapy
   d. All of the above
246. Which of the following opioids is the best choice of analgesic for an ER patient for whom vomiting and/or abdominal contractions are contraindicated?
   a. Methadone
   b. Midazolam
   c. Morphine
   d. Hydromorphone

247. Which of the following opioids would be the best choice for ER patients who have experienced some sort or head trauma and may need serial neurological exams?
   a. Morphine
   b. Methadone
   c. Fentanyl
   d. Remifentanil
248. Epidurals are contraindicated in which of the following patients?
   a. Patients with hind-limb trauma
   b. Patients undergoing surgery of the urogenital tract
   c. Diabetic patients
   d. Patients with a coagulation disorder such as von Willebrand's
249. For patients that have to be hospitalized long term, what is meant by keeping them in a "physiologic position"?
   a. Left lateral recumbency
   b. Right lateral recumbency
   c. Sternal recumbency with head elevated
   d. Standing
250. Chronic pain is often divided into what two categories?
   a. Nociceptive pain and neuropathic pain
   b. Somatic and visceral pain
   c. Deep pain and superficial pain
   d. Acute pain and chronic pain
251. Which drug class acts by preventing the loss of bone mass by blocking osteoclasts and helping to manage osteosarcoma pain?
   a. Opioids
   b. Bisphosphonates
   c. Gabapentinoids
   d. Neurokinin-1 inhibitors
252. Which of the following analgesic adjuncts is commonly applied topically?
   a. Gabapentin
   b. Amantadine
   c. Capsaicin
   d. Bisphosphonates
253. Which of the following demonstrates a nonpharmacological modality to treat dogs with chronic osteoarthritis?
   a. Weight loss
   b. Extra padding in sleeping areas
   c. Regular low-impact exercise
   d. All of the above
254. Which of the following neurotransmitters plays a role in the process of pain perception as well as in the vomiting reflex?
   a. Substance P
   b. TrpV1
   c. Epinephrine
   d. Norepinephrine
255. Which of the following analgesic adjuncts works to block NK-1 receptors and subsequent activation of substance P?
   a. Gabapentin
   b. Amantadine
   c. Maropitant
   d. Bisphosphonates
256. Of the inhalant anesthetics, which is the only one thought to have analgesic properties?
   a. Nitrous oxide
   b. Isoflurane
   c. Sevoflurane
   d. None of the above
257. Corticosteroids act as powerful agents in chronic pain management when used for their ____________________ effects.
   a. Opioid
   b. Anti-inflammatory
   c. Anti-nausea
   d. NMDA receptor antagonism
258. Which is the best wavelength for pain management with laser?
   a. 800–1100 nm
   b. 810–980 nm
   c. 600–800 nm
   d. 380–400 nm
259. Health Related Quality of Life is a subjective evaluation of circumstances that include ______________ and ______________.
   a. Pain and movement
   b. Pain and structure
   c. Altered health state and related interventions
   d. Anecdotal evidence and recent studies
260. How are the domains of pain evaluated in feline practice?
   a. Patient observation and physical exam
   b. Owner questionnaires
   c. Pain scales
   d. All of the above
261. What does COSM stand for?
   a. Client Specific Outcome Measures
   b. Client Standard Observation Measures
   c. Chronic Specific Outcome Measures
   d. None of the above
262. What is the first step in development of neuropathic pain?
   a. A surgical procedure to induce pain
   b. Development of a lesion in the somatosensory system
   c. Long term pain development from disease
   d. All of the above

SECTION

14 Exotic Animals

Jody Nugent-Deal

QUESTIONS

1. Which of the following may help decrease dental abrasions in pet ferrets?
   a. Housing the ferret in a wire cage
   b. Offering a raw diet consisting of bones, chicken, and green vegetables
   c. Offering a natural-prey diet or moistening dry kibble
   d. Annual periodontal treatments
2. Which of the following diagnostic tools is best used to evaluate real-time GI motility in ferrets?
   a. Magnetic resonance imaging
   b. Computed tomography
   c. Radiography
   d. Fluoroscopy
3. Which of the following is/are common presenting signs in a ferret with ibuprofen toxicity?
   a. Arrhythmia and vomiting
   b. Generalized neurologic signs
   c. Heart failure
   d. Excessive drooling and tachycardia
4. Which of the listed diseases best fits the statement that follows? It is most commonly transmitted by aerosol exposure, but it can also be spread by direct contact with conjunctival and nasal exudates, urine, feces, skin, and sometimes fomites. The incubation period is generally 7 to 10 days in the ferret. The disease spreads by viremia after it is in the body and it is almost always fatal.
   a. Canine distemper virus
   b. Influenza B
   c. *Pneumocystis carinii*
   d. Cryptococcosis
5. In ferrets, the heart is best auscultated between which of the following ribs?
   a. 5th and 7th
   b. 6th and 8th
   c. 2nd and 4th
   d. 1st and 3rd
6. Ferrets with vestibular signs demonstrate all of the following *except*:
   a. Ataxia
   b. Circling
   c. Left- or right-sided head tilt
   d. Head pressing
7. Which of the following areas contains more than half of all lymphoid tissue in the rabbit?
   a. Nervous system
   b. GI tract
   c. Urinary tract
   d. Heart and lungs
8. Which of the following is a microsporidium obligate intracellular protozoan parasite that causes neurologic disease in rabbits?
   a. *Encephalitozoon cuniculi*
   b. *Baylisascaris procyonis*
   c. *Toxoplasma gondii*
   d. *Pasteurella multocida*
9. Which of the following tools is the most useful option to help diagnose syncope in a rabbit?
   a. Thoracic radiographs
   b. Echocardiogram
   c. Computed tomography of the thorax
   d. Electrocardiogram
10. A lactating doe presents to the clinic for anorexia, depression, lethargy, and fever. What is the most likely cause of her symptoms?
    a. Septic mastitis
    b. Nonseptic cystic mastitis
    c. GI stasis
    d. Cellulitis
11. Which of the following methods definitively diagnoses *Treponema paraluiscuniculi*?
    a. Complete blood count
    b. Skin biopsy with silver staining
    c. ELISA testing
    d. PCR testing
12. A rabbit presents with a 2-day history of anorexia. You take radiographs and notice an ingesta-filled stomach with large amounts of gas in the intestines and cecum. This is suggestive of which condition?
    a. Acute GI dilation
    b. GI foreign-body obstruction
    c. GI stasis
    d. GI neoplasia
13. Which of the following can be used specifically to diagnose porphyrins in a rabbit's urine?
    a. Wood's lamp
    b. Urine dipstick
    c. Microscopic examination
    d. Urine sedimentation examination
14. In rabbits, pregnancy toxemia is most likely to occur during which week(s) of gestation?
    a. During the first 2 weeks
    b. During the last week
    c. During the 6th week
    d. During the 5th week

15. Which of the following bacteria are most often associated with antibiotic-associated enterotoxemia in guinea pigs?
a. *Escherichia coli*
b. *Pseudomonas aeruginosa*
c. *Clostridium difficile*
d. *Salmonella typhimurium*

16. Poor husbandry conditions, along with a humid environment, predispose guinea pigs to which of the following conditions?
a. *Demodex caviae*
b. *Trixacarus caviae*
c. *Gyropus ovalis*
d. *Bordetella bronchiseptica*

17. A 5-year-old intact male chinchilla presents with a 1-week history of excessive grooming, straining to urinate, repeatedly cleaning its penis, and production of several small spots of urine in the litter box. What is the most likely cause of these signs?
a. Acute renal failure
b. Urinary calculi
c. Penile fur ring
d. Urinary tract infection

18. What is the most common cause of alopecia and dermatitis in a pet mouse?
a. Fur mites
b. Dermatophytes
c. Contact dermatitis caused by pine shavings
d. Endoparasites

19. Which of the following factors does not contribute to cannibalism of the young by female hamsters?
a. Lean diet
b. Increased ambient temperature
c. Low body weight
d. Handling the mother and/or the young

20. Hypocalcemia in the sugar glider is primarily caused by an imbalance in which of the following?
a. Blood calcium, vitamin A, and phosphorus
b. Dietary calcium, vitamin B, and phosphorus
c. Blood calcium, vitamin C, and phosphorus
d. Dietary calcium, vitamin D, and phosphorus

21. An intact male African hedgehog of unknown age presents to the clinic with a 3-day history of lethargy, inappetence, icterus, and diarrhea. Which of the following diseases is most likely to cause these symptoms?
a. Acute renal failure
b. Hepatic lipidosis
c. Bacterial pneumonia
d. Glomerulosclerosis

22. Which of the following vessels is primarily used for blood collection in an African hedgehog?
a. Lateral saphenous
b. Cephalic
c. Femoral
d. Jugular

23. An Amazon parrot presents to the hospital with the following clinical signs: blunted choanal papillae, plantar erosions on the planter surfaces of the feet, poor-quality feathering, and poor skin. Its diet consists of seeds only. Which of the following diseases is most likely to cause these signs?
a. Hypovitaminosis C
b. Hypovitaminosis A
c. Hypocalcemia
d. Candidiasis

24. Which of the following values is used to evaluate renal function in an avian patient?
a. Uric acid
b. BUN
c. Creatinine
d. BUN, creatinine, and uric acid

25. For proper metabolization, ultraviolet lighting is necessary for which of the following?
a. Vitamin D3
b. Magnesium
c. Calcium and vitamin D3
d. Magnesium and calcium

26. Which of the following is not present in the reptilian urinary system?
a. Loop of Henle
b. Nephrons
c. Glomerulus
d. Ureters

27. Many species of lizards can "drop" or detach their tails if they are grabbed or restrained too tightly. This natural predatory response is referred to as:
a. Autolysis
b. Autotomy
c. Amputation
d. Dysecdysis

28. Which of the following is most commonly used to obtain a heart rate in a reptilian patient?
a. Ultrasound
b. Doppler
c. Stethoscope
d. Palpation of pulse

29. Which of the following vessels is most commonly used for blood collection in a lizard?
a. Cephalic vein
b. Jugular vein
c. Ventral abdominal vein
d. Caudal tail vein

30. Total blood volume in a reptilian patient is approximately what percentage of the body weight?
a. 5%–8%
b. 4%–6%
c. 8%–10%
d. 10%–12%

31. Total blood volume in the avian patient is approximately what percentage of the body weight?
a. 5%
b. 7%
c. 10%
d. 12%

32. A snake presents to the clinic for anorexia, striking at the owner, hissing, and a blue-opaque coloring to the eyes and skin. What is probably the cause?
   a. Contact dermatitis
   b. Fungal dermatoses
   c. Paramyxovirus
   d. It is about to shed its skin.
33. Oral examinations are most commonly performed in snakes using which of the following?
   a. Plastic spatula
   b. Gauze strips
   c. Tape strips
   d. Metal specula
34. Which of the following sites are commonly used for venipuncture in snakes?
   a. Heart and ventral abdominal vein
   b. Heart and caudal tail vein
   c. Heart only
   d. Caudal tail vein and ventral abdominal vein
35. The bones of a tortoise shell are covered with structures called scutes. What are scutes made of?
   a. Bone
   b. Epidermis
   c. Dermis
   d. Keratin
36. Which of the following species does not have a diaphragm?
   a. African hedgehog
   b. Sugar glider
   c. Box turtle
   d. Golden hamster
37. Sexing a tortoise is generally easy. The plastron in the male tortoise is usually:
   a. Convex
   b. Concave
   c. Wider and thicker compared with the female
   d. Narrower compared with the female
38. Which of the following is a condition in which uric acid is deposited into the joints and visceral organs and is caused by dehydration, kidney disease, and a high-protein diet?
   a. Hypovitaminosis A
   b. Metabolic bone disease
   c. Gout
   d. Hypocalcemia
39. A female tortoise presents to the clinic with the following clinical signs: straining, lethargy, anorexia, and bloody discharge from the cloaca. What is the most common cause of these symptoms?
   a. GI foreign body
   b. Internal parasites
   c. Hypervitaminosis A
   d. Dystocia
40. A complete radiographic series in turtles and tortoises includes which of the following views?
   a. Dorsoventral and lateral
   b. Ventrodorsal and lateral
   c. Anterior–posterior, dorsoventral, and lateral
   d. Anterior–posterior, ventrodorsal, and lateral
41. The normal feces of a parrot contain which of the following?
   a. Primarily Gram-positive organisms
   b. Primarily Gram-negative organisms
   c. An equal mixture of Gram-positive and Gram-negative organisms
   d. The feces are mostly sterile and do not contain bacteria.
42. You have been asked to obtain a blood sample for a CBC and chemistry panel from a 100-g cockatiel. Which of the following vessels is most commonly used in this species?
   a. Medial metatarsal vein
   b. Cutaneous ulnar vein
   c. Cephalic vein
   d. Jugular vein
43. A healthy bird can only lose ≤10% of its blood volume safely. You have been asked to draw a blood sample from a 1-kg macaw. What is the maximum amount of blood that can be taken from this patient safely?
   a. 1 mL
   b. 10 mL
   c. 15 mL
   d. 5 mL
44. In an avian patient, into which of the following muscles are intramuscular injections generally administered?
   a. Pectoral
   b. Epaxial
   c. Biceps
   d. Quadriceps
45. A figure-8 bandage is used for immobilization of which of the following bones?
   a. Femur, tibiotarsus, and tarsometatarsus
   b. Femur and tibiotarsus
   c. Ulna, radius, and metacarpals
   d. Humerus, radius, and ulna
46. Which of the following vessels is most commonly used for blood collection in chinchillas?
   a. Cephalic
   b. Lateral saphenous
   c. Auricular
   d. Jugular
47. Which of the following vessels is most commonly used for intravenous catheterization in a larger lizard such as an iguana?
   a. Femoral
   b. Cephalic
   c. Caudal tail vein
   d. Jugular
48. An iguana presents to the clinic with the following clinical signs: seizures, tremors, anorexia, kyphosis, pliable long bones, and a chronic femoral fracture. The patient has been housed without the proper UV lighting and has been given a diet of dog food, iceberg lettuce, and tofu. From which of the following diseases is this patient likely suffering?
   a. Gout
   b. Metabolic bone disease
   c. Hypercalcemia
   d. Hypervitaminosis A

49. A snake presents to the clinic 12 hours after suspected ingestion of a foreign body. Which of the following diagnostics should be performed first?
   a. Computed tomography
   b. Complete blood count
   c. Chemistry panel
   d. Whole-body radiographs
50. Atropine is not suggested for use in which of the following species?
   a. Birds
   b. Snakes
   c. Rabbits
   d. Lizards
51. The hydration status in an avian patient is best evaluated by assessing which of the following?
   a. Capillary refill time
   b. Venous refill time
   c. Mucous membranes for tacky saliva
   d. Quality of the feathers
52. Which of the following bones is pneumatic in the avian patient?
   a. Ulna
   b. Radius
   c. Tibiotarsus
   d. Femur
53. What percentage of body weight can be tube fed at any given time to a bird?
   a. 2%
   b. 5%
   c. 10%
   d. 12%
54. Which of the following are daily maintenance fluid amounts for an avian patient?
   a. 50–60 mL/kg/day
   b. 10–20 mL/kg/day
   c. 75–100 mL/kg/day
   d. 100–150 mg/kg/day
55. Which of the following two metals most commonly cause heavy metal toxicity after ingestion by birds?
   a. Lead and gold
   b. Zinc and copper
   c. Lead and zinc
   d. Cast iron and copper
56. A bird presents to the clinic after chewing on a galvanized wire cage for the previous several days. Clinical signs include weight loss, polyuria, polydipsia, anemia, weakness, and seizures. What are these signs and history indicative of?
   a. Lead toxicity
   b. Zinc toxicity
   c. Iron toxicity
   d. Copper toxicity
57. The pupil in birds and reptiles is made up of which type of muscle?
   a. Smooth muscle
   b. Cardiac muscle
   c. Striated skeletal muscle
   d. A mix of smooth and skeletal muscle
58. The most common cause of penile prolapse in a chinchilla is:
   a. Malnutrition
   b. Fur ring formation
   c. Improper breeding with female
   d. Bacterial infection
59. A hamster presents to the clinic with the following symptoms: diarrhea, matting around the tail, lethargy, and a hunched abdomen. Which of the following diseases is most likely the causative agent?
   a. GI stasis
   b. Cystic calculi
   c. Wet tail
   d. Dental disease
60. Which of the following drugs is contraindicated for use in a rabbit that presented for GI stasis and moderate-to-severe dental pain?
   a. Buprenorphine
   b. Fentanyl
   c. Butorphanol
   d. Hydromorphone
61. An owner calls the clinic regarding their sick guinea pig. They tell you that their pet has not eaten in 16 hours and has been "picky" with its food during the previous few weeks. They have noticed drooling, overgrooming, and small-sized feces. It sounds as if the veterinarian should examine the guinea pig. Although a diagnosis cannot be made on the phone, what is the most likely cause of the animal's signs?
   a. Cystic ovaries
   b. Dental disease
   c. *Pasteurella multocida*
   d. Trichobezoar
62. The most common neoplasia in an unspayed female rabbit is:
   a. Uterine adenocarcinoma
   b. Mast cell tumors
   c. Squamous cell carcinoma
   d. Osteosarcoma
63. Which of the following diseases causes upper respiratory tract signs including sinusitis, rhinitis, excessive tearing, snorting, sniffling, and nasal exudate?
   a. Pasteurella multocida
   b. Bacterial enteritis
   c. Allergic dermatitis
   d. Pneumonia
64. You have been asked to obtain 10 mL of blood from one ferret for blood donation to another ferret. Which of the following vessels is most likely the best choice for venipuncture?
   a. Cephalic
   b. Lateral saphenous
   c. Auricular
   d. Cranial vena cava
65. In an avian patient, what is the choana?
   a. Part of the urinary system where the ureter connects to the kidney
   b. Opening at the roof of the mouth that connects the trachea to sinuses and the nares
   c. The common holding area for urine, urates, and feces before being excreted from the body
   d. Small metacarpal bone in the distal wing

66. Which of the following bones are considered pneumatic in most avian species?
 a. Humerus and ulna
 b. Femur and tibiotarsus
 c. Tibiotarsus and tarsometatarsus
 d. Humerus and femur

67. Which of the following is *not* considered a potential complication of intraosseous catheterization?
 a. Difficulty maintaining patency
 b. Bone infection
 c. Pain
 d. Hematoma formation

68. Which of the following is the most common and largest space used for subcutaneous fluid administration in an avian patient?
 a. Wing web
 b. Between the shoulder blades
 c. Inguinal area
 d. Over the back, behind the pelvis

69. Moldy peanuts are a common cause of which of the following in an avian patient?
 a. Myotoxicity
 b. *Salmonella*
 c. *Escherichia coli*
 d. *Clostridium difficile*

70. In birds, air sac cannulas are placed into which of the following?
 a. Cervicocephalic air sac
 b. Clavicular air sac
 c. Caudal thoracic and abdominal air sacs
 d. Cranial thoracic air sac

71. Alopecia at the tail tip, symmetrical alopecia along the trunk of the body, intense pruritus, and enlarged vulva are symptoms in ferrets that indicate which disease?
 a. Green slime disease
 b. Insulinoma
 c. External parasites
 d. Adrenal disease

72. A ferret presents to the emergency clinic with anorexia, vomiting, lethargy, diarrhea, and generalized weakness. The owner stated that these symptoms started 36 hours earlier. A GI foreign body is suspected. Which of the following diagnostics would be used to determine whether a foreign body is present?
 a. Magnetic resonance imaging
 b. Chemistry panel
 c. Radiography
 d. Complete blood count

73. Which of the following is a common cause of upper respiratory disease in prairie dogs?
 a. Odontoma
 b. Mast cell tumor
 c. Adenocarcinoma
 d. Spindle cell sarcoma

74. Which of the following vessels is most commonly used for collection of a complete blood count and chemistry panel in prairie dogs?
 a. Cephalic vein
 b. Lateral saphenous vein
 c. Jugular vein
 d. Caudal tail vein

75. Which of the following vessels are most commonly used for collection of a complete blood count (CBC) and chemistry panel in the sugar glider?
 a. Jugular vein, cranial vena cava, medial tibial artery
 b. Lateral saphenous vein, femoral vein, medial tibial artery
 c. Cranial vena cava, cephalic vein, and lateral saphenous vein
 d. Jugular vein, femoral vein, lateral tail veins

76. Which of the following diseases causes an acute onset of hind limb paresis or paralysis in the captive sugar glider?
 a. Lymphoid neoplasia
 b. Cardiomyopathy
 c. Nutritional osteodystrophy
 d. Obesity

77. Which of the following species is considered arboreal?
 a. Chinchilla
 b. Prairie dog
 c. Guinea pig
 d. Sugar glider

78. Which of the following mammals has a cloaca where the gastrointestinal, urinary, and reproductive tract empty?
 a. Chinchilla
 b. Prairie dog
 c. Guinea pig
 d. Sugar glider

79. The captive diet of sugar gliders includes all of the following *except*:
 a. Chicken
 b. Insects
 c. Fruits
 d. Nectar

80. Pet skunks should be vaccinated against all of the following diseases *except*:
 a. Rabies
 b. Feline panleukopenia
 c. Canine distemper
 d. Canine parvovirus

81. A captive obese pet skunk presents with the following clinical signs: exercise intolerance, weight loss, lethargy, dyspnea, anorexia, coughing, ascites, pale mucous membranes, and cold extremities. Which disease is most likely?
 a. Hepatic lipidosis
 b. Dental disease
 c. Cardiomyopathy
 d. Canine distemper virus

82. Hedgehogs are which of the following, requiring a high-protein diet?
 a. Insectivores
 b. Strict carnivores
 c. Herbivores
 d. Nectarivores

83. A hospitalized hedgehog is offered part of a hardboiled egg as a treat. He suddenly becomes stiff and contorted, starts making licking motions with his tongue and heavily salivating. What is occurring?
 a. A seizure
 b. Self-anointing behavior
 c. Anxiety toward caretaker
 d. Wobbling hedgehog syndrome

84. You have been asked to obtain a complete blood count and chemistry panel for a pet hedgehog. Which vessels are most commonly used?
a. Lateral saphenous and jugular
b. Cephalic and cranial vena cava
c. Femoral and medial saphenous
d. Jugular and cranial vena cava

85. Which of the following diseases in hedgehogs is characterized by progressive ataxia, weight loss, paralysis, and eventual death?
a. Wobbling hedgehog syndrome
b. Tubulointerstitial nephritis
c. Hepatic adenocarcinoma
d. Plasmacytoma

86. Which of the following is the causative agent of Tyzzer's disease?
a. *Clostridium piliforme*
b. *Escherichia coli*
c. *Lawsonia intracellularis*
d. *Francisella tularensis*

87. Which statement about tularemia in rabbits is true?
a. Wild rabbits are highly susceptible.
b. Wild rabbits are the cause of most epizootic infections.
c. *Francisella tularensis* is the etiologic agent.
d. All of the above

88. Which is the correct order in the avian gastrointestinal tract descending from the oral cavity?
a. Crop, gizzard, proventriculus
b. Proventriculus, gizzard, crop
c. Gizzard, proventriculus, crop
d. Crop, proventriculus, gizzard

89. The feathered tracts in birds from which feathers originate are called:
a. Barbules
b. Rectrices
c. Pterylae
d. Remiges

90. The pectoral muscles in a bird attach to which of the following anatomical structures?
a. Keel
b. Pygostyle
c. Notarium
d. Synsacrum

91. What is the function of the operculum found in some psittacines?
a. To prevent the inhalation of foreign bodies
b. To humidify the air
c. To absorb saline from the nostrils
d. To connect the sinuses to the choanal slit

92. Which of the following is responsible for sound generation in birds?
a. Infraorbital sinus
b. Glottis
c. Syrinx
d. Larynx

93. Which of the following species lacks an epiglottis?
a. Amazon parrot
b. German shepherd
c. Persian cat
d. New Zealand white rabbit

94. Which of the following in birds is the final holding area for urine, urates, feces, and eggs before excretion from the body?
a. Choana
b. Cloaca
c. Cecum
d. Vent

95. Because of a lack of diaphragm in an avian patient, which of the following organs surrounds the apex of the heart?
a. Pancreas
b. Cecum
c. Liver
d. Kidneys

96. Bird diets that include only seeds are often deficient in which of the following?
a. Vitamin C
b. Vitamin D
c. Vitamin B
d. Vitamin A

97. Clinical signs in a bird that include loose green feces, green urates, lethargy, inappetence, ascites, abnormal beak and nails, and poor feather quality are often indicative of:
a. Renal failure
b. Hepatic disease
c. Fungal overgrowth
d. Cardiac disease

98. Most gas exchange in fish takes place in which of the following?
a. Operculum
b. Lungs
c. Bronchi
d. Gills

99. How many chambers does a fish heart contain?
a. 4
b. 2
c. 3
d. 5

100. Why is it important to maintain a reptile within its preferred optimal temperature zone (POTZ)?
a. The POTZ enables animals to metabolize drugs.
b. The POTZ enables animals to digest food properly.
c. The POTZ enables animals to heal after an injury or surgery.
d. All of the above

101. The term gravid is used for reptiles that are:
a. Oviparous
b. Viviparous
c. Ovoviviparous
d. Sterile

102. In the skin of chameleons, which of the following allows reflectivity of visible light that results in a color change?
a. Melanocytes
b. Heterophils
c. Azurophils
d. Chromatophores

103. Iguanas have teeth that are replaced many times throughout life. The teeth do not have roots but are attached to the jaw. This type of dentition is called:
a. Hypsodont
b. Elodont
c. Pleurodont
d. Monophyodont

104. Large femoral pores in the iguana are indicative of:
a. Male lizard
b. Systemic infection
c. Juvenile lizard
d. Breeding female

105. The reproductive organ in the male lizard consists of:
a. Single phallus
b. Paired hemipenes
c. External testicles
d. Bilobed phallus

106. Which of the following anatomical structures is located on the dorsal portion of the head and acts as a photoreceptor, helping to regulate hormone production and thermoregulatory behavior in the lizard species?
a. Thyroid gland
b. Jacobson's organ
c. Spectacle
d. Parietal eye

107. Which of the following species is arboreal?
a. Leopard gecko
b. Jackson's chameleon
c. Bearded dragon
d. Savannah monitor

108. Which of the following statements is true regarding carnivorous lizards?
a. They do not require calcium as part of their diets.
b. They do not require vitamin A in their diets.
c. They do not require UV-B lighting.
d. They require live prey.

109. Why is UV-B lighting so important for herbivorous, insectivorous, and omnivorous lizards?
a. UV-B lighting helps to keep these patients warm.
b. UV-B lighting helps with absorption of phosphorus and conversion of vitamin A.
c. UV-B lighting is required for absorption of vitamin C and normal behavior.
d. UV-B lighting is required for absorption of calcium and Vitamin D3 synthesis.

110. Heating a reptile cage safely can be accomplished by all of the following *except*:
a. Heat rock
b. Heater under tank
c. Ceramic radiant heating element outside the cage
d. Incandescent light bulb placed outside the cage

111. Rostral abrasions in captive lizards are most commonly caused by:
a. Fungal infections
b. Facial impact with terrarium walls
c. Trauma from cage mates
d. Trauma from feeding live prey

112. Dysecdysis is the abnormal shedding of skin in a reptile. Which of the following is a common complication resulting from dysecdysis?
a. Fungal infection of the dermis
b. Subsequent systemic bacterial infection
c. Extremity necrosis, especially of the toes or tail tip
d. Constipation caused by eating the shed skin

113. Cloacal prolapse in lizards is caused by all of the following *except*:
a. Egg laying
b. Foreign-body impaction
c. Straining to defecate
d. Septicemia

114. Diets high in purines cause which of the following?
a. Gout
b. Heart failure
c. Salmonellosis
d. Liver failure

115. Ferrets are vaccinated annually for which of the following diseases?
a. Rabies and feline panleukopenia
b. Rabies and canine distemper
c. Rabies and canine parvovirus
d. Rabies and canine coronavirus

116. The normal lifespan of a domestic ferret is:
a. 2–4 years
b. 7–10 years
c. 10–12 years
d. 5–7 years

117. You have been asked to place an intraosseous catheter in a very critical ferret. Which bone is most commonly used?
a. Radius
b. Ulna
c. Fibula
d. Femur

118. Which of the following white blood cells are predominant in rabbits?
a. Monocytes and neutrophils
b. Lymphocytes and heterophils
c. Metamyelocytes and azurophils
d. Eosinophils and bands

119. What percentage of body weight is composed of bone in rabbits?
a. 13%
b. 20%
c. 8%
d. 5%

120. Night feces in rabbits are also referred to as:
a. Cecotropes
b. Cecumliths
c. Fusustrophs
d. Colonoliths

121. Why is hay an important part of a rabbit's diet?
a. High in calories and vitamin C
b. High in digestible fiber and helps wear the teeth
c. Contains indigestible fiber that helps with weight management, dental disease, and gut health
d. Helps maintain gut motility and is high in vitamins A, D, and E

122. Oblique skull radiographs are used to evaluate which of the following in a rabbit?
a. Incisors
b. Lower dental arcade only
c. Upper dental arcade only
d. Tooth roots

123. Pain in a rabbit is often exhibited by all of the following *except*:
a. Moaning
b. Bruxism
c. Anorexia
d. Reduced grooming and activity

124. Female rabbits are referred to as:
a. Jill
b. Bitch
c. Doe
d. Hobb

125. Male rabbits are referred to as:
a. Bucks
b. Hobbs
c. Toms
d. Colts

126. What is the range of the gestational period in a rabbit?
a. 30–35 days
b. 34–38 days
c. 31–32 days
d. 28–30 days

127. What is the normal rectal temperature range in rabbits?
a. 101–104°F
b. 99.5–102.5°F
c. 100–103°F
d. 98.5–100.5°F

128. What is the normal percentage range for packed cell volume (PCV) in the rabbit?
a. 25%–35%
b. 33%–45%
c. 44%–50%
d. 50%–57%

129. Which of the following animals does not have molars that grow continuously throughout life?
a. Rats
b. Rabbits
c. Chinchillas
d. Guinea pigs

130. To keep its skin and coat healthy, a chinchilla should be offered a daily:
a. Multivitamin
b. Dust bath
c. Vitamin C tablet
d. Handful of dried papaya

131. Suitable bedding for the chinchilla includes all of the following *except*:
a. Newspaper
b. Recycled newspaper products
c. Aspen shavings
d. Pine shavings

132. Chinchillas are prone to all of the following diseases *except*:
a. Dental disease
b. Heat stroke
c. Back fractures
d. Choke

133. The average weight of an adult chinchilla ranges between:
a. 400–600 g
b. 200–400 g
c. 600–900 g
d. 800–1200 g

134. Female guinea pigs are referred to as:
a. Hen
b. Sow
c. Queen
d. Doe

135. A guinea pig presents with hind leg lameness. Physical examination findings include obesity, plantar thinning, and mild ulceration. These findings are indicative of which of the following diseases?
a. Gout
b. Vitamin C deficiency
c. Pododermatitis
d. *Streptobacillus* spp. infection

136. Scruffing is not recommended in chinchillas because of which of the following potential issues:
a. It is painful for them.
b. Fur slip
c. Scruffing is actually fine in chinchillas.
d. Chinchillas do not have enough skin around the neck region to scruff them properly.

137. Which of the following is not a sign of dental disease in chinchillas, rabbits, and guinea pigs?
a. Discharge from the ears
b. Drooling
c. Anorexia
d. Overgrooming

138. Which of the following diets is most appropriate for a ferret?
a. Oxbow Herbivore Care
b. Oxbow Carnivore Care
c. Ground alfalfa pellets
d. Sweet potato baby food

139. Which of the following species has a duplex uterus and two cervices?
a. Ferret
b. Guinea pig
c. Rat
d. Rabbit

140. The proper diet in a ferret contains:
a. 30%–40% protein and 15%–30% fat
b. 50%–60% protein and 15%–30% fat
c. 40%–50% protein and 15%–30% carbohydrates
d. 25%–30% protein and 50% carbohydrates

141. Which of the following feathers are trimmed as part of an avian wing trim?
a. Primary feathers
b. Secondary feathers
c. Tertiary feathers
d. Tail feathers

142. Which of the following does not contribute to pododermatitis in an avian patient?
a. Obesity
b. Hypovitaminosis A
c. Improper perch surfaces
d. Psittacine beak and feather virus

143. A blue-and-gold macaw presents to the clinic with the following signs: depression, lethargy, anorexia, dyspnea, nasal and ocular discharge, conjunctivitis, and biliverdinuria (green urates). Which disease should be at the top of the differential diagnosis list?
a. Papillomatosis
b. Psittacine beak and feather disease
c. Proventricular dilation disease
d. Avian chlamydophila

144. Which of the following leukocytes are usually the most numerous cells in avian blood?
a. Eosinophils
b. Heterophils
c. Basophils
d. Lymphocytes

145. Azurophils are leukocytes that are only found in which group of animals?
a. Amphibians
b. Mammals
c. Birds
d. Reptiles

146. Clinical signs of dystocia in the chelonian include all of the following *except*:
a. Anorexia
b. Lethargy
c. Straining
d. Seizures

147. The upper and lower shells of a turtle are referred to as:
a. Plastron and carapace
b. Anterior shell and posterior shell
c. Epiplastral and endoplastral
d. Hypoplastral and xiphiplastral

148. Where is the heart located in a snake?
a. In the middle of the body, similar to a monitor lizard
b. About 25% down the length of the body from the nares
c. Just below the base of the skull
d. About 2 inches below the skull

149. Which of the following statements is correct regarding the snake respiratory tract?
a. Snakes have air sacs similar to those in birds.
b. Snakes have complete cartilaginous tracheal rings.
c. Most species have a single right lung and a nonfunctioning left lung.
d. The lungs run the entire length of the snake's body.

150. Which of the following is *not* considered an appropriate bedding substrate for a snake?
a. Indoor/outdoor carpet
b. Newspaper
c. Gravel/corncob bedding
d. Cypress mulch

Answers

SECTION 1

1. d Both cardiac and skeletal muscles have a striped or striated appearance because of their alternating light and dark bands. The stomach wall, uterus, urinary bladder, and ciliary body of the eye are all composed of smooth muscles. Colville TP, Bassert JM, Clinical Anatomy and Physiology for Veterinary Technicians, ed 3, Mosby, 2016, pp. 212, 223.
2. a Blood going through the systemic circulation is under higher pressure than blood in the pulmonary circulation. Blood traveling away from the heart is under higher pressure because of the further distance it travels. The pulmonary circulation is a short distance and requires a lower pressure to complete. Equilibrium is anything balanced or the same. Partial pressure is the pressure of each individual gas. The circulatory system uses different pressures to contract blood throughout the body and cannot be at equilibrium. Colville TP, Bassert JM, Clinical Anatomy and Physiology for Veterinary Technicians, ed 3, Mosby, 2016, p. 346.
3. c In horses and pigs, diffuse attachment sites are spread diffusely over the entire surface of the placenta and the lining of the uterus. Dogs and cats have zonary attachment, where the placenta attaches to the uterus in a belt-shaped area that encircles the placenta. Cotyledons are attachments of numerous small, separate areas and are found in ruminants. Discoid attachment is located between the placenta and uterus in a single disk-shaped area and is found in humans, rabbits, and rodents. Colville TP, Bassert JM, Clinical Anatomy and Physiology for Veterinary Technicians, ed 3, Mosby, 2016, p. 492.
4. c Systolic pressure occurs when the heart muscle contracts, during which time blood is ejected from the atria to the ventricles and then from the ventricles to the systemic arteries, creating high pressure. Diastolic pressure occurs when the ventricles relax and refill with blood to be ejected during the next systolic contraction, thus creating low pressure. Osmotic pressure is the force of fluid moving from a level of higher solute concentration to a level of lower solute concentration, thus creating equal concentration on either side of the membrane. Colville TP, Bassert JM, Clinical Anatomy and Physiology for Veterinary Technicians, ed 3, Mosby, 2016, p. 357.
5. d Copulation causes the hormone oxytocin to be released from the pituitary gland of the female. Oxytocin causes the smooth muscle of the estrogen-primed female reproductive tract to contract, aiding the spermatozoa to move further into the oviducts. Estrogen and progesterone, which are produced by the developing ovarian follicles and corpus luteum, are responsible for the physical and behavioral changes in the female that are associated with the estrous cycle. Prolactin is produced by the anterior pituitary gland and is responsible for initiating lactation. Colville TP, Bassert JM, Clinical Anatomy and Physiology for Veterinary Technicians, ed 3, Mosby, 2016, p. 488.
6. b Cardiac muscle is known as involuntary striated muscle. It is considered striated because of the striped appearance of the cells. Cardiac muscles are considered involuntary because the contractions are not under conscious control. Nonstriated involuntary, nonstriated voluntary, and striated voluntary are all incorrect answers, because the function of the muscle does not occur under conscious control and the cardiac muscles contain striations. Colville TP, Bassert JM, Clinical Anatomy and Physiology for Veterinary Technicians, ed 3, Mosby, 2016, p. 223.
7. b During the conduction system of the heart, specialized cardiac muscle cells within the wall rapidly conduct an electrical impulse throughout the myocardium. This signal is initiated by the SA node and spreads to the rest of the atrial myocardium and to the AV node. The AV node then initiates a signal that is conducted through the ventricular myocardium by way of the AV bundle of His, which travels down the interventricular septum to the bottom end of the left and right ventricles, and the Purkinje fibers carry the impulses from the bundle of His up into the ventricular myocardium. Colville TP, Bassert JM, Clinical Anatomy and Physiology for Veterinary Technicians, ed 3, Mosby, 2016, p. 348.
8. a Pregnant cats (queens) and dogs (bitches) have zonary attachment, in which the placenta attaches to the uterus in a belt-shaped area that encircles the placenta. A cotyledon is the attachment of numerous small, separate areas and are found in ruminants. Diffuse attachments are attachment sites that are spread diffusely over the whole surface of the placenta and the whole lining of the uterus and are found in horses and pigs. Discoid attachment is located between the placenta and uterus is a single disk-shaped area and is found in rodents and rabbits. Colville TP, Bassert JM, Clinical Anatomy and Physiology for Veterinary Technicians, ed 3, Mosby, 2016, p. 494.
9. c Melanocyte-stimulating hormone (MSH) is associated with the control of color changes in the pigment cells of reptile, fish, and amphibians. Follicle-stimulating hormone (FSH) stimulates the growth and development of follicles in the ovaries. Luteinizing hormone (LH) completes the process of follicle development in the ovary that was started by FSH. Thyroid-stimulating hormone (TSH) stimulates the growth and development of the thyroid gland and causes it to produce hormones. Colville TP, Bassert JM, Clinical Anatomy and Physiology for Veterinary Technicians, ed 3, Mosby, 2016, p. 281.
10. d The electrocardiogram measures electrical current using metal electrodes attached to the skin in which the electrical current causes the stylus to move, creating a graph. When the SA node generates an electrical impulse and the impulse spreads across the atria, the

stylus is deflected from the resting position, creating a bump on the graph. This bump is associated with the depolarization of the atria and is called the P wave. The following waves on the graph are created by ventricular depolarization known as the QRS complex followed by repolarization of the ventricles known as the T wave. The PR interval is the time from the onset of the P wave to the start of the QRS complex. Colville TP, Bassert JM, Clinical Anatomy and Physiology for Veterinary Technicians, ed 3, Mosby, 2016, p. 357.

11. c The impulse for a heartbeat comes from the sinoatrial node (SA node), which is located within the wall of the right atrium of the heart. The signal is initiated by the SA node and then spreads to the rest of the atrial myocardium and to the AV node. The left atrium receives oxygenated blood from the lungs and pumps it into the left ventricle by means of the mitral valve. The right ventricle receives deoxygenated blood from the right atrium by means of the tricuspid valve. Colville TP, Bassert JM, Clinical Anatomy and Physiology for Veterinary Technicians, ed 3, Mosby, 2016, p. 223.

12. a In animals, a monogastric stomach is divided into five different areas. The pylorus is the muscular sphincter that regulates the movement of digested stomach contents, known as chyme, from the stomach into the duodenum. The cardia immediately surrounds the opening from the esophagus into the stomach. Rugae are multiple long folds located in the stomach. Colville TP, Bassert JM, Clinical Anatomy and Physiology for Veterinary Technicians, ed 3, Mosby, 2016, p. 393.

13. c Neurons are the nerve cells that are the basic, functional units of the nervous system and are responsible for conducting impulses from one part of the cell to another. Neuroglia cells support and protect the neurons. Schwann cells are glial cells associated with the peripheral nerves whose cellular membrane forms the myelin sheath for axons in the PNS. Oligodendrocytes are glial cells in the brain and spinal cord whose cellular membrane forms the myelin sheath for axons in the CNS. Colville TP, Bassert JM, Clinical Anatomy and Physiology for Veterinary Technicians, ed 3, Mosby, 2016, p. 142.

14. c Dogs are considered to have diestrous cycles because they only cycle twice per year in the spring and fall. Polyestrous animals cycle continuously throughout the year. Seasonally, polyestrous animals cycle continuously at certain times of the year and not at all during others. Monoestrous animals only cycle once per year. Colville TP, Bassert JM, Clinical Anatomy and Physiology for Veterinary Technicians, ed 3, Mosby, 2016, p. 483.

15. a The nervous system can be anatomically divided into two different components, the central nervous system and the peripheral nervous system. The central nervous system is anatomically composed of the brain and the spinal cord. The peripheral nervous system is made up of components of the nervous system that extend away from the central axis outward, toward the periphery of the body. The parasympathetic nervous system and the sympathetic nervous system are components of the autonomic nervous system. These two systems generally have opposite effects on organs or tissues. The sympathetic nervous system emerges from the thoracic and lumbar vertebral regions and the parasympathetic nervous system emerges from the brain and sacral vertebral regions. Colville TP, Bassert JM, Clinical Anatomy and Physiology for Veterinary Technicians, ed 3, Mosby, 2016, p. 228.

16. d The GI tract functions under unconscious control of the parasympathetic and sympathetic nervous systems, which are a division of the autonomic nervous system. The sympathetic nervous system can control the blood supply to the GI tract, whereas the parasympathetic nervous system controls the digestion and absorption of nutrients in the GI tract. The somatic nervous system provides conscious, voluntary control of the skeletal muscles. The central nervous system is composed of the brain and spinal cord, whereas the peripheral nervous system extends away from the central axis toward the periphery of the body. Colville TP, Bassert JM, Clinical Anatomy and Physiology for Veterinary Technicians, ed 3, Mosby, 2016, p. 231.

17. b The peripheral nervous system (PNS) is made up of components of the nervous system that extend away from the central axis outward, toward the periphery of the body. Cranial nerves are nerves of the PNS that originate directly from the brain and spinal nerves are PNS nerves that emerge directly from the spinal cord. The central nervous system consists of the brain and spinal cord. The parasympathetic nervous system and the sympathetic nervous system are components of the autonomic nervous system, which controls organ function and tissues. Colville TP, Bassert JM, Clinical Anatomy and Physiology for Veterinary Technicians, ed 3, Mosby, 2016, p. 230.

18. d Sensory nerves are also known as afferent nerves because they carry sensations from the skin and other locations toward the central nervous system (CNS). Efferent nerves conduct impulses away from the CNS. Efferent nerves are also known as motor nerves or efferent motor nerves because they are responsible for sending impulses to the skeletal muscles, causing muscle contraction and movement. Colville TP, Bassert JM, Clinical Anatomy and Physiology for Veterinary Technicians, ed 3, Mosby, 2016, p. 230.

19. a An initial stimulus must be sufficient to make the neuron respond, and when the stimulus is strong enough to cause complete depolarization, it has reached threshold. Repolarization is the change of a cell's charge back toward the net negative resting membrane potential. When a neuron is in the refractory period it is insensitive to new stimuli until it recovers from the previous nerve impulse. Action potential is a strong influx of sodium ions during depolarization, which results in a significant change in electrical charge from negative to positive. Colville TP, Bassert JM, Clinical Anatomy and Physiology for Veterinary Technicians, ed 3, Mosby, 2016, p. 233.

20. d Local anesthetics prevent sensory nerves from depolarizing despite the painful stimulation. If these sensory nerves do not depolarize, the brain is unaware of any sensation occurring in that area of the body. Local anesthetics prevent the sensory neuron from depolarizing by blocking the sodium channels preventing sodium from traveling inside the neuronal cell. If the sodium channels are blocked, this results in no positive charge to flow within the neuron, the charge remains negative, and threshold is not obtained. Potassium gates open when repolarization occurs, which results in a net negative charge inside the cell. Colville TP, Bassert JM, Clinical Anatomy and Physiology for Veterinary Technicians, ed 3, Mosby, 2016, p. 234.

21. b Smooth muscles are found all over the body in places such as the stomach, intestines, urinary bladder, blood vessels, reproductive tract, and eyes. Cardiac muscles are striated muscles. Pelvic limb consists of skeletal muscles that aid in movement of the bones of the skeleton. Voluntary striated skeletal muscles are in charge of breathing, swallowing, and posture, and may be found in the diaphragm. Colville TP, Bassert JM, Clinical Anatomy and Physiology for Veterinary Technicians, ed 3, Mosby, 2016, p. 140.

22. c Both smooth and cardiac muscles contain single nuclei, whereas skeletal muscles contain multiple nuclei. Colville TP, Bassert JM, Clinical Anatomy and Physiology for Veterinary Technicians, ed 3, Mosby, 2016, p. 140.

23. a Cattle and swine have polyestrous cycles because they cycle continuously throughout the year if they are not pregnant; as soon as one cycle ends, another begins. Seasonally polyestrous is an estrous cycle that occurs at certain times of the year. Diestrous cycles are animals that have two cycles per year. Monoestrous animals cycle only once per year. Colville TP, Bassert JM, Clinical Anatomy and Physiology for Veterinary Technicians, ed 3, Mosby, 2016, p. 483.

24. d In most species, ovulation occurs near the end of estrus. However, cats, ferrets, and rabbits only ovulate when breeding occurs. These animals are known as induced ovulators because they remain in a prolonged state of estrous if they are not bred. For bovine, equine, and canine animals, ovulation occurs near the end of estrus regardless of being bred. Colville TP, Bassert JM, Clinical Anatomy and Physiology for Veterinary Technicians, ed 3, Mosby, 2016, p. 483.

25. c Metestrus is the period after ovulation and is the stage of the estrous cycle when the corpus luteum develops. The corpus luteum is a solid structure that results when the granulosa cells left in the empty follicle multiply. Proestrus is the period of follicular development in the ovary. Estrus is the heat period or the period of sexual receptivity in the female. Diestrous is the active, luteal stage, when the corpus luteum has reached maximum size and exerts its maximum effect. Colville TP, Bassert JM, Clinical Anatomy and Physiology for Veterinary Technicians, ed 3, Mosby, 2016, p. 483.

26. b Pupil dilation results from sympathetic system stimulation. The heart rate decreases as a result of parasympathetic nervous system stimulation. Decreased GI motility results from sympathetic system stimulation. Bronchodilations result from sympathetic system stimulation. Colville TP, Bassert JM, Clinical Anatomy and Physiology for Veterinary Technicians, ed 3, Mosby, 2016, p. 246.

27. a The hormones produced in the ovaries fall into two categories: estrogen and progestins. The cell of developing ovarian follicles produces estrogen. Progestins, or progesterone, are produced by the corpus luteum, which develops from the empty follicle after ovulation. Prolactin is produced by the anterior pituitary gland. Oxytocin is produced by the posterior pituitary gland. Colville TP, Bassert JM, Clinical Anatomy and Physiology for Veterinary Technicians, ed 3, Mosby, 2016, p. 480.

28. a Implantation is the means by which the blastocyst makes itself a home by attaching itself to the lining of the uterus, known as the endometrium. The placenta is a complex structure that begins to form as soon as the blastocyst implants into the uterus. Spermatozoa travel to the oviducts to prepare for capacitation before fertilization with the ovum. The cervix is located in the upper level of the vaginal canal and is the opening to the uterus. Colville TP, Bassert JM, Clinical Anatomy and Physiology for Veterinary Technicians, ed 3, Mosby, 2016, p. 491.

29. a Parturition is the birth process. Gestation is the period and duration of pregnancy. Lactation is milk production by the mammary gland. Estrous is the heat period, which is the stage of the estrous cycle when the female is sexually receptive to the male, which will allow breeding to take place. Colville TP, Bassert JM, Clinical Anatomy and Physiology for Veterinary Technicians, ed 3, Mosby, 2016, p. 482.

30. c Estrogen is produced first by the developing ovarian follicles and prepares the animal for breeding and pregnancy. Progesterone comes next and is produced by the corpus luteum and prepares the uterus for implantation and maintains the pregnancy. Last, oxytocin causes contractions for parturition. Colville TP, Bassert JM, Clinical Anatomy and Physiology for Veterinary Technicians, ed 3, Mosby, 2016, p. 495.

31. d The area where the chorion attaches to the lining of the uterus is where the fetal and maternal blood vessels intertwine with each other. The exchange of nutrients and wastes takes place here, between the fetal and maternal bloodstreams. The type of attachment varies among species but can be categorized into one of four general types: diffuse, cotyledonary, zonary, or discoid. Colville TP, Bassert JM, Clinical Anatomy and Physiology for Veterinary Technicians, ed 3, Mosby, 2016, p. 492.

32. a Dogs and cats have zonary attachment, in which the placenta attaches to the uterus in a belt-shaped area that encircles the placenta. Cotyledonary is an attachment of numerous small, separate areas and found in ruminants. Diffuse attachments are sites that are spread diffusely over the whole surface of the placenta and the whole lining of the uterus and they are found in horses and pigs. Discoid attachment is located between the placenta and uterus is a single disk-shaped area and is found in humans, rabbits, and rodents. Colville TP, Bassert JM, Clinical Anatomy and Physiology for Veterinary Technicians, ed 3, Mosby, 2016, p. 493.

33. b In common domestic animals, including canines, the uterus is Y-shaped, with the uterine body forming the base of the Y and the two uterine horns forming the arms. Colville TP, Bassert JM, Clinical Anatomy and Physiology for Veterinary Technicians, ed 3, Mosby, 2016, p. 482.

34. a The number of mammary glands varies but there are usually 10: four thoracic glands, four abdominal glands, and two inguinal glands. Pigs typically have 14 mammary glands. Cattle typically have 4 mammary glands. Colville TP, Bassert JM, Clinical Anatomy and Physiology for Veterinary Technicians, ed 3, Mosby, 2016, p. 497.

35. d The heart rate decreases as a result of parasympathetic nervous system stimulation. Bronchodilation results from sympathetic system stimulation. Pupil dilation results from sympathetic system stimulation. Decreased GI motility results from sympathetic system stimulation. Colville TP, Bassert JM, Clinical Anatomy and Physiology for Veterinary Technicians, ed 3, Mosby, 2016, p. 224.

36. a Epinephrine is released primarily from the adrenal medulla and plays more of a role as a hormone in the fight-or-flight reactions of the sympathetic nervous system. Acetylcholine is either an excitatory or an inhibitory neurotransmitter and stimulates muscle fibers to contract. This affects the heart rate. Dopamine is involved with autonomic functions and muscle control. Serotonin is a neurotransmitter that is involved in the transmission of nerve impulses. Colville TP, Bassert JM, Clinical Anatomy and Physiology for Veterinary Technicians, ed 3, Mosby, 2016, p. 237.

37. a The impulse for a heartbeat comes from the sinoatrial node or SA node and is referred to as the pacemaker of the heart. Purkinje fibers are specialized fibers located in the ventricles and receive impulses from the AV nodes. The AV node initiates a signal that is conducted through the ventricular myocardium by way of the AV bundle of His and Purkinje fibers. The vagus nerve is a nerve of the parasympathetic nervous system that is involved in regulating GI motility and secretion. Colville TP, Bassert JM, Clinical Anatomy and Physiology for Veterinary Technicians, ed 3, Mosby, 2016, p. 223.

38. d The T wave on an electrocardiogram is associated with ventricular repolarization. The P wave is associated with atrial depolarization. The QRS complex is associated with ventricular depolarization. Colville TP, Bassert JM, Clinical Anatomy and Physiology for Veterinary Technicians, ed 3, Mosby, 2016, p. 358.

39. a The pressure within the thorax is negative compared with atmospheric pressure. Without negative intrathoracic pressure, normal breathing cannot take place. On inspiration, air is pulled into the lungs and blown back out with expiration. Colville TP, Bassert JM, Clinical Anatomy and Physiology for Veterinary Technicians, ed 3, Mosby, 2016, p. 372.

40. a As the CO_2 level in the blood rises, the pH of the blood goes down, indicating that the blood is becoming more acidic. If the chemical system detects a rise in the blood level of CO_2 and a decrease in the blood pH, the respiratory center is triggered to increase the rate and depth of respiration so that more CO_2 can be eliminated. Colville TP, Bassert JM, Clinical Anatomy and Physiology for Veterinary Technicians, ed 3, Mosby, 2016, p. 363.

41. d The packed cell volume (PCV) can be used as a screening for dehydration, which causes polycythemia and hemoconcentration. A decrease in PCV is indicative of anemia. Leukocytosis is an increase in the number of white blood cells. Colville TP, Bassert JM, Clinical Anatomy and Physiology for Veterinary Technicians, ed 3, Mosby, 2016, p. 300.

42. c Apnea is the cessation of breathing for a period of time, which will result in an increase in blood level of CO_2 and a decrease in blood pH, resulting in respiratory acidosis. Respiratory alkalosis is a rise in pH and a decrease in CO_2 because of hyperventilation. Metabolic acidosis results from the blood being too acidic. Metabolic alkalosis results from the blood being too alkaline. Colville TP, Bassert JM, Clinical Anatomy and Physiology for Veterinary Technicians, ed 3, Mosby, 2016, p. 376.

43. b Gluconeogenesis is the production of glucose from amino acids, which occurs in the liver. Long-chain fatty acids help to build cell membrane structure, produce energy, or form nerve cells. Vitamin C helps the growth and repair of tissues in all parts of the body. Iron aids in many functions, such as helping muscle to store and use oxygen and is part of hemoglobin in the blood. Colville TP, Bassert JM, Clinical Anatomy and Physiology for Veterinary Technicians, ed 3, Mosby, 2016, p. 402.

44. c A cataract is an abnormal condition of the eye whereby the lens becomes opaque. The lens of the eye normally has a transparent appearance and when a cataract is present the lens appears milky. The cornea is a transparent window that admits light to the interior of the eye, which consists of an orderly arrangement of collagen fibers and contains no blood vessels. Vitreous humor is the clear gelatinous fluid within the vitreous compartment located behind the lens and ciliary body. Aqueous humor is a clear watery fluid within the aqueous compartment located in front of the lens and ciliary body. Colville TP, Bassert JM, Clinical Anatomy and Physiology for Veterinary Technicians, ed 3, Mosby, 2016, p. 268.

45. a The choroid is located between the sclera and retina. It consists mainly of pigment and blood vessels that supply blood to the retina. The iris is located toward the front of the eye, lies in the middle vascular layer, and is the colored part of the eye. The pupil is centered within the iris of the eye and is controlled by the iris. The cornea is the outer fibrous layer and is the transparent window that admits light to the interior. The optic nerve is located in the back of the eye and carries visual information to the brain. The fovea centralis is located in the center of the retina in humans and is not part of the animal anatomy. Colville TP, Bassert JM, Clinical Anatomy and Physiology for Veterinary Technicians, ed 3, Mosby, 2016, p. 266.

46. d Lipids are organic molecules that are soluble in other lipids and in organic solvents and can be divided into four major categories: neutral fats, phospholipids, steroids, and other lipoid substances. Colville TP, Bassert JM, Clinical Anatomy and Physiology for Veterinary Technicians, ed 3, Mosby, 2016, p. 34.

47. d The hormone insulin is essential for life and causes glucose, amino acids, and fatty acids in the bloodstream to be absorbed through cell membranes into body cells and it is used for energy. Increased blood pressure is not a function of insulin. Colville TP, Bassert JM, Clinical Anatomy and Physiology for Veterinary Technicians, ed 3, Mosby, 2016, p. 287.

48. a The main endocrine cells of the pancreatic islets are alpha cells, which produce glucagon. Beta cells produce insulin. Delta cells produce somatostatin. Colville TP, Bassert JM, Clinical Anatomy and Physiology for Veterinary Technicians, ed 3, Mosby, 2016, p. 287.
49. c Glucocorticoid drugs are commonly used for their anti-inflammatory effect and can mimic the natural glucocorticoid hormones but can have the following long-term effects: suppression of the immune response because it can lower an animal's defenses and make it more susceptible to infection; white blood cell count alteration because neutrophil numbers increase and lymphocyte, eosinophil, and monocyte numbers decrease; premature parturition; hyperglycemia; suppression of the adrenal cortex stimulation; catabolic effects; slowing of wound healing; and iatrogenic hyperadrenocorticism. Colville TP, Bassert JM, Clinical Anatomy and Physiology for Veterinary Technicians, ed 3, Mosby, 2016, p. 286.
50. d Nociceptors are also known as pain receptors and are the most common and widely distributed sensory receptor inside the body and on its surface. Their purpose is to protect the body from damage by alerting the CNS to potentially harmful stimuli. Color, warmth, and lactic acid do not fall under the categories of harmful stimuli. Colville TP, Bassert JM, Clinical Anatomy and Physiology for Veterinary Technicians, ed 3, Mosby, 2016, p. 256.
51. d Visceral sensations include interior body sensations such as hunger, thirst, and full urinary bladder. Tactile sensations include touch and pressure sensation to the outside of the body. Proprioception is the sense of body position and movement. Colville TP, Bassert JM, Clinical Anatomy and Physiology for Veterinary Technicians, ed 3, Mosby, 2016, p. 254.
52. a The vagus nerve is classified as nerve X out of XII cranial nerves. Colville TP, Bassert JM, Clinical Anatomy and Physiology for Veterinary Technicians, ed 3, Mosby, 2016, p. 242.
53. c The brainstem's role is to maintain the basic support functions of the body and many of the cranial nerves originate from here. The cerebellum is located caudal to the cerebrum and allows the body to have coordinated movement, balance, posture, and complex reflexes. The spinal cord is the caudal continuation of the brainstem outside the skull and conducts sensory information and motor instructions between the brain and the periphery of the body. The cerebrum is made up of gray matter of the cerebral cortex and white matter fibers beneath the cortex, including the corpus callosum, and constitutes functions of higher-order behaviors. Colville TP, Bassert JM, Clinical Anatomy and Physiology for Veterinary Technicians, ed 3, Mosby, 2016, p. 242.
54. c Glaucoma is characterized as a group of diseases that cause increased intraocular pressure within the anterior chamber of the eye. Glaucoma results when there is insufficient drainage of aqueous humor, rather than overproduction, within the anterior chamber, which leads to the increased internal pressure. Colville TP, Bassert JM, Clinical Anatomy and Physiology for Veterinary Technicians, ed 3, Mosby, 2016, p. 267.
55. a Aqueous humor is formed in the posterior chamber of the eye by cells of the ciliary body. It slowly circulates through the pupil into the anterior chamber and is drained by the canal of Schlemm. The cornea is the front surface of the eye that provides a transparent window to the inside of the eye. Colville TP, Bassert JM, Clinical Anatomy and Physiology for Veterinary Technicians, ed 3, Mosby, 2016, p. 267.
56. d The tympanic membrane is commonly referred to as the eardrum and is a paper-thin tissue membrane that is stretched across the opening between the external auditory canal and the middle ear cavity. The oval window and round window are parts of the inner ear structure and are located behind the tympanic membrane at the base of the cochlea. The cochlea is part of the inner ear located behind the tympanic membrane and is contained in a spiral cavity shaped like a snail shell in the temporal bone and is the hearing portion of the inner ear. Colville TP, Bassert JM, Clinical Anatomy and Physiology for Veterinary Technicians, ed 3, Mosby, 2016, p. 258.
57. d Hypothyroidism results from a deficiency of thyroid hormone. Common clinical signs of hypothyroidism are weight gain, reluctance to exercise, lethargy, dry skin, alopecia, and increased appetite. Excessive water consumption is not associated with hypothyroidism. Colville TP, Bassert JM, Clinical Anatomy and Physiology for Veterinary Technicians, ed 3, Mosby, 2016, p. 284.
58. d Milk letdown is the immediate effect of nursing or milking. When nursing or milking occurs, sensory nerve impulses are sent to the brain in which the hypothalamus stimulates the anterior pituitary gland to produce the hormones necessary to maintain lactation. The hypothalamus releases oxytocin from the posterior pituitary gland, which travels to the mammary gland and causes muscle-like myoepithelial cells around the alveoli and small ducts to contract and squeeze milk down into the large ducts and sinuses. Adrenalin, norepinephrine, and dopamine are not associated with milk letdown. Colville TP, Bassert JM, Clinical Anatomy and Physiology for Veterinary Technicians, ed 3, Mosby, 2016, p. 282.
59. b Prolactin helps to trigger and maintain lactation. After lactation has begun, prolactin production and release by the anterior pituitary gland continue as long as the teat or nipple continues to be stimulated by nursing or milking. Follicle-stimulating hormone (FSH) stimulates the growth and development of follicles in the ovaries. Luteinizing hormone (LH) completes the process of follicle development in the ovary that was started by FSH. Thyroid-stimulating hormone (TSH) stimulates the growth and development of the thyroid gland and causes it to produce its hormones. Colville TP, Bassert JM, Clinical Anatomy and Physiology for Veterinary Technicians, ed 3, Mosby, 2016, p. 280.
60. c Mandibular lymph nodes are located behind each side of the jaw in the neck region and drain the nasal cavity, mouth, and pharynx. Popliteal nodes are located posterior to the knee. Inguinal nodes are located in the groin area. Prescapular nodes are located in front of the scapular region. Aspinall V, Cappello M, Introduction to Veterinary Anatomy and Physiology Textbook, ed 2, Butterworth Heinemann, 2009, p. 87.

61. d Discoid attachment is located between the placenta and uterus is a single disk-shaped area and is found in rodents and rabbits. Dogs and cats have zonary attachments that the placenta attaches to the uterus in a belt-shaped area that encircles the placenta. Cotyledonary is an attachment of numerous small, separate areas and found in ruminants. Diffuse attachment sites that are spread diffusely over the whole surface of the placenta and the whole lining of the uterus are found in horses and pigs. Colville TP, Bassert JM, Clinical Anatomy and Physiology for Veterinary Technicians, ed 3, Mosby, 2016, p. 494.
62. a The pituitary gland contains two sections, the anterior pituitary and the posterior pituitary. The caudal portion of the pituitary gland is called the posterior pituitary or the neurohypophysis. The hypothalamus is part of the diencephalon of the brain. The adrenal gland is located near the cranial ends of the kidneys and contains the adrenal cortex and adrenal medulla. The pancreas is a long, flat, abdominal organ near the duodenum. Colville TP, Bassert JM, Clinical Anatomy and Physiology for Veterinary Technicians, ed 3, Mosby, 2016, p. 279.
63. b Blood flows directly to the liver via the hepatic portal vein. The portal vein does not attach to the spleen or the heart. The spleen acts as storage for excess blood. Kidneys receive their blood via the renal arteries attached to the aorta. Blood travels from the heart to the lungs to become oxygenated before being circulated through the rest of the body. Colville TP, Bassert JM, Clinical Anatomy and Physiology for Veterinary Technicians, ed 3, Mosby, 2016, p. 405.
64. a Using anatomical directional terms, movement from a point between the eyes to the tip of the dog's nose would be known as moving rostrally. Movement cranially is any movement toward the animal's head. Movement caudally is any movement toward the animal's tail. Movement laterally is any movement away from the median plane. Colville TP, Bassert JM, Clinical Anatomy and Physiology for Veterinary Technicians, ed 3, Mosby, 2016, p. 5.
65. c On average, blood makes up between 6% and 8% of an animal's total lean body weight. Colville TP, Bassert JM, Clinical Anatomy and Physiology for Veterinary Technicians, ed 3, Mosby, 2016, p. 315.
66. b A dog that weighs 10 kg or 22 lb would have approximately 880 mL of total blood volume. 22 lb × 8% = 1.76 lbs. 1 pt of water = 1 lb. 1.76 lb = 1.76 pt. 2 pt = 1 qt, then 1.76 pt × 2 = 0.88 qt or 0.88 L. By converting L into mL, this animal has a blood volume of 880 mL. Colville TP, Bassert JM, Clinical Anatomy and Physiology for Veterinary Technicians, ed 3, Mosby, 2016, p. 315.
67. a In common domestic animals, the thoracic limb has no direct, bony connection with the axial skeleton. The forelegs support the weight of the body by a sling-like arrangement of muscles and tendons; therefore, an incision can be made in this location without cutting through a bone-to-bone joint. The hind/pelvic limb is directly connected to the axial skeleton through the sacroiliac joint. The vertebral column is made up of a series of individual irregular bones called vertebrae that extend from the skull to the tip of the tail. The tail is a continuance of the spinal column. Colville TP, Bassert JM, Clinical Anatomy and Physiology for Veterinary Technicians, ed 3, Mosby, 2016, p. 193.
68. a The occipital bone is a single bone that forms the caudoventral portion or base of the skull. The frontal bone forms the forehead region of the skull. The temporal bones are located below or ventral to the parietal bones. The parietal bones form the dorsolateral walls of the cranium. Colville TP, Bassert JM, Clinical Anatomy and Physiology for Veterinary Technicians, ed 3, Mosby, 2016, p. 182.
69. a Glycogenesis is the process of glucose absorbed from the GI tract stored in the liver as glycogen. Gluconeogenesis is the process of glucose being made in the liver from amino acids. Glycogenolysis is the breakdown of glycogen by the liver back into glucose and moved to the blood. Fatty acid synthesis is the initial process of converting glucose into fat. Colville TP, Bassert JM, Clinical Anatomy and Physiology for Veterinary Technicians, ed 3, Mosby, 2016, p. 408.
70. b Voice production is called phonation and it typically begins in the larynx, also known as the voice box. Other structures such as the thorax, nose, mouth, pharynx, and sinuses may contribute resonance and other characteristics to the vocal cords. Colville TP, Bassert JM, Clinical Anatomy and Physiology for Veterinary Technicians, ed 3, Mosby, 2016, p. 363.
71. c A nutrient is a substance derived from food that is used by the body to perform all of its normal functions. Nutrients are divided into six categories: water, carbohydrates, lipids, proteins, vitamins, and minerals. Colville TP, Bassert JM, Clinical Anatomy and Physiology for Veterinary Technicians, ed 3, Mosby, 2016, p. 417.
72. a Efferent nerves conduct nerve impulses away from the CNS out toward muscles and other organs. Afferent nerves conduct impulses toward the CNS; they conduct sensations from the sensory receptors in the skin and other locations in the body to the CNS. Colville TP, Bassert JM, Clinical Anatomy and Physiology for Veterinary Technicians, ed 3, Mosby, 2016, p. 231.
73. b Pancreatic lipases penetrate the bile acid coating and digest the fat molecules to produce glycerol, fatty acids, and monoglycerides. This results in the droplet fragmenting into even smaller pieces called micelles. These bile acid–lipid component micelles allow the lipid components to diffuse readily through the water contents of the intestine and to come in contact with the brush border of the intestinal wall, where they are absorbed. Low-density lipoproteins (LDL) are molecules that are a combination of lipid and protein and transport lipids in the blood. Very low-density lipoproteins (VLDL) move cholesterol, triglycerides, and other lipids around the body. Lymph from the digestive system is called chyle. After a meal, the chyle contains microscopic particles of fat known as chylomicrons that cause the lymph to appear white or pale yellow and cloudy. Colville TP, Bassert JM, Clinical Anatomy and Physiology for Veterinary Technicians, ed 3, Mosby, 2016, p. 406.
74. d There are only three types of RNA that have unique roles in protein synthesis. Transfer RNA copies the information in the DNA molecule, messenger RNA

carries the information out of the nucleus, and ribosomal RNA uses the information to create the proteins needed by the body. Colville TP, Bassert JM, Clinical Anatomy and Physiology for Veterinary Technicians, ed 3, Mosby, 2016, p. 42.

75. c Bile acids have a hydrophilic (water-loving) and a hydrophobic (water-fearing, fat-loving) end. The bile acids stick the hydrophobic end into the fat droplet, leaving the hydrophilic end exposed to the environment of the intestinal tract, aiding in the digestion of fat. Carbohydrates are broken down and digested by means of the enzyme amylase. Electrolytes are absorbed intact into the small intestine wall. Proteins are large molecules that must be reduced by proteases to their elemental form of amino acids or dipeptides before they can be absorbed, in which gastric pepsin breaks apart some of the protein chains. Colville TP, Bassert JM, Clinical Anatomy and Physiology for Veterinary Technicians, ed 3, Mosby, 2016, p. 406.

76. a Insulin is released in response to elevated blood glucose levels; its action is to move the glucose from the blood into the tissues of the body, thereby effectively supplying the cells with the nutrition they need to function and lowering the concentration of glucose in the blood. Glucagon, produced by the alpha cells in the pancreas, antagonizes insulin by mobilizing glucose from the liver via gluconeogenesis and glycogenolysis. Epinephrine is released in the body by the adrenal medulla as part of the flight-or-fight response. Glucocorticoids are hormones released by the adrenal cortex, which increases blood glucose and plays a role in blood pressure maintenance. Colville TP, Bassert JM, Clinical Anatomy and Physiology for Veterinary Technicians, ed 3, Mosby, 2016, p. 280.

77. a The integument is one of the largest and most extensive organ systems in the body and is composed of all four tissue types that cover and protect the underlying structures of the body. The cardiovascular system involves the pumping of the heart, which pumps oxygen and nutrients throughout the body but is not considered the largest system. The digestive system, involving multiple organs aiding in the digestion and absorption of essential nutrients, is also not the largest. The CNS, although it is a complex communication and control system in the animal body, is also not the largest. Colville TP, Bassert JM, Clinical Anatomy and Physiology for Veterinary Technicians, ed 3, Mosby, 2016, p. 148.

78. d The nucleotide thymine is only found in DNA. Adenine, cytosine, and guanine are all found in both DNA and RNA. Colville TP, Bassert JM, Clinical Anatomy and Physiology for Veterinary Technicians, ed 3, Mosby, 2016, p. 67.

79. a The SA node generates an electrical impulse and the impulse spreads across the atria. The bump in the graph associated with the depolarization of the atria creating atrial contraction is called the P wave. The QRS complex is created by ventricular depolarization and by repolarization of the ventricles corresponding with the T wave. Electrical current generated by the SA node travels through the AV node and Purkinje fibers and, after it passes through the cardiac muscle, the muscle contracts. Colville TP, Bassert JM, Clinical Anatomy and Physiology for Veterinary Technicians, ed 3, Mosby, 2016, p. 358.

80. b The endocrine portion of the pancreas is organized into thousands of tiny clumps of cells scattered throughout the organ. These clumps of cells are called pancreatic islets or islets of Langerhans. These endocrine cells include alpha cells, beta cells, and delta cells. The spleen, liver, and kidney are not associated with islets of Langerhans. Colville TP, Bassert JM, Clinical Anatomy and Physiology for Veterinary Technicians, ed 3, Mosby, 2016, p. 287.

81. a The kidney is made up of hundreds of thousands of microscopic filtering, reabsorbing, and secreting systems called nephrons and is the basic functional unit of the kidneys. The calyces are funnels that direct fluids into the renal pelvis. The hilus is the indented area on the medial side of the kidney where the blood and lymph vessels and ureters enter and leave the kidney. The medulla is the inner portion of the kidney around the renal pelvis. Colville TP, Bassert JM, Clinical Anatomy and Physiology for Veterinary Technicians, ed 3, Mosby, 2016, p. 450.

82. c The kidneys are located retroperitoneal to the abdominal cavity outside the parietal peritoneum and they are considered to be outside the abdominal cavity. They are located between the peritoneum and the dorsal abdominal muscles. Colville TP, Bassert JM, Clinical Anatomy and Physiology for Veterinary Technicians, ed 3, Mosby, 2016, p. 449.

83. c Blood traveling through the systemic circulating system is under higher pressure than the pulmonary and coronary system. It takes more pressure to carry blood the far distance to every extremity than it does to carry it through the shorter pulmonary and coronary routes. Colville TP, Bassert JM, Clinical Anatomy and Physiology for Veterinary Technicians, ed 3, Mosby, 2016, p. 374.

84. b Lymph from the digestive system is called chyle. After a meal, the chyle contains microscopic particles of fat known as chylomicrons that cause the lymph to appear white or pale yellow and cloudy. Pancreatic lipases penetrate the bile acid coating and digest the fat molecules to produce glycerol, fatty acids, and monoglycerides. This results in the droplet fragmenting into even smaller pieces called micelles. These bile acid–lipid component micelles allow the lipid components to diffuse readily through the water contents of the intestine and to come in contact with the brush border of the intestinal wall, where they are absorbed. Very low-density lipoproteins (VLDL) move cholesterol, triglycerides, and other lipids around the body. Low-density lipoproteins (LDL) are a molecule that is a combination of lipid and protein and transport lipids in the blood. Colville TP, Bassert JM, Clinical Anatomy and Physiology for Veterinary Technicians, ed 3, Mosby, 2016, p. 313.

85. b Each broad ligament has segments that are named according to the organ they directly support within the female reproductive tract. The mesovarium supports the ovary. The mesosalpinx supports the oviduct. The mesometrium supports the uterus. Colville TP, Bassert JM, Clinical Anatomy and Physiology for Veterinary Technicians, ed 3, Mosby, 2016, p. 477.

86. b The most obvious clinical sign associated with hypocalcemia is disturbance in skeletal muscle function, which is known as milk fever in cattle. The primary treatment for this condition is with IV calcium to raise rapidly the level of blood calcium. Glucose is not associated with milk fever. Atropine is a drug that aids in heart rate and decreases salivation. Antibiotics are used to treat infection and milk fever is a deficiency of calcium. Colville TP, Bassert JM, Clinical Anatomy and Physiology for Veterinary Technicians, ed 3, Mosby, 2016, p. 284.

87. a Normal CRT is 1 to 2 seconds. In animals with high blood pressure resulting from compensation for anemia, the CRT would be shortened. In animals that have compromised cardiac output, low blood pressure, and peripheral vasoconstriction, the CRT time would be prolonged. Colville TP, Bassert JM, Clinical Anatomy and Physiology for Veterinary Technicians, ed 3, Mosby, 2016, p. 130.

88. a The principal artery of the hind limb is the external iliac artery, which arises close to the termination of the aorta and branches into the femoral artery, supplying each of the hind limbs, and it is felt beginning in the inguinal region. The subclavian artery winds around the first rib to enter the forelimbs through the axilla and becomes the axillary artery. The popliteal artery is located posterior to the patella. The saphenous artery runs along the lateral surface of the hind limbs. Aspinall V, Cappello M, Introduction to Veterinary Anatomy and Physiology Textbook, ed 2, Butterworth Heinemann, 2009, p. 84.

89. b The carpus joint is known as the knee joint in horses on the forelimbs and is equivalent to the human wrist joint. The hip joint and knee joint in humans would be located on the forelimbs of horses. The finger joint of humans would be similar to that distal of the metacarpus in horses. Aspinall V, Cappello M, Introduction to Veterinary Anatomy and Physiology Textbook, ed 2, Butterworth Heinemann, 2009, p. 190, 191.

90. a The linea alba, or white line, is the combined aponeuroses of the three lateral abdominal muscles and it extends along the ventral midline from the xiphoid process of the sternum to the pubic symphysis. Aspinall V, Cappello M, Introduction to Veterinary Anatomy and Physiology Textbook, ed 2, Butterworth Heinemann, 2009, p. 49.

91. b The outer layer of arteries is the tunica adventitia, made up of collagen and elastic fibers. The middle layer is the tunica media, made up of smooth muscle and elastic fibers. The inner layer is the tunica intima, an endothelial lining. Aspinall V, Cappello M, Introduction to Veterinary Anatomy and Physiology Textbook, ed 2, Butterworth Heinemann, 2009, p. 83.

92. b A yellow tinge to the mucous membranes, known as jaundice, is indicative of increased levels of bilirubin related to hepatic disease. Renal disease does not affect the level of bilirubin in the blood. Shock would result in a pale mucous membrane resulting from low blood pressure and/or anemia. Dehydration would result in tacky mucous membranes. Colville TP, Bassert JM, Clinical Anatomy and Physiology for Veterinary Technicians, ed 3, Mosby, 2016, p. 130.

93. c Normal CRT is 1–2 seconds. Animals with anemia will have a shortened CRT. In animals that have compromised cardiac output, low blood pressure, or peripheral vasoconstriction, the CRT time would be prolonged. Colville TP, Bassert JM, Clinical Anatomy and Physiology for Veterinary Technicians, ed 3, Mosby, 2016, p. 130.

94. b The head of the femur is joined to the shaft by a neck. Lateral to the head is a projection called the greater trochanter and on the medial side is another smaller projection called the lesser trochanter. The trochanteric fossa is a depression on the medial side of the greater trochanter on its posterior surface where the great trochanter joins the neck. A tubercle is a protrusion of the bone that is usually for the attachment of muscles. Aspinall V, Cappello M, Introduction to Veterinary Anatomy and Physiology Textbook, ed 2, Butterworth Heinemann, 2009, p. 40.

95. b The femur has a strong shaft and on its distal extremity it has two caudally projecting condyles, the medial condyle and the lateral condyle, which articulate with the tibia at the stifle joint. The hip joint is cranial to the femur and stifle. The tarsal joint is distal to the stifle. The shoulder joint is located at the forelimb. Aspinall V, Cappello M, Introduction to Veterinary Anatomy and Physiology Textbook, ed 2, Butterworth Heinemann, 2009, p. 40.

96. c Proximal refers to structures or part of the structure that lies close to the main mass of the body and it also refers to parts that lie near the origin of a structure or point of attachment. Distal structures lie away from the main mass of the body or origin. Lateral structures lie toward the side of the animal. Superficial means near the surface of the body. Aspinall V, Cappello M, Introduction to Veterinary Anatomy and Physiology Textbook, ed 2, Butterworth Heinemann, 2009, p. 4.

97. c Palmar refers to the rear surface of the forepaw that bears the footpads. Plantar refers to the rear surface of the hind paw that bears the footpads; the opposite surface is the dorsal surface. Sagittal divides the body into equal left and right planes. Longitudinal divides the body into left and right halves. Aspinall V, Cappello M, Introduction to Veterinary Anatomy and Physiology Textbook, ed 2, Butterworth Heinemann, 2009, p. 4.

98. a Between the diaphysis and epiphyses a narrow band of cartilage persists. This is the growth plate or epiphyseal plate. The metaphysis is the wide portion of a long bone between the epiphysis and the narrow diaphysis. The diaphysis is the main or midsection of a long bone that contains bone marrow and adipose tissue. The periosteal plane is the outer covering of the cortex of the bone. Aspinall V, Cappello M, Introduction to Veterinary Anatomy and Physiology Textbook, ed 2, Butterworth Heinemann, 2009, p. 30.

99. a A membrane called the periosteum to which ligaments and tendons attach covers the outer surfaces of bones. The endosteum lines the hollow interior surfaces of bones and contains osteoblasts. Cartilage is a tough, specialized connective tissue that is commonly called gristle and is found in joints and helps prevent bone rubbing. Meniscus is a cartilaginous structure on the proximal surface of the tibia that helps support the condyles of the femur. Colville TP, Bassert JM, Clinical Anatomy and Physiology for Veterinary Technicians, ed 3, Mosby, 2016, p. 178.

100. d Except for their articular or joint surfaces, a membrane called the periosteum covers the outer surfaces of bones. The endosteum lines the hollow interior surfaces of bones and contains osteoblasts. Ligaments are bands of connective tissue that help stabilize the bones and hold the joint together. Colville TP, Bassert JM, Clinical Anatomy and Physiology for Veterinary Technicians, ed 3, Mosby, 2016, p. 176.

101. c Blood flows from the right atrium to the right ventricle through the right atrioventricular valve, also called the right AV valve or tricuspid valve. Blood that has collected in the left atrium flows through the left atrioventricular valve, also called the mitral valve, into the left ventricle. The pulmonary valve, also known as the pulmonic valve, prevents backward flow of blood from the pulmonary arteries. The last heart valve through which oxygenated blood passes on its way to the systemic and coronary arteries is the aortic valve, which has three flaps attached to an annulus. Colville TP, Bassert JM, Clinical Anatomy and Physiology for Veterinary Technicians, ed 3, Mosby, 2016, p. 343.

102. b The aortic and pulmonary valves are both called semilunar valves. The last heart valve through which oxygenated blood passes on its way to the systemic and coronary arteries is the aortic valve. The pulmonary valve, also known as the pulmonic valve, prevents the backward flow of blood from the pulmonary arteries. Blood flows from the right atrium to the right ventricle through the right atrioventricular valve, also called the right AV valve or tricuspid valve. Blood that has collected in the left atrium flows through the left atrioventricular valve, also called the mitral valve, into the left ventricle. Colville TP, Bassert JM, Clinical Anatomy and Physiology for Veterinary Technicians, ed 3, Mosby, 2016, p. 343.

103. a The normal dentition pattern for an adult cat is: Incisor 3/3, Canine 1/1, Premolar 3/2, and Molar 1/1. Feline deciduous teeth are: Incisor 3/3, Canine 1/1, Premolar 3/2, Molar 3/2. Canine normal adult dentition is: Incisor 3/3, Canine 1/1, Premolar 4/4, Molar is 2/3. Canine deciduous teeth are: Incisor 3/3, Canine 1/1, Premolar 3/3, Molar 0. Aspinall V, Cappello M, Introduction to Veterinary Anatomy and Physiology Textbook, ed 2, Butterworth Heinemann, 2009, p. 102.

104. b The esophagus is thin-walled and distensible to allow the passage of relatively large pieces of food. The crop is a diverticulum of the esophagus, lying outside the body cavity on the right side of the cranial thoracic inlet. The proventriculus is lined by gastric glands, which secrete pepsin, hydrochloric acid, and mucus, and is located caudal to the crop. The gizzard is a thick-walled muscular organ in which mechanical digestion occurs and it is located caudal to the proventriculus. Food leaves the gizzard by the pylorus and enters the small intestine, which consists of the duodenum and ileum. Aspinall V, Cappello M, Introduction to Veterinary Anatomy and Physiology Textbook, ed 2, Butterworth Heinemann, 2009, p. 160.

105. d Leading from various bronchi within the lungs are thin-walled air sacs. Most birds have nine air sacs, which penetrate the spaces of the body cavity and the inside of many bones. Aspinall V, Cappello M, Introduction to Veterinary Anatomy and Physiology Textbook, ed 2, Butterworth Heinemann, 2009, p. 158.

106. d The rectum is short and terminates at the cloaca. A pair of ureters carries urine to the outside via the cloaca. The female tract comprises a pair of ovaries and oviducts leading to the cloaca. The large intestine consists of a pair of blind-ending caeca, originating at the junction of the small and large intestines. Sometimes referred to as a wattle, a cleft palate is a fleshy appendage that suspends from the head in some species of birds. Aspinall V, Cappello M, Introduction to Veterinary Anatomy and Physiology Textbook, ed 2, Butterworth Heinemann, 2009, p. 161.

107. b In birds, the gizzard is also referred to as ventriculus, which is a thin-walled muscular organ in which mechanical digestion occurs. Gastric glands that secrete pepsin, hydrochloric acid, and mucus line the proventriculus. Food passes down through the esophagus on the right side of the neck and into the crop. Aspinall V, Cappello M, Introduction to Veterinary Anatomy and Physiology Textbook, ed 2, Butterworth Heinemann, 2009, p. 160.

108. b The diaphragm is a sheet of muscle that separates the thoracic and abdominal cavities and is the main muscle for inspiration. The epaxial muscles are a group of muscles that lie dorsal to the transverse processes of the vertebrae and support the spine. The internal abdominal oblique muscles are the intermediate muscles of the lateral abdominal wall, which also terminates in an aponeurosis on the linea alba. The hypaxial muscles are a group of muscles that lie ventral to the transverse processes of the vertebrae and flex the neck, the tail, and the vertebral column. Aspinall V, Cappello M, Introduction to Veterinary Anatomy and Physiology Textbook, ed 2, Butterworth Heinemann, 2009, p. 48.

109. d The uvea, a vascular pigmented layer, is firmly attached to the sclera at the exit of the optic nerve and is made up of the choroid, tapetum lucidum, ciliary body, suspensory ligament, and iris. The neural tunic is the inner layer of the avian eye and consists of the retina. The fibrous tunic is the outermost layer of the avian eye. The anterior chamber lies between the iris and the cornea and contains aqueous humor. Aspinall V, Cappello M, Introduction to Veterinary Anatomy and Physiology Textbook, ed 2, Butterworth Heinemann, 2009, p. 65.

110. b The lens of the eye is a soft, transparent structure made up of layers of microscopic fibers that are arranged like the layers of an onion. The front surface of the lens is in contact with aqueous humor and its back surface is in contact with vitreous humor. The retina is the inner, nervous layer that lines the back of the eye. The sclera is the white of the eye that is a dense, fibrous connective tissue making up the outer layer of the eye. Colville TP, Bassert JM, Clinical Anatomy and Physiology for Veterinary Technicians, ed 3, Mosby, 2016, p. 267.

111. c The chordae tendineae connect the free edges of the valvular flaps to the papillary muscles, which attach inside the ventricle on the interventricular septum that separates the right and left ventricles. The sternum is part of the components of the axial skeleton. The coronary muscle is the main heart muscle responsible for contraction and ejection of blood from the atria to the ventricles and then from the ventricles to the arteries. The myocardium is a cardiac muscle located inside the sac that is formed by the pericardium and is the thickest layer of heart tissue. Colville TP, Bassert JM, Clinical Anatomy and Physiology for Veterinary Technicians, ed 3, Mosby, 2016, p. 342.

112. a The myocardium is the cardiac muscle with the thickest layer of tissue making up the majority of the heart mass. The endocardium is located between the myocardium and the chambers of the heart and is a thin membranous lining. The myometrium is a muscle of the uterus in the female reproductive tract. The pericardium is the outer layer of the heart and consists of two layers including the fibrous pericardium and the serous pericardium. Colville TP, Bassert JM, Clinical Anatomy and Physiology for Veterinary Technicians, ed 3, Mosby, 2016, p. 341.

113. d The aorta emerges from the left ventricle into the aortic arch to supply the body with arterial blood. It is the largest artery in the body and the site of the highest blood pressure. The subclavian artery is a branch of the aorta that supplies blood to the cranial portion of the body into the forelimbs. The carotid artery is a branch of the aorta traveling up the neck supplying the head with blood. The pulmonary artery receives blood from the right ventricle. Colville TP, Bassert JM, Clinical Anatomy and Physiology for Veterinary Technicians, ed 3, Mosby, 2016, p. 346.

114. d The femoral vein that is found in the hind limbs merges into the right and left iliac veins, which return blood to the cauda vena cava, not the cranial vena cava. The brachiocephalic vein, thoracic duct, and azygos vein are located in the cranial portion of the body and all return blood to the cranial vena cava. Colville TP, Bassert JM, Clinical Anatomy and Physiology for Veterinary Technicians, ed 3, Mosby, 2016, p. 359.

115. b The hepatic portal vein takes blood straight from the digestive tract to the liver so that the product of digestion can be processed immediately. The hepatic veins drain the liver. The hepatic artery supplies the liver with oxygenated blood from a branch off the aorta. A portosystemic shunt is a congenital malformation where venous blood coming from the digestive system bypasses the liver and does not enter the hepatic portal system. Aspinall V, Cappello M, Introduction to Veterinary Anatomy and Physiology Textbook, ed 2, Butterworth Heinemann, 2009, p. 84.

116. b The venous return from the heart itself is via the coronary veins; these join to form the coronary sinus, which then empties into the right atrium further traveling into the right ventricle. The left atrium receives blood from the lungs and then travels into the left ventricle. Aspinall V, Cappello M, Introduction to Veterinary Anatomy and Physiology Textbook, ed 2, Butterworth Heinemann, 2009, p. 84.

117. b Blood going through the systemic circulation is under higher pressure than blood in the pulmonary circulation. Blood traveling away from the heart is under higher pressure because of the further distance it travels. The pulmonary circulation is a short distance and requires a lower pressure to complete. Equilibrium is anything balanced or the same. Partial pressure is the pressure of each individual gas. The circulatory system uses different pressures to contract blood throughout the body and cannot be at equilibrium. Colville TP, Bassert JM, Clinical Anatomy and Physiology for Veterinary Technicians, ed 3, Mosby, 2016, p. 342.

118. c An adult dog has 42 teeth. A young dog or puppy has 28 deciduous teeth. An adult human has 32 teeth. Primitive marsupials have 50 teeth. Aspinall V, Cappello M, Introduction to Veterinary Anatomy and Physiology Textbook, ed 2, Butterworth Heinemann, 2009, p. 100.

119. b The small intestine is divided into the following segments: duodenum, jejunum, ileum. The ilium (with an i) is a structure of the bony pelvis. Colville TP, Bassert JM, Clinical Anatomy and Physiology for Veterinary Technicians, ed 3, Mosby, 2016, p. 402.

120. b Neither the horse nor the rat has a gallbladder. The function of the gallbladder is to store bile. The horse and rat both contain kidneys, a pancreas, and a cecum as part of the abdominal organs. Aspinall V, Cappello M, Introduction to Veterinary Anatomy and Physiology Textbook, ed 2, Butterworth Heinemann, 2009; and Chapter 11, Clinical Anatomy and Physiology for Veterinary Technicians, ed 2.

121. a Ruminants do not have any upper incisors or upper canine teeth. Instead they have a dental pad, which is a flat, thick, connective-tissue structure on the maxilla opposite the lower incisors and canine teeth. Ruminants rely heavily on high concentrations of sodium bicarbonate and phosphate buffers found in their saliva to neutralize acids formed in the rumen. Ruminants do have molar teeth but do not have incisors. Colville TP, Bassert JM, Clinical Anatomy and Physiology for Veterinary Technicians, ed 3, Mosby, 2016, p. 385.

122. a Ruminants have a true stomach known as the abomasum and have three forestomachs that are the reticulum, rumen, and omasum. The forestomachs are compartments of differing sizes and functions, through which swallowed material must pass before reaching the abomasum. Colville TP, Bassert JM, Clinical Anatomy and Physiology for Veterinary Technicians, ed 3, Mosby, 2016, p. 396.

123. d The narrow pelvic flexure and small colon are areas of potential impaction/obstruction. Ingesta flow cranially, from the right to left ventral colon, through the sternal flexure. Ingesta are moved caudally in the left ventral colon and at the caudal end of the peritoneal cavity, the left ventral colon narrows into the pelvic flexure, which reflects on itself and opens into the left dorsal colon. Colville TP, Bassert JM, Clinical Anatomy and Physiology for Veterinary Technicians, ed 3, Mosby, 2016, p. 413.

124. c The contents of the digestive tract are moved and mixed by muscle contractions known as peristalsis. Mastication is the mechanical grinding and breaking down of food in the oral cavity. Prehension is the grasping of food with the lips or teeth. Elimination is the expulsion of waste products. Colville TP, Bassert

JM, Clinical Anatomy and Physiology for Veterinary Technicians, ed 3, Mosby, 2016, p. 391.

125. d The most distal portion of the monogastric stomach is the pylorus, which acts as a sphincter and opens into the first portion of the small intestine. The fundus is the largest and most cranial aspect of the stomach that expands to hold food particles. The antrum is the distal end of the stomach that grinds up swallowed food and regulates the hydrochloric acids and it is cranial to the pylorus. The cardia is the portion where the esophagus enters the stomach. Colville TP, Bassert JM, Clinical Anatomy and Physiology for Veterinary Technicians, ed 3, Mosby, 2016, p. 393.

126. c The gastric glands contain three key cells that are found in the fundus and body of the stomach: parietal cells that produce hydrochloric acid, chief cells that produce an enzyme precursor called pepsinogen, and mucous cells, which produce the protective mucus. G cells are found in the antrum of the stomach. Colville TP, Bassert JM, Clinical Anatomy and Physiology for Veterinary Technicians, ed 3, Mosby, 2016, p. 393.

127. d The thyroid gland produces two hormones: thyroid hormone and calcitonin. The pituitary gland produces luteinizing hormone, oxytocin, and growth hormones. Colville TP, Bassert JM, Clinical Anatomy and Physiology for Veterinary Technicians, ed 3, Mosby, 2016, p. 278.

128. b The basic units of the endocrine system are endocrine glands, also called ductless glands, because they secrete tiny amounts of hormones directly into the bloodstream. The exocrine system secretes their products onto epithelial surfaces through tiny tubes called ducts. The lymphatic system is a series of vessels or ducts that carries excess tissue fluid to blood vessels near the heart. Colville TP, Bassert JM, Clinical Anatomy and Physiology for Veterinary Technicians, ed 3, Mosby, 2016, p. 275.

129. d Progesterone is a hormone secreted by the corpus luteum, which develops from the remaining follicular tissue after the follicle has ovulated. The corpus luteum develops as a result of the production of luteinizing hormone (LH) from the anterior pituitary gland. Progesterone prepares the reproductive tract for pregnancy and maintains the pregnancy. Oxytocin is secreted by the posterior pituitary gland during the last hours of pregnancy to trigger milk letdown. LH is stimulated by the presence of estrogen and stimulates the follicles within the ovary. Estrogen is produced by the wall of the developing ovarian follicles, causes the behavior associated with estrous cycle, and prepares the reproductive tract for mating. Aspinall V, Cappello M, Introduction to Veterinary Anatomy and Physiology Textbook, ed 2, Butterworth Heinemann, 2009, p. 74.

130. b Luteinizing hormone stimulates the ripe follicles in the ovary to rupture and release their ova. The remaining tissue becomes luteinized to form the corpus luteum. The corpus callosum is a tract of white matter whose nerve fibers run across the brain between the right and left hemispheres. Corpus albicans is the regressed corpus luteum when no pregnancy occurs. The Graafian follicle is the primary follicle in advance of rupture. Aspinall V, Cappello M, Introduction to Veterinary Anatomy and Physiology Textbook, ed 2, Butterworth Heinemann, 2009, p. 72.

131. a A deficiency of antidiuretic hormone (ADH) in the body causes the disease diabetes insipidus. Affected animals produce large quantities of very dilute urine and drink large quantities of water. The condition is treated by administering a drug with ADH activity for the rest of the animal's life. Diabetes mellitus is a disease caused by a deficiency of the hormone glycosuria, or glucose, in the urine. Cushing's syndrome is a condition that results from too much glucocorticoid hormone being produced by the adrenal cortex. Pancreatic insufficiency is a disease in which the ability of the pancreas to secrete digestive enzymes is markedly reduced. Colville TP, Bassert JM, Clinical Anatomy and Physiology for Veterinary Technicians, ed 3, Mosby, 2016, p. 282.

132. c Kidneys produce the hormone erythropoietin, which stimulates red bone marrow to increase production of oxygen-carrying red blood cells. Antidiuretic hormone is produced by the hypothalamus. Adrenocorticotropic hormone is produced by the anterior pituitary gland. Adrenal cortex hormone production is regulated by feedback from the hormones of the adrenal cortex. Colville TP, Bassert JM, Clinical Anatomy and Physiology for Veterinary Technicians, ed 3, Mosby, 2016, p. 289.

133. a The main endocrine cells of the pancreatic islets are alpha cells, which produce glucagon, beta cells that produce insulin, and delta cells that produce somatostatin. Glycogen is the storage form of glucose in the liver. Colville TP, Bassert JM, Clinical Anatomy and Physiology for Veterinary Technicians, ed 3, Mosby, 2016, p. 287.

134. b Adrenocorticotropic hormone (ACTH) stimulates the growth and development of the cortex of the adrenal gland and the release of some of its hormones. Thyroid-stimulating hormone (TSH) stimulates the growth and development of the thyroid gland and causes it to produce hormones. Prolactin triggers lactations. Follicle-stimulating hormone (FSH) stimulates the growth and development of follicles in the ovaries. Colville TP, Bassert JM, Clinical Anatomy and Physiology for Veterinary Technicians, ed 3, Mosby, 2016, p. 281.

135. d The pineal body is a part of the brain located at the caudal end of the deep cleft that separates the two cerebral hemispheres and produces a hormonelike substance called melatonin that affects moods and wake–sleep cycles. The pituitary gland is an endocrine gland that is attached to the hypothalamus and produces the antidiuretic hormone oxytocin and is known as the master gland of the body. The spleen is responsible for storing blood and releasing blood into the circulatory system when needed. The thymus is an organ that helps kickstart the immune system. Colville TP, Bassert JM, Clinical Anatomy and Physiology for Veterinary Technicians, ed 3, Mosby, 2016, p. 290.

136. c The lymphatic system has four primary functions: removal of excess tissue fluid, waste material transport, filtration of lymph, and protein transport. Carbohydrate is not transported by the lymphatic system. Colville

TP, Bassert JM, Clinical Anatomy and Physiology for Veterinary Technicians, ed 3, Mosby, 2016, p. 311.

137. d Lymph from the digestive system is called chyle. After a meal, chyle contains microscopic particles of fat known as chylomicrons that cause the lymph to appear white or pale yellow. GALT is gut-associated lymph tissue. Haustra are the longitudinal bands that separate the colon into a series of lined-up sacs. Colville TP, Bassert JM, Clinical Anatomy and Physiology for Veterinary Technicians, ed 3, Mosby, 2016, p. 313.

138. b In the villi of the small intestine, the lymph capillaries are called lacteals and are responsible for collecting the products of fat digestion. Afferent lymphatic vessels carry lymph to each lymph node and enter the node on its convex surface. Trabeculae are a network of tissues that extends from the capsule and provides support for the entire node. The spleen is responsible for storage of blood, destruction of worn out RBCs, removal of particulate matter from the circulation, and the production of lymphocytes. Aspinall V, Cappello M, Introduction to Veterinary Anatomy and Physiology Textbook, ed 2, Butterworth Heinemann, 2009, p. 86.

139. d Tonsils are rings of lymphoid tissue around the junction of the pharynx with the oral cavity. Bile ducts are the ductwork connected to the gallbladder. Islets of Langerhans are the cellular structures of the pancreas responsible for secretion of hormones. The thyroid is an endocrine gland and is responsible for stimulating and releasing the thyroid hormones. Aspinall V, Cappello M, Introduction to Veterinary Anatomy and Physiology Textbook, ed 2, Butterworth Heinemann, 2009, p. 87.

140. c The forebrain consists of the cerebrum, thalamus, and hypothalamus. The midbrain, pons, and medulla oblongata are all structures of the brain that can be found as part of the brainstem. Aspinall V, Cappello M, Introduction to Veterinary Anatomy and Physiology Textbook, ed 2, Butterworth Heinemann, 2009, p. 56.

141. b The kidneys are a characteristic bean shape with an indented area known as the hilus, where the blood vessels, nerves, and ureters enter and leave the kidneys. The medulla is the inner portion of the kidneys that contains the pyramids. The cortex is the outermost layer of the kidney containing the renal corpuscles and convoluted tubules of the nephrons. The pelvis is the basin-shaped area into which urine formed by the nephrons drains. Aspinall V, Cappello M, Introduction to Veterinary Anatomy and Physiology Textbook, ed 2, Butterworth Heinemann, 2009, p. 111.

142. b Horses produce approximately 20 mL/kg/day of urine that is usually pale yellow in color and may be clear or cloudy depending on the amount of calcium carbonate being excreted. Aspinall V, Cappello M, Introduction to Veterinary Anatomy and Physiology Textbook, ed 2, Butterworth Heinemann, 2009, p. 204.

143. a Ruminants have a cotyledonary type of placental attachment. Horses and pigs have diffuse attachment. Dogs and cats have zonary attachment. Primates, rodents, and rabbits have discoid attachment. Colville TP, Bassert JM, Clinical Anatomy and Physiology for Veterinary Technicians, ed 3, Mosby, 2016, p. 492.

144. c Oxytocin is a hormone released from the posterior pituitary gland of the female that causes the smooth muscle of the estrogen-primed female reproductive tract to contract, giving the spermatozoa a free ride. Luteinizing hormone, follicle-stimulating hormone, and growth hormone are secreted by the anterior pituitary gland. Colville TP, Bassert JM, Clinical Anatomy and Physiology for Veterinary Technicians, ed 3, Mosby, 2016, p. 279.

145. a Spermatozoa, the male sex cells, are produced in the seminiferous tubules of the testes through a process called spermatogenesis. The epididymis is a storage site for spermatozoa and a place for them to mature before they are expelled by ejaculation. The vas deferens, also known as the ductus deferens, is a muscular tube that connects the tail of the epididymis with the pelvic portion of the urethra. The seminal vesicles are ducts that are sometimes called vesicular glands and they enter the pelvic urethra in the same area as the vas deferens. Colville TP, Bassert JM, Clinical Anatomy and Physiology for Veterinary Technicians, ed 3, Mosby, 2016, p. 468.

146. c The bulbourethral gland is an accessory gland seen only in tomcats, equines, and bovines. The canine male reproductive system consists of testis, epididymis, deferent duct, urethra, penis, and prostate gland. Aspinall V, Cappello M, Introduction to Veterinary Anatomy and Physiology Textbook, ed 2, Butterworth Heinemann, 2009, p. 123.

147. b The females of all these species of rodent are polyestrous and spontaneous ovulators. The rabbits, cat, and ferret are induced ovulators. Aspinall V, Cappello M, Introduction to Veterinary Anatomy and Physiology Textbook, ed 2, Butterworth Heinemann, 2009, p. 170.

148. a The estrous cycle is defined as the time from the beginning of one heat period to the beginning of the next. Estrus is the heat period or period of sexual receptivity in the female. Ovulation is the rupture of the mature follicle with a release of the reproductive cell into the oviduct. The mating cycle is the period of sexual receptivity or copulation. Colville TP, Bassert JM, Clinical Anatomy and Physiology for Veterinary Technicians, ed 3, Mosby, 2016, p. 483.

149. b The cremaster muscle passes down through the inguinal ring and attaches to the scrotum and can adjust the position of the testes relative to the body. The retractor penis muscle originates at the base of the tail and functions like a small bungee cord when an erection straightens out the sigmoid flexure the muscle stretches. Kegel muscles are part of the pelvic floor. The cremaster muscle is in charge of retracting the testicles. Colville TP, Bassert JM, Clinical Anatomy and Physiology for Veterinary Technicians, ed 3, Mosby, 2016, p. 471.

150. b Follicular atresia is when not all the follicles that were activated in a particular ovarian cycle fully develop and ovulate and the rest may degenerate at any stage of their development. Ovulation is the rupture of the mature follicle with the release of the reproductive cell into the oviduct. Graafian follicle is also known as a mature follicle. The corpus albicans is the regenerative form of the corpus luteum if pregnancy does not occur. Colville TP, Bassert JM, Clinical Anatomy and Physiology for Veterinary Technicians, ed 3, Mosby, 2016, p. 482.

151. a As a follicle grows, it produces increasing amounts of estrogen that feed back to the anterior pituitary. The placenta secretes chorionic gonadotropin and small amounts of estrogen and progesterone. The corpus hemorrhagicum is a blood-filled empty follicle. The corpus luteum produces progestin hormones, known as progesterone. Colville TP, Bassert JM, Clinical Anatomy and Physiology for Veterinary Technicians, ed 3, Mosby, 2016, p. 480.

152. c The gestational period is the interval between fertilization of the ovum and the birth of the offspring. For the bitch and the queen, the gestational period is approximately 63 days. Aspinall V, Cappello M, Introduction to Veterinary Anatomy and Physiology Textbook, ed 2, Butterworth Heinemann, 2009, p. 133.

153. b The gestational period is the interval between fertilization of the ovum and the birth of the offspring. The gestational period for ferrets is 42 days. Aspinall V, Cappello M, Introduction to Veterinary Anatomy and Physiology Textbook, ed 2, Butterworth Heinemann, 2009, p. 174.

154. c Some animals can have an exaggerated diestrous period, resulting in pseudocyesis or pseudopregnancy. Anestrus is a period of temporary ovarian inactivity seen in seasonally polyestrous, diestrous, and monoestrous animals. Metestrus is the period after ovulation when the corpus luteum develops. Proestrus is the period of follicular development in the ovary. Aspinall V, Cappello M, Introduction to Veterinary Anatomy and Physiology Textbook, ed 2, Butterworth Heinemann, 2009, p. 405.

155. d The pressure within the thorax is negative with respect to atmospheric pressure. The partial volume pulls the lungs tightly out against the thoracic wall. The negative pressure in the thorax also aids the return of blood to the heart. Colville TP, Bassert JM, Clinical Anatomy and Physiology for Veterinary Technicians, ed 3, Mosby, 2016, p. 472.

156. a Skeletal muscles are controlled by the conscious mind and move the bones of the skeleton so that the animal can move around. Skeletal muscles are striated and are attached to bones. Colville TP, Bassert JM, Clinical Anatomy and Physiology for Veterinary Technicians, ed 3, Mosby, 2016, p. 212.

157. c Calcium and phosphorus are the most abundant minerals in the body and together they compose three-fourths of the minerals by weight. Together these harden the teeth and form the rigid, hard material that gives bone its strength. Magnesium works together with calcium and phosphorus to harden teeth and give bones their strength. Potassium is included as a macromineral but calcium and phosphorus are responsible for the strength of bones. Colville TP, Bassert JM, Clinical Anatomy and Physiology for Veterinary Technicians, ed 3, Mosby, 2016, p. 173.

158. d Bones have the following functions: support, protection, leverage, and storage. Metabolism is not part of bone function. Colville TP, Bassert JM, Clinical Anatomy and Physiology for Veterinary Technicians, ed 3, Mosby, 2016, p. 173.

159. b Two hormones, calcitonin from the thyroid gland and parathyroid hormone from the parathyroid glands, act as "cashiers" at the calcium bank. Calcitonin helps prevent hypercalcemia, whereas the parathyroid hormone helps prevent hypocalcemia, which is a low level of calcium in the blood, in part by withdrawing calcium from the bones. T4 is a hormone produced by the thyroid gland and it helps with the body's metabolic rate. Vitamin D is essential for blood clotting and bone and tooth formation. Colville TP, Bassert JM, Clinical Anatomy and Physiology for Veterinary Technicians, ed 3, Mosby, 2016, p. 173.

160. a Osteoclasts are like the "evil twins" of osteoblasts; instead of forming bone, they eat it away. Osteoclasts are necessary for remodeling to take place by removing bone from where it is not needed, and osteoblasts form new bone in areas where it is needed. Chondroblasts are fixed cells that form cartilage. Chondroclasts are cells that destroy and resorb cartilage. Colville TP, Bassert JM, Clinical Anatomy and Physiology for Veterinary Technicians, ed 3, Mosby, 2016, p. 176.

161. d Except for their articular or joint surfaces, a membrane called the periosteum covers the outer surfaces of bones. Joint surfaces are not covered by the periosteum. The marrow cavity of bones is filled with bone marrow where blood cell formation takes place. The outer layer of the heart is lined with the pericardium. Colville TP, Bassert JM, Clinical Anatomy and Physiology for Veterinary Technicians, ed 3, Mosby, 2016, p. 176.

162. c Bones come in four basic shapes: long, short, flat, and irregular. Bones do not come in a "regular" shape. Colville TP, Bassert JM, Clinical Anatomy and Physiology for Veterinary Technicians, ed 3, Mosby, 2016, p. 176.

163. d The shaft of the bone is known as the diaphysis where bone begins developing. The trunk of the skeleton is part of the axial skeleton because the bones are along the central axis of the body. The epiphysis is the end of the bones. The periosteum is the outer covering of bones. Colville TP, Bassert JM, Clinical Anatomy and Physiology for Veterinary Technicians, ed 3, Mosby, 2016, p. 176.

164. b Short bones are shaped like small cubes or marshmallows. They consist of a core of spongy bone covered by a thin layer of compact bone. An example would be tarsal bones or carpal bones. Vertebrae are an example of irregular bones. Scapula is an example of a flat bone. Patella is an example of an irregular bone. Colville TP, Bassert JM, Clinical Anatomy and Physiology for Veterinary Technicians, ed 3, Mosby, 2016, p. 177.

165. c The occipital bone is a single bone that forms the caudoventral portion or base of the skull. It is the most caudal skull bone and is very important because it is where the spinal cord exits the skull and it is the skull bone that articulates with the first cervical vertebra. Parietal bones form the dorsolateral walls of the cranium. Temporal bones are located below or ventral to the parietal bones. The frontal bone forms the forehead region of the skull. Colville TP, Bassert

JM, Clinical Anatomy and Physiology for Veterinary Technicians, ed 3, Mosby, 2016, p. 180.

166. a The three tiny pairs of ear bones are known as ossicles and include the malleus, incus, and stapes. Sphenoid bones forming the ventral part of the cranium contain a depression and are located just rostral to the occipital bone. Colville TP, Bassert JM, Clinical Anatomy and Physiology for Veterinary Technicians, ed 3, Mosby, 2016, p. 187.

167. b Cervical vertebrae are in the neck region and are found in all common domestic animals and all of these animals have seven cervical vertebrae. This is the only group of vertebrae that has a constant number across most species. Colville TP, Bassert JM, Clinical Anatomy and Physiology for Veterinary Technicians, ed 3, Mosby, 2016, p. 189.

168. b The first cervical vertebra, C1, is known as the atlas because, like the mythical figure Atlas who holds up the world, this vertebra holds up the head. C2 is known as the axis. An arch is the hollow region of vertebrae where the spinal cord travels. An auricle is the external portion of the ears. Colville TP, Bassert JM, Clinical Anatomy and Physiology for Veterinary Technicians, ed 3, Mosby, 2016, p. 189.

169. d The sternum is also known as the breastbone, which forms the floor of the thorax. The hyoid bone is also known as the hyoid apparatus and is located high in the neck. A septum, also known as a nasal septum, is the central wall between the left and right nasal passages. Tubercles are large processes opposite the head on the proximal end where muscles attach. Colville TP, Bassert JM, Clinical Anatomy and Physiology for Veterinary Technicians, ed 3, Mosby, 2016, p. 192.

170. a The most caudal sternebra is called the xiphoid or xiphoid process. The coccyx is a portion of the pelvic bones. The manubrium is the most cranial sternebra. The costal is also known as the rib. Colville TP, Bassert JM, Clinical Anatomy and Physiology for Veterinary Technicians, ed 3, Mosby, 2016, p. 192.

171. a The integumentary system includes hair, hooves, horns, claws, and various skin-related glands and it is derived from living germinal layers. The outer shell of an animal is entirely dead; cells gave up vital organelles and nuclei to make room for the tough, protective substance called keratin in which they become keratinized. Agglutinated refers to antigens that are stuck together to make large clumps that are phagocytized by macrophages. Calcified is hardening of organic tissue by the deposit of lime and calcium salts. Crystallized is the formation of crystals. Colville TP, Bassert JM, Clinical Anatomy and Physiology for Veterinary Technicians, ed 3, Mosby, 2016, p. 167.

172. d External structures of the hoof include: frog, sole, bulbs of heel, seat of corn, bars, and coronet of coronary band. Internal structures of the hoof include: bones, digital cushion, lateral cartilages, and corium. Aspinall V, Cappello M, Introduction to Veterinary Anatomy and Physiology Textbook, ed 2, Butterworth Heinemann, 2009, p. 197.

173. c Adult cattle do not have any upper incisors or upper canine teeth. Instead they have a dental pad, which is a flat, thick, connective-tissue structure on the maxilla opposite the lower incisors and canine teeth. Colville TP, Bassert JM, Clinical Anatomy and Physiology for Veterinary Technicians, ed 3, Mosby, 2016, p. 387.

174. d The anatomic term for synovial joint is *diarthroses*, which are freely movable joints. Fibroarthroses are not a type of joint. Amphiarthroses are known as cartilaginous joints. Synarthroses are known as fibrous joints. Colville TP, Bassert JM, Clinical Anatomy and Physiology for Veterinary Technicians, ed 3, Mosby, 2016, p. 205.

175. c The following are types of synovial joints: hinge joints, gliding joints, pivot joints, and ball-and-socket joints. A swinging joint is not a type of joint. Colville TP, Bassert JM, Clinical Anatomy and Physiology for Veterinary Technicians, ed 3, Mosby, 2016, p. 205.

176. a The renal pelvis is a chamber where urine collection occurs before entering the ureters. The hilus is the area where blood and lymph vessels, nerves, and ureters enter and leave the kidney. The cortex is the outer portion of the kidney. The medulla is the inner portion of the kidney. Colville TP, Bassert JM, Clinical Anatomy and Physiology for Veterinary Technicians, ed 3, Mosby, 2016, p. 450.

177. d The collecting ducts play an important role in urine volume because they are the primary sites of action of the antidiuretic hormone. The loop of Henle continues from the PCT and descends into the medulla of the kidney where the glomerular filtrate continues its journey. The proximal convoluted tubule is a continuation of the capsular space of Bowman's capsule where the glomerular filtrate begins its journey. The glomerulus is a tuft of glomerular capillaries. Colville TP, Bassert JM, Clinical Anatomy and Physiology for Veterinary Technicians, ed 3, Mosby, 2016, p. 451.

178. d The renal corpuscle is located in the cortex of the kidney and is made up of the glomerulus and Bowman's capsule. The hilus of the kidney is where the blood and lymph vessels, nerves, and ureters leave and enter. The medulla is the inner portion of the kidney where urine formation takes place. The cortex is the outer layer of the kidney. Colville TP, Bassert JM, Clinical Anatomy and Physiology for Veterinary Technicians, ed 3, Mosby, 2016, p. 451.

179. a The renal corpuscle is located in the cortex of the kidney and is made up of the glomerulus and Bowman's capsule. The collecting ducts are distal to the convoluted tubules. The descending and ascending loops of Henle are continuous from the proximal convoluted tubule. The afferent arteriole is where the blood enters the glomerulus. Colville TP, Bassert JM, Clinical Anatomy and Physiology for Veterinary Technicians, ed 3, Mosby, 2016, p. 451.

180. b The function of the urinary bladder is to collect, store, and release urine. The kidneys constantly produce and filter urine. Colville TP, Bassert JM, Clinical Anatomy and Physiology for Veterinary Technicians, ed 3, Mosby, 2016, p. 459.

181. d The bones of the skeleton are divided into two groups, the bones of the head and trunk and the bones of the limbs. The bones of the head and trunk are referred to the axial skeleton because they are located along the central axis of the body, which would include the thorax and abdomen. Colville TP, Bassert JM, Clinical Anatomy and Physiology for Veterinary Technicians, ed 3, Mosby, 2016, p. 180.

182. d The middle phalanx is located proximal to the distal phalanx and distal to the proximal phalanx. There are no structures attached lateral or medial to the middle or distal phalanx. Aspinall V, Cappello M, Introduction to Veterinary Anatomy and Physiology Textbook, ed 2, Butterworth Heinemann, 2009, p. 39.

183. d The humerus, radius, and ulnar bones are all jointed at the elbow proximal to the carpus. Distal to the carpus are the metacarpal bones. There are no bones lateral or medial to the carpus. Colville TP, Bassert JM, Clinical Anatomy and Physiology for Veterinary Technicians, ed 3, Mosby, 2016, p. 193.

184. d The liver is the largest gland in the body and is divided into several lobes. Colville TP, Bassert JM, Clinical Anatomy and Physiology for Veterinary Technicians, ed 3, Mosby, 2016, p. 405.

185. a The fibula is a thin but complete bone in dogs and cats that parallels the tibia but does not support any significant weight; it mainly serves as a muscle attachment site. The femur is the long bone of the thigh with its proximal end being the ball portion of the ball-and-socket joint. The tibia is the main weight-bearing bone of the lower leg. The humerus is the long bone of the upper limb with its proximal end being the "ball" of the ball-and-socket joint. Colville TP, Bassert JM, Clinical Anatomy and Physiology for Veterinary Technicians, ed 3, Mosby, 2016, p. 202.

186. d The calcaneal tuberosity of the fibular tarsal bone projects upward and backward to form the point of the hock. It acts as the point of attachment for the tendon of the large gastrocnemius muscle and corresponds to our heel. The tibialis anterior runs from the proximal end of the tibia to the tarsus. The gracilis forms the caudal half of the medial surface of the thigh. The semimembranosus is part of the hamstring muscles that include the biceps, femoris, and the semitendinosus muscle. Colville TP, Bassert JM, Clinical Anatomy and Physiology for Veterinary Technicians, ed 3, Mosby, 2016, p. 202.

187. c The following muscles are included as part of the abdominal wall: external oblique, internal oblique, transversus abdominis, and the rectus abdominis. The latissimus dorsi is a large, fan-shaped muscle, which has a very broad origin on the thoracic spine and inserts on the humerus. Aspinall V, Cappello M, Introduction to Veterinary Anatomy and Physiology Textbook, ed 2, Butterworth Heinemann, 2009, p. 49.

188. b The number of heads refers to the number of sites that a muscle has attached to its origin. Biceps brachii has two heads, triceps brachii has three heads, and quadriceps femoris has four heads. Colville TP, Bassert JM, Clinical Anatomy and Physiology for Veterinary Technicians, ed 3, Mosby, 2016, p. 214.

189. b Fascia is an arrangement of dense regular connective tissue that lies over muscle. This layer helps to support, separate, and connect muscle to other structures. Colville TP, Bassert JM, Clinical Anatomy and Physiology for Veterinary Technicians, ed 3, Mosby, 2016, p. 126.

190. a The term *deltoid* means triangular and the deltoid muscle is a triangular muscle of the shoulder region. The gluteal muscles and the hamstring muscle group are extensor muscles of the hip joint. The biceps brachii and triceps brachii allow for movements of the elbow. The masseter muscle controls the opening and closing of the jaw. Colville TP, Bassert JM, Clinical Anatomy and Physiology for Veterinary Technicians, ed 3, Mosby, 2016, p. 214.

191. c The larynx is suspended from the skull by the hyoid apparatus, which allows it to swing backward and forward. The pharynx is a region at the back of the mouth that is shared by the respiratory and digestive systems and where inspired air passes. The epiglottis is composed of elastic cartilage and is responsible for sealing off the entrance to the larynx or glottis when an animal swallows. The mediastinum is a double layer of connective tissue that lies within the thoracic cavity. Aspinall V, Cappello M, Introduction to Veterinary Anatomy and Physiology Textbook, ed 2, Butterworth Heinemann, 2009, p. 90.

192. b Food enters the esophagus via the cardiac sphincter and leaves from the pyloric sphincter. The last sphincter is the anal sphincter, which allows for passage of feces. Aspinall V, Cappello M, Introduction to Veterinary Anatomy and Physiology Textbook, ed 2, Butterworth Heinemann, 2009, p. 103.

193. a The dorsal plane divides the body into upper and lower halves or dorsal and ventral portions. The median plane divides the body longitudinally into symmetrical left and right halves. Transverse planes divide the body into cranial and caudal portions or distal and proximal portions. Aspinall V, Cappello M, Introduction to Veterinary Anatomy and Physiology Textbook, ed 2, Butterworth Heinemann, 2009, p. 4.

194. a The middle portion of the small intestine is known as the jejunum. Following correct terminology, the "e" at the beginning of the word stands for "eat." The other answers are misspellings of the word. Aspinall V, Cappello M, Introduction to Veterinary Anatomy and Physiology Textbook, ed 2, Butterworth Heinemann, 2009, p. 97.

195. d The word visceral describes the serous membrane that covers all the organs within the cavity. Parietal describes the serous membrane that lines the boundaries or sides of the cavities. Viscous describes a substance as having a thick consistency. Aspinall V, Cappello M, Introduction to Veterinary Anatomy and Physiology Textbook, ed 2, Butterworth Heinemann, 2009, p. 25.

196. d The maxillary sinus is not a true sinus in the dog but a recess at the caudal end of the nasal cavity. The frontal sinus lies within the frontal bone of the skull. The external nares are the external opening of the nose. Paranasal sinuses lie within the facial bones of the skull. Aspinall V, Cappello M, Introduction to Veterinary Anatomy and Physiology Textbook, ed 2, Butterworth Heinemann, 2009, p. 89.

197. d The trapezius muscle is a triangular-shaped muscle that originates from the dorsal midline and inserts on the scapula. The latissimus dorsi muscle is a fan-shaped muscle that originates on the thoracic spine and inserts on the humerus. The brachiocephalicus is the muscle that travels from the base of the skull to an insertion of the cranial aspect of the humerus. The external intercostals are superficial muscles that originate on the caudal side of one rib and insert on the cranial side of the posterior rib. Aspinall V, Cappello M, Introduction to Veterinary Anatomy and Physiology Textbook, ed 2, Butterworth Heinemann, 2009, p. 49.

198. d The cardiovascular system includes the heart, blood, circulation, and blood vessels. The lungs are part of the respiratory system. Colville TP, Bassert JM, Clinical Anatomy and Physiology for Veterinary Technicians, ed 3, Mosby, 2016, p. 339.

199. c The pelvic girdle is part of the appendicular skeleton. The os cordis, ribs, and clavicles are all part of the visceral skeleton. Colville TP, Bassert JM, Clinical Anatomy and Physiology for Veterinary Technicians, ed 3, Mosby, 2016, p. 193.

200. d The os penis is a bone of the penis found in dogs and similar species such as cats, beavers, and raccoons, and it partially surrounds the penile portion of the urethra. The os penis is not found in hooved animals. Colville TP, Bassert JM, Clinical Anatomy and Physiology for Veterinary Technicians, ed 3, Mosby, 2016, p. 476.

201. b Short bones are shaped like cubes and consist of a core of spongy bone covered by a thin layer of compact bone. Long bones are longer than they are wide, are also covered by a thin layer of compact bone, and are filled with bone marrow. Vertebrae fall within the irregular bone category because of their irregular shape. Colville TP, Bassert JM, Clinical Anatomy and Physiology for Veterinary Technicians, ed 3, Mosby, 2016, p. 177.

202. c Flat bones consist of two thin plates of compact bone separated by a layer of cancellous bone. The scapula, skull bones, and pelvic bones are all examples of flat bones. Long bones are longer than they are wide and are found in the limbs. Short bones are cube shaped and are found in the carpal and tarsal bones. Irregular bones are irregularly shaped and consist of bones such as the vertebrae. Colville TP, Bassert JM, Clinical Anatomy and Physiology for Veterinary Technicians, ed 3, Mosby, 2016, p. 177.

203. a Irregular bones are known as such because of their irregular shape and include the vertebrae. Metacarpal bones fall under the short bones category. The ulna is an example of a long bone. The scapula is an example of a flat bone. Colville TP, Bassert JM, Clinical Anatomy and Physiology for Veterinary Technicians, ed 3, Mosby, 2016, p. 177.

204. b The axial skeleton consists of the skull, hyoid bones, spinal column, ribs, and sternum. The appendicular skeleton consists of the bones of the limbs. The scapula falls under the appendicular skeleton. Colville TP, Bassert JM, Clinical Anatomy and Physiology for Veterinary Technicians, ed 3, Mosby, 2016, p. 180.

205. b Synarthrosis is an immovable fibrous joint, such as the suture that unites the skull bones. Diarthrosis is a freely movable joint. Amphiarthrosis is a slightly movable cartilaginous joint. Cartilaginous joints are joints in which the bones are united by cartilage, which are also called amphiarthrosis joints. Colville TP, Bassert JM, Clinical Anatomy and Physiology for Veterinary Technicians, ed 3, Mosby, 2016, p. 180.

206. d Pivot joints are also known as trochoid joints and only allow for rotation. There is only one true pivot joint known as the atlantoaxial joint and it is located between the first and second cervical vertebrae. The spheroidal joint is also known as a ball-and-socket joint; the hip and shoulder are examples of this. The elbow joint is an example of a hinge joint. The carpus is an example of a gliding joint. Colville TP, Bassert JM, Clinical Anatomy and Physiology for Veterinary Technicians, ed 3, Mosby, 2016, p. 209.

207. a The trochanter is a large process only located on the femur where hip and thigh muscles attach. Tuberosity is located on the humerus and ischium. Spinal process is located on the vertebrae. Epicondyles are joint-forming processes. Colville TP, Bassert JM, Clinical Anatomy and Physiology for Veterinary Technicians, ed 3, Mosby, 2016, p. 201.

208. d A facet is a flat articular surface and is found on many bones. The meatus, sinus, and foramen all consist of holes or channels that allow the passage of nerves or blood vessels. Colville TP, Bassert JM, Clinical Anatomy and Physiology for Veterinary Technicians, ed 3, Mosby, 2016, p. 180.

209. c The meaning of costo is rib and the meaning of chondral is cartilage; therefore, the correct term is *costochondral junction*, which is the joint between the bony rib and the cartilaginous portion of the rib. The cartilaginous junction only consists of cartilage. Chondralcartilaginous is an incorrect term that would be defined as cartilage and cartilage. The costicartilaginous junction is an incorrect and misspelled term. Colville TP, Bassert JM, Clinical Anatomy and Physiology for Veterinary Technicians, ed 3, Mosby, 2016, p. 192.

210. d A normal dog has 7 cervical, 13 thoracic, and 7 lumbar vertebrae. Cattle have 7 cervical, 13 thoracic, and 6 lumbar vertebrae. The rest are incorrect numbers of vertebrae found in common species. Colville TP, Bassert JM, Clinical Anatomy and Physiology for Veterinary Technicians, ed 3, Mosby, 2016, p. 189.

211. b A normal horse has 7 cervical vertebrae, 18 thoracic vertebrae, and 7 lumbar vertebrae. Normal dogs, cats, and goats have 7, 13, and 7 cervical, thoracic, and lumbar vertebrae. The other choices are incorrectly ordered. Colville TP, Bassert JM, Clinical Anatomy and Physiology for Veterinary Technicians, ed 3, Mosby, 2016, p. 189.

212. b The adult bovine has the following dental formula: I 0/3, C 0/1 P 3/3 M 3/3. The adult canine has M 2/3 and the adult feline has M 1/1. Colville TP, Bassert JM, Clinical Anatomy and Physiology for Veterinary Technicians, ed 3, Mosby, 2016, p. 386.

213. d Aortic and pulmonary valves are also known as semilunar valves and they prevent the backflow of blood from the arteries to the ventricles. The tricuspid, bicuspid, and mitral valves are all located within the heart. Colville TP, Bassert JM, Clinical Anatomy and Physiology for Veterinary Technicians, ed 3, Mosby, 2016, p. 343.

214. b Purkinje fibers carry the impulses from the bundle of His up into the ventricular myocardium, causing contraction of the ventricles. The other options are misspellings of the fiber. Colville TP, Bassert JM, Clinical Anatomy and Physiology for Veterinary Technicians, ed 3, Mosby, 2016, p. 349.

215. a During systole, the heart muscles contract and blood is ejected from the atria to the ventricles and then from the ventricles to the arteries. During diastole, relaxation occurs. Contraction and relaxation cannot occur at the same time. Colville TP, Bassert JM, Clinical Anatomy and Physiology for Veterinary Technicians, ed 3, Mosby, 2016, p. 349.

216. a The aorta begins after it leaves the left ventricle. Then it extends into the aortic arch and travels down the length of the body. The other options are incorrect because the aorta begins on the left side of the body and is the main artery of the body. The inferior vena cava empties into the right atrium. After blood becomes oxygenated it is delivered into the left atrium. Colville TP, Bassert JM, Clinical Anatomy and Physiology for Veterinary Technicians, ed 3, Mosby, 2016, p. 343.

217. c After blood becomes oxygenated, it travels through the pulmonary veins and is delivered into the left atrium. Blood is emptied into the right atrium via the inferior vena cava. Blood leaves the heart into the aorta via the left ventricle. Blood flows through the right atrium into the right ventricle. Colville TP, Bassert JM, Clinical Anatomy and Physiology for Veterinary Technicians, ed 3, Mosby, 2016, p. 346.

218. b Blood traveling through the systemic circulation is under higher pressure compared with the coronary and pulmonary circulation because it takes more pressure to carry blood along the long distance to the farthest extremity. Colville TP, Bassert JM, Clinical Anatomy and Physiology for Veterinary Technicians, ed 3, Mosby, 2016, p. 342.

219. d The foramen ovale is the opening in the septum between the right and left atria and ventricles. This opening closes shortly after birth. An aortic hiatus is the opening between the diaphragm that allows the passage of the aorta, thoracic duct, and azygous vein from the thoracic cavity into the abdominal cavity. A foramen is an opening into or through a bone that allows the passage of blood vessels and nerves. A fossa is a hollow or depressed area on a bone. Aspinall V, Cappello M, Introduction to Veterinary Anatomy and Physiology Textbook, ed 2, Butterworth Heinemann, 2009, p. 84.

220. b Fluid that is carried by the lymphatic system is known as lymph and starts out as excess tissue fluid. Lymph contains mostly lymphocytes, proteins, fats, and hormones. Neutrophils are a type of white blood cell. Colville TP, Bassert JM, Clinical Anatomy and Physiology for Veterinary Technicians, ed 3, Mosby, 2016, p. 312.

221. c After the blood is collected in the right atrium it passes through the right tricuspid valve into the right ventricle of the heart. After blood has collected in the left atrium it travels through the mitral valve into the left ventricle. Colville TP, Bassert JM, Clinical Anatomy and Physiology for Veterinary Technicians, ed 3, Mosby, 2016, p. 343.

222. b The thymus is a lymphoid organ that helps fight off foreign invaders such as bacteria and viruses. The thymus is larger in young animals, begins to atrophy after puberty, and is very small in adults. This organ is located at the level of the heart and extends cranially through the thorax into the neck region on both sides of the trachea. The thymus is separate from the thyroid gland. Colville TP, Bassert JM, Clinical Anatomy and Physiology for Veterinary Technicians, ed 3, Mosby, 2016, p. 290.

223. b The medical term for the eardrum is the *tympanic membrane*. The ear pinna is the outer portion of the ear seen from the outside. The eustachian tube is the connection of the middle cavity to the pharynx. The cochlea is the snail-shaped cavity in the temporal bone of the skull that contains the hearing portion of the inner ear. Colville TP, Bassert JM, Clinical Anatomy and Physiology for Veterinary Technicians, ed 3, Mosby, 2016, p. 260.

224. a Hematopoiesis is the production of all blood cells and takes place in the liver as well as the spleen if necessary. The spleen is responsible for phagocytosis, storage of blood in the splenic pulp, and hematopoiesis. The pancreas is responsible for hormone production to control the metabolism and the use of glucose. The lungs are responsible for respirations. The prostate is a structure that surrounds the urethra in males and carries secretions into the urethra. Colville TP, Bassert JM, Clinical Anatomy and Physiology for Veterinary Technicians, ed 3, Mosby, 2016, p. 296.

225. a Efferent neurons are part of the motor system and afferent neurons are part of the sensory nervous system. Efferent neurons respond to afferent stimulus. Interneurons play a role in integrating incoming sensory impulses. Extraneuron is not part of any system. Colville TP, Bassert JM, Clinical Anatomy and Physiology for Veterinary Technicians, ed 3, Mosby, 2016, p. 244.

226. c Afferent neurons are part of the sensory system. Afferent neurons create the stimulus, and efferent neurons respond to the stimulus. Interneurons play a role in integrating the incoming sensory impulse. Extraneurons are not part of any system. Colville TP, Bassert JM, Clinical Anatomy and Physiology for Veterinary Technicians, ed 3, Mosby, 2016, p. 244.

227. c Oxygen is carried in the hemoglobin in red blood cells (RBCs). White blood cells provide a defense from foreign invaders into the body through phagocytosis. Platelets are responsible for clotting the blood. Colville TP, Bassert JM, Clinical Anatomy and Physiology for Veterinary Technicians, ed 3, Mosby, 2016, p. 15.

228. b The pulmonary artery carries deoxygenated blood from the heart to the lungs where it becomes oxygenated. The aorta leaves the heart and is the main artery that carries oxygenated blood to the rest of the body. Blood travels from the aortic valve into the coronary artery then to the aorta. The carotid artery is located in the neck and supplies the head with blood. Colville TP, Bassert JM, Clinical Anatomy and Physiology for Veterinary Technicians, ed 3, Mosby, 2016, p. 346.

229. d Albumin is a plasma protein. Phospholipids are fatty acids. A lipoprotein is a macromolecule composed of proteins and lipids. An enzyme is a protein molecule. Colville TP, Bassert JM, Clinical Anatomy and Physiology for Veterinary Technicians, ed 3, Mosby, 2016, p. 300.

230. a Albumin is a protein manufactured by the liver and it maintains the osmotic fluid balance between blood and tissues. Red bone marrow is responsible for the formation and the production of different red blood cells. Lymph nodes are responsible for filtering lymph and fluid throughout the body and they aid in the fight against infections. The pancreas is an endocrine and exocrine organ and it produces hormones and pancreatic juices for excretion. Colville TP, Bassert JM, Clinical Anatomy and Physiology for Veterinary Technicians, ed 3, Mosby, 2016, p. 76.

231. b The production of platelets is also known as thrombopoiesis. Hemostasis is the process that causes bleeding to stop. Homeostasis is the physiological balance of all body systems to maintain life. Colville TP, Bassert JM, Clinical Anatomy and Physiology for Veterinary Technicians, ed 3, Mosby, 2016, p. 298.

232. c There are five different types of white blood cells: lymphocytes, neutrophils, eosinophils, basophils, and monocytes. Antibody production and cellular immunity are performed by lymphocytes. Phagocytosis is done by neutrophils, basophils, and monocytes. Colville TP, Bassert JM, Clinical Anatomy and Physiology for Veterinary Technicians, ed 3, Mosby, 2016, p. 310.

233. c Leukocytosis is an increase in white blood cells. Leukopenia is a decrease in white blood cells. Anemia is a decrease in red blood cells. Thrombocytopenia is low blood platelet count. Colville TP, Bassert JM, Clinical Anatomy and Physiology for Veterinary Technicians, ed 3, Mosby, 2016, p. 303.

234. c The liver is the largest gland in the body and is divided into several different hepatic lobes. The pancreas, thyroid, and spleen are all much smaller than the liver. Colville TP, Bassert JM, Clinical Anatomy and Physiology for Veterinary Technicians, ed 3, Mosby, 2016, p. 405.

235. b Bile is produced by hepatic cells and the gallbladder is responsible for storage of bile. The pancreas and spleen are not related to bile production or storage. Colville TP, Bassert JM, Clinical Anatomy and Physiology for Veterinary Technicians, ed 3, Mosby, 2016, p. 406.

236. a Stimulation of the gallbladder occurs when the hormone CCK (cholecystokinin) is released during digestion. Glucagon is a hormone produced by the pancreas. Bile is produced by the liver and is stored in the gallbladder. Filling of the gallbladder does not determine its contraction. Colville TP, Bassert JM, Clinical Anatomy and Physiology for Veterinary Technicians, ed 3, Mosby, 2016, p. 404.

237. a Erythropoietin is a hormone produced by the kidney and is the process of red blood cell production. This hormone is released when the kidneys detect hypoxia in the blood. *Hypoxia* is a term that means deprivation of oxygen. Thrombocytes are simply platelets. Fibrinogen aids in blood clotting. Acetylcholine is a neurotransmitter found in the central and peripheral nervous system. The term *leukocytes* means white blood cells. Colville TP, Bassert JM, Clinical Anatomy and Physiology for Veterinary Technicians, ed 3, Mosby, 2016, p. 289.

238. d The sinoatrial (SA) node is located in the right atrium and is the pacemaker of the heart. The atrioventricular (AV) node initiates a signal that is conducted through the ventricular myocardium via the bundle of His and Purkinje fibers. Colville TP, Bassert JM, Clinical Anatomy and Physiology for Veterinary Technicians, ed 3, Mosby, 2016, p. 347.

239. c Cardiac output is the amount of blood that leaves the heart. This is determined by stroke volume or volume of blood with each cardiac contraction and heart rate, which is how often the heart contracts. CO = SV × HR. Colville TP, Bassert JM, Clinical Anatomy and Physiology for Veterinary Technicians, ed 3, Mosby, 2016, p. 351.

240. c The QRS complex waves are created by ventricular depolarization. The entire ECG cycle consists of the P wave, QRS complex, and the T wave. The P wave is created by atrial depolarization. The T wave is created by repolarization of the ventricles. Colville TP, Bassert JM, Clinical Anatomy and Physiology for Veterinary Technicians, ed 3, Mosby, 2016, p. 358.

241. b Fluid that leaks from the capillaries of the liver can cause free fluid to accumulate in the abdominal cavity, which is termed *ascites*. Pleural effusion is fluid in the thorax. An abscess is an infectious, purulent fluid that can occur anywhere in the body. Pneumothorax is a collapsed lung. Colville TP, Bassert JM, Clinical Anatomy and Physiology for Veterinary Technicians, ed 3, Mosby, 2016, p. 83.

242. c Horses do not have a gallbladder. Dogs and cats both have gallbladders for storage of bile to aid in digestion. Colville TP, Bassert JM, Clinical Anatomy and Physiology for Veterinary Technicians, ed 3, Mosby, 2016, p. 406.

243. c The pancreas is both an exocrine and endocrine gland. The pancreas secretes substances outside the body and produces hormones that are secreted directly into the blood without traveling through a duct. The thyroid is considered an endocrine gland. The kidneys and small intestines are considered endocrine glands. Colville TP, Bassert JM, Clinical Anatomy and Physiology for Veterinary Technicians, ed 3, Mosby, 2016, p. 287.

244. a The pancreas is divided into many different cells. The clumps of cells that form it are known as pancreatic islets or islets of Langerhans. The islets of Langerhans are not associated with the liver, kidneys, and adrenal glands. Colville TP, Bassert JM, Clinical Anatomy and Physiology for Veterinary Technicians, ed 3, Mosby, 2016, p. 287.

245. b Beta cells produce insulin. Alpha cells produce glucagon. Delta cells produce somatostatin. Colville TP, Bassert JM, Clinical Anatomy and Physiology for Veterinary Technicians, ed 3, Mosby, 2016, p. 287.

246. c Relaxin is a hormone produced by the ovaries late in pregnancy that causes the ligaments surrounding the birth canal to relax for parturition. Estrogen and progesterone are hormones produced by the ovaries throughout their cycles. Testosterone is a male hormone. Colville TP, Bassert JM, Clinical Anatomy and Physiology for Veterinary Technicians, ed 3, Mosby, 2016, p. 288.

247. d Diabetes mellitus can present with many different symptoms such as polyuria, polydipsia, polyphagia, weight loss, and weakness. Colville TP, Bassert JM, Clinical Anatomy and Physiology for Veterinary Technicians, ed 3, Mosby, 2016, p. 287.

248. b The urinary system is the single most important route of waste-product removal because it removes nearly all the soluble waste products from blood and transports them out of the body. It is also the major route of elimination of excess water in the body. The respiratory system removes carbon dioxide from the body but is not considered a waste-product removal system. The digestive system removes waste products from the body through stools but it is not considered the most important removal system. Colville TP, Bassert JM, Clinical Anatomy and Physiology for Veterinary Technicians, ed 3, Mosby, 2016, p. 446.

249. c The correct path in which urine is formed and travels through the body for elimination is: kidneys, ureters, bladder, and urethra. Urine is formed in the kidneys and travels to the bladder via the ureters. After the bladder is full, urine will leave the bladder via the urethra to the outside of the body. The other options are in the incorrect order. Colville TP, Bassert JM, Clinical Anatomy and Physiology for Veterinary Technicians, ed 3, Mosby, 2016, p. 447.

250. b The kidneys help maintain acid-base homeostasis by their ability to remove hydrogen and bicarbonate ions from the blood and excrete them in the urine. The lungs are responsible for taking in oxygen and expelling carbon dioxide. The liver is responsible for many different functions, such as bile production, protein production, breaking down of lipids, but acid-base balance is not one of them. The spleen is responsible for storage of blood, phagocytosis, and filtering of blood. Colville TP, Bassert JM, Clinical Anatomy and Physiology for Veterinary Technicians, ed 3, Mosby, 2016, p. 448.

251. b The indented area on the medial side of the kidney is termed the *hilum* and is the area where the blood vessels, nerves, and ureter enter and leave the kidney. The porta hepatis is where the portal triad (proper hepatic artery, portal vein, and common bile duct) enters the liver. The opposite side of the kidney is convex in shape. The cortex is the outermost portion of the kidney. Colville TP, Bassert JM, Clinical Anatomy and Physiology for Veterinary Technicians, ed 3, Mosby, 2016, p. 450.

252. b The basic function unit of the kidney is the nephron. Each kidney is made up of thousands of nephrons. The cortex is the outermost area of the kidney. The Bowman's capsule surrounds the glomerulus and is part of the renal corpuscle, which is within a nephron. The loop of Henle is also part of the nephron through which urine travels before entering the collecting duct. Colville TP, Bassert JM, Clinical Anatomy and Physiology for Veterinary Technicians, ed 3, Mosby, 2016, p. 450.

253. d Cows have approximately 4,000,000 nephrons per kidney. Sheep, pigs, and humans have approximately 1,000,000 nephrons per kidney. Dogs have approximately 700,000 nephrons per kidney. Colville TP, Bassert JM, Clinical Anatomy and Physiology for Veterinary Technicians, ed 3, Mosby, 2016, p. 450.

254. a The renal corpuscle, part of a nephron, is located in the cortex of the kidney. The descending loop of Henle is located in the renal medulla. The renal sinus is where urine is collected before entering the ureter. The hilum is the portion of the kidney that contains the ureter, vasculature, and nerves. Colville TP, Bassert JM, Clinical Anatomy and Physiology for Veterinary Technicians, ed 3, Mosby, 2016, p. 451.

255. c The kidneys are a very vascular organ because of their major function in the body and approximately 25% of the blood pumped from the heart travels to the kidneys. The other blood supply options are either not sufficient or are too much. Colville TP, Bassert JM, Clinical Anatomy and Physiology for Veterinary Technicians, ed 3, Mosby, 2016, p. 453.

256. d There are three main mechanisms by which the kidney performs its waste elimination role: filtration of the blood, reabsorption of useful substances back into the bloodstream, and secretion of waste products from the blood into the tubules of the nephrons. Colville TP, Bassert JM, Clinical Anatomy and Physiology for Veterinary Technicians, ed 3, Mosby, 2016, p. 453.

257. d The two hormones responsible for urine volume regulation are: antidiuretic hormone (ADH) released from the posterior pituitary gland and aldosterone secreted by the adrenal cortex. Glucagon is a hormone secreted by the pancreas. Colville TP, Bassert JM, Clinical Anatomy and Physiology for Veterinary Technicians, ed 3, Mosby, 2016, p. 454.

258. c The ureters are tubes composed of three layers, an outer fibrous layer, a middle, muscular layer of smooth muscle, and an inner epithelial layer lined with transition epithelium. Colville TP, Bassert JM, Clinical Anatomy and Physiology for Veterinary Technicians, ed 3, Mosby, 2016, p. 458.

259. d Prerenal uremia is associated with decreased blood flow to the kidneys and may be caused by dehydration, congestive heart failure, and/or shock. Colville TP, Bassert JM, Clinical Anatomy and Physiology for Veterinary Technicians, ed 3, Mosby, 2016, p. 461.

260. d The testes are the male gonads and have two main functions: spermatogenesis and hormone production. Spermatogenesis is the production of spermatozoa. Testosterone is the main hormone produced by the testes. Urine formation occurs within the kidneys. Colville TP, Bassert JM, Clinical Anatomy and Physiology for Veterinary Technicians, ed 3, Mosby, 2016, p. 469.

261. b The term *cryptorchidism* refers to a condition in which one or both of the testes do not descend into the scrotum. This results in the recommended surgical removal of both testes because of the potential development of testicular carcinoma of the undescended testis resulting from inappropriate conditions such as excessive heat. Torsion occurs when the testicle rotates about its axis within the scrotal sac causing disruption or cessation of vascularity flow and drainage resulting in testicular death. The surgical removal of the testicles is referred to as neutering. Many inflammatory conditions can develop within the testicles or reproductive tract; however, cryptorchidism does not relate to this condition. Colville TP, Bassert JM, Clinical Anatomy and Physiology for Veterinary Technicians, ed 3, Mosby, 2016, p. 472.

262. c The epididymis is a flat ribbon-like structure that lies along the surface of the testes, which connects the efferent ducts of the testes with the vas deferens. The cremaster muscle is a band-like muscle that passes down through the inguinal ring and attaches to the scrotum. The vas deferens is a tube-like structure that connects the testes with the urethra. The seminiferous tubules are the site of the germination, maturation, and transportation of the sperm cells within the male testes. Colville TP, Bassert JM, Clinical Anatomy and Physiology for Veterinary Technicians, ed 3, Mosby, 2016, p. 473.

263. b There are two bulbourethral glands, also known as the Cowper's glands, which secrete a mucinous fluid just before ejaculation. They are responsible for clearing and lubricating the urethra for the passage of semen and are present in all common domestic animals except dogs. Colville TP, Bassert JM, Clinical Anatomy and Physiology for Veterinary Technicians, ed 3, Mosby, 2016, p. 474.

264. c The broad ligaments are sheets of peritoneum that are divided into different segments based on the organ they support. The mesosalpinx ligament supports the oviduct, the uterus is supported by the mesometrium, and the ovaries are supported by the mesovarium. The vagina is the structure that connects the vulva with the cervix. Colville TP, Bassert JM, Clinical Anatomy and Physiology for Veterinary Technicians, ed 3, Mosby, 2016, p. 477.

265. c The number of follicles involved in each cycle depends on the species. Uniparous species, which include cattle, horses, and humans, give birth usually to only one offspring. Multiparous species, including cats, dogs, and sows, give birth to litters of offspring. Colville TP, Bassert JM, Clinical Anatomy and Physiology for Veterinary Technicians, ed 3, Mosby, 2016, p. 480.

266. a Anestrus refers to the period of temporary ovarian inactivity. Diestrus refers to the active, luteal stage, when the corpus luteum has reached its maximum size. Pseudocyesis, also known as pseudopregnancy or false pregnancy, is an exaggerated diestrous period. Heat is the period when pets are in estrous and is the time that they can become pregnant. Colville TP, Bassert JM, Clinical Anatomy and Physiology for Veterinary Technicians, ed 3, Mosby, 2016, p. 484.

267. d The placenta is known for providing the life-support system for the developing fetus and is connected to the fetus via the umbilical cord. The ovum is the egg that is released from the ovary and after fertilization by the sperm develops into the fetus. The uterus is the structure that houses the growing fetus. The amnion is the area located around the growing fetus. Colville TP, Bassert JM, Clinical Anatomy and Physiology for Veterinary Technicians, ed 3, Mosby, 2016, p. 290.

268. a The gestational period for cats is typically 56–69 days or 2 months, for cattle it is 271–291 days, for ferrets it is 42 days, and for hamsters it is 19–20 days. Colville TP, Bassert JM, Clinical Anatomy and Physiology for Veterinary Technicians, ed 3, Mosby, 2016, p. 494.

269. c The gestational period for elephants is 615–650 days, for horses it is 321–346 days, for sheep it is 143–151 days, and for cattle it is 271–291 days. Colville TP, Bassert JM, Clinical Anatomy and Physiology for Veterinary Technicians, ed 3, Mosby, 2016, p. 494.

270. b An infection that might occur in the mammary glands is known as mastitis. The production of colostrum is what occurs just before or immediately after birth has taken place. Mammary glands are present in both males and females and are simply known as mammary glands. A hormone that aids in the production of milk is known as prolactin. Colville TP, Bassert JM, Clinical Anatomy and Physiology for Veterinary Technicians, ed 3, Mosby, 2016, p. 497.

271. c The anterior pituitary gland is an endocrine gland that is responsible for producing several hormones such as prolactin, growth hormone, thyroid-stimulating, adrenocorticotropic, follicle-stimulating, luteinizing, and melanocyte-stimulating hormones. The posterior pituitary gland is responsible for producing antidiuretic hormone and oxytocin. The thyroid gland secretes thyroid hormone and calcitonin. The ovaries secrete estrogen and progestins. Colville TP, Bassert JM, Clinical Anatomy and Physiology for Veterinary Technicians, ed 3, Mosby, 2016, p. 280.

272. b The testes are responsible for secreting androgens. The ovaries are responsible for secreting estrogen and progestins. The adrenal cortex is responsible for the secretion of sex hormones. Colville TP, Bassert JM, Clinical Anatomy and Physiology for Veterinary Technicians, ed 3, Mosby, 2016, p. 469.

273. b Insulin is produced by the pancreas and is responsible for the movement of glucose into cells and its use for energy. Progestins are produced by the ovary and are responsible for the maintenance of pregnancy. Glucagon is produced by the pancreas and is responsible for increasing blood glucose. Calcitonin is produced in the thyroid and helps prevent hypercalcemia. Colville TP, Bassert JM, Clinical Anatomy and Physiology for Veterinary Technicians, ed 3, Mosby, 2016, p. 287.

274. d The following organs and glands are part of the endocrine system: pancreas, kidneys, stomach, small intestine, ovaries, testis, pituitary gland, thyroid gland, parathyroid gland, adrenal gland, thymus, pineal body, and placenta. Colville TP, Bassert JM, Clinical Anatomy and Physiology for Veterinary Technicians, ed 3, Mosby, 2016, p. 276.

275. d There are seven known hormones that are secreted by the anterior pituitary gland, including the growth hormone, prolactin, thyroid-stimulating hormone, adrenocorticotropic hormone, follicle-stimulating hormone, luteinizing hormone, and melanocyte-stimulating hormone. Colville TP, Bassert JM, Clinical Anatomy and Physiology for Veterinary Technicians, ed 3, Mosby, 2016, p. 279.

276. d Prolactin is secreted by the anterior pituitary gland and is responsible for triggering and maintaining lactation in the female. Follicle-stimulating hormone is also secreted by the anterior pituitary gland and is responsible for the growth of the follicle within the ovary for preparation of ovulation. Luteinizing hormone completes the process of follicle development within the ovary in advance of ovulation and helps to produce the corpus luteum, which is responsible for maintaining pregnancy. Mineralocorticoid hormone regulates the levels of electrolytes within the body. Colville TP, Bassert JM, Clinical Anatomy and Physiology for Veterinary Technicians, ed 3, Mosby, 2016, p. 276.

277. d There are four different routes responsible for waste excretion. The respiratory system removes carbon dioxide and water vapor, the sweat glands remove water, salts, and urea, the digestive system removes bile salts and pigments, the urinary system removes urea, salts, and water. Colville TP, Bassert JM, Clinical Anatomy and Physiology for Veterinary Technicians, ed 3, Mosby, 2016, p. 79.

278. b The kidneys are located retroperitoneal to the abdominal cavity. They are outside the parietal peritoneum, which is between the peritoneum and the dorsal abdominal muscles. The pelvic cavity is below the abdominal cavity and contains the genitals and urinary bladder. The thoracic cavity is above the diaphragm and contains the heart and lungs. Colville TP, Bassert JM, Clinical Anatomy and Physiology for Veterinary Technicians, ed 3, Mosby, 2016, p. 449.

279. c In all domestic animals (with the exception of cattle), the kidneys are smooth on the surface. Cattle kidneys are divided into 12 lobes, which give them a lumpy appearance. Colville TP, Bassert JM, Clinical Anatomy and Physiology for Veterinary Technicians, ed 3, Mosby, 2016, p. 449.

280. b The renal artery branches off the abdominal aorta and enters at the hilum of the kidney. The interlobar arteries are located within the kidney. The aorta is the main artery located in the midline of the body. The iliac arteries are the distal branch of the aorta before entering the hind limbs. Colville TP, Bassert JM, Clinical Anatomy and Physiology for Veterinary Technicians, ed 3, Mosby, 2016, p. 451.

281. b The renal vein leaves the hilum of the kidney to enter the vena cava. The aorta is the main artery of the body. The hepatic vein and portal vein are part of the liver anatomy. Colville TP, Bassert JM, Clinical Anatomy and Physiology for Veterinary Technicians, ed 3, Mosby, 2016, p. 452.

282. d There are five different types of white blood cells: basophil, neutrophil, eosinophil, lymphocytes, and monocyte. Colville TP, Bassert JM, Clinical Anatomy and Physiology for Veterinary Technicians, ed 3, Mosby, 2016, p. 306.

283. c Monocytes and lymphocytes do not contain cytoplasmic granules and are referred to as agranulocytes. Basophils, eosinophils, and neutrophils are called granulocytes because they contain cytoplasmic granules. Colville TP, Bassert JM, Clinical Anatomy and Physiology for Veterinary Technicians, ed 3, Mosby, 2016, p. 306.

284. a The preen gland or uropygial gland secretes an oily/fatty substance. During the act of preening the gland is stimulated and the oil is spread throughout the feathers to protect and clean them. Colville TP, Bassert JM, Clinical Anatomy and Physiology for Veterinary Technicians, ed 3, Mosby, 2016, p. 503.

285. a The vane is the flattened part of the feather that appears web-like and is located on either side of the rachis. The rachis is the main feather shaft. The superior umbilicus is the opening on the feather shaft. The inferior umbilicus is the opening at the base of the feather. Colville TP, Bassert JM, Clinical Anatomy and Physiology for Veterinary Technicians, ed 3, Mosby, 2016, p. 506.

286. b Flight feathers of birds are known as remiges. Tail feathers are known as retrices. Small contour feathers are known as auriculars. Down feathers are located under the contour feathers and are responsible for insulation. Colville TP, Bassert JM, Clinical Anatomy and Physiology for Veterinary Technicians, ed 3, Mosby, 2016, p. 506.

287. a The gizzard is the muscular portion of the stomach that contains bands of striated muscles that are responsible for grinding food. The proventriculus is the anterior glandular stomach and is where chemical digestion occurs. Colville TP, Bassert JM, Clinical Anatomy and Physiology for Veterinary Technicians, ed 3, Mosby, 2016, p. 525.

288. c Small birds less than 25 g typically have a restrained heart rate of 400–600 bpm. Birds more than 10,000 g have 100–150 bpm, birds around 200 g have 300–500 bpm, and birds around 2000 g have 110–175 bpm. Colville TP, Bassert JM, Clinical Anatomy and Physiology for Veterinary Technicians, ed 3, Mosby, 2016, p. 529.

289. a The cloaca is located at the end of the digestive tract. Colville TP, Bassert JM, Clinical Anatomy and Physiology for Veterinary Technicians, ed 3, Mosby, 2016, p. 525.

290. b The skin is primarily composed of two different layers. The epidermis is the most superficial layer, and the dermis is just beneath the epidermis. The hypodermis is beneath the skin. Aspinall V, Cappello M, Introduction to Veterinary Anatomy and Physiology Textbook, ed 2, Butterworth Heinemann, 2009, p. 143.

291. b The epidermis is composed of multiple layers of stratified squamous epithelium cells that are continually renewed. The dermis is composed of dense connective tissue of collagen and elastin fibers. The hypodermis lies beneath the actual skin and is composed of loose connective tissue and fat and gives the skin flexibility. Aspinall V, Cappello M, Introduction to Veterinary Anatomy and Physiology Textbook, ed 2, Butterworth Heinemann, 2009, p. 144.

292. a The dermis is composed of dense connective tissue of collagen and elastic fibers and houses the hair follicles, sebaceous glands, and sweat glands. The epidermis is composed of stratified squamous epithelium cells and continually renews itself. The hypodermis lies beneath the actual skin layer and is composed of loose connective tissue. Aspinall V, Cappello M, Introduction to Veterinary Anatomy and Physiology Textbook, ed 2, Butterworth Heinemann, 2009, p. 144.

293. c Epithelium cells are typically described by shape and are three basic shapes: flattened, cubic, column-shaped. Aspinall V, Cappello M, Introduction to Veterinary

Anatomy and Physiology Textbook, ed 2, Butterworth Heinemann, 2009, p. 15.

294. c Squamous cells are flattened. Cuboidal cells are square or cube. Columnar cells are column-shaped. These cells describe the three basic cell shapes seen within epithelium cells. Aspinall V, Cappello M, Introduction to Veterinary Anatomy and Physiology Textbook, ed 2, Butterworth Heinemann, 2009, p. 15.

295. b Ciliated epithelium cells contain tiny hair-like projections called cilia that move foreign particles along the epithelial surface. Simple columnar epithelium has tall narrow cells and is only one layer thick. Stratified epithelium is composed of multiple layers of cells and is thicker and tougher than the other types. Transitional epithelium cells are specialized stratified cells lining parts of the urinary system. Aspinall V, Cappello M, Introduction to Veterinary Anatomy and Physiology Textbook, ed 2, Butterworth Heinemann, 2009, p. 16.

296. d There are several types of connective tissue that differ based on the type of extracellular matrix in which it belongs. The following types of connective tissue are listed based on increasing order: blood, hemopoietic tissue, areolar tissue, adipose tissue, fibrous connective tissue, cartilage, and bone. Aspinall V, Cappello M, Introduction to Veterinary Anatomy and Physiology Textbook, ed 2, Butterworth Heinemann, 2009, p. 17.

297. a Hemopoietic tissue is the connective tissue that forms the bone marrow within the long bones and is also responsible for the formation of the blood. Areolar tissue is a loose connective tissue distributed across the entire body. Cartilage is a rigid but flexible tissue found throughout the body and contains no blood. Bone is a living tissue that can remodel and repair itself and provides the framework of the body. Aspinall V, Cappello M, Introduction to Veterinary Anatomy and Physiology Textbook, ed 2, Butterworth Heinemann, 2009, p. 18.

298. c Two hormones, calcitonin from the thyroid gland and parathyroid hormone from the parathyroid glands, act as "cashiers" at the calcium bank. Calcitonin helps prevent hypercalcemia, whereas parathyroid hormone helps prevent hypocalcemia, which is a low level of calcium in the blood, in part by withdrawing calcium from the bones. T4 is a hormone produced by the thyroid gland, which helps with the body's metabolic rate. Vitamin D is essential for blood clotting and bone and tooth formation. Colville TP, Bassert JM, Clinical Anatomy and Physiology for Veterinary Technicians, ed 3, Mosby, 2016, p. 173.

299. d Mammary glands contain compound alveolar or multiple alveolar tissues. Single and multiple alveolar tissues can be found in sebaceous glands. Single tubular cells can be found within the stomach and intestines. Tubular multiple cells can be found in the stomach, mouth, tongue, esophagus, and the bulbourethral glands. Aspinall V, Cappello M, Introduction to Veterinary Anatomy and Physiology Textbook, ed 2, Butterworth Heinemann, 2009, p. 19.

300. d The cancellous bone is also known as spongy bone and it contains the internal meshwork of trabeculae that has the spaces filled with red bone marrow. Compact bone is a solid and hard substance found in the outer layer of the bone. Aspinall V, Cappello M, Introduction to Veterinary Anatomy and Physiology Textbook, ed 2, Butterworth Heinemann, 2009, p. 20.

301. c The periosteum is a fibrous membrane that covers the outer surface of all types of bones. Cartilage is found in different areas throughout the body but does not cover the bone surface. The bone marrow is found within long bones. The lamellae are concentric cylinders of matrix material within the haversian canal. Aspinall V, Cappello M, Introduction to Veterinary Anatomy and Physiology Textbook, ed 2, Butterworth Heinemann, 2009, p. 21.

302. a The mediastinum is a connective tissue septum that separates the thorax into right and left sides. The pericardium is a double-layered membranous sheath that surrounds the heart. The pulmonary pleura cover the lungs. The sternum is the bony structure that lies in the middle of the thorax and protects the chest cavity. Aspinall V, Cappello M, Introduction to Veterinary Anatomy and Physiology Textbook, ed 2, Butterworth Heinemann, 2009, p. 25.

303. b The abdominal cavity lies immediately caudal to the thoracic cavity and contains the abdominal viscera. The pelvic cavity is caudal to the abdominal cavity and the abdominal cavity separates the thoracic and pelvic cavity. The pleural cavity is part of the thoracic cavity. The term *caudal* refers to the direction toward the tail. Aspinall V, Cappello M, Introduction to Veterinary Anatomy and Physiology Textbook, ed 2, Butterworth Heinemann, 2009, p. 26.

304. b Pneumatic bones contain the air-filled spaces that help to reduce the weight of the bones. The sesamoid bones are sesame-shaped bones that develop with a tendon. Splanchnic bones develop in a soft organ and are not attached to the rest of the skeleton. Irregular bones are not uniform in shape and include the vertebrae. Aspinall V, Cappello M, Introduction to Veterinary Anatomy and Physiology Textbook, ed 2, Butterworth Heinemann, 2009, p. 29.

305. a Osteoblasts are the cells that are responsible for laying down new bone. Osteoclasts are the cells that destroy the bones. Ossification is the process by which bone is formed. Hemopoiesis is responsible for forming the bone marrow. Aspinall V, Cappello M, Introduction to Veterinary Anatomy and Physiology Textbook, ed 2, Butterworth Heinemann, 2009, p. 29.

306. b The formation of one bone connecting to another bone forms an arthrosis or joint. A hinge is a type of joint. Cartilage is a rigid but flexible tissue found throughout the body and contains no blood. Ossification is the process by which bone is formed. Aspinall V, Cappello M, Introduction to Veterinary Anatomy and Physiology Textbook, ed 2, Butterworth Heinemann, 2009, p. 41.

307. a Fibrous joints are immovable joints that connect bones through a dense fibrous connective tissue. Cartilaginous joints allow very little or no movement and are connected to bone by cartilage. Synovial joints allow movement to occur because of the joint cavity that is filled with synovial fluid. Aspinall V, Cappello M, Introduction to Veterinary Anatomy and Physiology Textbook, ed 2, Butterworth Heinemann, 2009, p. 42.

308. c The mandibular symphysis joins the two halves of the mandible together. The two hip bones are joined by the symphysis pubis. Each vertebra within the spinal column is joined by a cartilaginous joint. The occipital and parietal bones are within the skull and are connected by sutures or synovial joints. Aspinall V, Cappello M, Introduction to Veterinary Anatomy and Physiology Textbook, ed 2, Butterworth Heinemann, 2009, p. 42.

309. d Synovial joints allow many different types of movements. The following are all possible movements within a synovial joint: abduction/adduction, retraction, protraction, circumduction, flexion/extension, rotation, and gliding/sliding. Aspinall V, Cappello M, Introduction to Veterinary Anatomy and Physiology Textbook, ed 2, Butterworth Heinemann, 2009, p. 43.

310. b Circumduction is defined as the movement of an extremity of one end of a bone in a circular pattern. Rotation describes a body part that twists on its own axis. Retraction describes an animal moving the limb back toward the body. Protraction describes an animal moving the limb cranially. Aspinall V, Cappello M, Introduction to Veterinary Anatomy and Physiology Textbook, ed 2, Butterworth Heinemann, 2009, p. 43.

311. d All of the following are different types of synovial joints: plane/gliding, hinge, pivot, condylar, and ball and socket. Plane/gliding allows for sliding of one body surface over the other. Condylar consists of a convex surface inside a concave surface and allows for a movement in two planes. Pivot joints allow rotation and ball and socket joints allow a great range of movement. Aspinall V, Cappello M, Introduction to Veterinary Anatomy and Physiology Textbook, ed 2, Butterworth Heinemann, 2009, p. 44.

312. c The stifle is an example of a hinge joint because it allows movement to occur in only one plane. The hip is an example of a ball-and-socket joint. The shoulder is also an example of a ball-and-socket joint. The atlantoaxial joint is located between C1 and C2. Aspinall V, Cappello M, Introduction to Veterinary Anatomy and Physiology Textbook, ed 2, Butterworth Heinemann, 2009, p. 44.

313. a With an isotonic contraction, the muscle actually moves or shortens. Muscle tone describes skeletal muscles that are always in a state of tension. Isometric contraction describes when tension is generated in the muscles, muscle tone is increased, but the muscle does not shorten. Aspinall V, Cappello M, Introduction to Veterinary Anatomy and Physiology Textbook, ed 2, Butterworth Heinemann, 2009, p. 45.

314. b Sphincter muscles are muscles that form a circular ring that serves to control the entrance or exit to a structure. Muscle tone describes the skeletal muscles always being in a state of tension. A bursa is a connective tissue sac lined with synovial membrane and filled with synovial fluid. Extrinsic muscles run from one region of the body to another and alter the position of the whole part. Aspinall V, Cappello M, Introduction to Veterinary Anatomy and Physiology Textbook, ed 2, Butterworth Heinemann, 2009, p. 46.

315. b Intrinsic muscles are responsible for moving the lips, cheeks, nostrils, eyelids, and external ears. Sphincter muscles form a circular ring and control the entrance or exit of a structure. Extrinsic muscles run from one region of the body to another and alter the position of the whole part. Digastricus is the muscle that opens the jaw. Aspinall V, Cappello M, Introduction to Veterinary Anatomy and Physiology Textbook, ed 2, Butterworth Heinemann, 2009, p. 47.

316. b During the gestational development process, the male testes begin to develop within the abdominal cavity near the kidneys and they later travel down to their final placement within the scrotal sac outside the body. The stomach and gallbladder are not related to the urinary tract system and are located too far cranially for this development to occur. The urinary bladder is located within the pelvis where the testes will travel past during their descent into the scrotal sac, but they do not begin development at this location. Colville TP, Bassert JM, Clinical Anatomy and Physiology for Veterinary Technicians, ed 3, Mosby, 2016, p. 471.

317. d The scrotum is the sac of skin that houses the testes and is also responsible for regulating the temperature of the testes. The production of sperm occurs within the testes itself. Colville TP, Bassert JM, Clinical Anatomy and Physiology for Veterinary Technicians, ed 3, Mosby, 2016, p. 471.

318. c The spermatic cord is a tube-like connective tissue structure that contains blood vessels, nerves, lymphatic vessels, and the vas deferens. The scrotum contains the testes. The vaginal tunics are layers of connective tissue that surround the testes. The pampiniform plexus is a network of tiny veins derived from the testicular vein. Colville TP, Bassert JM, Clinical Anatomy and Physiology for Veterinary Technicians, ed 3, Mosby, 2016, p. 471.

319. b The pampiniform plexus is a network of tiny veins derived from the testicular vein and surrounds the testicular artery. The spermatic cord links the testes with the rest of the body and houses the blood vessels, nerves, lymphatic, and vas deferens. The vas deferens is the duct that passes sperm from the testicle to the urethra. Colville TP, Bassert JM, Clinical Anatomy and Physiology for Veterinary Technicians, ed 3, Mosby, 2016, p. 471.

320. a After sperm detach from the Sertoli cells, they travel to the storage location within the epididymis. The vas deferens is the duct that passes sperm from the testes to the urethra. The visceral vaginal tunic is the thin inner layer of peritoneum that coats the testes as they develop in the abdomen. The pampiniform plexus is a network of tiny veins derived from the testicular vein and surrounding the testicular artery. Colville TP, Bassert JM, Clinical Anatomy and Physiology for Veterinary Technicians, ed 3, Mosby, 2016, p. 473.

321. c The two layers of connective tissue that surround the testes in the scrotum and spermatic cord are known as the vaginal tunics. The parietal vaginal tunic is the thick outer layer. The visceral vaginal tunic, also known as the proper vaginal tunic, is the thin, inner layer. Colville TP, Bassert JM, Clinical Anatomy and Physiology for Veterinary Technicians, ed 3, Mosby, 2016, p. 472.

322. b The tunica albuginea is a heavy fibrous connective tissue capsule that surrounds each testis beneath the tunics. The common vaginal tunic is also known as the parietal vaginal tunic and is the thick outer layer of connective tissue. The pampiniform plexus includes the testicular veins on the surface of the testes that surround the testicular artery. Septa are small partitions that extend into the testis from the capsule that surrounds and supports the soft contents of the testes. Colville TP, Bassert JM, Clinical Anatomy and Physiology for Veterinary Technicians, ed 3, Mosby, 2016, p. 472.

323. a Spermatogenesis is the process by which spermatozoa are produced from male primordial germs cells by mitosis and meiosis and it takes place within the seminiferous tubules. The epididymis is the duct adjacent to the testis that allows sperm to pass through to the vas deferens and allows the sperm to mature. The spermatic cord is the cord-like structure that is formed by the vas deferens and surrounds the tissue that travels from the inguinal ring into the testicles. The pampiniform plexus includes the testicular veins on the surface of the testes, which surround the testicular artery. Colville TP, Bassert JM, Clinical Anatomy and Physiology for Veterinary Technicians, ed 3, Mosby, 2016, p. 472.

324. c The vas deferens is responsible for propelling spermatozoa and fluid from the epididymis to the urethra. The sperm mature within the epididymis before ejaculation. The epididymis is also responsible for the storage of sperm before ejaculation. Spermatozoa are produced within the seminiferous tubules. Colville TP, Bassert JM, Clinical Anatomy and Physiology for Veterinary Technicians, ed 3, Mosby, 2016, p. 474.

325. d The accessory reproductive glands produce alkaline fluid to surround the spermatozoa, which helps to counteract the acidity of the female reproductive tract and contains the following substances: electrolytes, fructose, and prostaglandins. Colville TP, Bassert JM, Clinical Anatomy and Physiology for Veterinary Technicians, ed 3, Mosby, 2016, p. 474.

326. d Seminal vesicles are glands located behind the bladder and they make up most of the content of semen. Dogs and cats do not have seminal vesicles. The following animals do have seminal vesicles: boar, bull, ram, and stallion. Colville TP, Bassert JM, Clinical Anatomy and Physiology for Veterinary Technicians, ed 3, Mosby, 2016, p. 474.

327. e All of the following animals have prostate glands; dogs, cats, boars, stallion, bull, ram, and humans. Colville TP, Bassert JM, Clinical Anatomy and Physiology for Veterinary Technicians, ed 3, Mosby, 2016, p. 474.

328. c The prostate gland is a single structure that completely surrounds the urethra and contains multiple ducts that carry secretion into the urethra. The prostate gland is not located within the scrotum and therefore it does not cover the testis, epididymis, or spermatic cord. Colville TP, Bassert JM, Clinical Anatomy and Physiology for Veterinary Technicians, ed 3, Mosby, 2016, p. 474.

329. b The bulbourethral glands are also known as the Cowper's glands because they were first documented by anatomist William Cowper. The prostate is a separate gland from the bulbourethral gland. The root of the penis is the connection to the brim of the pelvis. The seminal gland does not exist. Colville TP, Bassert JM, Clinical Anatomy and Physiology for Veterinary Technicians, ed 3, Mosby, 2016, p. 474.

330. d The tip of the glans of the penis varies among species. Cats contain short spines on the gland. Horses contain a large amount of erectile tissue of the glans. In ruminants, the glans is small and not well defined. The dog contains the os penis and an erectile structure to aid in reproduction. Colville TP, Bassert JM, Clinical Anatomy and Physiology for Veterinary Technicians, ed 3, Mosby, 2016, p. 475.

331. a The os penis is a bone structure that lies within the penis and is only found in dogs and wildlife. No other domestic animals have the os penis. Colville TP, Bassert JM, Clinical Anatomy and Physiology for Veterinary Technicians, ed 3, Mosby, 2016, p. 475.

332. b The bulb of the glans of dogs become enlarged toward the rear of the glans, which can tightly clamp in place by contractions of the muscles surrounding the vagina and vulva causing the two animals to become "tied" together or stuck until the glands reduce in size. The testicles do not cause an issue during breeding. The os penis is a bone structure located within the penis of dogs. Colville TP, Bassert JM, Clinical Anatomy and Physiology for Veterinary Technicians, ed 3, Mosby, 2016, p. 475.

333. b The sagittal plane is a plane that runs the length of the body separating it into left and right parts. A median plane is also a sagittal plane but runs directly down the center of the body separating left and right into two equal halves. The dorsal plane is a plane at right angles to the sagittal and transverse plane, dividing the body into dorsal and ventral parts. The transverse plane runs across the body, dividing it into cranial and caudal parts. Colville TP, Bassert JM, Clinical Anatomy and Physiology for Veterinary Technicians, ed 3, Mosby, 2016, p. 3.

334. b The thoracic cavity is cranial to the abdomen, meaning that it is toward the head. The term *caudal* refers to the direction toward the tail. *Dorsal* is the term toward the back of the animal. The term *ventral* is toward the sternum. Colville TP, Bassert JM, Clinical Anatomy and Physiology for Veterinary Technicians, ed 3, Mosby, 2016, p. 5.

335. b The duodenum is the first portion of the small intestine that exits the stomach on the right side of the animal's abdomen. The cranial direction is toward the animal's head and the caudal direction is toward the animal's tail; both are incorrect locations of the duodenum. Colville TP, Bassert JM, Clinical Anatomy and Physiology for Veterinary Technicians, ed 3, Mosby, 2016, p. 5.

336. b The horses' shoulder is located cranial to the hip, meaning it is located toward the animal's head. Caudal refers to the direction toward the animal's tail. Proximal is located closer toward the body. Ventral is located toward the animal's belly. Colville TP, Bassert JM, Clinical Anatomy and Physiology for Veterinary Technicians, ed 3, Mosby, 2016, p. 5.

337. a The xiphoid process is the caudal end of the sternum. The trochanter is the part of the femur that connects to the hip bone. The calcaneus is the bone in the hind leg of the horse. The cannon bone is a bone located in the forelimb of a horse. Colville TP, Bassert JM, Clinical Anatomy and Physiology for Veterinary Technicians, ed 3, Mosby, 2016, p. 5.

338. a The back of the hind leg distal to the tarsus is known as the plantar surface or the ground surface. The palmar surface refers to the back or caudal surface of the front leg. Lateral refers to anything located toward the outer edges of the body or away from the midline. Medial refers to anything located toward the center of the body or toward the midline. Colville TP, Bassert JM, Clinical Anatomy and Physiology for Veterinary Technicians, ed 3, Mosby, 2016, p. 5.

339. b The animal's body consists of two main body cavities, the dorsal cavity and the ventral cavity. These two cavities contain other smaller cavities such as the cranial cavity, spinal cavity, thoracic cavity, and abdominal cavity. Colville TP, Bassert JM, Clinical Anatomy and Physiology for Veterinary Technicians, ed 3, Mosby, 2016, p. 6.

340. d The dorsal body cavity contains the brain and the spinal cord. The ventral cavity contains the chest. Colville TP, Bassert JM, Clinical Anatomy and Physiology for Veterinary Technicians, ed 3, Mosby, 2016, p. 6.

341. d The ventral body cavity is the largest body cavity and contains most of the soft organs within the body. The dorsal cavity, which contains the brain and spinal cord, cranial, and spinal cavity, are much smaller compared with the ventral cavity. Colville TP, Bassert JM, Clinical Anatomy and Physiology for Veterinary Technicians, ed 3, Mosby, 2016, p. 7.

342. d The thoracic cavity contains the following major structures: the heart, lungs, esophagus, and major blood vessels. Colville TP, Bassert JM, Clinical Anatomy and Physiology for Veterinary Technicians, ed 3, Mosby, 2016, p. 7.

343. b A thin membrane known as pleura covers all organs within the thoracic cavity. The thorax is the chest cavity. The peritoneum is a membrane that covers organs within the intestinal tract. Colville TP, Bassert JM, Clinical Anatomy and Physiology for Veterinary Technicians, ed 3, Mosby, 2016, p. 7.

344. d The abdomen contains the digestive, urinary, and reproductive organs, which are all covered by a thin membrane called the peritoneum. Colville TP, Bassert JM, Clinical Anatomy and Physiology for Veterinary Technicians, ed 3, Mosby, 2016, p. 7.

345. c Animals' bodies contain four different types of tissues: epithelial, connective, muscle, and nervous. Colville TP, Bassert JM, Clinical Anatomy and Physiology for Veterinary Technicians, ed 3, Mosby, 2016, p. 8.

346. b Epithelial tissues are composed of cells and are responsible for covering the body's surfaces. The connective tissue provides support and the muscle tissue provides movement. Colville TP, Bassert JM, Clinical Anatomy and Physiology for Veterinary Technicians, ed 3, Mosby, 2016, p. 8.

347. a Every cell specializes in different things. Red blood cells carry oxygen throughout the body. White blood cells are involved with protecting the immune system. Nerve cells are involved in organizing and controlling body functions. Not all cells within the body carry oxygen. Colville TP, Bassert JM, Clinical Anatomy and Physiology for Veterinary Technicians, ed 3, Mosby, 2016, p. 8.

348. d Epithelial tissue covers body surfaces and forms glands such as sweat glands, salivary glands, and mammary glands. Connective tissue provides support to surrounding structures. Muscle tissue moves the body inside and out, such as skeletal muscle, cardiac muscle, and smooth muscle. Nervous tissue transmits information from the body to the brain. Colville TP, Bassert JM, Clinical Anatomy and Physiology for Veterinary Technicians, ed 3, Mosby, 2016, p. 8.

349. c Muscle tissue is involved in moving the body inside and out and exists in three types of tissues: skeletal, cardiac, and smooth. Striated muscles are found throughout the body but are not a type of muscle tissue. Colville TP, Bassert JM, Clinical Anatomy and Physiology for Veterinary Technicians, ed 3, Mosby, 2016, p. 8.

350. e Smooth muscle is an automatic muscle that is found in internal organs such as the digestive tract and urinary bladder. The heart is made up of cardiac muscle. Colville TP, Bassert JM, Clinical Anatomy and Physiology for Veterinary Technicians, ed 3, Mosby, 2016, p. 8.

351. c The first indication that the heart is beginning to fail is a drop in cardiac output, which is the amount of blood that the heart pumps per minute. Shortly after the drop in cardiac output, the blood pressure begins to drop (it does not rise in heart failure). Oxygen saturation is the level of oxygen found in the blood and it begins to drop once the heart has begun to fail. Colville TP, Bassert JM, Clinical Anatomy and Physiology for Veterinary Technicians, ed 3, Mosby, 2016, p. 9.

352. d Nitrogen makes up 3.3% of the body mass and it is the component of all proteins and nucleic acid. Hydrogen is a component of water and organic molecules. Oxygen is necessary for cellular energy. Calcium is a component of bones and teeth. Colville TP, Bassert JM, Clinical Anatomy and Physiology for Veterinary Technicians, ed 3, Mosby, 2016, p. 14.

353. d Calcium is a component of bones and teeth and is required for muscle contraction, nerve impulse transmission, and blood clotting. Nitrogen is a component of all proteins and nucleic acids. Oxygen is necessary for cellular energy. Phosphorus is the principal component in the backbone of nucleic acids and is important in energy transfer. Colville TP, Bassert JM, Clinical Anatomy and Physiology for Veterinary Technicians, ed 3, Mosby, 2016, p. 14.

354. a Major elements in the body are oxygen, carbon, hydrogen, and nitrogen. Calcium, magnesium, and potassium are considered minor elements of the body. Colville TP, Bassert JM, Clinical Anatomy and Physiology for Veterinary Technicians, ed 3, Mosby, 2016, p. 14.

355. c Oxygen makes up approximately 65% of the body mass. Carbon makes up approximately 18.5% of the body mass. Hydrogen makes up approximately 9.5% of the body mass. Nitrogen makes up approximately 3.3% of the body mass. Colville TP, Bassert JM, Clinical

Anatomy and Physiology for Veterinary Technicians, ed 3, Mosby, 2016, p. 14.

356. d A chemical bond is a bond between two atoms that share electrons. There are three types of chemical bonds: covalent, ionic, and hydrogen bonds. Colville TP, Bassert JM, Clinical Anatomy and Physiology for Veterinary Technicians, ed 3, Mosby, 2016, p. 21.

357. b An ionic bond is formed when electrons are transferred from one atom to another and are most often formed between two types of atoms. A covalent bond is a bond formed when atoms share electrons. A hydrogen bond is a bond between hydrogen atoms already covalently bonded in a molecule to oppositely charged particles. The triple covalent bond is when the bond is formed with three electrons. Colville TP, Bassert JM, Clinical Anatomy and Physiology for Veterinary Technicians, ed 3, Mosby, 2016, p. 21.

358. b A synthesis reaction is a new and more complex chemical that is made from multiple, simpler chemicals. It occurs in the body during the digestive process and joins the chemicals into larger molecules that are needed by cells for life processes. A decomposition reaction is a single, complex chemical that is broken into multiple, simpler chemicals. An exchange reaction occurs when certain atoms are exchanged between molecules. Colville TP, Bassert JM, Clinical Anatomy and Physiology for Veterinary Technicians, ed 3, Mosby, 2016, p. 24.

359. d All living organisms are made up of inorganic and organic compounds. Inorganic compounds consist of water, salts, acids, and bases. Colville TP, Bassert JM, Clinical Anatomy and Physiology for Veterinary Technicians, ed 3, Mosby, 2016, p. 26.

360. b Organic compounds that make up living organisms include carbohydrates, lipids, proteins, and nucleic acids. Inorganic compounds include water, salts, bases, and acids. Colville TP, Bassert JM, Clinical Anatomy and Physiology for Veterinary Technicians, ed 3, Mosby, 2016, p. 31.

361. a Chemicals that dissolve or mix well in water are known as hydrophilic. Chemicals that do not dissolve well in water are known as hydrophobic. Solutes are chemicals that are added to water. A solvent is the water in which chemicals are dissolved. Colville TP, Bassert JM, Clinical Anatomy and Physiology for Veterinary Technicians, ed 3, Mosby, 2016, p. 26.

362. d Electrolytes are substances that have the ability to transmit electrical charges throughout the body. The following are examples of electrolytes: sodium, potassium, and calcium. Colville TP, Bassert JM, Clinical Anatomy and Physiology for Veterinary Technicians, ed 3, Mosby, 2016, p. 28.

363. a Acidity and alkalinity are measured on the pH scale that ranges from 1 to 14 with 7 being neutral: 1–6 is considered acidic and 8–14 is considered alkaline. Of these numbers, 2.5 is the most acidic. Colville TP, Bassert JM, Clinical Anatomy and Physiology for Veterinary Technicians, ed 3, Mosby, 2016, p. 28.

364. c Buffering the solution means to keep the pH in the neutral range close to 7. An acidic solution is anything less than 7 on the pH scale and an alkaline solution is anything greater than 7. Colville TP, Bassert JM, Clinical Anatomy and Physiology for Veterinary Technicians, ed 3, Mosby, 2016, p. 28.

365. b A buffer is a substance that keeps a solution close to the neutral zone of 7 on the pH scale and carbonic acid is an example of a buffer. Lemons and vinegar are examples of acidic solutions. Ammonia is an example of an alkaline solution. Colville TP, Bassert JM, Clinical Anatomy and Physiology for Veterinary Technicians, ed 3, Mosby, 2016, p. 28.

366. c Distilled water has a neutral pH of 7. Examples of the other pH levels would be: gastric fluid is 1, coffee is 5 , and milk of magnesia is 11. Colville TP, Bassert JM, Clinical Anatomy and Physiology for Veterinary Technicians, ed 3, Mosby, 2016, p. 28.

367. d Carbohydrates are molecules used for energy, storage of energy, and cellular structures. Examples of carbohydrates are sugar, starch, and cellulose. Colville TP, Bassert JM, Clinical Anatomy and Physiology for Veterinary Technicians, ed 3, Mosby, 2016, p. 31.

368. b Monosaccharides are the simplest form of a carbohydrate and contain 3–7 carbon atoms in a chain. Colville TP, Bassert JM, Clinical Anatomy and Physiology for Veterinary Technicians, ed 3, Mosby, 2016, p. 31.

369. b A sugar that contains five carbons is known as a pentose sugar. A hexose sugar contains six carbons. Montose and tritose sugars are not molecules. Colville TP, Bassert JM, Clinical Anatomy and Physiology for Veterinary Technicians, ed 3, Mosby, 2016, p. 31.

370. a Triglycerides, prostaglandins, steroids, and phospholipids are all lipid molecules. Ribose is a carbohydrate. Colville TP, Bassert JM, Clinical Anatomy and Physiology for Veterinary Technicians, ed 3, Mosby, 2016, p. 34.

371. d Triglycerides are lipids that store energy in body fat. Ribose is a carbohydrate that acts as the backbone of DNA and RNA. Globular proteins regulate chemical reactions. Prostaglandins are lipids that regulate hormone synthesis. Colville TP, Bassert JM, Clinical Anatomy and Physiology for Veterinary Technicians, ed 3, Mosby, 2016, p. 34.

372. d DNA, RNA, and adenosine triphosphate are all nucleic acids. Colville TP, Bassert JM, Clinical Anatomy and Physiology for Veterinary Technicians, ed 3, Mosby, 2016, p. 39.

373. d Prostaglandins are lipids that are responsible for regulating hormone synthesis, enhancing the immune response, and providing inflammatory response. Prostaglandins do not block the COX-2 pathway, which would block pain. Colville TP, Bassert JM, Clinical Anatomy and Physiology for Veterinary Technicians, ed 3, Mosby, 2016, p. 290.

374. a A synthesis reaction is a new and more complex chemical that is made from multiple, simpler chemicals. It occurs in the body during the digestive process and the chemicals made are joined into larger molecules needed by cells for life processes. When two monosaccharides are joined together, there is a synthesis reaction. A hydrolysis reaction is when water is used to break down a molecule. A decomposition reaction is a single, complex chemical broken into multiple, simpler chemicals. An exchange reaction occurs when certain atoms are exchanged between molecules. Colville TP, Bassert JM, Clinical Anatomy and Physiology for Veterinary Technicians, ed 3, Mosby, 2016, p. 24.

375. b Water is created during a synthesis reaction. It is extracted from the saccharides and is known as dehydration synthesis. A hydrolysis reaction is when water is used to break down a molecule. A decomposition reaction is a single, complex chemical that is broken into multiple, simpler chemicals. A synthesis reaction is a new and more complex chemical made from multiple, simpler chemicals; it occurs in the body during the digestive process and is joined into larger molecules needed by cells for the life processes. Colville TP, Bassert JM, Clinical Anatomy and Physiology for Veterinary Technicians, ed 3, Mosby, 2016, p. 31.

376. d Lipids are made of carbon, hydrogen, oxygen, and phosphorus, are used in the body for energy, and are stored in fat for future energy. Colville TP, Bassert JM, Clinical Anatomy and Physiology for Veterinary Technicians, ed 3, Mosby, 2016, p. 34.

377. b Lipoproteins are macromolecules composed of proteins and lipids and are used to transport fats within the body. Lipids are used for energy. Globular proteins regulate chemical reactions. Prostaglandins are lipids that regulate hormone synthesis. Colville TP, Bassert JM, Clinical Anatomy and Physiology for Veterinary Technicians, ed 3, Mosby, 2016, p. 34.

378. a Steroids are lipids that take the form of four interlocking hydrocarbon rings. Triglycerides consist of glycerol and three fatty acids. Prostaglandins consist of 20-carbon unsaturated fatty acids with a 5-carbon ring. Phospholipids consist of glycerol, three fatty acids, and phosphate. Colville TP, Bassert JM, Clinical Anatomy and Physiology for Veterinary Technicians, ed 3, Mosby, 2016, p. 34.

379. d Cholesterol is used by the adrenal glands, testes, and ovaries for the creation of steroid hormones such as cortisone, estrogen, progesterone, and testosterone. Colville TP, Bassert JM, Clinical Anatomy and Physiology for Veterinary Technicians, ed 3, Mosby, 2016, p. 34.

380. c Proteins have the widest variety of function and are the most abundant organic molecule found in the body. Amino acids, lipids, and prostaglandins are important molecules within the body, are all involved in different functions, but are not considered the most abundant organic molecule. Colville TP, Bassert JM, Clinical Anatomy and Physiology for Veterinary Technicians, ed 3, Mosby, 2016, p. 35.

381. c The shape of protein molecules directly determines their function. Size and location of proteins does not determine function. Colville TP, Bassert JM, Clinical Anatomy and Physiology for Veterinary Technicians, ed 3, Mosby, 2016, p. 35.

382. d Structural proteins are stable, rigid, water-insoluble proteins that are used for adding strength to tissues or cells. Proteins do not have any steroid properties. Colville TP, Bassert JM, Clinical Anatomy and Physiology for Veterinary Technicians, ed 3, Mosby, 2016, p. 35.

383. b Functional proteins are water-soluble with a flexible three-dimensional shape and are also known as globular proteins. Structural proteins are also known as fibrous proteins. Colville TP, Bassert JM, Clinical Anatomy and Physiology for Veterinary Technicians, ed 3, Mosby, 2016, p. 35.

384. c The largest molecules in the body are nucleic acids, which are composed of carbon, oxygen, hydrogen, nitrogen, and phosphorus. Lipids, proteins, and carbohydrates are important molecules within the body, but nucleic acids are the largest. Colville TP, Bassert JM, Clinical Anatomy and Physiology for Veterinary Technicians, ed 3, Mosby, 2016, p. 40.

385. d Nucleic acids consist of only two classes of DNA and RNA. Ribose is a carbohydrate that is the backbone of RNA and DNA. Colville TP, Bassert JM, Clinical Anatomy and Physiology for Veterinary Technicians, ed 3, Mosby, 2016, p. 40.

386. b Nucleotides are the molecular building blocks of nucleic acids and consist of five different ones that all have the same basic structure. Chromosomes are formed when a long chain of genes combines with a protein. Proteins and carbohydrates are part of the organic molecule group. Colville TP, Bassert JM, Clinical Anatomy and Physiology for Veterinary Technicians, ed 3, Mosby, 2016, p. 40.

387. c There are five basic nucleotides: adenine, guanine, cytosine, uracil, and thymine. Thiamine is a vitamin. Colville TP, Bassert JM, Clinical Anatomy and Physiology for Veterinary Technicians, ed 3, Mosby, 2016, p. 40.

388. b Only three of the five nucleotides occur in both DNA and RNA: adenine, guanine, and cytosine. Thiamine is a vitamin. Colville TP, Bassert JM, Clinical Anatomy and Physiology for Veterinary Technicians, ed 3, Mosby, 2016, p. 40.

389. d The nucleotide uracil occurs only in RNA. Adenine, guanine, and cytosine occur in both DNA and RNA. Colville TP, Bassert JM, Clinical Anatomy and Physiology for Veterinary Technicians, ed 3, Mosby, 2016, p. 40.

390. b The aorta is the largest and main artery of the body, originates from the left ventricle of the heart, and carries oxygenated blood to various body tissues. The right ventricle receives blood from the right atrium through the AV opening and the pulmonary artery originates from the right ventricle. The left atrium receives blood from the pulmonary veins. The inferior vena cava originates from the right atrium. Sirois M, Elsevier's Veterinary Assisting Textbook, ed 2, 2017, Elsevier, p. 80.

391. b Arteries carry blood away from the heart to the capillaries. Veins carry blood from the capillaries back to the heart. The capillaries permit substances to move freely between the extracellular fluid and the blood. The vena cava is the largest vein in the body, which courses along with the aorta and carries blood back toward the heart. Sirois M, Elsevier's Veterinary Assisting Textbook, ed 2, 2017, Elsevier, p. 79.

392. b Veins contain one-way valves that help propel blood back toward the heart and stop blood from flowing in the wrong direction. Arteries carry blood from the heart to various organs in the body and do not contain valves. Capillaries are porous and are composed of a single layer of epithelium that permits substances to move freely between the extracellular fluid and the blood. The aorta is the main artery of the body; it leaves the heart and branches off to carry blood to other organs in the body and does not contain valves. Sirois M, Elsevier's Veterinary Assisting Textbook, ed 2, 2017, Elsevier, p. 79.

393. d The pulmonary artery carries CO_2-rich blood from the right ventricle of the heart to the lungs for oxygenation. The aorta leaves the left ventricle of the heart and carries blood to the rest of the body. The inferior vena cava enters the right atrium bringing blood back to the heart. The pulmonary vein brings oxygenated blood from the lungs to the left atrium of the heart. Sirois M, Elsevier's Veterinary Assisting Textbook, ed 2, 2017, Elsevier, p. 80.

394. b The brachiocephalic artery is the first main branch off the aorta followed by the left common carotid artery, then the left subclavian artery. The superior mesenteric artery is located below the celiac axis and supplies a portion of the GI system with blood. Sirois M, Elsevier's Veterinary Assisting Textbook, ed 2, 2017, Elsevier, p. 80.

395. b Plasma contains approximately 92% water, 7% protein, and 1% other substances and electrolytes. Sirois M, Elsevier's Veterinary Assisting Textbook, ed 2, 2017, Elsevier, p. 81.

396. c Red blood cells are the most numerous blood cells in the body and typically number in the millions per μL of blood. White blood cells are also known as leukocytes and number in the tens of thousands per μL of blood. Plasma is the fluid portion of blood, and red cells, white cells, and platelets make up the cellular portion. Sirois M, Elsevier's Veterinary Assisting Textbook, ed 2, 2017, Elsevier, p. 81.

397. b The protein hemoglobin is responsible for giving erythrocytes their red color. Granulocytes are a division of white blood cells and eosinophils are granulocytes. Fibrinogen is a protein in the plasma that contains a meshwork of fibrin strands creating blood clots. Sirois M, Elsevier's Veterinary Assisting Textbook, ed 2, 2017, Elsevier, p. 81.

398. d Blood makes up approximately 7% of body weight and other fluids and tissues make up approximately 93% of body weight. Plasma makes up 55% of the blood volume and 45% is formed by elements such as platelets, leukocytes, and erythrocytes. Sirois M, Elsevier's Veterinary Assisting Textbook, ed 2, 2017, Elsevier, p. 81.

399. b White blood cells are divided into granulocytes and agranulocytes. Granulocytes consist of neutrophils, eosinophils, and basophils. Agranulocytes consist of lymphocytes and monocytes. A reticulocyte is an immature red blood cell. Sirois M, Elsevier's Veterinary Assisting Textbook, ed 2, 2017, Elsevier, p. 81.

400. b The trachea carries air to the lungs and is composed of several C-shaped incomplete rings of hyaline cartilage that prevent it from collapsing during inspiration. The esophagus is a muscular tube that connects the pharynx with the stomach to allow food to pass. The pharynx is the throat, which connects the mouth to the esophagus. Sirois M, Elsevier's Veterinary Assisting Textbook, ed 2, 2017, Elsevier, p. 85.

401. b Gas exchange within the lungs occurs in the alveolus, which consists of tiny, thin-walled sacs surrounded by elastic fibers and a network of capillaries. The bronchi are a continuation of the trachea into the lungs that eventually lead to the alveolus. The alveolar duct is the end of the bronchi that forms the grape-like clusters of alveoli where gas exchange takes place. The larynx is the tube that connects the pharynx with the trachea. Sirois M, Elsevier's Veterinary Assisting Textbook, ed 2, 2017, Elsevier, p. 85.

402. b The thoracic cavity is located above the diaphragm below the neck containing the heart and lungs. The thoracic cavity normally has negative pressure that allows the lungs to conform to the shape of the cavity. A small amount of pleural fluid lubricates the lung surfaces and pleural lining, allowing the lungs to move. Sirois M, Elsevier's Veterinary Assisting Textbook, ed 2, 2017, Elsevier, p. 85.

403. c The bulk of a tooth is made up of dense material called dentin. The enamel covers the crown of the tooth and is the hardest substance in the body. The crown is the exposed portion of the tooth. The root anchors the tooth in the boney socket and is covered by cementum. Sirois M, Elsevier's Veterinary Assisting Textbook, ed 2, 2017, Elsevier, p. 86.

404. d The incisors are the most rostral teeth in the mouth. The four canine teeth are located at the rostral lateral corners of the mouth. The premolars are the rostral cheek teeth and the molars are the caudal cheek teeth. Sirois M, Elsevier's Veterinary Assisting Textbook, ed 2, 2017, Elsevier, p. 86.

405. b The hypoglossal nerve key function is tongue movement. The abducent nerve controls eye movement. The olfactory nerve transmits information relating to smell. The vestibulocochlear nerve transmits information relating to balance. Sirois M, Elsevier's Veterinary Assisting Textbook, ed 2, 2017, Elsevier, p. 88.

406. c The cardiac sphincter functions as a valve to seal the esophagus off from the stomach and regulates the size of the opening of the esophagus into the stomach. The duodenum is a segment of the small intestine located past the stomach. The pyloric sphincter is located between the stomach and the duodenum and controls the release of food into the small intestines. The epiglottis is the flap of cartilage that acts as a trap door to cover the opening of the larynx during swallowing. Sirois M, Elsevier's Veterinary Assisting Textbook, ed 2, 2017, Elsevier, p. 87.

407. b After food has been mechanically broken down by the stomach and enters the small intestines, it is converted to a semiliquid homogenous material called chyme. Rugae are the folds within the stomach that aid in the movement of food. Cattle are ruminants because they have more than one stomach. Bile is the substance produced by the liver that is stored in the gallbladder and is excreted into the intestinal tract to aid in the digestion of food. Sirois M, Elsevier's Veterinary Assisting Textbook, ed 2, 2017, Elsevier, p. 87.

408. c The jejunum is the longest portion of the small intestines and is where most nutrient absorption occurs. The duodenum is the shortest segment of the small intestine and is the first segment that leaves the stomach. The ileum is also a short segment of the small intestine and leads to the cecum, which is considered to be the beginning of the large intestine. Sirois M, Elsevier's Veterinary Assisting Textbook, ed 2, 2017, Elsevier, p. 87.

409. b The colon is the second and longest segment of the colon. The first segment is the cecum. The final segment is the rectum, which carries contents to the anus for excretion from the body. The ileum is a portion of the small intestines. Sirois M, Elsevier's Veterinary Assisting Textbook, ed 2, 2017, Elsevier, p. 87.

410. b The portal vein carries nutrient-rich blood from the intestines directly to the liver. The inferior vena cava is the main vein of the body that carries deoxygenated blood back to the heart. The hepatic veins are responsible for carrying blood from the liver back to the heart. The splenic vein carries blood from the spleen to the portal confluence to join the portal vein. Sirois M, Elsevier's Veterinary Assisting Textbook, ed 2, 2017, Elsevier, p. 88.

411. c The liver is located just caudal to the diaphragm and is the largest organ in the body. The spleen is located caudal to the stomach and is smaller than the liver unless diseased. The pancreas is located near the duodenum and is significantly smaller than the liver. The gallbladder is located adjacent to the liver, is responsible for storage of bile, and is significantly smaller than the liver. Sirois M, Elsevier's Veterinary Assisting Textbook, ed 2, 2017, Elsevier, p. 87.

412. e The diencephalon of the brain consists of both the thalamus and hypothalamus. The brainstem consists of the midbrain, pons, and medulla. Sirois M, Elsevier's Veterinary Assisting Textbook, ed 2, 2017, Elsevier, p. 88.

413. b The largest, most rostral part of the brain is the cerebrum. The cerebellum is located caudal to the cerebrum and is smaller than the cerebrum. The thalamus is located within the diencephalon. The brainstem is located posterior to the brain and connects the cerebrum, cerebellum, and spinal cord. Sirois M, Elsevier's Veterinary Assisting Textbook, ed 2, 2017, Elsevier, p. 88.

414. a The term *gyri* refers to the systems of folds located on the surface of the cerebrum. Sulci are grooves within the cerebrum. The arachnoid villi are small protrusions of the arachnoid through the dura matter surrounding the brain. The meninges are the membranous coverings of the brain. Sirois M, Elsevier's Veterinary Assisting Textbook, ed 2, 2017, Elsevier, p. 88.

415. c The brainstem is considered the most primitive part of the brain. It forms the stem to which the cerebellum, cerebrum, and spinal cord are attached and maintains the vital functions of the body. The cerebellum coordinates movements of the body. The cerebrum is the center of higher learning and intelligence. The gray matter is the outer layer of the cerebrum and consists of nerve cell bodies. Sirois M, Elsevier's Veterinary Assisting Textbook, ed 2, 2017, Elsevier, p. 88.

416. b The cervical portion of the spinal cord is the most cranial end exiting the brain stem. Travel from cranial to caudal of the spinal cord is as follows: cervical, thoracic, lumbar, and sacral. Sirois M, Elsevier's Veterinary Assisting Textbook, ed 2, 2017, Elsevier, p. 73.

417. b Spinal nerves from the sacral region carry parasympathetic nerve fibers. Spinal nerves from the thoracic and lumbar region carry sympathetic nerve fibers. Sirois M, Elsevier's Veterinary Assisting Textbook, ed 2, 2017, Elsevier, p. 89.

418. d There are 12 pairs of cranial nerves that arise from the ventral surface of the brain. The following are the 12 cranial nerves: olfactory, optic, oculomotor, trochlear, trigeminal, abducent, facial, vestibulocochlear, glossopharyngeal, vagus, accessory, and hypoglossal. Sirois M, Elsevier's Veterinary Assisting Textbook, ed 2, 2017, Elsevier, p. 89.

419. b Cranial nerve VIII, known as the vestibulocochlear nerve, is responsible for balance and hearing. Cranial nerve IV, known as the trochlear nerve, is responsible for eye movement. Cranial nerve XI, known as the accessory nerve, is responsible for head movement. Cranial nerve II, known as the optic nerve, is responsible for vision. Sirois M, Elsevier's Veterinary Assisting Textbook, ed 2, 2017, Elsevier, p. 89.

420. d Cranial nerve IX, known as the glossopharyngeal nerve, is responsible for tongue movement, swallowing, salivation, and taste. Cranial nerve V, known as the trigeminal nerve, is responsible for sensation from the head and teeth and chewing. Cranial nerve VI is known as the abducens nerve; cranial nerve IV is known as the trochlear nerve; and cranial nerve III is known as the oculomotor nerve and is responsible for eye movement. Cranial nerve VIII is known as the facial nerve and is responsible for face and scalp movement, salivation, tears, and taste. Sirois M, Elsevier's Veterinary Assisting Textbook, ed 2, 2017, Elsevier, p. 89.

421. a Cranial nerve VIII, known as the vestibulocochlear nerve, is considered a sensory nerve and is responsible for balance and hearing. The accessory, trochlear, and hypoglossal nerves are all considered motor nerves. The accessory nerve is responsible for head movement. The trochlear nerve is responsible for eye movement. The hypoglossal nerve is responsible for tongue movement. Sirois M, Elsevier's Veterinary Assisting Textbook, ed 2, 2017, Elsevier, p. 89.

422. c The vagus nerve, known as cranial nerve X, is the longest cranial nerve, which innervates many organs of the body. It provides sensory function for the GI tract and respiratory tree and it provides motor functions for the larynx, pharynx, parasympathetic, abdominal, and thoracic organs. The trigeminal nerve is responsible for sensation from the head and teeth and chewing. The vestibulocochlear nerve is responsible for balance and hearing. The hypoglossal nerve is responsible for tongue movement. Sirois M, Elsevier's Veterinary Assisting Textbook, ed 2, 2017, Elsevier, p. 89.

423. b Visceral sensation is considered a general sense and includes the sensation of hunger and thirst. Heat and cold are temperature sensations. Touch and pressure are touch sensations. Odor is the sense of smell. Sirois

M, Elsevier's Veterinary Assisting Textbook, ed 2, 2017, Elsevier, p. 92.

424. d Proprioception is part of the general senses and it senses body position and movement. Taste, hearing, equilibrium, smell, and vision are all considered to be special senses. Sirois M, Elsevier's Veterinary Assisting Textbook, ed 2, 2017, Elsevier, p. 92.

425. a The ear pinna, also known as the earflap, is the cartilaginous funnel that collects sound waves and directs them medially into the external auditory canal. The eustachian tube links the middle ear with the pharynx. The cochlea is the fluid-filled space shaped like a spiral snail shell that absorbs vibrations of the sound waves. The tympanic membrane is the air-filled middle ear cavity that transmits vibrations of the tympanic membrane to the inner ear. Sirois M, Elsevier's Veterinary Assisting Textbook, ed 2, 2017, Elsevier, p. 92.

426. a The inner ear consists of the cochlea, vestibule, and the semicircular canals. The middle ear consists of the tympanic membrane, malleus, incus, and stapes. Sirois M, Elsevier's Veterinary Assisting Textbook, ed 2, 2017, Elsevier, p. 92.

427. b The organ of Corti runs along the cochlea and contains receptor cells for hearing. The tympanic membrane is the air-filled middle ear cavity that transmits vibrations of the tympanic membrane to the inner ear. The vestibule is part of the inner ear and is responsible for monitoring balance and head position. The incus is a bone located in the middle ear. Sirois M, Elsevier's Veterinary Assisting Textbook, ed 2, 2017, Elsevier, p. 92.

428. b The vestibular sense is responsible for balance and head position. The olfactory sense is responsible for smell. The visual sense is responsible for vision. The auditory sense is responsible for hearing. Sirois M, Elsevier's Veterinary Assisting Textbook, ed 2, 2017, Elsevier, p. 92.

429. b The clear window on the rostral portion of the eye is referred to as the cornea. The eyelids are the dorsal and ventral folds of skin lined by conjunctiva that cover and protect the eye when the animal blinks or sleeps. The iris is a muscular diaphragm that controls the size of the pupil. The sclera is the white portion of the eye. Sirois M, Elsevier's Veterinary Assisting Textbook, ed 2, 2017, Elsevier, p. 94.

430. c The anterior chamber is a fluid-filled space located caudal to the cornea and is also known as the aqueous humor. The lens is located caudal to the iris and is an elastic, crystalline structure responsible for focusing light rays. The iris is a muscular diaphragm that controls the size of the pupil. The vitreous humor is the transparent gelatinous substance located caudal to the lens. Sirois M, Elsevier's Veterinary Assisting Textbook, ed 2, 2017, Elsevier, p. 94.

431. d The retina is where visual images are formed and is a complex multilayered structure that lines most of the interior of the eye caudal to the lens. The lens is responsible for focusing light rays. The cornea is the clear window on the rostral portion of the eye where light rays enter. The vitreous humor, located caudal to the lens, is a transparent gelatinous substance where light rays pass before reaching the retina. Sirois M, Elsevier's Veterinary Assisting Textbook, ed 2, 2017, Elsevier, p. 94.

432. b Rods and cones are photoreceptor cells located within the retina. The cornea is the clear window on the rostral portion of the eye where light rays enter. The iris is the muscular diaphragm that controls the size of the pupil. The vitreous humor is the transparent gelatinous substance located anterior to the retina. Sirois M, Elsevier's Veterinary Assisting Textbook, ed 2, 2017, Elsevier, p. 94.

433. b The area of the retina where nerve fibers converge to form the optic nerve is referred to as the optic disc and is the blind spot of the eye because there are no rods or cones present there. The optic nerve is connected to the brain and relays visual images for the brain to interpret. The rods are sensitive to light and the cones are sensitive to details and colors. Sirois M, Elsevier's Veterinary Assisting Textbook, ed 2, 2017, Elsevier, p. 94.

434. c The lacrimal puncta are located at the medial canthus of the eye and are two small openings responsible for drainage of tears from the eye. The lacrimal glands are responsible for the production of tears. The conjunctiva is the thin membrane that lines the underside of the eyelids and covers the outer aspect of the eyeball. The membrana nictitans is also known as the third eyelid and is a plate of cartilage covered by conjunctiva. Sirois M, Elsevier's Veterinary Assisting Textbook, ed 2, 2017, Elsevier, p. 94.

435. a In dim light the muscular iris relaxes, allowing the pupil to dilate to allow more light to enter the eye. In bright light the pupil constricts, blocking the light protecting the photoreceptor cells. The pupil never fully closes. Sirois M, Elsevier's Veterinary Assisting Textbook, ed 2, 2017, Elsevier, p. 94.

436. b The ciliary body contains muscles responsible for changing the shape of the lens, which is required to focus light rays. The diameter of the iris changes with exposure to light. The lacrimal gland produces tears. The drainage of tears is produced by the lacrimal puncta. Sirois M, Elsevier's Veterinary Assisting Textbook, ed 2, 2017, Elsevier, p. 94.

437. c The corpus luteum is what remains after ovulation has occurred. If the animal becomes pregnant, the corpus luteum remains and produces the progesterone that is necessary to maintain the pregnancy. FSH is the follicle-stimulating hormone that stimulates the ovaries to develop follicles. Estrogen is produced by the developing follicles and is responsible for signs of heat and estrus. Sirois M, Elsevier's Veterinary Assisting Textbook, ed 2, 2017, Elsevier, p. 96.

438. a The testes produce two hormones; the main hormone is testosterone. The testes produce small amounts of estrogen. Luteinizing hormone causes the follicle within the ovary to rupture, known as ovulation. Progesterone is the hormone produced by the corpus luteum and is necessary to maintain pregnancy. Sirois M, Elsevier's Veterinary Assisting Textbook, ed 2, 2017, Elsevier, p. 96.

439. c The coccygeal vertebra forms the tail of the horse. The cervical vertebra forms the neck. The sacrum is the distal vertebra before becoming the coccygeal. The lumbar vertebra is cranial to the sacrum. Aspinall V, Cappello M, Introduction to Veterinary Anatomy and Physiology Textbook, ed 2, Butterworth Heinemann, 2009, p. 190.

440. a The humerus is located immediately distal to the scapula and cranial to the radius and ulna. The metacarpus is distal to the radius and ulna. The femur is a bone in the hind limb of the horse. Aspinall V, Cappello M, Introduction to Veterinary Anatomy and Physiology Textbook, ed 2, Butterworth Heinemann, 2009, p. 190.

441. d The carpus is located proximal to the metacarpus. The humerus, radius, and ulna are all located proximal to the carpus. Aspinall V, Cappello M, Introduction to Veterinary Anatomy and Physiology Textbook, ed 2, Butterworth Heinemann, 2009, p. 190.

442. c The metatarsal is located distal to the tarsal bone in the horse. The femur, patella, and fibula are located proximal to the tarsal bone. Aspinall V, Cappello M, Introduction to Veterinary Anatomy and Physiology Textbook, ed 2, Butterworth Heinemann, 2009, p. 190.

443. c The average horse has approximately 18 ribs. There are typically 15–20 coccygeal vertebrae in horses. There are five fused sacra in horses. There are normally six lumbar vertebrae in horses. Aspinall V, Cappello M, Introduction to Veterinary Anatomy and Physiology Textbook, ed 2, Butterworth Heinemann, 2009, p. 190.

444. d The thoracic vertebrae have large spinous processes in which T4–T9 make up the withers of the horse. The C1 vertebra is the first vertebrae in the neck and contains a large wing-shaped process. The C2 vertebra contains the prominent cranial process known as the dens. C3–C7 are the remaining vertebrae of the cervical region. Aspinall V, Cappello M, Introduction to Veterinary Anatomy and Physiology Textbook, ed 2, Butterworth Heinemann, 2009, p. 189.

445. a The humerus is one of the strongest bones in the body and lies at an angle that allows for great shock absorption during movement. The carpus contains eight small bones and helps to absorb shock and to distribute the concussion. The scapula is the large, flat, triangular bone that joints the humerus. The patella is located at the stifle joint and acts as a pulley for the tendons that run over the stifle joint between the femur and the tibia. Aspinall V, Cappello M, Introduction to Veterinary Anatomy and Physiology Textbook, ed 2, Butterworth Heinemann, 2009, p. 192.

446. c The metacarpals consist of three different bones; the large metacarpal bone is referred to as the cannon bone. The two small metacarpal bones are referred to as the splint bones. The phalanges are referred to as the pasterns and pedal bones. The carpus is referred to as the knee. The femur is the proximal bone in the hind limb. Aspinall V, Cappello M, Introduction to Veterinary Anatomy and Physiology Textbook, ed 2, Butterworth Heinemann, 2009, p. 192.

447. b The fetlock joint lies between the cannon bone and the long pastern. The stifle joint is formed by the distal femur, proximal tibia, and patella. The pastern joint lies between the long and the short pastern. The coffin joint lies between the short pastern and the pedal bone and it incorporates the navicular bone. Aspinall V, Cappello M, Introduction to Veterinary Anatomy and Physiology Textbook, ed 2, Butterworth Heinemann, 2009, p. 192.

448. c The middle phalanx is referred to as the pedal bone and is encased in a horse's hoof. The cannon bone is the large metacarpal bone. The navicular bone is the distal sesamoid that lies at the back of the pedal bone. The sesamoid bones contain three bones that are located at the back of the metacarpophalangeal or fetlock joint. Aspinall V, Cappello M, Introduction to Veterinary Anatomy and Physiology Textbook, ed 2, Butterworth Heinemann, 2009, p. 192.

449. b The glenoid cavity is located immediately proximal to the humerus and distal to the scapula. The ulna is located distal to the humerus and proximal to the carpal joint. The cannon bone is located distal to the carpus and proximal to the phalanx bones. Aspinall V, Cappello M, Introduction to Veterinary Anatomy and Physiology Textbook, ed 2, Butterworth Heinemann, 2009, p. 192.

450. c The deltoid tuberosity is located on the humerus of the horse. The ulna is distal to the humerus and contains the tubercle for lateral collateral ligament. The radius fuses together with the ulna and is distal to the humerus. The scapula is proximal to the humerus and contains the tuberosity of scapular spine. Aspinall V, Cappello M, Introduction to Veterinary Anatomy and Physiology Textbook, ed 2, Butterworth Heinemann, 2009, p. 192.

451. a The pubis is the bone that forms the floor of the pelvis. The ischium lies caudal to the pubis bone. The ilium forms the upper vertical portion of the pelvis. The tuber coxae form the points of the hip. Aspinall V, Cappello M, Introduction to Veterinary Anatomy and Physiology Textbook, ed 2, Butterworth Heinemann, 2009, p. 192.

452. b The ilium is the largest bone in the pelvis and is the upper, vertical position. The ischium lies caudal to the pubis bone and the pubis bone forms the pelvic floor. The acetabulum is the socket of the hipbone in which the head of the femur lies. Aspinall V, Cappello M, Introduction to Veterinary Anatomy and Physiology Textbook, ed 2, Butterworth Heinemann, 2009, p. 192.

453. b The interosseous space is located between the radius and ulna. This is the only major interosseous space located in the limb of a horse. Aspinall V, Cappello M, Introduction to Veterinary Anatomy and Physiology Textbook, ed 2, Butterworth Heinemann, 2009, p. 192.

454. b The femoral condyle is located at the distal end of the femur. The femoral head is at the proximal end of the femur. Aspinall V, Cappello M, Introduction to Veterinary Anatomy and Physiology Textbook, ed 2, Butterworth Heinemann, 2009, p. 193.

455. c The coxal tuber is located at the proximal end of the hip bone. The talus is located within the tarsal joint distal to the tibia. The metatarsal bones are located distal to the tarsal joint and proximal to the sesamoid bones. The femur is immediately distal to the hipbone. Aspinall V, Cappello M, Introduction to Veterinary Anatomy and Physiology Textbook, ed 2, Butterworth Heinemann, 2009, p. 193.

456. c The calcaneus bone forms the point of the hock in horses and it is where the Achilles tendon attaches. The fetlock lies between the cannon bone and the long pastern. The pastern bones are part of the phalanges. Aspinall V, Cappello M, Introduction to Veterinary Anatomy and Physiology Textbook, ed 2, Butterworth Heinemann, 2009, p. 192.

457. d The tarsus of horses, also known as the hock, has six small bones that are arranged in three rows. The upper row is the talus and the calcaneus, the central tarsus makes up the middle row, and the third row is the first and second tarsal bones, which are fused together with the third tarsal bone; the fourth tarsal bone is housed in spaces in the middle and lower rows. Aspinall V, Cappello M, Introduction to Veterinary Anatomy and Physiology Textbook, ed 2, Butterworth Heinemann, 2009, p. 193.

458. a The metatarsal IV bone is also referred to as the lateral splint bone. Metatarsal III is referred to as the cannon bone. The talus remains as the talus. The tarsus is referred to as the hock. Aspinall V, Cappello M, Introduction to Veterinary Anatomy and Physiology Textbook, ed 2, Butterworth Heinemann, 2009, p. 193.

459. c The forelimbs of the horse can carry approximately 60% of the weight and absorb most of the shock during movement. The hind limbs are angled and provide the main propulsive force and carry the remaining 40% of the weight. Aspinall V, Cappello M, Introduction to Veterinary Anatomy and Physiology Textbook, ed 2, Butterworth Heinemann, 2009, p. 193.

460. b The brachiocephalicus muscle is responsible for moving the head and neck. The rhomboideus raises the shoulder. The splenius elevates and flexes the neck. The deltoid abducts the forelimb and flexes the shoulder. Aspinall V, Cappello M, Introduction to Veterinary Anatomy and Physiology Textbook, ed 2, Butterworth Heinemann, 2009, p. 195.

461. a The sternocephalicus muscle inserts at the mandible of the horse. The latissimus dorsi, brachiocephalicus, infraspinatus, pectoral, and supraspinatus all attach to the humerus. The trapezius muscle inserts at the spine of the scapula. The semitendinosus inserts at the proximal tibia. Aspinall V, Cappello M, Introduction to Veterinary Anatomy and Physiology Textbook, ed 2, Butterworth Heinemann, 2009, p. 195.

462. c The longissimus dorsi muscle flexes the back and trunk, supports the head and neck, and supports the rider's weight. The pectoral muscle protracts and retracts the forelimb and abducts the forelimb. The semitendinosus extends the hip, flexes the stifle, and extends the hock. The rhomboideus raises the shoulder. Aspinall V, Cappello M, Introduction to Veterinary Anatomy and Physiology Textbook, ed 2, Butterworth Heinemann, 2009, p. 195.

463. d The point of origin of the pectoral muscle is the sternum and it inserts on the humerus and the scapula. The point of origin for the infraspinatus and triceps muscle is at the scapula. The semimembranosus muscle's point of origin is the pelvis. The latissimus dorsi muscle's point of origin is at the thoracic vertebrae. Aspinall V, Cappello M, Introduction to Veterinary Anatomy and Physiology Textbook, ed 2, Butterworth Heinemann, 2009, p. 195.

464. b The gastrocnemius, semitendinosus, and biceps femoris all extend the hock. The semimembranosus extends the hip and flexes the stifle. Aspinall V, Cappello M, Introduction to Veterinary Anatomy and Physiology Textbook, ed 2, Butterworth Heinemann, 2009, p. 195.

465. d The point of origin for the superficial gluteal muscle is at the tuber coxae of the pelvis. The gastrocnemius muscle originates at the femur. The infraspinatus muscle originates at the caudal aspect of the scapula. The latissimus dorsi muscle originates at the thoracic and lumbar vertebrae. Aspinall V, Cappello M, Introduction to Veterinary Anatomy and Physiology Textbook, ed 2, Butterworth Heinemann, 2009, p. 195.

466. d The triceps is responsible for the extension of the elbow. The infraspinatus abducts and rotates the forelimb. The gastrocnemius flexes the stifle and extends the hock. The pectoral muscle protracts and retracts the forelimb and abducts the limb. Aspinall V, Cappello M, Introduction to Veterinary Anatomy and Physiology Textbook, ed 2, Butterworth Heinemann, 2009, p. 195.

467. b The splenius muscle originates behind the poll (at the base of the skull). The trapezius originates at the occipital bone, the last cervical vertebrae, and the first 10 thoracic vertebrae. The sternocephalicus originates at the sternum. The brachiocephalicus originates at the wing of the atlas. Aspinall V, Cappello M, Introduction to Veterinary Anatomy and Physiology Textbook, ed 2, Butterworth Heinemann, 2009, p. 195.

468. d The semimembranosus muscle inserts at the distal femur and tibia. The gastrocnemius inserts at the hock. The semitendinosus inserts at the proximal tibia. The biceps femoris inserts at the femur, patella, and proximal tibia. Aspinall V, Cappello M, Introduction to Veterinary Anatomy and Physiology Textbook, ed 2, Butterworth Heinemann, 2009, p. 195.

469. b Tendons attach muscles to bone. Ligaments attach bone to bone. Blood vessels travel throughout the body. Aspinall V, Cappello M, Introduction to Veterinary Anatomy and Physiology Textbook, ed 2, Butterworth Heinemann, 2009, p. 195.

470. b The deep digital flexor tendon flexes the toe. The suspensory ligaments support and suspend the fetlock and prevent overextension. The superficial digital flexor tendon flexes the pastern joint. The lateral digital extensor tendon extends the pastern joint. Aspinall V, Cappello M, Introduction to Veterinary Anatomy and Physiology Textbook, ed 2, Butterworth Heinemann, 2009, p. 196.

471. c The cheek ligaments prevent strain and overextension of the joint. The suspensory ligament supports and suspends the fetlock and prevents overextension. The lateral digital extensor tendon assists in the extension of the pastern joint. The deep digital flexor tendon flexes the toe. Aspinall V, Cappello M, Introduction to Veterinary Anatomy and Physiology Textbook, ed 2, Butterworth Heinemann, 2009, p. 196.

472. b The stay apparatus locks the limbs and joints into position, enabling the horse to rest and sleep in a standing position. The cheek ligaments prevent strain and overextension of the joint. The deep digital flexor tendon flexes the toe. The superficial digital flexor tendon flexes the pastern joint. Aspinall V, Cappello M, Introduction to Veterinary Anatomy and Physiology Textbook, ed 2, Butterworth Heinemann, 2009, p. 196.

473. b A protective external capsule (the hoof) surrounds the internal structures of the foot of a horse. The frog is a small triangular wedge that aids in blood circulation, absorption, and concussion. A horseshoe is the manmade apparatus placed on the bottom side of a hoof for added protection. The sole supports and protects the structures within the foot. Aspinall V, Cappello M, Introduction to Veterinary Anatomy and Physiology Textbook, ed 2, Butterworth Heinemann, 2009, p. 197.

474. a The bars within the hoof allow for expansion of the foot and provide strength. The frog aids in blood circulation and absorption of concussion. The sole provides support and protects the structures within the foot. The coronet is the point from which the horn tissue grows and extends. Aspinall V, Cappello M, Introduction to Veterinary Anatomy and Physiology Textbook, ed 2, Butterworth Heinemann, 2009, p. 197.

475. c It takes approximately 9–12 months for the horn to grow from the coronet to the tip of the toe on the ground surface. Aspinall V, Cappello M, Introduction to Veterinary Anatomy and Physiology Textbook, ed 2, Butterworth Heinemann, 2009, p. 197.

476. d The periople forms the outer layer to protect the hoof and to maintain the moisture level to prevent it from becoming dry and brittle. The hoof surrounds the internal structures of the foot. The sole provides support and protects the structures within the foot. The frog aids in blood circulation and absorption of concussion. Aspinall V, Cappello M, Introduction to Veterinary Anatomy and Physiology Textbook, ed 2, Butterworth Heinemann, 2009, p. 197.

477. b The frog corium provides nourishment to the digital cushion and functions within the frog. The sole corium attaches to the sole of the pedal bone to the horny sole of the foot. The laminar corium consists of the sensitive laminae attached to the periosteum of the pedal bone. The perioplic corium supplies the periople with nutrients. Aspinall V, Cappello M, Introduction to Veterinary Anatomy and Physiology Textbook, ed 2, Butterworth Heinemann, 2009, p. 198.

478. b The gait is the sequence in which the horse lifts its feet from the ground. A trot, gallop, and canter are all types of gaits. Aspinall V, Cappello M, Introduction to Veterinary Anatomy and Physiology Textbook, ed 2, Butterworth Heinemann, 2009, p. 199.

479. c The floating phase occurs within the gallop, in which none of the feet touch the ground; they are gathered underneath the horse. A walk is the slowest gait during which each foot comes down separately and weight is taken equally on all four feet. A trot is when the body is alternately balanced on diagonally opposite feet. A canter is a slower form of a gallop in which the hind feet are still on the ground when the first forefoot returns to the ground. Aspinall V, Cappello M, Introduction to Veterinary Anatomy and Physiology Textbook, ed 2, Butterworth Heinemann, 2009, p. 198.

480. d During a gallop there are never more than two legs on the ground at the same time. A walk is the slowest gait during which each foot comes down separately and weight is taken equally on all four feet. A trot is when the body is alternately balanced on diagonally opposite feet. A canter is a slower form of a gallop in which the hind feet are still on the ground when the first forefoot returns to the ground. Aspinall V, Cappello M, Introduction to Veterinary Anatomy and Physiology Textbook, ed 2, Butterworth Heinemann, 2009, p. 199.

481. b A horse's vision is primarily monocular because each eye is situated on the lateral sides of the head. This aids in the ability to watch for predators. There are limited areas of binocular and 3D vision. Aspinall V, Cappello M, Introduction to Veterinary Anatomy and Physiology Textbook, ed 2, Butterworth Heinemann, 2009, p. 199.

482. b The blind spot of a horse lies directly behinds the ears or behind the head. In front of the muzzle there is limited 3D vision or binocular vision. On both sides of the head is a wide range of 2D or monocular vision. Aspinall V, Cappello M, Introduction to Veterinary Anatomy and Physiology Textbook, ed 2, Butterworth Heinemann, 2009, p. 199.

483. d The corpora nigra provides additional shading for the retina to limit the entry of light. The iris is responsible for contracting the pupil. The cornea is a transparent layer forming the front of the eye. The ciliary muscle is responsible for altering the shape of the lens to focus images on to the retina. Aspinall V, Cappello M, Introduction to Veterinary Anatomy and Physiology Textbook, ed 2, Butterworth Heinemann, 2009, p. 199.

484. a The normal resting heart rate for a horse is 24–42 bpm. The heart rate of dogs is 40–140 bpm. The heart rate for cattle is 48–84 bpm. The heart rate for gerbils is 260–600 bpm. Aspinall V, Cappello M, Introduction to Veterinary Anatomy and Physiology Textbook, ed 2, Butterworth Heinemann, 2009, p. 200.

485. c The alar fold forms the ventral margin of each nostril. The external nares are the two large flexible nostrils. The false nostrils are the blind ending pouch on the dorsal end. The ethmoturbinates are delicate coiled bones covered by olfactory mucosa. Aspinall V, Cappello M, Introduction to Veterinary Anatomy and Physiology Textbook, ed 2, Butterworth Heinemann, 2009, p. 200.

486. a The front sinus lies in the dorsal part of the skull medial to the orbit. The two maxillary sinuses occupy a large proportion of the upper jaw. The oropharynx and the nasopharynx are part of the pharynx. Aspinall V, Cappello M, Introduction to Veterinary Anatomy and Physiology Textbook, ed 2, Butterworth Heinemann, 2009, p. 200.

487. d The hyoid apparatus is the structure that suspends the larynx from the skull. The epiglottis is a flap lying on the rostral part of the larynx that covers the glottis. The arytenoid cartilage is part of the larynx. The laryngopharynx extends from the oropharynx to the opening of the esophagus. Aspinall V, Cappello M, Introduction to Veterinary Anatomy and Physiology Textbook, ed 2, Butterworth Heinemann, 2009, p. 201.

488. d The trachea, bronchi, and lungs are all part of the lower respiratory tract. The pharynx is part of the upper respiratory tract. Aspinall V, Cappello M, Introduction to Veterinary Anatomy and Physiology Textbook, ed 2, Butterworth Heinemann, 2009, p. 201.

489. d Most ruminants, sheep, cattle, and goats have a cotyledonary placental attachment in which the areas of attachment are small, separate, and numerous. Horses and pigs have a diffuse attachment of the placenta in which the attachment sites are spread diffusely over the whole surface of the placenta and the whole lining of the uterus. Dogs and cats have a zonary attachment where the placenta attaches to the uterus in a belt-shaped area. Colville TP, Bassert JM, Clinical Anatomy and Physiology for Veterinary Technicians, ed 3, Mosby, 2016, p. 493.

490. a On an electrocardiogram, the P wave is associated with atrial depolarization. The T wave is associated with ventricular repolarization. The QRS complex is associated with ventricular depolarization. Colville TP, Bassert JM, Clinical Anatomy and Physiology for Veterinary Technicians, ed 3, Mosby, 2016, p. 358.

491. a The popliteal lymph node is located on the caudal aspect of the leg at the level of the patella. Inguinal lymph nodes are located in the groin region of the hind limbs. Mandibular lymph nodes are located in the caudal part of the jaw. Prescapular lymph nodes are located in front of the scapular region. Aspinall V, Cappello M, Introduction to Veterinary Anatomy and Physiology Textbook, ed 2, Butterworth Heinemann, 2009, p. 87.

492. b Permanent teeth in the horse begin to erupt around the age of 2½ years. At the age of 1 year the deciduous teeth are still in use. By the age of 5 years the deciduous teeth are discarded. By the age of 6 years the permanent teeth are fully erupted. Aspinall V, Cappello M, Introduction to Veterinary Anatomy and Physiology Textbook, ed 2, Butterworth Heinemann, 2009, p. 202.

493. c An adult male horse has 40 permanent teeth. An adult female horse has 36 permanent teeth. There are 24 deciduous teeth in horses. Any count greater than 36 (for females) or 40 (for males) is considered an abnormal count of teeth in a horse. Aspinall V, Cappello M, Introduction to Veterinary Anatomy and Physiology Textbook, ed 2, Butterworth Heinemann, 2009, p. 202.

494. b A horse develops wolf teeth between the ages of 18 months and 5 years. Permanent teeth are fully erupted by 6 years. Deciduous teeth are erupted at birth and discarded by 5 years. Aspinall V, Cappello M, Introduction to Veterinary Anatomy and Physiology Textbook, ed 2, Butterworth Heinemann, 2009, p. 202.

495. a The occlusal surfaces of horse teeth are worn down approximately 1–2 mm every year because of the mastication process. Aspinall V, Cappello M, Introduction to Veterinary Anatomy and Physiology Textbook, ed 2, Butterworth Heinemann, 2009, p. 202.

496. b The term *hypsodontic* refers to the lack of enamel over the occlusal surfaces of the horse teeth. The horse enamel casing of the sides is folded, which increases the amount of hard wearable material. Horses' teeth have a large crown reserve, which enables all the teeth to grow continuously. Aspinall V, Cappello M, Introduction to Veterinary Anatomy and Physiology Textbook, ed 2, Butterworth Heinemann, 2009, p. 202.

497. c The section between the canine teeth and the first premolar is termed the *diastema*. Wolf teeth are the first premolar teeth that may erupt between 18 months and 5 years. The term *hypsodontic* refers to the lack of enamel on the occlusal surface. The infundibulum is a portion inside the tooth. Aspinall V, Cappello M, Introduction to Veterinary Anatomy and Physiology Textbook, ed 2, Butterworth Heinemann, 2009, p. 202.

498. d The average length of the esophagus of an average sized horse is approximately 1.5 m. This structure is a muscular tube that extends from the throat to the horse's stomach. The other options include incorrect units. Aspinall V, Cappello M, Introduction to Veterinary Anatomy and Physiology Textbook, ed 2, Butterworth Heinemann, 2009, p. 203.

499. c The volume that a horse's stomach can hold is approximately 7–14 L. Aspinall V, Cappello M, Introduction to Veterinary Anatomy and Physiology Textbook, ed 2, Butterworth Heinemann, 2009, p. 203.

500. c Food passes from the esophagus to the stomach by means of the cardiac sphincter. The pyloric sphincter from the stomach to the small intestines is by means of the pyloric sphincter. The epiglottis is the cartilage flap that covers the trachea during swallowing. The duodenum is the first portion of the small intestines. Aspinall V, Cappello M, Introduction to Veterinary Anatomy and Physiology Textbook, ed 2, Butterworth Heinemann, 2009, p. 203.

501. c The stomach of the horse empties when it is approximately ⅔ full, resulting in a minimal amount of time that food spends in the stomach, which causes minimal digestion. Aspinall V, Cappello M, Introduction to Veterinary Anatomy and Physiology Textbook, ed 2, Butterworth Heinemann, 2009, p. 203.

502. d The digestion and absorption of food takes places at the ileocecal junction. The duodenum, jejunum, and ileum are all parts of the small intestine that end at the ileocecal junction. Aspinall V, Cappello M, Introduction to Veterinary Anatomy and Physiology Textbook, ed 2, Butterworth Heinemann, 2009, p. 203.

503. c The microbial digestion of cellulose takes place within the small intestines. The small intestine is responsible for the digestion of food products, which mainly occurs at the ileocecal junction. The stomach is responsible for the mechanical breakdown of food products. Aspinall V, Cappello M, Introduction to Veterinary Anatomy and Physiology Textbook, ed 2, Butterworth Heinemann, 2009, p. 203.

504. a The duodenum, jejunum, and ileum are all part of the small intestine. The cecum is part of the large intestine. Aspinall V, Cappello M, Introduction to Veterinary Anatomy and Physiology Textbook, ed 2, Butterworth Heinemann, 2009, p. 204.

505. d The cecum of a horse can hold up to 35 L of ingesta. Aspinall V, Cappello M, Introduction to Veterinary Anatomy and Physiology Textbook, ed 2, Butterworth Heinemann, 2009, p. 204.

506. d The colon of a horse can hold up to 100 L of ingesta. Aspinall V, Cappello M, Introduction to Veterinary

Anatomy and Physiology Textbook, ed 2, Butterworth Heinemann, 2009, p. 204.

507. d The colon of a horse holds food for approximately 36–65 hours. Aspinall V, Cappello M, Introduction to Veterinary Anatomy and Physiology Textbook, ed 2, Butterworth Heinemann, 2009, p. 204.

508. b The left kidney of a horse lies caudal to the right kidney and is located ventral to the last rib and near the first two or three transverse processes. The right kidney lies cranial to the left and ventral to the last two or three ribs and the first transverse process. The kidneys lie on opposite sides of the abdomen; lateral and medial would not be appropriate terms. Aspinall V, Cappello M, Introduction to Veterinary Anatomy and Physiology Textbook, ed 2, Butterworth Heinemann, 2009, p. 204.

509. b The kidney of an average sized horse weighs approximately 400–600 g. The kidneys vary in size and weight among every animal and every size of horse. Aspinall V, Cappello M, Introduction to Veterinary Anatomy and Physiology Textbook, ed 2, Butterworth Heinemann, 2009, p. 204.

510. b The average sized horse produces approximately 20 mL/kg/day of urine. The other amounts would be considered either too much or too little urine production. Aspinall V, Cappello M, Introduction to Veterinary Anatomy and Physiology Textbook, ed 2, Butterworth Heinemann, 2009, p. 204.

511. d The normal urine pH of the horse is alkaline–greater than 9 because of the high potassium content of fresh vegetation. A pH less than 6 is considered acidic. Aspinall V, Cappello M, Introduction to Veterinary Anatomy and Physiology Textbook, ed 2, Butterworth Heinemann, 2009, p. 204.

512. c Around 2 years of age testicles reach their full adult size of 8–12 cm and are then mature enough to produce spermatozoa and testosterone. Aspinall V, Cappello M, Introduction to Veterinary Anatomy and Physiology Textbook, ed 2, Butterworth Heinemann, 2009, p. 205.

513. b The seminal vesicles are a pair of smooth-surfaced, pear-shaped glands located on either size of the bladder. The bulbourethral glands are paired glands that lie dorsal to the urethra. The adrenal glands lie near the kidneys. The thyroid gland lies in the neck around the trachea of the horse. Aspinall V, Cappello M, Introduction to Veterinary Anatomy and Physiology Textbook, ed 2, Butterworth Heinemann, 2009, p. 205.

514. d The prostate gland is responsible for secreting clear fluid that cleans the urethra in advance of ejaculation as well as neutralizing the acidity of any remaining urine. Aspinall V, Cappello M, Introduction to Veterinary Anatomy and Physiology Textbook, ed 2, Butterworth Heinemann, 2009, p. 205.

515. c Fertilization normally occurs in the fallopian tubes of a horse. The beginning of the fallopian tubes after leaving the ovary is termed the *infundibulum*. Fertilization does not occur in the ovaries or testicles. Aspinall V, Cappello M, Introduction to Veterinary Anatomy and Physiology Textbook, ed 2, Butterworth Heinemann, 2009, p. 205.

516. b The unfertilized ova are reabsorbed back into the body; only fertilized ova pass through the uterotubular junction into the uterus. They do not remain in the fallopian tube until fertilization occurs and they are not expelled from the body. Aspinall V, Cappello M, Introduction to Veterinary Anatomy and Physiology Textbook, ed 2, Butterworth Heinemann, 2009, p. 205.

517. b The ovaries of the mare are largely inactive until sexual maturity occurs at around 1–2 years of age. Aspinall V, Cappello M, Introduction to Veterinary Anatomy and Physiology Textbook, ed 2, Butterworth Heinemann, 2009, p. 205.

518. b The mare is a uniparous animal, which is defined as only naturally giving birth to one foal at a time. The term *nulliparity* is defined as the absence of having reproduced. The term *multiparous* is defined as the number of pregnancy occurrences. Aspinall V, Cappello M, Introduction to Veterinary Anatomy and Physiology Textbook, ed 2, Butterworth Heinemann, 2009, p. 205.

519. b The typical breeding season of a mare is between the seasons of early spring to late summer. The normal breeding season can be manipulated with the use of drugs. Aspinall V, Cappello M, Introduction to Veterinary Anatomy and Physiology Textbook, ed 2, Butterworth Heinemann, 2009, p. 20.

520. a A mare is considered a spontaneous ovulator, which means she will ovulate without the stimulus of mating. Polyestrous refers to having multiple estrous cycles. The term *anestrous* refers to not having any estrous cycle. The term *multiparous* refers to having multiple pregnancies. Aspinall V, Cappello M, Introduction to Veterinary Anatomy and Physiology Textbook, ed 2, Butterworth Heinemann, 2009, p. 206.

521. c The typical estrous cycle of a mare usually lasts 17–21 days, although some mares have had cycles that last as long as 35 days. Aspinall V, Cappello M, Introduction to Veterinary Anatomy and Physiology Textbook, ed 2, Butterworth Heinemann, 2009, p. 206.

522. b During the estrus phase, a horse is said to be "in heat" or "in season," which lasts approximately 3–5 days (ovulation, as well as mating, also occurs). Follicle development and secretion of estrogen occurs during the diestrus phase. Aspinall V, Cappello M, Introduction to Veterinary Anatomy and Physiology Textbook, ed 2, Butterworth Heinemann, 2009, p. 206.

523. c The diestrus phase typically lasts 14–16 days. The estrous cycle lasts 17–21 days but can last up to 35 days. The estrus cycle lasts 3–5 days. Aspinall V, Cappello M, Introduction to Veterinary Anatomy and Physiology Textbook, ed 2, Butterworth Heinemann, 2009, p. 206.

524. b The sternum of birds is extended into a laterally flattened keel, which provides a large surface area of the attachment of the major flight muscles. The coracoid is a large bone between the keel and shoulder joint that supports the wings. The beak replaces a boney mandible. The quadrate bone lies between the mandible and the skull. Aspinall V, Cappello M, Introduction to Veterinary Anatomy and Physiology Textbook, ed 2, Butterworth Heinemann, 2009, p. 151.

525. d Pneumatic bones refer to the large bones of birds that are filled with air in membranous sacs that connect with the respiratory system. Compact, long, and irregular bones are not typical bones found in birds but rather in mammals. Aspinall V, Cappello M, Introduction to Veterinary Anatomy and Physiology Textbook, ed 2, Butterworth Heinemann, 2009, p. 151.

526. b Birds are missing a diaphragm, which separates the thorax from the abdomen. The keel is the large flattened bone in the chest area, which represents the sternum. Lungs and liver are both present in the bird population. Aspinall V, Cappello M, Introduction to Veterinary Anatomy and Physiology Textbook, ed 2, Butterworth Heinemann, 2009, p. 151.

527. b The digital flexor tendon is responsible for bringing about the perching reflex so that birds can land on a branch without falling off. The tibiotarsus is a fused bone in the leg. A craniofacial hinge is a joint between the upper beak and the skull. The supracoracoid muscle is responsible for the upstroke during flight. Aspinall V, Cappello M, Introduction to Veterinary Anatomy and Physiology Textbook, ed 2, Butterworth Heinemann, 2009, p. 151.

528. c Most birds have three toes pointing forward and one toe pointing backward. Aspinall V, Cappello M, Introduction to Veterinary Anatomy and Physiology Textbook, ed 2, Butterworth Heinemann, 2009, p. 152.

529. b The pygostyle is located distal to the coccygeal vertebrae of birds, forming the tail. The sternum is on the anterior side of birds distal to the coracoid. The tibiotarsus is distal to the femur in the leg. The hallux is part of the foot distal to the tarsometatarsus. Aspinall V, Cappello M, Introduction to Veterinary Anatomy and Physiology Textbook, ed 2, Butterworth Heinemann, 2009, p. 152.

530. a The alula is the first digit in birds. The major metacarpal is proximal to the second digit. The tarsometatarsus is proximal to the hallux. The hallux is the foot of birds and is distal to the tarsometatarsus. Aspinall V, Cappello M, Introduction to Veterinary Anatomy and Physiology Textbook, ed 2, Butterworth Heinemann, 2009, p. 152.

531. c The primary feathers are located on digit 3 (the main digit) and are fused to the metacarpal bones. Digit 1 is also known as the alula and carries few feathers. Aspinall V, Cappello M, Introduction to Veterinary Anatomy and Physiology Textbook, ed 2, Butterworth Heinemann, 2009, p. 152.

532. d The central shaft of a bird's feather is also referred to as the rachis. The dentary is part of the lower beak. The talon is part of the foot. The hallux is the foot of birds. Aspinall V, Cappello M, Introduction to Veterinary Anatomy and Physiology Textbook, ed 2, Butterworth Heinemann, 2009, p. 153.

533. b The rachis of a feather is filled with blood capillaries during growth but as it matures it becomes hollow. Molting refers to the loss of old feathers. Aspinall V, Cappello M, Introduction to Veterinary Anatomy and Physiology Textbook, ed 2, Butterworth Heinemann, 2009, p. 153.

534. b Secretions from the preen gland at the base of the tail keeps the feathers waterproof. The alula is the first digit of the wing. The gizzard is part of the digestive tract in some animals. The coracoid is the bone located on the anterior surface cranial to the sternum. Aspinall V, Cappello M, Introduction to Veterinary Anatomy and Physiology Textbook, ed 2, Butterworth Heinemann, 2009, p. 153.

535. c The secondary feathers are attached to the ulna and are shorter than the primaries. The primary feathers are attached to digit 3. There are a few feathers attached to digit 1 that control takeoff and landing. The hallux is the foot of birds. Aspinall V, Cappello M, Introduction to Veterinary Anatomy and Physiology Textbook, ed 2, Butterworth Heinemann, 2009, p. 152.

536. c The contour feathers cover the outermost layer of the body to produce a smooth outline. The primary and secondary feathers provide thrust for flight and are fused to the metacarpal bones. The filoplume feathers are close to the body below the contour feathers and provide insulation. Aspinall V, Cappello M, Introduction to Veterinary Anatomy and Physiology Textbook, ed 2, Butterworth Heinemann, 2009, p. 153.

537. c All adult birds go through a molting process once a year, typically after the breeding season. Aspinall V, Cappello M, Introduction to Veterinary Anatomy and Physiology Textbook, ed 2, Butterworth Heinemann, 2009, p. 153.

538. b The dorsal surface of the wing is longer and convex and the ventral surface is shorter and more concave. The wing is slightly curved to provide lift and to aid in landing; therefore, the dorsal and ventral sides are shaped differently for this purpose. The wing is a long structure but is not curved differently from proximal to distal. Aspinall V, Cappello M, Introduction to Veterinary Anatomy and Physiology Textbook, ed 2, Butterworth Heinemann, 2009, p. 153.

539. a Air passing over the dorsal surface travels faster than air passing under the ventral surface, generating lift. The speed of air passing over the proximal or distal side does not alter the lift of the bird. Aspinall V, Cappello M, Introduction to Veterinary Anatomy and Physiology Textbook, ed 2, Butterworth Heinemann, 2009, p. 153.

540. c The lift force must equal the weight of the bird for flight to occur. The size of the bird, shape of the wings, and gravity are unrelated to lift force. Aspinall V, Cappello M, Introduction to Veterinary Anatomy and Physiology Textbook, ed 2, Butterworth Heinemann, 2009, p. 153.

541. b If the angle of the tilt of the wing is greater than 15 degrees, lift is reduced and the bird may fall out of the sky. At 5 degrees the bird is still able to have lift. Aspinall V, Cappello M, Introduction to Veterinary Anatomy and Physiology Textbook, ed 2, Butterworth Heinemann, 2009, p. 154.

542. a To land, the tail is used as a brake and the wings are extended into a stall position. The tail is not used as a guide for landing or perching. For a bird to land, thrust is not needed or generated by the tail. Aspinall V, Cappello M, Introduction to Veterinary Anatomy and Physiology Textbook, ed 2, Butterworth Heinemann, 2009, p. 155.

543. c Sight and hearing are well developed in birds for survival. The special senses of touch, taste, and smell are underdeveloped. Aspinall V, Cappello M, Introduction to Veterinary Anatomy and Physiology Textbook, ed 2, Butterworth Heinemann, 2009, p. 155.

544. c A bird has to move its head to view an image because it has few eye muscles. The optic lobes are large and occupy the majority of the midbrain but do not assist eye movement. The eye fills the orbits, leaving little room for eye muscles. Aspinall V, Cappello M, Introduction to Veterinary Anatomy and Physiology Textbook, ed 2, Butterworth Heinemann, 2009, p. 155.

545. b A predator-type bird has forward-pointing eyes, producing binocular vision to locate its prey. Seed-eating birds have laterally placed eyes, creating monocular vision to locate their predators. 3D vision occurs in some animals such as a small section of the visual field in horses. Aspinall V, Cappello M, Introduction to Veterinary Anatomy and Physiology Textbook, ed 2, Butterworth Heinemann, 2009, p. 155.

546. b The sclerotic ring helps to reinforce the large circumference of the eye. The cornea is the transparent layer on the front of the eye. The optic lobe is located in the brain and is the vision control center. The optic nerve connects the eye to the brain, relaying visual images to be interpreted. Aspinall V, Cappello M, Introduction to Veterinary Anatomy and Physiology Textbook, ed 2, Butterworth Heinemann, 2009, p. 155.

547. b The iris of a bird's eye is formed by the striated muscle, which enables the bird to control the size of the pupil voluntarily. Mammals have smooth muscle in the iris, which is controlled involuntarily. The cardiac muscle is only located in the heart. Aspinall V, Cappello M, Introduction to Veterinary Anatomy and Physiology Textbook, ed 2, Butterworth Heinemann, 2009, p. 156.

548. b The vitreous humor in the posterior chamber of the eye contains a ribbon-like structure attached to the retina known as pectin, which provides nutrition for the inner eye structures. The nictitating membrane is similar to the third eyelid in dogs and cats and is located on the upper and lower lid. The optic nerve connects the eye to the brain, relaying images for interpretation. Aspinall V, Cappello M, Introduction to Veterinary Anatomy and Physiology Textbook, ed 2, Butterworth Heinemann, 2009, p. 156.

549. d The photoreceptor cells contain rods that provide night vision and cones that provide color vision. Nocturnal birds have more rods than cones. Monocular and binocular vision is dependent on the placement of the eye and the visual field. Aspinall V, Cappello M, Introduction to Veterinary Anatomy and Physiology Textbook, ed 2, Butterworth Heinemann, 2009, p. 156.

550. d Avian species do not have ear pinnae. Owls appear to have ear pinnae, but they are just tufts of feathers. Aspinall V, Cappello M, Introduction to Veterinary Anatomy and Physiology Textbook, ed 2, Butterworth Heinemann, 2009, p. 156.

551. d The columella bone is located in the ear and transmits sound to the inner ear. The sternum is caudal to the clavicle. The humerus is proximal to the ulna. The coracoid is cranial to the sternum. Aspinall V, Cappello M, Introduction to Veterinary Anatomy and Physiology Textbook, ed 2, Butterworth Heinemann, 2009, p. 156.

552. c The free spaces in birds are located within the major bones of the body, which are filled with membranous air sacs connected to the respiratory system. Birds do not have a diaphragm separating the thorax from the abdomen. The free spaces are within the humerus of the wings. Aspinall V, Cappello M, Introduction to Veterinary Anatomy and Physiology Textbook, ed 2, Butterworth Heinemann, 2009, p. 156.

553. b The combined effect of air passing through the larynx and syrinx produces the characteristic sounds associated with the bird species. The glottis is part of the larynx, which covers the airway when a bird swallows food. The trachea divides into the right and left bronchi, which is where the syrinx is located. The choana is a cleft in the hard palate that connects the oral and nasal cavities. Aspinall V, Cappello M, Introduction to Veterinary Anatomy and Physiology Textbook, ed 2, Butterworth Heinemann, 2009, p. 157.

554. d The average bird contains nine air sacs that penetrate the spaces of the body cavity and the insides of multiple bones. Aspinall V, Cappello M, Introduction to Veterinary Anatomy and Physiology Textbook, ed 2, Butterworth Heinemann, 2009, p. 158.

555. b The nine different air sacs in birds are responsible for lightening the weight of the skeleton, the bellows effect, and to act as a reservoir for air. These air sacs do not participate in gaseous exchange. Aspinall V, Cappello M, Introduction to Veterinary Anatomy and Physiology Textbook, ed 2, Butterworth Heinemann, 2009, p. 158.

556. a During respiration, the air circulates continuously and passes through the lungs twice. Aspinall V, Cappello M, Introduction to Veterinary Anatomy and Physiology Textbook, ed 2, Butterworth Heinemann, 2009, p. 158.

557. a The air in the cranial air sac passes straight through the lungs and out. Air passes through the remaining air sacs during the normal respiratory cycle after passing through the lungs. Aspinall V, Cappello M, Introduction to Veterinary Anatomy and Physiology Textbook, ed 2, Butterworth Heinemann, 2009, p. 158.

558. d The avian heart contains four chambers, similar to that of mammals. Aspinall V, Cappello M, Introduction to Veterinary Anatomy and Physiology Textbook, ed 2, Butterworth Heinemann, 2009, p. 159.

559. c The pericardial sac covers the heart of the bird. The bronchi are not covered by anything. The keel is a bone located cranial to the sternum. The syrinx is part of the larynx of birds and is not surrounded by a covering. Aspinall V, Cappello M, Introduction to Veterinary Anatomy and Physiology Textbook, ed 2, Butterworth Heinemann, 2009, p. 158.

560. e There is a large blood supply to the flight muscles and wings via the pectoral and brachial arteries. The carotid artery carries blood to the head of birds. Aspinall V, Cappello M, Introduction to Veterinary Anatomy and Physiology Textbook, ed 2, Butterworth Heinemann, 2009, p. 159.

561. d The pudendal artery is located near the rectum in birds. The ulnar artery is located distal to the humerus. The brachiocephalic artery is located as a branch of the aorta. Aspinall V, Cappello M, Introduction to Veterinary Anatomy and Physiology Textbook, ed 2, Butterworth Heinemann, 2009, p. 159.

562. d The carotid artery is the main artery that runs parallel to the trachea. The brachial artery runs along the length of the humerus. The jugular runs parallel to the trachea and carotid but is a vein not an artery. The subclavian artery courses perpendicular to the trachea across the chest and becomes the brachial artery. Aspinall V, Cappello M, Introduction to Veterinary Anatomy and Physiology Textbook, ed 2, Butterworth Heinemann, 2009, p. 159.

563. b The ulnar artery runs parallel to the radial artery in the wing. The brachial artery is proximal to the bifurcation of the ulnar and radial artery. The femoral artery is located in the legs. The ischiatic artery courses posterior to the external iliac artery entering the legs. Aspinall V, Cappello M, Introduction to Veterinary Anatomy and Physiology Textbook, ed 2, Butterworth Heinemann, 2009, p. 159.

564. d The femoral artery is distal to the external iliac artery in the leg. The coeliac artery is the first branch of the distal aorta. The renal artery branches off the aorta to supply the kidneys. The pectoral artery branches off the subclavian artery. Aspinall V, Cappello M, Introduction to Veterinary Anatomy and Physiology Textbook, ed 2, Butterworth Heinemann, 2009, p. 159.

565. b In birds, food passes down the esophagus on the right side of the neck and enters the crop, which acts as a storage organ. The gizzard is a thick-walled muscular organ in which mechanical digestion occurs and it is part of the stomach. Food leaves the gizzard and enters the duodenum of the small intestines. The proventriculus is part of the stomach and is where food is stored and mixed with digestive juices. Aspinall V, Cappello M, Introduction to Veterinary Anatomy and Physiology Textbook, ed 2, Butterworth Heinemann, 2009, p. 160.

566. b The cloaca is located distal to the cecum of birds. The gizzard is distal to the proventriculus. The proventriculus is distal to the crop. The crop is distal to the esophagus. Aspinall V, Cappello M, Introduction to Veterinary Anatomy and Physiology Textbook, ed 2, Butterworth Heinemann, 2009, p. 160.

567. b Food leaves the gizzard by means of the pylorus and enters the duodenum of the small intestine. The cloaca is the most distal part of the digestive tract in birds. The proventriculus is distal to the crop and proximal to the gizzard. The ileum is part of the small intestine and is distal to the duodenum. Aspinall V, Cappello M, Introduction to Veterinary Anatomy and Physiology Textbook, ed 2, Butterworth Heinemann, 2009, p. 160.

568. c The pancreas of birds has three lobes, which are connected to the duodenal lobe by three pancreatic ducts. Aspinall V, Cappello M, Introduction to Veterinary Anatomy and Physiology Textbook, ed 2, Butterworth Heinemann, 2009, p. 161.

569. c The ureters carry urine to the outside of the body via the cloaca in birds. The isthmus is located cranial to the uterus. The vagina is distal to the uterus and enters the cloaca. The proventriculus is distal to the crop. Aspinall V, Cappello M, Introduction to Veterinary Anatomy and Physiology Textbook, ed 2, Butterworth Heinemann, 2009, p. 161.

570. d The cloaca is the common external opening in birds in which the reproductive, digestive, and urinary system all enter before producing excretions from the body. Aspinall V, Cappello M, Introduction to Veterinary Anatomy and Physiology Textbook, ed 2, Butterworth Heinemann, 2009, p. 161.

571. d One ovum is released approximately every 24 hours in female birds during the breeding season until the clutch is complete. Aspinall V, Cappello M, Introduction to Veterinary Anatomy and Physiology Textbook, ed 2, Butterworth Heinemann, 2009, p. 161.

572. b The magnum of the oviduct in birds is the largest and most glandular oviduct. The infundibulum is funnel shaped and catches the ovum when it is released into the oviduct. The isthmus is distal to the magnum and enters the uterus. The cloaca is the external opening, which is where the reproductive tract exits the body. Aspinall V, Cappello M, Introduction to Veterinary Anatomy and Physiology Textbook, ed 2, Butterworth Heinemann, 2009, p. 161.

573. c The majority of the albumen is added to the egg as it travels down the magnum of the oviduct. The first layer of albumen is added in the infundibulum. The cloaca is the external opening to the body, which the reproductive tract enters, and the egg passes thorough before being excreted. The isthmus is where the inner and outer shell membranes are formed. Aspinall V, Cappello M, Introduction to Veterinary Anatomy and Physiology Textbook, ed 2, Butterworth Heinemann, 2009, p. 161.

574. d It takes approximately 15 hours for eggs to calcify in the bird. It takes 5 hours for pigmentation to occur. Aspinall V, Cappello M, Introduction to Veterinary Anatomy and Physiology Textbook, ed 2, Butterworth Heinemann, 2009, p. 161.

575. a The testes are connected to the cloaca via the vas deferens. The magnum and infundibulum are part of the female reproductive tract. The ureters are connected directly to the cloaca in both male and female birds. Aspinall V, Cappello M, Introduction to Veterinary Anatomy and Physiology Textbook, ed 2, Butterworth Heinemann, 2009, p. 162.

576. d The testes in birds are located cranial to the kidneys inside the body cavity and are attached to the body wall. Aspinall V, Cappello M, Introduction to Veterinary Anatomy and Physiology Textbook, ed 2, Butterworth Heinemann, 2009, p. 162.

577. c The spermatozoa of birds are stored in the ductus deferens. Spermatozoa are produced in the seminiferous tubules, pass through the convoluted tubules, are stored in the ductus deferens, and travel to the cloaca by the vas deferens. Aspinall V, Cappello M, Introduction to Veterinary Anatomy and Physiology Textbook, ed 2, Butterworth Heinemann, 2009, p. 162.

578. c During mating the phallus of male birds becomes engorged with lymph fluid. Blood, air, and water do not engorge the phallus. Aspinall V, Cappello M, Introduction to Veterinary Anatomy and Physiology Textbook, ed 2, Butterworth Heinemann, 2009, p. 162.

579. a Rabbits' eyes are set on either side of the head, creating monocular vision to watch for prey and predators. Binocular vision occurs when the eyes are set together in the front of the head. 3D vision occurs in small areas of some animals, such as the horse. Aspinall V, Cappello M, Introduction to Veterinary Anatomy and Physiology Textbook, ed 2, Butterworth Heinemann, 2009, p. 163.

580. b Female rabbits develop a large fold of skin under the chin known as a dewlap. The upper lip is divided by a philtrum that helps when rabbits eat short grass. Crepuscular refers to the fact that the activity of the rabbit is mostly at dawn and at dusk. Aspinall V, Cappello M, Introduction to Veterinary Anatomy and Physiology Textbook, ed 2, Butterworth Heinemann, 2009, p. 163.

581. d The scent glands of rabbits are located under the chin, on either side of the perineum, and at the anus. Aspinall V, Cappello M, Introduction to Veterinary Anatomy and Physiology Textbook, ed 2, Butterworth Heinemann, 2009, p. 163.

582. d The forelegs of rabbits have five toes. The hind feet of rabbits have four toes. Aspinall V, Cappello M, Introduction to Veterinary Anatomy and Physiology Textbook, ed 2, Butterworth Heinemann, 2009, p. 163.

583. a There are 7 cervical vertebrae in rabbits. Dogs have 8 cervical vertebrae. Birds have 13–25 cervical vertebrae. Aspinall V, Cappello M, Introduction to Veterinary Anatomy and Physiology Textbook, ed 2, Butterworth Heinemann, 2009, p. 163.

584. b Rabbits have 12–13 thoracic vertebrae. Rabbits have 7 cervical and lumbar vertebrae and 4 sacral vertebrae. Dogs have 8 cervical vertebrae. Aspinall V, Cappello M, Introduction to Veterinary Anatomy and Physiology Textbook, ed 2, Butterworth Heinemann, 2009, p. 163.

585. d The fibula of rabbits is half the length of tibia and is completely fused together. Aspinall V, Cappello M, Introduction to Veterinary Anatomy and Physiology Textbook, ed 2, Butterworth Heinemann, 2009, p. 163.

586. c The average life span of a rabbit is 6–8 years. The life span of a rat is 3–4 years. The life span of a mouse is 2–3 years. The life span of a chinchilla is 10 years. Aspinall V, Cappello M, Introduction to Veterinary Anatomy and Physiology Textbook, ed 2, Butterworth Heinemann, 2009, p. 164.

587. b The normal body temperature of rabbits is 38.3°C. The normal body temperature of the golden hamster is 36.2–37.5°C. The normal body temperature of dogs is 38.3–39.2°C. Aspinall V, Cappello M, Introduction to Veterinary Anatomy and Physiology Textbook, ed 2, Butterworth Heinemann, 2009, p. 164.

588. a The normal respiratory rate of rabbits is 35–60 breaths/min. The normal respiratory rate of a chinchilla is 40–80 breaths/min. The normal respiratory rate of a mouse is 100–250 breaths/min. The normal respiratory rate of a guinea pig is 90–150 breaths/min. Aspinall V, Cappello M, Introduction to Veterinary Anatomy and Physiology Textbook, ed 2, Butterworth Heinemann, 2009, p. 164.

589. b The average heart rate of rabbits is 220 bpm. The average heart rate of a gerbil is 250–500 bpm. The average heart rate of guinea pigs is 130–190 bpm. The average heart rate of rats is 260–450 bpm. Aspinall V, Cappello M, Introduction to Veterinary Anatomy and Physiology Textbook, ed 2, Butterworth Heinemann, 2009, p. 164.

590. d The average adult weight of rabbits is 1000–8000 g. The average weight of rats is 400–800 g. The average weight of gerbils is 50–60 g. The average weight of golden hamsters is 100 g. Aspinall V, Cappello M, Introduction to Veterinary Anatomy and Physiology Textbook, ed 2, Butterworth Heinemann, 2009, p. 164.

591. a The length of the estrous cycle of rabbits is every 4 days. The estrous cycle of chinchillas is every 30–35 days. The estrous cycle of guinea pigs is 15–16 days. The estrous cycle of gerbils is 4–6 days. Aspinall V, Cappello M, Introduction to Veterinary Anatomy and Physiology Textbook, ed 2, Butterworth Heinemann, 2009, p. 164.

592. a The gestational period of rabbits is 28–32 days. The gestational period for a chinchilla is 111 days. The gestational period for guinea pigs is 63 days. The gestational period for mice is 19–21 days. Aspinall V, Cappello M, Introduction to Veterinary Anatomy and Physiology Textbook, ed 2, Butterworth Heinemann, 2009, p. 164.

593. c The average litter size for rabbits is 2–7 offspring. The average litter size for chinchillas is 2–3. The average litter size for horses is 1–2. The average litter size for mice and rats is 6–12. Aspinall V, Cappello M, Introduction to Veterinary Anatomy and Physiology Textbook, ed 2, Butterworth Heinemann, 2009, p. 164.

594. c The weaning age of rabbits is 4–6 weeks. The weaning age for chinchillas is 6–8 weeks. The weaning age for gerbils, guinea pigs, and hamsters is 3–4 weeks. The weaning age for rats is only 18 days. Aspinall V, Cappello M, Introduction to Veterinary Anatomy and Physiology Textbook, ed 2, Butterworth Heinemann, 2009, p. 164.

595. d The age of sexual maturity for rabbits is 5–8 months. The age of sexual maturity for mice is 3–4 months. The age of sexual maturity for gerbils is 10–12 weeks. The age of sexual maturity for chipmunks is 12 months. Aspinall V, Cappello M, Introduction to Veterinary Anatomy and Physiology Textbook, ed 2, Butterworth Heinemann, 2009, p. 164.

596. d Rabbits do not have canine teeth. Both dogs and cats have four canine teeth. Aspinall V, Cappello M, Introduction to Veterinary Anatomy and Physiology Textbook, ed 2, Butterworth Heinemann, 2009, p. 165.

597. c The premolars of rabbits are also known as cheek teeth. The incisors of rabbits do not have another name. Rabbits do not have canine teeth. The diastema is the space between the incisors and the cheek teeth. Aspinall V, Cappello M, Introduction to Veterinary Anatomy and Physiology Textbook, ed 2, Butterworth Heinemann, 2009, p. 165.

598. c Rabbits are unable to vomit because of the arrangement of the cardia in relation to the stomach. The esophagus is the tubular structure that allows the passage of food from the mouth to the stomach. The pylorus is the sphincter that allows food to pass from the stomach to the small intestine. The duodenum is the first section of small intestine. Aspinall V, Cappello M, Introduction to Veterinary Anatomy and Physiology Textbook, ed 2, Butterworth Heinemann, 2009, p. 166.

599. b The ileum in rabbits terminates at the cecum. The ileocecal tonsil is an arranged network of lymph follicles inside the mucosa. The rectum is distal to the colon. The duodenum is distal to the stomach and proximal to the ileum. Aspinall V, Cappello M, Introduction to Veterinary Anatomy and Physiology Textbook, ed 2, Butterworth Heinemann, 2009, p. 166.

600. c The largest organ in the abdominal cavity of rabbits is the cecum. The liver and spleen are smaller than the cecum in rabbits. The colon is distal to the cecum and is narrow. Aspinall V, Cappello M, Introduction to Veterinary Anatomy and Physiology Textbook, ed 2, Butterworth Heinemann, 2009, p. 166.

601. a Rabbits are not omnivores; they are herbivores. Rabbits are monogastric hindgut fermenters. Omnivores eat food of both plant and animal origin. Herbivores eat food of plant material. Aspinall V, Cappello M, Introduction to Veterinary Anatomy and Physiology Textbook, ed 2, Butterworth Heinemann, 2009, p. 166.

602. b Hard fibrous pellets are produced within 4 hours of eating. Soft pellets are produced within 3–8 hours of eating. Aspinall V, Cappello M, Introduction to Veterinary Anatomy and Physiology Textbook, ed 2, Butterworth Heinemann, 2009, p. 167.

603. d Food material passes through the digestive system of rabbits twice within 24 hours. Aspinall V, Cappello M, Introduction to Veterinary Anatomy and Physiology Textbook, ed 2, Butterworth Heinemann, 2009, p. 167.

604. c Rabbits are an obligate nose breather and when rabbits breathe through their mouth it is a poor prognostic sign. Aspinall V, Cappello M, Introduction to Veterinary Anatomy and Physiology Textbook, ed 2, Butterworth Heinemann, 2009, p. 167.

605. d The nose of a rabbit twitches approximately 20–120 times when it is under general anesthesia. Aspinall V, Cappello M, Introduction to Veterinary Anatomy and Physiology Textbook, ed 2, Butterworth Heinemann, 2009, p. 167.

606. a Rabbits have one medullary pyramid of the kidney that drains into the renal pelvis and ureter. Aspinall V, Cappello M, Introduction to Veterinary Anatomy and Physiology Textbook, ed 2, Butterworth Heinemann, 2009, p. 167.

607. c The testes of rabbits descend at around 12 weeks of age. Testes of dogs usually descend between 8 and 10 weeks of age. Testes of horses descend within 10 days of birth. Aspinall V, Cappello M, Introduction to Veterinary Anatomy and Physiology Textbook, ed 2, Butterworth Heinemann, 2009, p. 167.

608. a The uterus of a rabbit is bicornuate, which means it has two separate uterine horns designed to hold litters of young. A unicornuate uterus contains only one uterine horn. The didelphys uterus contains two separate uterine horns, two separate cervixes, and two different vaginal canals. The septate uterus contains a partition of the uterus by a long septum. Aspinall V, Cappello M, Introduction to Veterinary Anatomy and Physiology Textbook, ed 2, Butterworth Heinemann, 2009, p. 167.

609. d When applied to newborn rabbits, the term *altricial* includes hairless, deaf, and blind, and means they are totally dependent on their mother for a few weeks. Aspinall V, Cappello M, Introduction to Veterinary Anatomy and Physiology Textbook, ed 2, Butterworth Heinemann, 2009, p. 167.

610. c A male guinea pig is known as a boar. A female guinea pig is called a sow. A female rabbit is called a doe and a male rabbit is known as a buck. Aspinall V, Cappello M, Introduction to Veterinary Anatomy and Physiology Textbook, ed 2, Butterworth Heinemann, 2009, p. 172.

611. b The gestational period of guinea pigs is approximately 63 days. The gestational period of chinchillas is 111 days. The gestational period of mice is 19–21 days. The gestational period of rabbits is 28–32 days. Aspinall V, Cappello M, Introduction to Veterinary Anatomy and Physiology Textbook, ed 2, Butterworth Heinemann, 2009, p. 172.

612. b Ferrets' eyes point forward on the head, resulting in binocular vision. Monocular vision would result if the eyes were located on either side of the head. 3D vision is limited to some animals, such as horses. Aspinall V, Cappello M, Introduction to Veterinary Anatomy and Physiology Textbook, ed 2, Butterworth Heinemann, 2009, p. 173.

613. b The main source of a ferret's body odor is from the well-supplied sebaceous glands located all over its body. The fur is thick but does not produce the foul smell of ferrets. The anal glands are also scent glands that secrete a yellow serous secretion with a strong smell; however, the sebaceous glands secrete the most odor. Aspinall V, Cappello M, Introduction to Veterinary Anatomy and Physiology Textbook, ed 2, Butterworth Heinemann, 2009, p. 173.

614. b Ferrets have 15 thoracic vertebrae, 7 cervical vertebrae, 5–6 lumbar vertebrae, and 3 sacral vertebrae. Aspinall V, Cappello M, Introduction to Veterinary Anatomy and Physiology Textbook, ed 2, Butterworth Heinemann, 2009, p. 173.

615. d The coccygeal vertebrae of a ferret are 18 vertebrae located in its tail. The cervical vertebrae are located in the neck region. The thoracic vertebrae are located in the thoracic or chest region. The sacral vertebrae are located in the pelvic region. Aspinall V, Cappello M, Introduction to Veterinary Anatomy and Physiology Textbook, ed 2, Butterworth Heinemann, 2009, p. 173.

616. d The spine of the ferret is flexible and allows the ferret to bend at an angle of at least 180 degrees. Aspinall V, Cappello M, Introduction to Veterinary Anatomy and Physiology Textbook, ed 2, Butterworth Heinemann, 2009, p. 173.

617. a The lumbar vertebra is located distal to the thoracic vertebrae in ferrets. The sacrum, also referred to as the pelvis, and the coccygeal vertebrae are located distal to the lumbar vertebrae. Aspinall V, Cappello M, Introduction to Veterinary Anatomy and Physiology Textbook, ed 2, Butterworth Heinemann, 2009, p. 173.

618. c The average litter size of ferrets is about 8–10; however, a litter of up to 18 has been reported. A litter of fewer than 6 can occur in other animals, such as dogs, cats, etc. Aspinall V, Cappello M, Introduction to Veterinary Anatomy and Physiology Textbook, ed 2, Butterworth Heinemann, 2009, p. 174.

619. c After mating has occurred in ferrets, ovulation occurs within 30–40 hours. Anything before or after that time results in the lack of ovulation. Aspinall V, Cappello M, Introduction to Veterinary Anatomy and Physiology Textbook, ed 2, Butterworth Heinemann, 2009, p. 174.

620. b The average gestational period for ferrets is 42 days. The gestational period for guinea pigs is 63 days. The gestational period for rabbits is 28–32 days. The gestational period for chinchillas is approximately 111 days. Aspinall V, Cappello M, Introduction to Veterinary Anatomy and Physiology Textbook, ed 2, Butterworth Heinemann, 2009, p. 174.

621. b When a ferret is castrated it is referred to as a hobble. A female ferret is referred to as a jill. A male ferret is referred to as a hob. A castrated male horse is referred to as a gelding. Aspinall V, Cappello M, Introduction to Veterinary Anatomy and Physiology Textbook, ed 2, Butterworth Heinemann, 2009, p. 174.

622. b The lungs of a tortoise are located on the dorsal side below the carapace and above all of the internal organs. The ventral surface contains the heart and intestines. The liver, spleen, and intestines are caudal to the stomach. Caudal to the heart is a portion of the stomach, pancreas, and intestines. Aspinall V, Cappello M, Introduction to Veterinary Anatomy and Physiology Textbook, ed 2, Butterworth Heinemann, 2009, p. 178.

623. c The testes of a male tortoise are located adjacent to the kidneys. The stomach is cranial to the testes and located alongside the liver and small intestines. The urinary bladder is located on the ventral side above the pelvic bone. The liver is cranial to the testes and is located next to the stomach and lungs. Aspinall V, Cappello M, Introduction to Veterinary Anatomy and Physiology Textbook, ed 2, Butterworth Heinemann, 2009, p. 180.

624. d The zygomatic bones, pterygoid bones, and vomer bones are all part of the face of small animals. The sphenoid bone is a bone of the cranium. Colville TP, Bassert JM, Clinical Anatomy and Physiology for Veterinary Technicians, ed 3, Mosby, 2016, p. 187.

625. a The incus, malleus, and stapes are all bones in the ear. The bones of the face include incisive, lacrimal, mandible, maxillary, nasal, zygomatic, palatine, pterygoid, turbinates, and vomer bones. The foot includes the phalanx bones. Bones of the cranium include the frontal, interparietal, occipital, parietal, temporal, ethmoid, and sphenoid bones. Colville TP, Bassert JM, Clinical Anatomy and Physiology for Veterinary Technicians, ed 3, Mosby, 2016, p. 187.

626. b The most caudal bone of the skull is the occipital bone. The parietal bones are on the dorsolateral walls. The interparietal bone is located on the dorsal midline. The temporal bone is located ventral to the parietal bones. Colville TP, Bassert JM, Clinical Anatomy and Physiology for Veterinary Technicians, ed 3, Mosby, 2016, p. 180.

627. c The spinal cord exits through the foramen magnum on the occipital bone. On either side of the foramen magnum are the occipital condyles that are articular surfaces, which join the first cervical vertebrae (known as the atlas). The temporal bones are located ventral to the parietal bones. Colville TP, Bassert JM, Clinical Anatomy and Physiology for Veterinary Technicians, ed 3, Mosby, 2016, p. 180.

628. b The calcaneus of dogs is also referred to as the point of hock. The manubrium is the cranial end of the sternum. The olecranon is also referred to as the point of elbow. Colville TP, Bassert JM, Clinical Anatomy and Physiology for Veterinary Technicians, ed 3, Mosby, 2016, p. 202.

629. e Cattle and sheep are the only animals that have an os cordis, which is a bone in the heart that helps to support the valves of the heart. Colville TP, Bassert JM, Clinical Anatomy and Physiology for Veterinary Technicians, ed 3, Mosby, 2016, p. 203.

630. c The tibia and fibula are located immediately proximal to the tarsal bones. The metatarsal bones are distal to the tarsal bones. The metacarpal bones are located in the forelimb. The olecranon is in the forelimb and is the point of the elbow. Colville TP, Bassert JM, Clinical Anatomy and Physiology for Veterinary Technicians, ed 3, Mosby, 2016, p. 202.

631. b The sacrum is cranial to the coccygeal. The ligamentum nuchae is between the axis and first thoracic vertebra. The lumbar vertebra is cranial to the sacrum. The atlas is the first cervical vertebra connected to the base of the skull. Colville TP, Bassert JM, Clinical Anatomy and Physiology for Veterinary Technicians, ed 3, Mosby, 2016, p. 199.

632. b The mental foramen is an opening located on the mandible bone. The foramen magnum is located on the occipital bone. The external acoustic meatus is located on the tympanic bulla. The nasal passages are located below the nasal bone. Colville TP, Bassert JM, Clinical Anatomy and Physiology for Veterinary Technicians, ed 3, Mosby, 2016, p. 187.

633. c The incisive bone is located on the rostral surface of the cranium. The caudal end of the cranium includes the occipital bone. The interparietal bone is located on the caudal end above the occipital bone. The lacrimal bones are located in the medial portion of the orbit. Colville TP, Bassert JM, Clinical Anatomy and Physiology for Veterinary Technicians, ed 3, Mosby, 2016, p. 187.

634. a The lacrimal space within the lacrimal bones houses the lacrimal sac, which is the tear drainage system of the eye. The maxillary sinuses are part of the maxillary bone. The maxillary bones form the hard palate. The nasal bone forms the dorsal side of the nasal cavity. Colville TP, Bassert JM, Clinical Anatomy and Physiology for Veterinary Technicians, ed 3, Mosby, 2016, p. 187.

635. c The zygomatic bones are also referred to as the malar bones. The premaxillary bones are also known as the incisive bones. The maxillary bones form the hard palate. The cochlea is part of the inner ear. Colville TP, Bassert JM, Clinical Anatomy and Physiology for Veterinary Technicians, ed 3, Mosby, 2016, p. 187.

636. b The shaft of the mandible is the horizontal portion that houses all the teeth. The ramus of the mandible is the caudal end and vertical portion. The palate is known as the hard palate and is formed by the maxillary bones. The malar bone is also known as the zygomatic bone. Colville TP, Bassert JM, Clinical Anatomy and

Physiology for Veterinary Technicians, ed 3, Mosby, 2016, p. 187.

637. d The vomer, palatine, and pterygoid bones are all part of the inner face of small animals. Colville TP, Bassert JM, Clinical Anatomy and Physiology for Veterinary Technicians, ed 3, Mosby, 2016, p. 188.

638. a The two pterygoid bones support the lateral wall of the pharynx. The mandibular symphysis is the cartilaginous joint that joins each mandible. The nasal septum is the central wall between the right and left nasal passages. The nasal conchae are four thin bones that fill most of the space in the nasal cavity. Colville TP, Bassert JM, Clinical Anatomy and Physiology for Veterinary Technicians, ed 3, Mosby, 2016, p. 188.

639. a Horses have five sacral vertebrae. Dogs and cats have three sacral vertebrae. Pigs have four sacral vertebrae. Colville TP, Bassert JM, Clinical Anatomy and Physiology for Veterinary Technicians, ed 3, Mosby, 2016, p. 188.

640. b Cats have approximately 7 cervical vertebrae, 3 sacral vertebrae, 13 thoracic vertebrae, and 5–23 coccygeal vertebrae. Colville TP, Bassert JM, Clinical Anatomy and Physiology for Veterinary Technicians, ed 3, Mosby, 2016, p. 188.

641. c The bodies of adjacent vertebrae are separated by intervertebral disks. The spinal canal is located within the vertebral foramen and houses the spinal cord. The articular process is located on the cranial and caudal ends of the vertebral arches and helps form the joints between adjacent vertebrae. The ligamentum nuchae is the ligament located between the cervical axis and the first thoracic vertebrae. Colville TP, Bassert JM, Clinical Anatomy and Physiology for Veterinary Technicians, ed 3, Mosby, 2016, p. 188.

642. a The junction between the bone and the cartilage of ribs is referred to as the costochondral junction. The xiphoid process is the caudal end of the sternum. The asternal ribs join the adjacent costal cartilage and make up the caudal part of the thorax. The manubrium is the cranial end of the sternum. Colville TP, Bassert JM, Clinical Anatomy and Physiology for Veterinary Technicians, ed 3, Mosby, 2016, p. 192.

643. c The most proximal bone of the thoracic limb is the scapula. The ulna is distal to the humerus. The humerus is also known as the brachium and is distal to the scapula. Colville TP, Bassert JM, Clinical Anatomy and Physiology for Veterinary Technicians, ed 3, Mosby, 2016, p. 193.

644. e Organic molecules are molecules that contain carbon and are divided into four groups: carbohydrates, lipids, proteins, and nucleic acids. Colville TP, Bassert JM, Clinical Anatomy and Physiology for Veterinary Technicians, ed 3, Mosby, 2016, p. 306.

645. b Steroids, triglycerides, and prostaglandins are all lipids. Glycogen is a carbohydrate. Colville TP, Bassert JM, Clinical Anatomy and Physiology for Veterinary Technicians, ed 3, Mosby, 2016, p. 34.

646. c A sugar that contains five carbons is referred to as a pentose sugar. A monosaccharide is known as a simple sugar. A hexose sugar contains six carbon atoms. A disaccharide is a sugar composed of two monosaccharides. Colville TP, Bassert JM, Clinical Anatomy and Physiology for Veterinary Technicians, ed 3, Mosby, 2016, p. 31.

647. a The nucleus is the part of the cell that contains and processes genetic information and controls cell metabolism. The cell membrane is the boundary between extracellular and intracellular compartments. The cilia are fine hair-like structures on the surface of cells that provide a rhythmic beating that propels mucus and debris across the luminal surface of cells. The chromatin regulates protein synthesis and other molecular interactions. Colville TP, Bassert JM, Clinical Anatomy and Physiology for Veterinary Technicians, ed 3, Mosby, 2016, p. 46.

648. c The organelle lysosome is responsible for the digestion of absorbed material. Peroxisomes detoxify various molecules such as alcohol and formaldehyde and remove free radicals. Ribosomes are the site of protein synthesis. The mitochondria are the site of adenosine triphosphate production from respiration. Colville TP, Bassert JM, Clinical Anatomy and Physiology for Veterinary Technicians, ed 3, Mosby, 2016, p. 65.

649. a Flagella are long structures that propel cells through fluid. Cilia move fluid across cell surfaces. Both cilia and flagella originate from a pair of centrioles called basal bodies, which are located at the periphery of the cell under the plasma membrane. Colville TP, Bassert JM, Clinical Anatomy and Physiology for Veterinary Technicians, ed 3, Mosby, 2016, p. 58.

650. b The fluid inside the cell is referred to as cytosol. The cytoplasm is the inner substance of the cell. The cytoskeleton is the three-dimensional frame for the cell. The tubulins are spherical molecules that make up microtubules. Colville TP, Bassert JM, Clinical Anatomy and Physiology for Veterinary Technicians, ed 3, Mosby, 2016, p. 60.

651. d Glucose that is not immediately used by cells is converted to glycogen and is stored in the liver. The gallbladder stores bile produced by the liver. The pancreas produces hormones and pancreatic enzymes for secretions. The spleen stores blood cells. Colville TP, Bassert JM, Clinical Anatomy and Physiology for Veterinary Technicians, ed 3, Mosby, 2016, p. 408.

652. b The term *ectothermic* refers to cold-blooded animals such as amphibians and reptiles. The term *endothermic* refers to warm-blooded animals. Behavioral thermoregulation refers to the self-regulation of body temperatures according to metabolic need. Colville TP, Bassert JM, Clinical Anatomy and Physiology for Veterinary Technicians, ed 3, Mosby, 2016, p. 542.

653. b The term *ecdysis* refers to the shedding of the skin of reptiles. The term *ectothermic* refers to being cold-blooded. The term *hibernation* is also known as brumation and is a state of inactivity and metabolic depression. The term *nocturnal* refers to being active at night. Colville TP, Bassert JM, Clinical Anatomy and Physiology for Veterinary Technicians, ed 3, Mosby, 2016, p. 544.

654. b Isometric contraction is tension generated in the muscle or when muscle tone increases but the muscle does not shorten. Isotonic contraction is when the muscle actually moves or shortens. Muscle tone is the muscle being in a slight state of tension. Aspinall V,

Cappello M, Introduction to Veterinary Anatomy and Physiology Textbook, ed 2, Butterworth Heinemann, 2009, p. 45.

655. c The digastricus muscle is located on the caudoventral surface of the mandible and is responsible for opening the jaw. The temporalis muscle closes the jaw. The masseter muscle closes the jaw. The dorsal rectus muscle is part of the extrinsic muscle of the eye. Aspinall V, Cappello M, Introduction to Veterinary Anatomy and Physiology Textbook, ed 2, Butterworth Heinemann, 2009, p. 47.

656. c The medial and lateral pterygoids are responsible for side-to-side movements of the mouth. The masseter muscle closes the jaw. The temporalis muscle also closes the jaw. The digastricus muscle opens the jaw. Aspinall V, Cappello M, Introduction to Veterinary Anatomy and Physiology Textbook, ed 2, Butterworth Heinemann, 2009, p. 47.

657. c The tone in the muscles of the jaw is responsible for closure and is what keeps the mouth closed when it is not in use. The shape and length of the muscle does not aid in involuntary closure. Atrophy refers to the loss of muscle mass. Aspinall V, Cappello M, Introduction to Veterinary Anatomy and Physiology Textbook, ed 2, Butterworth Heinemann, 2009, p. 47.

658. b The masseter muscle originates at the zygomatic arch and inserts on the masseteric fossa on the lateral surface of the mandible. The temporalis muscle fills the temporal fossa of the skull and inserts on the coronoid process of the mandible. The digastricus muscle originates at the jugular process of the occipital bone and inserts on the angle and ventral surface of the mandible. The medial and lateral pterygoids are deep muscles that lie medial to the mandible. Aspinall V, Cappello M, Introduction to Veterinary Anatomy and Physiology Textbook, ed 2, Butterworth Heinemann, 2009, p. 47.

659. d There are four extrinsic muscles of the eye that are responsible for movement of the eye within the socket. The four muscles are dorsal rectus, ventral rectus, medial rectus, and lateral rectus. Aspinall V, Cappello M, Introduction to Veterinary Anatomy and Physiology Textbook, ed 2, Butterworth Heinemann, 2009, p. 47.

660. d The dorsal oblique and the ventral oblique muscles are responsible for rotating the eye about its visual axis. The dorsal rectus muscle aids in the movement of the eye upward. Aspinall V, Cappello M, Introduction to Veterinary Anatomy and Physiology Textbook, ed 2, Butterworth Heinemann, 2009, p. 47.

661. d The retractor bulbi muscle pulls the eye deeper in the socket. The dorsal rectus muscle moves the eye upward. The ventral rectus muscle moves the eye downward. The lateral rectus turns the eye outward. Aspinall V, Cappello M, Introduction to Veterinary Anatomy and Physiology Textbook, ed 2, Butterworth Heinemann, 2009, p. 48.

662. a The epaxial muscles lie dorsal to the transverse process of the vertebrae. The hypaxial muscles lie ventral to the transverse process of the vertebrae. The diaphragm lies between the thoracic and abdominal cavity. The rectus abdominis muscle lies on each side of the linea alba. Aspinall V, Cappello M, Introduction to Veterinary Anatomy and Physiology Textbook, ed 2, Butterworth Heinemann, 2009, p. 48.

663. b The external intercostal muscles originate from the caudal border of one rib and insert on the cranial border of the rib behind it. The internal intercostals lie below the external intercostal within the intercostal spaces. The external abdominal oblique muscles originate from the lateral surfaces of the ribs and lumbar fascia. The internal abdominal oblique muscle is the intermediate muscle of the lateral abdominal wall and terminates in an aponeurosis on the linea alba. Aspinall V, Cappello M, Introduction to Veterinary Anatomy and Physiology Textbook, ed 2, Butterworth Heinemann, 2009, p. 48.

664. d The aortic hiatus allows the passage of the aorta, thoracic duct, and azygous vein from the thorax to the abdominal cavity. The vagal nerve passes through the esophageal hiatus. Aspinall V, Cappello M, Introduction to Veterinary Anatomy and Physiology Textbook, ed 2, Butterworth Heinemann, 2009, p. 48.

665. b The caval foramen is the opening that lies within the central tendon and transmits the caudal vena cava. The aortic hiatus allows passage of the aorta, azygous vein, and thoracic duct. The esophageal hiatus allows passage of the esophagus and the vagal nerve. The foramen magnum is where the spinal cord originates and passes through the occipital bone. Aspinall V, Cappello M, Introduction to Veterinary Anatomy and Physiology Textbook, ed 2, Butterworth Heinemann, 2009, p. 48.

666. b The trapezius muscle originates from the dorsal midline from C2 to C7 and inserts on the spine of the scapula. The pectoralis muscle runs from the ribs and sternum and inserts on the humerus. The latissimus dorsi originates on the thoracic spine and inserts on the humerus. The brachiocephalicus runs from the base of the skull to an insertion on the cranial aspect of the humerus. Aspinall V, Cappello M, Introduction to Veterinary Anatomy and Physiology Textbook, ed 2, Butterworth Heinemann, 2009, p. 49.

667. c The latissimus dorsi is responsible for retracting the forelimb of dogs. The pectoralis adducts the limb and holds the forelimb against the body wall. The trapezius draws the leg forward and protracts the limb. The supraspinatus muscle extends and stabilizes the shoulder. Aspinall V, Cappello M, Introduction to Veterinary Anatomy and Physiology Textbook, ed 2, Butterworth Heinemann, 2009, p. 49.

668. b The infraspinatus muscle helps to stabilize and flex the shoulder joint. The supraspinatus extends the shoulder and stabilizes the shoulder joint. The triceps brachii extends the elbow joint. The biceps brachii flexes the elbow joint. Aspinall V, Cappello M, Introduction to Veterinary Anatomy and Physiology Textbook, ed 2, Butterworth Heinemann, 2009, p. 50.

669. b The gluteal muscles extend the hip joint and abduct the thigh. The sartorius muscles adduct the hind limb. The quadriceps femoris extends the stifle joint. The gastrocnemius extends the hock and flexes the stifle. Aspinall V, Cappello M, Introduction to Veterinary Anatomy and Physiology Textbook, ed 2, Butterworth Heinemann, 2009, p. 51.

670. c The semimembranosus muscle is the most medial muscle of the hamstring and runs from the pelvis to the femur and tibia. The semitendinosus runs from the pelvis and inserts on the tibia and calcaneus. The gastrocnemius muscle originates from the caudal aspect of the femur and inserts on the calcaneus of the hock. The quadriceps femoris runs down the cranial aspect of the thigh. Aspinall V, Cappello M, Introduction to Veterinary Anatomy and Physiology Textbook, ed 2, Butterworth Heinemann, 2009, p. 51.

671. b The anterior tibialis muscle flexes the hock and rotates the paw medially. The gastrocnemius extends the hock and flexes the stifle. The pectineus muscle adducts the hind limb. The gracilis muscle adducts the hind limb. Aspinall V, Cappello M, Introduction to Veterinary Anatomy and Physiology Textbook, ed 2, Butterworth Heinemann, 2009, p. 51.

672. d The biceps femoris, quadriceps femoris, and semitendinosus are all muscles of the hind limb. The biceps brachii is a muscle of the forelimb. Aspinall V, Cappello M, Introduction to Veterinary Anatomy and Physiology Textbook, ed 2, Butterworth Heinemann, 2009, p. 50.

673. b The epicondyle is a projection of bone on the lateral edge above its condyle. The foramen is an opening or passage into or through a bone. The head of the bone is the end of a long bone. The periosteum is the outer covering of bones. Aspinall V, Cappello M, Introduction to Veterinary Anatomy and Physiology Textbook, ed 2, Butterworth Heinemann, 2009, p. 31.

674. c The tuberosities are the protuberances on bones that are used for the attachment of muscles. The fossa is a hollow or depressed area on a bone. The tendon connects muscle to bone. The shaft is the longest portion of long bones. Aspinall V, Cappello M, Introduction to Veterinary Anatomy and Physiology Textbook, ed 2, Butterworth Heinemann, 2009, p. 31.

675. c The trochlea are bony structures through or which tendons pass and they allow tendons to act as pulleys. The fossa is a hollow or depressed area on a bone. Ligaments connect one bone to another bone. The epicondyle is a projection of bone on the lateral edge above its condyle. Aspinall V, Cappello M, Introduction to Veterinary Anatomy and Physiology Textbook, ed 2, Butterworth Heinemann, 2009, p. 31.

676. c The mesaticephalic head is the normal or average-shaped head in dogs such as a beagle. Boxers and bulldogs are examples of dogs with a brachycephalic head in which the cranium is rounded and the nose is short. Greyhounds have a dolichocephalic head in which the nose is long and narrow. Aspinall V, Cappello M, Introduction to Veterinary Anatomy and Physiology Textbook, ed 2, Butterworth Heinemann, 2009, p. 34.

677. a The pulmonary artery carries deoxygenated blood to the lungs. The carotid artery carries blood toward the head. The subclavian artery carries blood to the forelimbs. The renal artery carries blood to the kidneys. Aspinall V, Cappello M, Introduction to Veterinary Anatomy and Physiology Textbook, ed 2, Butterworth Heinemann, 2009, p. 83.

678. b The azygous vein drains venous blood from the thoracic body wall. The jugular vein drains blood from the head. The iliac vein drains blood from the hind limbs. The hepatic veins drain blood from the liver. Aspinall V, Cappello M, Introduction to Veterinary Anatomy and Physiology Textbook, ed 2, Butterworth Heinemann, 2009, p. 84.

679. c The portal veins receive blood from the digestive tract such as the stomach, intestines, and pancreas. The hepatic veins drain the liver. The hepatic arteries supply the liver with blood. The iliac veins drain the hind limbs of blood. Aspinall V, Cappello M, Introduction to Veterinary Anatomy and Physiology Textbook, ed 2, Butterworth Heinemann, 2009, p. 84.

680. d The celiac artery branches off the aorta and supplies the stomach, spleen, and liver with blood. The renal artery supplies the kidneys with blood. The portal vein supplies the liver with blood from the digestive tract. The hepatic veins drain the liver. Aspinall V, Cappello M, Introduction to Veterinary Anatomy and Physiology Textbook, ed 2, Butterworth Heinemann, 2009, p. 84.

681. b The cranial mesenteric artery supplies the small intestines with blood. The caudal mesenteric arteries supply the large intestines with blood. The celiac artery supplies the stomach, spleen, and liver with blood. The femoral artery supplies the hind limb with blood. Aspinall V, Cappello M, Introduction to Veterinary Anatomy and Physiology Textbook, ed 2, Butterworth Heinemann, 2009, p. 84.

682. a The caudal vena cava returns deoxygenated blood from the pelvic region, hind limbs, and abdominal viscera. The aorta is the main blood vessel that has multiple branches supplying organs with blood. The iliac veins are located in the groin and drain blood to the vena cava from the hind limbs. The pulmonary vein supplies the heart with oxygenated blood. Aspinall V, Cappello M, Introduction to Veterinary Anatomy and Physiology Textbook, ed 2, Butterworth Heinemann, 2009, p. 84.

683. b The smallest veins are called venules. Capillaries are the smallest arteries. Iliacs are the veins in the groin that drain the hind limbs. The term *vessel* refers to a tubular structure that carries a substance throughout the body. Aspinall V, Cappello M, Introduction to Veterinary Anatomy and Physiology Textbook, ed 2, Butterworth Heinemann, 2009, p. 84.

684. b Capillaries are present in all organs/tissues and are the sites of exchange between blood and tissue fluid. Venules are the smallest veins that drain blood from tissues. Valves are found within veins, not arteries, and help to propel blood toward the heart. Lymph fluid circulates throughout the body by means of the lymphatic system. Aspinall V, Cappello M, Introduction to Veterinary Anatomy and Physiology Textbook, ed 2, Butterworth Heinemann, 2009, p. 85.

685. a The ductus venosus is a venous shunt within the liver that connects the umbilical vein to the caudal vena cava. The ligamentum arteriosus is the remnant of the ductus arteriosus that closes shortly after birth. The foramen ovale is an opening in the septum between the right and left atria and ventricles. The ductus arteriosus is a vessel that forms a connection between the pulmonary artery and the aorta. Aspinall V,

Cappello M, Introduction to Veterinary Anatomy and Physiology Textbook, ed 2, Butterworth Heinemann, 2009, p. 85.

686. c Blood leaves the right ventricle to enter the cranial vena cava to travel onto the pulmonary artery. Blood leaves the left ventricle to enter the aorta. Blood does not cross over from the right to the left atrium. The caudal vena cava carries blood from the caudal end of the body toward the right atrium. Aspinall V, Cappello M, Introduction to Veterinary Anatomy and Physiology Textbook, ed 2, Butterworth Heinemann, 2009, p. 85.

687. b Blood leaves the lungs via the pulmonary veins and enters the left atrium of the heart. The left atrium opens into the left ventricle where blood then leaves the heart toward the aorta. Blood enters the right atrium via the caudal vena cava. Blood leaves the right atrium to enter the cranial vena cava. Aspinall V, Cappello M, Introduction to Veterinary Anatomy and Physiology Textbook, ed 2, Butterworth Heinemann, 2009, p. 85.

688. d The spleen is the largest lymphoid organ. The liver does not produce lymph fluid. The cisterna chyli is the main lymphatic duct of the abdomen, receiving lymph from the abdomen, pelvis, and hind limbs. The lymph nodes are masses of lymphoid tissue situated in intervals along the lymphatic vessels. Aspinall V, Cappello M, Introduction to Veterinary Anatomy and Physiology Textbook, ed 2, Butterworth Heinemann, 2009, p. 86.

689. a Dehydration can be detected in a patient through a packed cell volume (PCV). Dehydration results in polycythemia and hemoconcentration; therefore, there would be an increase in both the hematocrit and PCV. Colville TP, Bassert JM, Clinical Anatomy and Physiology for Veterinary Technicians, ed 3, Mosby, 2016, p. 300.

690. a The larynx, also known as the voice box, is a short irregular tube of cartilage and muscles that connect the pharynx with the trachea. The epiglottis is a flap of cartilage that acts as a trap door to cover the opening of the larynx during swallowing. The bronchi branch off the trachea into each lung and then they branch into smaller air passageways that lead to the alveoli. The esophagus is a long tube-like structure that carries food from the mouth to the stomach. Colville TP, Bassert JM, Clinical Anatomy and Physiology for Veterinary Technicians, ed 3, Mosby, 2016, p. 363.

691. b The ribosomes are the site of protein synthesis. The Golgi apparatus is responsible for packaging and altering substances for secretion or internal use. The endoplasmic reticulum is responsible for transport and storage of materials in the cell. The mitochondria are the site of adenosine triphosphate production from respiration. Colville TP, Bassert JM, Clinical Anatomy and Physiology for Veterinary Technicians, ed 3, Mosby, 2016, p. 63.

692. b The linea alba extends along the ventral midline from the xiphoid process of the sternum to the pubic symphysis. The spinal cord extends from the base of the skull to the pelvic region along the spinal column on the dorsal surface. The diaphragm is the muscular structure that separates the thoracic and abdominal cavity. The transversus abdominis is a lateral abdominal muscle that terminates on the linea alba. Aspinall V, Cappello M, Introduction to Veterinary Anatomy and Physiology Textbook, ed 2, Butterworth Heinemann, 2009, p. 49.

693. d The gracilis muscle forms the caudal half of the medial surface of the thigh. The sartorius inserts on the cranial border of the tibia with the gracilis muscle. The semitendinosus muscle runs from the pelvis and inserts on the tibia and calcaneus. The biceps femoris originates from the pelvis and runs over the femur to the tibia and inserts on the calcaneus of the hock. Aspinall V, Cappello M, Introduction to Veterinary Anatomy and Physiology Textbook, ed 2, Butterworth Heinemann, 2009, p. 51.

694. d The three types of cells that make up bone are osteoblasts, osteocytes, and osteoclasts. Osteoblasts are the cells that form bone. Colville TP, Bassert JM, Clinical Anatomy and Physiology for Veterinary Technicians, ed 3, Mosby, 2016, p. 173.

695. a The bones of the skeleton can be conveniently divided into two main groups: the bones of the head and trunk and the bones of the limbs. Because the bones of the head and trunk are located along the central axis of the body, they are referred to as the axial skeleton. The limbs are appendages of the trunk and their bones are collectively called the appendicular skeleton. Some animals may have a third category of bones called the visceral skeleton. These are bones formed in the viscera or soft organs. The metacarpal bones extend distally from the distal row of carpal bones to the proximal phalanges of the digits. Colville TP, Bassert JM, Clinical Anatomy and Physiology for Veterinary Technicians, ed 3, Mosby, 2016, p. 180.

696. a The ethmoid bone is an internal bone of the cranium located just rostral to the sphenoid bone. The temperal bones form the lateral walls of the cranium. The incisive bone is the most rostral skull bone. The parietal bones form the dorsolateral walls of the cranium. Colville TP, Bassert JM, Clinical Anatomy and Physiology for Veterinary Technicians, ed 3, Mosby, 2016, p. 182.

697. d The lacrimal bones are two small bones that form part of the medial portion of the orbit of the eye. The three tiny but very important pairs of ear bones are hidden away in the middle ear. Known as the ossicles, these bones are–starting from the outside–the malleus or hammer, the incus or anvil, and the stapes or stirrup. Colville TP, Bassert JM, Clinical Anatomy and Physiology for Veterinary Technicians, ed 3, Mosby, 2016, p. 187.

698. d The anconeal process is a beak-shaped process located at the proximal end of the trochlear notch. The antebrachium is the two bones of the forearm. The olecranon process forms the point of the elbow. The styloid process is located at the distal end of the ulna. Colville TP, Bassert JM, Clinical Anatomy and Physiology for Veterinary Technicians, ed 3, Mosby, 2016, p. 194.

699. c The turbinates are also called the nasal conchae. They are four, thin, scroll-like bones that fill most of the space in the nasal cavity. Each side has a dorsal and a ventral turbinate. The moist, very vascular soft-tissue lining of the nasal passages covers the turbinates. The scroll-like shape of the turbinates forces air inhaled through the nose around many twists and turns as it passes through the nasal cavity. This helps warm and humidify the air and also helps trap any tiny particles of inhaled foreign material in the moist surface of the nasal epithelium. This process helps condition the inhaled air before it reaches the delicate lungs. The two palatine bones make up the caudal portion of the hard palate (the bony part of the roof of the mouth), which separates the mouth from the nasal cavity. The rest of the hard palate (the rostral portion) is made up of part of the maxillary bones. The two small pterygoid bones support part of the lateral walls of the pharynx (throat). The single vomer bone is located on the midline of the skull and forms part of the nasal septum, which is the central "wall" between the left and right nasal passages. Colville TP, Bassert JM, Clinical Anatomy and Physiology for Veterinary Technicians, ed 3, Mosby, 2016, p. 188.

700. b The ribs that join the adjacent costal cartilage are called asternal ribs and they make up the caudal part of the thorax. Each rib has two parts: a dorsal part made of bone and a ventral part made of cartilage. The term for rib is *costal*, and the cartilaginous part is therefore called the costal cartilage and its junction with the bony part is called the *costochondral junction*. The costal cartilages either join the sternum directly or join the costal cartilage ahead of them. The ribs whose cartilages join the sternum are called the sternal ribs and they make up the cranial part of the thorax. The cartilages of the last ribs, two on each side, may not join anything at all; they may just end in the muscles of the thoracic wall. These unattached ribs are called floating ribs. Colville TP, Bassert JM, Clinical Anatomy and Physiology for Veterinary Technicians, ed 3, Mosby, 2016, p. 192.

SECTION 2

1. c A credentialed veterinary technician is allowed to perform certain duties under the direct supervision of a licensed veterinarian who is on the premises and is readily available. An office manager, lead veterinary technician, and/or practice owner do not provide supervision of medical-related activities for credentialed veterinary technicians, as outlined by state veterinary practice acts. Prendergast H, Front Office Management for the Veterinary Team, ed 3, Saunders, 2020, p. 5.

2. a A licensed veterinarian is the only health care team member who is allowed to diagnose, prescribe medication, and perform surgery. An office manager does not hold the proper credentials to perform these duties. A credentialed veterinary technician and a veterinary technologist are allowed to perform certain duties under the direct supervision of a licensed veterinarian but are not allowed to diagnose, to prescribe medication, or to perform surgery. Prendergast H, Front Office Management for the Veterinary Team, ed 3, Saunders, 2020, p. 9.

3. d Of the tasks listed, a veterinary assistant is responsible for maintaining legible and accurate medical records. A credentialed veterinary technician or technologist is responsible for performing dental prophylaxis and calculating drug dosages. A licensed veterinarian is responsible for performing surgical procedures. Prendergast H, Front Office Management for the Veterinary Team, ed 3, Saunders, 2020, p. 4.

4. b The term *petty cash* refers to cash that is set aside in the practice to purchase items needed for business when a check is not available. Change that is owed back to a client on a bill is the difference of the bill owed and what was paid to the practice. The cash balance in the drawer at the start and end of every day is the cash flow available to receive cash and to provide change back as needed. Prendergast H, Front Office Management for the Veterinary Team, ed 3, Saunders, 2020, p. 54.

5. b The human voice contains four different components: volume, tone, rate, and quality. Prendergast H, Front Office Management for the Veterinary Team, ed 3, Saunders, 2020, p. 36.

6. b The mission is defined as the purpose of the hospital; it is the fundamental reason that the practice exists. The vision statement is the desired future of the practice. The core values are the guiding principles that are not to be compromised during change. Prendergast H, Front Office Management for the Veterinary Team, ed 3, Saunders, 2020, p. 15.

7. d Characteristics of effective leaders include the following: self-confident, team player, innovator, effective communicator, effective listener, sincere, problem solver, and many more. Prendergast H, Front Office Management for the Veterinary Team, ed 3, Saunders, 2020, p. 16.

8. d All of the following are methods that can be used to decrease loss: implement internal controls to prevent employee theft, use travel sheets to decrease missed charges, manage inventory appropriately, implement electronic medical records, and set appropriate fees. Prendergast H, Front Office Management for the Veterinary Team, ed 3, Saunders, 2020, p. 30.

9. c To avoid loss of interest and to maximize the value of time spent, staff meetings should not last longer than 45 minutes (unless training information is included). Prendergast H, Front Office Management for the Veterinary Team, ed 3, Saunders, 2020, p. 25.

10. b There are four branches of veterinary ethics: descriptive, official, administrative, and normative. Prendergast H, Front Office Management for the Veterinary Team, ed 3, Saunders, 2020, p. 143.

11. a Descriptive ethics refers to the study of ethical views of veterinarians and veterinary professionals regarding their behavior and attitudes. Official veterinary ethics refers to the creation of the official ethical standards adopted by organizations of professionals and imposed on their members. Normative ethics refers to the search for correct principles of good and bad, right and wrong, justice or injustice. Administrative ethics involves the actions by administrative government bodies that regulate veterinary practice and activities in which veterinarians engage. Prendergast H, Front Office Management for the Veterinary Team, ed 3, Saunders, 2020, p. 143.

12. b A law generally consists of established rules, statutes, and administrative agency rules that can be enforced to establish limits of conduct for governments and individuals in society. It is divided into two categories: civil and criminal. Prendergast H, Front Office Management for the Veterinary Team, ed 3, Saunders, 2020, p. 147.
13. a A noncompete agreement falls under the division of the civil law. A civil law relates to the duties between people and the government. A contract law deals with duties established by individuals as a result of contractual agreement. A criminal law deals with the unlawful activity against a member of the public and is prosecuted by a public official. Prendergast H, Front Office Management for the Veterinary Team, ed 3, Saunders, 2020, p. 148.
14. b Animal abuse falls under the division of a criminal law. A crime is an unlawful activity against a member of the public and is prosecuted by a public official. A civil law relates to the duties between people and the government. Prendergast H, Front Office Management for the Veterinary Team, ed 3, Saunders, 2020, p. 148.
15. c Negligence is the performance of an act that a reasonable person under the same circumstance would not perform. A tort is a civil offense to an opposing party in which harm has occurred. An intentional tort is defined as an intentional action that has taken place in which harm has occurred to another member of society. A crime is an unlawful activity against a member of the public that is prosecuted by a public official. Prendergast H, Front Office Management for the Veterinary Team, ed 3, Saunders, 2020, p. 150.
16. c Lawsuits against veterinarians are almost always based on neglect versus breach of contract, defamation, or breach of warranty. Negligence is defined as performing an act that a person of ordinary prudence would not have done under similar circumstances. Prendergast H, Front Office Management for the Veterinary Team, ed 3, Saunders, 2020, p. 150.
17. e Acts of malpractice include the following: incorrect drug administration, incorrect strength of drug administration, failure to clean animals that have defecated and/or urinated on themselves, abandonment, leaving foreign objects in a patient after surgery, failure to exercise good judgment, failure to communicate, loss or damage to patients' personal property, disease transmission, a patient attacking another while in the veterinary practice, use of defective equipment or medication. Prendergast H, Front Office Management for the Veterinary Team, ed 3, Saunders, 2020, p. 148.
18. c When a mistake is written in the medical record, a single line should be drawn through the mistake, should be initialed, and then the correction should be written legibly. Erasing, using white-out, or scratching out the mistake should not be done because these could all be considered as altering the medical record. Prendergast H, Front Office Management for the Veterinary Team, ed 3, Saunders, 2020, p. 152.
19. b The Fair Labor and Standards Act was created to establish minimum wage and overtime pay standards as well as to regulate the employment of minors. The Family and Medical Leave Act was created to protect and preserve the integrity of the family. The Equal Employment Opportunity was created to prohibit discrimination against employees based on race, color, sex, religion, or national origin. The Occupational Safety and Health Administration sets safety standards to protect employees. Prendergast H, Front Office Management for the Veterinary Team, ed 3, Saunders, 2020, p. 103.
20. d All veterinary facilities have to comply with all of the following laws/acts: Uniformed Services Employment and Reemployment Rights Act, Immigration Reform and Control Act, Employee Polygraph Protection Act, Family and Medical Leave Act (practices with 50+ employees). Prendergast H, Front Office Management for the Veterinary Team, ed 3, Saunders, 2020, p. 103.
21. d The following are examples of employee benefits: health insurance, dental/vision insurance, continuing education, vacation, sick leave, holiday pay, professional liability insurance, disability insurance, life insurance, retirement plans, dues and licenses, veterinary care. Prendergast H, Front Office Management for the Veterinary Team, ed 3, Saunders, 2020, p. 113.
22. c Employee discounts on services greater than 20% are reported as fringe benefits and must be reported to the IRS as pay. Prendergast H, Front Office Management for the Veterinary Team, ed 3, Saunders, 2020, p. 115.
23. d Incorporeal property is defined as something that a person or corporation can have ownership of and can transfer ownership to another person or corporation, but has no physical substance. Practice goodwill is the reputation within the community, with colleagues and staff, and in doctor and client/patient relationships, and it is an example of incorporeal property or intangible property. Tangible property is anything that can be touched and includes both real and personal property such as buildings, equipment, and vehicles. Prendergast H, Front Office Management for the Veterinary Team, ed 3, Saunders, 2020, p. 116.
24. d A practice cannot discriminate against pregnant team members. They should be counseled on the safety issues but the team member is responsible for deciding what safety level they should obtain. Prendergast H, Front Office Management for the Veterinary Team, ed 3, Saunders, 2020, p. 117.
25. c The following are examples of questions that should NOT be asked during an interview: Do you have any children? What is your national origin? What is your maiden name? What is your religion? Do you have any physical disabilities? What holidays do you observe? The following are examples of questions that should be asked during an interview: Are you currently employed? What is your salary requirement? What are some areas you feel you need improvement on? Prendergast H, Front Office Management for the Veterinary Team, ed 3, Saunders, 2020, p. 121.
26. a Compassion fatigue results in the following symptoms; Cognitive, behavioral, emotional, spiritual, interpersonal, and physical. Examples of social symptoms include isolation, intolerance, and mistrust. Pain is a physical symptom. Depression is an emotional symptom. Nightmares are a behavioral symptom. Prendergast H, Front Office Management for the Veterinary Team, ed 3, Saunders, 2020, p. 158.
27. c Compassion fatigue is a natural result of being a caregiver and occurs only in caregiving roles and has

a short and sudden onset of symptoms. Compassion fatigue can be resolved by time spent away from the caregiving role. Burn-out is an overall decrease in job satisfaction, can occur in any job industry, and occurs over a longer period of time. Prendergast H, Front Office Management for the Veterinary Team, ed 3, Saunders, 2020, p. 157.

28. c Every business has a life cycle that consists of four stages; introduction, growth, maturity, and decline. Prendergast H, Front Office Management for the Veterinary Team, ed 3, Saunders, 2020, p. 176.

29. a There are many different signs of compassion fatigue. Decreased concentration and/or ability to concentrate is an example of a cognitive sign of compassion fatigue. Questioning life's meaning is a spiritual sign of compassion fatigue. Failure to develop non–work-related aspects of life is an interpersonal sign of compassion fatigue. Dread of working with certain co-workers is a work-related sign of compassion fatigue. Prendergast H, Front Office Management for the Veterinary Team, ed 3, Saunders, 2020, p. 158.

30. b Ergonomics refers to the science that studies the relationship between people and their work environments. The organization of material in a logical sequence, positioning of objects as close to the point of use as possible, and the amount of time and degree of motion required to perform a given task all refer to motion economy. Prendergast H, Front Office Management for the Veterinary Team, ed 3, Saunders, 2020, p. 344.

31. b PASS is the correct acronym to remember when using a fire extinguisher. PASS stands for Pull, Aim, Squeeze, and Sweep. Prendergast H, Front Office Management for the Veterinary Team, ed 3, Saunders, 2020, p. 345.

32. b The lead aprons, gloves, and thyroid collars, which are the PPE used when taking radiographs, should be radiographed yearly to ensure that no cracks have occurred. These radiographs should be compared year on year. Lead PPEs should always be stored flat or hung to prevent cracking. Prendergast H, Front Office Management for the Veterinary Team, ed 3, Saunders, 2020, p. 81.

33. c The Occupational Safety and Health Administration (OSHA) provides guidelines and laws for employee safety with radiation exposure. The Americans with Disabilities Act (ADA) protects employees and/or clients with disabilities and allows full access to the facility, including parking lots, restrooms, exam rooms, and so forth. The sale and distribution of pharmaceuticals is monitored by the FDA. Prendergast H, Front Office Management for the Veterinary Team, ed 3, Saunders, 2020, p. 81.

34. a A dosimetry badge is used to measure the amount of radiation an individual receives and is assigned to each individual employee who partakes is obtaining radiographs. Lead is worn as PPE to protect the body against radiation. A Cathode is a mechanical part of the x-ray machine. A MPD refers to the maximum permissible dose of radiation an individual may receive per year. Prendergast H, Front Office Management for the Veterinary Team, ed 3, Saunders, 2020, p. 81.

35. c The abbreviation OU indicates "both eyes." The abbreviation BID indicates "twice daily." The abbreviation OD indicates "right eye." The abbreviation AU indicates "both ears." Prendergast H, Front Office Management for the Veterinary Team, ed 3, Saunders, 2020, p. 87.

36. b Magnetic resonance imaging (MRI) uses a magnet to produce images. Ultrasound uses soundwaves to produce images. Radiographs and CT scans use radiation to produce images. Prendergast H, Front Office Management for the Veterinary Team, ed 3, Saunders, 2020, p. 82.

37. a Ethylenediamine tetraacetic acid is an anticoagulant added to blood collection tubes in advance of collection. Serum separator is added to a blood collection tube to aid in the separation process of serum. Ethylene glycol is rubbing alcohol often added to the skin for aseptic purposes before collection. Prendergast H, Front Office Management for the Veterinary Team, ed 3, Saunders, 2020, p. 69.

38. c When submitting a tissue sample for pathology that requires the use of formalin, the sample should contain 10% formalin at 10 times the volume of the tissue, creating a 10:1 ratio. Prendergast H, Front Office Management for the Veterinary Team, ed 3, Saunders, 2020, p. 69.

39. d A clean read top tube should be used for the collection of serum to monitor the following therapeutic levels: phenobarbital, theophylline, and digoxin. Prendergast H, Front Office Management for the Veterinary Team, ed 3, Saunders, 2020, p. 69.

40. d The following are common anticoagulant agents included within blood collections tubes: potassium citrate, lithium heparin, sodium heparin, and ethylenediaminetetraacetic acid (EDTA). ETDA does not exist. Prendergast H, Front Office Management for the Veterinary Team, ed 3, Saunders, 2020, p. 69.

41. d An anaerobic culture is a culture that requires the absence of air and should be kept at room temperature and processed within 48 hours of collection. Prendergast H, Front Office Management for the Veterinary Team, ed 3, Saunders, 2020, p. 71.

42. d A SWOT analysis is used in the marketing aspect and is an acronym for strengths, weaknesses, opportunities, and threats. A coordinated SWOT analysis is used to evaluate all of these areas to help improve the practice from a marketing standpoint. Prendergast H, Front Office Management for the Veterinary Team, ed 3, Saunders, 2020, p. 178.

43. a A Web page or social media are examples of internal marketing. Yellow pages and newspaper advertisements are examples of direct marketing. Client education is an example of indirect marketing. Prendergast H, Front Office Management for the Veterinary Team, ed 3, Saunders, 2020, p. 189.

44. e Recalls should be performed on every patient that has attended the practice regardless of the reason. Prendergast H, Front Office Management for the Veterinary Team, ed 3, Saunders, 2020, p. 193.

45. d Client education is an example of internal marketing. External marketing includes outdoor building sign, lectures, media advertising, and much more. Prendergast H, Front Office Management for the Veterinary Team, ed 3, Saunders, 2020, p. 189.

46. b A message has three components when being developed. Nonverbal skills or body language contribute about 55% of the message. Verbal skills or word choice contribute about 7%, and paraverbal skills, the way the words are spoken, contribute about 38% to the message. Prendergast H, Front Office Management for the Veterinary Team, ed 3, Saunders, 2020, p. 254.
47. a Nonverbal skills are referred to as body language. Folded arms are a form of nonverbal communication. Pitch and tone are paraverbal skills. Slang word choice and using the phrase of "yeah" instead of "yes" are examples of verbal skills. Prendergast H, Front Office Management for the Veterinary Team, ed 3, Saunders, 2020, p. 256.
48. c Veterinary technicians should be the team members presenting treatment plans to owners. They are the team members familiar with the pet and should be able to discuss the treatment options with confidence. Receptionists should handle the financial transaction but should not present the treatment plan because of the lack of scientific knowledge. The kennel assistant should not deliver a treatment plan because of the lack of scientific knowledge to support the discussion. The veterinarian should not discuss financial issues with the client; veterinarians should only diagnose, prescribe medication, and perform procedures. Prendergast H, Front Office Management for the Veterinary Team, ed 3, Saunders, 2020, p. 5.
49. d Client compliance is defined as the percentage of clients who accept recommendations given by the veterinary health care team. Client retention refers to the ability to keep clients long term. Quantity refers to the total number of clients. Turnover refers to the occurrence of having new employees because of the continual loss of current employees. Prendergast H, Front Office Management for the Veterinary Team, ed 3, Saunders, 2020, p. 258.
50. b Client grievances should be handled immediately on occurrence. Any grievance that is handled later will result in a decrease in client retention and compliance and may make it more difficult to acquire new clients (clients who are upset do not refer friends and family). Prendergast H, Front Office Management for the Veterinary Team, ed 3, Saunders, 2020, p. 268.
51. b When a client is not present to sign a euthanasia form, the owner must tell two team members that he or she wishes to euthanize the pet. Both team members must document the conversation in the medical record. Prendergast H, Front Office Management for the Veterinary Team, ed 3, Saunders, 2020, p. 271.
52. d Euthanasia comes from the Greek terms *eu* meaning good and *thanatos* meaning death. Prendergast H, Front Office Management for the Veterinary Team, ed 3, Saunders, 2020, p. 270.
53. e Different cultures have different communication structures and these can therefore be barriers when two different cultures are trying to communicate. Examination room tables, reception desks, and lack of eye contact are all barriers to communication and detract from the message being delivered. Prendergast H, Front Office Management for the Veterinary Team, ed 3, Saunders, 2020, p. 257.
54. b A mass cremation is a cremation of multiple animals at the same time without the return of ashes. A private cremation can be performed with either private ashes returned or no ashes returned. Prendergast H, Front Office Management for the Veterinary Team, ed 3, Saunders, 2020, p. 272.
55. c An animal should be presented to an owner after euthanasia within a waterproof body bag. A box, trash bag, or no covering at all is not acceptable to present a deceased pet to an owner. Prendergast H, Front Office Management for the Veterinary Team, ed 3, Saunders, 2020, p. 271.
56. a Barbiturates are commonly used as a euthanasia solution. Morphine, acepromazine, and Telazol are drugs commonly used for surgery induction, tranquilization, or pain management. Prendergast H, Front Office Management for the Veterinary Team, ed 3, Saunders, 2020, p. 271.
57. d When scheduling appointments, many factors need to be considered: number of veterinarians seeing appointments, veterinary technician appointments, nonsterile procedures, length of time for client education, dental and surgical procedures, holidays, and vacation times. Prendergast H, Front Office Management for the Veterinary Team, ed 3, Saunders, 2020, p. 283.
58. c Nonsterile procedures include any procedure that does not require aseptic techniques. Examples of nonsterile procedures include abscess debridement, dental procedures, anal sac expression, and ear flushes. Spay, orthopedic, and exploratory surgeries are all examples of sterile procedures. Prendergast H, Front Office Management for the Veterinary Team, ed 3, Saunders, 2020, p. 286.
59. c To help reduce client overload at the front desk, appointments should be staggered every 5 minutes. Appointments can be set for every 15–30 minutes or more depending on the type of appointment; however, multiple appointments can be seen around the same time, therefore staggering them is ideal. Prendergast H, Front Office Management for the Veterinary Team, ed 3, Saunders, 2020, p. 282.
60. d Appointment lengths may vary for many reasons such as specific clients, type of appointment, and the veterinarian. The length of appointments usually does not vary because of the type of patient (versus the appointment type). Prendergast H, Front Office Management for the Veterinary Team, ed 3, Saunders, 2020, p. 283.
61. d Medical records must be legible and be able to be read by everybody. An illegible medical record is perceived as incompetency in veterinary practitioners. Prendergast H, Front Office Management for the Veterinary Team, ed 3, Saunders, 2020, p. 293.
62. d Computerized records, also known as paperless records, are filed under the client's last name and client number. The pet name is too generic to locate records. Prendergast H, Front Office Management for the Veterinary Team, ed 3, Saunders, 2020, p. 295.
63. c A disadvantage to using computerized medical records includes the lack of medical details. Computerized records are legible, can target specific clients quickly and efficiently when promoting specific services, and clients perceive progressive and higher-quality medicine.

Prendergast H, Front Office Management for the Veterinary Team, ed 3, Saunders, 2020, p. 297.

64. b Medical record entries should follow the standard SOAP format, which includes: subjective, objective, assessment, and plan. Prendergast H, Front Office Management for the Veterinary Team, ed 3, Saunders, 2020, p. 298.

65. c The term *prognosis* refers to the prediction of the outcome of the disease. The surgical procedure and medication prescribed fall under the treatment plan and all depend on the prognosis. Prendergast H, Front Office Management for the Veterinary Team, ed 3, Saunders, 2020, p. 299.

66. b The objective portion of the examination includes information gathered directly from the patient, physical examination, or diagnostic workup. The subjective portion is the reason for the visit, history, and observations made by the client. The assessment is the conclusion reached along with a definitive diagnosis. The plan includes treatment, surgery, medication, and diagnostics recommended. Prendergast H, Front Office Management for the Veterinary Team, ed 3, Saunders, 2020, p. 299.

67. b Surgical patients must be examined within 12 hours of anesthesia being administered and the examination must be documented in the medical record. Prendergast H, Front Office Management for the Veterinary Team, ed 3, Saunders, 2020, p. 83.

68. c The correct form to enter medication into a record is: 0.4 mL Cefazolin (100 mg/mL) IV. Choices a and b do not include a dose strength. Choice d does not indicate which route to administer and also needs a zero placeholder in front of the decimal so that this amount is not confused. Prendergast H, Front Office Management for the Veterinary Team, ed 3, Saunders, 2020, p. 299.

69. a When a medication is being dispensed to an owner, all of the following must be clearly written in the medical record: drug name, strength, administration route, duration of treatment, and frequency. Drug lot numbers do not need to be recorded. Prendergast H, Front Office Management for the Veterinary Team, ed 3, Saunders, 2020, p. 300.

70. b An inactive medical record is defined as a client who has not been seen by that practice for a year or more. Prendergast H, Front Office Management for the Veterinary Team, ed 3, Saunders, 2020, p. 301.

71. a Records must be written in blue or black ink only. The following are rules for medical records: the author of the entry must date and initial each time an entry is made, correction fluid may never be used, standard and approved abbreviations must be used, records must be legible, and when correcting a mistake a single line may be drawn through it and then it may be rewritten and initialed. Prendergast H, Front Office Management for the Veterinary Team, ed 3, Saunders, 2020, p. 300.

72. d Losses associated with poor inventory management include theft, backorders, shrinkage, frequent ordering, expired products, wrong products, too much product on the shelf, or not enough product on the shelf. Prendergast H, Front Office Management for the Veterinary Team, ed 3, Saunders, 2020, p. 310.

73. b The number of times a specific product turns over in a practice is referred to as the turnover rate. Each product will have its own turnover rate. The more popular the product is, the more often it will turn over per year. Product expiration dates change and vary from product to product. The time it takes to receive a product after it has been purchased depends on the distributor and the shipping agreement. Prendergast H, Front Office Management for the Veterinary Team, ed 3, Saunders, 2020, p. 313.

74. c Expired drugs must be dissolved in an appropriate pouch that inactivates the medication, rendering them irretrievable, then disposed of in the trash. Expired drugs cannot be thrown away whole, flushed down the drain, or prescribed to owners. Prendergast H, Front Office Management for the Veterinary Team, ed 3, Saunders, 2020, p. 85.

75. d Dispensing fees are added to a product after the markup has been determined to cover costs associated with filling the prescription such as the label on the bottle, the vial used to package the medication, the wear and tear on the label writer machine, and the technician's time it takes to fill it. Prendergast H, Front Office Management for the Veterinary Team, ed 3, Saunders, 2020, p. 319.

76. b Missed charges account for approximately 10% of gross revenue. By managing inventory and investigating discrepancies managers should be able to determine why there are missed charges. Prendergast H, Front Office Management for the Veterinary Team, ed 3, Saunders, 2020, p. 226.

77. b Pharmaceutical drugs that are controlled substances will have the letter "C" on the bottle, followed by a Roman numeral. The letters A, D, and S do not denote any type of pharmaceutical. Prendergast H, Front Office Management for the Veterinary Team, ed 3, Saunders, 2020, p. 324.

78. b Controlled substance prescriptions for classes III, IV, and V for a 30-day supply can have five refills that are available for 6 months. After 6 months, there must be a new prescription submitted to the pharmacy. Usually a 30-day supply is allowed with refills that can follow, but it still cannot exceed 6 months. Prendergast H, Front Office Management for the Veterinary Team, ed 3, Saunders, 2020, p. 324.

79. a Controlled substance class I holds the highest level for abuse potential. Classes IV and V hold the lowest levels of abuse potential. There are not any classes of controlled substances past level V. The lower the Roman numeral, the higher the level is for abuse. Prendergast H, Front Office Management for the Veterinary Team, ed 3, Saunders, 2020, p. 324.

80. d Class II controlled substances are allowed to be filled for 30 days but are not allowed to have refills on the original script; there must be a new script written for the next 30 days if needed. Classes III and IV can have up to five refills, therefore 1 or 3 are acceptable as well. Prendergast H, Front Office Management for the Veterinary Team, ed 3, Saunders, 2020, p. 324.

81. d Class V controlled substances do not contain any DEA dispensing limits because it holds the lowest level of abuse potential. Class I is labeled for research only. Class II is written prescription only with no refills. Class IV is written prescription with five refills. Prendergast H, Front Office Management for the Veterinary Team, ed 3, Saunders, 2020, p. 324.

82. b Class II controlled substances must have their own separate log and invoices kept from classes III, IV, and V.

Class I controlled substances are for research only and are not found in the veterinary hospitals. Prendergast H, Front Office Management for the Veterinary Team, ed 3, Saunders, 2020, p. 325.

83. d Drugs logs should include the following information: client name and address, patient name, reason for use, amount of drug administered, balance of drug after use, and initials. Drug lot numbers are not required. Prendergast H, Front Office Management for the Veterinary Team, ed 3, Saunders, 2020, p. 327.

84. c All of the following must be included on an inventory log: product name, strength and count in a full bottle, date of purchase, name and address of vendor, date and time of inventory, log quantity, physical quantity, any discrepancy found, and initials. Client and patient names will not be included on the inventory log. Prendergast H, Front Office Management for the Veterinary Team, ed 3, Saunders, 2020, p. 327.

85. c If a drug loss or theft takes place, both the DEA and local police need to be notified. In some states, the pharmacy and veterinary boards may also need to be notified. Prendergast H, Front Office Management for the Veterinary Team, ed 3, Saunders, 2020, p. 329.

86. b Formerly controlled substances had to be submitted through a reverse distributor for destruction; however, the DEA recently updated this requirement using the DEA form 41, which includes logging of destroyed inventory, method of destruction and requires two witnesses who must sign off on the destruction of the substances. Prendergast H, Front Office Management for the Veterinary Team, ed 3, Saunders, 2020, p. 329.

87. c A loss of 3% or higher for any controlled substance must be reported to the DEA. The loss of less than 3% of a controlled substance does not need to be reported. Prendergast H, Front Office Management for the Veterinary Team, ed 3, Saunders, 2020, p. 328.

88. b The law requires controlled substance logs. Laboratory logs are not required by law but are helpful for maintaining reference records for certain tests. Compliance logs are used for internal monitoring. Prendergast H, Front Office Management for the Veterinary Team, ed 3, Saunders, 2020, p. 327.

89. b Controlled substance logs must be kept for 2 years beyond the last recorded entry date and should remain retrievable for inspection. Some facilities may want to keep them longer for added reassurance, but the DEA requires 2 years. Prendergast H, Front Office Management for the Veterinary Team, ed 3, Saunders, 2020, p. 327.

90. a Accounts receivable is defined as the money owed to a business for services rendered or products that are sold and not paid for at the time of service. Accounts receivable should NOT exceed 1.5% of gross revenue. Anything greater than 1.5% can decrease the cash flow of the practice. Prendergast H, Front Office Management for the Veterinary Team, ed 3, Saunders, 2020, p. 216.

91. c The Fair Debt Collection Practices Act of 1996 protects the public from unethical collection procedures. It only allows phone calls to be placed between 8 AM and 9 PM. Collecting agencies are not allowed to impersonate lawyers or government agencies. The business is allowed to use collecting agencies on past-due accounts, but they must follow what the law allows. Prendergast H, Front Office Management for the Veterinary Team, ed 3, Saunders, 2020, p. 241.

92. d All of the following are allowed to be given to a collection agency: client's full name, address and telephone number, client's occupation, client's driver's license number, client's employment address if known, total balance due on the account, copy of client information sheet, and signature of client guaranteeing payment for services rendered. Prendergast H, Front Office Management for the Veterinary Team, ed 3, Saunders, 2020, p. 240.

93. c Indemnity insurance provides compensation of injured or sick pets paid directly to the client after services are rendered, according to their insurance policy. The client still pays for services in full and submits receipts to retrieve compensation. A contract for physicians to provide medical services at set prices is seen with HMOs or PPOs typically with human health care. Prendergast H, Front Office Management for the Veterinary Team, ed 3, Saunders, 2020, p. 244.

94. b A per-incident limit is the maximum dollar amount an insurance company will pay out per incident filed. A lifetime limit is the maximum dollar amount a company will pay out on one policy for the lifetime of the pet. A preexisting condition is an injury or illness contracted, manifested, or incurred before the policy effective date. A rider is an extension of coverage that can be purchased and added to a base medical policy. Prendergast H, Front Office Management for the Veterinary Team, ed 3, Saunders, 2020, p. 244.

95. a An eyewash station must be within 10 seconds from any team member potentially exposed to a chemical. If the practice is large, multiple eyewash stations must be available to allow access within 10 seconds. Prendergast H, Front Office Management for the Veterinary Team, ed 3, Saunders, 2020, p. 352.

96. c The minimum PPE required to perform x-rays is a lead gown, thyroid collar, and lead gloves. Some practices may recommend the use of goggles, but OSHA does not require it. Prendergast H, Front Office Management for the Veterinary Team, ed 3, Saunders, 2020, p. 81.

97. c Dosimeter badges measure the radiation exposure of the individual team member and they should be worn on the outside of the PPE. Under the PPE or in pockets is not acceptable to measure the amount of radiation exposure. Dosimeter badges should be kept in a separate location than the x-ray room when a team member is not participating in the imaging procedures. Prendergast H, Front Office Management for the Veterinary Team, ed 3, Saunders, 2020, p. 81.

98. d OSHA states that dosimetry reports be kept on hand for 30 years. Team members should always have access to the information regarding how much radiation they have been exposed to. Prendergast H, Front Office Management for the Veterinary Team, ed 3, Saunders, 2020, p. 81.

99. b Hearing protection should be available for team members when the noise levels reach 85 dB and greater. OSHA standards require noise measurement, noise protection, and hearing testing when noise measurement exceeds 85 dB. Noise loudness is measured in decibel units. Prendergast H, Front Office Management for the Veterinary Team, ed 3, Saunders, 2020, p. 346.

100. b Safety data sheets are fact lists for chemicals and the following information is included: identity of the chemical, physical and chemical characteristics, health hazards, permissible exposure limits, whether the product is a carcinogen, emergency first aid procedures, and specific hazards. SDS sheets do not list the nearest emergency facility; however, this should be included in the safety book. Prendergast H, Front Office Management for the Veterinary Team, ed 3, Saunders, 2020, p. 348.

101. b A spill kit should include all of the following: cat litter, dustpan and broom, nitrile gloves, eye protection, and a laminated copy of the cleanup procedure. Water is not included in a spill kit. Prendergast H, Front Office Management for the Veterinary Team, ed 3, Saunders, 2020, p. 352.

102. d The skull and crossbones HCS pictogram indicates acute toxicity (fatal or toxic). Explosives will be found under the exploding bomb pictogram. Skin irritant will be found under the explanation mark pictogram. Flammables will be found under the flame pictogram. Prendergast H, Front Office Management for the Veterinary Team, ed 3, Saunders, 2020, p. 352.

103. d Urine sediments check for the following: white blood cells, red blood cells, epithelial cells, bacterial, casts, and crystals. Prendergast H, Front Office Management for the Veterinary Team, ed 3, Saunders, 2020, p. 68.

104. c Urine dipstick tests check for all of the following: glucose, pH, leukocytes, blood, ketones, bilirubin, and nitrates. Bacteria are only seen at the microscopic level with a urine sediment. Prendergast H, Front Office Management for the Veterinary Team, ed 3, Saunders, 2020, p. 68.

105. d Sonography, also known as ultrasound, uses sound waves to provide imaging. MRI uses very strong magnets to provide images. Fluoroscopy uses a continuous x-ray beam to provide images. Prendergast H, Front Office Management for the Veterinary Team, ed 3, Saunders, 2020, p. 82.

106. b The abbreviation QOD is defined as "every other day." The abbreviation QID stands for four times daily. The abbreviation BID stands for twice daily. The abbreviation OD stands for right eye. Prendergast H, Front Office Management for the Veterinary Team, ed 3, Saunders, 2020, p. 87.

107. c Anti-inflammatories reduce the amount of inflammation within various locations of the body. Anthelmintics are antiparasitic drugs. Antimicrobials are drugs that kill or inhibit bacteria, protozoa, viruses, or fungi. Antifungal drugs specifically target fungal agents. Prendergast H, Front Office Management for the Veterinary Team, ed 3, Saunders, 2020, p. 87.

108. c Insulin is responsible for the movement of glucose from the blood into the tissue cells and is an endocrine drug. Anthelmintics are antiparasitic drugs. Gastric drugs affect the gastrointestinal tract. Anesthetic drugs are examples of drugs that affect the nervous system. Prendergast H, Front Office Management for the Veterinary Team, ed 3, Saunders, 2020, p. 87.

109. c A positive practice culture is warm and welcoming to all who enter the practice, including clients. In addition, teamwork and etiquette are fostered. Gossip contributes to a negative culture. Prendergast H, Front Office Management for the Veterinary Team, ed 3, Saunders, 2020, p. 16.

110. a When a caller is placed on hold, team members should pick up the phone when 1 minute has passed and let the client know they are still locating the requested information. If the caller is going to be on hold for more than 2 minutes, the team member should offer to call the client back. Prendergast H, Front Office Management for the Veterinary Team, ed 3, Saunders, 2020, p. 39.

111. c Seventy percent of phone shoppers should become clients of the practice. Prendergast H, Front Office Management for the Veterinary Team, ed 3, Saunders, 2020, p. 40.

112. d Clients, when entering the practice for the first time, or with a new pet, are expected to complete a client and patient information sheet. Team members are responsible for filling out rabies certificates, spay and neuter certificates, as well as medical records. Prendergast H, Front Office Management for the Veterinary Team, ed 3, Saunders, 2020, p. 43.

113. a The Privacy Act of 1974 states, in part: "No agency shall disclose any record which is contained in a system of records by any means of communication to any person, or to another agency, except pursuant to a written request by, or with the prior written consent of, the individual to whom the record pertains." Many practices request that owners fill out medical release forms and return them to the clinic either by mail, email, or fax. The FMLA act applies to employees taking time off and the Fair Credit Act applies to collecting funds from clients when they have a balance owed to the practice. Prendergast H, Front Office Management for the Veterinary Team, ed 3, Saunders, 2020, p. 48.

114. b The Red Flags Rule was established to decrease fraud and identity theft in the United States. Therefore, any business should check the identity of a person who presents a credit card for payment. The Fairness to Pets Act gives clients the option to purchase their medication wherever they choose. Practices must verify the citizenship of all potential employees through the use of an I-9 form. Prendergast H, Front Office Management for the Veterinary Team, ed 3, Saunders, 2020, p. 52.

115. d Most practices will accept cash, check, credit cards, and vendors such as Care Credit, for services rendered. Prendergast H, Front Office Management for the Veterinary Team, ed 3, Saunders, 2020, p. 52.

116. b Animal restraint in a reception area is vitally important to ensure the welfare of both clients and patients. Placing every client and pet in an examination room as they arrive may be an ideal situation but is far from practical. Signage regarding restraint policies is important but will not ensure safety. Separating ill and healthy patients does not ensure the safety of clients or pets. Prendergast H, Front Office Management for the Veterinary Team, ed 3, Saunders, 2020, p. 35.

117. d Staff interactions contribute to team culture, which in this example is negative. Etiquette is defined as the rules that society has set for the proper way to behave around other people. The disagreement may cause a job description discussion at a staff meeting to clarify roles but will not change staff duties. Cleaning product selection is unaffected by staff interaction. Prendergast H, Front Office Management for the Veterinary Team, ed 3, Saunders, 2020, p. 36.

SECTION 3

1. b A 25% solution contains 250 mg of drug/mL. Because this concentration is in mg/mL, we need to convert the 5 g to mg. There are 1000 mg in 1 g, therefore 5 g is equal to 5000 mg (1000 mg/g × 5 g = 5000 mg) and 5000 mg is the total dose required. We can divide that by 250 mg/mL and obtain 20 mL (5000 mg ÷ 250 mg/mL = 20 mL). This patient requires 20 mL of mannitol to administer 5 g of the drug. Mannitol will crystallize and therefore a filter should always be used during administration.
2. c "Percent" indicates parts of active drug/100 parts of a solution; a 1.0% solution is therefore equal to 1.0 parts/100 parts of a solution. The solution weighs 1 g/mL, therefore there is 1.0 g of active drug in 100 g of solution or 1.0 g in 100 mL of solution. Because the strength of most liquid medications is measured in mg/mL, this is broken down further to 1000 mg (which is equal to 1.0 g) in 100 mL of solution, which can be broken down further to 10 mg/mL. This means a 1.0% solution is 10 mg/mL. Lake T, Green N, Essential Calculations for Veterinary Nurses and Technicians, ed 3, Elsevier, 2017, p. 64-65.
3. b 1 tbs = 3 tsp
4. a 30 mL/h ÷ 3600 s/h × 60 drops/mL = 0.49 s/drop
Therefore by applying the equation: 1 ÷ 0.49 s/drop = 1 drop/2 s
5. c 5% solution = 50 mg/mL
50 mg/mL ÷ 0.5 mL = 25 mg
6. c 75 lb × 1 mg/lb = 75 mg
75 mg ÷ 100 mg/mL = 0.75 mL
7. c There are 5 mL in 1 tsp. Bill RL, Clinical Pharmacology and Therapeutics for the Veterinary Technician, ed 4, Elsevier, 2017, p. 34.
8. b 3 mL × 2 doses/day = 6 mL
6 mL × 30 days = 180 mL
30 mL = 1 oz of fluid
180 mL ÷ 30 mL = 6 oz
9. a 60 lb × 70 kcal/lb/day = 4200 kcal/day
4200 kcal ÷ 420 kcal/cup = 10 cups
10 cups ÷ 2 feedings/day = 5 cups/feeding
10. a 80 g ÷ 1000 g/kg = 0.08 kg
0.08 kg × 100 mg/kg = 8 mg
8 mg ÷ 100 mg/mL = 0.08 mL
11. c 8 lb ÷ 2.2 lb/kg = 3.6 kg
3.6 kg × 300 μg/kg = 1080 μg
1% Ivomec = 10 mg/mL
1080 μg ÷ 1000 μg/mg = 1.08 mg ÷ 10 mg/mL = 0.1 mL
12. d 5% dextrose solution = 50 mg/mL × 1000 mL/L = 50,000 mg/L
50% dextrose solution = 500 mg/mL
50,000 mg/L ÷ 500 mg/mL = 100 mL
(100 mL of 50% dextrose solution + 900 mL of water = 1000 mL of 5%)
13. b 12 oz ÷ 16 oz/lb = 0.75 lb
0.75 lb × 1 mL/lb = 0.75 mL
0.75 mL × 6 puppies = 4.5 mL
14. b 3 μg/kg/h × 50 kg = 150 μg/h
150 μg/h ÷ 50 μg/mL = 3 mL/h
15. d 30 g × 1000 mg/g = 30,000 mg
30,000 mg ÷ 15 mg/mL = 2000 mL
16. d Tab: tablets; q4h: every 4 hours; po: per os (by mouth); prn: as needed; until gone: until all tablets are gone. Four times a day would be every 6 hours or QID and the prescription does not indicate it should be taken with food or water or that it should be taken for pain. Bill RL, Clinical Pharmacology and Therapeutics for the Veterinary Technician, ed 4, Elsevier, 2017, p. 22-27.
17. c 1.5 tablets × 3 doses/day = 4.5 tablets/day
4.5 tablets/day × 30 days = 135 tablets total
18. d 1 g × 1000 mg/g = 1000 mg
1000 mg ÷ 20 mg/mL = 50 mL
19. d 6 vials × 10 mL = 60 mL × (50 mg/mL) = 3000 mg
20 mL × 10 mg/mL = 200 mg
3000 mg ÷ 200 mg = 15 vials
20. d 120 mL/h × 20% = 24 mL
120 mL - 24 mL = 96 mL/h
21. c One ounce is equal to 2 tablespoons, which is equal to 30 mL (15 mL are in one tablespoon).
22. b 0.1 mL × 10 mg/mL = 1 mg
1 mg ÷ 5 kg = 0.2 mg/kg
23. c 5 mg ÷ 10 kg = 0.5 mg/kg
24. c 50 g ÷ 1000 g/kg = 0.05 kg
0.05 kg × 4 mg/kg = 0.2 mg
0.2 mg ÷ 2 doses = 0.1 mg
25. b 50 lb ÷ 2.2 lb/kg = 22.7 kg
22.7 kg × 1 mg/kg = 22.7 mg
26. c 60 mL ÷ 2 mL/min = 30 min
27. a 6 + 5 + (7 × 0.5) = 14.5 tablets
28. b To help solve the problem, know that:
    - 50% dextrose = 500 mg/mL
    - 2.5% dextrose = 25 mg/mL
    - 1 L = 1000 mL

    500 mg/mL × 50 mL = 25,000 mg
25 mg/mL × 1000 mL = 25,000 mg
25,000 mg + 25,000 mg = 50,000 mg of dextrose
50,000 mg ÷ 1050 mL = 47.6 mg/mL or 4.76%
29. c 5 bowls × 100 mL= 500 mL
500 mL - 475 mL = 25 mL
30. a 70 kVp × 20% = 14
70 + 14 = 84
31. b 15 mL/kg × 10 kg = 150 mL/breath
150 mL/breath × 10 breaths/min= 1500 mL/min
32. a 15 mL/kg × 10 kg = 150 mL/breath; 150 mL/breath × 10 breaths/min = 1500 mL/min for a normal pet;
10 kg × 10 mL/kg = 100 mL/kg for diaphragmatic hernia patient;
1500 mL/min ÷ 100 mL/min = 15 breaths/min
33. d Because this drug is enterically coated, it should not be split. The enteric coating prevents the tablet from being broken down in the stomach and allows it to move into the intestine where it will be absorbed. Administrating 50 mg is an overdose for the patient and may lead to toxicity. This medication should be ordered or a prescription should be written so that the correct dose can be administered. Sirois M, Principles and Practice of Veterinary Technology, ed 4, Elsevier, 2017, p. 245.
34. d 3% = 30 mL/1 L
1 L = 1000 mL

30 mL of isoflurane/1000 mL of oxygen × 60 min = 1800 mL of isoflurane will be delivered

35. d 2 mL/100 g × 300 g = 6 mL
6 mL × 3 times/day = 18 mL
1 g = 15 mL; therefore, 18 mL ÷ 15 mL = 1.2 mL

36. c 1500 kcal/15 oz = 100 kcal/oz
300 kcal/day are needed = 3 oz/day will be needed
1 oz = 30 mL; therefore, 3 oz = 90 mL
90 mL diluted 50:50 with water = 180 mL/day to be administered
180 mL ÷ 45 mL = 4 feedings/day

37. a 160 mL ÷ 45 mL = 3.5mL additional boluses of water must be given.

38. c 14 + 15 + 19 + 14 + 18 = 80
80 ÷ 5 = 16

39. c 3 units ÷ 100 units/mL = 0.03 mL

40. a 3 units ÷ 30 units/mL = 0.1 mL

41. b 0.1 mL × 50% = 0.05 mL
1 mL/0.05 mL = 20 tubes

42. d 300 mL × 40% = 120 mL
120 mL ÷ 50% = 240 mL
240 mL - 120 mL = 120 mL of saline

43. b 10 beats/5 s × 60 s/min = 120 beats/min

44. d 115 + 120 + 123 + 121 + 121 + 112 = 712 ÷ 6 = 119

45. d 2.5 cm/in × 2 in = 5 cm

46. c 8 × 5 = 40 cm

47. a 1 oz = 30 mL
16 oz × 30 mL = 480 mL

48. b 400 lb ÷ 2.2 kg/lb = 182 kg

49. a 18 g/lb × 60% = 10.8 g/lb
10.8 g/lb × 2000 lb/ton = 21,600 g/ton

50. c "Percent" indicates the percentage of a solution that is active drug. This is measured in g/100 mL. 24% is equal to 24 g of active drug in 100 mL of solution. Because we measure concentrations as mg/mL, we can break this down further to 24,000 mg (or 24 g) in 100 mL of solution. This can be broken down to mg/mL by dividing both sides of the equation by 100, which becomes 240 mg/mL (24,000/100 = 240 mg and 100/100 = 1 mL). So a 24% solution has a concentration of 240 mg/mL. The quick way to do this is to move the decimal point one space to the right. Wanamaker BP, Massey KL, Applied Pharmacology for Veterinary Technicians, ed 5, Elsevier, 2015, p. 59-60.

51. d 20 + 5 + 1 + 2 = 28 lb total
20 lb (corn) ÷ 28 lb (total) = 0.71 × 100 = 71%

52. b 32 oz/qt × 4 qt/gal = 128 oz/gal
128 oz × 30% = 38.4 oz

53. b 30 mEq/L = 0.03 mEq/mL
2 mEq ÷ 0.03 mEq/mL = 67 mL/h

54. b 1000 U/mL is a concentration of a medication. Mg/kg indicates a dose (how much of a drug to give per kilogram of weight), gr/mg is impossible because grains and milligrams are either weights or concentrations, and g/lb also refers to a dose. Prendergast H, Front Office Management for the Veterinary Team, ed 3, Elsevier, 2020, p. 372-374.

55. c 4 mg/h at 30 mL/h = 4 mg ÷ 30 mL = 133.3 mg/1000 mL
133.3 mg ÷ 30 mg/mL = 4.4 mL

56. c 5% Dextrose = 50 mg/mL × 100 mL = 5000 mg
5000 mg ÷ 140 mL = 35.7 mg/mL × 100 = 3.6%

57. b One grain is equal to 64.8 mg.

58. a 0.005 mL × 10 = 0.05 mL

59. b 100 g = 0.1 kg
0.1 kg × 10 mg/kg/day = 1 mg/day × 10 cockatiels = 10 mg/day total

60. b Metronidazole can be halved and you can therefore use the 500-mg tablets and cut them in half to provide a 250-mg dose. BID indicates it should be administered twice daily. Half a tablet twice daily for 6 days is equal to 6 tablets (0.5 tablets × 2 times daily × 6 days = 6 tablets).

61. a Average weight per cow = 825 lb + 1050 lb = 1875 ÷ 2 = 938 lb
1 mL/100 lb × 938 lb = 9.38 mL/cow
9.38 mL × 100 head = 938 mL total dewormer
938 mL ÷ 250 mL = 3.75 bottles; round up to 4

62. c 450 mL remains in the bag.

63. a 700 mL remains in the bag.

64. d There are 2.2 pounds in a kilogram, therefore a 10-kg dog weighs 22 lb (10 kg × 2.2 lb/kg).

65. c 50% Dextrose = 50 mg/mL

66. d CRI stands for constant rate infusion. Fentanyl has a short half-life and will only last 30 to 40 minutes after injection. For this reason, it is best used for analgesia during short procedures or as a CRI.

67. b French size ÷ 3 = diameter in millimeters, therefore 12 French ÷ 3 = 4 mm

68. c 28 lb ÷ 2.2 lb/kg = 12.7 kg
12.7 kg × 0.1 mg/kg = 1.27 mg
1.27 mg ÷ 1 mg/mL = 1.3 mL

69. d 28 lb ÷ 2.2 lb/kg = 12.7 kg
12.7 kg × 0.1 mg/kg = 1.27 mg

70. a 7 lb ÷ 2.2 lb/kg = 3.18 kg
3.18 kg × 1 mg = 3.18 mg and 3.18 kg × 5 mg = 15.9 mg

71. d 7 lb ÷ 2.2 lb/kg = 3.18 kg
3.18 kg × 1 mg = 3.18 mg and 3.18 kg × 5 mg = 15.9 mg
3.18 mg ÷ 20 mg/mL = 0.2 mL and 15.9 mg ÷ 20 mg/mL = 0.8 mL

72. b 8 lb ÷ 20 lb = 0.4 mL of the whole mixture
0.4 mL ÷ 2 = 0.2 mL

73. b 10 lb ÷ 2.2 lb/kg = 4.55 kg
4.55 kg × 25 to 50 mL/kg/min = 113 to 227 mL/min
4.55 kg × 130 to 300 mL/kg/min = 591 to 1365 mL/min
The nonrebreathing system would be used because of the animal's size.

74. c 32 lb ÷ 2.2 lb/kg = 14.55 kg
14.55 kg × 25 to 50 mL/kg/min = 363 to 727 mL/min
The rebreathing system would be used because of the animal's size.
14.55 kg × 130 to 300 mL/kg/min = 1892 to 4365 mL/min

75. b 0.2 mL × 10 mg = 0.2 mg

76. d 1 gr = 64.8 mg

77. c 64.8 mg ÷ 4 = 16.2 mg

78. c 37.5 kg × 10 mg/kg = 375 mg
375 mg/250 mg tablets = 1.5 tablets/dose
BID (twice a day) for 7 days = 14 total doses (2 times a day for 7 days = 2 × 7 = 14). Therefore 14 doses × 1.5 tablets/dose = 14 × 1.5 = 21 total tablets

79. c 2% = 20 mg/mL
13 lb ÷ 2.2 lb/kg = 5.9 kg
5.9 kg × 2 mg/kg = 11.8 mg
11.8 mg ÷ 20 mg/mL = 0.6 mL

80. b 1.2 mL × 300,000 U/mL
81. b mEq is the common measurement for anything related to potassium whether it is being administered or measured.
82. b 42 lb ÷ 2.2 lb/kg = 19 kg
19 kg × 0.3 mg/kg = 5.7 mg
5.7 mg ÷ 5 mg/mL = 1.1 mL
83. c 42 lb ÷ 2.2 lb/kg = 19 kg
19 kg × 0.3 mg/kg = 5.7 mg
84. c 12 lb ÷ 2.2 lb/kg = 5.45 kg
5.45 kg × 1 unit/kg = 5.5 units
85. d 12 lb ÷ 2.2 lb/kg = 5.45 kg
5.45 kg × 1 unit/kg = 5.5 units
5.5 units ÷ 100 u/mL = 0.05 mL
86. c 1000 mL ÷ 100 mL = 10 units
87. d 1 unit/100 mL
88. d 6 unit × 100 mL = 600 mL
600 mL × 60 gtt/mL= 36,000 gtt
3600 gtt ÷ 7200 s = 5 gtt/s
89. a 5.5 lb ÷ 2.2 lb/kg = 2.5 kg
2.5 kg × 100 u/kg = 250 units
90. c 25 units ÷ 2000 units/mL = 0.01 mL
91. d 10 lb ÷ 2.2 lb/kg = 4.54 kg
¼ tsp/4.5 kg
1 tsp = 5 mL; therefore, 5 mL ÷ 4 = 1.25 mL
1.25 mL × 2 = 2.5 mL total
92. a 5 mEq/5 mL = 1 mEq/1 mL; therefore, 2 mL = 2 mEq.
93. c Square meters – conversion from body weight to body surface area
94. b 33 lb ÷ 2.2 kg = 15 kg
15 kg × 9% = 1.35 kg of fluid loss
1.35 kg × 1000 mL/kg of fluid = 1350 mL
95. d 128 oz × 30 mL/oz = 3480 mL
3480 mL ÷ 8 = 480 mL of iodine
3480 mL is total volume – 480 mL of iodine = 3360 mL of alcohol
96. c 10 lb ÷ 2.2 kg = 4.54 kg 4.54 kg × 12% = 0.54 kg of fluid loss
0.54 kg × 1000 mL/kg of fluid = 545 mL
97. b 1 cup = 8 oz × 30 mL/oz = 240 mL
240 mL ÷ 7 total parts = 34.3 mL of milk
240 mL total – 34.3 mL = 205.7 mL of water
98. a Glucose 5% = 50 mg/mL
450 mL × 50 mg/mL = 2250 mg
2250 mg ÷ 500 mg/mL = 45 mL of 50% glucose
500 mL of sterile – 45 mL = 405 mL of sterile water
99. b Sulfamethazine 25% = 250 mg/mL
100. d 0.85% solution = 8.5 mg/mL
8.5 mg/mL × 5000 mL = 42,500 mg
42,500 mg ÷ 1000 mg/g = 42.5 g
101. a NaOH 1.2% = 120 mg/mL or 1.2 g/100 mL or 1200 mg/100 mL. Therefore, 600 mg of NaOH = 50 mL.
102. b 2.5% = 25 mg/mL or 0.025 g/mL or 2.5 g/100 mL. Therefore, 5 g/200 mL will create a 2.5% solution.
103. c (1:5) × (1:3) × (1:2) × (1:6) = 1:180
Total dilution factor (DF) = 180
Original concentration = Final concentration × DF
0.4 mg/mL (final concentration × 180 [DF]) = 72 mg/mL = 7.2%
104. b C1V1 = C2V2
6% × 12.5 mL = 0.5% × V2
V2 (final volume) = 150 mL
150 mL – 12.5 mL stock = 137.5 mL water
105. d (1:5) × (1:10) × (1:3) × (1:4) = 1:600
[F] = [O] × 1/D = 30% × 1/600 = 0.05%
106. d C1V1 = C2V2
45 mg/mL × V1 = 9 mg/mL × 750 mL
V1 (volume of stock) = 150 mL
107. b 2.50 g ÷ 400 mL = 0.625 g/100 mL = 0.00625
0.00625 × 100 = 0.625%
108. a 4.5% solution = 45 mg/mL
45 mg × 500 mL = 22,500 mg
22,500 mg ÷ 1000 mg/g = 22.5 g
109. a 22 lb ÷ 2.2 kg = 10 kg
10 kg × 0.2 mg/kg = 2 mg
110. b Total dilution = (1:10) × (1:3) × (1:5) × (1:3) = 1:450
Total dilution factor = 450
[O] = [F] × DF = 100 µg/mL × 450 = 45,000 µg/mL = 45 mg/mL = 4.5%
111. a 12% v/v solution = 12 mL/100 mL = X mL/275 mL
100X = 12 × 275
12 × 275 = 3300/100 = 33 mL
112. c 4500 mg/3.6 L = 4.5 g/3600 mL = 0.125 g/100 mL = 0.125%.
113. b There are 15 cubic centimeters (cc), or milliliters (mL), in a tablespoon. Another way to think of this is that there are 5 mL in a teaspoon and 3 teaspoons (or 15 mL) in a tablespoon.
114. b The gram is the basic unit of mass in the metric system; 1 kilogram = 103 g; 1 milligram = 10^{-3} g; 1 microgram = 10^{-6} g.
115. c 1200 mg ÷ 375 mg/mL = 3.2 mL
116. b 1 kg = 1000 g
117. d pg = picogram
1 pg = 10^{-12} g
24.3 pg = 24.3 × 10^{-12} g
118. a fl = femtoliter
1 fl = 10 –15 L
66.5 fl = 66.5 × 10 –15 L
119. c The meter is the basic unit of length in the metric system; 1 millimeter = 10^{-3} meters; 1 centimeter = 10^{-2} meters; 1 kilometer = 10^{3} meters.
120. c 1 km = 10^{3} m or 10^{6} mm; so 485 km = 4.85 × 10^{8} mm
121. b 250 cc = 250 mL = 0.25 L
122. c 1 ton = 1000 kg
1 kg = 2.2 lb
2.2 lb × 1000 = 2200 lb
123. c 1 cm = 10 mm = 10,000 µ (microns)
124. d 55 lb ÷ 2.2 lb/kg = 25 kg
125. a 1 oz = 28.4 g
1 g = 1000 mg
1000 mg × 28.4 g = 28,400 mg
28,400 mg × 8 = 227,200 mg
126. c 1 in = 2.5 cm
2.5 cm × 10 = 25 cm
127. b 3.5 L = 3500 mL
3500 mL ÷ 40 = 87.5 mL
128. b C1V1 = C2V2
2.2 mg/mL × V1 = 0.5 mg/mL × 40 mL; V1 = 9.1 mL
129. b 20 kg × 2 mg/kg/day = 40 mg/day (40 mg will be added to the 1-L bag of fluids)
40 mg/day ÷ 5 mg/mL = 8 mL
130. a 150 mL × 25 = 3750 mL

131. a 20 mL + 380 mL = 400 mL
Dilution = 20:400 = 1:20
[O] = [F] × DF = 0.75% × 20 = 15%
132. d 1:10,000 = 0.01 = 0.1 mg/mL
133. b The calculation is the same regardless of what type of fluid is delivered.
134. c 20 mL/h ÷ 60 min/h × 60 drops/mL = 20 drops/min
135. b 1 L = 1000 mL
1000 mL ÷ 8 h = 125 mL/h
125 mL/h ÷ 60 min/h × 20 drops/mL = 42 drops/min
136. b Know your metric conversions and watch your decimal places. 1 mg = 1000 μg.
137. c 1 mg = 103 μg
138. c Study apothecary and household measurements, as well as the metric system. 1 gr = 64 mg, so ½ gr = 32 mg.
139. d Don't confuse abbreviations. g = gram; gr = grain; 1 gr = 64 mg.
140. d 7.5 kg × 2 mg/kg = 15 mg
15 mg ÷ 5 mg = 3 tablets
141. c 35 kg × 2.2 lb/kg = 15.9 kg
15.9 kg × 2.2 mg/kg = 35 mg
1/2 gr = 32.4 mg; therefore, you would administer 1 half grain tablet.
142. a 750 mg ÷ 500 mg tablets = 1.5 tablets/dose
1.5 tablets × 2 = 3 tablets/day
3 tablets × 10 days = 30 tablets
143. c 12.5 mg ÷ 5 mL = 2.5 mg/mL
25 mg ÷ 2.5 mg/mL = 10 mL
144. c Mannitol = 200 mg/mL or 0.2 g/mL
0.5 g/kg = 500 mg/kg
44 ÷ 2.2 = 20 kg
20 kg × 500 mg/kg = 10,000 mg
10,000 mg ÷ 200 mg/mL = 50 mL
145. c % means "grams per hundred milliliters." Therefore, 10% = 10 g/100 mL or 100 mg/mL.
146. b The order tells you what volume to draw up.
147. c 4% = 40 mg/mL or 4 g/100 mL
4 g/100 mL = 5X
X = 124 mL
148. c 0.2 mg = 200 μg
200 μg ÷ 400 μg/mL= 0.5 mL
149. a 20 mg ÷ 25 mg/mL = 0.8 mL
150. a 30 mEq/15 mL = 2 mEq/mL
2X = 20 mEq
X = 10 mL
151. c 50 mL/h ÷ 1 h/60 min × 60 drops/mL = 50 drops/min
152. c 3 L= 3000 mL ÷ 24 h = 125 mL/h
125 mL/h ÷ 1 h/60 min × 15 drops/mL = 31 drops/min
153. b Current drip rate is 7 drops/15 s or 28 drops/min. Therefore, double the drip rate to obtain 60 drops/min.
154. b 1000 mL ÷ 650 mL = 350 mL remain
10 h – 5 h = 5 h remain
350 mL ÷ 5 h × 1 h/60 min × 15 drops/mL = 17.5 drops/min
155. d 750 mL –300 mL = 450 mL remain
6 h – 2 h = 4 h remain
450 mL ÷ 4 h × 1 h/60 min × 20 drops/mL = 37.5 drops/min
156. d 500 mL – 150 mL = 350 mL remain
6 h – 4 h = 2 h remain
350 mL ÷ 2 h × 1 h/60 min × 20 drops/mL = 58 drops/min
157. d C1V1 = C2V2
50 × X = 5 × (1000 + X); solve for X
158. b 25 mg/5 mL = 12.5 mg/2.5 mL
2.5 mL × 3 doses/day = 7.5 mL/day total
30 mL ÷ 7.5 mL = 4 days
159. a 4 IU/mL × 250 mL = 1000 IU
1000 IU/1 mL is available; therefore, 1 mL will be added to 250 mL.
160. d 1 L = 1000 mL
161. b cc and mL are equivalent.
162. d 1 kg = 2.2 lb; 5 kg × 2.2 lb/kg = 11 lb
163. b 1 kg = 1000 g; 354 g ÷ 1000 g/kg = 0.354 kg
164. d 1,000,000 μg = 1 g; 450 μg ÷ 1,000,000 μg/g = 0.00045 g
165. d 3700 cc = 3700 mL = 3.7 L
166. b 11 lb ÷ 2.2 lb/kg = 5 kg
167. c 1 g = 1,000,000 μg; 6.2 g = 6,200,000 μg
168. b 0.5 g/mL = 50 g/100 mL
169. c 500 kg × 2.2 lb/kg = 1100 lb
170. c 1 dram = ⅛ oz
20 dram × ⅛ oz = 2.5 oz
171. d 1 gr = 65 mg
120 gr × 65 mg = 7800 mg
172. a 1 gr = 65 mg
45 gr × 65 mg = 2925 mg/30 mL
2925 mg ÷ 30 mL = 97.5 mg/mL; round up to 100 mg/mL.
173. b 1 dram = ⅛ oz
12 dram × ⅛ oz = 1.5 oz
1 oz = 20 mL
1.5 oz x 30 mL = 45 mL
174. c 1 gr = 65 mg; 120 ÷ 65 mg = 0.5 mg
175. d 2 qt = 64 oz
176. a 1 oz = 30 mL; therefore, 14 oz × 30 mL = 420 mL.
177. c 1 tbs = 15 mL × 6 tbs = 90 mL × 2 = 180 mL or 1.8 L
178. c 1 tbs = 15 mL and 1 oz = 30 mL. Therefore, ½ oz or 7 oz = 15 mL.
179. b 1 tbs = 15 mL or ½ oz
16 oz = 1 pt
32 oz = 1 qt
2 tbs bid = 4 tbs daily or 15 mL × 4 = 60 mL
60 mL ÷ 30 mL/oz = 2 oz
2 oz/day × 16 days = 32 oz or 1 qt
180. d 1.5 tsp × 2 = 3 tsp/day
3 tsp × 14 days = 42 tsp total
3 tsp = 1 tbs
42 tsp ÷ 3 tsp = 14 tbs
181. c 1 tsp = 5 mL; 5 mL × 3 = 15 mL or 3 tsp
182. c 1 tbs = 15 mL
There are 7 days in "every other day dosing" for 2 weeks. 15 mL × 7 = 105 mL.
183. d 40% = 400 mg/mL
554 kg × 2.2 lb/kg = 1218.8 lb
121.8 × 10 mg/lb = 12,1808 g
12,188 mg ÷ 400 mg/mL = 30.5 mL
184. c 22.2% = 222 mg/mL
45 lb × 50 mg/lb = 2250 mg
2250 mg ÷ 222 mg/mL = 10 mL
1 tsp = 5 mL
10 mL ÷ 5 mL = 2 tsp
185. b 900 lb ÷ 2.2 lb/kg = 409 kg

409 kg × 20,000 IU/kg = 8,181,818 IU
8,181,818 IU ÷ 300,000 IU/mL = 27 mL

186. b 0.22% solution = 2.2 mg/mL
990 lb ÷ 2.2 lb/kg = 450 kg
450 kg × 0.044 mg/kg = 19.8 mg
19.8 mg ÷ 2.2 mg/mL = 9 mL
9 mL × 15 days = 135 mL

187. a 65 lb ÷ 2.2 lb/kg = 29.5 kg
Butorphanol: 29.5 kg × 0.2 mg/kg = 5.9 mg
5.9 mg ÷ 10 mg/mL= 0.59 mL

188. a 65 lb ÷ 2.2 lb/kg = 29.5 kg
Acepromazine: 29.5 kg × 0.05 mg/kg = 1.48 mg
1.48 mg ÷ 10 mg/mL = 0.15 mL

189. b 65 lb ÷ 2.2 lb/kg = 29.5 kg
Atropine: 29.5 kg × 0.02 mg/kg = 0.59 mg
0.59 mg ÷ 0.2 mg/mL= 3.0 mL

190. a 700 lb ÷ 2.2 lb/kg = 318 kg
Butorphanol: 318 g × 0.02 mg/kg = 6.36 mg
6.36 mg ÷ 10 mg/mL = 0.6 mL

191. b 700 lb ÷ 2.2 lb/kg = 318 kg
Xylazine: 318 g × 0.2 mg/kg = 63.6 mg
63.6 mg ÷ 10 mg/mL= 6.4 mL

192. b 700 lb ÷ 2.2 lb/kg = 318 kg
Ketamine: 318 g × 2.2 mg/kg = 700 mg
700 mg ÷ 100 mg/mL = 7 mL

193. b 100 mg ÷ 50 mg = 2 tablets

194. b 35 mg ÷ 100 mg/mL = 0.35 mL

195. a 10 lb ÷ 2.2 lb/kg = 4.54 kg
4.54 kg × 5 mg = 22.7 mg; 1 tablet will be administered.

196. b 25 lb ÷ 2.2 lb/kg = 11.36 kg
11.36 kg × 100 mg/kg = 1136 mg
1136 mg ÷ 100 mg/mL = 11 mL

197. c 25 mg ÷ 20 mg/mL = 1.25 mL

198. d 4 lb ÷ 2.2 lb/kg = 1.8 kg
1.8 kg × 0.04 mg/kg = 0.07 mg
0.07 mg ÷ 10 mg/mL = 0.1 mL

199. d 1 tablet every 8 hours = 3 tablets/day
3 tablets/day × 5 days = 15 tablets to be dispensed

200. c 25 lb ÷ 2.2 lb/kg = 11.36 kg
11.36 kg × 5 mg/kg = 56.8 mg on day 1
56.8 mg ÷ 125 mg = 0.45 tablets or ½ tablet for day 1
11.36 kg × 2.5 mg/kg = 28.4 mg on days 2–6
28.4 mg ÷ 125 mg = 0.22 tablets or ¼ tablet for days 2–6
Dispense 2 tablets.

201. c 22 lb ÷ 2.2 lb/kg = 10 kg
10 kg × 66 mL/kg/24 h = 660 mL/24 h
660 mL ÷ 24 h = 27.5 mL/h

202. d 7 lb ÷ 2.2 lb/kg = 3.18 kg
3.18 kg × 11 mL/kg/h = 35 mL/h

203. c 120 lb ÷ 2.2 lb/kg = 54.54 kg
54.54 kg × 132 mL/kg/24 h = 7199 mL/24 h
7199 mL ÷ 24 h = 300 mL/h

204. d 32 lb ÷ 2.2 lb/kg = 14.54 kg
14.54 kg × 11 mL/kg/h = 160 mL/h

205. d 50 lb ÷ 2.2 lb/kg = 22.7 kg
22.7 kg × 132 mL/kg/24 h = 3000 mL/24 h

206. c 4.5 lb ÷ 2.2 lb/kg = 2 kg
2 kg × 66 mL/kg/24 h = 132 mL/24 h

207. a 2% = 20 mg/mL
33 lb ÷ 2.2 lb/kg = 15 kg
15 kg × 2 mg/kg = 30 mg
30 mg ÷ 20 mg/mL = 1.5 mL

208. a 3.2 mL × 300,000 U/mL

209. d 66 lb ÷ 2.2 lb/kg = 30 kg
30 kg × 0.6 mg/kg = 18 mg
18 mg ÷ 5 mg/mL = 3.6 mL

210. a 66 lb ÷ 2.2 lb/kg = 30 kg
30 kg × 0.6 mg/kg = 18 mg

211. d 12 lb ÷ 2.2 lb/kg = 5.45 kg
5.45 kg × 2 units/kg = 11 u

212. a 12 lb 2.2 lb/kg = 5.45 kg
5.45 kg × 2 units/kg = 11 units
11 u ÷ 40 units/mL = 0.27 mL

213. b 20 mL/h ÷ 3600 s/h × 60 drops/mL = 0.33 drops/s
Apply the equation: 1 ÷ 0.33 drops/s = 1 drops/3 s.

214. b 10% solution = 100 mg/mL
100 mg/mL ÷ 1.2 mL = 83 mg

215. d 60 lb × 3 mg/lb = 180 mg
180 mg ÷ 200 mg/mL = 0.9 mL

216. b 3 mL × 3 doses/day = 9 mL
9 mL × 30 days = 270 mL
30 mL = 1 oz of fluid
270 mL/30 mL = 9 oz

217. a 5 lb × 40 kcal/lb/day = 200 kcal/day
200 kcal ÷ 120 kcal/cup = 1.66 cups
1.66 cups ÷ 2 feedings/day = 0.8 cups/feeding

218. a 30 g ÷ 1000 g/kg = 0.03 kg
0.03 kg × 100 mg/kg = 3 mg
3 mg ÷ 100 mg/mL = 0.03 mL

219. b 40 mEq/L = 0.04 mEq/mL
1 mEq ÷ 0.04 mEq/mL = 25 mL/h

220. c 5 mg/h at 50 mL/h = 5 mg ÷ 50 mL = 100 mg/1000 mL
100 mg ÷ 50 mg/mL = 2 mL

221. c 45 kg × 2.2 lb/kg = 99 lb

222. c 50% Dextrose = 50 mg/mL
50 mg/mL × 6 mL = 300 mg

SECTION 4

1. b An intact male cat is referred to as a tom. A sire is the male parent of his offspring. A dam is the female parent to her offspring. A stud is an intact male dog. Colville JL, Oien SA, Clinical Veterinary Language, ed 1, Elsevier, 2014, p. 2.
2. b Poly- is a prefix that is correctly defined as many. The word root arthr refers to a joint. The suffix -pathy refers to disease. The term *chondro-* refers to cartilage. Colville JL, Oien SA, Clinical Veterinary Language, ed 1, Elsevier, 2014, p. 19.
3. b A group of turkeys is referred to as a rafter. A poult is a young turkey of either sex. A paddling is a group of ducks. A gaggle is a group of geese. Colville JL, Oien SA, Clinical Veterinary Language, ed 1, Elsevier, 2014, p. 6.
4. a Etiopathology refers to the cause of disease. Neogenic refers to new growth or regeneration. Pathology refers to the study of disease. Idiopathic refers to a disease of unknown origin. Colville JL, Oien SA, Clinical Veterinary Language, ed 1, Elsevier, 2014, p. 23.
5. c The prefix osteo- refers to bone. The prefix myelo- refers to bone marrow. The prefix corpo- refers to body. The prefix cerebro- refers to the brain. Colville JL, Oien SA, Clinical Veterinary Language, ed 1, Elsevier, 2014, p. 388.

6. d Kaliopenia refers to less than the normal amount of potassium. Hypernatremia refers to the excess amount of sodium in the blood. Hyperkalemia refers to the excess amount of potassium. Natriuresis refers to the excretion of an abnormal amount of sodium in the urine. Colville JL, Oien SA, Clinical Veterinary Language, ed 1, Elsevier, 2014, p. 342.
7. d The terms *clowder, cluster*, and *pounce* all refer to a group of cats. Colville JL, Oien SA, Clinical Veterinary Language, ed 1, Elsevier, 2014, p. 2.
8. c A murmur is an atypical heart sound associated with a functional or structural valve abnormality. An arrhythmia is an abnormal heart rate or rhythm. Fibrillation is the rapid, irregular myocardial contractions resulting in loss of a simultaneous heartbeat and pulse. Infarct is a localized area of tissue that is dying or dead because of a lack of blood supply. Colville JL, Oien SA, Clinical Veterinary Language, ed 1, Elsevier, 2014, p. 176.
9. c A whelp or pup is a young canine. A bitch is an intact female dog. A kitten is a young female cat. A sire is the male parent of his offspring. Colville JL, Oien SA, Clinical Veterinary Language, ed 1, Elsevier, 2014, p. 2.
10. b The prefix myring- refers to eardrum. The prefix oto- refers to ear. The prefix embryo- refers to embryo. The prefix vacu- refers to empty. Colville JL, Oien SA, Clinical Veterinary Language, ed 1, Elsevier, 2014, p. 390.
11. d An intact male horse that is older than 4 years is referred to as a stallion. A gelding is a castrated male horse. A mare is an intact female horse older than 4 years. A colt is an intact male horse younger than 4 years. Colville JL, Oien SA, Clinical Veterinary Language, ed 1, Elsevier, 2014, p. 3.
12. a An equine that is around 1 year of age is referred to as a yearling. Foaling is the process of giving birth to a colt or filly. A weanling is a young equine that has been weaned from its mother. A filly is an intact female younger than 4 years. Colville JL, Oien SA, Clinical Veterinary Language, ed 1, Elsevier, 2014, p. 3.
13. c An intact male donkey is referred to as a jack, whereas a jenny is an intact female donkey. A dam is the female parent of her offspring and a sire is the male parent of his offspring. Colville JL, Oien SA, Clinical Veterinary Language, ed 1, Elsevier, 2014, p. 3.
14. b A female calf (usually sterile) that is born twin to a bull calf is referred to as a freemartin. Freshening refers to the process of a dairy-cow calving. A heifer is a young cow that has not yet had her first calf. A cow is an intact female bovine. Colville JL, Oien SA, Clinical Veterinary Language, ed 1, Elsevier, 2014, p. 5.
15. d A castrated/neutered male ovine is referred to as a wether, whereas an intact male sheep is known as a ram. A young ovine is referred to as a lamb and the process of giving birth to lambs is referred to as lambing. Colville JL, Oien SA, Clinical Veterinary Language, ed 1, Elsevier, 2014, p. 5.
16. c Farrowing is the process of giving birth to pigs. Freshening is the process whereby dairy goats give birth to kids. A stag is a male that is castrated/neutered after sexual maturity. Kidding is the process of giving birth to kids. Colville JL, Oien SA, Clinical Veterinary Language, ed 1, Elsevier, 2014, p. 5.
17. b A young female pig that has not yet given birth is referred to as a gilt. A dam is the female parent of her offspring. A sow is an intact female pig. A stag is a male that has been castrated after sexual maturity. Colville JL, Oien SA, Clinical Veterinary Language, ed 1, Elsevier, 2014, p. 5.
18. b A cockerel is a young male chicken between 10 and 32 weeks of age. A rooster is an intact male chicken, whereas a capon is a castrated male chicken. A pullet is an immature female chicken between 10 and 32 weeks of age. Colville JL, Oien SA, Clinical Veterinary Language, ed 1, Elsevier, 2014, p. 6.
19. b An egg-type chicken more than 32 weeks of age is referred to as a layer. A roaster is a meat-type chicken sent to the market between 9 and 11 weeks of age. A hen is an intact female chicken, and a chick is a very young chicken. Colville JL, Oien SA, Clinical Veterinary Language, ed 1, Elsevier, 2014, p. 6.
20. a An intact male duck is referred to as a drake, whereas an intact female duck is referred to as a duck. An immature duck of either sex is referred to as a duckling and a poult is a young turkey. Colville JL, Oien SA, Clinical Veterinary Language, ed 1, Elsevier, 2014, p. 7.
21. d An intact male ferret is referred to as a hob. A gib is a castrated male ferret, whereas a jill is an intact female ferret. A sprite is a spayed female ferret. Colville JL, Oien SA, Clinical Veterinary Language, ed 1, Elsevier, 2014, p. 8.
22. b The prefix blephar- refers to eyelid. The prefixes oculo-, opthalm-, and opt- all refer to the eye. The prefixes adipo-, lip-, and steat- all refer to fat. The prefix pseudo- refers to false. Colville JL, Oien SA, Clinical Veterinary Language, ed 1, Elsevier, 2014, p. 390.
23. b A zoonotic disease is transmitted from animals to humans. Zoology is the study of animal life. Enzootic is a disease found in nearly every animal of a species within a limited geographical area. Epizootic is a disease that appears suddenly and spreads rapidly throughout a large geographical area. Colville JL, Oien SA, Clinical Veterinary Language, ed 1, Elsevier, 2014, p. 16.
24. a Morbidity is the number of animals in a population that become sick. Mortality is the number of animals in a population that die from a disease. Chronic is the slow onset of an abnormal condition that lasts a long time. Acute is the sudden onset of an abnormal condition with a short duration. Colville JL, Oien SA, Clinical Veterinary Language, ed 1, Elsevier, 2014, p. 17.
25. b The suffix -itis refers to inflammation. The suffix -pathy refers to disease. Pseudo- is a prefix referring to false. Osteo- is a prefix referring to bone. Colville JL, Oien SA, Clinical Veterinary Language, ed 1, Elsevier, 2014, p. 17.
26. c Chondro- refers to cartilage, whereas osteo- refers to bone. Poly- refers to many and -itis refers to inflammation. Colville JL, Oien SA, Clinical Veterinary Language, ed 1, Elsevier, 2014, p. 18.
27. b The prefix hyster- refers to uterus. The term *salping-* refers to oviduct. The term *oophor-* refers to ovary. The suffix -ectomy refers to surgical removal. Colville JL, Oien SA, Clinical Veterinary Language, ed 1, Elsevier, 2014, p. 19.
28. a The suffix -ac refers to pertaining to. The suffix -ate refers to act on. The suffix -ium refers to a structure or a thing. The suffix -ation refers to a condition. Colville JL, Oien SA, Clinical Veterinary Language, ed 1, Elsevier, 2014, p. 21.

29. b In vivo refers to something within a living body. In vitro refers to something within a glass, test tube, or container outside the living body. Benign refers to a condition that does not recur and has a favorable outlook for recovery. Infection is an invasion and multiplication of a disease-causing organism in a body tissue. Colville JL, Oien SA, Clinical Veterinary Language, ed 1, Elsevier, 2014, p. 22.

30. b The term *malignant* refers to becoming progressively worse, recurring, and leading to death. Remission refers to improvement in or absence of signs of disease. Exacerbation refers to worsening severity of a disease. Idiopathic refers to a disease of unknown origin. Colville JL, Oien SA, Clinical Veterinary Language, ed 1, Elsevier, 2014, p. 22.

31. a Chondro- refers to cartilage, and -ology refers to the study of something. Therefore, chondrology refers to the study of cartilage. Oncology refers to the study of malignancy. Cardiology refers to the study of the cardiovascular system. Osteology refers to the study of bones. Colville JL, Oien SA, Clinical Veterinary Language, ed 1, Elsevier, 2014, p. 22.

32. c The term *neoplasm* refers to any new or abnormal growth. Dysplasia refers to the process of abnormal or difficult growth. A malignant neoplasm is a malignant growth of tissue; the term *neoplasm* by itself only refers to any new growth of tissue. Death of tissue is termed *necrosis*. Colville JL, Oien SA, Clinical Veterinary Language, ed 1, Elsevier, 2014, p. 25.

33. a The term *diastole* refers to the resting phase of a heartbeat that occurs between the filling of the lower chambers of the heart and the start of contraction. Systole refers to the period of ventricular contraction of the cardiac cycle. Arrhythmia is the improper beating of the heart either irregular, too fast, or too slow. Tachycardia refers to an abnormally fast heartbeat. Colville JL, Oien SA, Clinical Veterinary Language, ed 1, Elsevier, 2014, p. 25.

34. a Medial refers to toward the median plane. Lateral refers to away from the median plane. Anterior refers to toward the ventral or front surface. Posterior refers to toward the dorsal or back surface. Colville JL, Oien SA, Clinical Veterinary Language, ed 1, Elsevier, 2014, p. 32.

35. b Rostral refers to toward the nose when referring to the head. Cranial refers to toward the head end of the body. Caudal refers to toward the tail end of the body. The posterior surface of the body is also known as the dorsal surface. Colville JL, Oien SA, Clinical Veterinary Language, ed 1, Elsevier, 2014, p. 33.

36. b The transverse plane divides the body into cranial and caudal parts. The coronal plane divides the body into anterior and posterior parts. The longitudinal plane divides the body into left and right parts. Proximal refers to a position on a limb closer to the point of attachment. Colville JL, Oien SA, Clinical Veterinary Language, ed 1, Elsevier, 2014, p. 33.

37. c Hemothorax refers to a collection of blood in the cranial portion of the ventral cavity. Pneumothorax refers to a collapsed lung. Pneumonia refers to fluid within the lungs. Hemostasis refers to an interruption of the blood flow to a part of the body. Colville JL, Oien SA, Clinical Veterinary Language, ed 1, Elsevier, 2014, p. 50.

38. b Histiocytosis refers to an abnormal presence of tissue cells in the blood. Histology is the study of tissues. Karyogenic refers to producing a nucleus. Homeostasis refers to the self-regulating process by which the systems maintain stability. Colville JL, Oien SA, Clinical Veterinary Language, ed 1, Elsevier, 2014, p. 50.

39. c Myelodysplasia refers to an abnormal development of muscles. An adipocyte refers to cells specialized for the storage of fat. Neoplasm refers to an abnormal growth of tissue. Bradycardia refers to a heartbeat that is slower than normal. Colville JL, Oien SA, Clinical Veterinary Language, ed 1, Elsevier, 2014, p. 51.

40. d An abrasion is a skin scrape. An abscess is a localized collection of pus. Alopecia refers to the loss of hair, wool, or feathers. A carbuncle is a group of furuncles in adjacent hairs. Colville JL, Oien SA, Clinical Veterinary Language, ed 1, Elsevier, 2014, p. 70.

41. b Ecchymosis refers to blood leaking from a ruptured vessel into subcutaneous tissue. Cicatrix is a scar. Eschar is dried serum, blood, pus, or a scab. Fissure is a crack-like lesion in the skin. Colville JL, Oien SA, Clinical Veterinary Language, ed 1, Elsevier, 2014, p. 70.

42. a Excoriate refers to scratching the skin. A furuncle is a boil or skin abscess. Eschar is dried serum, blood, or pus. A scar is referred to as a cicatrix. Colville JL, Oien SA, Clinical Veterinary Language, ed 1, Elsevier, 2014, p. 70.

43. d A keloid is an overgrowth of scar tissue at the site of injury. A papule is a small, solid, usually pointed elevation of the skin. A petechia consists of tiny bleeds or bruising within the dermal layer. A laceration refers to a rough or jagged skin tear. Colville JL, Oien SA, Clinical Veterinary Language, ed 1, Elsevier, 2014, p. 70.

44. c An ulcer is a circumscribed crater-like lesion of the skin or mucous membrane. A wheal is a circumscribed, elevated papule caused by localized edema. Suppurate means to produce or to discharge pus. A papule is a small, solid pointed elevation of the skin. Colville JL, Oien SA, Clinical Veterinary Language, ed 1, Elsevier, 2014, p. 70.

45. b The suffix -emia refers to a blood condition that is usually abnormal. The suffix -staxis refers to bleeding. The suffix -clast refers to breaking into pieces. The suffix -pnea refers to breath or respiration. Colville JL, Oien SA, Clinical Veterinary Language, ed 1, Elsevier, 2014, p. 388.

46. b A callus is a bridge that forms as part of the healing process across the two halves of a bone. A condyle is the smooth end of a bone that forms part of a joint. A crest is a raised ridge along the surface of a bone. Cull refers to the removal of an animal from a herd. Colville JL, Oien SA, Clinical Veterinary Language, ed 1, Elsevier, 2014, p. 113.

47. b Luxation refers to a joint dislocation in which the joint is displaced or goes out of alignment. Subluxation refers to a partial dislocation of a joint. A fracture is a break or rupture. Olecranon refers to the large process on the proximal end of the ulna that forms the point of the elbow. Colville JL, Oien SA, Clinical Veterinary Language, ed 1, Elsevier, 2014, p. 113.

48. c A rough projection on a bone is known as a tuberosity. A suture is the line of the junction of two bones forming an immovable joint. A wing is a transverse process on the first cervical vertebrae. Trochanter refers to two knobs at the proximal end of the femur where the muscles of the thigh and pelvis attach. Colville JL, Oien SA, Clinical Veterinary Language, ed 1, Elsevier, 2014, p. 113.

49. b Osteomalacia refers to the softening of bones. Osteopetrosis refers to the hardening of bone. A multiple myeloma refers to the collection of abnormal cells that accumulate within the bones. Pachydermia refers to thickened skin. Colville JL, Oien SA, Clinical Veterinary Language, ed 1, Elsevier, 2014, p. 114.

50. b Hypoplasia is an incomplete development of an organ or tissue. Hyperplasia is an overgrowth of tissue. Osteoporosis refers to the thinning of bones. Ankylosis is a condition of stiffness. Colville JL, Oien SA, Clinical Veterinary Language, ed 1, Elsevier, 2014, p. 114.

51. b A small opening or perforation is referred to as a foramen. A fossa is a depression, trench, or hollow area. An exacerbation is an increase in the severity of a disease or in clinical signs. A process is a natural overgrowth or projection. Colville JL, Oien SA, Clinical Veterinary Language, ed 1, Elsevier, 2014, p. 113.

52. b Tendons connect muscles to bones. Ligaments connect bones to bones. A foramen refers to an opening or perforation. A process is a natural overgrowth or projection. Colville JL, Oien SA, Clinical Veterinary Language, ed 1, Elsevier, 2014, p. 113.

53. a Cartilage provides a smooth joint surface so that bones can move freely over one another. Ligaments connect bones to bones. A callus is a bridge that forms as part of the healing process across two halve of a bone fracture. A fossa is a depression or hollow area. Colville JL, Oien SA, Clinical Veterinary Language, ed 1, Elsevier, 2014, p. 113.

54. c The prefix chondro- refers to cartilage. The prefix osteo- refers to bone. The prefix myelo- refers to muscle. The prefix bucco- refers to cheek. Colville JL, Oien SA, Clinical Veterinary Language, ed 1, Elsevier, 2014, p. 389.

55. b Rhabdomyoma refers to a rare benign tumor derived from striated muscle. Cervicomuscular refers to muscles of the neck. Myopathology is the study of muscle diseases. Rhabdomyosarcoma is a malignant tumor that starts in muscle. Colville JL, Oien SA, Clinical Veterinary Language, ed 1, Elsevier, 2014, p. 125.

56. b Myofibrosis refers to an abnormal condition of muscle fibers. Myospasm refers to spasms of the muscles. Myotonia refers to a disorder in which muscles are slow to relax. An electromyography is a technique used for evaluating and recording the electrical activity produced by skeletal muscles. Colville JL, Oien SA, Clinical Veterinary Language, ed 1, Elsevier, 2014, p. 125.

57. b Endomysium is a connective tissue membrane that surrounds each muscle fiber. Epimysium is a connective tissue membrane that covers and defines the entire muscle. Myopathy is a muscle disease. Sarcoma is a tumor of skeletal muscle. Colville JL, Oien SA, Clinical Veterinary Language, ed 1, Elsevier, 2014, p. 126.

58. b The prefix cephal- refers to the head. The prefix scler- refers to hard. The prefix acous- refers to hearing. The prefix cardio- refers to the heart. Colville JL, Oien SA, Clinical Veterinary Language, ed 1, Elsevier, 2014, p. 391.

59. a Skeletal muscle is also known as striated muscle. Smooth muscles are found in hollow organs such as blood vessels, GI tract, bladder, and uterus. Cardiac muscle is an involuntary striated muscle found only in the heart. Colville JL, Oien SA, Clinical Veterinary Language, ed 1, Elsevier, 2014, p. 127.

60. b The term *ipsilateral* refers to something that is located on or affects the same side of the body. Contralateral refers to something that is on the opposite side of the affected side of the body. Admaxillary refers to something that is near or connected to the maxilla or jawbone. Abductor refers to movement away from the point of origin. Colville JL, Oien SA, Clinical Veterinary Language, ed 1, Elsevier, 2014, p. 132.

61. b Hemialgia refers to pain that is affecting only half of the body. Semiconscious refers to being only half awake. Analgesia refers to the inability to feel pain. Bicaudal refers to having two tails. Colville JL, Oien SA, Clinical Veterinary Language, ed 1, Elsevier, 2014, p. 134.

62. a Tetradactyly refers to the presence of four digits on a foot. Polydactyl refers to the congenital anomaly of having more than the normal number of toes on one or more paws. Multiarticular pertains to having too many joints. Quadrilateral refers to having four sides. Colville JL, Oien SA, Clinical Veterinary Language, ed 1, Elsevier, 2014, p. 135.

63. a Panosteitis refers to inflammation of all bones or inflammation of every part of one bone. Polypathia refers to the presence of many diseases at the same time. Pandemic refers to a widespread disease across a region, across continents, or worldwide. Osteoporosis refers to weak or brittle bones. Colville JL, Oien SA, Clinical Veterinary Language, ed 1, Elsevier, 2014, p. 135.

64. c The word root digitorum refers to digit. The word root costals refers to ribs. The word root carpi refers to wrist. The word root femoris refers to thigh. Colville JL, Oien SA, Clinical Veterinary Language, ed 1, Elsevier, 2014, p. 137.

65. c The word root brachii refers to the upper foreleg. The word root tibialis refers to the shin bone. The word root femoris refers to the thigh bone. The word root scapularis refers to the shoulder blade. Colville JL, Oien SA, Clinical Veterinary Language, ed 1, Elsevier, 2014, p. 137.

66. b Extrinsic muscles attach the limb to the body. Intrinsic muscles originate and insert on the limb. Adductor muscles move the limb toward the body. Abductor muscles move the limb away from the body. Colville JL, Oien SA, Clinical Veterinary Language, ed 1, Elsevier, 2014, p. 139.

67. a Amyoplasia refers to the lack of muscle formation or development. Myoplegia refers to the paralysis of muscles. Hemiparesis refers to muscular weakness or partial paralysis restricted to one side of the body. Myopathy refers to any muscle disease. Colville JL, Oien SA, Clinical Veterinary Language, ed 1, Elsevier, 2014, p. 142.

68. b Rhabdomyolysis is the destruction of the rod-shaped muscle cells. Hypertrophy is the increase in the volume of an organ or tissue resulting from the enlargement of its component cells. Hypoplasia is the underdevelopment or incomplete development of a tissue or organ. Necrosis refers to the death of body tissue. Colville JL, Oien SA, Clinical Veterinary Language, ed 1, Elsevier, 2014, p. 143.

69. d Aponeurosis is a sheet-like dense fibrous collagenous connective tissue that binds muscles together or connects muscle to bone. Avulsion is an acute tendon injury in which the tendon is forcibly torn away from its attachment side on the bone. Rigor mortis is the temporary muscular stiffening that follows death. Shivers refer to the rapid involuntary muscle contractions that release waste heat. Colville JL, Oien SA, Clinical Veterinary Language, ed 1, Elsevier, 2014, p. 146.

70. a The prefix onych- refers to claw or nail. The prefix cyt- refers to the cell. The prefix coagul- refers to the clotting process. The prefix corne- refers to cornea. Colville JL, Oien SA, Clinical Veterinary Language, ed 1, Elsevier, 2014, p. 389.

71. c Clonic spasm refers to alternating spasm and muscle relaxation. Spasm refers to an acute involuntary muscle contraction. Tonic spasm refers to a continuous spasm. Tetanus refers to the painful, sustained muscle contractions caused by toxins. Colville JL, Oien SA, Clinical Veterinary Language, ed 1, Elsevier, 2014, p. 146.

72. b The term *atrophy* refers to wasting away. Appendicular skeleton refers to all four limbs. The term *myotatic* refers to muscle stretch. Myositis refers to inflammation of muscles. Colville JL, Oien SA, Clinical Veterinary Language, ed 1, Elsevier, 2014, p. 152.

73. a Tetraparesis refers to the muscular weakness in all four limbs. Neuritis refers to the inflammation of nerves. Polymyositis refers to the inflammation of many muscles. Tonic spasm refers to a continuous spasm. Colville JL, Oien SA, Clinical Veterinary Language, ed 1, Elsevier, 2014, p. 152.

74. b The suffix -rrhage refers to excessive flow. The suffix -rrhea refers to flow or flowing. The suffix -esthesia refers to sensation. The suffix -extasis refers to expansion or dilation. Colville JL, Oien SA, Clinical Veterinary Language, ed 1, Elsevier, 2014, p. 390.

75. c Acardia refers to the absence of a heart. Cardiomyopathy refers to a disease affecting the muscles of the heart. Auricular hyperplasia refers to the excessive growth of the auricles. Cardiovascular refers to the heart and blood vessels. Colville JL, Oien SA, Clinical Veterinary Language, ed 1, Elsevier, 2014, p. 157.

76. b Atrioventricular refers to the upper and lower chambers of the heart. Atriotomy refers to the surgical incision into the upper chamber of the heart. Valvulosis refers to the diseased condition of a valve. Avascular necrosis is the death of body tissue because the blood supply has been cut off. Colville JL, Oien SA, Clinical Veterinary Language, ed 1, Elsevier, 2014, p. 158.

77. b Hydremia refers to a disorder in which there is an excess of fluid in the blood. Ischemia refers to an inadequate supply of blood to a part of the body. Anemia refers to a low red blood cell count in the body. Apex refers to the narrow pointed bottom of the heart. Colville JL, Oien SA, Clinical Veterinary Language, ed 1, Elsevier, 2014, p. 157.

78. c The prefix eu- refers to good or normal. The prefix aden- refers to a gland. The prefix gluco- refers to glucose. The prefix trich- refers to hair. Colville JL, Oien SA, Clinical Veterinary Language, ed 1, Elsevier, 2014, p. 391.

79. c Interventricular groove or sulcus is the demarcation line that separates the left and right ventricles of the heart. The interventricular septum is the stout wall separating the lower chambers of the heart. The atrium is one of two of the four chambers of the heart. The auricles are the flaps that lie on top of the heart. Colville JL, Oien SA, Clinical Veterinary Language, ed 1, Elsevier, 2014, p. 160.

80. c The pulmonary artery is the vessel responsible for carrying blood to the lungs. The aorta is the main artery leaving the heart that supplies the body with blood. The inferior vena cava is the main vein that returns blood back from the body to the heart. The carotid artery carries blood from the heart to the head. Colville JL, Oien SA, Clinical Veterinary Language, ed 1, Elsevier, 2014, p. 161.

81. b The endocardium is a thin membrane that lines the inside surface of the chamber of the heart. The pericardium is the fibrous connective tissue that covers the outer surface of the heart. The atrium is one of two of the four chambers of the heart. The epicardium is the inner layer of the pericardial sac. Colville JL, Oien SA, Clinical Veterinary Language, ed 1, Elsevier, 2014, p. 162.

82. c The bicuspid valve is also known as the mitral valve because it has two flaps that resembled a bishop's miter or hat. The tricuspid valve has three flaps, not two. The semilunar valve resembles the half-moon or crescent shape. The atrioventricular valve is the valve located between the atria and the ventricle on both sides of the heart. Colville JL, Oien SA, Clinical Veterinary Language, ed 1, Elsevier, 2014, p. 162.

83. a The suffix -tripsy refers to crushing or grinding. The suffix -lytic refers to destruction or dissolving. The suffix -osis refers to disease or an abnormal condition. The suffix -pathy refers to disease. Colville JL, Oien SA, Clinical Veterinary Language, ed 1, Elsevier, 2014, p. 389.

84. a A hemangioma is a benign tumor composed of newly formed blood vessels. A hamartoma is a benign tumor made up of cartilage, muscle, fat, and bone. Hepatoma is a benign tumor of the liver. A hepatocellular carcinoma is a primary malignant tumor of the liver. Colville JL, Oien SA, Clinical Veterinary Language, ed 1, Elsevier, 2014, p. 164.

85. b A rupture of an artery is known as arteriorrhexis. Venostasis refers to the slowing or stopping of the flow of blood in a vein. Arteriostasis refers to the slowing or stopping of the flow of blood in an artery. Hemorrhage refers to the abnormal severe internal or external discharge of blood. Colville JL, Oien SA, Clinical Veterinary Language, ed 1, Elsevier, 2014, p. 165.

86. c The largest artery in an animal's body is known as the aorta, which leaves the heart and travels the length of the body with multiple branches. The carotid artery is a branch of the aorta that carries blood to the brain. The pulmonary artery carries blood from the right ventricle of the heart to the lungs. The inferior vena cava is the main vein in the body that carries blood back to the heart. Colville JL, Oien SA, Clinical Veterinary Language, ed 1, Elsevier, 2014, p. 166.

87. a The prefix ultra- refers to beyond or in excess of. The prefix sub- refers to below or to a decrease. The prefix melano- refers to the color black. The prefix plantar- refers to the back surface of the rear limb. Colville JL, Oien SA, Clinical Veterinary Language, ed 1, Elsevier, 2014, p. 388.

88. a Bradycardia is a slower than normal heart rate. Tachycardia is an abnormally rapid heart rate. An arrhythmia is an irregular rate or rhythm. Arteriostenosis is the narrowing of the arteries. Colville JL, Oien SA, Clinical Veterinary Language, ed 1, Elsevier, 2014, p. 170.

89. b Enlargement of the heart is known as cardiomegaly. Agnathia is the absence of the lower jaw. Dactyledema is the swelling of a digit, finger, or toe. Pericarditis is the inflammation of the pericardium. Colville JL, Oien SA, Clinical Veterinary Language, ed 1, Elsevier, 2014, p. 171.

90. c Ascites is the accumulation of fluid in the abdominal cavity. To auscultate is to evaluate by listening with the aid of a stethoscope. Infarct is a localized area of tissue that is dying or dead because of a lack of blood supply. Edema is the excess fluid accumulation around the cells of connective tissue. Colville JL, Oien SA, Clinical Veterinary Language, ed 1, Elsevier, 2014, p. 176.

91. c Phlebitis is the inflammation of a vein. Arteritis is the inflammation of an artery. Venostasis is an abnormally slow or completely stopped blood flow through a vein. Stenosis is the impedance of the flow of blood through a vessel. Colville JL, Oien SA, Clinical Veterinary Language, ed 1, Elsevier, 2014, p. 177.

92. a An increase in arterial blood pressure is known as hypertension. A decrease in arterial blood pressure is known as hypotension. Edema is the buildup of fluid in tissue. Pleural effusion is fluid within the thoracic cavity. Colville JL, Oien SA, Clinical Veterinary Language, ed 1, Elsevier, 2014, p. 177.

93. d The removal of fluid via a needle inserted into the pericardial sac is known as pericardiocentesis. Effusion is the abnormal buildup of fluid within a space. Pericardial effusion is the buildup of fluid between the layer of the pericardial sac and the epicardium. Cardiac tamponade is when the pericardial sac is so full of fluid that the heart can no longer beat. Colville JL, Oien SA, Clinical Veterinary Language, ed 1, Elsevier, 2014, p. 177.

94. b The suffix -ptosis refers to downward placement. The suffix -ate refers to act on. The suffix -ase refers to enzyme. The suffix -ize refers to engage in a specific activity. Colville JL, Oien SA, Clinical Veterinary Language, ed 1, Elsevier, 2014, p. 390.

95. b The extensive loss of blood resulting from bleeding is termed *exsanguination*. Hematology is the study of the function of diseases of the blood. Electrohemostasis is the stopping of bleeding by means of an electrical device. Anemia is an abnormal red blood cell count. Colville JL, Oien SA, Clinical Veterinary Language, ed 1, Elsevier, 2014, p. 187.

96. a Plasmacytoma refers to an abnormal new growth of plasma cells. A plasmocyte is a plasma cell. Serosanguineous pertains the serum that contains both blood and serous fluid. Polycythemia refers to a condition involving many cells in the blood. Colville JL, Oien SA, Clinical Veterinary Language, ed 1, Elsevier, 2014, p. 187.

97. c Karyoclastic refers to the breaking up of a cell nucleus. The rupture of a nucleus is known as karyorrhexis. Cells that break down cartilage are known as chondroclasts. The condition of many cells in the blood is referred to as polycythemia. Colville JL, Oien SA, Clinical Veterinary Language, ed 1, Elsevier, 2014, p. 188.

98. b Redness of the skin is referred to as erythematous. An erythrocyte is a red blood cell, whereas a leukocyte is a white blood cell. Leukocytosis refers to an abnormally high white blood cell count. Colville JL, Oien SA, Clinical Veterinary Language, ed 1, Elsevier, 2014, p. 188.

99. d The prefix steth- refers to the chest. The prefix baso- refers to chemically basic. The prefix chyl- refers to chyle. The prefix col- refers to colon. Colville JL, Oien SA, Clinical Veterinary Language, ed 1, Elsevier, 2014, p. 389.

100. b A neutrophil is a blood cell that has both pale red and blue granules visible within the cytoplasm. A basophil is a blood cell seen with blue granules in the cytoplasm. An eosinophil is a white blood cell that is stained by eosin. An agranulocyte refers to a type of blood cell that has no colored granules seen within the cytoplasm. Colville JL, Oien SA, Clinical Veterinary Language, ed 1, Elsevier, 2014, p. 189.

101. b Lymphangitis is referred to as the inflammation of lymph vessels. Leukocytosis refers to a high white blood cell count. Lymphoma is cancer of the lymph system. An immunocyte is a cell involved in immunity. Colville JL, Oien SA, Clinical Veterinary Language, ed 1, Elsevier, 2014, p. 189.

102. a Dysphagia refers to difficulty in eating or swallowing. Dystocia refers to a difficult labor or birth. Dysraphism refers to congenital anomalies of the fetus. Aphagia refers to the inability to swallow. Colville JL, Oien SA, Clinical Veterinary Language, ed 1, Elsevier, 2014, p. 190.

103. b A hematoblast is a primitive blood cell. The formation of blood or blood cells in the living body is known as hematopoiesis. Hemoglobin is the protein found in red blood cells. Hemolysis is the destruction of red blood cell membranes. Colville JL, Oien SA, Clinical Veterinary Language, ed 1, Elsevier, 2014, p. 196.

104. c Leukopenia refers to an abnormally low white blood cell count. *Normocytic* is a descriptive term applied to a normal red blood cell size. Leukocytosis refers to a high white blood cell count. Anemia refers to a low red blood cell count. Colville JL, Oien SA, Clinical Veterinary Language, ed 1, Elsevier, 2014, p. 196.

105. b Idiopathic refers to a disease that has an unknown cause. A general term for abnormality is *cytopenia*. Ataxia describes an uncoordinated and dehydrated animal. A blood clot that forms and adheres to the wall of a blood vessel is a thrombus. Colville JL, Oien SA, Clinical Veterinary Language, ed 1, Elsevier, 2014, p. 199.

106. b The prefix cox- refers to the hip. The prefix pyro- refers to heat. The prefix herni- refers to hernia. The prefix humer- refers to the humerus. Colville JL, Oien SA, Clinical Veterinary Language, ed 1, Elsevier, 2014, p. 392.

107. b Hemolytic anemia refers to the increased destruction of erythrocytes, which may occur in the vascular system. Macrocytic anemia refers to red blood cells that are larger than normal. Polychromasia refers to the variation of hemoglobin content within erythrocytes. Hypochromic anemia refers to a condition in which the decrease in hemoglobin is proportionately much greater than the decrease in the number of erythrocytes. Studdert VP, Gay CC, Blood DC, Saunders Comprehensive Veterinary Dictionary, ed 4, Saunders, 2012, p. 54.

108. b Neutropenia refers to an abnormally low number of neutrophils. Pancytopenia refers to an abnormally low number of all blood cells. Monocytosis refers an abnormally high number of monocytes in the blood. Eosinophilia refers to an abnormally high number of eosinophils in the blood. Colville JL, Oien SA, Clinical Veterinary Language, ed 1, Elsevier, 2014, p. 201.

109. d A hematocrit and packed cell volume refers to the measure of the percentage of red blood cells in a volume of blood. Total protein refers to the protein measurement in serum. Colville JL, Oien SA, Clinical Veterinary Language, ed 1, Elsevier, 2014, p. 203.

110. a Hematopoiesis refers to the formation of blood cells in the body. Neutropenia refers to an abnormally low number of neutrophils in the blood. Leukocytosis refers to a high number of white blood cells. Leukocytoid refers to a resemblance to a white blood cell. Colville JL, Oien SA, Clinical Veterinary Language, ed 1, Elsevier, 2014, p. 206.

111. c Thrombolysis refers to the destruction of a blood clot. Exsanguination refers to the condition in which a massive loss of blood occurs. Monocyte refers to a white blood cell with only one nucleus. Leukemia refers to an overabundance of white blood cells in the blood. Colville JL, Oien SA, Clinical Veterinary Language, ed 1, Elsevier, 2014, p. 206.

112. c Neutropenia refers to an abnormally low number of neutrophils in the blood. Leukocytosis is defined as too many white blood cells. The formation of blood cells in the body is known as hematopoiesis and thrombocytosis refers to an abnormally increased number of platelets. Colville JL, Oien SA, Clinical Veterinary Language, ed 1, Elsevier, 2014, p. 206.

113. b Hypercapnia refers to an increased amount of carbon dioxide in the blood. Olfaction pertains to the sense of smell. Hyperemia refers to an excess of blood in the vessels supplying an organ. Hypoxia refers to a deficiency in the amount of oxygen reaching the tissues. Colville JL, Oien SA, Clinical Veterinary Language, ed 1, Elsevier, 2014, p. 211.

114. a Apnea refers to the absence of breathing. A collection of air in the chest from a wound or tear in the lung is known as a pneumothorax. A surgical puncture of the lung is termed *pneumocentesis*. Alveolar dysplasia refers to the abnormal development of the air sacs of the lungs. Colville JL, Oien SA, Clinical Veterinary Language, ed 1, Elsevier, 2014, p. 215.

115. b Agonal breathing pertains to the last breaths taken near or at death. Emphysema refers to the overexpansion of alveolar walls, causing the walls to break down and block other airways, resulting in less oxygen/carbon dioxide exchange in the lungs. Asthma refers to a chronic disease that often causes bronchoconstriction. Furcation refers to being divided or branched. Colville JL, Oien SA, Clinical Veterinary Language, ed 1, Elsevier, 2014, p. 216.

116. b Epistaxis refers to a nosebleed. Cardiectasis refers to the dilation of the heart. Atelectasis refers to the incomplete expansion of the lungs at birth. Tussiculation refers to a short, dry hacking cough such as seen in kennel cough. Colville JL, Oien SA, Clinical Veterinary Language, ed 1, Elsevier, 2014, p. 228.

117. b Apepsia refers to a lack of digestion. Bradypeptic pertains to slow digestion. Monogastric refers to having a single digestion system (also referred to as a simple stomach). Anastomosis refers to a surgical connection of two hollow organs or joining of blood vessels. Colville JL, Oien SA, Clinical Veterinary Language, ed 1, Elsevier, 2014, p. 236.

118. d Stomatomalacia refers to a pathological softening of any of the structures of the mouth. Hyperphagia refers to overeating or gluttony. Polydipsia refers to an excessive or abnormal thirst. Cheilophagia refers to excessive biting of the lips. Colville JL, Oien SA, Clinical Veterinary Language, ed 1, Elsevier, 2014, p. 239.

119. a The term *buccal* pertains to a direction toward the side of the mouth or cheek. Lingual refers to an orientation toward the tongue. Rostral pertains to toward the nose. Lateral refers to away from the midline of the body. Colville JL, Oien SA, Clinical Veterinary Language, ed 1, Elsevier, 2014, p. 240.

120. b The term *hemoptysis* refers to the act of spitting up blood. Esophagoplegia pertains to the paralysis of the esophagus. Xerostomia refers to a dry mouth that may or may not be associated with a lack of saliva. Hypoptyalism refers to the abnormal decrease in the amount of saliva, leading to xerostomia. Colville JL, Oien SA, Clinical Veterinary Language, ed 1, Elsevier, 2014, p. 241.

121. b Abomasopexy refers to the surgical fixation of the stomach of a ruminant to the body wall. Gastropexy refers to the surgical fixation of the stomach of a simple-stomached animal to the body wall. Omasal stenosis refers to the inability of food to move from the reticulum into the omasum because of a narrowed opening. Laparosplenotomy refers to a surgical incision into the abdominal wall to gain access to the spleen. Colville JL, Oien SA, Clinical Veterinary Language, ed 1, Elsevier, 2014, p. 242.

122. c The term *cholangitis* refers to an infection of the common bile duct, which is the tube that carries bile from the liver to the gallbladder and intestines. Hepatitis refers to an inflammation of the liver. Pancreatitis refers to an inflammation of the pancreas. Cholecystitis refers to an inflammation of the gallbladder itself. Colville JL, Oien SA, Clinical Veterinary Language, ed 1, Elsevier, 2014, p. 243.

123. d Cachexia refers to the generalized wasting of the body as a result of disease. Eructation refers to a burp or the method by which ruminants continually rid fermentation gases. Anemia refers to an abnormally low red blood cell count. Necrosis refers to the death of tissue. Colville JL, Oien SA, Clinical Veterinary Language, ed 1, Elsevier, 2014, p. 245.

124. a The term *melena* refers to the passing of dark, tarry feces containing blood that have been acted on by bacteria in the intestines. Chyme refers to a semifluid mass of partially digested food that enters the small intestine from the stomach. An enzyme is a protein produced by living cells that initiates a chemical reaction but is not affected by the reaction. Relapse refers to falling back into a disease state after an apparent recovery. Colville JL, Oien SA, Clinical Veterinary Language, ed 1, Elsevier, 2014, p. 245.

125. d Peristalsis refers to the progressive wave of contraction and relaxation of the smooth muscles in the wall of the digestive tract that moves food through the digestive tract. Ingesta refers to ingested material, especially food taken into the body via the mouth. Rumination is bringing ingesta from the reticulorumen back to the mouth, followed by remastication and reswallowing. Retrograde refers to being inverted, to being reversed, to moving backward, to receding, or to deteriorating.

Colville JL, Oien SA, Clinical Veterinary Language, ed 1, Elsevier, 2014, p. 245.

126. b Incisor teeth are the most rostral teeth used for grasping food. Canine teeth are next to the incisors and are used for tearing food. Molar teeth are the most caudal teeth in the mouth and are used for grinding food. Deciduous teeth are temporary or baby teeth. Colville JL, Oien SA, Clinical Veterinary Language, ed 1, Elsevier, 2014, p. 246.

127. b Steatorrhea refers to a large amount of fat in the feces. Lipase is an enzyme used to break down the fat in food so that it can be absorbed in the intestines. Lipolysis refers to the breaking down of fat and malodorous refers to something that is smelly or stinky. Colville JL, Oien SA, Clinical Veterinary Language, ed 1, Elsevier, 2014, p. 252.

128. b Lithiasis refers to the pathological condition that results from a stone. Enteroptosis refers to an abnormal downward placement of the intestines in the abdominal cavity. Lipolysis refers to the breaking down of fat. Lithogenesis refers to the production or formation of stones. Colville JL, Oien SA, Clinical Veterinary Language, ed 1, Elsevier, 2014, p. 253.

129. b Tube feeding through a stomach tube is referred to as gavage. The term *emesis* refers to the vomiting of food from the stomach. Emetic refers to a substance that causes vomiting. An enema refers to an injection of fluid into the rectum to stimulate a bowel movement. Colville JL, Oien SA, Clinical Veterinary Language, ed 1, Elsevier, 2014, p. 258.

130. c Intussusception refers to the slipping or telescoping of one part of a tubular organ into a lower portion, causing the sort of obstruction typically seen in the intestines. Impaction is a physical blockage of one part of the digestive tract by abnormal amounts of material. Nosocomial is a hospital-acquired infection. Ileus is the lack of neuromuscular control of the intestines. Colville JL, Oien SA, Clinical Veterinary Language, ed 1, Elsevier, 2014, p. 258.

131. a Ruminal tympany refers to the overdistention of the reticulorumen as a result of rumen gas being trapped in the rumen when the ruminant is unable to eructate. Retch refers to involuntary spasms of ineffective vomiting or dry heaves. Volvulus is the abnormal twisting of the intestines causing an obstruction, whereas torsion is the twisting or rotating on a long axis. Colville JL, Oien SA, Clinical Veterinary Language, ed 1, Elsevier, 2014, p. 258.

132. b Total parenteral nutrition refers to nutrition that must be administered by means other than the mouth. Nil per os or NPO is a fasting condition where no food or water is given. Prescription diet is a specialized doctor-ordered diet for certain diseases. An ad lib diet refers to the provision of food as needed or as desired. Colville JL, Oien SA, Clinical Veterinary Language, ed 1, Elsevier, 2014, p. 260.

133. b Alopecia refers to hair loss on any portion of the body. Abrasion is a scrape of the superficial skin layer. Proud flesh refers to exuberant granulation tissue at the site of injury. Aphagia refers to the inability or refusal to swallow. Colville JL, Oien SA, Clinical Veterinary Language, ed 1, Elsevier, 2014, p. 264.

134. c Rhabdomyolysis refers to the destruction of skeletal muscle. A papule is an inflamed, small, solid, pointed elevation of the skin with no pus. Osteochondritis refers to inflammation of bone and cartilage. Pneumothorax refers to air within the thoracic cavity. Colville JL, Oien SA, Clinical Veterinary Language, ed 1, Elsevier, 2014, p. 264.

135. a Neuropathy is a disease of the nerves. Enchondroma refers to a slow-growing tumor of cartilage growing into bone tissue. Poliomyelitis is a highly infectious viral disease that causes inflammation of the gray matter of the spinal cord and brainstem. Neuromyelitis is a neuritis combined with inflammation of the spinal cord. Colville JL, Oien SA, Clinical Veterinary Language, ed 1, Elsevier, 2014, p. 269.

136. a The prefix sarc- refers to flesh. The prefix femor- refers to femur. The prefix lapar- refers to flank. The prefix prim- refers to first. Colville JL, Oien SA, Clinical Veterinary Language, ed 1, Elsevier, 2014, p. 391.

137. b Cerebroatrophy refers to the wasting away of the brain tissue. Meningocele is a hernia protrusion of the meninges through a defect in the cranium or the vertebral column. Necrosis refers to the death of tissue. Neuromyelitis refers to inflammation of the spinal cord. Colville JL, Oien SA, Clinical Veterinary Language, ed 1, Elsevier, 2014, p. 269.

138. c Leptocephaly refers to an abnormally small or thin head. Ataxia is a lack of coordination. Arachnoid is a resemblance to a spider web. Hydrocephalus is a buildup of fluid within the deep cavities of the brain. Colville JL, Oien SA, Clinical Veterinary Language, ed 1, Elsevier, 2014, p. 270.

139. b The term *aberrant* refers to a deviation from the usual or ordinary. Afferent refers to carrying to or bringing toward a place. Efferent refers to carrying out or taking away from a place. Kyphosis refers to an abnormal convex curvature of the spine. Colville JL, Oien SA, Clinical Veterinary Language, ed 1, Elsevier, 2014, p. 271.

140. d The cerebellum is referred to as the little brain because it is the second largest portion of the brain. The corpus callosum is the bundle of nerve fibers that connect the right and left hemisphere of the cerebrum. The cortex is the outer layer of nervous tissue in the brain. The cerebrum is the largest portion of the brain. Colville JL, Oien SA, Clinical Veterinary Language, ed 1, Elsevier, 2014, p. 271.

141. b A syrinx refers to a pathological tube-shaped lesion in the brain or spinal cord. The thalamus is the part of the brain that relays sensory impulses to the cerebral cortex. A synapse is the junction across which a nerve impulse passes from an axon to another neuron, a muscle cell, or a gland cell. Potential space is the space or cavity that can exist between two adjacent body parts that are not tightly adjoined. Colville JL, Oien SA, Clinical Veterinary Language, ed 1, Elsevier, 2014, p. 271.

142. a Dendrites are short, fine-branching fibers extend from the cell body. A perikaryon is the cell body. The axon is the single long fiber that extends from the cell body, which can extend to several feet long. Microglial cells are macrophages of the central nervous system. Colville JL, Oien SA, Clinical Veterinary Language, ed 1, Elsevier, 2014, p. 272.

143. b Albumin is a protein manufactured by the liver that maintains the osmotic fluid balance between capillaries and tissues. Aldosterone is a mineralocorticoid hormone secreted by the cortex of the adrenal gland. Alkaline refers to a basic solution that is at a pH level above 7. Acetylcholine is a neurotransmitter associated with somatic nerves and with the parasympathetic nervous system. Colville T, Bassert JM, Clinical Anatomy and Physiology for Veterinary Technicians, ed 3, MO Mosby Elsevier, 2016, p. 273.

144. a Nociperception is the recognition by the nervous system of an injury or painful stimulus. Proprioception refers to the physical feeling of your body moving. Anesthesia pertains to the lack of sensation produced by medications. Visceral sensations are sensations produced in the hollow visceral organs such as the GI tract, urinary tract, and reproductive tract. Colville JL, Oien SA, Clinical Veterinary Language, ed 1, Elsevier, 2014, p. 291.

145. a Allodynia is the painful response to a normally nonpainful stimulus. Nociperception is the recognition by the nervous system of an injury or painful stimulus. Proprioception refers to the physical feeling of your moving body. Tactile agnosia refers to the inability to recognize objects by handling them. Colville JL, Oien SA, Clinical Veterinary Language, ed 1, Elsevier, 2014, p. 291.

146. b Normal digestion is referred to as eupepsia. Rhinitis refers to the inflammation of the upper respiratory tract. Malodorous refers to a bad smell or odor. Anosmia refers to the inability to smell. Colville JL, Oien SA, Clinical Veterinary Language, ed 1, Elsevier, 2014, p. 292.

147. d Myringectomy is the surgical removal of the eardrum. Splenectomy is the removal of the spleen. Cholecystectomy is the removal of the gallbladder. Nephrectomy is the removal of a kidney. Colville JL, Oien SA, Clinical Veterinary Language, ed 1, Elsevier, 2014, p. 293.

148. b Oculocutaneous pertains to the eyes and the skin. Ophthalmology refers to the study of the eyes. Audiology refers to the study of hearing disorders. Blepharospasm refers to an abnormal contraction of the eyelid. Colville JL, Oien SA, Clinical Veterinary Language, ed 1, Elsevier, 2014, p. 294.

149. a Palpebration refers to an abnormal contraction of the eyelid. Palpation refers to the method of feeling with fingers or hands during the physical examination. Inflammation of the cornea is referred to as keratitis. Dacryopyorrhea refers to the flow of tears mixed with pus. Colville JL, Oien SA, Clinical Veterinary Language, ed 1, Elsevier, 2014, p. 294.

150. d Corectasis refers to the abnormal dilation of the pupil of the eye. Iridocele refers to the protrusion of a portion of the iris through a defect in the cornea. Keratitis refers to inflammation of the cornea. Corneitis refers to inflammation of the cornea. Colville JL, Oien SA, Clinical Veterinary Language, ed 1, Elsevier, 2014, p. 295.

151. a Neuroretinitis refers to an inflammation affecting both the optic nerve and the retina. Conjunctivitis is an inflammation of the conjunctiva of the eye, also referred to as pink eye. Cholecystitis is defined as inflammation of the gallbladder, whereas hepatitis is defined as an inflammation of the liver. Colville JL, Oien SA, Clinical Veterinary Language, ed 1, Elsevier, 2014, p. 295.

152. c Miosis refers to the prolonged constriction of the pupil of the eye. Canthus refers to the corner of each eye, each of which is formed by the junction of the upper and lower eyelids. Mydriasis refers to the prolonged dilation of the pupil of the eye. Iridocele refers to the protrusion of a portion of the iris through a defect in the cornea. Colville JL, Oien SA, Clinical Veterinary Language, ed 1, Elsevier, 2014, p. 295.

153. d A pheromone is a liquid substance released in small quantities by an animal, which causes a specific response if it is detected by another animal of the same species. Sensory receptors are nerve endings that respond to a stimulus, found in the internal or external environment of an animal. Nocturnal refers to an animal that is active at night. A matrix refers to a surrounding substance in which something else is contained. Colville JL, Oien SA, Clinical Veterinary Language, ed 1, Elsevier, 2014, p. 295.

154. a An ear flap is also known as a pinna. A papilla refers to a small, round, or cone-shaped projection on top of the tongue that may contain taste buds. A callus is a bridge that forms as part of the healing process across the two halves of a bone fracture. A canthus refers to the corner of each eye, which is formed by the junction of the upper and lower eyelids. Colville JL, Oien SA, Clinical Veterinary Language, ed 1, Elsevier, 2014, p. 295.

155. a The study of cells is called cytology. Morphology is the study of organisms, whereas zoology is the study of animals. Oncology is the study of different malignancies. Colville JL, Oien SA, Clinical Veterinary Language, ed 1, Elsevier, 2014, p. 300.

156. d Dyspnea refers to difficult or labored breathing. Epistaxis refers to a nosebleed. Lysis refers to destruction or breakage. Leukopenic refers to the lack or deficiency of white blood cells. Colville JL, Oien SA, Clinical Veterinary Language, ed 1, Elsevier, 2014, p. 300.

157. b Red blood cells are cells that carry oxygen to the body. White blood cells are involved with the immune system. Neutrophils are white blood cells with granulocytes and they aid in the immune response. Eosinophils are also white blood cells that are specialized in aiding the immune system. Colville JL, Oien SA, Clinical Veterinary Language, ed 1, Elsevier, 2014, p. 192.

158. d A gastrolith refers to a stone found in the stomach. A hepatolith refers to a stone found within the liver, and a cholelith refers a stone found in the gallbladder. A coprolith refers to a stone formed around fecal matter. Colville JL, Oien SA, Clinical Veterinary Language, ed 1, Elsevier, 2014, p. 310.

159. a An arteriolith refers to a stone in the artery. A cardiolith refers to a stone in the heart, a hysterolith refers to a stone found in the uterus, and a broncholith refers to a stone found within the bronchus. Colville JL, Oien SA, Clinical Veterinary Language, ed 1, Elsevier, 2014, p. 310.

160. b Colpocentesis refers to the surgical puncture of the vagina. Vaginodynia refers to pain in the vagina.

Paracentesis refers to the draining of fluid from the abdominal cavity. Cystocentesis refers to the removal of urine directly from the bladder with the use of a needle. Colville JL, Oien SA, Clinical Veterinary Language, ed 1, Elsevier, 2014, p. 359.

161. d Lithoclasty refers to the crushing of a stone into fragments. Lithogenesis refers to the process of the formation or beginning of a stone. Lithologist refers to a person who studies or has knowledge of stones. Lithiasis refers to the pathological condition that results from a stone. Colville JL, Oien SA, Clinical Veterinary Language, ed 1, Elsevier, 2014, p. 310.

162. a A hormone is a substance produced by one tissue or by one group of cells that is carried by the bloodstream to another tissue or organ to affect its physiological functions such as metabolism or growth. An endorphin is a compound produced in the brain and in other body tissues that reduces the sensation of pain. A protein is a biological molecule consisting of one or more long chains of amino acids. An enzyme is a biological molecule that acts on catalysts and helps complex reactions to occur. Colville JL, Oien SA, Clinical Veterinary Language, ed 1, Elsevier, 2014, p. 315.

163. b Adenopathy refers to any disease of a gland. Amyotrophy refers to the muscular degeneration of muscles. Adrenomegaly refers to the enlargement of the adrenal gland. Cardiomyopathy refers to the disease of the muscles of the heart. Colville JL, Oien SA, Clinical Veterinary Language, ed 1, Elsevier, 2014, p. 315.

164. c Thyroidectomy refers to the surgical removal of the thyroid gland. Splenectomy refers to the surgical removal of the spleen. Oophorectomy refers to the surgical removal of the ovaries, and cholecystectomy refers to the surgical removal of the gallbladder. Colville JL, Oien SA, Clinical Veterinary Language, ed 1, Elsevier, 2014, p. 315.

165. d Luteinizing hormone is responsible for the production of testosterone in males and estrogen in females and also for ovulation in females. Prolactin hormone stimulates the production of milk after the animal has given birth. Thyroid-stimulating hormone stimulates the thyroid gland to make thyroid hormones that help regulate the animal's metabolism. Follicle-stimulating hormone regulates sperm production in males and stimulates egg production from the ovaries in females. Colville JL, Oien SA, Clinical Veterinary Language, ed 1, Elsevier, 2014, p. 318.

166. b A nephroblastoma refers to a rapidly developing malignant tumor of the kidney. A renogram refers to a record made of the kidneys, such as an x-ray. A hepatoblastoma refers to a tumor found within the liver. A sarcoma is a tumor found in the soft tissue or muscle. Colville JL, Oien SA, Clinical Veterinary Language, ed 1, Elsevier, 2014, p. 331.

167. c The term *uremia* refers to urine constituents that are found in the blood. Dysuria refers to painful urination. Surgical repair of the kidney pelvis is known as pyeloplasty. Blood found in the urine is referred to as hematuria. Colville JL, Oien SA, Clinical Veterinary Language, ed 1, Elsevier, 2014, p. 331.

168. b Ureteralgia refers to pain within the ureter. Cystitis refers to an inflammation of the bladder. Dysuria refers to painful urination. Menorrhagia refers to pain felt during menstruation. Colville JL, Oien SA, Clinical Veterinary Language, ed 1, Elsevier, 2014, p. 331.

169. b Lithotripsy refers to the crushing or grinding of stones. Lithogenesis refers to the process of the formation or beginning of a stone. Lithiasis refers to the pathological condition that results from a stone. Lithology refers to the study of stones. Colville JL, Oien SA, Clinical Veterinary Language, ed 1, Elsevier, 2014, p. 331.

170. b Nephroptosis refers to the downward displacement or prolapse of the kidney. Nephrectomy refers to the surgical removal of the kidney. Nephrostomy refers to the placement of a drainage tube within the renal pelvis that leads to the outer skin surface to allow urine to drain. Nephrology refers to the study of the kidneys. Colville JL, Oien SA, Clinical Veterinary Language, ed 1, Elsevier, 2014, p. 331.

171. a A concretion is a solid or calcified mass formed by disease found in a body cavity or tissue. A stone is referred to as a calculus. An electrolyte is a chemical element that carries an electrical charge when dissolved in water. The parenchyma is the functional tissue of an organ. Colville JL, Oien SA, Clinical Veterinary Language, ed 1, Elsevier, 2014, p. 332.

172. d The act of urination is also referred to as micturition and voiding. Concretion refers to a solid or calcified mass formed by disease found in a body cavity or tissue. Colville JL, Oien SA, Clinical Veterinary Language, ed 1, Elsevier, 2014, p. 332.

173. c The term *denude* refers to the loss of epidermis, caused by exposure to urine, feces, body fluids, drainage, or friction. The process in the kidney whereby blood pressure forces material through a filter is known as filtration. The end product of muscle metabolism, which is the waste produced excreted in urine, is referred to as creatinine. Colville JL, Oien SA, Clinical Veterinary Language, ed 1, Elsevier, 2014, p. 332.

174. b Stranguria refers to painful urination resulting from muscle spasms in the urinary bladder and urethra. Dysuria refers to painful urination. Urea is the water-soluble, nitrogen-based compound that is in the waste material of protein metabolism from the body's cells. Slough refers to a mass or layer of necrotic tissue that separates from the underlying healthy tissue. Colville JL, Oien SA, Clinical Veterinary Language, ed 1, Elsevier, 2014, p. 332.

175. c Incontinence refers to the lack of voluntary urination or defecation. Urolithiasis refers to the presence of urinary calculi within the urinary system. Uremia refers to a buildup of nitrogenous waste material in the blood. Anuria refers to the lack of urine passage. Colville JL, Oien SA, Clinical Veterinary Language, ed 1, Elsevier, 2014, p. 342.

176. d Azotemia refers to the buildup of nitrogenous waste material in the blood. The presence of urinary calculi is referred to as urolithiasis. Incontinence refers to the lack of voluntary urination and diuresis refers to the increased production of urine. Colville JL, Oien SA, Clinical Veterinary Language, ed 1, Elsevier, 2014, p. 342.

177. c The excess dilution of urine, which results in a low specific gravity, is referred to as hydruria. Oliguresis refers to the excretion of a small amount of urine.

Albuminuria refers to the presence of albumin in the urine. Hydrocephalus refers to the buildup of water within the cavities of the brain. Colville JL, Oien SA, Clinical Veterinary Language, ed 1, Elsevier, 2014, p. 342.

178. b Azotemia refers to the higher than normal blood level of nitrogen-containing compounds. Bilirubinuria refers to the presence of bilirubin in urine. Hydruria refers to the excess dilution of urine. Natriuresis refers to the excretion of an abnormal amount of sodium in the urine. Colville JL, Oien SA, Clinical Veterinary Language, ed 1, Elsevier, 2014, p. 343.

179. c Ketosis refers to a depleted amount of glycogen in the liver. Hypoglycemia refers to low blood sugar. Hyperglycemia refers to high blood sugar. Sepsis refers to an infection of the bloodstream. Colville JL, Oien SA, Clinical Veterinary Language, ed 1, Elsevier, 2014, p. 343.

180. a Ureteropyosis refers to a diseased condition in which there is pus within a ureter. Bacterium refers to one single-cell microorganism that can exist independently. Ketonuria refers to the presence of ketone bodies in the urine. Pyometra refers to the presence of pus within the uterus. Colville JL, Oien SA, Clinical Veterinary Language, ed 1, Elsevier, 2014, p. 343.

181. b Nephrolithotomy refers to the surgical incision into the kidney to remove a stone. Cholecystectomy refers to the surgical removal of the gallbladder. Nephrectomy refers to the surgical removal of a kidney. Splenectomy refers to the surgical removal of the spleen. Colville JL, Oien SA, Clinical Veterinary Language, ed 1, Elsevier, 2014, p. 343.

182. b Cystocentesis refers to the collection of urine directly from the bladder through a surgical puncture. The microscopic examination of a urine sample is referred to as urinalysis. The surgical incision into the bladder is referred to as cystotomy. A paracentesis refers to the drainage of free fluid from the abdominal cavity. Colville JL, Oien SA, Clinical Veterinary Language, ed^1, Elsevier, 2014, p. 344.

183. d Hypokalemia refers to a low potassium level. Hypernatremia refers to a high sodium level, whereas hyponatremia refers to a low sodium level. Hypokalemia refers to a low potassium level. Colville JL, Oien SA, Clinical Veterinary Language, ed 1, Elsevier, 2014, p. 344.

184. a The surgical removal of a testicle is referred to as an orchiectomy. Oophorectomy refers to the surgical removal of the ovary. Cryptorchidism refers to the failure of one or both of the testicles to descend into the scrotum. A hysterectomy refers to the surgical removal of the uterus. Colville JL, Oien SA, Clinical Veterinary Language, ed 1, Elsevier, 2014, p. 353.

185. b Spermaturia refers to the presence of sperm in the urine. Spermous pertains to sperm. Hematuria refers to the presence of blood in the urine. Dysuria refers to painful urination. Colville JL, Oien SA, Clinical Veterinary Language, ed 1, Elsevier, 2014, p. 353.

186. b The surgical removal of the penis is referred to as penectomy. Castration is the surgical removal of both testicles. Hysterectomy is the surgical removal of the uterus. Oophorectomy is the surgical removal of the ovaries. Colville JL, Oien SA, Clinical Veterinary Language, ed 1, Elsevier, 2014, p. 353.

187. a Priapitis refers to the inflammation of the penis. Megalopenis refers to hypertrophy of the penis. Micropenis refers to hypoplasia of the penis. Hypospadias refers to a urethra opening on the ventral surface of the penis. Colville JL, Oien SA, Clinical Veterinary Language, ed 1, Elsevier, 2014, p. 353.

188. c Phimosis refers to the inability to extend the penis, which is most often caused by a stenosis of the urethral opening. Priapism refers to the persistent erection of the penis. Paraphimosis refers to the idiopathic protrusion of the nonerect penis with the inability to retract it. Colville JL, Oien SA, Clinical Veterinary Language, ed 1, Elsevier, 2014, p. 357.

189. b The release of an egg from the ovary is termed *ovulation*. An ovum is a mature female gamete cell that has been released from its ovarian follicle. An oocyte is a developing egg inside an ovarian follicle. Paraphimosis is the idiopathic protrusion of the nonerect penis with the inability to retract it. Colville JL, Oien SA, Clinical Veterinary Language, ed 1, Elsevier, 2014, p. 357.

190. b Oophorrhagia refers to bleeding from the ovary. Ovariectomy refers to the removal of one or both ovaries. Menorrhagia refers to abnormally heavy uterine bleeding. Vaginodynia refers to pain within the vagina. Colville JL, Oien SA, Clinical Veterinary Language, ed 1, Elsevier, 2014, p. 358.

191. a Vulvitis refers to the inflammation of the vulva. Cystitis refers to the inflammation of the bladder. Vaginitis refers to the inflammation of the vagina. Pyometra refers to an infection of the uterus. Cha Colville JL, Oien SA, Clinical Veterinary Language, ed 1, Elsevier, 2014, p. 359.

192. c The term *corpus* refers to the body. The term *cornus* refers to the horn. The flared end of a funnel-shaped duct is referred to as the infundibulum. The clitoris is a sensitive female external organ homologous to the penis. Colville JL, Oien SA, Clinical Veterinary Language, ed 1, Elsevier, 2014, p. 360.

193. b The fimbria is a fringe-like structure of the infundibulum of the oviduct. The caruncles are permanently raised areas where an embryo will attach to the uterus. The oviduct (also called uterine tubes) catches the ova as they are released from their follicles. A follicle is a small cavity or sac. Colville JL, Oien SA, Clinical Veterinary Language, ed 1, Elsevier, 2014, p. 360.

194. c The prefix hetero- refers to different. The prefixes pepto- and peps- refer to digestion. The prefix digit- refers to digits. The prefix patho- refers to disease. Colville JL, Oien SA, Clinical Veterinary Language, ed 1, Elsevier, 2014, p. 390.

195. c Embryectomy is the surgical removal of an animal in the early stages of development in the womb. Hysterectomy is the surgical removal of the uterus. Oophorectomy is the surgical removal of the ovaries. Penectomy is the surgical removal of the penis. Colville JL, Oien SA, Clinical Veterinary Language, ed 1, Elsevier, 2014, p. 362.

196. b Pseudocyesis refers to a false pregnancy. Primigravida refers to the first pregnancy. Pseudoaneurysm refers to a false aneurysm resulting from a leaking hole in an artery. Uniparous refers to giving birth to only one offspring. Colville JL, Oien SA, Clinical Veterinary Language, ed 1, Elsevier, 2014, p. 363.

197. c A female that has given birth twice in two separate pregnancies is termed *bipara.* Postpartum refers to the period of time just after the birth of offspring. A false pregnancy is known as pseudocyesis. A female that has never given birth is referred to as nulliparous. Colville JL, Oien SA, Clinical Veterinary Language, ed 1, Elsevier, 2014, p. 363.

198. d The term *fecund* refers to the capability of producing offspring. Fetus pertains to an animal in the later stages of development within the uterus. The term *natal* refers to birth. Perineum refers to the region between the scrotum and the anus in males or the region between the vulva and the anus in females. Colville JL, Oien SA, Clinical Veterinary Language, ed 1, Elsevier, 2014, p. 364.

199. c The placenta is the vascular membranous organ between a mother and her offspring in the womb. Fecund is the capability of producing offspring. The perineum refers to the region between the scrotum and the anus in males or the region between the vulva and the anus in females. The umbilical cord is the attachment from the fetus to the placenta from which the fetus receives all nutrients. Colville JL, Oien SA, Clinical Veterinary Language, ed 1, Elsevier, 2014, p. 364.

200. d Artificial insemination refers to the injection of semen into the vagina or uterus by the use of a syringe. Copulation is the natural act of reproduction. In vitro fertilization is the injection of an embryo into the uterus of a female. In vivo fertilization is the injection of the sperm and ovum into the uterus of a female. Colville JL, Oien SA, Clinical Veterinary Language, ed 1, Elsevier, 2014, p. 364.

201. c Diestrous refers to a species that has two estrous cycles per year. Monestrous refers to species that have only one estrous cycle per year. Polyestrous refers to species that have numerous estrous cycles per year. Anestrous refers to lack of estrous cycles. Colville JL, Oien SA, Clinical Veterinary Language, ed 1, Elsevier, 2014, p. 364.

202. b Dystocia refers to an abnormally slow or difficult birth. Dysuria refers to painful urination. Ectopic refers to an abnormal development of an embryo occurring somewhere other than within the uterus. Pyometra refers to an accumulation of pus within the uterus. Colville JL, Oien SA, Clinical Veterinary Language, ed 1, Elsevier, 2014, p. 367.

203. b An animal that is not able to produce offspring is referred to as being sterile. A stillborn is a fetus that is born dead. Pseudocyesis refers to a false pregnancy. Hermaphroditism refers to a condition whereby an animal has both male and female reproductive organs. Colville JL, Oien SA, Clinical Veterinary Language, ed 1, Elsevier, 2014, p. 367.

204. d The term *zoodermic* pertains to the skin of animals. Zoogenous refers to animal origin. Zoogamous refers to animals that reproduce sexually. Endozoic refers to one animal living within another animal. Colville JL, Oien SA, Clinical Veterinary Language, ed 1, Elsevier, 2014, p. 372.

205. d The term *zoophagy* refers to feeding on animals. Zoophile refers to being a lover of animals. Zooplasty refers to the surgical repair of an animal organ. Zooid refers to a resemblance to an animal. Colville JL, Oien SA, Clinical Veterinary Language, ed 1, Elsevier, 2014, p. 372.

206. c Zoonosis refers to any human disease that is transmitted from an animal. Zooscopy is a hallucination where a person believes he sees animals. Zootomy refers to the dissection of animals. Zootrophic refers to providing nutrition to animals for growth. Colville JL, Oien SA, Clinical Veterinary Language, ed 1, Elsevier, 2014, p. 372.

207. b An anticoagulant is a substance that prevents blood from clotting when it is added to the blood. An anticodon is the triplet pair of nucleotides in tRNA that corresponds to the triplet bases or codons of mRNA. Antigens are cells or organisms that are "not self." An anticonvulsant refers to a drug that stops seizures from occurring. Colville T, Bassert JM, Clinical Anatomy and Physiology for Veterinary Technicians, ed 3, Mosby Elsevier, 2016, p. 294.

208. a Apteria refers to the bare area of the skin of birds where feathers do not originate. Aponeurosis refers to a broad sheet of fibrous connective tissue that attaches certain muscles to bones. Anuria refers to the lack of urination. Ataxia refers to the incoordination of spastic movements. Colville T, Bassert JM, Clinical Anatomy and Physiology for Veterinary Technicians, ed 3, Mosby Elsevier, 2016, p. 507.

209. c Atony refers to the lack of normal muscle tone. Atrophy is the shrinkage or loss of something. Auricle is the ear-shaped appendage of either atrium of the heart. Ataxia refers to the incoordination of spastic movements. Colville T, Bassert JM, Clinical Anatomy and Physiology for Veterinary Technicians, ed 3, Mosby Elsevier, 2016, p. 570.

210. d Avascular refers to without a blood supply. A blood clot is referred to as a thrombus. Hypervascular refers to an increased amount of blood supply. Hypovascular refers to a decreased amount of blood supply. Colville T, Bassert JM, Clinical Anatomy and Physiology for Veterinary Technicians, ed 3, Mosby Elsevier, 2016, p. 570.

211. b Bronchitis is a lower respiratory tract infection affecting the lining of the larger air passageways in the lungs. Pneumonia is the presence of fluid within the lungs. Pleural effusion is the presence of fluid within the thoracic cavity. Conjunctivitis refers to an inflammation of the conjunctiva of the eyes. Colville T, Bassert JM, Clinical Anatomy and Physiology for Veterinary Technicians, ed 3, Mosby Elsevier, 2016, p. 371.

212. c The carapace refers to the dorsal shell of turtles and tortoises. The canthus refers to the corner of the eyelids where they come together. Capsular space refers to the space between the visceral and parietal layers of the Bowman's capsule. Cardia refers to the part of the stomach where the esophagus enters. Colville T, Bassert JM, Clinical Anatomy and Physiology for Veterinary Technicians, ed 3, Mosby Elsevier, 2016, p. 573.

213. b Chemotaxis refers to the movement of white blood cells into an area of inflammation in response to chemical mediators released at the site by injured tissue. Leukocytosis refers to the increased number of white blood cells. Anemia refers to the low number of red blood cells. Leukopenia refers to the low number of white blood cell counts. Colville T, Bassert JM, Clinical Anatomy and Physiology for Veterinary Technicians, ed 3, Mosby Elsevier, 2016, p. 574.

214. b Circumduction refers to a joint motion whereby the distal end of an extremity moves in a circle. The removal of the male testicle is known as castration. A cisterna is a reservoir that stores fluid. Abduction is the movement of a joint where the distal end of the extremity moves away from the body. Colville T, Bassert JM, Clinical Anatomy and Physiology for Veterinary Technicians, ed 3, Mosby Elsevier, 2016, p. 575.

215. c Colostrum is the initial secretion of the mammary gland before milk is produced. Colloidal is gelatinous and viscous fluid. Columella is the middle ear bone in birds. Cisterna is a reservoir that stores fluid. Colville T, Bassert JM, Clinical Anatomy and Physiology for Veterinary Technicians, ed 3, Mosby Elsevier, 2016, p. 335.

216. b Coping is the process of trimming and shaping a bird's beak. Culling refers to the selection from a large group or to reducing the size. The term *crop* refers to the dilation of the esophagus in some species of birds that acts as a storage pouch for food. Corium refers to the dermis of the skin. Colville T, Bassert JM, Clinical Anatomy and Physiology for Veterinary Technicians, ed 3, Mosby Elsevier, 2016, p. 576.

217. b Diapedesis refers to the process by which white blood cells leave the blood vessel and enter tissue by squeezing through the tiny spaces between the cells' lining. Leukopenia refers to low white blood cell count. Leukocytosis refers to a high white blood cell count. Chemotaxis refers to the movement of white blood cells into an area of inflammation in response to chemical mediators released at the site by injured tissue. Colville T, Bassert JM, Clinical Anatomy and Physiology for Veterinary Technicians, ed 3, Mosby Elsevier, 2016, p. 578.

218. c Diarthrosis refers to a freely moveable joint. Diastole refers to the part of the cardiac cycle associated with relaxation of the atria and ventricles. Diestrous refers to animals that have two estrous cycles per year. Diaphysis refers to the shaft portion of a long bone. Colville T, Bassert JM, Clinical Anatomy and Physiology for Veterinary Technicians, ed 3, Mosby Elsevier, 2016, p. 578.

219. b The prefix dys- refers to painful or defective. The prefix pro- refers to before or anterior. The prefix infra- refers to below or beneath. The prefix inter- refers to between. Colville JL, Oien SA, Clinical Veterinary Language, ed 1, Elsevier, 2014, p. 388.

220. c A gosling is an immature goose of either sex. A poult is a young turkey of either sex. A rafter is a group of turkeys. A gander is an intact male goose. Colville JL, Oien SA, Clinical Veterinary Language, ed 1, Elsevier, 2014, p. 7.

221. d Ovariohysterectomy refers to the complete removal of the uterus and ovaries/oviducts. Hysterectomy is the removal of the uterus only. Oophorectomy is the removal of the ovaries. Castration is the removal of the male testicles. Colville JL, Oien SA, Clinical Veterinary Language, ed 1, Elsevier, 2014, p. 19.

222. b Pruritus refers to itching. Edema refers to swelling of tissue. Purulent refers to containing or consisting of pus. A keloid is an overgrowth of scar tissue. Colville JL, Oien SA, Clinical Veterinary Language, ed 1, Elsevier, 2014, p. 70.

223. a Hypochromic refers to pale red blood cells after they have been stained. Hemoglobin is the protein found in red blood cells. An agranulocyte is a type of blood cell that has no colored granules seen within the cytoplasm. Anucleate is a mature mammalian red blood cell. Colville JL, Oien SA, Clinical Veterinary Language, ed 1, Elsevier, 2014, p. 192.

224. c The auditory canal is also referred to as the eustachian tube. The humerus is a long bone found is the fore extremity. The cochlea is the spiral organ in the inner ear that turns sound waves into sensory impulses. The pinna refers to the ear flap. Colville JL, Oien SA, Clinical Veterinary Language, ed 1, Elsevier, 2014, p. 295.

225. c A tracheotomy refers to the surgical incision into the windpipe. The glottis is the vocal cords and the space between them. Epistaxis refers to a nosebleed. An endoscope refers to the instrument used to view the inner part of a body. Colville JL, Oien SA, Clinical Veterinary Language, ed 1, Elsevier, 2014, p. 300.

226. b Diuresis refers to an increased production of urine. Dysuria refers to painful urination. Polyuria refers to an increased passage of urine. Anuria refers to a lack of urine passage. Colville JL, Oien SA, Clinical Veterinary Language, ed 1, Elsevier, 2014, p. 341.

227. b Natriuresis refers to the excretion of an abnormal amount of sodium in the urine. Hypernatremia refers to an excessive amount of sodium found in the blood. Hydruria refers to the excess dilution of urine. Albuminuria refers to the presence of albumin in the urine. Colville JL, Oien SA, Clinical Veterinary Language, ed 1, Elsevier, 2014, p. 342.

228. b Orchialgia refers to pain within one or both testicles. Orchiectomy refers to the surgical removal of the testicles. Menorrhagia refers to abnormally heavy bleeding during menstruation. Myalgia refers to pain of the muscles. Colville JL, Oien SA, Clinical Veterinary Language, ed 1, Elsevier, 2014, p. 353.

229. c The myometrium is the thickest layer of the uterine wall and it is composed of smooth muscle cells. The perimetrium is the outer layer of the uterus. The endometrium is the inner epithelial layer that contains mucus. Caruncles are numerous, permanently raised areas typically found in ruminants where the developing embryo will attach to the uterus. Colville JL, Oien SA, Clinical Veterinary Language, ed 1, Elsevier, 2014, p. 361.

230. c The prefix atel- refers to being incomplete. The prefix noci- refers to injury. The prefix enter- refers to intestines. The prefixes em- and en- refer to inward. Colville JL, Oien SA, Clinical Veterinary Language, ed 1, Elsevier, 2014, p. 392.

SECTION 5

1. d A neonate's liver may not be completely functional until several weeks of age. Because of this, the biotransformation of drugs is decreased. Bill RL, Clinical Pharmacology and Therapeutics for the Veterinary Technician, ed 4, Mosby, 2016, p. 74-75.
2. b The liver is the primary organ involved in biotransformation. The kidney, spleen, and pancreas are involved to a much lesser degree. Bill RL, Clinical Pharmacology and Therapeutics for the Veterinary Technician, ed 4, Mosby, 2016, p. 74-76.
3. d The generic name is also called the nonproprietary name or the compendial name. This is the name found in the United States Pharmacopoeia (USP). The generic name is usually the active ingredient of the drug (such as metronidazole). The trade name and proprietary name both refer to the name given to the medication by the drug company and these names vary from company to company (such as Flagyl or Metro for metronidazole). The chemical name describes the chemical structure of the drug 2-(2-methyl-5-nitro-1H-imidazol1-1yl) ethanol for metronidazole. Wanamaker BP, Massey KL, Applied Pharmacology for Veterinary Technicians, ed 5, Elsevier, 2015, p. 16.
4. d Because this drug is enterically coated, it should not be split. The enteric coating prevents the tablet from being broken down in the stomach and allows it to move into the intestine, where it will be absorbed. Administrating 50 mg is an overdose for the patient and may lead to toxicity. This medication should be ordered or a prescription should be written so that the correct dose can be administered. Sirois M, Principles and Practice of Veterinary Technology, ed 3, Elsevier, 2011, p. 250.
5. d Tab: tablets; q4hr: every 4 hours; po: per os (by mouth); prn: as needed; until gone: until all tablets are gone. Four times a day would be every 6 hours or QID and the prescription does not indicate it should be taken with food or water or that it should be taken for pain. Bill RL, Clinical Pharmacology and Therapeutics for the Veterinary Technician, ed 4, Mosby, 2016, p. 25-26.
6. c Percent indicates parts of active drug per 100 parts of a solution, therefore 2.5% is equal to 2.5 parts per 100 parts of a solution. The solution weighs 1 g/mL therefore there are 2.5 g of active drug in 100 g of solution or 2.5 g in 100 mL of solution. Because the strength of most liquid medications is measured in mg/mL, this is broken down further to 2500 mg (which is equal to 2.5 g) in 100 mL of solution, which can be broken down further to 25 mg/mL. This means a 2.5% solution is 25 mg/mL and 10 mL of this solution will contain 250 mg of thiopental. Lake T, Green N, Essential Calculations for Veterinary Nurses and Technicians, ed 3, Butterworth Heinemann, 2016, p. 62-65.
7. b Bioavailability determines how much of the drug actually reaches the plasma. Absorption indicates how much of the drug is absorbed or moved into the cell. Distribution refers to how the drug is carried from the site of absorption to the blood, and clearance indicates how long it takes for a certain volume of the drug to be eliminated from the body. Wanamaker BP, Massey KL, Applied Pharmacology for Veterinary Technicians, ed 5, Saunders, 2014, p. 8.
8. c Cholinergic agents can be used to decrease intraocular pressure. Cholinergic agents also increase gastrointestinal motility, act as antiemetics, and increase contractions of the uterus (in swine). Side effects of cholinergic agents can include bradycardia. Wanamaker BP, Massey KL, Applied Pharmacology for Veterinary Technicians, ed 5, Elsevier, 2015, p. 76-77.
9. b Although none of these NSAIDs are appropriate to use in cats, acetaminophen is especially toxic because of a cat's limited supply of glutathione, which is required for metabolism. Even the smallest dose will cause methemoglobinemia and death. Bill RL, Clinical Pharmacology and Therapeutics for the Veterinary Technician, ed 3, Mosby, 2006, p. 360; Thomas J, Lerche P, Anesthesia and Analgesia for Veterinary Technicians, ed 5, Mosby, 2014, p. 228.
10. b Aminoglycosides accumulate in the kidney (causing tubular necrosis) and the ear (leading to ototoxicity and damage to the 8th cranial nerve). Aminoglycosides can cause neurological signs but this is much less common than renal damage and hearing loss. Wanamaker BP, Massey KL, Applied Pharmacology for Veterinary Technicians, ed 5, Saunders, 2014, p. 14 and 233.
11. c Tetracyclines are bacteriostatic (slowing bacterial growth), but not bactericidal (killing bacteria). They are able to penetrate the cell wall through pores or via active transport, where they bind the bacterial ribosomes, preventing protein synthesis. Bacteria have developed a resistance to tetracyclines. Wanamaker BP, Massey KL, Applied Pharmacology for Veterinary Technicians, ed 5, Saunders, 2014, p. 247.
12. c Cephalosporins and penicillins are both beta-lactam antibiotics. Tetracyclines are macrolides, sulfas are antibacterial sulfonamides, and fluoroquinolones are quinolones. Bill RL, Clinical Pharmacology and Therapeutics for the Veterinary Technician, ed 4, Mosby, 2016, p. 223-224.
13. b The kidneys excrete sulfonamides, which leads to high concentrations in the urine. For this reason they are ideal for urinary tract infections. Joint capsules and nervous tissue are not involved with excretion. Some drugs can be excreted via the skin through sweat, but this is not the case with sulfonamides. Bill RL, Clinical Pharmacology and Therapeutics for the Veterinary Technician, ed 4, Mosby, 2016, p. 232-233.
14. c Because of possible danger to the public, fluoroquinolones should not be used in food animals. Bill RL, Clinical Pharmacology and Therapeutics for the Veterinary Technician, ed 4, Mosby, 2016, p. 229-230.
15. d Chloramphenicol has been known to cause aplastic anemia in humans and the FDA bans its use. Lincosamides are used in cattle, but withdrawal times must be strictly enforced. Cephalexin can be used in food animals and enrofloxacin is not used in poultry. Bill RL, Clinical Pharmacology and Therapeutics for the Veterinary Technician, ed 4, Mosby, 2016, p. 236.
16. c Penicillin is a beta-lactam, which is excreted by the kidneys. Some beta-lactams are excreted via the liver through the bile, but only a small portion, hence the liver is not the primary method of excretion. The

stomach and small intestine are not involved in the excretion of medications. Boothe DM, Small Animal Clinical Pharmacology and Therapeutics, ed 2, Elsevier, 2012, p. 215.

17. d Acepromazine is known to cause penile relaxation in horses. If this is prolonged, it will increase the chances of injury. For this reason it should be used with caution in breeding stallions. This is also true of breeding bulls, although there is no contraindication for its use in bitches, tomcats, or heifers. Holtgrew-Bohling K, Large Animal Clinical Procedures for Veterinary Technicians, ed 3, Elsevier, 2014, p. 350.

18. c Ketamine can cause muscle rigidity in cats and is therefore often administered with Valium to counteract these effects. Another advantage is that ketamine and Valium can be placed in the same syringe and will work together to provide mild analgesia and minimal cardiac depression. Droperidol, morphine, and xylazine are not commonly used in conjunction with diazepam. Thomas J, Lerche P, Anesthesia and Analgesia for Veterinary Technicians, ed 5, Mosby, 2016, p. 64.

19. c Diazepam will be absorbed by the plastic and should not be drawn up until you are ready to administer it to the patient. This is not known to occur with acepromazine, atropine, or ketamine. Thomas J, Lerche P, Anesthesia and Analgesia for Veterinary Technicians, ed 5, Mosby, 2016, p. 64.

20. d Xylazine is an alpha-2 agonist. These are reversed with yohimbine, which is an alpha-2 antagonist. Naloxone is a reversal for opioids, whereas flumazenil is used to reverse benzodiazepines. Atropine is an anticholinergic and is not used to reverse any medications, although it can be used to treat organophosphate toxicity. Bassert JM, Thomas JA, McCurnin's Clinical Textbook for Veterinary Technicians, ed 9, Elsevier, 2017, p. 1015.

21. d Griseofulvin is an fungistatic antibiotic used to treat dermatophyte fungal infections in dogs and cats, as well as ringworm in horses. Wanamaker BP, Massey KL, Applied Pharmacology for Veterinary Technicians, ed 5, Elsevier, 2015, p. 259.

22. c Sulfonamides commonly cause keratoconjunctivitis sicca (KCS), thrombocytopenia, and crystalluria. Other side effects include allergic skin reactions, liver dysfunction, leukopenia, and anemia. Seizures are not associated with sulfonamide use. Bill RL, Clinical Pharmacology and Therapeutics for the Veterinary Technician, ed 4, Mosby, 2016, p. 233-234.

23. b Fluoroquinolones can cause lesions in the joint cartilage of rapidly growing animals. This is not known to occur with the use of cephalosporins, macrolides, or penicillins. Wanamaker BP, Massey KL, Applied Pharmacology for Veterinary Technicians, ed 4, Saunders, 2009, p. 238.

24. c Bacteria that contain the beta-lactamase enzyme inactivate penicillin. They do this by attacking the beta-lactam ring of the penicillin, which causes it to be ineffective. Potentiated penicillins are penicillins combined with another drug that will inactivate the beta-lactamase enzyme. This is seen in Clavamox (amoxicillin and clavulanic acid) and Unasyn (ampicillin and sulbactam). These drugs will have a wider spectrum of action because of the resistance to beta-lactamase bacteria. Penicillin is commonly used to treat mastitis and cephalosporins are not penicillins. Bill RL, Clinical Pharmacology and Therapeutics for the Veterinary Technician, ed 4, Mosby, 2016, p. 220-221.

25. c IP is short for intraperitoneal, which means you will be injecting the medication into the abdominal cavity. An injection into a vein is IV (intravenous), into a muscle is IM (intramuscular), and medications are not injected into an artery. Bassert JM, Thomas JA, McCurnin's Clinical Textbook for Veterinary Technicians, ed 9, Elsevier, 2017, p. 556.

26. c Xylazine has been known to cause gastric distention in some deep-chested breeds therefore it is not considered safe in all breeds. Naloxone is a reversal for opioids and ketamine is reversed with yohimbine. Xylazine does provide some short-acting analgesia and is usually combined with an opioid. Xylazine is not known to cause priapism in stallions. Bill RL, Clinical Pharmacology and Therapeutics for the Veterinary Technician, ed 3, Mosby, 2006, p. 214-216.

27. d Propofol is a hypnotic and does not provide any analgesia. It should only be given IV and never as a bolus because of the possibility of causing seizure activity. Propofol will only last 2–5 minutes and is therefore ideal to use in incremental doses for short procedures. Wanamaker BP, Massey KL, Applied Pharmacology for Veterinary Technicians, ed 5, Elsevier, 2015, p. 91.

28. b Butorphanol is a synthetic opioid that is used as an analgesic in dogs and cats, as well as being used in dogs for its antitussive activity. Because it is an opioid, it is reversed with naloxone and not yohimbine. Wanamaker BP, Massey KL, Applied Pharmacology for Veterinary Technicians, ed 5, Elsevier, 2015, p. 105.

29. a An iodophor is made up of iodine and a carrier that allows the iodine to be released with time, providing prolonged activity (although it may need to be applied more than once to provide adequate disinfection). Organic materials can inactivate it and the area should be thoroughly cleaned before application. It should also be diluted before use to avoid irritation of the tissues. Sirois M, Principles and Practice of Veterinary Technology, ed 3, Elsevier, 2011, p. 274.

30. c Ivermectin is used to treat many parasites (excluding tapeworms), but when used in Heartgard it is meant to prevent heartworm infection. Ivermectin will not prevent the development of congestive heart failure caused by adult worms; however, studies have shown that if ivermectin is administered before treating adult heartworms with melarsomine, patients will experience fewer pulmonary problems caused by the presence of dead adult worms. Ivermectin can be given orally, subcutaneously, and intramuscularly. Papich MG, Saunders Handbook of Veterinary Drugs: Small and Large Animal, ed 4, Elsevier, 2015, p. 420-422; 2014 American Heartworm Society Canine-Guidelines.

31. c Moxidectin is an antiparasitic in the class milbemycin, which include macrolides used as antiparasitic agents. They are closely related to avermectins. Arsenicals are used to treat adult heartworms and include melarsomine (Immiticide) and thiacetarsamide (Carparsolate). Pyrantel is used to treat intestinal nematodes and belongs in the drug class tetrahydropyrimidines. Organophosphates are toxic. Papich MG, Saunders

Handbook of Veterinary Drugs: Small and Large Animal, ed 4, Elsevier, 2015, p. 545-546.

32. d Prostaglandins cause bronchoconstriction and may induce an asthma attack in people who have a history of asthma. Prostaglandins also cause smooth muscle contractions and may therefore cause abortions. Acne, liver failure, and kidney damage have not been associated with prostaglandins. Wanamaker BP, Massey KL, Applied Pharmacology for Veterinary Technicians, ed 5, Elsevier, 2015, p. 179.

33. d Potassium excretion is increased with furosemide and chronic use will cause hypokalemia. Diuretics are often used in patients with pulmonary edema to pull fluid out of the lung tissue. ACE inhibitors are commonly used in conjunction with diuretics to treat heart failure and normal animals with free access to water should not become dehydrated when administered diuretics. Boothe DM, Small Animal Clinical Pharmacology and Therapeutics, ed 2, Elsevier, 2012, p. 633-635.

34. a Nociceptors are located throughout the body and are stimulated by a variety of noxious stimuli. C fibers are unmyelinated fibers that carry the signal from the nociceptors to the brain. Proprioceptors tell the body where it is in space and prostaglandins are associated with inflammation and pain but are not pain receptors. Boothe DM, Small Animal Clinical Pharmacology and Therapeutics, ed 2, Elsevier, 2012, p. 994-995.

35. c Lidocaine, if administered too quickly, will cause sinus arrest as a result of cardiac suppression. It will cause numbness when injected locally, but this will not be body wide. Lidocaine is not associated with seizures or polyuria. Boothe DM, Small Animal Clinical Pharmacology and Therapeutics, ed 2, Elsevier, 2012, p. 506-509.

36. c Agonists bind and stimulate the receptor causing an effect, whereas antagonists bind or block the binding site of the receptor and inhibit the effect. Oxymorphone, meperidine, and fentanyl are pure opioid agonists whereas butorphanol acts as an agonist on kappa receptors and as an antagonist on mu receptors. Thomas J, Lerche P, Anesthesia and Analgesia for Veterinary Technicians, ed 5, Mosby, 2016, p. 259-260.

37. c Acepromazine is a phenothiazine tranquilizer that will cause relaxation of vascular smooth muscle, which can lead to hypotension. Because it is a tranquilizer, it will not cause tachycardia and is not known to cause respiratory depression or a decrease in salivation. Bill RL, Clinical Pharmacology and Therapeutics for the Veterinary Technician, ed 4, Mosby, 2016, p. 185.

38. d The LD50 is the dose that will be lethal in 50% of patients, whereas the ED50 is the dose that will produce the desired effect in 50% of patients. The toxic index does not exist. The therapeutic index is calculated by dividing the LD50 by the ED50 (LD50/ED50). Drugs with a low therapeutic index have a narrow margin of safety, whereas drugs with a high therapeutic index will have a wide margin of safety. Wanamaker BP, Massey KL, Applied Pharmacology for Veterinary Technicians, ed 5, Elsevier, 2015, p. 14.

39. d The half-life of aspirin is very different in dogs (8 hours) than it is in cats (40 hours). Bonagura JD, Twedt DC, Kirk's Current Veterinary Therapy XV, Elsevier, 2014, p. 115.

40. c *Insect growth regulators* is a broad term encompassing anything that interferes with the development of the insect. Because of this, they will not affect adults or prevent the laying of eggs. Insects develop differently from mammals and insect growth regulators will therefore not be toxic to mammals. Bill RL, Clinical Pharmacology and Therapeutics for the Veterinary Technician, ed 4, Mosby, 2016, p. 286-287.

41. d Anipryl is used for canine cognitive dysfunction (also known as old dog senility) and works by increasing the dopamine in the brain. Clomipramine is used for obsessive-compulsive disorders, separation anxiety, or aggression. Meloxicam is an NSAID, and diazepam is used as an anticonvulsant or antianxiety drug. Bill RL, Clinical Pharmacology and Therapeutics for the Veterinary Technician, ed 4, Mosby, 2016, p. 206.

42. d Corticosteroids are known to have several short-term side effects, including polyuria and immunosuppression (which would cause a delay in healing). Osteoporosis can be a long-term effect of corticosteroid therapy. Bassert JM, Thomas JA, McCurnin's Clinical Textbook for Veterinary Technicians, ed 9, Elsevier, 2017, p. 685.

43. b There are multiple histamine receptors in the body including H1 found in smooth muscle and the endothelium, H2 found in the gastric cells, H3 found in the central nervous system, and H4 found in the cells of the immune system. Antihistamines cause sedation via blocking of H3 receptors in the central nervous system. They are also used to treat pruritus and are not known to cause panting or polyuria. Wanamaker BP, Massey KL, Applied Pharmacology for Veterinary Technicians, ed 5, Elsevier, 2015, p. 156.

44. a H2 receptors are found in the parietal cells in the gastric mucosa. These receptors are not found in saliva, the carotid arteries, or the aortic arch. Bassert JM, Thomas JA, McCurnin's Clinical Textbook for Veterinary Technicians, ed 8, Elsevier, 2014, p. 1014.

45. b Barbiturates move down a greyhound's concentration gradient from the brain to the blood and then to the adipose tissue. When there is less adipose tissue available, more of the drug will stay in the blood, which decreases the concentration gradient preventing the drug from moving out of the brain. Sight hounds (greyhounds, whippets) have less adipose tissue and will require a lower dose. Bill RL, Clinical Pharmacology and Therapeutics for the Veterinary Technician, ed 3, Mosby, 2006, p. 217-220.

46. a Chloramphenicol is an antibiotic and is not used to treat glaucoma, although it may be used postoperatively to prevent infection if the glaucoma is treated surgically. Carbachol and pilocarpine are parasympathomimetics used to induce miosis in glaucoma, whereas latanoprost is used to decrease intraocular pressure. Wanamaker BP, Massey KL, Applied Pharmacology for Veterinary Technicians, ed 5, Elsevier, 2015, p. 198-200.

47. b A chronotropic agent will either increase (positive chronotropic) or decrease (negative chronotropic) the rate of contraction. Inotropic agents change the force of the contraction. A lusitropic agent will affect the rate of diastolic relaxation. Silverstein D, Hopper K, Small Animal Critical Care Medicine, ed 1, Saunders, 2009, p. 27.

48. d Doxapram is a respiratory stimulant that can be placed under the tongue of neonates to stimulate respirations. Dobutamine is a positive inotropic agent that will increase contractility and digitalis is used to increase cardiac contractility, treat arrhythmias, and decrease the heart rate, none of which should be needed in a newborn. Diazepam will cause sedation and should not be used in a patient that is not breathing well. Tear M, Small Animal Surgical Nursing: Skills and Concepts, ed 3, Elsevier, 2016, p. 147.

49. d If phenylbutazone is administered subcutaneously, intramuscularly, or intradermally, it will cause sloughing of the tissue. For this reason it should only be given intravenously. Wanamaker BP, Massey KL, Applied Pharmacology for Veterinary Technicians, ed 5, Elsevier, 2015, p. 303.

50. a Allergy testing includes intradermal injections of possible allergens followed by monitoring of the reaction. Intradermal injections are also used to test for tuberculosis. Insulin and vaccinations are administered subcutaneously, whereas antibiotics can be given intramuscularly, subcutaneously, or intravenously. Sirois M, Principles and Practice of Veterinary Technology, ed 4, Elsevier, 2016, p. 250, 647.

51. a Biotransformation occurs in many organs including the liver, lungs, skin, and kidneys. Of these, the liver is where the majority of the biotransformation occurs. Wanamaker BP, Massey KL, Applied Pharmacology for Veterinary Technicians, ed 5, Elsevier, 2015, p. 11.

52. c When a drug company develops a new drug, it also has a patent for that drug. Companies invest a large amount of money and time in the development of a drug and the patent allows them to be the only ones manufacturing the drug, allowing them to recover costs. After the patent expires, other drug companies are allowed to manufacture that drug. Because other companies did not incur the cost of development, they are able to sell it at a reduced price. Generic drugs do not use less expensive ingredients and they are as effective as the original drug. Wanamaker BP, Massey KL, Applied Pharmacology for Veterinary Technicians, ed 5, Elsevier, 2015, p. 15-16.

53. b A repository drug is one that is designed to produce a sustained, long-lasting release of medication. Medications composed of plant or animal parts are called biologics, whereas the coating on a drug that protects it from the environment of the stomach is called the enteric coating. Bill RL, Clinical Pharmacology and Therapeutics for the Veterinary Technician, ed 4, Mosby, 2016, p. 11.

54. d Drugs are eliminated via the kidneys (in urine), liver (in bile), and lungs. The spleen is not involved with elimination of drugs. Bill RL, Clinical Pharmacology and Therapeutics for the Veterinary Technician, ed 4, Mosby, 2016, p. 76.

55. b A solution is a drug in a liquid that dissolves and will not precipitate. If a drug is dissolved in liquid sugar, it is considered to be a syrup. An emulsion is a suspension made with oil or fat. Elixirs and tinctures are alcohol-based solutions. Syrups, elixirs, and tinctures are given orally. Bill RL, Clinical Pharmacology and Therapeutics for the Veterinary Technician, ed 4, Mosby, 2016, p. 9-10.

56. a The therapeutic range is the concentration range in which most animals will have the desired response. A narrow range means the range of concentration at which the blood or serum levels need to be to achieve the desired effect is small, and the possibility of overdosing or underdosing is high. The therapeutic range does not refer to what the drug treats, the dosage, or the concentration. Boothe DM, Small Animal Clinical Pharmacology and Therapeutics, ed 2, Elsevier, 2012, p. 215.

57. b The EPA (Environmental Protection Agency) regulates medications applied topically. The FDA (Food and Drug Administration) approves new medications as well as anything taken orally, the USDA (United States Department of Agriculture) regulates vaccines, and the DEA (Drug Enforcement Agency) regulates controlled substances. Bowman DD, Georgi's Parasitology for Veterinarians, ed 10, Elsevier, 2014, p. 40.

58. a The classification for controlled substances numbers drugs from C-I to C-V. The lower the number, the more potential there is for abuse of the drug. A classification of C-I indicates extreme potential and includes drugs with no medical use. Illegal drugs (heroin, LSD, and marijuana) fall into this category. The lowest category including drugs approved for medical use is C-II. These drugs have a high potential for abuse. Drugs classified as C-IV have a low potential for abuse, whereas drugs classified as C-V also have a low potential for abuse but are controlled by the state or local government. Bill RL, Clinical Pharmacology and Therapeutics for the Veterinary Technician, ed 3, Mosby, 2006, p. 25-26.

59. d Drugs given orally, intramuscularly, or subcutaneously have to reach the blood before the peak plasma concentration can be achieved. A drug administered intravenously does not have to take time to reach the blood because it is injected directly into the vein and it will reach peak plasma concentration faster than any other route. Thomas J, Lerche P, Anesthesia and Analgesia for Veterinary Technicians, ed 5, Mosby, 2016, p. 73-74.

60. d Antifungal drugs (also called azole drugs) are imidazole derivatives and interfere with ergosterol synthesis of the fungi. Sulfadimethoxine is combined with other compounds, which are then used as anti-inflammatory drugs and antibacterial drugs. Bill RL, Clinical Pharmacology and Therapeutics for the Veterinary Technician, ed 4, Mosby, 2016, p. 237-238.

61. b Some bacteria contain an enzyme (beta-lactamase) that will render antibiotics ineffective by attacking the beta-lactam ring on the antibiotic. Drugs can be combined with a beta-lactamase inhibitor to prevent this and to make the antibiotic more effective. Some examples include clavulanic acid (combined with amoxicillin to make Clavamox) and sulbactam (combined with ampicillin to make Unasyn). Bill RL, Clinical Pharmacology and Therapeutics for the Veterinary Technician, ed 4, Mosby, 2016, p. 223.

62. a Cells in the inner ear and kidney take up aminoglycosides. Patients receiving drugs in this class should be monitored closely for hearing loss and renal damage. Barbiturates, dissociative anesthetics, and phenothiazine tranquilizers do not have these effects.

Bill RL, Clinical Pharmacology and Therapeutics for the Veterinary Technician, ed 4, Mosby, 2016, p. 225-226.

63. b The only way to know whether the correct antibiotic is being used is to run a culture and sensitivity test of the infected area. Not all infections require 2 weeks of an antibiotic and a broad-spectrum antibiotic should only be used if a culture and sensitivity test are not options or until the culture results are received from the laboratory. The highest dose is not always required and should not be used unless necessary Bonagura JD, Twedt DC, Kirk's Current Veterinary Therapy XV, Elsevier, 2014, p. 23.

64. d Chloramphenicol is known to cause aplastic anemia and it has been fatal in humans; for this reason, it is no longer used in food animals. Gentamicin, tetracycline, and erythromycin are not associated with aplastic anemia. Bill RL, Clinical Pharmacology and Therapeutics for the Veterinary Technician, ed 4, Mosby, 2016, p. 236.

65. a Sulfonamides can cause crystals to form in the kidneys leading to hematuria and can also decrease tear production causing keratoconjunctivitis sicca (KCS). Doberman pinschers are more sensitive to developing allergic reactions and long-term use has been known to cause the development of thrombocytopenia and leukopenia. Tetracyclines will cause chelation of calcium, leading to yellow, mottled teeth and slow bone development in young animals. Fluoroquinolones will cause lesions in the joint cartilage of young animals, whereas patients taking macrolides might develop abdominal cramping, pain, and diarrhea. Bill RL, Clinical Pharmacology and Therapeutics for the Veterinary Technician, ed 4, Mosby, 2016, p. 232-233.

66. d Tetracyclines will chelate with calcium, leading to yellow, mottled teeth and slow bone development in young animals. For the same reason, they should not be given with food (chelating with the calcium will cause a decrease in absorption). Tetracyclines are bacteriostatic, not bactericidal, and they are not nephrotoxic or ototoxic. Bill RL, Clinical Pharmacology and Therapeutics for the Veterinary Technician, ed 4, Mosby, 2016, p. 230-232.

67. b There are 2.2 pounds (lb) in a kilogram (kg). A 50-lb dog will weigh 22.7 kg (50 lb/2.2 lb/kg). 22.7 kg × 1 mg/kg = 22.7 mg. Lake T, Green N, Essential Calculations for Veterinary Nurses and Technicians, ed 3, Butterworth Heinemann, 2016, p. 55-58.

68. c Unlike other aminopenicillins, amoxicillin is absorbed well with food and so should be given with a meal. All antibiotics should be given until the prescription is finished and Amoxi-Drops should be refrigerated. Owners should always be encouraged to call with any questions or concerns. Boothe DM, Small Animal Clinical Pharmacology and Therapeutics, ed 2, Elsevier, 2012, p. 216.

69. a Fluoroquinolones generally end with the suffix -oxacin (enrofloxacin, marbofloxacin, orbifloxacin). Penicillins usually end with -in (ampicillin, amoxicillin), cephalosporins start with cef- or ceph- (cefazolin, cephalexin), and aminoglycosides can end in -cin (gentamicin, amikacin, neomycin). Bassert JM, Thomas JA, McCurnin's Clinical Textbook for Veterinary Technicians, ed 9, Elsevier, 2017, p. 962.

70. d Rabbits are sensitive to medications that are known to kill off the normal flora of the gastrointestinal tract, causing dysbiosis and/or enterotoxemia. Because of this, antibiotics that should be avoided include penicillins (Clavamox), cephalosporins (cefotaxime), lincosamides (clindamycin), and some macrolides (erythromycin). Enrofloxacin does not have this side effect and is therefore safe for use in rabbits. Carpenter JW, Exotic Animal Formulary, ed 4, Elsevier, 2013, p. 548, 673.

71. a Guaifenesin is used as a muscle relaxant, sedative, and expectorant. Expectorants increase the fluidity of mucus to make it more easily removed by the mucociliary apparatus. Decongestants decrease tissue edema in the nasal passages, bronchodilators will cause bronchodilation, and antitussives suppress coughing. Bonagura JD, Twedt DC, Kirk's Current Veterinary Therapy XV, Elsevier, 2014, p. 627.

72. b Codeine, hydrocodone, and butorphanol are all controlled drugs and therefore cannot be purchased over the counter. Common antitussives contain dextromethorphan, which is found in Robitussin, Thera-Flu, and NyQuil. Sirois M, Principles and Practice of Veterinary Technology, ed 3, Elsevier, 2011, p. 261.

73. c Theophylline, albuterol, and terbutaline are bronchodilators and will not stimulate respirations. Doxapram is a central nervous system stimulant and can be used to treat apnea or bradypnea. This can be placed under the tongue of a newborn to encourage breathing. Bill RL, Clinical Pharmacology and Therapeutics for the Veterinary Technician, ed 4, Mosby, 2016, p. 193-194.

74. a Butorphanol acts as both an analgesic and an antitussive. It is unlikely to cause vomiting and is therefore not used as an emetic. Butorphanol can cause sedation but is not a tranquilizer. It does not cause secretions in the respiratory tract and does not act as an expectorant. Bill RL, Clinical Pharmacology and Therapeutics for the Veterinary Technician, ed 4, Mosby, 2016, p. 146.

75. c A patient with a productive cough should not receive a cough suppressant (antitussive) because a cough is beneficial to remove excretions from the lungs and airway. An expectorant would be most beneficial because it would increase fluid excretion in the airway and would thin the mucus, making it easier to expel. An antihistamine would not benefit a patient with a productive cough and coughing should not be painful; hence the patient should not require analgesia. Bill RL, Clinical Pharmacology and Therapeutics for the Veterinary Technician, ed 4, Mosby, 2016, p. 148.

76. a Heparin is often added to sterile saline to produce a heparinized saline, which can be used to flush intravenous catheters. EDTA (ethylenediaminetetraacetic acid) is used as an anticoagulant in blood tubes or, if added to calcium disodium, to chelate zinc in a zinc toxicity case or lead in a lead toxicity case. Coumarin derivatives are used to treat thromboembolic diseases, but they are not appropriate for use in healthy patients. Acid citrate dextrose is used in blood collection bags used when collecting blood for transfusions. Bassert JM, Thomas JA, McCurnin's Clinical Textbook for Veterinary Technicians, ed 8, Elsevier, 2014, p. 596, 899; Peterson ME, Talcott PA, Small Animal Toxicology, ed 2, Elsevier, 2006, p. 461-462.

77. b Fibrinolytic drugs will break down clots in a controlled manner, which would be most beneficial in this patient.

Anticoagulant drugs are used to prevent or to decrease the formation of clots and may benefit this patient in the future but they will not treat a pre-existing clot. Hemostatic drugs are used to induce clotting and to stop hemorrhage, which would not be appropriate in this patient. Hematinic drugs increase the level of hemoglobin in the blood, which would not help this patient. Silverstein D, Hopper K, Small Animal Critical Care Medicine, ed 1, Saunders, 2009, p. 115.

78. d Furosemide is a loop diuretic and, of those listed here, is the most common diuretic used in congestive heart failure. Chlorothiazide is a thiazide diuretic that can be used in conjunction with furosemide if the patient becomes less responsive to furosemide alone. Spirolactone is a potassium-sparing diuretic and it can also be used in conjunction with furosemide. Mannitol is an osmotic diuretic and is used to address cerebral edema or to increase urine output in renal failure. Bill RL, Clinical Pharmacology and Therapeutics for the Veterinary Technician, ed 4, Mosby, 2016, p. 137-139.

79. a Epinephrine is an adrenergic agonist, meaning it will attach to and stimulate adrenergic receptors, which will cause an increase in the heart rate. Because it is an agonist and because it stimulates receptors, it will decrease neither the heart rate nor the blood pressure. Epinephrine is not a reversal agent and acepromazine is not reversible therefore it is not used for this purpose. Papich MG, Saunders Handbook of Veterinary Drugs: Small and Large Animal, ed 4, Elsevier, 2015, p. 291-292.

80. d Vasodilators dilate blood vessels through several mechanisms including relaxation of the smooth muscle found in the vessel wall. The vasodilation of the vessels can lead to hypotension, which is a common side effect. Tachycardia (not bradycardia) will occur to increase the blood pressure. Vasodilators do not have a direct effect on the heart and do not cause cardiac arrhythmias. Anorexia, vomiting, and diarrhea can occur but are not the most common side effects. Wanamaker BP, Massey KL, Applied Pharmacology for Veterinary Technicians, ed 5, Elsevier, 2015, p. 122.

81. a Inotropes affect the contractility (the force of the contraction) of the heart, whereas chronotropic drugs will affect the heart rate. A positive inotrope will increase contractility and a negative chronotropic drug will decrease the heart rate. Neither of these drug classes directly affects blood pressure by changing peripheral vascular resistance. Silverstein D, Hopper K, Small Animal Critical Care Medicine, ed 1, Saunders, 2009, p. 27.

82. a Drugs used in cardiac arrest will depend on the cause and any arrhythmias that may be present. Epinephrine will cause arterial vasoconstriction, which will increase blood flow to the heart and kidneys and, of the drugs listed, is the drug of choice. Atropine is used in the presence of ventricular asystole or bradyarrhythmia. The other drugs listed are used post-arrest: lidocaine is used to address ventricular arrhythmias, dobutamine will be used to support blood pressure, and sodium bicarbonate will be used to address acidosis that may be present after the patient is resuscitated. Battaglia AM, Small Animal Emergency and Critical Care for Veterinary Technicians, ed 3, Saunders, 2015, p. 240.

83. d Warfarin is used in anticoagulant rodenticides and acts by preventing the recycling of vitamin K, which is required to synthesize clotting factors II, VII, IX, and X. These clotting factors are involved with the formation of fibrin and are essential for the clotting cascade to function correctly. Vitamin K can be administered subcutaneously or orally to replace the vitamin K while the rodenticide is active. Streptokinase is a fibrinolytic and will break down clots, coumarin binds vitamin K and so will be contraindicated, and protamine sulfate is given to reverse heparin by binding with it to form a molecule that does not have anticoagulant activity. This may be beneficial in a patient with a heparin overdose but it will not benefit this patient. Peterson ME, Talcott PA, Small Animal Toxicology, ed 2, Elsevier, 2006, p. 569-573.

84. b Chemotherapeutics have a low or narrow margin of safety and doses should therefore be checked and then double-checked by both the doctor and the technician. These drugs can be administered orally, intravenously, intramuscularly, or intradermally. They are not available over the counter because they must be provided under the supervision of a veterinarian. Few chemotherapeutics are nephrotoxic. More commonly, they will cause bone marrow suppression, vomiting, anorexia, and diarrhea. Bassert JM, Thomas JA, McCurnin's Clinical Textbook for Veterinary Technicians, ed 8, Elsevier, 2014, p. 714-717.

85. b Chemotherapeutics act against cancer cells and normal cells in the body. Because they target quickly dividing cells, the bone marrow is commonly affected, which causes bone marrow suppression and immunosuppression. Chemotherapeutics do not cause hyperphagia, constipation, or hyperglycemia and instead are more likely to cause anorexia, diarrhea, and hypoglycemia. Bassert JM, Thomas JA, McCurnin's Clinical Textbook for Veterinary Technicians, ed 9, Elsevier, 2017, p. 732-738.

86. c Hypersensitivity (which may manifest itself as pruritus) is a rare side effect of chemotherapy. Because chemotherapeutics target quickly dividing cells (e.g., bone marrow, the gastrointestinal tract, and hair follicles), you are more likely to see immunosuppression, vomiting, diarrhea, or alopecia. Bassert JM, Thomas JA, McCurnin's Clinical Textbook for Veterinary Technicians, ed 9, Elsevier, 2017, p. 741-742.

87. d Microorganisms found in the rumen will limit the bioavailability or effectiveness of medications administered orally. The medication will dissolve quickly and eructation will therefore not be a factor and the size of the rumen or the presence of gas will not have any bearing on the effectiveness of the medications. Bassert JM, Thomas JA, McCurnin's Clinical Textbook for Veterinary Technicians, ed 8, Elsevier, 2014, p. 1011.

88. a Some drugs will stay in the tissue until the concentration in the blood drops to create a concentration gradient. When this happens, the drug will move into the blood. Common organs in which drugs will accumulate include the liver, kidney, bone, and fat. This does not occur in the pancreas. Wanamaker BP, Massey KL, Applied Pharmacology for Veterinary Technicians, ed 5, Elsevier, 2015, p. 10-11.

89. b Hyperadrenocorticism (Cushing's disease) results from an increase in cortisol, either because of a lesion in the pituitary gland causing excessive production or because of chronic high doses of glucocorticoids. When there are high levels of cortisol in the blood, negative feedback occurs, which decreases production of adrenocorticotropic hormone (ACTH) and thus cortisol. This results in atrophy of the adrenal cortex and hypoadrenocorticism (Addison's disease). Hypothyroidism is a result of thyroid atrophy of the thyroid gland, whereas hyperthyroidism is secondary to an excess production of T3 and T4. Bill RL, Clinical Pharmacology and Therapeutics for the Veterinary Technician, ed 4, Mosby, 2016, p. 302.

90. c Glucocorticoids can cause immunosuppression and should not be used to treat infections. They are commonly used to treat immune-mediated diseases in which the immune system attacks cells of the body. In these diseases, suppression of the immune system is advantageous. Musculoskeletal problems are often painful because of inflammation and glucocorticoids can therefore be beneficial. Allergies will also respond to glucocorticoids. Bill RL, Clinical Pharmacology and Therapeutics for the Veterinary Technician, ed 4, Mosby, 2016, p. 298-303.

91. a Glucocorticoids are classified by their duration of activity. Most topical steroids will last 12 hours, prednisone and triamcinolone will last 12–36 hours, and dexamethasone will last 48 hours or longer. Bill RL, Clinical Pharmacology and Therapeutics for the Veterinary Technician, ed 4, Mosby, 2016, p. 299.

92. d Glucocorticoids are steroids (they do not fall under the category of NSAIDs) and are not safer than NSAIDs. They commonly cause suppression of the immune system and so are used to treat immune-medicated diseases. With long-term use, the body decreases production of glucocorticoids, therefore steroids should not be discontinued quickly; instead, they should be tapered. Bill RL, Clinical Pharmacology and Therapeutics for the Veterinary Technician, ed 4, Mosby, 2016, p. 298-303.

93. a Prednisone is a glucocorticoid, not an NSAID. All other options are NSAIDs. Bill RL, Clinical Pharmacology and Therapeutics for the Veterinary Technician, ed 4, Mosby, 2016, p. 303-309.

94. b Because of its effectiveness in addressing visceral pain, flunixin is commonly used for pain associated with colic in horses. It is an NSAID and does not have anticoagulant activity and, although it may help in reducing fever and treating chronic osteoarthritis pain, these are not the most common uses. Bassert JM, Thomas JA, McCurnin's Clinical Textbook for Veterinary Technicians, ed 9, Elsevier, 2017, p. 1002.

95. b NSAIDs have a longer half-life in cats because of the deficiency in glucuronic acid in this species. This is added to a substrate (usually a toxin) to allow metabolism of the substrate (glucuronidation). For this reason, NSAIDs should not be used in cats or the dose and dosing interval should be adjusted. Ford RB, Mazzaferro F, Kirk and Bistner's Handbook of Veterinary Procedures and Emergency Treatment, ed 9, Elsevier, 2012, p. 73-74.

96. a Aspirin is eliminated via conjugation with glucuronic acid (glucuronidation). Cats have a relative deficiency in glucuronic acid, hence the half-life of aspirin is prolonged in cats. For this reason, the dosing interval should be longer than that in other species. Ibuprofen, carprofen, and naproxen should never be given to cats. Bassert JM, Thomas JA, McCurnin's Clinical Textbook for Veterinary Technicians, ed 9, Elsevier, 2017, p. 913.

97. b NSAIDs work by blocking production of prostaglandins via inhibition of cyclooxygenase (COX). COX-1 synthesizes prostaglandins that protect the gastric mucosa, whereas COX-2 synthesizes prostaglandins involved with inflammation and pain. Unless the NSAID is specific to COX-2, it can cause ulcerations. Thomas J, Lerche P, Anesthesia and Analgesia for Veterinary Technicians, ed 4, Mosby, 2011, p. 423.

98. d DMSO is a solvent added to topical medications to allow the medications to penetrate the skin. Because of this, gloves should be worn to prevent penetration of the skin of the person applying the medication. DMSO does have an odor, but the fumes are nontoxic and a mask is not required and a bandage does not need to cover the area.

99. d Nitrous oxide will diffuse into the alveoli and take the place of oxygen. For this reason, the patient should be maintained on 100% oxygen for 5–10 minutes after the gas is shut off to allow time for the nitrous oxide to leave the alveoli and oxygen to take its place, which will ensure diffusion hypoxia does not occur. There is no reversal for nitrous oxide and the patient should be closely monitored. Thomas J, Lerche P, Anesthesia and Analgesia for Veterinary Technicians, ed 5, Mosby, 2016, p. 410, appendix C.

100. a Apomorphine is not a controlled substance and its use does not have to be tracked. Diazepam is classified as a C-IV drug, whereas ketamine is a C-III drug and hydromorphone is a C-II drug. Bassert JM, Thomas JA, McCurnin's Clinical Textbook for Veterinary Technicians, ed 8, Elsevier, 2014, p. 1033.

101. c Halothane (no longer available in the United States) has been known to cause malignant hyperthermia. Although the other inhalant anesthetics listed have the potential to cause malignant hyperthermia, the risk is highest with halothane. Thomas J, Lerche P, Anesthesia and Analgesia for Veterinary Technicians, ed 5, Mosby, 2016, p. 408, appendix B.

102. c Thiopental and phenobarbital are both barbiturates. Atropine is an anticholinergic, diazepam is a benzodiazepine tranquilizer, and ketamine is a dissociative anesthetic. Thomas J, Lerche P, Anesthesia and Analgesia for Veterinary Technicians, ed 5, Mosby, 2016, p. 404, appendix A.

103. a Fentanyl comes in several forms, including a solution for injection, tablets for oral administration, and a patch for transdermal application. Pentazocine is only in the injectable form, whereas meperidine and butorphanol come in the injectable and oral forms. Other medications available in the form of a transdermal patch include nitroglycerin and selegiline hydrochloride. Bassert JM, Thomas JA, McCurnin's Clinical Textbook for Veterinary Technicians, ed 9, Elsevier, 2017, p. 545.

104. c Diazepam is the first drug of choice for the emergency treatment of seizures. In addition to intravenous use, it can also be administered rectally and nasally. This allows the owner to give it at home in the event of a breakthrough seizure. Midazolam is not well absorbed when given rectally, acepromazine will not treat seizure activity (and may actually lower the seizure threshold), and pentobarbital, a common ingredient in euthanasia solutions, should not be given to an owner to take home. Silverstein D, Hopper K, Small Animal Critical Care Medicine, ed 1, Saunders, 2009, p. 417-418.

105. a Dexmedetomidine causes hypertension, resulting in a reflex bradycardia. Diazepam, ketamine, and acepromazine may lower the heart rate slightly but not to the extent of dexmedetomidine. Wanamaker BP, Massey KL, Applied Pharmacology for Veterinary Technicians, ed 5, Elsevier, 2015, p. 82.

106. b Detomidine is an alpha-2 agonist used in horses to provide sedation and analgesia. Naloxone is used to reverse opioids, flumazenil is used to reverse benzodiazepines, and yohimbine is used to reverse alpha-2 agonists. Bonagura JD, Twedt DC, Kirk's Current Veterinary Therapy XV, Elsevier, 2014, p. 30.

107. a How quickly the depth of anesthesia changes is a result of the blood–gas partition coefficient. Inhalants with a high blood–gas partition coefficient will more readily move into the tissue and blood, meaning less stays in the alveoli. This leaves a small difference in the drug concentration in the blood and alveoli (therefore there is a low concentration gradient), and the drug is slow to leave the blood (or move down its concentration gradient). This means it takes longer for the patient to react to changes in the percentage of gas being delivered as well as taking longer to recover. Inhalants with a low blood–gas partition coefficient will leave the alveoli more slowly, leaving a much higher concentration of drug in the alveoli than in the blood. This leaves a large difference in the concentration of the drug compared with the alveoli (therefore there is a high concentration gradient) and the drug more readily moves from the blood back to the alveoli. This means changes are seen very quickly and recovery is also quick. The blood–gas partition coefficients of the anesthetics listed (from lowest to highest) are: Desflurane (0.47), Sevoflurane (0.69), Isoflurane (1.1), and Halothane (2.36). This means Desflurane will produce very fast changes in the patient's status and will require the most intense monitoring. Bassert JM, Thomas JA, McCurnin's Clinical Textbook for Veterinary Technicians, ed 9, Elsevier, 2017, p. 1018.

108. b The nervous system consists of the central nervous system and the peripheral nervous system. The peripheral nervous system is divided into the sympathetic and parasympathetic nervous systems. The neurotransmitters listed are catecholamines and their main effect is in the sympathetic nervous system. The neurotransmitter for the parasympathetic nervous system is acetylcholine. Wanamaker BP, Massey KL, Applied Pharmacology for Veterinary Technicians, ed 5, Elsevier, 2015, p. 75-76.

109. b Pentobarbital is the main component of euthanasia solutions. If it is the only drug in the solution, it is classified as C-II. If it is combined with other agents (such as a dye to identify it as a euthanasia solution), it is classified as C-III. Phenobarbital is used to treat seizures. Methohexital and thiopental are both short-acting barbiturates used in anesthetic procedures. Wanamaker BP, Massey KL, Applied Pharmacology for Veterinary Technicians, ed 5, Elsevier, 2015, p. 95.

110. d Acepromazine has been known to cause persistent paraphimosis, increasing the chances of injury to the stallion. Detomidine, diazepam, and xylazine are commonly used in horses. Bassert JM, Thomas JA, McCurnin's Clinical Textbook for Veterinary Technicians, ed 9, Elsevier, 2017, p. 685.

111. c Propofol contains egg, lecithin, and soybean oil, all of which encourage bacterial growth. Because of this, it is ideal to keep it refrigerated after it has been opened and it should be discarded after 6 hours. One bottle of propofol contains enough drug to use in multiple patients and, unless blood is present in the vial, it is highly unlikely a contagious disease will be present in the vial. (It should be noted that Propofol-28 can be kept at room temperature for 28 days as long as aseptic technique is used when the bottle is punctured.) Thomas J, Lerche P, Anesthesia and Analgesia for Veterinary Technicians, ed 5, Mosby, 2016, p. 76.

112. d Ruminants are very sensitive to xylazine and may experience a decrease in rumen motility. Some cattle breeds (Herefords and Brahmas) are even more sensitive. A tenth of the normal dose used in horses should be used in cattle. Holtgrew-Bohling K, Large Animal Clinical Procedures for Veterinary Technicians, ed 3, Mosby, 2015, p. 465.

113. c Ketamine causes increased salivation and muscle rigidity and cats tend to keep their eyes open. For this reason, it is often combined with diazepam to promote muscle relaxation. Xylazine, propofol, and medetomidine will all cause muscle relaxation and do not promote salivation. Bassert JM, Thomas JA, McCurnin's Clinical Textbook for Veterinary Technicians, ed 9, Elsevier, 2017, p. 1017.

114. d Xylazine is an alpha-2 agonist and can be reversed with yohimbine. Epinephrine is not a reversal agent and naloxone reverses opioids. Cattle are sensitive to ketamine and should receive only a tenth of the dose given horses. Wanamaker BP, Massey KL, Applied Pharmacology for Veterinary Technicians, ed 5, Elsevier, 2015, p. 81.

115. a Acepromazine has been shown to lower the seizure threshold and might increase the chance of seizures occurring in a patient with a previous history of seizures. Acepromazine will be more potent, will last longer in geriatric patients, and should be used with caution, but it does not need to be avoided in these patients. Some breeds (e.g., giant breeds, Australian shepherds, collies, greyhounds, and boxers) may require a lower dose or might be more sensitive to the cardiovascular effects of the drug. Doberman pinschers are not known to be one of the more sensitive breeds. Unless it is contraindicated because of medical history, aggressive patients will benefit from sedation. Thomas J, Lerche P, Anesthesia and Analgesia for Veterinary Technicians, ed 4, Mosby, 2011, p. 60.

116. c Mirtazapine is a selective serotonin reuptake inhibitor that acts as an appetite stimulant and can be sent home with the patient. Diazepam (a benzodiazepine) may stimulate the appetite but cannot be sent home. Progestins and tricyclic antidepressants do not act as appetite stimulants. Wanamaker BP, Massey KL, Applied Pharmacology for Veterinary Technicians, ed 5, Saunders, 2009, p. 166-167.
117. a Megestrol acetate is a progestin used to treat inappropriate spraying in male cats. Oxazepam is a benzodiazepine, amitriptyline is a tricyclic antidepressant, and fluoxetine is a selective serotonin reuptake inhibitor. Papich MG, Saunders Handbook of Veterinary Drugs: Small and Large Animal, ed 4, Elsevier, 2015, p. 485.
118. d Of the drugs listed, clomipramine is the only tricyclic antidepressant. Buspirone is an azaperone agent, selegiline is a monoamine oxidase inhibitor, and paroxetine is a selective serotonin reuptake inhibitor. Wanamaker BP, Massey KL, Applied Pharmacology for Veterinary Technicians, ed 5, Saunders, 2009, p. 94.
119. c Bladder atony occurs when the patient is unable to empty the urinary bladder completely because of atony of the bladder muscles. Urinary incontinence occurs when the patient is unable to control urination. Phenylpropanolamine causes contraction of the bladder neck (increasing sphincter tone) and proximal urethra, which helps the patient control urination. Bonagura JD, Twedt DC, Kirk's Current Veterinary Therapy XV, Elsevier, 2014, p. 915.
120. a Erythropoietin is produced by the kidneys and stimulates the hemocytoblast to become a rubriblast, which eventually becomes a red blood cell. There is a decrease in the production of erythropoietin in renal disease, hence some cats will benefit from supplementation. A cardiomyopathy will not cause anemia and anemia secondary to rodenticide should be treated with a transfusion and vitamin K. Tylenol can cause methemoglobinemia but does not require erythropoietin. Sirois M, Principles and Practice of Veterinary Technology, ed 4, Elsevier, 2016, p. 126.
121. a Famotidine is an H2 receptor antagonist and will decrease gastric acid production by inhibiting histamine in the stomach. Sucralfate is a gastrointestinal protectant and requires an acidic environment to be most effective, omeprazole is a proton pump inhibitor that inhibits the transport of hydrogen ions into the stomach by binding to the parietal cells, and misoprostol inhibits gastric acid secretion from the parietal cell. Wanamaker BP, Massey KL, Applied Pharmacology for Veterinary Technicians, ed 5, Saunders, 2009, p. 157-158.
122. d Amphojel (aluminum hydroxide) and Basaljel (aluminum carbonate) are used both as phosphate binders and as antacids. They can be provided with a meal to bind the phosphorus in the food, preventing or treating hyperphosphatemia. Neither of these drugs will acidify the urine, nor will they address hypertension. Wanamaker BP, Massey KL, Applied Pharmacology for Veterinary Technicians, ed 5, Elsevier, 2015, p. 441.
123. d Selamectin will prevent heartworm disease and also treats or controls ear mites, fleas, and sarcoptic mange in dogs. Diethylcarbamazine does not treat any of these and ivermectin and milbemycin do not treat mites or mange. Wanamaker BP, Massey KL, Applied Pharmacology for Veterinary Technicians, ed 5, Saunders, 2009, p. 285.
124. c A coccidiostat is an antiprotozoal that acts against coccidia parasites. Ascarids, tapeworms, and flukes all require an antihelminth. Summers A, Common Diseases of Companion Animals, ed 3, Elsevier, 2014, p. 692.
125. a Phenylbutazone should only be administered intravenously. When given intramuscularly or subcutaneously it will cause sloughing of the tissue. Oxymorphone can be given intravenously, intramuscularly, or subcutaneously. Dexmedetomidine is most often used intravenously but can also be given intramuscularly. Ketamine can be given intravenously, intramuscularly, or orally in fractious cats. Wanamaker BP, Massey KL, Applied Pharmacology for Veterinary Technicians, ed 5, Saunders, 2009, p. 303.
126. d Organophosphates are used to control endo- and ectoparasites and have a very narrow margin of safety. They work by inhibiting acetylcholinesterase, which breaks down acetylcholine. When this occurs, there is overstimulation of the nicotinic receptors in the nervous system, making them neurotoxic. They have multiple side effects, including salivation, lacrimation, urination, defecation, dyspnea, and bronchospasm. Bonagura JD, Twedt DC, Kirk's Current Veterinary Therapy XV, Elsevier, 2014, p. 135; Bowman DD, Georgi's Parasitology for Veterinarians, ed 10, Elsevier, 2014, p. 272-273.
127. b Insulin can be administered intravenously or intramuscularly when treating diabetic ketoacidosis, but it is given subcutaneously when maintaining diabetes. Insulin is not given orally because it will be broken down in the stomach. Sirois M, Principles and Practice of Veterinary Technology, ed 4, Elsevier, 2016, p. 126.
128. c Because it is so important for a patient to receive the correct amount of insulin, it is measured in units per millimeter. This allows the measurement to be the same no matter where the patient travels internationally. Sirois M, Principles and Practice of Veterinary Technology, ed 4, Elsevier, 2016, p. 614-615.
129. b Glipizide may be used in cats that do not require insulin (Type II diabetes). One possible mechanism of action is the stimulation of beta cells to increase insulin secretion. Glipizide will be ineffective in the treatment of diabetic ketoacidosis and, because it increases the secretion of insulin, it will make hypoglycemia worse. Pancreatitis does not require treatment from insulin or glipizide. Summers A, Common Diseases of Companion Animals, ed 3, Elsevier, 2014, p. 66.
130. c Insulin decreases blood glucose by causing glucose uptake by cells. It is not involved with the regulation of gastrointestinal, reproductive, or metabolic processes throughout the body. Wanamaker BP, Massey KL, Applied Pharmacology for Veterinary Technicians, ed 5, Saunders, 2009, p. 185.
131. a The bottle should be rolled gently. Shaking or heating the vial will damage the proteins, rendering the insulin useless. The vial should be refrigerated, but this will not cause resuspension of the insulin. Bill RL, Clinical

Pharmacology and Therapeutics for the Veterinary Technician, ed 3, Mosby, 2006, p. 185-186.

132. c Altrenogest is an oral progestin. The main progestin in the body is progesterone, which prepares the uterus for pregnancy. Progestins are provided to delay the onset of estrus and to synchronize estrus in mares. Sirois M, Principles and Practice of Veterinary Technology, ed 4, Elsevier, 2016, p. 258.

133. c Excessive estrogen can lead to suppression of the bone marrow, leading to anemia. Gastric ulcers, arrhythmias, and hepatopathy are not known side effects of elevated estrogen levels and should therefore not be associated with DES. Papich MG, Saunders Handbook of Veterinary Drugs: Small and Large Animal, ed 4, Elsevier, 2015, p. 236-237.

134. d Kaolin, pectin, and bismuth subsalicylate are all gastrointestinal protectants. These cover the wall of the stomach and gastrointestinal tract to protect it from acid or irritating compounds. Kaolin and pectin are often used in combination because there is evidence that they absorb bacteria, which decreases hypersecretion in the gastrointestinal tract, which in turn decreases diarrhea. Bismuth subsalicylate acts the same way by decreasing secretions in the gastrointestinal tract. Be aware that subsalicylate is changed to salicylate, which is toxic to cats. Bill RL, Clinical Pharmacology and Therapeutics for the Veterinary Technician, ed 4, Mosby, 2016, p. 101-102.

135. b Metamucil is indigestible and moves through the gastrointestinal tract drawing fluid into the gastrointestinal tract and acting as a bulk laxative. Psyllium is a hydrophilic compound (absorbs water) and acts the same way. Irritants to the gastrointestinal tract will increase motility. Saline cathartics pull fluid into the gastrointestinal tract through oncotic pull, whereas lubricants will lubricate the stool to allow easier passage. Sirois M, Principles and Practice of Veterinary Technology, ed 4, Elsevier, 2016, p. 252-253.

136. b Phenothiazines act as tranquilizers and antiemetics. They will cause sedation, lower the seizure threshold, and cause vasodilation (leading to hypotension). Diarrhea is not a known side effect of phenothiazines. Papich MG, Saunders Handbook of Veterinary Drugs: Small and Large Animal, ed 4, Elsevier, 2015, p. 153-154.

137. a Docusate sodium succinate acts as a surfactant and decreases surface tension. This allows water to move into the stool, softening it and making it easier to pass. Bran will increase the bulk of the gastrointestinal contents and would be uncomfortable for the patient. Mineral oil acts as a lubricant but will not soften the stool and magnesium chloride is used in antacids and will not soften the stool. Wanamaker BP, Massey KL, Applied Pharmacology for Veterinary Technicians, ed 4, Saunders, 2009, p. 162-163.

138. a All of the drugs listed can be used for motion sickness, but phenothiazines are the most widely used. They act by blocking dopamine receptors. Some common phenothiazines used to treat motion sickness are chlorpromazine and prochlorperazine. Wanamaker BP, Massey KL, Applied Pharmacology for Veterinary Technicians, ed 5, Elsevier, 2015, p. 155-156.

139. a Xylazine is the most effective emetic in cats, with an approximate 60% success rate. Syrup of ipecac is not effective and can cause cardiotoxic arrhythmias. Apomorphine has only a 10% success rate in cats and hydrogen peroxide should not be used in cats because it can cause hemorrhagic gastritis. Peterson ME, Talcott PA, Small Animal Toxicology, ed 3, Elsevier, 2013, p. 74-76.

140. c In dogs, apomorphine works quickly, is very effective, and is reversible. Xylazine is not effective in dogs. Hydrogen peroxide and syrup of ipecac are both effective but are no longer recommended because of the possibility of gastric and esophageal ulcerations (hydrogen peroxide) and cardiotoxic arrhythmias (syrup of ipecac). Peterson ME, Talcott PA, Small Animal Toxicology, ed 3, Elsevier, 2013, p. 74-76.

141. c Apomorphine is available in both injectable and tablet form. The tablets can be crushed and placed in the conjunctival sac. Apomorphine must be rinsed from the eye to prevent continued vomiting. Xylazine is not effective in dogs. Syrup of ipecac and hydrogen peroxide should never be placed in the eye or they will cause severe irritation. Peterson ME, Talcott PA, Small Animal Toxicology, ed 3, Elsevier, 2013, p. 74-76.

142. b Sucralfate is a disaccharide that turns into a paste binding to ulcers, which protects them from the gastric contents. Kaopectate coats the stomach but will not adhere to the ulcer. Cimetidine is a histamine (H2) blocker and misoprostol is a prostaglandin that inhibits secretion of hydrogen from the parietal cells in the stomach. It also increases production of mucus and bicarbonate in the stomach, both of which provide some protection to the lining. Wanamaker BP, Massey KL, Applied Pharmacology for Veterinary Technicians, ed 5, Elsevier, 2015, p. 159.

143. c Sodium phosphate enemas can be absorbed through the gastrointestinal tract and into the blood, leading to hypernatremia and hypophosphatemia, which can result in death in cats or small dogs. Ford RB, Mazzaferro E, Kirk and Bistner's Handbook of Veterinary Procedures and Emergency Treatment, ed 9, Elsevier, 2012, p. 506.

144. a Biotransformation refers to the changing of a drug from the administered form to the usable form. The majority of this occurs in the liver. The kidneys and lungs are also involved with a small amount of biotransformation. The stomach and small intestine are not involved with biotransformation. Wanamaker BP, Massey KL, Applied Pharmacology for Veterinary Technicians, ed 5, Elsevier, 2015, p. 11.

145. d Maropitant citrate is a NK-1 antagonist that works by blocking substance P in the chemoreceptor trigger zone. Syrup of ipecac and apomorphine are emetics and will cause vomiting. Atropine is an anticholinergic and does not prevent nausea related to motion sickness. Wanamaker BP, Massey KL, Applied Pharmacology for Veterinary Technicians, ed 5, Elsevier, 2015, p. 156-157.

146. c In renal failure the kidneys are often damaged to the point that they no longer produce erythropoietin (or they produce a deceased amount), which is involved with the release of red blood cells from the bone marrow. Erythropoietin is not involved with fibrinolytic or immunosuppressive activity and is not involved with regulation of blood pressure. Colville TP, Bassert JM, Clinical Anatomy and Physiology for Veterinary Technicians, ed 3, Mosby, 2015, p. 297-298.

147. a Interferon (a biological response modifier) is produced by leukocytes, fibroblasts, and epithelial cells. Biological response modifiers have antitumor, antiviral, and immunoregulatory properties. Interferon is used to treat or to increase the life expectancy of cats with FIP or FeLV. The other drugs listed are not biologic response modifiers. Wanamaker BP, Massey KL, Applied Pharmacology for Veterinary Technicians, ed 5, Elsevier, 2015, p. 365-366.

148. c Atropine is an anticholinergic and blocks acetylcholine at the cholinergic receptors. This results in an increase in heart rate and a decrease in salivation, bronchial secretions, gastrointestinal motility, and tear production. It also will cause mydriasis and bronchodilation. Bassert JM, Thomas JA, McCurnin's Clinical Textbook for Veterinary Technicians, ed 9, Elsevier, 2017, p. 1012-1013.

149. c An antagonist binds to a receptor, blocking the action of another drug at that receptor. An agonist binds to a receptor and mimics another substance, stimulating a reaction. Agonists have a high affinity and efficacy and will cause a specific action. A principle agonist will increase the release of a neurotransmitter that binds to a receptor. Wanamaker BP, Massey KL, Applied Pharmacology for Veterinary Technicians, ed 5, Elsevier, 2015, p. 14.

150. a Aspirin is associated with all of these, but in this case it has been discontinued because of the decrease in platelet aggregation. With an upcoming surgery, it is advantageous to discontinue aspirin therapy to decrease the risk of bleeding associated with a decrease in platelet aggregation. Wanamaker BP, Massey KL, Applied Pharmacology for Veterinary Technicians, ed 5, Elsevier, 2015, p. 145.

151. d Fentanyl is an opioid used for pain. It will not be effective if used to control vomiting, diarrhea, or seizures. Bassert JM, Thomas JA, McCurnin's Clinical Textbook for Veterinary Technicians, ed 9, Elsevier, 2017, p. 545.

152. b Acetylcysteine is used in the treatment of acetaminophen toxicity. It acts as a precursor to glutathione, which is necessary to metabolize acetaminophen. Lidocaine toxicity has no specific treatment and should be addressed by discontinuing the drug and treating clinical signs. Digoxin toxicity requires the discontinuation of the drug for 48 hours and the treatment of cardiac arrhythmias with lidocaine. If the toxicity is life-threatening, it can be treated with Digibind, which contains digoxin antibodies. Opioids are reversed with naloxone. Peterson ME, Talcott PA, Small Animal Toxicology, ed 3, Elsevier, 2013, p. 1113.

153. b Expectorants will thin mucus in the respiratory tract by increasing the secretion of a thinner substance from the cells of the respiratory tract. This causes it to move more easily out of the airways and be expelled. An antitussive will suppress a cough, although a productive cough should never be suppressed. Suppression of inflammation is performed with an anti-inflammatory drug. The allergic component of respiratory disease is addressed with an antihistamine. Sirois M, Principles and Practice of Veterinary Technology, ed 3, Elsevier, 2011, p. 261-262.

154. a The therapeutic range refers to the range into which the plasma concentration can fall to achieve the desired effect. The relationship between the drug's therapeutic or toxic capacities is the therapeutic index and the adverse reactions associated with a drug refers to which and how often idiosyncratic reactions occur. Bill RL, Clinical Pharmacology and Therapeutics for the Veterinary Technician, ed 3, Mosby, 2006, p. 45.

155. c Acepromazine has been known to lower the seizure threshold and is therefore contraindicated in patients with a history of seizures. Diazepam treats seizures, whereas thiopental and fentanyl are not associated with seizure activity. Thomas J, Lerche P, Anesthesia and Analgesia for Veterinary Technicians, ed 5, Mosby, 2016, p. 63.

156. d The word nutraceutical is a combination of the words nutrition (or nutrient) and pharmaceutical and it describes something produced in a purified or extracted form that is used to improve health and well-being. Some examples include glucosamine, omega-3 fatty acids, and S-adenosylmethionine (Sam-e). Wanamaker BP, Massey KL, Applied Pharmacology for Veterinary Technicians, ed 5, Elsevier, 2015, p. 394.

157. d Xylazine is an alpha-2 agonist that is reversed by yohimbine. Fentanyl is an opioid that is reversed by naloxone; acepromazine is not a reversal agent. Thomas J, Lerche P, Anesthesia and Analgesia for Veterinary Technicians, ed 5, Mosby, 2016, p. 69.

158. a Opioids are reversed with naloxone. Yohimbine is used to reverse alpha-2 agonists and neither diazepam nor acetylcysteine are reversal agents. Thomas J, Lerche P, Anesthesia and Analgesia for Veterinary Technicians, ed 5, Mosby, 2016, p. 72.

159. c Opioids can cause bradycardia (but not arrhythmias), respiratory depression, excitement (but not seizures), vomiting, and hypotension (not hypertension). Thomas J, Lerche P, Anesthesia and Analgesia for Veterinary Technicians, ed 5, Mosby, 2016, p. 70.

160. c Thiobarbiturates will be redistributed from the blood to the patient's fat stores within the first 30 minutes after administration. In patients with lean body mass (and thus decreased fat), there is nowhere for the drug to be redistributed therefore it will stay in the blood for a longer period. For this reason, it should not be used in sight hounds because of their lean body conditions. Patients with respiratory alkalosis will have a decreased concentration of carbon dioxide in the blood. Because thiobarbiturates cause respiratory depression, they will cause a patient to retain carbon dioxide (because they are not breathing it off), which may help correct the alkalosis. Obese patients have a large amount of fat stores and thiobarbiturates can therefore be safely used in these patients. Thiobarbiturates are highly protein bound and patients with hyperproteinemia will require a higher dose because there is more protein available to bind the drug, leaving less available to generate an effect. For this reason, it should not be used in hypoproteinemic patients. Wanamaker BP, Massey KL,

Applied Pharmacology for Veterinary Technicians, ed 5, Elsevier, 2015, p. 372.

161. a Loop diuretics cause retention of sodium in the kidneys. When this occurs, potassium is excreted in an attempt to maintain homeostasis. This potassium is lost in the urine and can lead to hypokalemia with chronic use of a loop diuretic. Sirois M, Principles and Practice of Veterinary Technology, ed 4, Elsevier, 2016, p. 255.

162. a Amlodipine is a calcium channel blocker that causes vasodilation and is often used to treat hypertension. Erythromycin is a macrolide antibiotic, amitriptyline is a tricyclic antidepressant, and atropine is an anticholinergic. Bassert JM, Thomas JA, McCurnin's Clinical Textbook for Veterinary Technicians, ed 9, Elsevier, 2017, p. 644.

163. c Ketamine can cause tachycardia, hypertension, apneustic breathing, and muscle rigidity, . Bassert JM, Thomas JA, McCurnin's Clinical Textbook for Veterinary Technicians, ed 9, Elsevier, 2017, p. 1017.

164. b ACE (angiotensin-converting enzyme) inhibitors block the conversion of angiotensinogen I to angiotensinogen II. Angiotensinogen II causes vasoconstriction, which will increase blood pressure. By preventing the conversion of angiotensinogen I to angiotensinogen II, there will be vasodilation, leading to a decrease in blood pressure, increase in cardiac output (resulting from a decrease in preload and afterload), and a decrease in heart rate. Angiotensinogen II is also involved in the release of aldosterone. When this does not occur, there is an increase in urine output, which also helps decrease blood pressure by decreasing fluid retention. Wanamaker BP, Massey KL, Applied Pharmacology for Veterinary Technicians, ed 5, Elsevier, 2015, p. 141-143.

165. a Nitroglycerin is a vasodilator (not an ACE inhibitor) that causes vasodilation (not vasoconstriction) by relaxing the venous blood vessels. It is not effective against arrhythmias Sirois M, Principles and Practice of Veterinary Technology, ed 4, Elsevier, 2016, p. 254-255.

166. b Of the medications listed here, diltiazem is the only calcium channel blocker. Procainamide and lidocaine are antiarrhythmics and digoxin is a cardiac glycoside. Papich MG, Saunders Handbook of Veterinary Drugs: Small and Large Animal, ed 4, Elsevier, 2015, p. 244-245.

167. b Lidocaine is used to treat ventricular tachycardia by decreasing depolarization. Supraventricular tachycardia is a tachyarrhythmia that originates above the ventricles (in the atria, the atrioventricular junction, or above the bundle of His). These are treated with calcium channel blockers or beta blockers. If a supraventricular tachyarrhythmia resolves with lidocaine, it probably originated from the ventricles and not from the atria. Lidocaine will not treat hypertension or a supraventricular bradycardia. Silverstein D, Hopper K, Small Animal Critical Care Medicine, ed 1, Saunders, 2009, p. 202.

168. b The body produces glucocorticoids from the adrenal gland. When glucocorticoids are administered, there is negative feedback that decreases production from the adrenal cortex. If glucocorticoids are stopped abruptly, there is no time for the adrenal cortex to adjust and start producing glucocorticoids. This can cause hypoadrenocorticism (Addison's disease). Colville TP, Bassert JM, Clinical Anatomy and Physiology for Veterinary Technicians, ed 3, Mosby, 2015, p. 286.

169. c Hyperadrenocorticism results from an excessive production of glucocorticoids from the adrenal gland. If glucocorticoids are administered long term, it can cause the same symptoms that are associated with hyperadrenocorticism. Because this is caused by a treatment, it is considered iatrogenic. The thyroid is not associated with the production of glucocorticoids. Colville TP, Bassert JM, Clinical Anatomy and Physiology for Veterinary Technicians, ed 3, Mosby, 2015, p. 286.

170. d When prescribing steroids, the owner should be informed that common side effects include polyuria, polydipsia, polyphagia, and hyperglycemia. Vomiting is not a common side effect of glucocorticoid therapy and, if it occurs, is probably a result of the disease being treated. Wanamaker BP, Massey KL, Applied Pharmacology for Veterinary Technicians, ed 5, Elsevier, 2015, p. 313-314.

171. d Steroids are often used to suppress the immune system during treatment of autoimmune diseases, to decrease inflammation associated with asthma, and to shrink tumors, including those associated with lymphoma. The use of steroids might actually induce hyperadrenocorticism and their use is contraindicated unless treatment includes the destruction of the adrenal gland, at which point glucocorticoids are used as supplementation to replace what the adrenal gland would have produced. Bassert JM, Thomas JA, McCurnin's Clinical Textbook for Veterinary Technicians, ed 9, Elsevier, 2017, p. 972.

172. c Of the drugs listed, atropine is the only anticholinergic. Acetylcysteine, pilocarpine, and nicotine are all cholinergic drugs. Thomas J, Lerche P, Anesthesia and Analgesia for Veterinary Technicians, ed 5, Mosby, 2016, p. 61-62.

173. a Compounding relates to changing a medication (through dilution or combination) from the form approved by the FDA to a form used in treatment. This may be done to make administration easier (adding a flavor) or to make it into a different form (paste or patch). As a technician, you will do this many times when you dilute an antibiotic given intravenously (to decrease the chances of it causing nausea) or when you combine two medications into one syringe (such as ketamine and valium). Wanamaker BP, Massey KL, Applied Pharmacology for Veterinary Technicians, ed 4, Saunders, 2009, p. 21.

174. a Of the drugs listed, phenylpropanolamine (PPA) is used to treat urinary incontinence. Diethylcarbamazine is used as a daily preventative for heartworms and roundworms. Acepromazine is a phenothiazine and bethanechol is a cholinergic drug. Wanamaker BP, Massey KL, Applied Pharmacology for Veterinary Technicians, ed 5, Elsevier, 2015, p. 123-125.

175. c Of the drugs listed, mannitol is the only osmotic diuretic. Furosemide is a loop diuretic, chlorothiazide is a thiazide diuretic, and spironolactone is a potassium sparing diuretic. Wanamaker BP, Massey KL, Applied

Pharmacology for Veterinary Technicians, ed 5, Elsevier, 2015, p. 117-119.

176. d Apomorphine is used to induce vomiting in the face of ingestion of a toxic substance. Chlorpromazine blocks dopamine receptors in the chemoreceptor trigger zone. Metoclopramide acts both centrally and peripherally by blocking dopamine receptors in the chemoreceptor trigger zone, as well as decreasing gastric emptying time and increasing gastric contractions. Maropitant citrate is an NK-1 antagonist that acts on the chemoreceptor trigger zone. Wanamaker BP, Massey KL, Applied Pharmacology for Veterinary Technicians, ed 5, Elsevier, 2015, p. 155-157.

177. b Cephalosporins are similar to penicillins and should be avoided in patients that are allergic to penicillins. Bill RL, Clinical Pharmacology and Therapeutics for the Veterinary Technician, ed 4, Mosby, 2016, p. 223-224.

178. a Griseofulvin is used for dermatophyte fungal infections and is used to treat dermatophytosis. Staphylococcal pyoderma is not caused by a fungus and should be treated with antibiotics. Rickettsial diseases are tick-borne and are treated with antibiotics and nematodes are intestinal parasites that are treated with dewormers. Wanamaker BP, Massey KL, Applied Pharmacology for Veterinary Technicians, ed 5, Elsevier, 2015, p. 259.

179. d Of the drugs listed, only fentanyl is an opioid and provides analgesia. Acepromazine is a sedative and tranquilizer, diazepam is suited to treat seizures and as a sedative, and thiopental is an anesthetic. Wanamaker BP, Massey KL, Applied Pharmacology for Veterinary Technicians, ed 5, Elsevier, 2015, p. 307-308.

180. a Melarsomine is the only adulticide listed. Ivermectin, milbemycin, and moxidectin are all microfilaricides. Bowman DD, Georgi's Parasitology for Veterinarians, ed 10, Elsevier, 2014, p. 216-217.

181. c Warfarin is considered an anticoagulant rodenticide. Rodenticides work by preventing the recycling of vitamin K, which is used in the production of clotting factors II, VII, IX, and X. When this occurs, vitamin K supplementation should be started and continued until the effects of the rodenticide have worn off. Vitamin C is sometimes used to treat acetaminophen toxicity because it assists with the conversion of methemoglobin to hemoglobin. Naloxone is used to reverse the effects of opioids. 4-methylprayzole is used to treat ethylene glycol toxicity. Peterson ME, Talcott PA, Small Animal Toxicology, ed 3, Elsevier, 2013, p. 460-466.

182. a Propranolol works by blocking both beta-1 and beta-2 receptors, which changes the automaticity of cardiac cells and decreases the heart rate. Xylazine is an alpha-2 agonist, hydralazine is a calcium channel blocker and arteriolar dilator, and epinephrine is a catecholamine, which increases the contraction of the heart. Wanamaker BP, Massey KL, Applied Pharmacology for Veterinary Technicians, ed 5, Elsevier, 2015, p. 81.

183. c The wider the spectrum of a drug, the more microbes it is effective against. The effectiveness of a drug indicates how well it works, the efficacy of a drug indicates the degree to which the drug produces a response, and a drug's affinity is an indication of a drug's tendency to bind to the receptor. Bassert JM, Thomas JA, McCurnin's Clinical Textbook for Veterinary Technicians, ed 8, Elsevier, 2014, p. 1018.

184. d Ivermectin does not suppress the immune system. Cyclosporine, azathioprine, and prednisone are all used for immune suppression and are often used to treat immune-mediated diseases. Wanamaker BP, Massey KL, Applied Pharmacology for Veterinary Technicians, ed 5, Elsevier, 2015, p. 367-368.

185. c Neomycin is the only aminoglycoside listed. Although the others listed are also antibiotics, they fall into different classes. Ampicillin is a beta-lactam, erythromycin is a macrolide, and doxycycline is a tetracycline. Wanamaker BP, Massey KL, Applied Pharmacology for Veterinary Technicians, ed 5, Elsevier, 2015, p. 332-333.

186. a Cats have experienced retinal degeneration and blindness, therefore doses at the low end of the range are recommended. Bonagura JD, Twedt DC, Kirk's Current Veterinary Therapy XV, Elsevier, 2014, p. 467.

187. a Lidocaine toxicity causes central nervous signs as a result of the inhibition of excitatory neurons. These include a decreased responsiveness (drowsiness), ataxia, and muscle tremors. At even higher doses, the inhibitory neurons are affected, causing seizures. Clinical signs of lidocaine toxicity do not include renal, hepatic, or respiratory signs. Bill RL, Clinical Pharmacology and Therapeutics for the Veterinary Technician, ed 4, Mosby, 2016, p. 127.

188. d Theophylline acts as a bronchodilator and can be used in asthma to open the airways. Histamine is not administered but instead is released by the body in response to a hypersensitivity reaction. It causes vasodilation and increased vascular permeability, both of which will worsen asthma. Prednisone is an anti-inflammatory that is sometimes used as a long-term treatment for asthma (prednisolone should be used in cats). Digoxin is a positive inotrope and is not useful in treating asthma. Bill RL, Clinical Pharmacology and Therapeutics for the Veterinary Technician, ed 4, Mosby, 2016, p. 148-150.

189. a Tetracyclines are effective against mycoplasma, spirochetes, chlamydia, and rickettsial diseases. Penicillins, aminoglycosides, and sulfonamides all treat gram-positive and gram-negative bacteria. Wanamaker BP, Massey KL, Applied Pharmacology for Veterinary Technicians, ed 5, Elsevier, 2015, p. 297.

190. d Amikacin, banamine, and cisplatin are all known to be nephrotoxic. Oxymorphone does not cause nephrotoxicity but will cause respiratory depression, sedation, and excitement. Wanamaker BP, Massey KL, Applied Pharmacology for Veterinary Technicians, ed 5, Elsevier, 2015, p. 233, 304, 364.

191. a Cats lack adequate glucuronidation pathways to metabolize salicylates. For this reason, the half-life is much longer in cats and the doses and frequency for cats should be changed accordingly. Salicylates have the potential to cause vomiting, diarrhea, nausea, mentation changes, and an increase in the respiratory rate and effort. Peterson ME, Talcott PA, Small Animal Toxicology, ed 3, Elsevier, 2013, p. 338-339.

192. d Levothyroxine is a thyroid supplement that is used to treat hypothyroidism. Hyperthyroidism can be treated with surgery to remove the thyroid, radioactive iodine to decrease the production of thyroid hormone, or methimazole, which decreases the production of thyroid hormones by preventing the incorporation of iodine into the precursors T3 and T4. Summers A, Common Diseases of Companion Animals, ed 4, Mosby, 2019, p. 60-61.

193. b Common side effects of sulfonamides include thrombocytopenia, decreased tear production, and crystalluria. Triple sulfas were developed to decrease the formation of crystals in the urine and the incidence of crystalluria. Bill RL, Clinical Pharmacology and Therapeutics for the Veterinary Technician, ed 4, Mosby, 2016, p. 275-276.

194. a Diphenhydramine is a histamine blocker that is administered to prevent the effects seen from the massive histamine release that may be seen when a mast cell tumor is manipulated. In addition to surgery, this is also administered before the mass is aspirated. Methimazole is used to treat hyperthyroidism, vincristine is a chemotherapeutic often used to treat mast cell tumors but will not block the effects of histamine, and sulfasalazine is an anti-inflammatory. Wanamaker BP, Massey KL, Applied Pharmacology for Veterinary Technicians, ed 5, Elsevier, 2015, p. 309-310.

195. a Diazepam is a benzodiazepine that is used to stop seizure activity, to cause sedation, and to stimulate appetite in cats. Cyproheptadine is an appetite stimulant but does not stop or prevent seizures and, although it may cause mild sedation, it is not used as a sedative. Ketamine is used for sedation and potassium bromide is given daily to prevent seizures. Wanamaker BP, Massey KL, Applied Pharmacology for Veterinary Technicians, ed 5, Elsevier, 2015, p. 80-81.

196. a If the pH of the urine is altered, it would become more acidic or alkalotic (the pH is not associated with the concentration of the urine). Methionine will decrease the pH of the urine, making it more acidic. This will dissolve any stones present and prevent the formation of other stones. Wanamaker BP, Massey KL, Applied Pharmacology for Veterinary Technicians, ed 5, Elsevier, 2015, p. 122.

197. b Glargine, NPH, and Vetsulin are intermediate or long acting and regular insulin is short acting. Wanamaker BP, Massey KL, Applied Pharmacology for Veterinary Technicians, ed 4, Saunders, 2009, p. 186.

198. d Insulin should always be given after the patient has eaten. If the patient does not eat or only eats a partial meal, the owner should be directed to call the veterinarian to discuss whether insulin should be given and how much insulin to give. Otherwise, patients may become hypoglycemic and experience seizure activity. Insulin should be stored in the refrigerator and should never be shaken (unless the client is using Vetsulin, which should be shaken), which will damage the proteins and render the insulin useless. Injection sites can be rotated to prevent the formation of sores and the anticipation of pain by the patient. Wanamaker BP, Massey KL, Applied Pharmacology for Veterinary Technicians, ed 5, Elsevier, 2015, p. 188.

199. c Giardia and Eimeria are both protozoans and should be treated with an antiprotozoal. Bactericidal drugs treat bacteria, virucidal drugs treat viruses, and fungistatic drugs treat fungi. Bowman DD, Georgi's Parasitology for Veterinarians, ed 10, Elsevier, 2014, p. 92.

200. c MIC stands for minimum inhibitory concentration and indicates how susceptible an organism is when a drug is at the lowest effective dose. Wanamaker BP, Massey KL, Applied Pharmacology for Veterinary Technicians, ed 5, Elsevier, 2015, p. 232.

201. d The drugs listed are all aminoglycosides. Penicillins include amoxicillin and ampicillin, cephalosporins include cefazolin and cephalexin, and quinolones include enrofloxacin and ciprofloxacin. Wanamaker BP, Massey KL, Applied Pharmacology for Veterinary Technicians, ed 5, Elsevier, 2015, p. 232-235.

202. d Aminoglycosides accumulate in the kidney and inner ear, potentially causing damage. For this reason, a patient on an aminoglycoside should have urine sediment and specific gravity checked daily and should be monitored closely for hearing loss. Wanamaker BP, Massey KL, Applied Pharmacology for Veterinary Technicians, ed 5, Elsevier, 2015, p. 233.

203. a Failing to administer antibiotics for the full course prescribed, administrating low doses, or prescribing antibiotics that will not reach the site of infection will all contribute to bacterial resistance. Prolonged use of a high dose may allow some bacteria to develop resistance, but it is less likely than the other choices to cause significant resistance. Bill RL, Clinical Pharmacology and Therapeutics for the Veterinary Technician, ed 4, Mosby, 2016, p. 215-217.

204. c Although any medication can cause an allergic reaction, penicillins are known to cause this and it is a common side effect. Aminoglycosides, quinolones, and tetracyclines are not associated with allergic reactions to the extent of penicillins. Wanamaker BP, Massey KL, Applied Pharmacology for Veterinary Technicians, ed 5, Elsevier, 2015, p. 244-245.

205. a Some antifungals work by causing mutations in the DNA. There is also the possibility that they can cause mutations in mammalian DNA, causing birth defects. Antibacterial, antivirals, and antiprotozoal drugs may also affect the target organism's DNA but will not alter mammalian DNA. Bill RL, Clinical Pharmacology and Therapeutics for the Veterinary Technician, ed 4, Mosby, 2016, p. 218-219.

206. b Penicillin G is made inactive by gastric acid. Because it becomes ineffective, it will not cause gastrointestinal upset including vomiting, diarrhea, or cramping. It will never reach the gastrointestinal tract (beyond the stomach), hence it can neither be absorbed effectively nor ineffectively. Sirois M, Principles and Practice of Veterinary Technology, ed 4, Elsevier, 2016, p. 261.

207. d Penicillin will kill the normal flora of the gastrointestinal tract, which allows an overgrowth of *Clostridium* to develop. This will cause severe, life-threatening diarrhea in both rabbits and guinea pigs. Sirois M, Principles and Practice of Veterinary Technology, ed 4, Elsevier, 2016, p. 832.

208. b Some bacteria produce beta-lactamase, an enzyme that is able to deactivate the antibiotic by breaking down the beta-lactam ring. A beta-lactamase inhibitor can be combined with the antibiotic to prevent the breakdown of the beta-lactam ring, preventing bacterial resistance. Examples include Clavamox (amoxicillin and clavulanate acid) and Unasyn (ampicillin and sulbactam). Wanamaker BP, Massey KL, Applied Pharmacology for Veterinary Technicians, ed 5, Elsevier, 2015, p. 245.

209. b Clavulanic acid is combined with amoxicillin to make Clavamox, an antibiotic to which beta-lactamase–producing bacteria are not resistant. Trimethoprim is combined to sulfonamides to inhibit bacterial DNA synthesis. Piperonyl butoxide is a synergist that will increase the efficacy of pyrethrins. Ormetoprim is a coccidiostat that is sometimes combined with sulfonamides to prevent the breakdown of insecticides, which is a natural defense of the insect. Wanamaker BP, Massey KL, Applied Pharmacology for Veterinary Technicians, ed 5, Elsevier, 2015, p. 229.

210. b Procaine and benzathine will delay absorption (thus decreasing the rate at which it enters the blood), which extends the duration of the activity (although plasma concentrations will be lower). Procaine will extend the duration of activity by 24 hours and benzathine by up to 5 days. Neither will enhance the efficacy of the penicillin nor act as a local anesthetic. Bill RL, Clinical Pharmacology and Therapeutics for the Veterinary Technician, ed 4, Mosby, 2016, p. 221-222.

211. b Each generation (from first to fourth) is more resistant to beta-lactamase than the previous generation. The first generation (e.g., cefazolin, cephalexin) has good gram-positive and poor gram-negative coverage. The second generation (e.g., cefoxitin) has extended gram-negative coverage. The third generation (cefpodoxime, cefotaxime) has even better gram-negative coverage. Fourth-generation cephalosporins are not available in the United States. Plumb DC, Veterinary Drug Handbook, ed 4, Blackwell, 2002, p. 154-155.

212. a Aminoglycosides require an environment with a high oxygen tension to be transported into the bacteria. The aminoglycosides are effective against both gram-positive and gram-negative bacteria. Resistance to antibiotics is through a decrease in the antibiotic's ability to enter the bacteria, a change in the structure of the bacteria's ribosome, or the destruction of the antibiotic by enzymes (although this is not the reason aminoglycosides are ineffective in an anaerobic environment). Boothe DM, Small Animal Clinical Pharmacology & Therapeutics, ed 2, Elsevier, 2012, p. 223.

213. b Aminoglycosides are not absorbed systemically when given orally and are poorly absorbed when applied topically. It is unlikely that a species will be resistant to kidney damage if it is a known side effect. Even if excreted quickly, the drug will still be able to cause damage to the kidneys. Papich MG, Saunders Handbook of Veterinary Drugs: Small and Large Animal, ed 4, Elsevier, 2015, p. 559.

214. b Aminoglycosides will accumulate in the inner ear and kidneys and can cause hearing loss and renal failure. Amoxicillin is well known to cause vomiting, diarrhea, and allergic reactions. Enrofloxacin will cause the development of lesions in the joint cartilage of rapidly growing dogs, and tetracyclines will bind with calcium, causing of the teeth in young animals. Tetracyclines will also cause hepatotoxicity at high doses. Wanamaker BP, Massey KL, Applied Pharmacology for Veterinary Technicians, ed 4, Saunders, 2009, p. 286.

215. c By allowing the plasma concentration of the drug to drop between doses, you will allow the drug to move out of the cell, down its concentration gradient, and into the plasma. This prevents an accumulation of the drug in the kidney (and decreases the risk of nephrotoxicity) if you did not allow the plasma concentration to fall. If the drug is administered as a constant infusion, there would be no drop in plasma concentration, which would allow the drug to accumulate in the cell, thus increasing the risk of nephrotoxicity. Given orally, intramuscularly, or as an intravenous bolus will still allow the concentration to fall because these are not constant infusions. Bill RL, Clinical Pharmacology and Therapeutics for the Veterinary Technician, ed 4, Mosby, 2016, p. 225-226.

216. d Damage to the kidneys is first evident by the presence of casts and protein in the urine, which indicates damage to the renal tubules. The BUN and creatinine will not become elevated until the damage to the kidneys is extensive. The CBC and total protein levels will not be affected by early renal damage and there will be no change in the consistency of the feces unless the damage to the kidneys is severe. Bill RL, Clinical Pharmacology and Therapeutics for the Veterinary Technician, ed 4, Mosby, 2016, p. 226.

217. c Necrotic debris will bind aminoglycosides (attaching to the nucleic acids of the ribosomes of the dead white blood cells), causing them to be ineffective. Aminoglycosides prefer an alkaline environment and the enzymes that affect the drug are found inside the cell, not in the tissue. Bill RL, Clinical Pharmacology and Therapeutics for the Veterinary Technician, ed 4, Mosby, 2016, p. 227-228.

218. b Fluoroquinolones typically end with the suffix -floxacin (danofloxacin, enrofloxacin), tetracyclines end with the suffix -cycline (oxytetracycline, doxycycline), and sulfonamides start with the prefix sulfa- (sulfadimethoxine, sulfamethazine). Chloramphenicol is an amphicol and lincomycin is a lincosamide. Bassert JM, Thomas JA, McCurnin's Clinical Textbook for Veterinary Technicians, ed 8, Elsevier, 2014, p. 1019.

219. a The prostate has a blood–prostate barrier. This type of barrier is also found in the eye, testicle, brain, joint, and placenta (but not the thyroid, pancreas, or spleen). Peterson ME, Talcott PA, Small Animal Toxicology, ed 3, Elsevier, 2013, p. 23.

220. a Enrofloxacin does not kill the normal flora in the gastrointestinal tract and it is safe for use in rabbits. Enrofloxacin should be avoided in young, growing dogs because it will cause the development of lesions on the cartilage. This also occurs in horses along with oral lesions (if a concentrated oral solution is used). Cats are susceptible to retinal damage if the higher dose of enrofloxacin is used. Papich MG, Saunders Handbook of Veterinary Drugs: Small and Large Animal, ed 4, Elsevier, 2015, p. 287-288.

221. c Ticks (*Ixodes* sp.) are vectors for Lyme disease, which is caused by bacteria (*Borrelia burgdorferi*). Because it is caused by bacteria, an antibiotic (e.g., doxycycline) will be the drug of choice. An antifungal, antiviral, and antiprotozoal response will not be effective against a bacterial infection. Bowman DD, Georgi's Parasitology for Veterinarians, ed 10, Elsevier, 2014, p. 251; Summers A, Common Diseases of Companion Animals, ed 3, Elsevier, 2014, p. 175-176.

222. c Calcium will chelate tetracyclines, decreasing absorption, and owners should be told they should not hide the medication in a piece of cheese. Iron, aluminum, and magnesium should also be avoided. Sodium, potassium, and fat should not affect the absorption of tetracyclines. Papich MG, Saunders Handbook of Veterinary Drugs: Small and Large Animal, ed 4, Elsevier, 2015, p. 769.

223. b Because tetracycline binds calcium, it will bind to the bone of the developing fetus as well as to the teeth that appear later. Tetracyclines do not cause liver disease or impair the development of the liver or joints of the developing puppies. Papich MG, Saunders Handbook of Veterinary Drugs: Small and Large Animal, ed 4, Elsevier, 2015, p. 769.

224. b Prostaglandin F2 alpha is involved with causing uterine contractions, relaxation of the cervix, and lysis of the corpus luteum. It does not have any effect on ovulation and it does not stimulate follicle formation or corpus luteum formation. Wanamaker BP, Massey KL, Applied Pharmacology for Veterinary Technicians, ed 4, Saunders, 2009, p. 178.

225. d Chloramphenicol crosses the blood–brain barrier as well as the corneal barrier (although in the cornea it will only reach concentrations high enough to be bacteriostatic and not bactericidal). Oxytetracycline, enrofloxacin, and amoxicillin can be used for soft tissue infections, pneumonia, and urinary tract infections. Boothe DM, Small Animal Clinical Pharmacology and Therapeutics, ed 2, Elsevier, 2012, p. 254, 275.

226. a Because chloramphenicol will inhibit drug-metabolizing enzymes and hepatic metabolism of other drugs, it should be used with caution in patients taking medications metabolized by the liver, such as phenobarbital. Penicillin will enhance the activity of chloramphenicol (but the half-life is not prolonged). Tetracycline works on a different ribosomal site from chloramphenicol, hence combining these two medications can be beneficial. Sulfadimethoxine is excreted via the kidney and is not affected by chloramphenicol. Boothe DM, Small Animal Clinical Pharmacology and Therapeutics, ed 2, Elsevier, 2012, p. 255.

227. b Chloramphenicol has been known to cause circulatory collapse because of toxicity that occurs secondary to the inability of these patients to conjugate or to excrete the drug. Cats are also more susceptible to chloramphenicol-induced bone marrow suppression (which is reversible). The binding of calcium is not a reason to use chloramphenicol with caution. Cats will not have problems with the development of bone, cartilage, or enamel, and they do not experience fatal diarrhea. Boothe DM, Small Animal Clinical Pharmacology and Therapeutics, ed 2, Elsevier, 2012, p. 254-255; Plumb DC, Veterinary Drug Handbook, ed 4, Blackwell, 2002, p. 167.

228. b Chloramphenicol causes stem cell damage, leading to bone marrow suppression. This has also been seen in humans and it is therefore not used in food animals because it can be found in meat, milk, and eggs. Boothe DM, Small Animal Clinical Pharmacology and Therapeutics, ed 2, Elsevier, 2012, p. 255; Wanamaker BP, Massey KL, Applied Pharmacology for Veterinary Technicians, ed 5, Saunders, 2014, p. 254.

229. b Sulfonamides can cause the development of crystals in the kidneys, causing damage to renal tubules. A patient that is dehydrated will have decreased urine production, allowing the crystals to accumulate in the kidneys, causing further damage. A bladder infection or loss of a kidney will not contribute to the nephrotoxicity caused by chloramphenicol. Intravenous fluids will flush out the kidneys, decreasing build-up of crystals in the renal tubules. Wanamaker BP, Massey KL, Applied Pharmacology for Veterinary Technicians, ed 5, Elsevier, 2015, p. 253.

230. b Trimethoprim and ormetoprim are combined with sulfonamides to potentiate their effects by inhibiting a step in the folate synthesis pathway. They are not combined with penicillins and will not reduce liver damage. Sirois M, Principles and Practice of Veterinary Technology, ed 4, Elsevier, 2016, p. 262.

231. c Decreased tear production causing keratoconjunctivitis sicca (KCS) is a known side effect of sulfonamides. Increased urination, sudden liver failure, and cardiac arrest are not associated with the use of sulfonamides. Papich MG, Saunders Handbook of Veterinary Drugs: Small and Large Animal, ed 4, Elsevier, 2015, p. 749-750.

232. c Metronidazole is often used to treat diarrhea caused by *Giardia*. Clindamycin is an antibiotic but it does not treat *Giardia*. Monensin is coccidiostatic, hence it will be ineffective against *Giardia*, and griseofulvin is an antifungal. Bowman DD, Georgi's Parasitology for Veterinarians, ed 10, Elsevier, 2014, p. 285.

233. d Ketoconazole, miconazole, and griseofulvin are all antifungals. Viruses should be treated with antivirals such as acyclovir and interferon. Flukes are treated with antihelminths such as albendazole and praziquantel. Nematodes are roundworms and can be treated with ivermectin. Bassert JM, Thomas JA, McCurnin's Clinical Textbook for Veterinary Technicians, ed 9, Elsevier, 2017, p. 962.

234. c Diazepam is the drug of choice for treating status epilepticus. It works by binding to GABA receptors and decreasing neuronal firing. Phenobarbital is considered a maintenance drug. Potassium bromide is also a maintenance drug often used as an adjunct therapy to phenobarbital. Levetiracetam is used in patients that are not responding to treatment. It can be administered intravenously in the hospital if the patient does not respond to diazepam and then, if necessary, it can be administered orally at home. Silverstein D, Hopper K, Small Animal Critical Care Medicine, ed 1, Saunders, 2009, p. 417-418; Wanamaker BP, Massey KL, Applied Pharmacology for Veterinary Technicians, ed 5, Elsevier, 2015, p. 87-88.

235. b Primidone will be metabolized to phenobarbital. Diazepam is metabolized to nordazepam and oxazepam. Clonazepam is metabolized to aminoclonazepam and acetaminoclonazepam, and phenytoin is metabolized to hydroxyphenytoin. Wanamaker BP, Massey KL, Applied Pharmacology for Veterinary Technicians, ed 5, Elsevier, 2015, p. 87-88.

236. b Potassium bromide is often used as an adjunct therapy to phenobarbital. Diazepam is used for status epilepticus. Phenytoin has been used as an anticonvulsant in the past, but it has recently fallen out of favor. Strychnine is not used as a treatment for seizures. Wanamaker BP, Massey KL, Applied Pharmacology for Veterinary Technicians, ed 5, Elsevier, 2015, p. 88.

237. d Doxapram stimulates the respiratory center and can be used during anesthesia or in neonates to stimulate respirations. None of the other medications listed affects respiration. Oxytocin is used to aid in delivery by increasing contractions of the uterus. Dobutamine increases cardiac contractility and propranolol decreases the automaticity of the cardiac cells, which will decrease heart rate and blood pressure. Wanamaker BP, Massey KL, Applied Pharmacology for Veterinary Technicians, ed 5, Elsevier, 2015, p. 92.

238. c Antitussives are used for suppression of a nonproductive cough. Mucolytics and expectorants decrease the viscosity of respiratory secretions, allowing them to be more easily expelled. Decongestants will decrease congestion in the nasal tissue via vasoconstriction, which decreases edema by decreasing blood flow to the area. Wanamaker BP, Massey KL, Applied Pharmacology for Veterinary Technicians, ed 5, Elsevier, 2015, p. 85.

239. b Expectorants decrease the viscosity of secretions by increasing the fluid in the secretions, thinning them and making them easier to move out of the respiratory tract. Anti-inflammatories decrease inflammation and antitussives suppress the cough. Bill RL, Clinical Pharmacology and Therapeutics for the Veterinary Technician, ed 4, Mosby, 2016, p. 147-148.

240. a Bronchodilators cause dilation of the airways through several mechanisms. These include beta-receptor agonists, which cause relaxation of the smooth muscle in the airways, methylxanthines, which inhibit phosphodiesterases, causing bronchodilation, and anticholinergics, which decrease the sensitivity of receptors to irritants and prevent vagally mediated bronchoconstriction. Expectorants decrease the viscosity of airway secretions, causing them to be easier to expel, antitussives are used to suppress coughing, and antihistamines decrease allergic reactions. Boothe DM, Small Animal Clinical Pharmacology and Therapeutics, ed 2, Elsevier, 2012, p. 753-760.

241. c Butorphanol and hydrocodone are both used as cough suppressants. Neither of these drugs will act as mucolytics, expectorants, or antihistamines. Wanamaker BP, Massey KL, Applied Pharmacology for Veterinary Technicians, ed 5, Elsevier, 2015, p. 105-106.

242. d Beta-receptor agonists cause relaxation of smooth muscle (causing bronchodilation) and decrease histamine release through stabilization of the mast cell. They are not involved with changing the viscosity of airway secretions. Wanamaker BP, Massey KL, Applied Pharmacology for Veterinary Technicians, ed 5, Elsevier, 2015, p. 107-108

243. a Terbutaline, albuterol, and metaproterenol are bronchodilators that cause dilation of the airways. They are not used in shock because of the possibility of worsening vasodilation. Bronchodilators are not involved in stimulation of secretions and, if the patient has a productive cough, the use of a cough suppressant should be avoided because a productive cough will assist with expelling secretions from the airway. Battaglia AM, Small Animal Emergency and Critical Care for Veterinary Technicians, ed 2, Saunders, 2007, p. 264.

244. a Theophylline and aminophylline are methylxanthine. These inhibit phosphodiesterase, which is then used to inhibit cyclic AMP. By blocking phosphodiesterase, cyclic AMP is able to cause smooth muscle relaxation, which opens the airways. The other drugs listed are antitussives with the exception of propranolol, which is a bronchodilator. Wanamaker BP, Massey KL, Applied Pharmacology for Veterinary Technicians, ed 5, Elsevier, 2015, p. 108.

245. d Inotropes influence the myocardial contractility of the heart (the force of the contraction). Positive inotropes increase contractility and negative inotropes decrease contractility. Chronotropic drugs influence the heart rate, with positive chronotropes increasing the heart rate and negative chronotropes decreasing the heart rate. There is also a third class of drugs called dromotropic medications, which affect the rate of conduction through the heart. As with the others, positive dromotropes increase the rate of conduction and negative dromotropes decrease the rate of conduction. Boothe DM, Small Animal Clinical Pharmacology and Therapeutics, ed 2, Elsevier, 2012, p. 579.

246. b Lidocaine is a sodium channel blocker used to treat ventricular tachycardia by decreasing the automaticity of the cardiac cells. Propranolol is a beta blocker, procainamide is a sodium channel blocker that decreases myocardial excitability, and digoxin is a positive inotrope. Wanamaker BP, Massey KL, Applied Pharmacology for Veterinary Technicians, ed 5, Elsevier, 2015, p. 138-139.

247. b Beta blockers (such as atenolol and propranolol) can be used to treat these cats chronically (or until the hyperthyroidism is controlled) as well as postoperatively. Lidocaine, quinidine, and digoxin are not beta blockers. Wanamaker BP, Massey KL, Applied Pharmacology for Veterinary Technicians, ed5, Saunders, 2015, p. 139-140; B Bonagura JD, Twedt DC, Kirk's Current Veterinary Therapy XV, Elsevier, 2014, p. 749.

248. c The therapeutic index indicates a drug's therapeutic properties versus its toxic properties. The narrower the index, the smaller the margin of safety. Wanamaker BP, Massey KL, Applied Pharmacology for Veterinary Technicians, ed 5, Elsevier, 2015, p. 14.

249. c The side effects of digoxin toxicity include gastrointestinal signs (vomiting, diarrhea, anorexia) and cardiac arrhythmias. Digoxin toxicity is not known to cause renal signs (increased or decreased urination), respiratory signs (respiratory distress or coughing), or neurologic signs (ataxia, syncope). Wanamaker BP, Massey KL, Applied Pharmacology for Veterinary Technicians, ed 5, Elsevier, 2015, p. 135-136.

250. d Digoxin competes with potassium on digoxin receptors. Because of this, hypokalemia allows more digoxin to attach to receptors, which, in turn, causes a decrease in excretion (because it is attached to the receptors). Sodium and chloride does not affect digoxin. Silverstein D, Hopper K, Small Animal Critical Care Medicine, ed 1, Saunders, 2009, p. 364-365.

251. d Dermatophytes are fungal parasites found on the skin and should be treated with an antifungal. Of the medications listed, itraconazole is the only antifungal. Tylosin, enrofloxacin, and sulfadimethoxine are all antibiotics. Sirois M, Principles and Practice of Veterinary Technology, ed 4, Elsevier, 2016, p. 263-264.

252. b ACE (angiotensin-converting enzyme) inhibitors block the conversion of angiotensinogen I (the inactive form) to angiotensinogen II (the active form). Angiotensinogen II increases blood pressure by causing vasoconstriction. If an ACE inhibitor is used, the inactive form of angiotensinogen will not be converted to the active form and vasodilation will occur. ACE inhibitors will not directly affect the strength of cardiac contractions, the heart rate, or bronchodilation. Boothe DM, Small Animal Clinical Pharmacology and Therapeutics, ed 2, Elsevier, 2012, p. 494.

253. d Captopril is an ACE inhibitor, which will prevent the inactive form of angiotensinogen from conversion to the active form. This will cause vasodilation. Captopril does not act as a positive inotrope, antiarrhythmic, or bronchodilator. Wanamaker BP, Massey KL, Applied Pharmacology for Veterinary Technicians, ed 5, Elsevier, 2015, p. 142-143.

254. b Nitroglycerin is a venodilator that works by relaxing smooth muscle on the venous side of the circulatory system. It will decrease preload by causing pooling of blood in the periphery, which decreases blood returning to the heart. This will decrease both preload and afterload, decreasing the work of the heart. Nitroglycerin will not directly cause an increase in the strength of cardiac contractions, cause bronchodilation, or decrease the heart rate. Wanamaker BP, Massey KL, Applied Pharmacology for Veterinary Technicians, ed 5, Elsevier, 2015, p. 142.

255. a Spirolactone is a potassium-sparing diuretic, chlorothiazide is a thiazide diuretic, and furosemide is a loop diuretic. Wanamaker BP, Massey KL, Applied Pharmacology for Veterinary Technicians, ed 5, Elsevier, 2015, p. 143-144.

256. b Controlled drugs are divided into five schedules (C-I through C-V) under the Controlled Substances Act. The lower the number, the higher the potential is for abuse. Of the options listed, C-II indicates the highest potential for abuse. Drugs in this schedule include hydromorphone, oxycodone, morphine, fentanyl, and hydrocodone. Bassert JM, Thomas JA, McCurnin's Clinical Textbook for Veterinary Technicians, ed 9, Elsevier, 2017, p. 954.

257. c Apomorphine is an emetic that stimulates the chemoreceptor zone to cause vomiting. It does not influence blood pressure or renal function and has no analgesic properties. Wanamaker BP, Massey KL, Applied Pharmacology for Veterinary Technicians, ed 5, Elsevier, 2015, p. 154.

258. b Maropitant is a neurokinin receptor agonist that can be used to prevent or treat motion sickness. Apomorphine and xylazine are both emetics that are used in dogs and cats, respectively. Diphenhydramine can also be used to prevent motion sickness but is less effective than maropitant. Bill RL, Clinical Pharmacology and Therapeutics for the Veterinary Technician, ed 4, Mosby, 2016, p. 12.

259. b Although rarely recommended because of the possible complications including lethargy, prolonged vomiting, and cardiotoxicity, syrup of ipecac can be used to induce vomiting. Ipecac will not stimulate defecation or increase blood flow to the gastrointestinal tract. Peterson ME, Talcott PA, Small Animal Toxicology, ed 3, Elsevier, 2013, p. 129-130.

260. c Activated charcoal should not be administered until the effects of the apomorphine have passed to avoid making the patient vomit, and possibly aspirate, the charcoal. The combination of activated charcoal and apomorphine does not worsen vomiting and they each will not cancel the benefits of the other. Diarrhea and intestinal cramping are not side effects associated with apomorphine or activated charcoal. Peterson ME, Talcott PA, Small Animal Toxicology, ed 3, Elsevier, 2013, p. 55-56.

261. d Anticholinergics block acetylcholine at the cholinergic fibers in the nervous system. This causes a decrease in salivation, tear production, and gastrointestinal motility, and it inhibits bradycardia caused by vagal stimulation. Boothe DM, Small Animal Clinical Pharmacology and Therapeutics, ed 2, Elsevier, 2012, p. 887.

262. d Bismuth coats the gastrointestinal tract, acting as a protectant. Subsalicylate is converted to salicylate, which has anti-inflammatory properties and it also blocks prostaglandins that increase the absorption of fluids. This decreases fluid moving into the stool and decreases diarrhea. Bismuth will also decrease hypermotility of the stomach. Care should be taken when using this medication, especially in cats, to avoid salicylate toxicity. Sirois M, Principles and Practice of Veterinary Technology, ed 3, Elsevier, 2011, p. 257.

263. c NSAIDs are cyclooxygenase (COX) inhibitors. COX is involved with the production of prostaglandins that are involved with a multitude of activates. COX-1 blocks the formation of prostaglandins involved with renal perfusion, platelet aggregation, and maintenance of gastric mucosa. COX-2 blocks prostaglandins associated with pain and inflammation. NSAIDs that block COX-1 will result in gastric ulceration because of its involvement in the maintenance of gastric mucosa. NSAIDs do not affect gastrointestinal motility or the ability to digest fat. Sirois M, Principles and Practice of Veterinary Technology, ed 4, Elsevier, 2016, p. 265-266.

264. d Cimetidine and ranitidine are H2 receptor agonists that will inhibit histamine at the parietal cells in the stomach. This will prevent or reduce hydrochloride acid secretions in the stomach. Wanamaker BP, Massey KL, Applied Pharmacology for Veterinary Technicians, ed 5, Elsevier, 2015, p. 157-158.

265. a Sucralfate becomes a paste in the stomach and binds to the surface of the ulcer, protecting it from the acidic environment. Sucralfate is not a prostaglandin analog, proton pump inhibitor, or H2 receptor antagonist. Wanamaker BP, Massey KL, Applied Pharmacology for Veterinary Technicians, ed 5, Elsevier, 2015, p. 159.

266. c Hypothyroidism occurs because of a decrease in T4 (thyroxine) and T3 (triiodothyronine) from the thyroid gland. Because T3 is the deionized form of T4, it can be supplemented with just levothyroxine (T4) and liothyronine (T3) is not needed. Thyroid-stimulating hormone (TSH) will be ineffective because the thyroid is unable to produce thyroid hormone. Bonagura JD, Twedt DC, Kirk's Current Veterinary Therapy XV, Elsevier, 2014, p. 178-183.

267. c Methimazole is used to treat hyperthyroidism by preventing the incorporation of iodine into the precursors of T3 and T4. Hypothyroidism is treated with thyroid supplementation, such as thyroxine. Hyperadrenocorticism is treated with mitotane or trilostane and hypoadrenocorticism is treated with desoxycorticosterone pivalate (DOCP). Wanamaker BP, Massey KL, Applied Pharmacology for Veterinary Technicians, ed 5, Elsevier, 2015, p. 182-183.

268. c Prostaglandins cause lysis of the corpus luteum if the animal is not pregnant. Progesterone prevents the release of gonadotropin-releasing hormone to prevent the development of new follicles. Estrogen inhibits ovulation and gonadotropin mimics luteinizing hormone and will also cause ovulation. Wanamaker BP, Massey KL, Applied Pharmacology for Veterinary Technicians, ed 5, Elsevier, 2015, p. 175-176.

269. d Progestin suppresses estrous. After the medication is discontinued, the animal will begin cycling again with a return to proestrus. Estradiol cypionate is an estrogen that induces estrous whereas prostaglandin F2 alpha will start a new estrus cycle. Human chorionic gonadotropin acts as a luteinizing hormone or follicle-stimulating hormone and causes the formation of a corpus luteum and the growth of a follicle. Wanamaker BP, Massey KL, Applied Pharmacology for Veterinary Technicians, ed 5, Elsevier, 2015, p. 178.

270. b Megestrol acetate is a progestin used for behavioral problems in addition to its use as a reproductive drug. Altrenogest is also a progestin, but it is used in horses and pigs. Estradiol is an estrogen replacement and it induces abortions. Dinoprost induces estrus as well as causing abortions. Wanamaker BP, Massey KL, Applied Pharmacology for Veterinary Technicians, ed 5, Elsevier, 2015, p. 177.

271. a Aspirin is a nonselective COX inhibitor, therefore it will inhibit COX-1 (which is involved with the maintenance of the gastric mucosa) and COX-2 (which is involved with pain and inflammation). When both of these are blocked, inflammation resolves, but there is risk of gastric ulceration. The other drugs listed are COX-2 selective. These will block COX-2 (although will have little to no effect on COX-1). With long-term use, high doses, or toxicity there is a risk of gastric ulceration. Bonagura JD, Twedt DC, Kirk's Current Veterinary Therapy XV, Elsevier, 2014, p. 864.

272. b Prednisone (prednisolone in cats) is commonly sent home with patients that require glucocorticoid therapy for immune-mediated diseases. Hydrocortisone is not used for immune-mediated diseases. Dexamethasone may be used as an injection while the patient is in the hospital but it is not sent home for oral administration. Triamcinolone and hydrocortisone are not commonly used in immune-mediated diseases. Bonagura JD, Twedt DC, Kirk's Current Veterinary Therapy XV, Elsevier, 2014, p. 269.

273. a Prednisone commonly causes polyuria. Prednisone causes a decreased response to antidiuretic hormone, which is involved with reabsorption of water from the kidneys into the bloodstream. When the response to ADH is decreased, water is not reabsorbed and urine production increases. This makes the animal polyuric and, in response to the large loss of fluid, the animal drinks more water. Prednisone is not known to cause respiratory signs or skin irritation (although it may cause alopecia and thinning of the skin). Long-term therapy has the potential to cause gastrointestinal upset or ulcerations but this is not usually associated with short-term therapy. Plumb DC, Veterinary Drug Handbook, ed 4, Blackwell, 2002, p. 387-388.

274. c Glucocorticoids can cause an increase in platelets, neutrophils, and red blood cells. There will be a decrease in lymphocytes, monocytes, and eosinophils because these stay in, or are redistributed to, the lungs, spleen, and bone marrow. Plumb DC, Veterinary Drug Handbook, ed 4, Blackwell, 2002, p. 387.

275. c Chronic use of glucocorticoids causes an iatrogenic hyperadrenocorticism (Cushing's disease). Glucocorticoids cause polyuria and polydipsia but not renal failure. Iatrogenic hypoadrenocorticism (Addison's disease) is caused by the sudden discontinuation of glucocorticoid therapy, which does not allow time for the adrenal gland to begin producing steroids. Johne's disease is caused by bacteria (*Mycobacterium avium* ssp. *paratuberculosis*). Sirois M, Principles and Practice of Veterinary Technology, ed 4, Elsevier, 2016, p. 257-258.

276. a Administration of corticosteroids in mares or cows mimics elevated cortisol levels, which are found at the beginning of parturition. Because of this, dexamethasone can induce abortions. This is not known to occur in dogs, cats, or pigs. Sirois M, Principles and Practice of Veterinary Technology, ed 4, Elsevier, 2016, p. 258.

277. b Because some NSAIDs inhibit COX-1 (involved with renal perfusion and gastric mucosa maintenance) side effects can include renal failure and gastric ulceration. Pulmonary, cardiac, or hepatic effects are not normally seen. Wanamaker BP, Massey KL, Applied Pharmacology for Veterinary Technicians, ed 5, Elsevier, 2015, p. 301.

278. a If injected outside a vein, phenylbutazone can cause necrosis and sloughing of the skin. Etodolac and carprofen are used in dogs, whereas meclofenamic acid is no longer available in the United States and, when used, is given orally. Holtgrew-Bohling K, Large Animal Clinical Procedures for Veterinary Technicians, ed 23, Mosby, 2015, p. 285.

279. b Dimethyl sulfoxide (DMSO) is often used as a carrier for agents applied to the skin. Because it also carries other things with it when it penetrates the skin, the area must be cleaned well to avoid bacteria or other chemicals from entering the blood. Dexamethasone and flunixin meglumine are both administered orally and hydrocortisone does not act as a carrier. Bill RL, Clinical Pharmacology and Therapeutics for the Veterinary Technician, ed 4, Mosby, 2016, p. 309-310.

280. d Tramadol became classified as a schedule C-IV drug on 18 August 2014. Butorphanol (1997), buprenorphine (2002), and Fentanyl (1964) were controlled before Tramadol. Plumb DC, Veterinary Drug Handbook, ed 8, Wiley-Blackwell, 2015, p. 1055.

281. b Anticestodal drugs treat tapeworms. Ascarids require an anthelmintic, protozoa require an antiprotozoal, and flukes require flukicides. Wanamaker BP, Massey KL, Applied Pharmacology for Veterinary Technicians, ed 5, Elsevier, 2015, p. 279.

282. b Collies (along with several types of shepherds, whippets, and sheepdogs) are sensitive to ivermectin because of an MDR1 (multidrug resistance protein 1) mutation. MDR1 is also known P-glycoprotein 1 and is found throughout the body including the intestine, liver, kidney, and blood–brain barrier. This protein is involved in preventing drugs or toxins from entering cells or crossing the blood–brain barrier. Because these breeds might have this mutation, they are more susceptible to adverse drug reactions. The other breeds listed do not have this gene mutation. Bowman DD, Georgi's Parasitology for Veterinarians, ed 10, Elsevier, 2014, p. 291-292.

283. c There is no FDA-approved microfilaricide available, but ivermectin is often used to treat the presence of microfilaria. Thiacetarsamide and melarsomine are used to treat adult heartworms and piperazine is not used in the treatment or prevention of heartworms. Bowman DD, Georgi's Parasitology for Veterinarians, ed 10, Elsevier, 2014, p. 297.

284. d Organophosphates interfere with the breakdown of acetylcholine at cholinergic sites, causing muscarinic (salivation, lacrimation, urination, defecation, bradycardia, vomiting), nicotinic (weakness, paresis, stiffness, muscle tetany), and central nervous signs (anxiety, hyperactivity, seizures, coma). Atropine will address muscarinic signs and some central nervous signs. It will not address nicotine signs. Diphenhydramine and corticosteroids do not treat overdoses. Intravenous fluids may be used for supportive care but are not specific for organophosphate toxicity. Peterson ME, Talcott PA, Small Animal Toxicology, ed 3, Elsevier, 2013, p. 948-949.

285. b Amitraz is an acaricide used to treat demodicosis and is found in flea and tick collars. Pyrethrin and allethrin are both pyrethroids and are used to treat ticks, mites, and fleas. Fenoxycarb is an insect growth regulator and is used against flea larvae. Wanamaker BP, Massey KL, Applied Pharmacology for Veterinary Technicians, ed 5, Elsevier, 2015, p. 225.

286. c Insect growth regulators are absorbed by the flea and are passed into the egg. After they are hatched, the drug prevents the larvae from maturing into an adult flea. Insect growth regulators are commonly used in flea collars. Sirois M, Principles and Practice of Veterinary Technology, ed 4, Elsevier, 2016, p. 264-265.

287. d Prescriptions must include the name, address, telephone number, signature, and DEA number (if the drug is controlled) of the prescribing veterinarian, as well as the drug name, concentration, and quantity (mL or number of tablets). It must also include directions, name and address of the client, name and species of the patient, any cautionary information, and the number of refills. Bassert JM, Thomas JA, McCurnin's Clinical Textbook for Veterinary Technicians, ed 9, Elsevier, 2017, p. 977.

288. b PO stands for per os or by mouth. Administer as needed is indicated with PRN. There is no abbreviation for administer on an empty stomach or with a meal. Sirois M, Principles and Practice of Veterinary Technology, ed 3, Elsevier, 2011, p. 251.

289. b BID means that the medication should be administered every 12 hours or two times a day. Once a day would be Q24h, three times a day would be every 8 hours (or TID), and four times a day would be every 6 hours (or QID). Sirois M, Principles and Practice of Veterinary Technology, ed 4, Elsevier, 2016, p. 247.

290. c PRN is short for the Latin term *pro re nata* or give as needed. By mouth is indicated by PO and every other day is EOD. Sirois M, Principles and Practice of Veterinary Technology, ed 4, Elsevier, 2016, p. 247.

291. b OD stands for oculus dexter, or right eye, and OS stands for oculus sinister, or left eye. Other abbreviations would be by mouth (PO), per rectum (PR), every other day (EOD), every three days (Q3d), left ear (AS), and right ear (AD). Bill RL, Clinical Pharmacology and Therapeutics for the Veterinary Technician, ed 4, Mosby, 2016, p. 27.

292. a In this context, gr stands for grain and g stands for grams; this would therefore read 15 grains and 10 grams. Bill RL, Clinical Pharmacology and Therapeutics for the Veterinary Technician, ed 4, Mosby, 2016, p. 29.

293. b One grain is equal to 64.8 mg. Bill RL, Clinical Pharmacology and Therapeutics for the Veterinary Technician, ed 4, Mosby, 2016, p. 29.

294. c 100 mg PO TID is the dosing frequency. One tablet is the dose form, 100 mg is the dose, and 10–20 mg/kg is the dose range. Bill RL, Clinical Pharmacology and Therapeutics for the Veterinary Technician, ed 4, Mosby, 2016, p. 25-26.

295. c There are 5 mL in 1 tsp. Bill RL, Clinical Pharmacology and Therapeutics for the Veterinary Technician, ed 4, Mosby, 2016, p. 977.

296. b There are 15 cubic centimeters, or milliliters, in a tablespoon. Another way to think of this is that there are 5 mL in a teaspoon and 3 teaspoons (or 15 mL) in a tablespoon. Bill RL, Clinical Pharmacology and Therapeutics for the Veterinary Technician, ed 4, Mosby, 2016, p. 29.

297. b Q12h is equal to twice a day or BID, Q4h is equal to 5 times a day, and Q8h is equal to three times a day or

TID. Bill RL, Clinical Pharmacology and Therapeutics for the Veterinary Technician, ed 4, Mosby, 2016, p. 247.

298. d There are 2.2 pounds in a kilogram; a 10-kg dog therefore weighs 22 lb (10 kg × 2.2 lb/kg) Bill RL, Clinical Pharmacology and Therapeutics for the Veterinary Technician, ed 4, Mosby, 2016, p. 29.

299. d A suspension is a drug that does not dissolve in a liquid. It will settle out and must be shaken before using. A drug in a solution completely dissolves and will not settle out or precipitate. Ointment and gels are semisolids and cannot be mixed by shaking. Bill RL, Clinical Pharmacology and Therapeutics for the Veterinary Technician, ed 4, Mosby, 2016, p. 9-10.

300. b Extra-label use occurs when the medication is used in a way not recommended by the manufacturer. Extra-label use has been legal since the Animal Medical Drug Use Clarification Act was added to the Federal Food, Drug, and Cosmetic Act. This allows medications approved for use in animals and humans to be used in species not listed on the label and at doses, frequencies, and routes not listed on the label. The AVMA is not involved with the regulation of drugs and the manufacturer does not need to imply consent for this to happen. Bassert JM, Thomas JA, McCurnin's Clinical Textbook for Veterinary Technicians, ed 9, Elsevier, 2017, p. 998.

301. d A drug's withdrawal period is an important aspect of veterinary medicine and must be kept in mind when treating food animals. The half-life is the period for the serum concentration of the drug to decrease by half. The secretion period is the rate at which the drug is removed from the body and the refractory period is the window of time the patient becomes unresponsive to the medication or treatment. Bassert JM, Thomas JA, McCurnin's Clinical Textbook for Veterinary Technicians, ed 9, Elsevier, 2017, p. 974-975.

302. b The loading dose will bring the serum concentration to a therapeutic level quickly. The dose or frequency is then decreased to maintain the drug at this level in the serum. This is commonly done with phenobarbital. Wanamaker BP, Massey KL, Applied Pharmacology for Veterinary Technicians, ed 5, Elsevier, 2015, p. 5.

303. c Percent indicate parts of active drug per 100 parts of a solution, hence a 1.0% solution is equal to 1.0 parts per 100 parts of a solution. The solution weighs 1 g/mL, therefore there is 1.0 g of active drug in 100 g of solution or 1.0 g in 100 mL of solution. Because the strength of most liquid medications is measured in mg/mL, this is broken down further to 1000 mg (which is equal to 1.0 g) in 100 mL of solution, which can be broken down further to 10 mg/mL. This means a 1.0% solution is 10 mg/mL. Lake T, Green N, Essential Calculations for Veterinary Nurses and Technicians, ed 3, Butterworth Heinemann, 2016, p. 62-63

304. c Percentage indicates the percentage of a solution that is active drug. This is measured in g/100 mL. 24% is equal to 24 g of active drug in 100 mL of solution. Because we measure concentrations as mg/mL, we can break this down further to 24,000 mg (or 24 g) in 100 mL of solution. This can be broken down to mg/mL by dividing both sides of the equation by 100, which becomes 240 mg/mL (24,000/100 = 240 mg and 100/100 = 1 mL). Therefore, a 24% solution has a concentration of 240 mg/mL. The quick way to do this is to move the decimal point one space to the right. Wanamaker BP, Massey KL, Applied Pharmacology for Veterinary Technicians, ed 5, Elsevier, 2015, p. 57-58.

305. b Antineoplastics are used to treat cancer and can be teratogenic, mutagenic, and carcinogenic. This can occur in a patient receiving the drug or a technician handling the drug. Some drugs are excreted unchanged in the urine and feces and owners should be warned and educated how to handle waste. Antibiotic, antinematodal, and antiprotozoal drugs pose very little health risk to humans. Wanamaker BP, Massey KL, Applied Pharmacology for Veterinary Technicians, ed 4, Saunders, 2009, p. 357-358.

306. d Because most drugs are biotransformed by the liver and excreted by the kidneys, any impairment in function of these organs will increase the time it takes for the drug to go through biotransformation or to be eliminated. It will not decrease the absorption or volume of distribution of drugs. Wanamaker BP, Massey KL, Applied Pharmacology for Veterinary Technicians, ed 5, Elsevier, 2015, p. 5.

307. b The Drug Enforcement Agency classifies any drug that has potential for abuse as a controlled drug. The EPA (Environmental Protection Agency) regulates environmentally hazardous materials. The USDA (United States Department of Agriculture) regulates food animals. Bassert JM, Thomas JA, McCurnin's Clinical Textbook for Veterinary Technicians, ed 9, Elsevier, 2017, p. 954.

308. a Articular injections go into a joint. Injections into the bone marrow are called intramedullary, into the subdural space are called intrathecal, and into the heart are called intracardiac. Wanamaker BP, Massey KL, Applied Pharmacology for Veterinary Technicians, ed 5, Elsevier, 2015, p. 7.

309. d When this occurs, the injection should be stopped immediately. You should then withdraw as much of the drug as possible from the intravenous catheter. The area can be infiltrated with saline, sodium bicarbonate, or epinephrine to dilute the drug to constrict the vessels and to prevent the drug from spreading into nearby tissue. Bonagura JD, Twedt DC, Kirk's Current Veterinary Therapy XV, Elsevier, 2014, p. 333.

310. c One ounce is equal to 2 tablespoons, which is equal to 30 mL (15 mL are in 1 tbs). Lake T, Green N, Essential Calculations for Veterinary Nurses and Technicians, ed 3, Butterworth Heinemann, 2016, p. 51.

311. b Lufenuron prevents development of the chitin, which is necessary for the formation of eggs as well as the exoskeleton of the larva. Griseofulvin is fungistatic and is used for dermatophytes, methoprene is an insect growth regulator, and spinosad is a neurotoxin. Sirois M, Principles and Practice of Veterinary Technology, ed 4, Elsevier, 2016, p. 264-265.

312. a Diphenhydramine is the active ingredient in Benadryl, which is the trade name for the drug. Prozac is fluoxetine hydrochloride, Dulcolax is bisacodyl, and Panacur is fenbendazole. Wanamaker BP, Massey KL,

Applied Pharmacology for Veterinary Technicians, ed 5, Elsevier, 2015, p. 156.

313. a Calcium gluconate will protect the heart from the effects of the hyperkalemia but will not decrease the potassium. The other drugs listed will aid in bringing down the potassium. Dextrose causes a release of insulin, which causes glucose to move into the cells. The mechanism by which this occurs also causes potassium to move into the cell. Dextrose can be administered to cause a release of insulin or an injection of insulin can be given with the same result. Sodium bicarbonate will cause a change in the acid-base status of the blood, causing potassium to move into the cells to maintain the acid-base balance. Battaglia AM, Small Animal Emergency and Critical Care for Veterinary Technicians, ed 2, Saunders, 2007, p. 308.

314. a Alfaxalone was approved for use in the United States in 2014 and, like propofol, it is used for sedation for short procedures or for induction of anesthesia. It is compared with propofol not only because of this but also because of the similarities in response and recovery times. The other drugs listed have been in use in the United States for several years. Plumb DC, Veterinary Drug Handbook, ed 8, Wiley-Blackwell, 2015, p. 26-29.

315. b Malignant hyperthermia is seen with inhalant anesthetics and is secondary to changes in calcium metabolism, which can cause muscle tremors. Halothane is the only inhalant anesthetic listed here. Fentanyl, propofol, and etomidate have not been linked to malignant hyperthermia. Silverstein D, Hopper K, Small Animal Critical Care Medicine, ed 1, Saunders, 2009, p. 58.

316. b Dantrolene is specifically used for malignant hyperthermia. It is a muscle relaxant that will bind to receptors, preventing or decreasing the excitation and contraction seen in skeletal muscle. Dexmedetomidine and acepromazine may have sedative effects but will not stop the contraction of the muscle. Diazepam will stop seizures because of its activity in the brain, but it does not address the skeletal muscle. Silverstein D, Hopper K, Small Animal Critical Care Medicine, ed 1, Saunders, 2009, p. 58.

317. b Passive transport occurs when no energy is required to move the molecule across a cell membrane. One way this occurs is through diffusion caused by the difference in the concentration gradient. Molecules want to be evenly distributed on each side of the cell membrane and will therefore move from a high concentration to a low concentration through passive diffusion. Diffusive transport is not a medical term, and active transport requires energy because molecules are being moved from a low concentration to a high concentration. Facilitated transport does not require energy but does require a membrane channel or carrier protein. Wanamaker BP, Massey KL, Applied Pharmacology for Veterinary Technicians, ed 5, Elsevier, 2015, p. 8-9.

318. b Maropitant is an antiemetic and is the active ingredient in Cerenia. Carafate is the trade name for sucralfate, Flagyl is the trade name for metronidazole, and Reglan is the trade name for metoclopramide. Wanamaker BP, Massey KL, Applied Pharmacology for Veterinary Technicians, ed 5, Elsevier, 2015, p. 156-157.

319. d Studies have shown that following an oral medication with a syringe of water will decrease the risk of the tablet or capsule sitting in the esophagus and causing lesions. Oral medications are often sent home with owners, so not giving medications is not feasible. The ability to bring the cat into the clinic for medicating is also not feasible and the risk is still present no matter who gives the pill. Some medications should not be crushed when administering, therefore this is not an option. Boothe DM, Small Animal Clinical Pharmacology and Therapeutics, ed 2, Elsevier, 2012, p. 721.

320. d Lidocaine stabilizes the myocardial membrane (class IB). Class 1A will decrease myocardial excitability, class II includes beta blockers, and class IV includes calcium channel blockers. Wanamaker BP, Massey KL, Applied Pharmacology for Veterinary Technicians, ed 5, Elsevier, 2015, p. 138-141.

321. b A delta fibers are responsible for sharp, localized pain. C fibers are responsible for dull pain, A and C fibers carry impulses to the spinal cord, and C delta fibers do not exist. Wanamaker BP, Massey KL, Applied Pharmacology for Veterinary Technicians, ed 5, Elsevier, 2015, p. 299.

322. a COX-1 is involved with synthesis of prostaglandins that maintain physiological function, maintain gastric mucosa, and are involved with the regulation of blood flow to the kidneys. COX-1 is not associated with healing, inflammation, or pain. NSAIDs that block COX-1 can cause gastric ulcerations and renal failure. Thomas J, Lerche P, Anesthesia and Analgesia for Veterinary Technicians, ed 5, Mosby, 2016, p. 263-264.

323. c The myocardium's response to lidocaine (and other class 1 antiarrhythmic drugs) depends on the presence of potassium and hypokalemia will decrease its efficacy. Boothe DM, Small Animal Clinical Pharmacology and Therapeutics, ed 2, Elsevier, 2012, p. 509; Bonagura JD, Twedt DC, Kirk's Current Veterinary Therapy XV, Elsevier, 2014, p. 252.

324. a Affinity refers to the drug's tendency (how likely it is) to bind to a receptor, whereas its efficacy refers to the degree at which the drug produces the desired response. Specificity refers to how specific the drug is with regard to the receptor with which it will bind and effective dose refers to the dose at which the desired action occurs. Wanamaker BP, Massey KL, Applied Pharmacology for Veterinary Technicians, ed 5, Elsevier, 2015, p. 13-14.

325. c Pinocytosis (cell drinking) and phagocytosis (cell eating) are both forms of active transport. Phagocytosis involves the intake of solid particles. Pinocytosis involves the intake of liquid particles. Facilitated transport requires a carrier protein, whereas passive transport refers to molecules freely crossing the cell membrane. Bill RL, Clinical Pharmacology and Therapeutics for the Veterinary Technician, ed 4, Mosby, 2016, p. 53-55.

326. d Carprofen is the active ingredient in Rimadyl. Deracoxib is the active ingredient in Deramaxx, meloxicam is the active ingredient in Metacam, and firocoxib is the active ingredient in Previcox. Wanamaker BP, Massey KL, Applied Pharmacology for Veterinary Technicians, ed 5, Elsevier, 2015, p. 305.

327. c COX-2 is involved with the synthesis of prostaglandins that cause inflammation and pain. COX-1 is involved with the synthesis of prostaglandins that maintain physiological function, maintain gastric mucosa, and are involved with the regulation of blood flow to the kidneys. NSAIDs that specifically block COX-2 are less likely to cause gastric ulcerations or renal disease. Thomas J, Lerche P, Anesthesia and Analgesia for Veterinary Technicians, ed 5, Mosby, 2016, p. 263-264.

328. a Furosemide (a loop diuretic) is the active ingredient in Lasix, which is the trade name. Mannitol (an osmotic diuretic) is the active ingredient in Osmitrol, Spirolactone (a potassium-sparing diuretic) is the active ingredient in Aldactone, and hydrochlorothiazide (a thiazide diuretic) is the active ingredient in HydroDIURIL. Wanamaker BP, Massey KL, Applied Pharmacology for Veterinary Technicians, ed 5, Elsevier, 2015, p. 117-120.

329. d Metronidazole can cause ataxia, nystagmus, or seizures at high doses if there is an overdose. A carprofen overdose will cause gastrointestinal-related signs (vomiting, diarrhea, ulceration), furosemide overdosing has been associated with ototoxicity and can result in permanent hearing loss, and chloramphenicol can cause signs associated with bone marrow suppression (which is often reversible). Boothe DM, Small Animal Clinical Pharmacology and Therapeutics, ed 2, Elsevier, 2012, p. 92-93, 255.

330. a Levetiracetam is the active ingredient in Keppra. Valium is the trade name for diazepam, Luminal is the trade name for phenobarbital, and Zonegran contains zonisamide. Wanamaker BP, Massey KL, Applied Pharmacology for Veterinary Technicians, ed 5, Elsevier, 2015, p. 87-88.

331. b Fluoroquinolones work by directly inhibiting DNA. They are not involved with protein or cell wall synthesis and do not inhibit the metabolic pathway. Wanamaker BP, Massey KL, Applied Pharmacology for Veterinary Technicians, ed 5, Elsevier, 2015, p. 237.

332. a Facilitated diffusion requires a carrier molecule but does not require energy. Active transport also requires a carrier protein but, unlike facilitated diffusion, it requires and uses energy when transporting the molecule into the cell. Neither pinocytosis nor passive diffusion requires a carrier protein or energy. Bill RL, Clinical Pharmacology and Therapeutics for the Veterinary Technician, ed 4, Mosby, 2016, p. 53-58.

333. b Metronidazole can be halved, therefore you can use the 500-mg tablets and cut them in half to provide a 250-mg dose. BID indicates it should be given twice a day. Half a tablet twice a day for 6 days is equal to 6 tablets (0.5 tablets × 2 times a day × 6 days = 6 tablets) Lake T, Green N, Essential Calculations for Veterinary Nurses and Technicians, ed 3, Butterworth Heinemann, 2016, p. 33-37.

334. c Baytril is the trade name for enrofloxacin. Neurontin is one trade name for gabapentin, Keflex is a trade name for cephalexin, and acepromazine has several trade names including ProMACE and Aceprotabs. Sirois M, Principles and Practice of Veterinary Technology, ed 4, Elsevier, 2016, p. 262-263.

335. a When a patient has been on a drug long enough for it to be become therapeutic, the highest plasma concentration (reached sometime after receiving the dose) that a drug reaches is called its peak whereas the lowest concentration (reached sometime before the next dose is due) is called the trough. This is important for drug monitoring because sometimes the laboratory wants blood drawn at the peak and other times at the trough. Bill RL, Clinical Pharmacology and Therapeutics for the Veterinary Technician, ed 4, Mosby, 2016, p. 50-51.

336. c When the plasma concentration of a drug is consistently the same (or steady) at its highest concentration (peak) and lowest concentration (trough), it is said to be in a steady state. Steady state does not imply how long the patient has been taking the drug, the patient's response to the drug, or if the owner is being compliant and giving the drug as directed. Bill RL, Clinical Pharmacology and Therapeutics for the Veterinary Technician, ed 4, Mosby, 2016, p. 79-80.

337. a Acute inflammation causes vasodilation and increased blood flow to the area. Shock will cause the body to shunt blood to the vital organs, decreasing blood flow to the extremities, hemorrhage will decrease blood volume and an area of necrosis will not receive blood flow. Boothe DM, Small Animal Clinical Pharmacology and Therapeutics, ed 2, Elsevier, 2012, p. 168.

338. c Metronidazole is the active ingredient in Flagyl. Sucralfate is the active ingredient in Carafate, Cerenia is the trade name for maropitant (which is the active ingredient), and metoclopramide is the active ingredient in Reglan. Wanamaker BP, Massey KL, Applied Pharmacology for Veterinary Technicians, ed 5, Elsevier, 2015, p. 165.

339. b Because the patient is vomiting, any medication given orally will probably be vomited back up before it is absorbed. Metronidazole is not labeled for use IM or SQ. The best option for this patient would be to administer the metronidazole IV. This will ensure the medication is absorbed and it will also reach peak plasma concentrations much faster than IM, SQ, or PO. Papich MG, Saunders Handbook of Veterinary Drugs, ed 3, Elsevier, 2011, p. 505-506.

340. b Antibiotics should be continued for 2 weeks after signs of the pneumonia are no longer evident on radiographs. If they are only continued 2 weeks past resolution of the clinical signs, it is possible the pneumonia has not completely resolved and will return after the antibiotics are discontinued. Radiographs should always be rechecked before discontinuing antibiotics even if clinical signs are resolved. Ford RB, Mazzaferro E, Kirk and Bistner's Handbook of Veterinary Procedures and Emergency Treatment, ed 9, Elsevier, 2012, p. 150.

341. b Prophylactic antibiotics are given when a hollow viscous is entered (such as the gastrointestinal tract, gallbladder, or urinary bladder). The skin should be disinfected before any incision is made and the surgeon and instruments should both be sterile. Bassert JM, Thomas JA, McCurnin's Clinical Textbook for Veterinary Technicians, ed 9, Elsevier, 2017, p. 1142.

342. d Reglan is the trade name for metoclopramide. The trade name for metronidazole is Flagyl, the trade name for dolasetron is Anzemet, and the trade name for maropitant is Cerenia. Wanamaker BP, Massey KL, Applied Pharmacology for Veterinary Technicians, ed 5, Elsevier, 2015, p. 156.

343. d Antibiotics are usually used in surgeries that involve anything that may decrease the patients' ability to fight infection such as shock, trauma, or poor body condition. In these cases, antibiotics are given right before surgery or when surgery starts and then every 90–120 minutes during the surgery. Sirois M, Principles and Practice of Veterinary Technology, ed 4, Elsevier, 2016, p. 301.

344. c Metronidazole requires an anaerobic environment to be effective. Transport of aminoglycosides (chloramphenicol, clindamycin, and neomycin) into the bacterial cell requires a high oxygen tension environment and will not be effective in an anaerobic environment. Boothe DM, Small Animal Clinical Pharmacology and Therapeutics, ed 2, Elsevier, 2012, p. 245-246.

345. c First-tier antibiotics (clindamycin) are those that are known to have a wide spectrum of use. Second-tier antibiotics (fluroquinolones) are more specific to certain organisms that may not be susceptible to the first-tier antibiotics. Third-generation antibiotics (cefotaxime) are those used when bacteria have become resistant to other antibiotics. Negative-tier antibiotics do not exist. Boothe DM, Small Animal Clinical Pharmacology and Therapeutics, ed 2, Elsevier, 2012, p. 271; Bonagura JD, Twedt DC, Kirk's Current Veterinary Therapy XV, Elsevier, 2014, p. 438, 881.

346. a Ticks spread Rocky Mountain spotted fever. In the list given, Advantix is the only tick preventative. Heartgard will act as a heartworm preventative and also controls hookworms and roundworms. Revolution is effective against heartworm, fleas, ear mites, mange, hookworms, and roundworms. Interceptor is effective against heartworms, roundworms, and whipworm. Summers A, Common Diseases of Companion Animals, ed 4, Mosby, 2019, p. 104-105.

347. d Ketoconazole is in the drug class imidazole (antifungal agents). Amoxicillin is a penicillin, cephalexin is a cephalosporin, and enrofloxacin is a fluoroquinolone. Bill RL, Clinical Pharmacology and Therapeutics for the Veterinary Technician, ed 4, Mosby, 2016, p. 237-238.

348. b Malassezia is a yeast infection and is often treated topically. When it becomes chronic, systemic antifungals may also be required. Itraconazole or ketoconazole are the drugs of choice. Griseofulvin is ineffective against Malassezia. Metronidazole and tetracycline are antibiotics and are not effective in treating yeast infections. Bassert JM, Thomas JA, McCurnin's Clinical Textbook for Veterinary Technicians, ed 9, Elsevier, 2017, p. 1142.

349. d Acyclovir is an antiviral and fights viruses by preventing DNA synthesis. It has no action against bacteria, fungi, or parasites. Wanamaker BP, Massey KL, Applied Pharmacology for Veterinary Technicians, ed 5, Elsevier, 2015, p. 260-261.

350. a Chlorhexidine is ototoxic and is very irritating to the ear canal. It should not be used or should be diluted 1:100 with saline. Saline solution, a mix of vinegar and water, or an aural cleaning solution can clean the ear safely. Wanamaker BP, Massey KL, Applied Pharmacology for Veterinary Technicians, ed 4, Saunders, 2009, p. 205.

351. c Calcium gluconate will not change the level of potassium in the blood but it will antagonize the cardiotoxic effects of the potassium on the cells of the heart (prolonged depolarization/repolarization causing bradycardia and atrial standstill). Battaglia AM, Small Animal Emergency and Critical Care for Veterinary Technicians, ed 3, Saunders, 2015, p. 386.

352. b Tetanus favors anaerobic environments. Metronidazole works well in anaerobic environments and is best suited to treat tetanus because it will be bactericidal in these areas. Penicillin G can also be effective but less so than metronidazole. Enrofloxacin and neomycin are not effective in anaerobic environments. Silverstein D, Hopper K, Small Animal Critical Care Medicine, ed 1, Saunders, 2009, p. 437.

353. c Class IA drugs affect the heart by decreasing the automaticity of myocardial cells. Drugs that block beta receptors are in class II, drugs that block calcium channels are in class IV, and drugs that stabilize myocardial cells are in class IB. Wanamaker BP, Massey KL, Applied Pharmacology for Veterinary Technicians, ed 5, Elsevier, 2015, p. 137-140.

354. c Propranolol blocks both beta-1 and beta-2 receptors and is considered a nonselective beta blocker. Wanamaker BP, Massey KL, Applied Pharmacology for Veterinary Technicians, ed 5, Elsevier, 2015, p. 139.

355. c Diltiazem is a calcium channel blocker and is one of the most common calcium channel blockers used in veterinary medicine. It is used primarily for supraventricular tachycardia. Wanamaker BP, Massey KL, Applied Pharmacology for Veterinary Technicians, ed 5, Elsevier, 2015, p. 140.

356. d Vincristine will increase platelet numbers. The exact mechanism is unknown but might be caused by an increased number of platelets released from the bone marrow or fragmentation of megakaryocytes into functional platelets. Chlorambucil, doxorubicin, and vinblastine do not have this effect. Silverstein D, Hopper K, Small Animal Critical Care Medicine, ed 1, Saunders, 2009, p. 517-569.

357. d Oxyglobin is bovine hemoglobin and will provide oxygen-carrying capacity for up to 40 hours after administration. Plasma (fresh frozen or frozen) and cryoprecipitate do not contain hemoglobin and therefore have no oxygen-carrying capacity. Wanamaker BP, Massey KL, Applied Pharmacology for Veterinary Technicians, ed 5, Elsevier, 2015, p. 337-338.

358. c 1200 mg/375 mg/mL = 3.2 mL to be administered. Lake T, Green N, Essential Calculations for Veterinary Nurses and Technicians, ed 2, Butterworth Heinemann, 2009, p. 82-83.

359. d A drug is thought to be in a steady state when the amount of drug being eliminated is the same as the amount of drug being administered. When a drug is given, the half-life is the time it takes for the concentration to reach half the original concentration (50%). Each time the drug is given and it goes through a half-life, the concentration increases because it is added to the previous concentration reached. (Keep in mind that the doses given previously also continue to go through half-lives.) This continues until the drug has gone through a total of five half-lives, at which point the concentration is at a total of 97%: 1st dose given, reaches its half-life of 50% 2nd dose given, reaches its half-life of 50%, at which point the 1st dose is at 25% = 75% 3rd dose given, reaches its half-life of 50% + the 2nd dose at 25% + the 3rd dose at 12.5% = 87.5% 4th dose given, reaches its half-life of 50% + the 3rd dose at 25% + the 2nd dose at 12.5% + the 1st dose at 6.25 = 93.75 5th dose given, reaches its half-life of 50% + the 4th dose at 25% + the 3rd dose at 12.5% + the 2nd dose at 6.25% + the 1st dose at 3.125% = 96.875% or 97%. At this point the drug is at its steady state. Some drugs require a sixth half-life to reach steady state but five is more common. Bill RL, Clinical Pharmacology and Therapeutics for the Veterinary Technician, ed 4, Mosby, 2016, p. 78-80.

360. c 37.5 kg × 10 mg/kg = 375 mg. 375 mg/250 mg tablets = 1.5 tablets per dose. BID (twice a day) for seven days = 14 total doses (2 times a day for 7 days = 2 × 7 = 14). So 14 doses × 1.5 tablets per dose = 14 × 1.5 = 21 total tablets. Lake T, Green N, Essential Calculations for Veterinary Nurses and Technicians, ed 2, Butterworth Heinemann, 2009, p. 57-60.

361. a Class IB drugs affect the heart by stabilizing myocardial cells. Drugs that decrease the automaticity of myocardial cells belong in class IA. Drugs that block beta receptors are in class II, drugs that block calcium channels are in class IV. Wanamaker BP, Massey KL, Applied Pharmacology for Veterinary Technicians, ed 5, Elsevier, 2015, p. 137-140.

362. b D5W is dextrose 5% in water. It consists only of dextrose and water and does not contain sodium. The other fluids listed contain sodium (0.9% NaCl has 154 mEq/L, 0.45% NaCl has 77 mEq/L, and lactated ringers contain 130 mEq/L). Wanamaker BP, Massey KL, Applied Pharmacology for Veterinary Technicians, ed 5, Elsevier, 2015, p. 336.

363. a When administering calcium gluconate, you should monitor the patient's EKG closely because of the possibility of cardiotoxicity and the development of a prolonged PR interval, wide QRS, and bradycardia. Calcium gluconate should not directly affect the blood pressure, SpO_2, or temperature. Battaglia AM, Small Animal Emergency and Critical Care for Veterinary Technicians, ed 3, Saunders, 2015, p. 36, 360.

364. c Active transport requires a carrier molecule and also requires energy. Facilitated diffusion also requires a carrier protein but, unlike activated transport, it does not require energy. Neither pinocytosis nor passive diffusion requires a carrier protein. Bill RL, Clinical Pharmacology and Therapeutics for the Veterinary Technician, ed 4, Mosby, 2016, p. 54-55.

365. d Hetastarch is a synthetic (man-made) colloid. It contains larger molecules than a crystalloid and therefore stays in the circulation longer. An example of a natural colloid is a blood product. Crystalloids (e.g., lactated ringers, Plasmalyte) contain smaller molecules than colloids. Wanamaker BP, Massey KL, Applied Pharmacology for Veterinary Technicians, ed 5, Elsevier, 2015, p. 337.

366. b Spirolactone affects the collecting duct where it decreases excretion of potassium and reabsorption of sodium. Loop diuretics (furosemide) act at the loop of Henle, osmotic diuretics (mannitol) act at the proximal tubule, and there are no diuretics that act on Bowman's capsule. Silverstein D, Hopper K, Small Animal Critical Care Medicine, ed 1, Saunders, 2009, p. 766.

367. b Esmolol is a beta-1 blocker. It does not act on beta-2 receptors and is therefore not a nonselective beta blocker. Wanamaker BP, Massey KL, Applied Pharmacology for Veterinary Technicians, ed 5, Elsevier, 2015, p. 140.

368. a A positive inotrope will increase cardiac contractility whereas a negative inotrope will decrease contractility. A chronotropic agent will either increase (positive) or decrease (negative) the heart rate. Wanamaker BP, Massey KL, Applied Pharmacology for Veterinary Technicians, ed 5, Elsevier, 2015, p. 135.

369. d The patient will require 2 of the 25-mg tablets for each dose (50 mg per dose/25-mg tablets = 2 tablets per dose). TID means it should be given three times daily (or every 8 hours), hence 2 tablets per dose × 3 doses per day × 7 days = 2 × 3 × 7 = 42 total tablets. Lake T, Green N, Essential Calculations for Veterinary Nurses and Technicians, ed 2, Butterworth Heinemann, 2009, p. 57-60.

370. b Drugs in class II block beta receptors. Class IA drugs affect the heart by decreasing the automaticity of myocardial cells. Drugs that block calcium channels are in class IV and drugs that stabilize myocardial cells are in class IB. Wanamaker BP, Massey KL, Applied Pharmacology for Veterinary Technicians, ed 5, Elsevier, 2015, p. 137-140.

371. d Chronic inflammation will cause purulent discharge as well as an acidic and hypoxic environment, all of which can inhibit the efficacy of antibiotics. Acute inflammation increases delivery of the drug to the area because of the presence of vasodilation and an increase in blood flow to the area. Shock will cause the body to shunt blood to the vital organs thereby decreasing blood flow to the extremities, which will decrease delivery of the drug but not necessarily its efficacy. Necrosis will result in no delivery of drug to the area because of a complete lack of blood flow. Boothe DM, Small Animal Clinical Pharmacology and Therapeutics, ed 2, Elsevier, 2012, p. 168.

372. b Cisapride is a serotonergic prokinetic that acts on the whole gastrointestinal tract from (and including) the gastroesophageal sphincter to the colon. Cisapride does not act as an antiemetic, antidiarrheal, or gastrointestinal protectant. Wanamaker BP, Massey

KL, Applied Pharmacology for Veterinary Technicians, ed 5, Elsevier, 2015, p. 163.

373. a Dirlotapide is used for obesity in dogs and acts by preventing the release of lipoproteins into the blood. Dirlotapide is not used in cats and does not increase the appetite. Wanamaker BP, Massey KL, Applied Pharmacology for Veterinary Technicians, ed 5, Elsevier, 2015, p. 166.

374. d Ondansetron is a serotonin antagonist that acts on the chemoreceptor trigger zone. It is especially useful for nausea caused by chemotherapy. It is not classified as an anticholinergic, phenothiazine, or barbiturate. Bill RL, Clinical Pharmacology and Therapeutics for the Veterinary Technician, ed 4, Mosby, 2016, p. 97.

375. b Lactulose will pull ammonia into the colon where it will change ammonia to ammonium. Ammonium will not diffuse back into the blood, which results in a decrease of the ammonia concentrations in the blood. Lactulose also acts as a cathartic, increasing GI motility and acting as a laxative. Bonagura JD, Twedt DC, Kirk's Current Veterinary Therapy XV, Elsevier, 2014, p. 593.

376. a Of the drugs listed, cyclosporine is the only one used for both pruritus and autoimmune diseases (such as immune-mediated hemolytic anemia and immune-mediated thrombocytopenia). Bonagura JD, Twedt DC, Kirk's Current Veterinary Therapy XV, Elsevier, 2014, p. 269-270.

377. b Atopica is one of the brand names for cyclosporine. Anzemet is the brand name for dolasetron and Lasix is the brand name for furosemide. Wanamaker BP, Massey KL, Applied Pharmacology for Veterinary Technicians, ed 5, Elsevier, 2015, p. 367-368.

378. d Midazolam is the only benzodiazepine listed. Fentanyl is an opioid, ketamine is a dissociative agent, and medetomidine is an alpha-2 adrenergic agonist. Bassert JM, Thomas JA, McCurnin's Clinical Textbook for Veterinary Technicians, ed 9, Elsevier, 2016, p. 1013-1014.

379. b Osmotic diuretics (e.g., mannitol) are used to decrease intracranial pressure in cases of head trauma. Loop, thiazide, and potassium-sparing diuretics are used instead for diseases such as heart failure or conditions such as pulmonary edema. Sirois M, Principles and Practice of Veterinary Technology, ed 4, Elsevier, 2016, p. 428.; Battaglia AM, Small Animal Emergency and Critical Care for Veterinary Technicians, ed 3, Saunders, 2015, p. 36, 360.

380. a Of the medications listed, buprenorphine is the only opioid. Carprofen is a nonsteroidal anti-inflammatory drug, lidocaine is used as an antiarrhythmic and local anesthetic, and naloxone is reversal agent for opioids. Bassert JM, Thomas JA, McCurnin's Clinical Textbook for Veterinary Technicians, ed 9, Elsevier, 2016, p. 993-994.

381. d CRI stands for constant rate infusion. Fentanyl has a short half-life and will only last 30–40 minutes after injection. For this reason it is best used for analgesia during short procedures or as a CRI. Sirois M, Principles and Practice of Veterinary Technology, ed 3, Elsevier, 2011, p. 2; Thomas J, Lerche P, Anesthesia and Analgesia for Veterinary Technicians, ed 5, Mosby, 2014, p. 258.

382. d Tramadol is an oral analgesic that is a synthetic analog of codeine. The others are not synthetic derivatives of codeine, although dextromethorphan is a synthetic derivative of opium. Boothe DM, Small Animal Clinical Pharmacology and Therapeutics, ed 2, Elsevier, 2012, p. 1027.

383. b When administering chemotherapeutics it is extremely important that the catheter be placed with a clean stick. If this is not done, the catheter should be pulled and placed in a different vein to avoid any chances of extravasation of the drug. Bassert JM, Thomas JA, McCurnin's Clinical Textbook for Veterinary Technicians, ed 9, Elsevier, 2016, p. 554-555.

384. c L-asparaginase is used primarily for lymphoma and lymphoid leukemia. It works by preventing the cancer cells from using asparagine, which is essential for the lymphoma cells' survival. L-asparaginase is not used for mast cell tumors, hemangiosarcoma, or osteosarcoma. Boothe DM, Small Animal Clinical Pharmacology and Therapeutics, ed 2, Elsevier, 2012, p. 1231.

385. d A supersaturated solution contains more solute than can be dissolved by the solvent. A concentrated solution contains a large amount of solute, all of which is dissolved. A dilute solution contains very little solute and a saturated solution contains the maximum amount of solute that can be dissolved by the solvent. Wanamaker BP, Massey KL, Applied Pharmacology for Veterinary Technicians, ed 5, Elsevier, 2015, p. 57.

386. b The number of moles per liter of a solution is termed *molarity*, the amount of solute per kilogram is termed *molality*, the weight (in g) per liter of solution is termed *normality*, and the total number of solute particles per liter is termed *osmolarity*. Boothe DM, Small Animal Clinical Pharmacology and Therapeutics, ed 2, Elsevier, 2012, p. 1256-1257.

387. b The CRI is at 3 μg/kg/h and the dog weighs 50 kg, hence the total fentanyl used in 1 hour will be 150 μg (3 μg/kg/h × 50 kg = 150 μg/h). The fentanyl is 50 μg/mL so 3 mL/h will be required (150 μg/h ÷ 50 μg/mL = 3 mL/h). Lake T, Green N, Essential Calculations for Veterinary Nurses and Technicians, ed 3, Butterworth Heinemann, 2016, p. 97-103.

388. c Ketamine will increase cerebral blood flow and thus intracranial pressure, which would be detrimental in a patient with existing intracranial disease. The other drugs listed are all advantageous in a patient with intracranial disease: propofol decreases intracranial and cerebral perfusion pressures, whereas barbiturates and etomidate both decrease cerebral blood flow and oxygen consumption. Boothe DM, Small Animal Clinical Pharmacology and Therapeutics, ed 2, Elsevier, 2012, p. 891-892.

389. b A common side effect of phenobarbital is hepatotoxicity. If the patient has a pre-existing liver disease, this medication should be avoided. The other medications listed do not have an adverse effect on the liver. Bassert JM, Thomas JA, McCurnin's Clinical Textbook for Veterinary Technicians, ed 9, Elsevier, 2016, p. 971-972.

390. a Etomidate has few cardiorespiratory depressive effects. The other drugs listed commonly cause cardiorespiratory depression and should be used with caution and the respiratory and heart rates should be monitored closely. Thomas J, Lerche P, Anesthesia and Analgesia for Veterinary Technicians, ed 5, Mosby, 2016, p. 77-78.

391. b Methocarbamol is a muscle relaxant that is often used to treat muscle spasms associated with skeletal muscle trauma (such as a dog with back pain). It is not an anticonvulsant, but it can be used to control muscle tremors associated with toxicities. It will not directly address intracranial pressure or joint pain. Sirois M, Principles and Practice of Veterinary Technology, ed 4, Elsevier, 2016, p. 260.

392. c Myasthenia gravis is caused by a problem with the acetylcholine receptors. It can be congenital in which the receptors do not develop properly or acquired when the immune system attacks the receptors. A diagnosis can be confirmed by injecting Tensilon, which is a short-acting acetylcholinesterase. This makes more acetylcholine available to attach to receptors not occupied by an antibody. The patient will respond quickly and muscle weakness will resolve for a short period. Acepromazine, metoclopramide, and theophylline will not have this effect and are not used to diagnosis myasthenia gravis. Wanamaker BP, Massey KL, Applied Pharmacology for Veterinary Technicians, ed 5, Elsevier, 2015, p. 77.

393. a Bloat-Pac is an antifoaming agent that breaks down the bubbles in the rumen that are the cause of the bloat. This occurs in ruminants and is not seen in dogs, pigs, or horses because they are not ruminants. Wanamaker BP, Massey KL, Applied Pharmacology for Veterinary Technicians, ed 5, Elsevier, 2015, p. 165-166.

394. c 5-Fluorouacil should never be used in cats because of the side effects that include unprovoked aggression, dementia, and sudden death. Carboplatin, hydroxyurea, and procarbazine are all commonly used in cats to treat cancer. Wanamaker BP, Massey KL, Applied Pharmacology for Veterinary Technicians, ed 5, Elsevier, 2015, p. 364; Boothe DM, Small Animal Clinical Pharmacology and Therapeutics, ed 2, Elsevier, 2012, p. 1228.

395. b Robaxin-V is the brand name for methocarbamol. Gabapentin has the brand name Neurontin, methimazole has the brand name Tapazole, and methionine (S-Adenosyl) has the brand name SAM-e. Sirois M, Principles and Practice of Veterinary Technology, ed 4, Elsevier, 2016, p. 260.

396. d Drugs in class IV have their effect by blocking calcium channels. Class IA drugs affect the heart by decreasing the automaticity of myocardial cells. Drugs that block beta receptors are in class II and drugs that stabilize myocardial cells are in class IB. Wanamaker BP, Massey KL, Applied Pharmacology for Veterinary Technicians, ed 5, Elsevier, 2015, p. 137-141.

397. c The longer the abdomen is open to the air, the more likely it is that an infection will occur. Thus antibiotics should be administered 90 minutes after surgery begins and every 90 minutes after that. If the patient has a decreased immunity (e.g., related to disease, trauma), antibiotics should be given when surgery starts and every 90 minutes thereafter. Bassert JM, Thomas JA, McCurnin's Clinical Textbook for Veterinary Technicians, ed 9, Elsevier, 2016, p. 1142.

398. b A 25% solution contains 250 mg of drug/mL. Because this concentration is in mg/mL, we must convert the 5 g ordered to mg. There are 1000 mg in 1 g, hence 5 g is equal to 5000 mg (1000 mg/g × 5 g = 5000 mg.) 5000 mg is the total dose required. We can divide that total by 250 mg/mL and obtain 20 mL (5000 mg/250 mg/mL = 20 mL). This patient requires 20 mL of mannitol for administration of 5 g of the drug. Mannitol can crystallize and a filter should therefore always be used during administration. Lake T, Green N, Essential Calculations for Veterinary Nurses and Technicians, ed 2, Butterworth Heinemann, 2009, p. 61-66.

399. d Drugs that are used long term should be monitored to ensure that the dose the patient receives is a therapeutic dose. Of the medications listed, phenobarbital is most likely to be in long-term use. Bassert JM, Thomas JA, McCurnin's Clinical Textbook for Veterinary Technicians, ed 8, Elsevier, 2014, p. 1016-1017.

400. a An aerotolerant organism is one that can survive in an environment with or without oxygen. The other types of organisms are not seen in veterinary medicine. Organisms that can tolerate elevated temperatures are seen in volcanoes or hot springs and are referred to as hyperthermophiles. Organisms are termed *desiccation-tolerant* when they can live in an environment that lacks moisture (or is dehydrated). Boothe DM, Small Animal Clinical Pharmacology and Therapeutics, ed 2, Elsevier, 2012, p. 13.

401. b Some bacteria are able to produce a layer, much like a slime, that allows it to adhere to other bacteria or to a surface. If this layer becomes hard, it will provide additional protection to the bacteria. This does not replace the cell wall. Bill RL, Clinical Pharmacology and Therapeutics for the Veterinary Technician, ed 4, Mosby, 2016, p. 246-247.

402. a Beta-lactams interfere with synthesis of the cell wall. Aminoglycosides are examples of bacteria that interfere with protein synthesis. Quinolones interfere with DNA synthesis. Boothe DM, Small Animal Clinical Pharmacology and Therapeutics, ed 2, Elsevier, 2012, p. 202.

403. d Metoclopramide can be added to IV fluids and is also available in tablet form. Dolasetron is in injectable form but is not added to IV fluids and there is no oral form available. Maropitant is available in injectable and oral forms but the injectable form is not added to IV fluids. Diphenhydramine should not be added to intravenous fluids. Of the medications listed, metoclopramide is the only one that will increase gastrointestinal motility. Wanamaker BP, Massey KL, Applied Pharmacology for Veterinary Technicians, ed 5, Elsevier, 2015, p. 156.

404. b Sulfonamides prevent bacteria from synthesizing folic acid, which is important for metabolism of proteins and nucleic acids. The bacteria are able to adjust and use the host's folic acid, thus becoming resistant to the sulfonamide. Boothe DM, Small Animal Clinical Pharmacology and Therapeutics, ed 2, Elsevier, 2012, p. 248-249.

405. c By binding subunit 50s, macrolides impair a translocation step of protein synthesis. Macrolides do not bind to the other ribosomal subunits listed. Boothe DM, Small Animal Clinical Pharmacology and Therapeutics, ed 2, Elsevier, 2012, p. 259.

406. d A prodrug is one that is in an inactive form when provided to the patient. As it goes through biotransformation, the byproducts of the process are the active form of the drug. Examples are enalapril, which becomes the active form enalaprilat, or benazepril, which becomes the active form benazeprilat. Bill RL, Clinical Pharmacology and Therapeutics for the Veterinary Technician, ed 4, Mosby, 2016, p. 74.

407. c Buprenorphine is best given transmucosally (TM). If given orally (po) so that the patient is allowed to swallow it, the drug will be ineffective. Because buprenorphine is very effective when given transmucosally, there is no reason for an owner give it IM or SQ. Bassert JM, Thomas JA, McCurnin's Clinical Textbook for Veterinary Technicians, ed 9, Elsevier, 2016, p. 993.

408. d Glycopyrrolate crosses the placental barrier (although minimally) and is safe to use in pregnant dogs. Atropine, fentanyl, and acepromazine all cross the placental barrier and should be avoided in pregnant dogs. Thomas J, Lerche P, Anesthesia and Analgesia for Veterinary Technicians, ed 5, Mosby, 2016, p. 60-63.

409. b Geriatric patients may not have the ability to biotransform or to eliminate drugs as well as younger patients, therefore drug doses are generally decreased or the dose interval increased. Thomas J, Lerche P, Anesthesia and Analgesia for Veterinary Technicians, ed 4, Mosby, 2011, p. 370-371.

410. a Digoxin prefers to bind to Na,K-ATPase at the same place that potassium binds. When hypokalemia is present, there is less potassium binding to these sites and there are therefore more available binding sites for digoxin, which can lead to toxicity (because more of the drug is binding and having an effect). Boothe DM, Small Animal Clinical Pharmacology and Therapeutics, ed 2, Elsevier, 2012, p. 523; Bassert JM, Thomas JA, McCurnin's Clinical Textbook for Veterinary Technicians, ed 8, Elsevier, 2014, p. 1015.

411. b Amikacin can develop a pale yellow discoloration, which has no bearing on its efficacy. It does not need to be discarded or diluted. Wanamaker BP, Massey KL, Applied Pharmacology for Veterinary Technicians, ed 5, Elsevier, 2015, p. 233.

412. c Because the nitroglycerin will be absorbed by anyone who gets it on their skin, it is important to wear gloves and to make a note of where it has been placed so that other people know to avoid that area. Nitroglycerin should be placed on the patient's skin and it should be applied thinly. Wanamaker BP, Massey KL, Applied Pharmacology for Veterinary Technicians, ed 5, Elsevier, 2015, p. 142.

413. b Low molecular weight heparin will not block the activity of thrombin, hence it is less likely to cause hemorrhage than unfractionated heparin. Low molecular weight heparin is purer and more expensive than unfractionated heparin. Papich MG, Saunders Handbook of Veterinary Drugs: Small and Large Animal, ed 4, Elsevier, 2015, p. 285-286

414. a Clopidogrel is the active ingredient in Plavix. Sildenafil is Viagra, and tadalafil is Cialis. The brand name for nitroprusside is Nitropress. Wanamaker BP, Massey KL, Applied Pharmacology for Veterinary Technicians, ed 4, Saunders, 2009, p. 143.

415. d Sotalol is a beta blocker that has a similar action as propranolol and can be sent home with the patient as an oral form. Pimobendan is a positive inotrope used to treat dilated cardiomyopathy, hydralazine is an arteriole dilator, and prazosin is used as an adjunct therapy for congestive heart failure therapy. Wanamaker BP, Massey KL, Applied Pharmacology for Veterinary Technicians, ed 5, Elsevier, 2015, p. 140.

416. a Of the medications listed, digoxin is the only one used for atrial fibrillation. Hydralazine is used for congestive heart failure, lidocaine is used to treat ventricular tachycardia, and pimobendan is used to treat dilated cardiomyopathy. Wanamaker BP, Massey KL, Applied Pharmacology for Veterinary Technicians, ed 5, Elsevier, 2015, p. 135-136.

417. c Potassium phosphate can be added to the patient's intravenous fluids in response to hypophosphatemia. It is important to note that you will also be adding potassium to the fluids and it should be taken into consideration so that the patient does not receive too high a dose of potassium, which can result in cardiac arrest. Dexamethasone sodium phosphate is a steroid. It will not increase the phosphorus and should not be administered as a constant infusion. Amphojel is a phosphorus binder and will lower the phosphorus further. Tums is calcium carbonate and is used to increase calcium. It will not increase phosphorus. Ford RB, Mazzaferro E, Kirk and Bistner's Handbook of Veterinary Procedures and Emergency Treatment, ed 9, Elsevier, 2012, p. 277.

418. d Feline asthma is commonly treated with terbutaline, which is a bronchodilator and acts to open the airways. Amphotericin B is used in the treatment of blastomycosis and hydralazine and digoxin are both used to treat dilated cardiomyopathy. Summers A, Common Diseases of Companion Animals, ed 3, Elsevier, 2014, p. 89.

419. a Aminophylline is a bronchodilator. It does not have any expectorant, decongestant, or mucolytic properties. Sirois M, Principles and Practice of Veterinary Technology, ed 4, Elsevier, 2016, p. 255-256.

420. c Of the medications listed, sucralfate is the only one that is not absorbed systemically. It coats the esophagus and stomach and is not absorbed into the blood. Dolasetron, diphenhydramine, and tramadol are available in both injectable and oral forms (injectable tramadol is not currently available in the United States) and are absorbed systemically when given orally. Any medication given IV, IM, or SQ will be absorbed systemically. Sirois M, Principles and Practice of Veterinary Technology, ed 4, Elsevier, 2016, p. 253.

421. a Tums is a brand name for calcium carbonate. It can be used to treat hypocalcemia in patients that have had a parathyroidectomy or in pregnant or lactating bitches. Bonagura JD, Twedt DC, Kirk's Current Veterinary Therapy XV, Elsevier, 2014, p. 180.

422. d Vitamin B1 is thiamine. Ascorbic acid is vitamin C, cyanocobalamin is vitamin B12, and riboflavin is vitamin B2. Wanamaker BP, Massey KL, Applied Pharmacology for Veterinary Technicians, ed 5, Elsevier, 2015, p. 343-344, 483.

423. c Calcitriol will cause an increase in calcium levels by increasing uptake from the gastrointestinal tract, increasing uptake from the bone, and decreasing excretion from the kidneys. Alendronate and calcitonin will inhibit osteoclast activity and decrease bone resorption, which will decrease calcium levels. Calcimimetics is a class of drugs that interacts with calcium receptors causing negative feedback that will decrease PTH levels leading to a decrease in calcium levels. Bonagura JD, Twedt DC, Kirk's Current Veterinary Therapy XV, Elsevier, 2014, p. e33.

424. a Prednisone is metabolized to prednisolone by the liver. Cats do not metabolize prednisone well and there will be very little active drug available. For this reason they should be given prednisolone to avoid the need to metabolize prednisone. This also occurs in horses. Papich MG, Saunders Handbook of Veterinary Drugs, ed 3, Elsevier, 2011, p. 666-667.

425. b A 20-kg dog receiving 2 mg/kg/day will require 40 mg/day (20 kg × 2 mg/kg/day = 40 mg/day). The 1-L bag of fluids will last 24 hours (1 day), hence you will need to add 40 mg to the bag of fluids. Metoclopramide is 5 mg/mL. 40 mg/day divided by 5 mg/mL is equal to 8 mL of metoclopramide added to the fluids (40 mg/5mg/mL). Lake T, Green N, Essential Calculations for Veterinary Nurses and Technicians, ed 2, Butterworth Heinemann, 2009, p. 99-105.

426. a Mannitol decreases the vitreous humor via dehydration. This decreases the intraocular pressure. Methazolamide is a carbonic anhydrase inhibitor and decreases the production of aqueous humor. Pilocarpine causes miosis, which opens the iridocorneal angle and increases the outflow of aqueous humor. Timolol is a beta blocker and decreases the production of aqueous humor. Bonagura JD, Twedt DC, Kirk's Current Veterinary Therapy XV, Elsevier, 2014, p. 1172-1174.

427. b Because IV injections are injected directly into the bloodstream, high concentrations are reached rapidly, which can cause adverse effects such as vomiting or seizures. Medications given IM, SQ, or IP are absorbed more slowly and are less likely to cause similar problems. Thomas J, Lerche P, Anesthesia and Analgesia for Veterinary Technicians, ed 4, Mosby, 2011, p. 60.

428. c Potassium should not be delivered at a rate of more than 0.5 mEq/kg/h. A rate higher than this can cause cardiac arrest. Bassert JM, Thomas JA, McCurnin's Clinical Textbook for Veterinary Technicians, ed 9, Elsevier, 2016, p. 827-828.

429. c Spinal epidurals often decrease the ability of the patient to urinate. Because of this, urination and bladder size should be monitored closely until the patient urinates and empties the bladder (this should not be confused with the patient experiencing an overflow of urine. This is why it is also important to monitor bladder size). An epidural should not cause any changes in the patient's appetite, attitude, or ability to walk. Thomas J, Lerche P, Anesthesia and Analgesia for Veterinary Technicians, ed 4, Mosby, 2011, p. 221.

430. b Dexmedetomidine is used primarily as a sedative. When combined with morphine as an epidural, it has been shown to increase the length of analgesia. Bupivacaine, hydromorphone, and morphine, although they may cause some sedation, are primarily used for their analgesic properties. Thomas J, Lerche P, Anesthesia and Analgesia for Veterinary Technicians, ed 4, Mosby, 2011, p. 266.

431. b Reperfusion injury occurs when oxygen delivery is restored to tissue after a period of ischemia (lack of oxygen). This period of ischemia causes damage and when blood flow returns, it brings inflammatory factors and free radicals that do further damage. Lidocaine has been shown to act as a free radical scavenger and is used in reperfusion injury to prevent or decrease damage. Bassert JM, Thomas JA, McCurnin's Clinical Textbook for Veterinary Technicians, ed 8, Elsevier, 2014, p. 927.

432. b Glucosamine/Chondroitin are often combined as a supplement and are used to treat arthritis. They work together to increase cartilage production and inhibit cartilage breakdown. They do not have any effect on anemia, pruritus, or urinary incontinence. Wanamaker BP, Massey KL, Applied Pharmacology for Veterinary Technicians, ed 5, Elsevier, 2015, p. 927.

433. c Metronidazole has been shown to have anti-inflammatory properties in the gastrointestinal tract and is sometimes used as the sole treatment for inflammatory bowel disease. Ciprofloxacin, enrofloxacin, and tetracycline are not known to have these properties. Silverstein D, Hopper K, Small Animal Critical Care Medicine, ed 1, Saunders, 2009, p. 578; Bonagura JD, Twedt DC, Kirk's Current Veterinary Therapy XV, Elsevier, 2014, p. 521.

434. b Famotidine is an H2 receptor agonist that should be administered up to 1 hour after sucralfate to prevent changing the acidic environment of the stomach, which would inhibit or decrease the binding of sucralfate to ulcers. The other medications listed should not change the acidity of the stomach. Cisapride is a prokinetic, Lactulose is used for constipation, and metoclopramide is an antiemetic. Wanamaker BP, Massey KL, Applied Pharmacology for Veterinary Technicians, ed 5, Elsevier, 2015, p. 159.

435. c The toxic dose of lidocaine is 6–8 mg and you should take care not to exceed this amount. Neurological or cardiac signs of toxicity include seizures, coma, and cardiovascular collapse. Bassert JM, Thomas JA, McCurnin's Clinical Textbook for Veterinary Technicians, ed 8, Elsevier, 2014, p. 1280.

436. c Controlled drugs that are scheduled as C-II require a written prescription and cannot be called in by phone. Of the medications listed, morphine is the only C-II drug included. Buprenorphine is scheduled as C-III and phenobarbital and diazepam are scheduled as C-IV. Sirois M, Principles and Practice of Veterinary Technology, ed 4, Elsevier, 2016, p. 249.

437. b Vetmedin is the brand name for pimobendan. This is a veterinary drug and will not be available at a human pharmacy unless the pharmacy has veterinary drugs available. Atenolol's brand name is Tenormin, procainamide has several brand names including Pronestyl, and quinidine also has several brand names including Cin-Quin and Cardioquin. Wanamaker BP, Massey KL, Applied Pharmacology for Veterinary Technicians, ed 5, Elsevier, 2015, p. 159.

438. d Lidocaine can be diluted with sodium bicarbonate at a ratio of 9 parts lidocaine to 1 part sodium bicarbonate, which will change the acidity of the lidocaine and decrease the burning associated with injection. Silverstein D, Hopper K, Small Animal Critical Care Medicine, ed 1, Saunders, 2009, p. 710.

439. d Morphine has a longer onset of action (90 minutes) but will last longest with a duration of action up to 24 hours. Bupivacaine lasts up to 6 hours, butorphanol lasts up to 3 hours, and ketamine lasts only 1.5 hours. Boothe DM, Small Animal Clinical Pharmacology and Therapeutics, ed 2, Elsevier, 2012, p. 1013.

440. a Alpha-tocopherol is the most active form of vitamin E. Vitamin D2 is ergocalciferol, vitamin D3 is cholecalciferol, and vitamin B2 is riboflavin. Bassert JM, Thomas JA, McCurnin's Clinical Textbook for Veterinary Technicians, ed 9, Elsevier, 2016, p. 301.

441. c DMSO can cause histamine release from mast cells in the skin causing inflammation in the skin. This reaction can be much worse in a patient with mast cell tumors and it should therefore be avoided in these patients. Hemangiosarcoma, lymphoma, and osteosarcoma are not associated with mast cells and this reaction does not occur. Bill RL, Clinical Pharmacology and Therapeutics for the Veterinary Technician, ed 4, Mosby, 2016, p. 309-310.

442. d A toxoid is a vaccine that produces an immunity to a toxin. Some examples include the tetanus toxoid. The other vaccine types listed are not effective against toxins. Wanamaker BP, Massey KL, Applied Pharmacology for Veterinary Technicians, ed 5, Elsevier, 2015, p. 376.

443. c An ointment is considered a semisolid. An implant is a solid form, whereas syrup and injectable are both considered liquid forms. Sirois M, Principles and Practice of Veterinary Technology, ed 4, Elsevier, 2016, p. 246.

444. a Because cardiac disease affects blood flow to the gastrointestinal tract (absorption), tissues (distribution), liver (metabolism), and kidneys (elimination), it can greatly affect the patient's reaction to the drug. Cardiac disease must be taken into consideration when choosing drugs and their doses. Kidney disease will only affect elimination and liver disease will only affect metabolism. Bassert JM, Thomas JA, McCurnin's Clinical Textbook for Veterinary Technicians, ed 9, Elsevier, 2016, p. 958.

445. b Idiosyncratic drug reactions are unpredictable. They do not affect many patients and are not dose dependent. Dose-dependent drug reactions are predictable and affect multiple patients. Idiosyncratic drug reactions are not affected by other reactions. Bassert JM, Thomas JA, McCurnin's Clinical Textbook for Veterinary Technicians, ed 9, Elsevier, 2016, p. 958.

446. c Room temperature includes a range of 60°–68° Fahrenheit. Anything less than 46°F is considered cold, temperatures ranging from 46°–59°F are considered cool, and anything from 87°–104°F is considered warm. It is important to ensure that medications are stored at the correct temperature. Sirois M, Elsevier's Veterinary Assisting Textbook, ed 1, Elsevier, 2013, p. 119.

447. c Insulin is sensitive and shaking the vial can cause the proteins to break down making it inactive. Clavamox, amoxicillin, and metronidazole should all be shaken to make sure any drug that has settled at the bottom of the bottle is resuspended. Sirois M, Principles and Practice of Veterinary Technology, ed 4, Elsevier, 2016, p. 248.

448. b Glycopyrrolate and atropine are both anticholinergics; however, glycopyrrolate is more predictable in rabbits. Acepromazine is a phenothiazine, whereas Diazepam is a benzodiazepine; both produce excellent sedation, not the effects of an anticholinergic. Thomas J, Lerche P, Anesthesia and Analgesia for Veterinary Technicians, ed 4, Mosby, 2011.

449. d Both diazepam and midazolam have marked sedative effects in rodents and rabbits, unlike their effects in dogs and cats. They can be administered by intraperitoneal, intramuscular, or intravenous injection and are often used in combination with other agents to produce balanced anesthesia. Thomas J, Lerche P, Anesthesia and Analgesia for Veterinary Technicians, ed 4, Mosby, 2011.

450. c Xylazine, medetomidine, and dexmedetomidine can be used to produce sedation with some analgesia in small mammals. A major advantage of these sedatives is that their action can be reversed by administration of specific antagonists. Both yohimbine and atipamezole have been used for this purpose in small mammals. Thomas J, Lerche P, Anesthesia and Analgesia for Veterinary Technicians, ed 4, Mosby, 2011.

451. b Atipamezole is preferable over yohimbine, because it has fewer side effects. It can be given through the subcutaneous, intraperitoneal, intramuscular, and intravenous routes. Absorption after subcutaneous injection is rapid; the drug generally acts within 5–10 minutes. Dose rates of 0.5–1.0 mg/kg are required, depending on the dose of medetomidine that has been administered. Thomas J, Lerche P, Anesthesia and Analgesia for Veterinary Technicians, ed 4, Mosby, 2011.

452. c Anticholinergic agents are used to decrease effects of parasympathetic nervous system (PNS) stimulation such as bradycardia and excessive salivation. Thomas J, Lerche P, Anesthesia and Analgesia for Veterinary Technicians, ed 4, Mosby, 2011.

SECTION 6

1. b Successful surgery depends on careful attention to the rules of asepsis. An item should be considered nonsterile if there is any uncertainty or if it is lying in the outer area of the sterile zone. Never rely on fellow team members as to whether an item is contaminated or not. Personnel who are not scrubbed in should never reach over the draped, sterile area. Tear M, Small Animal Surgical Nursing, ed 2, Elsevier, 2012, p. 102.

2. d Kelly forceps are hemostatic forceps that are used to occlude small to medium-sized vessels. Needle holders are used to hold a surgical needle, whereas the function of a towel clamp is to clamp sterile surgical towels to the patient. There are various types of surgical scissors that are used to obtain delicate tissue, cut suture, or perform other surgical tasks. Sonsthagen TF, Veterinary Instruments and Equipment: a Pocket Guide, ed 2, Elsevier, 2011, p. 441.
3. b -plasty is the suffix used to describe a surgical alteration of a shape. -pexy is the suffix used to describe a surgical fixation. -rrhapy is surgical repair by suturing. -ostomy is the surgical creation of an artificial opening. Sirois M, Principles and Practice of Veterinary Technology, ed 3, Mosby, 2011, p. 379.
4. a Steam sterilization in an autoclave is used most often for instruments and equipment that would not be damaged by moisture or heat. A typical surgical pack would be autoclaved, whereas forceps used to probe an abscess may be disinfected with a liquid chemical. Dry heat is not typically used in veterinary applications. Ethylene oxide would be used to sterilize plastics or any other surgical device that would be damaged by any other method. Bassert JM, Thomas JA, McCurnin's Clinical Textbook for Veterinary Technicians, ed 8, Elsevier, 2014, p. 1163.
5. d To destroy all living microorganisms, the correct relationship between temperature, pressure, and time must be achieved. The minimum temperature and exposure time for the steam of an autoclave to provide sterility is 250°F or 121°C for 13 minutes at 15 psi. Sirois M, Principles and Practice of Veterinary Technology, ed 3, Mosby, 2011, p. 385.
6. d The white lead is attached to the right foreleg, the red lead is attached to the left rear, the green lead is attached to the right rear, and the black lead is attached to the left front. "Green and white is always right; newspaper (white and black) comes in the morning (front); Christmas comes at the end of the year (back legs)." Sirois M, Principles and Practice of Veterinary Technology, ed 3, Mosby, 2011, p. 609.
7. c Scrubbing the surgical site reduces, but does not completely eliminate (or sterilize), normal microbial flora on the patient's skin. Reducing the contaminants on the skin can greatly reduce the risk of wound infection, postoperatively. It is not advised to provide antibiotics prophylactically before surgery, even when the patient's skin has been prepped for surgery. Tear M, Small Animal Surgical Nursing, ed 2, Elsevier, 2012, p. 70.
8. a The mask is donned before scrubbing and gowning and is therefore not considered sterile. The drape, instrument, and gloves must be sterile. Fossum TW, Small Animal Surgery, ed 3, Mosby, 2007, p. 38.
9. a A surgical scrub involves the mechanical removal of dirt, oil, and bacteria, and it inactivates any remaining bacteria by coming into contact with the antimicrobial solution. Different antimicrobial solutions have different requirements for contact time, but all have a required contact time for effectiveness. The amount of soap used is insignificant and scrubbing alone decreases efficacy. The temperature of the water has no bearing on the effectiveness of the scrub. Sirois M, Principles and Practice of Veterinary Technology, ed 3, Mosby, 2011, p. 394.
10. c First-intention wound healing occurs with no infection or suppuration (pus formation). First-intention wound healing occurs with skin edges held together and with minimal scar formation. Table 13-1, Sirois M, Principles and Practice of Veterinary Technology, ed 3, Mosby, 2011.
11. d The cautery unit is not sterilized; only the handle and adapter ends are sterilized. The nonsterile technician adjusts the settings on the unit. Bassert JM, Thomas JA, McCurnin's Clinical Textbook for Veterinary Technicians, ed 8, Elsevier, 2014, p. 1131.
12. a A No. 10 blade is commonly used for incisions. A No. 11 blade has a sharp point for making a small incision, just large enough for an arthroscope or cannula to enter the joint. The No. 12 blade resembles a hook, with the cutting edge on the inside curve, and it is frequently used to declaw a cat. A No. 15 blade has the appearance of a No. 10 blade, but with only half the No. 10's length. The larger scalpel blades (Nos. 20 to 29) are generally reserved for use in large animal surgery. Tear M, Small Animal Surgical Nursing, ed 2, Elsevier, 2012, p. 22.
13. d The packs of suture material should not be opened until they are needed and the nonsterile circulating nurse opens them. The remaining options are all steps that require sterility and are the jobs of the sterile surgical assistant. Tear M, Small Animal Surgical Nursing, ed 2, Elsevier, 2012, p. 131-127; Bassert JM, Thomas JA, McCurnin's Clinical Textbook for Veterinary Technicians, ed 8, Elsevier, 2014, p. 1188, 1193.
14. a Females do not have prostate glands. Prevention of pyometra, estrus, and sterilization are all reasons to perform an ovariohysterectomy. Tear M, Small Animal Surgical Nursing, ed 2, Elsevier, 2012, p. 149.
15. a A good rule of thumb is to schedule surgeries from cleanest to dirtiest. The cruciate would require the cleanest environment, followed by an OHE, compound fracture repair, and intestinal resection. Tear M, Small Animal Surgical Nursing, ed 2, Elsevier, 2012, p. 37.
16. b Not all bandages need to be removed 24 hours post application. A bandage should be checked three or four times daily for signs of swelling, slippage, moisture, or soiling. If any of these scenarios occurs, the bandage should be changed. Tear M, Small Animal Surgical Nursing, ed 2, Elsevier, 2012, p. 178.
17. a The hair coat of a puppy is always different from that of the adult; however, the quality of the coat will change no matter what the reproductive status of the dog. Shedding is always an issue. The remaining options are all true. Tear M, Small Animal Surgical Nursing, ed 2, Elsevier, 2012.
18. b Ovaries and the uterus will be removed from any patient experiencing a pyometra. In addition, the uterus could rupture before surgery, which enhances the risk associated with anesthesia. Bassert JM, Thomas JA, McCurnin's Clinical Textbook for Veterinary Technicians, ed 8, Elsevier, 2014, p. 1236.
19. a When the newborns are removed from the uterus, the circulation pattern in the body of the mother undergoes a drastic change, and she runs the risk of going into shock. The anesthesia-monitoring technician should be particularly vigilant during this time. A hysterotomy is also known as a cesarean section and a majority of the time bulldogs will need to have a cesarean scheduled to deliver the puppies. Always wait to place newborns

on the mother until she has recovered from anesthesia, preventing injury to the newborns. Tear M, Small Animal Surgical Nursing, ed 2, Elsevier, 2012, p. 153.

20. c The client should observe the surgical incision daily. The newborns can contribute to surgical-site problems by sucking on suture ends and kneading at the incision. Thus, it is important that the incision is monitored. Bloody vaginal discharge is common in postoperative cesarean section patients. Newborns must be immediately removed from the membranous sac or they could suffocate. Newborns are under the effect of anesthesia because the drugs generally cross the placenta barrier before the newborns are removed from the uterus. Tear M, Small Animal Surgical Nursing, ed 2, Elsevier, 2012, p. 156.

21. c A male dog does not experience a heat cycle. Technicians should always ensure that the patient is male, has two testicles that have descended into the scrotum, and that the phone number is verified to reach the client in case of emergency. Tear M, Small Animal Surgical Nursing, ed 2, Elsevier, 2012.

22. d Enteral nutrition is administered through a feeding tube, not an IV catheter. Having a catheter in place before surgical anesthesia is administered provides excellent benefits to the patient, including the provision of fluids, anesthesia, and emergency drugs if necessary. Tear M, Small Animal Surgical Nursing, ed 2, Elsevier, 2012.

23. d Aspirin is not given for preemptive analgesia before a surgery because of its effect on platelet function, which may diminish blood clotting during the procedure. Also, preemptive analgesics are generally given by injection before surgery and aspirin comes in an oral form only. Technicians should always ensure that the patient is female and should verify the phone number of the client in case of emergency. In addition, older female patients should be checked for an abdominal scar, which may indicate the pet is already spayed. Tear M, Small Animal Surgical Nursing, ed 2, Elsevier, 2012, p. 50.

24. b Follicular damage does not occur because of clipper burn. Irritation caused by clipper burn can lead to licking, adverse wound healing, and increased bacterial growth. Tear M, Small Animal Surgical Nursing, ed 2, Elsevier, 2012, p. 75.

25. c Canine castrations are usually performed through a prescrotal incision, as long as both testicles are descended. Occasionally, cryptorchid castration patients may have multiple incision areas, especially when the testicle has to be retrieved from the abdomen. Fossum TW, Small Animal Surgery, ed 3, Mosby, 2007, p. 714; Tear M, Small Animal Surgical Nursing, ed 2, Elsevier, 2012, p. 157.

26. c -ostomy is the surgical creation of an artificial opening. -ectomy is to remove. -otomy is to cut into. -rrhapy is surgical repair by suturing. Sirois M, Principles and Practice of Veterinary Technology, ed 3, Mosby, 2011, p. 379.

27. b Feline castrations are usually performed through a scrotal incision, as long as both testicles are descended. Occasionally, cryptorchid castration patients may have multiple incision areas, especially when the testicle has to be retrieved from the abdomen. Fossum TW, Small Animal Surgery, ed 3, Mosby, 2007, p. 715; Tear M, Small Animal Surgical Nursing, ed 2, Elsevier, 2012, p. 159.

28. d The ventral midline abdominal incision opens the abdomen at a location where the ovaries and the uterus can be removed through one incision. The remaining options may be used for male patients when retrieving testicles. Fossum TW, Small Animal Surgery, ed 3, Mosby, 2007, p. 710.

29. d The Brown-Adson is a tissue forceps used to pick up, hold, and maneuver delicate tissues. A retractor is used to retract tissue, a rongeur is used to trim bone, and a periosteal elevator is used to remove teeth. Sonsthagen TF, Veterinary Instruments and Equipment: a Pocket Guide, ed 2, Elsevier, 2011, p. 455.

30. c Technicians should clip against the grain of the hair with electrical clippers using a No. 40 blade. Plucking and scissoring will take too long. No. 10 blades have fewer teeth than No. 40 blades and thus do not cut as closely. Tighe MM, Brown M, Mosby's Comprehensive Review for Veterinary Technicians, ed 3, Mosby, 2008, p. 408.

31. d The patient will be in significant pain after the surgery, as with all surgeries. The animal may have difficulty eating and drinking, therefore necessitating the placement of a feeding tube. Fossum TW, Small Animal Surgery, ed 3, Mosby, 2007, p. 109.

32. b Immediately after feeding the patient with a gruel type of meal, the tube should be slowly flushed with water. The technician should never rapidly inject food or fluids because this could induce immediate vomiting. In addition, the tube should never be flushed with air. Patients should gradually be introduced to larger volumes of food after the initial placement; never administer the total caloric amount on the first postoperative day. Tear M, Small Animal Surgical Nursing, ed 2, Elsevier, 2012, p. 248.

33. c Physical therapy techniques enhance patient comfort, prevent complications from disuse, hasten healing, and decrease edema. Tear M, Small Animal Surgical Nursing, ed 2, Elsevier, 2012, p. 248.

34. d Feeding tubes are not placed through the mouth. The patient would chew through a tube placed through the mouth, rendering it useless. Nasogastric, pharyngostomy, and gastrostomy tubes all bypass the mouth. Bassert JM, Thomas JA, McCurnin's Clinical Textbook for Veterinary Technicians, ed 8, Elsevier, 2014, p. 330-331.

35. a Although having the patient fast before surgery is ideal, there are many instances where the surgery is performed on an emergency basis, such as an acute abdomen. An acute abdomen has sudden onset of clinical signs associated with the abdomen (trauma, abdominal masses) and in some cases can be life-threatening. The GI tract is not sterile; therefore, all precautions must be taken to keep GI contents out of the peritoneal cavity, including irrigation with sterile isotonic solution. Tear M, Small Animal Surgical Nursing, ed 2, Elsevier, 2012, p. 133.

36. c Appropriate analgesic therapy is necessary for patient comfort; however, it will not prevent decubital ulcers. Repositioning the patient, adequate padding, and massage will all reduce pressure and/or increase circulation to the pressure points, decreasing the likelihood of decubital ulcer formation. Sirois M,

Principles and Practice of Veterinary Technology, ed 3, Mosby, 2011, p. 638-639.

37. a Brachycephalic breeds of cats and dogs run the risk of proptosis (dislocation of the eye globe from the socket) when held too tightly around the neck. Proptosed eyes are always an emergency and are never the result of conjunctivitis. Dolichocephalic breeds rarely experience proptosed globes. Morgan RV, Small Animal Practice Client Handouts, Saunders, 2011.

38. d Abscesses are drained by lancing but are left open to continue draining and are not sutured closed. Abscesses are fluid-filled and are not solid infiltrates of inflammatory cells. The formation of an abscess is a common sequela of bite wounds, especially in cats. Bassert JM, Thomas JA, McCurnin's Clinical Textbook for Veterinary Technicians, ed 8, Elsevier, 2014, p. 997.

39. c If a Penrose drain is secured to the animal using percutaneous sutures, it will not fall out. Placing an Elizabethan collar and monitoring the patient will prevent premature removal of the drain. Drained fluid may accumulate, which prevents further drainage. The owner may need to clean around the drain to keep it open. Bassert JM, Thomas JA, McCurnin's Clinical Textbook for Veterinary Technicians, ed 8, Elsevier, 2014, p. 1199; Tear M, Small Animal Surgical Nursing, ed 2, Elsevier, 2012, p. 243.

40. d Activity is allowed but is limited when the animal is wearing a cast or splint. An animal should not be allowed to chew on a splint or cast and chewing can sometimes indicate swelling or pressure points that are creating sores under the bandage material. Therefore, clients should call the hospital if they notice chewing, moisture, or swelling above or below the cast or splint. Bassert JM, Thomas JA, McCurnin's Clinical Textbook for Veterinary Technicians, ed 8, Elsevier, 2014, p. 991; Tighe MM, Brown M, Mosby's Comprehensive Review for Veterinary Technicians, ed 3, Mosby, 2008, p. 445.

41. a It is important to keep a splint or bandage clean and dry; it should therefore not be washed at any time. Clients should inspect the bandage daily for any swelling, shifting, or moisture collection. Tighe MM, Brown M, Mosby's Comprehensive Review for Veterinary Technicians, ed 3, Mosby, 2008, p. 445.

42. b Trimming the pinna is done when tumors are removed from the pinna or when ears are cropped. The pinna is not trimmed when repairing an aural hematoma. Aural hematomas must be drained and they are bandaged by wrapping the head with the ear folded back across the top of the head. Hematomas are painful and bothersome to patients; therefore, pain medication and anti-inflammatories should be administered. Fossum TW, Small Animal Surgery, ed 3, Mosby, 2007, p. 313.

43. a A Balfour abdominal retractor is commonly used to hold open the abdomen and expose the contents. A Weitlaner is often used in orthopedic surgery; a Gelpi is fairly traumatic and has limited use in soft tissue surgery. A Senn retractor is not often used in abdominal exploratory surgery. Tear M, Small Animal Surgical Nursing, ed 2, Elsevier, 2012, p. 24.

44. c Suture material can be either braided or monofilament. Suture material is available in both absorbable and nonabsorbable forms. In addition, some suture is supplied with a needle, whereas others are not. Tear M, Small Animal Surgical Nursing, ed 2, Elsevier, 2012, p. 32-34.

45. b Instruments should be passed with the first ratchet closed, with the ring handles facing the floor, and the tips facing the ceiling, concave side up. Tear M, Small Animal Surgical Nursing, ed 2, Elsevier, 2012, p. 123.

46. c Blotting the surgical site to remove blood is preferred. Wiping may cause more bleeding and is irritating to the tissues. The technician should cut the sutures to the length that the surgeon suggests, usually ⅛–¼ inch beyond the knot. The tips of the scissors should be used to cut sutures. Scalpel blades are placed on the handle, using needle holders and not hemostats. Tear M, Small Animal Surgical Nursing, ed 2, Elsevier, 2012, p. 124.

47. a Metal clips and staples are inert and made of noncorrosive metal. Wounds closed with staples exhibit infection resistance similar to that of minimally reactive suture; however, staples often cause scarring. They must be applied with a special device and cannot be removed with scissors. Fossum TW, Small Animal Surgery, ed 3, Mosby, 2007, p. 57.

48. c Surgical instruments should be placed on surfaces, never dropped or thrown. They should be lubricated with instrument milk, not oil, and should be cleaned in water with nonabrasive cleansers. They must be dried completely to avoid rusting and should be lubricated with instrument milk after drying. Tear M, Small Animal Surgical Nursing, ed 2, Elsevier, 2012, p. 258-259.

49. c A bone plate is an example of an internal fixation device; it is a steel device that is screwed onto the bone to line up and stabilize a fracture site. Casts, splints, and K-E apparatuses are examples of external fixators. Tear M, Small Animal Surgical Nursing, ed 2, Elsevier, 2012, p. 182.

50. a Properly inflating the endotracheal tube and keeping it inflated while the patient's gag reflex is absent is the only way to guard against aspiration when the pet is under anesthesia. Overinflation of the ET cuff will damage the cells of the trachea. Underinflated ET cuffs will increase the levels of waste anesthetic gas in the surgical room and will inhibit proper anesthetic levels in patients. Box 8-4, "Complications of Endotracheal Intubation," Thomas JA, Lerche P, Anesthesia and Analgesia for Veterinary Technicians, ed 4, Mosby, 2011, p. 250.

51. d Pneumothorax is when air has been trapped in the chest cavity, between the lungs and the chest wall, and the lungs collapse because of increased pressure within the chest cavity. A chest tube can help evacuate the air and allow the lungs to expand. Pulmonary edema is fluid within the lungs (chest tubes are never placed within lungs). Ascites is fluid within the abdominal cavity. Subcutaneous emphysema is air trapped under the skin and a chest tube does not treat emphysema. Fossum TW, Small Animal Surgery, ed 3, Mosby, 2007, p. 899.

52. a The English bulldog has an elongated soft palate. If the endotracheal tube is pulled before the dog is awake, the soft palate may act as a respiratory obstruction. It is wise to keep the endotracheal tube in as long as possible in most brachycephalic breeds. Breeds with normal soft palates have less risk. Thomas JA, Lerche P, Anesthesia and Analgesia for Veterinary Technicians, ed 4, Mosby, 2011, p. 326.

53. c Dystocia is defined as difficult birth. Dyspnea is difficulty breathing, whereas dysuria is difficult urination. Bassert JM, Thomas JA, McCurnin's Clinical Textbook for Veterinary Technicians, ed 8, Elsevier, 2014, p. 379.
54. d Enucleation is removal of the eye. Otoplasty, bulla osteotomy, and aural hematomas are all procedures related to the ear. Fossum TW, Small Animal Surgery, ed 3, Mosby, 2007, p. 260.
55. c Onychectomy is defined as "declawing or removal of the entire nail." Entropion repair, keratectomy, and enucleation are all procedures that involve the eye. Fossum TW, Small Animal Surgery, ed 3, Mosby, 2007, p. 251.
56. a A cystotomy is a surgical procedure to open the urinary bladder. The entire abdomen should be clipped from the xyphoid to the pubis. The head and spine do not have any significance related to a cystotomy. Tear M, Small Animal Surgical Nursing, ed 2, Elsevier, 2012, p. 161.
57. c An ovariohysterectomy is the removal of the uterus and ovaries. This is usually performed through a midabdominal incision. The paw, chest wall, and ear do not have any significance in regard to an ovariohysterectomy. Tighe MM, Brown M, Mosby's Comprehensive Review for Veterinary Technicians, ed 3, Mosby, 2008, p. 408.
58. b A femoral head ostectomy is the removal of the proximal end of the femur, which is located in the hip. The head, shoulder, and spine are insignificant. Fossum TW, Small Animal Surgery, ed 3, Mosby, 2007, p. 1114.
59. b An orchidectomy is the removal of the testicles. The surgical site should be clipped from the tip of the prepuce to just above the scrotum. The abdomen would not be prepared unless the testicles have not descended to the scrotal sac. The paw and ear are insignificant. Tear M, Small Animal Surgical Nursing, ed 2, Elsevier, 2012, p. 157.
60. a The popliteal lymph nodes are located behind the knee; therefore, the stifle area would be prepped. Fossum TW, Small Animal Surgery, ed 3, Mosby, 2007, p. 617.
61. b An onychectomy is a declaw procedure. An orchidectomy is also known as castration or the removal of testicles. An ovariohysterectomy is the removal of the ovaries and uterus from female patients. An onychotomy is the incision into a toenail. Bassert JM, Thomas JA, McCurnin's Clinical Textbook for Veterinary Technicians, ed 8, Elsevier, 2014, p. 1225.
62. d The epididymis is not part of the spermatic cord. The pampiniform plexus, vas deferens, and testicular artery are all part of the spermatic cord, which connects the testicle to the body. Colville T, Bassert JM, Clinical Anatomy and Physiology for Veterinary Technicians, ed 2, Mosby, 2008, p. 393-395.
63. a The broad ligament is separated from the uterine horn in advance of the removal of the ovaries, uterine horn, and oviduct. Fossum TW, Small Animal Surgery, ed 3, Mosby, 2007, p. 713.
64. c Enucleation is indicated after severe ocular trauma or proptosis of the eye. A third eyelid can prolapse, but it is surgically repaired, not removed. A penile prolapse relates to the penis (not the eye) and an aural hematoma involves the ear. Fossum TW, Small Animal Surgery, ed 3, Mosby, 2007, p. 267.
65. a Olsen-Hegar devices are needle holders with scissors set behind the jaws. The Mayo-Hager is only a needle driver. Brown-Adson forceps are tissue holders and Rochester-Pean are hemostatic forceps. Sonsthagen TF, Veterinary Instruments and Equipment: a Pocket Guide, ed 2, Elsevier, 2011, p. 493.
66. a Rochester-Carmalt has both horizontal and vertical serrations, making it effective in clamping large vessels or large tissue masses, whereas the Crile forceps can be used to clamp small and medium vessels. Brown-Adson and Ochsner forceps hold tissue. Sonsthagen TF, Veterinary Instruments and Equipment: a Pocket Guide, ed 2, Elsevier, 2011, p. 443.
67. a Ethylene oxide is thought to be a human carcinogen. Bassert JM, Thomas JA, McCurnin's Clinical Textbook for Veterinary Technicians, ed 8, Elsevier, 2014, p. 122.
68. b Prolene is classified as a nonabsorbable suture. Polydioxanone, catgut, and Vicryl are all considered absorbable suture material. Bassert JM, Thomas JA, McCurnin's Clinical Textbook for Veterinary Technicians, ed 8, Elsevier, 2014, p. 1202-1203.
69. a Scrotal hematomas are common complications associated with canine castrations and they may result from a hemorrhaging vessel. Ascites is accumulation of fluid in the peritoneal cavity. Both hemangiomas and lipomas are types of tumors and are not related to orchidectomies. Tear M, Small Animal Surgical Nursing, ed 2, Elsevier, 2012, p. 158.
70. d Rat-tooth forceps are designed to grasp skin and other dense tissue. Surgical scissors do not hold tissue. Dressing forceps have no teeth; therefore, they cannot grasp tissue. Sponge forceps are designed to hold gauze sponges. Sonsthagen TF, Veterinary Instruments and Equipment: a Pocket Guide, ed 2, Elsevier, 2011, p. 451.
71. d The skin layer is closed with a continuous Ford interlocking pattern. It is wise to close the ventral aspect of the skin incision with two or three simple interrupted sutures. If incisional infection is obvious, drainage can be easily obtained by removing these ventral two or three sutures if necessary. Fubini S, Ducharme M, Farm Animal Surgery, Saunders, 2004, p. 191.
72. d The incision is closed in multiple layers starting with the peritoneum and then closing each muscle layer individually with a heavy absorbable suture material such a size 3 polydioxanone. Rocket J, Bosted S, Veterinary Clinical Procedures in Large Animal Practice, 2nd ed, Cengage Learning 2017, p. 298-299.
73. c Pyometras generally occur soon after a heat cycle and may be classified as open or closed. An open pyometra has purulent discharge, whereas a closed pyometra has no purulent discharge. PU/PD is not a clinical sign associated with pyometras. Onychectomies are a declaw procedure and are therefore insignificant. Tear M, Small Animal Surgical Nursing, ed 2, Elsevier, 2012, p. 155.
74. d Enucleation is indicated after severe ocular trauma, such as a proptosed eye. Orchidectomy (neuter), ovariohysterectomy (spay), and onychectomy (declaw) are all elective procedures. Fossum TW, Small Animal Surgery, ed 3, Mosby, 2007, p. 267.
75. b Nephr- is a prefix that indicates kidney; -ectomy is a suffix that indicates removal. -otomy is a suffix that

indicates incision. Appendix C, "Medical Terminology, Tighe MM, Brown M, Mosby's Comprehensive Review for Veterinary Technicians, ed 3, Mosby, 2008, p. 569-570.

76. d Clipping should take place after the animal is under anesthesia. The patient should be clipped in the position it will be in during surgery. Shaving before anesthesia does not save time, induces stress on the patient, and will probably result in patient injuries from the clippers. Tear M, Small Animal Surgical Nursing, ed 2, Elsevier, 2012, p. 67.

77. a Reduction of a fracture refers to bringing the opposing ends of the fracture back into alignment. Placing pins through the marrow cavity will help stabilize the fracture after it has been reduced, aiding in healing the injury. Tear M, Small Animal Surgical Nursing, ed 2, Elsevier, 2012, p. 182.

78. a -ectomy is to remove. -otomy is to cut into. -ostomy is the surgical creation of an artificial opening. -rrhapy is surgical repair by suturing. Sirois M, Principles and Practice of Veterinary Technology, ed 3, Mosby, 2011, p. 379.

79. b Caslick surgery is performed to prevent fecal contamination of the vagina and uterus. The guttural pouches are paired diverticulae of the eustachian tubes that communicate with the pharynx via slit-like openings and they are not cleaned out. Navicular disease is related to confirmation and lameness, not the uterus. Holtgrew-Bohling K, Large Animal Clinical Procedures for Veterinary Technicians, ed 2, Elsevier, 2012, p. 291.

80. c Isopropyl alcohol is the only compound listed that is used as both a disinfectant and an antiseptic. Quaternary ammonium, Roccal-D, mercurial chloride, bleach, and formaldehyde are all disinfectants. Bassert JM, Thomas JA, McCurnin's Clinical Textbook for Veterinary Technicians, ed 8, Elsevier, 2014, p. 1166-1169.

81. d Stay sutures are placed in hollow organs to allow the organ to be manipulated with minimal handling. It would be unnecessary to place them for a hepatic biopsy. During a cystotomy, stay sutures are placed to hold the bladder up and open while removing bladder stones. Stay sutures are placed in the gastrointestinal tract while manipulating the intestines. Bassert JM, Thomas JA, McCurnin's Clinical Textbook for Veterinary Technicians, ed 8, Elsevier, 2014, p. 1198.

82. d All knots should have a minimum or 4 throws (or 2 knots). Any fewer would put the knot at risk of untying. Sirois M, Principles and Practice of Veterinary Technology, ed 3, Mosby, 2011, p. 319.

83. b Hand ties are used in confined or hard-to-reach areas; however, they do waste suture material because the ends must be left longer than for an instrument tie. For all remaining options, instrument ties are advised. Fossum TW, Small Animal Surgery, ed 3, Mosby, 2007, p. 70.

84. a The chemical or mechanical destruction of pathogens is known as disinfection, whereas the cleaning and disinfecting or sterilization process is known as decontamination. A barrier is a material used to reduce or to inhibit the migration of microorganisms and aseptic technique is a method to prevent contamination by microorganisms. Fossum TW, Small Animal Surgery, ed 3, Mosby, 2007, p. 711-712.

85. d Monofilament material passes through tissue with less drag because it is not a braided material. Greater knot security and greater suture strength are advantages of multifilament suture material, which is braided. Suture reaction is a result of the suture material rather than any differences between monofilament and multifilament material. Tear M, Small Animal Surgical Nursing, ed 2, Elsevier, 2012, p. 34-35.

86. a Mayo-Hegar is a needle holder without scissors. There are various types of surgical scissors that are used to obtain delicate tissue, to cut suture, or to perform other surgical tasks. The function of a towel clamp is to clamp sterile surgical towels to the patient. Hemostatic forceps are used to grasp blood vessels or to clamp and hold tissue or vessels. Sonsthagen TF, Veterinary Instruments and Equipment: a Pocket Guide, ed 2, Elsevier, 2011, p. 491.

87. c The greater the number of zeros, the smaller the diameter. As the suture decreases in diameter, tensile strength also decreases. For ophthalmic surgeries, sutures should be small in diameter but should still have strength; therefore, 6-0 would be most appropriate. Size 0 may be used to ligate uterine vessels, whereas 3-0 might be used to suture skin. Bassert JM, Thomas JA, McCurnin's Clinical Textbook for Veterinary Technicians, ed 8, Elsevier, 2014, p. 1201.

88. c Drains implanted in a wound provide an escape path for unwanted air and/or wound fluids, thus preventing or reducing seroma or hematoma formation in tissue pockets or dead space. Accumulation of exudate in a wound favors infection. Excessive fluid prevents phagocytic cells from reaching bacteria within a wound and provides a medium for bacterial growth. Drains are needed when wounds produce fluids and exudates for several days after initial treatment. Sirois M, Principles and Practice of Veterinary Technology, ed 3, Mosby, 2011, p. 316.

89. a Polydioxanone is a synthetic, absorbable suture. Prolene is synthetic but nonabsorbable. Silk and cotton are natural but nonabsorbable. Sirois M, Principles and Practice of Veterinary Technology, ed 3, Mosby, 2011.

90. a Although tissue will heal faster in a younger animal, the material will still absorb at a predictable rate. Presence of infection will increase the rate of absorption of most materials. Sutures placed in areas such as the pancreas will be absorbed more quickly than those placed in the fascia. Finally, natural materials, such as catgut, are absorbed more rapidly than synthetic materials, such as polyglactin. Bassert JM, Thomas JA, McCurnin's Clinical Textbook for Veterinary Technicians, ed 8, Elsevier, 2014, p. 1201-1202.

91. a The cruciate surgery is the cleanest, least contaminated surgery of the options listed. Dental and gastrointestinal surgeries involve large amounts of bacteria and they should always be scheduled at the end of the surgery lineup. Tear M, Small Animal Surgical Nursing, ed 2, Elsevier, 2012, p. 37; Bassert JM, Thomas JA, McCurnin's Clinical Textbook for Veterinary Technicians, ed 8, Elsevier, 2014, p. 1160.

92. c Crile forceps are too traumatic to the edges of the incision and are used to occlude vessels. Rat-tooth, Brown-Adson, and Allis tissue forceps can be used to hold the edges of skin. Sonsthagen TF, Veterinary Instruments and Equipment: a Pocket Guide, ed 2, Elsevier, 2011, p. 439.

93. d Lembert is a type of rongeur, an orthopedic instrument; it is also known as the Ruskin rongeur. Mayo, Metzenbaum, and iris instruments are all scissors. Sonsthagen TF, Veterinary Instruments and Equipment: a Pocket Guide, ed 2, Elsevier, 2011, p. 581.

94. a Sponge counts should be performed before any are used and again before the surgical site is closed. Tear M, Small Animal Surgical Nursing, ed 2, Elsevier, 2012, p. 125.

95. a A sterile technique is a method, whereas a sterile field is an area around the site of incision. Sterility would be free of living organisms and terminal sterilization is a procedure performed to destroy pathogens in the OR, after the patient has been removed. Fossum TW, Small Animal Surgery, ed 3, Mosby, 2007, p. 2.

96. a The respiratory rate increases with internal bleeding. Pale mucous membranes and slow capillary refill times are signs associated with internal bleeding. Slow recovery from anesthesia can be caused by poor perfusion or shock associated with internal hemorrhage. Tear M, Small Animal Surgical Nursing, ed 2, Elsevier, 2012, p. 233-234; Thomas JA, Lerche P, Anesthesia and Analgesia for Veterinary Technicians, ed 4, Mosby, 2011, p. 175.

97. d Other vital signs and reflexes must be assessed. Different anesthetic agents can affect eye position and pupil size. Tear M, Small Animal Surgical Nursing, ed 2, Elsevier, 2012, p. 114.

98. c Increased PaO_2 indicates that the hemoglobin is saturated. This would trigger the respiratory center to decrease respiratory rate. Increased blood CO_2 triggers increased respirations. If anesthesia is too light, the patient will begin waking, resulting in an increased RR. When a patient experiences hyperthermia, its temperature is increasing. Companion animals use panting as a cooling method. Therefore, hyperthermia will increase the RR. Colville T, Bassert JM, Clinical Anatomy and Physiology for Veterinary Technicians, ed 2, Mosby, 2008, p. 261-263.

99. a Debridement is the removal of tissue. Smooth edges are needed when suturing tissue together. Curettage is the cleansing of a diseased surface with a curette. Cauterization is the destruction of tissue with a cautery. Decoupage does not exist. Sirois M, Principles and Practice of Veterinary Technology, ed 3, Mosby, 2011, p. 315.

100. c The depth of the wound is not a factor in the formation of proud flesh or exuberant granulation tissue. Infection, missing tissue, and the location of the wound may increase the likelihood of the formation of exuberant granulation tissue. Sirois M, Principles and Practice of Veterinary Technology, ed 3, Mosby, 2011, p. 319.

101. b Serosanguineous discharge (contains both blood and serous fluid) from the incision site is an early sign of dehiscence. Mucopurulent material is an indicator of infection. Sirois M, Principles and Practice of Veterinary Technology, ed 3, Mosby, 2011, p. 382.

102. d Extracapsular repairs involve placement of sutures outside the stifle joint. The TPLO and TTA are both intracapsular repairs. An FHO is the removal of the femoral head and is not used to repair a cruciate tear. Tear M, Small Animal Surgical Nursing, ed 3, Elsevier, 2017, p. 176.

103. c Nonscrubbed personnel should always face the surgical field and should never walk between two sterile fields. Although asepsis is not broken when passing back to back, in situations when facing the back of the surgeon, the nonsterile person can more easily watch for instances that might lead to contamination. Tear M, Small Animal Surgical Nursing, ed 2, Elsevier, 2012, p. 103.

104. a The autoclave tape is on the outside of the sterile gown pack and is removed by the nonsterile person before scrubbing occurs. All of the other items listed are located inside the outer wrap and should only be handled by scrubbed personnel. Tear M, Small Animal Surgical Nursing, ed 2, Elsevier, 2012, p. 104.

105. a Silk has the highest tissue reactivity of the suture material listed. Nylon and Prolene have low tissue reactivity. Bassert JM, Thomas JA, McCurnin's Clinical Textbook for Veterinary Technicians, ed 8, Elsevier, 2014, p. 1202-1203.

106. c The hands are kept higher than the elbows to allow the water and scrub to drip from the elbows. Above the head would yield unproductive scrubbing. Procedure 15-3, "Surgical Personnel Scrub Procedure," Sirois M, Principles and Practice of Veterinary Technology, ed 3, Mosby, 2011, p. 395.

107. b The purpose of presoaking is to prevent blood from drying on the instruments or to soften dried blood. Surgical soap will not remove bacteria nor sterilize them. Excess blood should be removed before placing instruments in the ultrasonic cleaner. Tear M, Small Animal Surgical Nursing, ed 2, Elsevier, 2012, p. 257.

108. c Everting patterns are contraindicated because the mucosa would then be exposed. Everting and inverting suture patterns retard intestinal healing and may cause greater stricture formation. Fossum TW, Small Animal Surgery, ed 3, Mosby, 2007.

109. d Surgery packs must be labeled with the contents, date made, and the initials of the individual making the pack. Bassert JM, Thomas JA, McCurnin's Clinical Textbook for Veterinary Technicians, ed 8, Elsevier, 2014, p. 1163.

110. d Rochester-Carmalt are the only forceps in this group with longitudinal striations. Sonsthagen TF, Veterinary Instruments and Equipment: a Pocket Guide, ed 2, Elsevier, 2011, p. 443.

111. c The Lembert is an orthopedic instrument. Finochietto, Gelpi, and Balfour instruments are retractors. Sonsthagen TF, Veterinary Instruments and Equipment: a Pocket Guide, ed 2, Elsevier, 2011, p. 559-567, 581.

112. b Shearing refers to an injury in which a majority of the soft tissue is lost, exposing the bone, and in some cases, the bone is sheared away or missing. Fracture healing requires apposition (realignment) of the bones, reduction (correction) of the facture, and fixation (stabilization). Tear M, Small Animal Surgical Nursing, ed 2, Elsevier, 2012, p. 182.

113. d In the dissection method of the onychectomy procedure, the nail and third (distal) phalanx are removed. Fossum TW, Small Animal Surgery, ed 3, Mosby, 2007, p. 252.

114. d Adson is a type of tissue forceps. It is used to pick up, hold, and maneuver delicate tissues. A retractor is used to retract tissue, a rongeur is used to trim bone, and a periosteal elevator is used to remove teeth. Sonsthagen TF, Veterinary Instruments and Equipment: a Pocket Guide, ed 2, Elsevier, 2011, p. 453.

115. b Anterior drawer movement is used to detect cranial cruciate ligament (CCL) damage/rupture in the stifle joint. The anterior drawer movement test is not used with elbows, stifles, or hocks. Colville T, Bassert JM, Clinical Anatomy and Physiology for Veterinary Technicians, ed 2, Mosby, 2008, p. 186.

116. a Cystotomy is a surgical incision into the bladder. Cystectomy is the removal of a cyst. Cystocentesis is the withdrawal of fluid from the bladder. A cystostomy is the removal of stones from the bladder. Glossary, Tear M, Small Animal Surgical Nursing, ed 2, Elsevier, 2012, p. 308.

117. d Ileus refers to the temporary loss of intestinal motility, but it does not require surgical intervention. GDV, intussusception, and mesenteric torsion all require surgical repair. Bassert JM, Thomas JA, McCurnin's Clinical Textbook for Veterinary Technicians, ed 8, Elsevier, 2014, p. 1229.

118. a Laminectomy is the surgical excision of the dorsal arch of a vertebra and it is often performed to relieve the symptoms caused by ruptured intervertebral disks. Studdert, VP, Gay CC, Blood DC, Saunders Comprehensive Veterinary Dictionary, ed 4, Saunders, 2012, p. 361.

119. a The tibia articulates with the femur and the proximal tibia is distal to the femur. Colville T, Bassert JM, Clinical Anatomy and Physiology for Veterinary Technicians, ed 2, Mosby, 2008, p. 183.

120. c A ventral midline incision provides the best visualization of retained testicles. Proper visualization is imperative to prevent accidental prostatectomy and/or urethral and ureteral removal. Prescrotal and scrotal incisions are used for patients in which the testicles have fully descended into the scrotal sac. Perianal incisions are not used to remove testicles. KM, Johnston SA, Veterinary Surgery: Small Animal, Elsevier, 2012, p. 1914.

121. d Although incisions are commonly performed through the sternum in humans, lateral incisions perpendicular to the spine, and between the ribs, are more common in dogs. Sirois M, Principles and Practice of Veterinary Technology, ed 3, Mosby, 2011, p. 379.

122. d The ventilation system should provide 15–20 air exchanges per hour. Fossum TW, Small Animal Surgery, ed 3, Mosby, 2007, p. 15.

123. b Quaternary ammonium compounds can destroy enveloped viruses, but they are ineffective against nonenveloped viruses. Glutaraldehyde, formalin, and isopropyl alcohol are more effective against viruses. Sirois M, Principles and Practice of Veterinary Technology, ed 3, Mosby, 2011, p. 273.

124. d Mayo-Hegar is a type of needle holder that is without any cutting ability. Sonsthagen TF, Veterinary Instruments and Equipment: a Pocket Guide, ed 2, Elsevier, 2011, p. 491.

125. a Rongeurs are used to remove bone during orthopedic procedures. A curette is used to scrape out cancellous bone from the medullary cavity so as to perform bone grafts or to scrape osteochondrosis desiccans (OCD) lesions. A periosteal elevator is used to work under and lift the periosteum or soft tissues away from the bone. A trephine is used to drill holes in the cranium. Sonsthagen TF, Veterinary Instruments and Equipment: a Pocket Guide, ed 2, Elsevier, 2011, p. 581.

126. a Pleural effusion is the accumulation of fluid in the thoracic cavity. Treatment includes oxygen supplementation and thoracocentesis. Pulmonary edema is fluid in the lungs; ascites is fluid in the abdomen and a pyothorax is defined as pus in the thoracic cavity. Bassert JM, Thomas JA, McCurnin's Clinical Textbook for Veterinary Technicians, ed 8, Elsevier, 2014, p. 684.

127. b A rumenotomy is performed via a left-flank abdominal incision in a standing cow. Bassert JM, Thomas JA, McCurnin's Clinical Textbook for Veterinary Technicians, ed 8, Elsevier, 2014, p. 1281.

128. b The only piece of information that the autoclave tape provides is that steam has reached the tape and has resulted in a color change. It is by no means an indicator that adequate sterilization conditions (temperature and pressure) have been achieved. Bassert JM, Thomas JA, McCurnin's Clinical Textbook for Veterinary Technicians, ed 8, Elsevier, 2014, p. 1164.

129. d Flash sterilization is performed on single unwrapped instruments sterilized at 272°F for 4 minutes. Tear M, Small Animal Surgical Nursing, ed 2, Elsevier, 2012, p. 264.

130. d Puppies are not usually intubated following delivery. Their nasal and oral passages are suctioned and oxygen ventilation via mask is performed. Doxapram may be placed under the tongue to stimulate respiration. Puppies can be physically stimulated to begin breathing with vigorous rubbing and a gentle swinging motion. Minimizing anesthetic drugs that affect the puppies, the position of the bitch, and suctioning fluid from the puppy's nasal cavities are top priorities. Tear M, Small Animal Surgical Nursing, ed 2, Elsevier, 2012, p. 154.

131. d Ventricular arrhythmias are not commonly associated with pyometra surgeries. However, sepsis and renal damage secondary to *Escherichia coli* toxins are a major concern. Tear M, Small Animal Surgical Nursing, ed 2, Elsevier, 2012, p. 155-156.

132. d Gastric dilatation and volvulus status can usually be confirmed visually by passing an orogastric tube or via radiography. Hemodynamic shock, sepsis, and cardiac arrhythmias are possible sequelae. Fluids should be provided in shock doses and lidocaine should be readily available to treat ventricular arrhythmias. Bassert JM, Thomas JA, McCurnin's Clinical Textbook for Veterinary Technicians, ed 8, Elsevier, 2014, p. 1232-1233.

133. a In this list, only the No. 10 fits a No. 3 scalpel handle. Sonsthagen TF, Veterinary Instruments and Equipment: a Pocket Guide, ed 2, Elsevier, 2011, p. 473.

134. d No. 4 scalpel handles use No. 20 blades. Sonsthagen TF, Veterinary Instruments and Equipment: a Pocket Guide, ed 2, Elsevier, 2011, p. 473.

135. d -rrhapy is surgical repair by suturing. -ectomy means to remove. -otomy is to cut into. -ostomy is the surgical creation of an artificial opening. Sirois M, Principles and Practice of Veterinary Technology, ed 3, Mosby, 2011, p. 379.

136. b Pathogenic means that the bacteria cause disease. Microbial bacteria produce toxins. When bacteria live off and gain nutrients from a host, it is known as parasitism. Studdert, VP, Gay CC, Blood DC, Saunders Comprehensive Veterinary Dictionary, ed 4, Saunders, 2012, p. 824.

137. c The chamber is sealed before setting the timer for the cycle. Bassert JM, Thomas JA, McCurnin's Clinical Textbook for Veterinary Technicians, ed 8, Elsevier, 2014, p. 163.

138. a Sterile implies that there are no living organisms of any type. Studdert, VP, Gay CC, Blood DC, Saunders Comprehensive Veterinary Dictionary, ed 4, Saunders, 2012, p. 1047.

139. c All nonsterile personnel entering the operating room are required to wear a cap, mask, booties, and clean scrubs. The surgeon and the assistant would also wear sterile gowns. Tear M, Small Animal Surgical Nursing, ed 2, Elsevier, 2012, p. 86-87.

140. c A double-wrapped pack can be stored in this manner for 6 to 8 weeks. A single wrapped crepe-paper pack can be stored on an open shelf for 3 weeks. A pack that was opened, but not used, cannot be considered sterile for the next day's procedures. Any pouch that has a small perforation is considered nonsterile. Table 30-6, "Safe Storage Time for Sterile Packs," Bassert JM, Thomas JA, McCurnin's Clinical Textbook for Veterinary Technicians, ed 8, Elsevier, 2014, p. 1163.

141. b Instruments with hinges or box locks should remain in the unlocked position with ratchets open, allowing steam to penetrate the entire surface. Ratchets will not tear wrap material. Surgical trays help keep packs organized, but they are not required. Instruments can touch while being autoclaved without fear of corrosion. Technician Note, Bassert JM, Thomas JA, McCurnin's Clinical Textbook for Veterinary Technicians, ed 8, Elsevier, 2014, p. 1161.

142. d The Gelpi is a self-retaining retractor and does not require a surgical assistant to hold it in place. The Gelpi retractor is available in sizes both larger and smaller than the Senn retractor and cost is relative to size. The Senn retractor does not have to be molded to fit the position required. Sonsthagen TF, Veterinary Instruments and Equipment: a Pocket Guide, ed 2, Elsevier, 2011, p. 559.

143. a -rrhapy is surgical repair by suturing. -ectomy means to remove. -otomy is to cut into. -ostomy is the surgical creation of an artificial opening. Sirois M, Principles and Practice of Veterinary Technology, ed 3, Mosby, 2011, p. 379.

144. c Aseptic technique does not create a sterile environment. That would require the removal of ALL microorganisms, including spores. Tear M, Small Animal Surgical Nursing, ed 2, Elsevier, 2012, p. 101.

145. a The strip turns dark when a temperature of 121°C has been reached. Bassert JM, Thomas JA, McCurnin's Clinical Textbook for Veterinary Technicians, ed 8, Elsevier, 2014, p. 1164.

146. d Metzenbaum scissors are fine-edged scissors that are used to cut tissue only. They are too large to use on ophthalmic surgery and cutting paper drapes or suture will dull the blades quickly. Sonsthagen TF, Veterinary Instruments and Equipment: a Pocket Guide, ed 2, Elsevier, 2011, p. 494.

147. d The only areas of the gown considered sterile are from just below the shoulders, including the sleeves, to the waist/level of the table. Bassert JM, Thomas JA, McCurnin's Clinical Textbook for Veterinary Technicians, ed 8, Elsevier, 2014, p. 1182.

148. b The larger the diameter of the suture, the greater its tensile strength. In the options provided, 1 chromic gut is the largest suture and 600 silk is the smallest. Fossum TW, Small Animal Surgery, ed 3, Mosby, 2007, p. 57.

149. c Cleaning the instruments reduces the lubrication in the box lock; therefore, it must be replaced after ultrasonic cleaning. Instrument milk does not clean or complete the sterilization process, nor will it prevent rust spots. Bassert JM, Thomas JA, McCurnin's Clinical Textbook for Veterinary Technicians, ed 8, Elsevier, 2014, p. 1158.

150. d Eyed needles can be reautoclaved and reused because they are not attached to any suture. Swaged-on needles are manufactured with suture. Taper-point needles lose the ability to move atraumatically through tissue after the surgery and should therefore not be considered reusable. Trocar needles are manufactured for single use only. Fossum TW, Small Animal Surgery, ed 3, Mosby, 2007, p. 61.

151. c All personnel in the surgical suite should face the sterile field, decreasing the risk of contamination. Tear M, Small Animal Surgical Nursing, ed 2, Elsevier, 2012, p. 103.

152. b Capillarity is the process by which fluid and bacteria are carried into the interstices of multifilament fibers. Because neutrophils and macrophages are too large to enter the interstices of the fiber, infection may persist, particularly in nonabsorbable sutures. All braided materials (e.g., polyglycolic acid, silk) have degrees of capillarity, whereas monofilament sutures are considered noncapillary. Coating reduces the capillarity of some sutures, but, regardless, capillary suture materials should not be used in contaminated or infected sites. Polypropylene is a monofilament suture. Fossum TW, Small Animal Surgery, ed 3, Mosby, 2007, p. 64.

153. a Braided suture has more friction and better knot security than the same material in a monofilament. Braided suture does not have more tensile strength, is more tissue reactive than monofilament, and also hides bacteria. Tear M, Small Animal Surgical Nursing, ed 2, Elsevier, 2012, p. 35.

154. c The white lead is attached to the right foreleg, the red lead is attached to the left rear, the green lead is attached to the right rear, and the black lead is attached to the left front. "Green and white is always right; newspaper (white and black) comes in the morning (front); Christmas comes at the end of the year (back legs)." Sirois M, Principles and Practice of Veterinary Technology, ed 3, Mosby, 2011, p. 609.

155. c The suffix -cidal means to kill. The prefix viru- indicates viruses. A sporicidal kills spores. Saunder Studdert VP, Gay CC, Blood DC, Saunders Comprehensive Veterinary Dictionary, ed 4, Saunders, 2012, p. 1178.

156. c The purpose of the surgical drape is to create a sterile field. A circulating warm water blanket or Bear Hugger would be used to keep the patient warm. A drape is not needed to keep the surgeon focused, nor does it protect the table and mayo stand from contamination. Tear M, Small Animal Surgical Nursing, ed 2, Elsevier, 2012, p. 102.

157. b The minimum temperature and exposure time to the steam of an autoclave to provide sterility is 250°F or 121°C for 13 minutes at 15 psi. Bassert JM, Thomas JA, McCurnin's Clinical Textbook for Veterinary Technicians, ed 8, Elsevier, 2014, p. 1164.

158. a Disinfectants are used on inanimate objects and antiseptics are used on living tissue. Bassert JM, Thomas JA, McCurnin's Clinical Textbook for Veterinary Technicians, ed 8, Elsevier, 2014, p. 1166.

159. b Strike through occurs when liquids soak through a drape from a sterile area to a nonsterile area and vice versa. Therefore, you should prevent drapes and the surgical gowns from becoming wet during surgery. The location of the fenestration and type of needle used has nothing to do with strike through. Tear M, Small Animal Surgical Nursing, ed 2, Elsevier, 2012, p. 102.

160. c Ethylene oxide is the most commonly used agent in gas sterilization. Glutaraldehyde is used in cold sterile trays. Chlorhexidine is a disinfectant and formaldehyde is used to preserve tissue samples. Bassert JM, Thomas JA, McCurnin's Clinical Textbook for Veterinary Technicians, ed 8, Elsevier, 2014, p. 1165.

161. a Olsen-Hegar needle holders have a cutting surface, whereas Mayo-Hager needle holders do not. Metzenbaums do not hold needles; they are used to cut tissue. Crile-Wood are forceps and are not used to hold needles. Sonsthagen TF, Veterinary Instruments and Equipment: a Pocket Guide, ed 2, Elsevier, 2011, p. 491-493.

162. d Rochester-Pean forceps are generally large with transverse longitudinal serrations along the entire length. Allen clamps have longitudinal serrations with interdigitating teeth at the tips. Rochester-Carmalt forceps have longitudinal serrations with a crosshatched pattern at the tips. Sonsthagen TF, Veterinary Instruments and Equipment: a Pocket Guide, ed 2, Elsevier, 2011.

163. a A Buhner needle is used to correct vaginal and uterine prolapses in cows. A Buhner is designed for large animals and thick tissues and is therefore too large for an eye enucleation, for intestinal anastomosis, or for orthopedic surgeries. Bassert JM, Thomas JA, McCurnin's Clinical Textbook for Veterinary Technicians, ed 8, Elsevier, 2014, p. 1290; Sonsthagen TF, Veterinary Instruments and Equipment: a Pocket Guide, ed 2, Elsevier, 2011, p. 273.

164. b A Snook hook is typically used to elevate the uterus during an ovariohysterectomy or spay. It would serve no purpose in a castration or declawing procedure and would not be used in a diaphragmatic hernia repair. Sonsthagen TF, Veterinary Instruments and Equipment: a Pocket Guide, ed 2, Elsevier, 2011, p. 476.

165. c Ovario- means ovaries; hyster- refers to uterus; -ectomy indicates to remove. Tear M, Small Animal Surgical Nursing, ed 2, Elsevier, 2012, p. 149.

166. a A patient experiencing pyometra will have purulent discharge accumulate within the uterus. This is a serious condition that might exist with a closed or an open cervix. Mastitis is inflammation of the mammary gland(s). Peritonitis is inflammation of the serosa (peritoneum) that lines the walls of the abdominal cavity and covers the abdominal organs and mesenteries. Vaginitis is inflammation of the vagina. Tear M, Small Animal Surgical Nursing, ed 2, Elsevier, 2012, p. 155.

167. c A pack double wrapped in muslin can be kept in a closed cabinet for about 6 to 7 weeks, as long as the cabinet has doors and not open shelving. Open shelving shortens the life span to roughly half. Table 30-6, "Safe Storage Times for Sterile Packs," Bassert JM, Thomas JA, McCurnin's Clinical Textbook for Veterinary Technicians, ed 8, Elsevier, 2014, p. 1163.

168. c Operating scissors, scissors on Olsen-Hegar needle holders, and Mayo scissors can be used to cut suture. Mayo-Hegar needle holders do not have scissors and Metzenbaum scissors are never used to cut suture. Tear M, Small Animal Surgical Nursing, ed 2, Elsevier, 2012, p. 19-21.

169. a IM stands for intramedullary because these pins are often placed into the medullary cavity of long bones. Sonsthagen TF, Veterinary Instruments and Equipment: a Pocket Guide, ed 2, Elsevier, 2011, p. 591.

170. c Normal wound healing causes inflammation, which causes minor increases in skin temperature and erythema. Purulent discharge, edema, or seromas are of concern and should be seen by a veterinarian. Colville T, Bassert JM, Clinical Anatomy and Physiology for Veterinary Technicians, ed 2, Mosby, 2008, p. 129.

171. a Premedication can help relax the patient for the placement of the IV catheter; having the catheter in place allows for induction. After the animal is induced, clipping and prepping should occur out of the surgery suite. After the animal is moved into surgery, the final preparation is applied. Tear M, Small Animal Surgical Nursing, ed 2, Elsevier, 2012, p. 54-65.

172. c It is not necessary to have a sterile gown when working as a nonsterile assistant; however, a mask, cap, shoe covers, and clean scrubs should be worn. Tear M, Small Animal Surgical Nursing, ed 2, Elsevier, 2012, p. 86-87.

173. b The nonsterile assistant must approach from the back so that the front of the gown will not be contaminated. Never use a nonsterile piece of gauze to adjust the mask. Tear M, Small Animal Surgical Nursing, ed 2, Elsevier, 2012, p. 102-103 .

174. b Roccal, a quaternary ammonium, is a disinfectant not intended for use on living tissue. Chlorhexidine, alcohol, and povidone-iodine can all be used to prepare a surgical patient. Bassert JM, Thomas JA, McCurnin's Clinical Textbook for Veterinary Technicians, ed 8, Elsevier, 2014, p. 1168.

175. b Second-intention healing is indicated for heavily contaminated wounds. Primary intention is used for surgically induced incisions. Third intention is healing of a wound that has already formed granulation tissue and has undergone secondary closure. Fourth intention does not exist. Bassert JM, Thomas JA, McCurnin's Clinical Textbook for Veterinary Technicians, ed 8, Elsevier, 2014, p. 1433.

176. d A ventral midline incision is made along the linea alba and extends from the xiphoid process to the umbilicus. Incisions of this type are often used when exploring the upper abdomen. A flank incision would be made in the lower quad of the abdomen, and it is usually used when looking for a retained testicle in a male dog or cat. A paracostal incision is a smaller incision in the upper quad of the abdomen that can be used to expose the kidneys and adrenal glands. A paramedian incision simply refers to off the midline. Tear M, Small Animal Surgical Nursing, ed 2, Elsevier, 2012, p. 134.

177. c Cesarean sections in cattle are most commonly performed through the left paralumbar fossa; this approach is often called a left-flank incision. Fubini S, Ducharme M, Farm Animal Surgery, Saunders, 2004, p. 81.

178. a Emasculators are used to crush and cut the spermatic cord during large-animal castrations and are not used in any small-animal procedure. Sonsthagen TF, Veterinary Instruments and Equipment: a Pocket Guide, ed 2, Elsevier, 2011, p. 241.

179. b The rumen is located on the left side of the body; therefore, the left paralumbar fossa would be prepped. Bassert JM, Thomas JA, McCurnin's Clinical Textbook for Veterinary Technicians, ed 8, Elsevier, 2014, p. 1281.

180. a Tilting the table more than 15 degrees may cause the abdominal contents to put pressure on the diaphragm; therefore, this position should be avoided in animals with breathing difficulties. Tilting the table will not initiate defecation or gastric volvulus and it actually helps to visualize the caudal abdomen. Thomas JA, Lerche P, Anesthesia and Analgesia for Veterinary Technicians, ed 4, Mosby, 2011, p. 253.

181. b 4-0 silk should be chosen to meet the veterinarian's request. Chromic gut is absorbable, and 0 and 00 are too large. Table 9-2, "Characteristics of Suture Materials Commonly Used in Veterinary Medicine," Fossum TW, Small Animal Surgery, ed 3, Mosby, 2007, p. 60.

182. d In cats undergoing a castration procedure, the hair is plucked until the scrotum is free of hair and then the surgical scrub is performed. If the patient was a flank cryptorchid, the abdomen may be clipped and prepped from the umbilicus to the scrotum with a No. 40 clipper blade. Tear M, Small Animal Surgical Nursing, ed 2, Elsevier, 2012, p. 158.

183. c A ventral midline is not used for the correction of a left-displaced abomasum. All other approaches are used in left-displaced abomasum (LDA) surgeries. Fubini S, Ducharme M, Farm Animal Surgery, Saunders, 2004, p. 216-217.

184. d 24 hours after postop surgery, exercise is required in horses to promote drainage from the surgical site and to prevent excessive swelling. It is not advised for horses to be strictly confined because drainage does need to occur. Antibiotics are not routinely prescribed post castration and sutures are not generally placed because the scrotal incision is commonly stretched, allowing drainage to occur. Bassert JM, Thomas JA, McCurnin's Clinical Textbook for Veterinary Technicians, ed 8, Elsevier, 2014, p. 1266.

185. a A laparotomy can also be called a celiotomy. A pleurotomy is an incision of the pleura. A thoracotomy is an incision of the chest wall and a cystotomy is an incision into the bladder. Bassert JM, Thomas JA, McCurnin's Clinical Textbook for Veterinary Technicians, ed 8, Elsevier, 2014, p. 1228.

186. c The pulse oximeter measures how much of the available hemoglobin is saturated with oxygen and it also monitors the pulse rate. Tear M, Small Animal Surgical Nursing, ed 2, Elsevier, 2012, p. 115.

187. c The ECG indicates electrical activity only; it does not measure the contractility or perfusion of the heart. Sirois M, Principles and Practice of Veterinary Technology, ed 3, Mosby, 2011, p. 370, 609.

188. b External fixators are used in orthopedic sutures to stabilize fractures and they can also be called a Kirschner-Ehmer apparatus. Rush pins and Steinmann pins are placed within the bones and a bone plate is applied on the outside surface of the bone, but not on the external areas of the skin. Tear M, Small Animal Surgical Nursing, ed 2, Elsevier, 2012, p. 186-187.

189. c Nosocomial infections are acquired in hospital. Sirois M, Principles and Practice of Veterinary Technology, ed 3, Mosby, 2011, p. 382.

190. a Electric heating pads can cause severe burns and should not be used. Warm water circulating pads and warm air convection blankets help keep the patient warm, along with a towel placed between the surgery table and the patient. Plastic bubble wrap can be wrapped around the patient's extremities. Tear M, Small Animal Surgical Nursing, ed 3, Elsevier, 2012, p. 82-83.

191. d The Jacobs bone chuck is used to place IM pins in orthopedic procedures and it is also called the intramedullary pin chuck. The Jacob's bone pin would not be used for onychectomies, celiotomies, or thoracotomies. Tear M, Small Animal Surgical Nursing, ed 2, Elsevier, 2012, p. 183; Sonsthagen TF, Veterinary Instruments and Equipment: a Pocket Guide, ed 2, Elsevier, 2011, p. 593.

192. c Neutering a dog will not prevent him from lifting his leg to urinate. It is a normal, learned behavior. Neutering will decrease the risks of perineal hernias, the need to roam, and some aggression toward other dogs. Bassert JM, Thomas JA, McCurnin's Clinical Textbook for Veterinary Technicians, ed 8, Elsevier, 2014.

193. b Chlorhexidine scrub can be used to prep a patient. Solutions cannot be used as surgical scrubs and alcohol is commonly used as a rinse agent. Bassert JM, Thomas JA, McCurnin's Clinical Textbook for Veterinary Technicians, ed 8, Elsevier, 2014, p. 1170.

194. d It is not necessary to have a complete tail wrap unless the tail will cause contamination because of its proximity to the surgical site. Bassert JM, Thomas JA, McCurnin's Clinical Textbook for Veterinary Technicians, ed 8, Elsevier, 2014, p. 1261.

195. a Padding is one of the measures that helps prevent myositis in horses, which is defined as severe inflammation of the muscles that can be life-threatening. Hypothermia does not have anything to do with myositis, although it is important to maintain temperature. Overinflating the ET cuff does not have anything to do with myositis, but it should not be done. Before surgery, NPO is not indicated for horses. Bassert JM, Thomas JA, McCurnin's Clinical Textbook for Veterinary Technicians, ed 8, Elsevier, 2014, p. 1262.

196. c The primary task for a lone technician is the careful and constant monitoring of the patient. Attaching the monitoring devices first will allow the individual to assess the patient's status while performing the remaining duties. Tear M, Small Animal Surgical Nursing, ed 2, Elsevier, 2012, p. 107.

197. b Compartment syndrome may occur to the "up" side if the limbs are not positioned properly or if prolonged hypotension is allowed to occur. It can affect one or several muscle compartments, can occur even if all precautions are followed, and euthanasia is not an uncommon outcome. Holtgrew-Bohling K, Large Animal Clinical Procedures for Veterinary Technicians, ed 2, Elsevier, 2012, p. 277.

198. c A gastrotomy refers to a surgical incision into the stomach. Tear M, Small Animal Surgical Nursing, ed 2, Elsevier, 2012, p. 137.

199. b After the scrub has been started, nonsterile items cannot be handled without breaking sterility. If your hands or arms inadvertently touch a nonsterile object (including surgical personnel), repeat the scrub. During and after scrubbing, keep the hands higher than the elbows. This allows water and soap to flow from the cleanest area (hands) to a less clean area (elbows). Sirois M, Principles and Practice of Veterinary Technology, ed 3, Mosby, 2011, p. 397.

200. c Although the remaining statements are important, the main reason for the aseptic technique is to protect the animal from microbes entering through the surgical site. Tear M, Small Animal Surgical Nursing, ed 2, Elsevier, 2012, p. 101.

201. a A fenestration is a window; therefore, the correct answer is a window opening in the middle of a drape through which surgery can be performed. Any drape or towel is folded in accordion style, with the goal of maintaining asepsis when lying on top of the patient. A drape can be made of cloth that can be washed and reused or of material designed for one-time use. Tear M, Small Animal Surgical Nursing, ed 2, Elsevier, 2012, p. 12.

202. c To destroy all living microorganisms, the correct relationship between temperature, pressure, and time must be achieved. The minimum temperature and exposure time for the steam of an autoclave to provide sterility is 250°F or 121.5°C for 13 minutes at 15 psi. Tear M, Small Animal Surgical Nursing, ed 2, Elsevier, 2012, p. 263.

203. a The basic requirements for first-intention healing are minimal tissue damage and apposition of the wound edges, usually with sutures. Second-intention healing is when a wound is not sutured, but it heals by contraction and epithelialization. Excessive granulation tissue is called proud flesh. Third-intention healing occurs 305 days after cleaning and debridement, but before granulation tissue forms. Sirois M, Principles and Practice of Veterinary Technology, ed 3, Mosby, 2011, p. 278.

204. d The basic functional unit of the nervous system, the neuron, is incapable of reproduction; consequently, damage to the nervous system is often repaired by scar tissue. The gastrointestinal tract, liver, and bone have excellent healing potential. Colville T, Bassert JM, Clinical Anatomy and Physiology for Veterinary Technicians, ed 2, Mosby, 2008, p. 315.

205. c Caudal epidural anesthesia is routinely used for analgesia of the tail, perineum, anus/rectum, vulva, and vagina. Caudal epidural analgesia is easily performed on large animals. The site of injection is between the first and second coccygeal vertebrae on the dorsal midline. Holtgrew-Bohling K, Large Animal Clinical Procedures for Veterinary Technicians, ed 2, Elsevier, p. 273.

206. c An electric drill must be sterilized by ethylene oxide gas because it would be damaged or inadequately sterilized by any other method. A typical surgical pack would be autoclaved, whereas forceps used to probe an abscess may be disinfected with a liquid chemical. Dry heat is not typically used in veterinary applications. Bassert JM, Thomas JA, McCurnin's Clinical Textbook for Veterinary Technicians, ed 8, Elsevier, 2014, p. 122.

207. b Chemical autoclave indicators are the only type listed that can provide immediate information on all three of the basic criteria for autoclave sterilization: (1) the presence of steam at the proper combination, (2) exposure time, and (3) temperature. Bassert JM, Thomas JA, McCurnin's Clinical Textbook for Veterinary Technicians, ed 8, Elsevier, 2014, p. 1164.

208. a Microorganisms in a wound during surgery are considered contaminants until, or unless, they multiply and cause damage. Contamination of an object or a wound implies the presence of microorganisms within or on it. Contamination of a wound can, but does not necessarily, lead to infection. With infection, microorganisms in the body or in a wound multiply and cause harmful effects. Infection can lead to septicemia (systemic disease associated with the presence and persistence of pathogenic microorganisms and their toxins in the blood). Debridement is the cleaning of a wound and the removal of necrotic tissue. Sirois M, Principles and Practice of Veterinary Technology, ed 3, Mosby, 2011, p. 382.

209. d A surgical mask does not come in contact with anything sterile during a surgical procedure; therefore, it has only to be clean. Drapes, gloves, and gowns must be sterile. Sirois M, Principles and Practice of Veterinary Technology, ed 3, Mosby, 2011, p. 394-399.

210. d An autoclave sterilizes by exposing packs to high-temperature steam under pressure. Chemical disinfectant is generally used in cold sterile trays; ethylene oxide is used in gas sterilization units. Dry heat is not used in the veterinary practice. Tear M, Small Animal Surgical Nursing, ed 2, Elsevier, 2012, p. 262-263.

211. d A No. 40 clipper blade is a surgical blade. It clips the hair off at the skin surface. The larger the numbered blade is, the closer the shave. No. 10 blades are often used for grooming. Tighe MM, Brown M, Mosby's Comprehensive Review for Veterinary Technicians, ed 3, Mosby, 2008, p. 408.

212. b Curettage involves scraping a tissue or cavity. Crushing, ligation, and pressure are all methods of achieving mechanical hemostasis. Crushing forceps are used to crush tissue. Suture material is used to ligate vessels and pressure can be applied to an area of hemorrhage to help control bleeding. Sirois M, Principles and Practice of Veterinary Technology, ed 3, Mosby, 2011, p. 405.

213. d Using overly large suture material would not cause a wound to break down. It would actually have greater holding power than a smaller size of suture material. Excessive physical activity, wound infection, and a difficult surgical recovery could cause surgical wound dehiscence. Fossum TW, Small Animal Surgery, ed 3, Mosby, 2007, p. 57; Tear M, Small Animal Surgical Nursing, ed 2, Elsevier, 2012.

214. b Contaminated items look identical to sterile items; if there is any doubt about the sterility of an item, it must be considered contaminated. Sirois M, Principles and Practice of Veterinary Technology, ed 3, Mosby, 2011, p. 382.

215. b Exuberant granulation tissue (proud flesh) inhibits wound healing and epithelial regeneration. Debridement involves the removal of unhealthy tissue, therefore enhancing wound healing. A normal amount of granulation tissue enhances wound healing, just as wound flushing does. Sirois M, Principles and Practice of Veterinary Technology, ed 3, Mosby, 2011, p. 319.

216. d One of the most important characteristics of wound healing by first intention is approximation of the wound edges. A wound can be contaminated with or without minimal tissue damage, but it can be cleaned and debrided, allowing first-intention wound healing. Sirois M, Principles and Practice of Veterinary Technology, ed 3, Mosby, 2011, p. 278.

217. d The ventral midline approach provides the most extensive access to the abdominal cavity. A flank incision is off the midline and is too caudal to serve the needs of an exploratory laparotomy. Paracostal and paramedian incisions are off the midline; neither incision would allow a complete exploratory laparotomy. Fossum TW, Small Animal Surgery, ed 3, Mosby, 2007, p. 319.

218. a As a result of normal inflammation, a slight elevation of body temperature that lasts for a day or two is normal after major surgery. Serosanguineous discharge, a swollen incision, or heated incisions are all early indicators of wound dehiscence. Colville T, Bassert JM, Clinical Anatomy and Physiology for Veterinary Technicians, ed 2, Mosby, 2008, p. 129.

219. d Prevention of surgical wound contamination is the whole purpose of aseptic technique in the operating room; all the other choices contribute to the main goal. Tear M, Small Animal Surgical Nursing, ed 2, Elsevier, 2012, p. 101.

220. a The number of microorganisms entering the wound can be influenced by aseptic technique. Proper aseptic techniques can decrease the microorganism load. Pathogenicity, route of exposure, and susceptibility are inherent of the microorganisms in the environment, the surgical procedure being performed, and the immunity of the patient. Tear M, Small Animal Surgical Nursing, ed 2, Elsevier, 2012, p. 101.

221. b Occasionally when recovering from general anesthesia, the animal exhibits signs of excitement, possibly with exaggerated and uncontrolled movements. The patient may thrash around in the cage, cry out, or paddle with all four legs. This phenomenon is called emergence delirium. Tear M, Small Animal Surgical Nursing, ed 3, Elsevier, 2012, p. 213.

222. a Ehmer slings are used to stabilize a hip luxation, Robert Jones bandages are used to stabilize long bone fractures, spica splints are used to stabilize humeral fractures, and Velpeau slings are used for scapula fractures. Tear M, Small Animal Surgical Nursing, ed 3, Elsevier, 2012, p. 163.

223. a The surgical cap does not come in contact with the tissues of the patient either directly or indirectly. It therefore needs to be clean but not sterile. Drapes, gowns, and the scrub brush used to scrub hands must be sterile. Sirois M, Principles and Practice of Veterinary Technology, ed 3, Mosby, 2011, p. 394-399.

224. b Endoscopic instruments are routinely cleaned with chemical sterilization agents such as glutaraldehyde. These instruments should be rinsed before coming into contact with patient tissue. Electrical equipment should not be immersed in liquid. Orthopedic equipment and drapes are autoclaved to achieve sterility. Fossum TW, Small Animal Surgery, ed 3, Mosby, 2007, p. 3.

225. d Warming the solution speeds up the chemical reactions necessary to kill microorganisms. Cooling the solution can prolong the time needed to achieve the disinfectant state. Diluting the solution will reduce efficacy; however, increasing the strength of the solution will not increase the speed of kill. Sirois M, Principles and Practice of Veterinary Technology, ed 3, Mosby, 2011, p. 357.

226. d Cloth and paper drapes are subject to capillary action; plastic drapes are not. Bassert JM, Thomas JA, McCurnin's Clinical Textbook for Veterinary Technicians, ed 8, Elsevier, 2014, p. 1183.

227. d A well-trained, educated, and alert technician is the best monitoring device. The technician can monitor changes in respiration, heart rate, mucous membrane color, and can assess pulses to determine changes in blood pressure. The technician can also make immediate corrections to any abnormalities. Surgical monitors are also important, but they aid the technician in monitoring and do not replace the technician. Tear M, Small Animal Surgical Nursing, ed 2, Elsevier, 2012, p. 115.

228. b Isotonic saline is a sterile solution that can be used to flush wounds, abdominal cavities, or instruments that have been soaking in a cold sterile solution. Tap water could be contaminated and should not be used. Povidone and hydrogen peroxide can be irritating to tissues and cannot be used in internal cavities. Bassert JM, Thomas JA, McCurnin's Clinical Textbook for Veterinary Technicians, ed 8, Elsevier, 2014, p. 975.

229. a Dehiscence of all layers of the body wall exposes abdominal viscera. Repair must be immediate to prevent serious damage to the abdominal organs and structures. Tear M, Small Animal Surgical Nursing, ed 2, Elsevier, 2012, p. 235.

230. d Inflammation results from any injury to the body, whether intentional (surgical) or unintentional (traumatic). The increased blood supply to an area of inflammation results in increased warmth to the area. Good surgical technique minimizes inflammation but does not eliminate it. Contamination, infection, and debridement itself would not cause an increase in temperature because the trauma to the tissue would have occurred days earlier, not recently, as asked in the question. Colville T, Bassert JM, Clinical Anatomy and Physiology for Veterinary Technicians, ed 2, Mosby, 2008, p. 129.

231. b It takes 4 to 6 days for production of collagen strands in a wound to reach a significant level. Until that time, the sutures are the main things holding the suture line together. Box 13-1, "Events in the Three Phases of Wound Healing," Sirois M, Principles and Practice of Veterinary Technology, ed 3, Mosby, 2011, p. 312.

232. c Wound contraction represents movement of the whole thickness of the skin toward the center of the wound. Fossum TW, Small Animal Surgery, ed 3, Mosby, 2007, p. 161.

233. b Gowns should be grasped from the inside portion of the gown to maintain asepsis. Gowns are commonly made of cloth or paper, but not plastic, and they are commonly sterilized using a steam autoclave. Sirois M, Principles and Practice of Veterinary Technology, ed 3, Mosby, 2011, p. 396.

234. a A patient in shock would be expected to show rapid, shallow breathing in an effort to oxygenate the blood as rapidly as possible. Slow capillary refill time, tachycardia, and weakness are all signs of hemorrhagic shock. Tear M, Small Animal Surgical Nursing, ed 2, Elsevier, 2012, p. 233-234; Thomas JA, Lerche P, Anesthesia and Analgesia for Veterinary Technicians, ed 4, Mosby, 2011, p. 175.

235. b Unless very large or ruptured, postoperative seromas are unsightly but of little importance to the animal's health. Tear M, Small Animal Surgical Nursing, ed 2, Elsevier, 2012, p. 235.

236. a Bones have excellent healing capacities, provided that the fragments are properly aligned and movement is minimized. Bones that are misaligned and mobile have a poor prognosis. Tobias KM, Johnston SA, Veterinary Surgery: Small Animal, Elsevier, 2012, p. 586.

237. d The internal reproductive tract of a patient is considered sterile and would not contribute to the transmission of microorganisms. The primary sources of microorganisms from inanimate objects are fomites and air. A fomite is any inanimate object capable of carrying infectious organisms, which includes the hospital structure (walls, floors, etc.), furniture, equipment, implants, cleaning equipment, and staff members' clothing, shoes, or skin. Fossum TW, Small Animal Surgery Textbook, ed 4, Mosby, 2013.

238. b A flank incision is most appropriate for a standing animal undergoing a cesarean section. If the animal were anesthetized, a ventral midline might be appropriate. A paracostal and paramedian incision would not be appropriate for a cesarean section, even for an anesthetized patient. Fubini S, Ducharme M, Farm Animal Surgery, Saunders, 2004, p. 81.

239. c Treating for shock, decompression of the stomach, and monitoring the patient for arrythmias are all common preoperative procedures for GDVs. Administration of oral medications would not be possible because of twisting of the stomach. Tear M, Small Animal Surgical Nursing, ed 3, Elsevier, 2012, p. 140-141.

240. c Inflammation is the first step in wound healing. Endothelial and fibroblast proliferation occur in the second phase, and the equilibrium of collagen synthesis occurs in the final phase. Box 13-1, "Events in the Three Phases of Wound Healing," Sirois M, Principles and Practice of Veterinary Technology, ed 3, Mosby, 2011, p. 312.

241. d Other than the sutures, a surgical wound has no appreciable strength until significant numbers of collagen fibers, fibrins, and granulation tissue are produced in about 4 to 6 days. Box 13-1, "Events in the Three Phases of Wound Healing," Sirois M, Principles and Practice of Veterinary Technology, ed 3, Mosby, 2011, p. 312.

242. d The linea alba, on the ventral midline of the abdominal wall, is the tendinous attachment of all of the ventral abdominal muscles. One layer of sutures in this area effectively closes the abdominal wall. Multiple layers of suture would be required to close a flank, paracostal, and paramedian incision. Tear M, Small Animal Surgical Nursing, ed 2, Elsevier, 2012.

243. b Anything outside the sterile zone in an operating room is considered contaminated. Objects within the sterile field and sterilized instruments are considered aseptic, as are freshly exposed tissues. Sirois M, Principles and Practice of Veterinary Technology, ed 3, Mosby, 2011, p. 382.

244. a Nonscrubbed personnel should touch only items that are not sterile. The inside of the patient's body is considered sterile, as well as within the sterile zone and sterile field. Sirois M, Principles and Practice of Veterinary Technology, ed 3, Mosby, 2011, p. 382.

245. c The hands of scrubbed personnel should always be held between waist level and shoulder level to help prevent inadvertent contamination. Clasping the hands when not otherwise occupied helps prevent fatigue from compromising the position of the hands and arms. The arms of scrubbed personnel should never be folded, held above shoulder level, or below the waistline. Bassert JM, Thomas JA, McCurnin's Clinical Textbook for Veterinary Technicians, ed 8, Elsevier, 2014, p. 1182.

246. a Nonscrubbed personnel should never violate the sterile zone in which scrubbed personnel are working. Tear M, Small Animal Surgical Nursing, ed 2, Elsevier, 2012, p. 103.

247. b Sterility is destroyed if a nonscrubbed person touches pack contents. The nonscrubbed person can remove the autoclave tape from the outside of the pack. The outside corners of the wrap can be touched to open the pack (being careful not to touch the inside contents). Nonscrubbed personnel can touch the instrument stand. Tear M, Small Animal Surgical Nursing, ed 2, Elsevier, 2012, p. 104.

248. c Ethylene oxide gas is very flammable and is toxic to tissues. Any exposure to ethylene oxide is considered a health risk. Bassert JM, Thomas JA, McCurnin's Clinical Textbook for Veterinary Technicians, ed 8, Elsevier, 2014, p. 1165.

249. d Leaving skin sutures in too long increases scarring but does not directly contribute to breakdown of the surgical wound. Chronic postoperative vomiting could contribute to wound dehiscence if the incision is located in the abdominal area. Infection will cause severe inflammation and dehiscence. If internal sutures are cut too short, the wound could open. Fossum TW, Small Animal Surgery, ed 3, Mosby, 2007, p. 57; Tear M, Small Animal Surgical Nursing, ed 2, Elsevier, 2012.

250. d Wet saline dressings are useful to help debride wounds with extensive tissue damage. They absorb and remove inflammatory products from the wound. Antiseptics do not have any wound debridement activity. Dry gauze may stick to a wound, but it does not contribute to debridement. Tear M, Small Animal Surgical Nursing, ed 2, Elsevier, 2012, p. 242.

251. d Redistribution of blood flow results in pale mucous membranes, poor capillary refill, and cold extremities, which are all symptoms seen in an animal experiencing shock. Acidosis, alkalosis, and cell death do not occur because of excessive blood loss. Bassert JM, Thomas JA, McCurnin's Clinical Textbook for Veterinary Technicians, ed 8, Elsevier, 2014, p. 912.

252. d A pus-filled uterus must be removed to return the animal to health without restoring normal reproductive function. A diagnosis is made before uterus removal and it is not done to confirm the diagnosis. Removing the uterus is not done as a prophylactic measure, but rather to remove infection. Tear M, Small Animal Surgical Nursing, ed 2, Elsevier, 2012, p. 155.

253. c After the dead and damaged tissue has been removed from a wound by inflammation, a bed of granulation tissue, consisting primarily of collagen fibers and capillaries, must form on the floor of the wound before wound contraction can begin. Scar tissue forms well after the second phase. Table 13-1, "Types of Wound Closure," Sirois M, Principles and Practice of Veterinary Technology, ed 3, Mosby, 2011, p. 318.

254. b If the outside of the glove is touched by anything that is not sterile, including freshly scrubbed fingers, it becomes contaminated and must not be used for surgery. Sirois M, Principles and Practice of Veterinary Technology, ed 3, Mosby, 2011, p. 397.

255. d A pack placed vertically in the autoclave receives the best circulation of steam around its contents. Sterilization failure may occur if packs are wrapped too tightly or are improperly loaded in the autoclave or the gas sterilizer container. Heavy packs should be placed at the periphery, where steam enters the chamber. A small amount of air space is allowed between packs to facilitate the flow of steam (1 to 2 inches between the packs and away from the surrounding walls). Linen packs are loaded so that the fabric layers are oriented vertically (i.e., on edge). These packs are not stacked, because increased thickness reduces the penetration of the steam. Close supervision and exact standards for preparing, packaging, and loading the supplies are necessary for effective steam and gas sterilization. Fossum TW, Small Animal Surgery, ed 3, Mosby, 2007, p. 12.

256. b Metzenbaum scissors are made for delicate tissue dissection only. They become dull or spring open if used on heavier tissue or material. Mayo scissors are used to cut thicker tissue, including the linea alba and fascia. Suture scissors are used to cut suture. Fossum TW, Small Animal Surgery Textbook, ed 4, Mosby, 2013.

257. d Gelpi retractors have a ratchet device to hold them in place during use. Deaver, Senn, and Rake retractors must be held to retract tissue. Sonsthagen TF, Veterinary Instruments and Equipment: a Pocket Guide, ed 2, Elsevier, 2011, p. 559.

258. d Cold sterilization is a misnomer; it is a high-level disinfection process. To achieve a level of sterility, most agents used in cold sterilization must be in contact with the instruments for a minimum of 10 hours. Tear M, Small Animal Surgical Nursing, ed 2, Elsevier, 2012, p. 266; Fossum TW, Small Animal Surgery, ed 3, Mosby, 2007, p. 13.

259. d An instrument that is wrapped in heat-sealed paper and transparent plastic pouches is considered sterile for 1 year. Table 30-6, "Safe Storage Times for Sterile Packs," Bassert JM, Thomas JA, McCurnin's Clinical Textbook for Veterinary Technicians, ed 8, Elsevier, 2014, p. 1161.

260. d There are no cleansing agents in instrument milk; however, it does lubricate, inhibit rust, and extend the life of an instrument. Bassert JM, Thomas JA, McCurnin's Clinical Textbook for Veterinary Technicians, ed 8, Elsevier, 2014, p. 1158.

261. c Backhaus towel forceps are used to secure and clamp the surgical drapes to the patient. The function of needle holders is to hold the surgical needle (Mayo-Hagar, for example), scissors cut tissue (Metzenbaums, for example), and hemostatic forceps hold or clamp blood vessels. Sonsthagen TF, Veterinary Instruments and Equipment: a Pocket Guide, ed 2, Elsevier, 2011, p. 465.

262. c A cesarean section is the surgical removal of the calf from the cow and OB chains are used to slip over the calf's hocks to help pull it out. Sonsthagen TF, Veterinary Instruments and Equipment: a Pocket Guide, ed 2, Elsevier, 2011, p. 255.

263. b Plastic pipette tips can be sterilized effectively in an autoclave, whereas all of the others would be damaged by the high heat or moisture. Bassert JM, Thomas JA, McCurnin's Clinical Textbook for Veterinary Technicians, ed 8, Elsevier, 2014, p. 1163.

264. a Ultrasonic cleaners are used to remove small particles of blood and tissue from instruments. Instrument milk is responsible for inhibiting rust and lubricating instruments. Disinfectant is used to disinfect instruments. Bassert JM, Thomas JA, McCurnin's Clinical Textbook for Veterinary Technicians, ed 8, Elsevier, 2014, p. 1158.

265. c Hyperthermia is not a sign of hypotension. Hypotension, or low blood pressure, may be associated with hypovolemia, drop in circulating blood volume, excessive vasodilation, allowing blood to pool decreasing venous return, and excessive anesthetic depth. Tear M, Small Animal Surgical Nursing, ed 2, Elsevier, 2012, p. 111-112.

266. d Incorrect labeling has no effect on the sterility of a pack. However, the sterilization date is important, as sterility does expire (length of sterility depends on the type of wrapping material). Indicator color change is important because color changes when the correct ratio of steam, pressure, and heat are achieved. Holes in a wrap or moisture in a pack render it nonsterile. Bassert JM, Thomas JA, McCurnin's Clinical Textbook for Veterinary Technicians, ed 8, Elsevier, 2014, p. 1163.

267. b Mayo scissors are heavy and can cut thicker skin and materials. If used on delicate tissue, they might crush the tissue instead of cleanly cutting it. Metzenbaum scissors are used to cut delicate tissue. Sonsthagen TF, Veterinary Instruments and Equipment: a Pocket Guide, ed 2, Elsevier, 2011, p. 497.

268. d A nonsterile member of the team should handle the administration of drugs during surgery. Passing of instruments, draping of patients, and identifying suture patterns are all duties that can be assigned to a sterile surgical assistant. Tear M, Small Animal Surgical Nursing, ed 2, Elsevier, 2012, p. 126-128.

269. d In preparation of the abdomen of a male dog, one task musk be done before the surgical site prep is started. After all of the hair has been removed from the prepuce, the sheath must be flushed to remove potential contaminants. Tear M, Small Animal Surgical Nursing, ed 2, Elsevier, 2012, p. 71.

270. b A No. 11 blade has a sharp point for making a small incision, just large enough for an arthroscope or cannula to enter the joint. A No. 10 blade is commonly used for incisions. The No. 12 blade resembles a hook, with the cutting edge on the inside curve, and is frequently used to declaw a cat. A No. 15 blade has the appearance of a No. 10 blade, but with only half the length of the No. 10. Tear M, Small Animal Surgical Nursing, ed 2, Elsevier, 2012, p. 22.

271. d Boiling does not sterilize instruments; it is a disinfectant only. It is acceptable only for contaminated or clean-contaminated surgery. Instruments can be gas or chemical sterilized and autoclaved. Bassert JM, Thomas JA, McCurnin's Clinical Textbook for Veterinary Technicians, ed 8, Elsevier, 2014, p. 1163.

272. b It is impossible to sterilize a surgeon's hands; however, surgical hand scrub can remove dirt and oil and reduce microorganisms. Tear M, Small Animal Surgical Nursing, ed 2, Elsevier, 2012, p. 88.

273. c Of the chemicals listed, chlorhexidine gluconate produces the greatest residual activity. Table 3-1, "Characteristics of Selected Antimicrobials Used in Surgical Scrub Solutions," Tear M, Small Animal Surgical Nursing, ed 2, Elsevier, 2012, p. 90.

274. d A rat-tooth forceps is used for grasping tissue, not to control bleeding. Electrocautery can be applied directly to the source of bleeding and a hemostat can clamp the vessel. Suction can be used to remove liquid contents from an area of bleeding, allowing the source of the bleeding to be better visualized. Sonsthagen TF, Veterinary Instruments and Equipment: a Pocket Guide, ed 2, Elsevier, 2011, p. 451.

275. c As long as an item remains sealed, it remains sterile indefinitely when subjected to gamma radiation. Tobias KM, Johnston SA, Veterinary Surgery: Small Animal, Elsevier, 2012, p. 151.

276. c A Senn retractor has no ratchet and must be held to be functional. Weitlaner, Alms, and Balfour retractors are self-retaining. Sonsthagen TF, Veterinary Instruments and Equipment: a Pocket Guide, ed 2, Elsevier, 2011, p. 555.

277. a Steam under pressure can permeate rapidly and then condense; this kills microorganisms most effectively. Gas can take several hours to kill microorganisms. Dry heat is less effective than moist heat. Radiation sterilization is not used in veterinary medicine. Tear M, Small Animal Surgical Nursing, ed 2, Elsevier, 2012, p. 262-265.

278. b Double wrapping provides longer sterility (up to 4 weeks) than that of a single wrap. Table 30-6, "Safe Storage Times for Sterile Packs," Bassert JM, Thomas JA, McCurnin's Clinical Textbook for Veterinary Technicians, ed 8, Elsevier, 2014, p. 1161.

279. c Ordinary hand soaps can leave behind insoluble alkaline residue, abrasive compounds can damage the surface of the instruments, and plain water is too slow and is less thorough than a low-sudsing detergent. In addition, a low-sudsing instrument detergent is formulated with the correct pH, reducing the potential for rusting on instruments and extending the lifetime of such instruments. Tear M, Small Animal Surgical Nursing, ed 2, Elsevier, 2012, p. 258.

280. b Vicryl (polyglactin 910) is an absorbable suture. Prolene (polypropylene), Mersilene (Prelone), and silk are nonabsorbable. Table 1-2, "Summary and Comparison of Common Suture Materials," Tear M, Small Animal Surgical Nursing, ed 2, Elsevier, 2012, p. 34.

281. c Skin staples are more expensive than skin sutures; however, they do save the surgeon time and provide excellent wound healing. In addition, with staples the skin is more resistant to abscess formation. Tear M, Small Animal Surgical Nursing, ed 2, Elsevier, 2012, p. 36-37.

282. c The interrupted horizontal mattress provides more strength than any of the other suture patterns. It also is the one most easily used, with rubber tubing for tension reduction. Tear M, Small Animal Surgical Nursing, ed 2, Elsevier, 2012, p. 129.

283. c Hyperglycemia does not contribute to prolonged recovery. It can be associated with breed predisposition (sight hounds are sensitive to barbiturate anesthetics), poor perfusion, which can prevent the injectable anesthetics from reaching the organs that will eliminate them, and hypothermia, which can decrease the rate at which drugs are metabolized. Tear M, Small Animal Surgical Nursing, ed 2, Elsevier, 2012, p. 129.

284. c Gut is an absorbable suture that breaks down rapidly and therefore it should not be used for skin closure. Bassert JM, Thomas JA, McCurnin's Clinical Textbook for Veterinary Technicians, ed 8, Elsevier, 2014, p. 1202.

285. b Placing subcuticular sutures eliminates the need for skin sutures; this prevents animals from self-mutilating by removing the sutures. Subcuticular patterns do not eliminate infection, are not more cost effective, and do not reduce the amount of suture material needed. Tear M, Small Animal Surgical Nursing, ed 2, Elsevier, 2012, p. 128.

286. a A Cushing suture pattern inverts the skin and is therefore not used to close the skin. Fossum TW, Small Animal Surgery, ed 3, Mosby, 2007, p. 69.

287. b A Cushing suture pattern is inverting. A cruciate pattern is a modification of the horizontal mattress and results in an everting pattern. A vertical mattress pattern can result in an eversion when the tension is pulled too tightly. Fossum TW, Small Animal Surgery, ed 3, Mosby, 2007, p. 69.

288. b A surgeon's knot has two throws on the first pass and one throw on the second pass; a square knot has one pass on each throw. Tobias KM, Johnston SA, Veterinary Surgery: Small Animal, Elsevier, 2012, p. 210.

289. c With mass ligation, the blood supply to the area may still be great enough to cause the suture to break. Fossum TW, Small Animal Surgery, ed 3, Mosby, 2007, p. 57.

290. d Transfixation ligatures may be placed on single vessels, usually arteries, or vascular pedicles. The suture penetrates the vessel or pedicle and encloses it. Security of placement is the primary advantage of a transfixation ligation compared with a circumferential ligation because the ligature is held in place at a given tissue level. Tobias K, Johnston S, Veterinary Surgery: Small Animal, Saunders, 2012.

291. c Instrument ties are not more accurate than hand ties; in fact, hand ties are more useful in confined or difficult-to-reach areas. Fossum TW, Small Animal Surgery, ed 3, Mosby, 2007, p. 172.

292. d The type of needle does not affect the strength of the suture and vice versa. Tear M, Small Animal Surgical Nursing, ed 2, Elsevier, 2012, p. 33.

293. c A cutting needle penetrates the skin with the least amount of trauma. Tear M, Small Animal Surgical Nursing, ed 2, Elsevier, 2012, p. 33.

294. c All of the answers are true; however, trauma to the tissues is the most important factor to consider. Tear M, Small Animal Surgical Nursing, ed 2, Elsevier, 2012, p. 32-33.

295. c Tendons and nerves should be sutured with tension sutures, whereas viscera should be closed with inverting sutures; therefore, the skin should be closed with appositional sutures. Fossum TW, Small Animal Surgery, ed 3, Mosby, 2007, p. 66.

296. c The larger the number (3), the larger the diameter of suture. 3-0 is the smallest listed size in this sequence. Tear M, Small Animal Surgical Nursing, ed 2, Elsevier, 2012.

297. b -rrhapy is surgical repair by suturing. -ectomy means to remove. -otomy is to cut into. -ostomy is the surgical creation of an artificial opening. Sirois M, Principles and Practice of Veterinary Technology, ed 3, Mosby, 2011, p. 379.

298. d Poor nutrition would contribute to wound dehiscence, not optimal nutrition. Suture failure can occur by loosening, untying, or breaking. Tissue weakness may result from the age of the animal (older or debilitated animals). Sirois M, Principles and Practice of Veterinary Technology, ed 3, Mosby, 2011, p. 382.

299. b Early signs of surgical wound dehiscence are frequently seen within the first 3 or 4 days after surgery. They may include a serosanguineous discharge from the incision, firm or fluctuant swelling deep to (under) the suture line, and palpation of a hernial ring or loop of bowel beneath the skin. Sirois M, Principles and Practice of Veterinary Technology, ed 3, Mosby, 2011, p. 382.

300. b If both the muscle layer and the skin sutures of an abdominal incision break down, the animal can eviscerate (abdominal organs protrude through suture line). If evisceration occurs, the involved organs can become bruised and grossly contaminated and the animal itself might even mutilate them. Sirois M, Principles and Practice of Veterinary Technology, ed 3, Mosby, 2011, p. 382.

301. d Four main factors determine whether infection occurs: number of microorganisms (there must be sufficient microorganisms to overcome the defenses of the animal); virulence of the microorganisms (their ability to cause disease); susceptibility of the animal (some individuals have a greater natural resistance to infection than others); route of exposure to the microorganisms (some routes of exposure are more likely to result in infection than others). Sirois M, Principles and Practice of Veterinary Technology, ed 3, Mosby, 2011, p. 382.

302. d Improper application of methods of sanitation, sterilization, and disinfection can lead to microbial resistance and increase the risk of nosocomial (hospital-acquired) infection. Sirois M, Principles and Practice of Veterinary Technology, ed 3, Mosby, 2011, p. 382.

303. c Sterile patient preparation consists of three rounds of alternating antiseptic solution with saline rinse. Sirois M, Principles and Practice of Veterinary Technology, ed 3, Mosby, 2011, p. 382.

304. d A patient would experience all of the clinical signs except hypotension. A patient in pain would experience hypertension. Sirois M, Principles and Practice of Veterinary Technology, ed 3, Mosby, 2011, p. 336.

305. c The No. 2 suture is the largest of these options and a cow's uterus, being large and heavy, requires larger suture material. The more zeros, the smaller the suture; therefore, it would be less likely keep such an incision closed. Largest to smallest suture of the options provided are 2, 1, 2-0, 3-0. Tear M, Small Animal Surgical Nursing, ed 2, Elsevier, 2012.

306. c Multifilament suture material has a greater chance of wicking bacteria than the single strand in a monofilament suture. A multifilament suture has better knot security than monofilament, is no more traumatic to tissue than monofilament, and can have more strength than a monofilament suture. Tear M, Small Animal Surgical Nursing, ed 2, Elsevier, 2012, p. 34-35.

307. c Polyethylene is a monofilament suture, whereas polyglactin, polyester, and cotton are multifilament suture material. Table 1-2 "Summary and Comparison of Common Suture Material," Tear M, Small Animal Surgical Nursing, ed 2, Elsevier, 2012, p. 34.

308. d Stainless steel wire would have the greatest tensile strength and least flexibility of any of the materials listed, making it the one that would present the least ease of use. Silk, braided polyglycolic, and chromic catgut all are handled easily. Tear M, Small Animal Surgical Nursing, ed 2, Elsevier, 2012, p. 34.

309. b A good suture material would not constitute a favorable environment for bacterial growth. Ideally, minimal tissue reaction, comfort when working with the material, and economically efficient would be characteristics to look for. Tear M, Small Animal Surgical Nursing, ed 2, Elsevier, 2012, p. 34-35.

310. a Inverted suture patterns turn tissue toward the lumen of a hollow organ, away from the surgeon. The purse-string pattern is the only one that fits that description. Simple interrupted, interrupted horizontal mattress, and simple continuous patterns turn the tissue edges outward toward the surgeon but away from the patient. Fossum TW, Small Animal Surgery, ed 3, Mosby, 2007, p. 66.

311. b Synthetic absorbable suture loses most of its breaking strength within 60 days of placement; they are absorbed by hydrolysis. At 30 days, the tensile strength would still be acceptable. Past 60 days, the suture strength would be negligible. Bassert JM, Thomas JA, McCurnin's Clinical Textbook for Veterinary Technicians, ed 8, Elsevier, 2014, p. 1201.

312. c Catgut is rapidly removed from infected sites or areas where it is exposed to digestive enzymes. It is a natural (not synthetic) suture type and is therefore more susceptible to phagocytic activity. Synthetic suture (Vicryl, PDS, and nylon) is more resistant to phagocytic activity. Fossum TW, Small Animal Surgery, ed 3, Mosby, 2007, p. 59.

313. d The age of the animal is not a consideration when choosing suture material. The surgeon's experience, the part of the body being sutured, and the size of the animal are all considerations when choosing suture material. Tear M, Small Animal Surgical Nursing, ed 2, Elsevier, 2012, p. 35.

314. b With each suture placed, the stress on the other sutures is decreased; thus, more sutures are better than fewer. Large sutures increase trauma that is induced during placement and they result in a greater quantity of foreign material left inside the patient. Bassert JM, Thomas JA, McCurnin's Clinical Textbook for Veterinary Technicians, ed 8, Elsevier, 2014, p. 1201.

315. c Surgical catgut is not recommended for internal use because of its rapid absorption and short duration of tensile strength. The rate of absorption is variable and unpredictable. This rapid loss of strength calls into question its use for securing support layers. Bassert JM, Thomas JA, McCurnin's Clinical Textbook for Veterinary Technicians, ed 8, Elsevier, 2014, p. 1202.

316. a This chemical reaction increases strength, decreases absorption, and reduces tissue reaction. Decreased strength, increased tissue reaction, and decreased absorption are not qualities associated with treatment using basic chromium salts. Sirois M, Principles and Practice of Veterinary Technology, ed 3, Mosby, 2011, p. 407.

317. c If a proper aseptic technique is used, antibiotics should not be administered for short, routine, uncomplicated procedures. The longer the procedure takes, the more likely contamination will occur and antibiotics should be given to prevent infection. Box 10-1, "Examples of Surgical Procedures that Warrant Prophylactic Antibiotics," Fossum TW, Small Animal Surgery, ed 3, Mosby, 2007, p. 86.

318. a The Balfour retractor is used to hold the abdominal wall open. A rongeur is used to trim bone, a periosteal elevator is used in dental procedures, and thumb forceps are used to hold and maneuver delicate tissue. Sonsthagen TF, Veterinary Instruments and Equipment: a Pocket Guide, ed 2, Elsevier, 2011, p. 561.

319. b The Lempert, also called a Ruskin, is used to break up or remove small pieces of bone. A retractor is used to retract skin, a periosteal elevator is used to remove teeth, and a thumb forceps is used to pick up, hold, and maneuver delicate tissues. Sonsthagen TF, Veterinary Instruments and Equipment: a Pocket Guide, ed 2, Elsevier, 2011, p. 581.

320. a Chlorhexidine does not stain the skin and hair coat. It is effective against *Pseudomonas* and *E. coli*, one of the trade names is Nolvasan, and rinsing with alcohol increases its residual activity. Tear M, Small Animal Surgical Nursing, ed 2, Elsevier, 2012, p. 70-71.

321. b After the gauze has touched hair or any other dirty or contaminated area, it must never return to the scrub area. Therefore, it must be discarded and replaced with a new sponge. Tear M, Small Animal Surgical Nursing, ed 2, Elsevier, 2012, p. 72.

322. b The target pattern is the most common scrub pattern; it is used to prepare surgical sites for abdominal, thoracic, and neurologic procedures. There should be a systematic pattern to ensure proper asepsis, moving from the site of the future incision outward, and there should be rinsing in between to remove any residual contamination between scrubs. Tear M, Small Animal Surgical Nursing, ed 2, Elsevier, 2012, p. 72.

323. b The purse-string suture is placed before preparing the area for perineal procedures. This prevents the evacuation of fecal material onto the surgical site during the procedure. It has no bearing on the tail or the urethra, nor does it affect the perianal skin. Tear M, Small Animal Surgical Nursing, ed 2, Elsevier, 2012, p. 74-75.

324. d The prepuce is flushed with weak povidone solution to remove potential contaminants. It would not be sutured closed; however, it is considered contaminated and therefore needs to be afforded special consideration. Flushing with alcohol while the animal is awake would be painful for the animal and would not provide appropriate antiseptic properties. Tear M, Small Animal Surgical Nursing, ed 2, Elsevier, 2012, p. 71.

325. c Unless contraindicated, the urinary bladder should be emptied to prevent the animal from urinating during the surgical procedure. Lying in urine during the surgery could lead to hypothermia and/or urine scald. The stomach and gallbladder cannot be emptied in advance of surgery. Expressing the anal glands is a good customer-service gesture, but it is not required before surgery. Tear M, Small Animal Surgical Nursing, ed 2, Elsevier, 2012, p. 70.

326. b Metzenbaum is a type of surgical scissor whose primary function is to cut delicate tissue or to assist in blunt dissection. Needle holders are used to hold a surgical needle, whereas the function of a towel clamp is to clamp sterile surgical towels to the patient. Hemostatic forceps are used to grasp blood vessels or to clamp and hold tissue or vessels. Sonsthagen TF, Veterinary Instruments and Equipment: a Pocket Guide, ed 2, Elsevier, 2011, p. 495.

327. c The purpose of the rongeur is to remove or break up small chunks of bone, cartilage, or fibrous tissue. Hemostatic forceps would be used to pinch off a bleeding vessel and a dressing forceps could be used to remove small pieces of bone. A periosteal elevator would elevate soft tissue away from bone. Sonsthagen TF, Veterinary Instruments and Equipment: a Pocket Guide, ed 2, Elsevier, 2011, p. 581.

328. b Talking and nonessential personnel should be kept to a minimum in the surgical suite to reduce distractions and to allow more careful monitoring of the patient. Talking with fellow team members would not inject bacteria into the operating suite, nor would it have a direct effect on expediting the surgery. Tear M, Small Animal Surgical Nursing, ed 2, Elsevier, 2012, p. 103.

329. a Operating scissors are used to cut inanimate materials, including suture and drape material. Metzenbaums are for cutting fine tissue only. Scalpel blades are used to cut tissue, whereas wire scissors are used to cut wire in orthopedic surgeries. Sonsthagen TF, Veterinary Instruments and Equipment: a Pocket Guide, ed 2, Elsevier, 2011, p. 499.

330. b The Army-Navy is the only handheld retractor listed. Sonsthagen TF, Veterinary Instruments and Equipment: a Pocket Guide, ed 2, Elsevier, 2011, p. 553.

331. a The purpose of the preoperative skin preparation is to remove soil and transient microorganisms, to reduce the resident microbial count to subpathogenic levels, and to inhibit rapid rebound growth of microorganisms. Scrubbed areas should not be touched with ungloved hands and scrubbing should be done in a consistent, fastidious manner. Alcohol has been shown to increase the residual activity and it is therefore recommended, regardless of the surgical prep solution chosen. Fossum TW, Small Animal Surgery, ed 3, Mosby, 2007, p. 34.

332. b Ethylene oxide can be used on objects that cannot withstand the heat or pressure of steam sterilization. Autoclaving and flash flaming would damage the item. An alcohol scrub would not provide sterilization. Fossum TW, Small Animal Surgery, ed 3, Mosby, 2007, p. 11.

333. b Asepsis is the absence of pathogenic microorganisms that cause infection. Uncontaminated, healthy, and clean do not refer to the lack of infection as it applies to surgical technique. Tear M, Small Animal Surgical Nursing, ed 2, Elsevier, 2012, p. 101.

334. d Filtration refers to the use of a filter to separate particulate material from liquids or gases. Pharmaceuticals are commonly sterilized by filtration. A nutrient solution is not an option because the question asks for surgical materials. Irrigation and surgical solutions are sterilized, but not by filtration. Bassert JM, Thomas JA, McCurnin's Clinical Textbook for Veterinary Technicians, ed 8, Elsevier, 2014, p. 1161.

335. c Autoclaves are designed to deliver saturated steam under pressure. The increased pressure causes steam to achieve a higher temperature. Ovens and crematoriums provide heat without steam. Plasma sterilization is a low-temperature sterilization technique that has become the method of choice for sterilizing heat-sensitive items. Bassert JM, Thomas JA, McCurnin's Clinical Textbook for Veterinary Technicians, ed 8, Elsevier, 2014, p. 1163.

336. b Sterilization indicators undergo color changes when subjected to saturated steam for adequate time periods. Because they are placed inside the pack, the color change ensures that the center of the pack reached the optimal temperature and pressure. Sterilization tape changes color, but it only indicates that the optimal temperature and pressure were reached on the outside of the pack. One cannot inspect surgical packs for microorganisms. Bassert JM, Thomas JA, McCurnin's Clinical Textbook for Veterinary Technicians, ed 8, Elsevier, 2014, p. 1164.

337. b Materials need to be packed as loosely as is practical to ensure good steam penetration in autoclaves. Autoclaves can be used for metal surgical instruments and implants and they are very economical for most veterinary clinics. Autoclaves should not be used to resterilize syringes for vaccines. Bassert JM, Thomas JA, McCurnin's Clinical Textbook for Veterinary Technicians, ed 8, Elsevier, 2014, p. 1161.

338. b Electrocautery can be used to cut or coagulate vessels; however, it does not sterilize skin. It can be used for surgical procedures, but it can be traumatic and should be used with caution. Tear M, Small Animal Surgical Nursing, ed 2, Elsevier, 2012, p. 16.

339. b Warming, stimulation through rubbing, and suctioning the airway are all correct procedures for resuscitating puppies and kittens following c-section. Swinging puppies and kittens is not considered a correct method for clearing the airway. Tear M, Small Animal Surgical Nursing, ed 3, Elsevier, 2012, p. 147.

340. b If a radiopaque sponge is missing, an x-ray may be taken to look for the sponge. The patient should not be re-explored because the sponges are detectable on x-ray and can save extra surgical time on the patient. Sponges are not absorbable and need to be removed if left in the patient. Tear M, Small Animal Surgical Nursing, ed 3, Elsevier, 2012, p. 122-123.

341. b If a proper aseptic technique is used, antibiotics should not be given for short, routine, uncomplicated procedures. Proper attire, scrubbing, and asepsis remove the need for prophylactic antibiotic use. Indiscriminate use of antibiotics can lead to antibiotic resistance. Box 10-1 " Examples of Surgical Procedures that Warrant Prophylactic Antibiotics," Fossum TW, Small Animal Surgery, ed 3, Mosby, 2007, p. 86.

342. b A disinfectant is an agent that destroys or kills bacteria. Bacterial static agents would slow proliferation. The mechanical action associated with scrubbing the area will remove organic debris, but not kill bacteria. Flushing bacteria from the site can be obtained with the use of a bacterial disinfectant, but it is not the main function of the disinfectant. Bassert JM, Thomas JA, McCurnin's Clinical Textbook for Veterinary Technicians, ed 8, Elsevier, 2014, p. 1164.

343. d To keep the surgical environment as free of microorganisms as possible, routine cleaning and disinfection should be performed throughout the hospital. The placement of the surgical suite within the practice can decrease contamination, but this does not preclude the need to keep the remaining environment clean. Although it is a good idea to keep the environment clean for good public relations, it is not the primary reason to keep the entire clinic clean (patient health is). AVMA does not mandate cleaning practices within the hospital, although they can make recommendations. Fossum TW, Small Animal Surgery, ed 3, Mosby, 2007, p. 19.

344. c The sterile drapes are used to establish a sterile field; therefore, only the draped field on the patient and instrument table are considered the sterile field. The shaved and prepped patient (when not draped) is not considered the sterile field. Tear M, Small Animal Surgical Nursing, ed 2, Elsevier, 2012, p. 102.

345. c All personnel moving within or around a sterile field should do so in a manner to maintain the integrity of the sterile field. A surgical nurse must be concerned with maintaining the aseptic technique and must wear sterile gloves while assisting the surgeon (passing instruments, gauze, etc.). An anesthesia nurse is responsible for keeping the animal anesthetized and monitoring vital signs. Tear M, Small Animal Surgical Nursing, ed 2, Elsevier, 2012, p. 103.

346. b Perineal urethrostomies are performed on male cats with recurrent urethral obstruction. Female cats do not have a urethra. Gastric torsions (stomach twist) and pyometras (pus-filled uterus) are not related to urethras. Sirois M, Principles and Practice of Veterinary Technology, ed 3, Mosby, 2011, p. 380.

347. a During surgery, the aseptic technique protects the exposed tissues of the patient from four main sources of potential contamination: the operative personnel, the surgical instruments and equipment, the patient itself, and the surgical environment. If a proper aseptic technique is followed, the patient would be the only source of contamination. Sirois M, Principles and Practice of Veterinary Technology, ed 3, Mosby, 2011, p. 382.

348. c Clean, freshly laundered scrub suits should be donned just before entry into the surgery room. Scrubs should not be worn from home, while treating other patients, or when checking in patients. To decrease the risk of contamination, the scrubs must be dedicated to surgery use only. Box 3-1, "Surgical Dress Code," Tear M, Small Animal Surgical Nursing, ed 2, Elsevier, 2012, p. 86.

349. b Masks filter droplets containing microorganisms that come from the mouth and nose and they should be changed frequently. After masks become wet, strike through can occur and this decreases their effectiveness. They do not prevent odors from reaching the wearer. Tear M, Small Animal Surgical Nursing, ed 2, Elsevier, 2012, p. 87.

350. d Surgical gowns must be folded so that they can be easily donned without breaking sterile technique. Tying the arms together would decrease the ease in which the gown could be donned. The inside of the gown should be on the outside so that if any of it is touched while gowning, the outer surface remains sterile. Sirois M, Principles and Practice of Veterinary Technology, ed 3, Mosby, 2011, p. 387.

351. c The back of the gown or the body is never considered sterile, regardless of the situation. Tear M, Small Animal Surgical Nursing, ed 2, Elsevier, 2012, p. 94.

352. b Bone wax as the name implies, is a hemostatic agent made of bees wax and a softening agent and is used on a cut bone surface to assist with hemorrhage control. Cautery is used to stop bleeding in vessels or soft tissues. Gelfoam is used to stop bleeding in a tissue defect such as the liver. Tear M, Small Animal Surgical Nursing, ed 3, Elsevier, 2012, p. 122-123.

353. c The counted brush stroke method addresses scrubbing hands and arms in a methodical, consistent manner. The anatomic timed method involves scrubbing hands and arms for a set time. Both methods, if performed correctly, provide appropriate asepsis. Procedure 15-3, "Surgical Personnel Scrub Procedures," Sirois M, Principles and Practice of Veterinary Technology, ed 3, Mosby, 2011, p. 395.

354. b The timed anatomic scrub should be a minimum of 5 minutes, 2–3 minutes per arm. Procedure 15-3, "Surgical Personnel Scrub Procedures," Sirois M, Principles and Practice of Veterinary Technology, ed 3, Mosby, 2011, p. 395.

355. b Closed gloving provides the least chance of glove contamination; the individual's fingers never extend past the sterile sleeve cuff, preventing contamination. In the open gloving technique, the fingers do extend past the sleeve cuffs, allowing accidental contamination. Assisted gloving allows the possibility of contamination. Double gloving does not routinely occur. Bassert JM, Thomas JA, McCurnin's Clinical Textbook for Veterinary Technicians, ed 8, Elsevier, 2014, p. 1176.

356. a Gowns are not worn as part of the open gloving process; this statement is therefore false because the question pertains to open gloving. All other statements are part of the open gloving procedure. Tear M, Small Animal Surgical Nursing, ed 3, Elsevier, 2012, p. 113-115.

357. b Povidone-iodine is bactericidal, virucidal, fungistatic, and fungicidal. Iodophors will stain clothing and fur, are tissue toxic, and have less residual activity than chlorhexidine. Tear M, Small Animal Surgical Nursing, ed 2, Elsevier, 2012, p. 70-71.

358. d Only essential personnel should be present and movement should be kept to a minimum to prevent contamination. Temperatures should remain as low as possible to reduce the likelihood of microorganism replication. Bassert JM, Thomas JA, McCurnin's Clinical Textbook for Veterinary Technicians, ed 8, Elsevier, 2014, p. 1182.

359. a The manual cleaning, or decontamination, of the instrument is done to help break down the biologic debris. Ultrasonic cleaners can then be used after the manual cleaning to reach inaccessible areas on the instruments. Tear M, Small Animal Surgical Nursing, ed 2, Elsevier, 2012, p. 258-259.

360. b Alcohols are used as disinfectants and antiseptic agents. Although they are bactericidal, they are ineffective against spores and fungi and therefore cannot be used to sterilize instruments. Alcohol has no residual activity. Bassert JM, Thomas JA, McCurnin's Clinical Textbook for Veterinary Technicians, ed 8, Elsevier, 2014, p. 1168.

361. c Quaternary ammonium products are effective against both gram-positive and gram-negative bacteria, have low toxicity, and do not require long contact times. Chlorhexidine must be in contact with the surface for at least 5 minutes to be effective. Isopropyl alcohol needs to be applied multiple times to be effective, and povidone-iodine are antiseptics, not disinfectants. Table 9-1, "Comparison of Different Types of Disinfectants," Tear M, Small Animal Surgical Nursing, ed 2, Elsevier, 2012, p. 257.

362. b A 10% diluted povidone-iodine solution would be acceptable to instill into the conjunctival sac before surgery. 10% chlorhexidine and 5% isopropyl alcohol would damage the tissues and diluted soapy water would initiate a burning sensation. Fossum TW, Small Animal Surgery, ed 3, Mosby, 2007, p. 260.

363. b Clean-contaminated wounds are identified when nonsterile luminal organs are entered without significant spillage of contents. A clean wound is classified as nontraumatic, noninflamed operative wounds in which the respiratory, gastrointestinal, genitourinary, and oropharyngeal tracts are not entered. A contaminated surgery is classified as an open, fresh, accidental wound; procedures in which gastrointestinal contents or infected urine is spilled; or a major break in aseptic technique. Fossum TW, Small Animal Surgery, ed 3, Mosby, 2007, p. 84.

364. a Exogenous organisms are those from sources outside the patient's body and would include those that come from the surgeon and those that come from the external surgical environment. They can originate from the patient's own body and can cause serious issues in surgical wounds. Tear M, Small Animal Surgical Nursing, ed 2, Elsevier, 2012, p. 86.

365. d Breaks will occur; it is important to have plans to remedy the situation. Any break in aseptic technique should be immediately reported and addressed or corrected. The surgery does not need to be stopped, but the break cannot be ignored because it can lead to serious complications, regardless of when it occurs. Although the break is serious, it does not mean the patient will die. Tear M, Small Animal Surgical Nursing, ed 2, Elsevier, 2012, p. 101.

366. a Daily cleaning should be done at the end of the day because cleaning creates airborne dust that takes several hours to settle. Bassert JM, Thomas JA, McCurnin's Clinical Textbook for Veterinary Technicians, ed 8, Elsevier, 2014, p. 1169.

367. b Performing a gastric lavage helps to dilute any pollutants and when warm lavage fluids are used, this will warm the patient. Sterile fluid should not provide a medium for bacteria growth and lavage can be done to help reduce the likelihood of sepsis. Tear M, Small Animal Surgical Nursing, ed 2, Elsevier, 2012, p. 138.

368. a Elective procedures are not necessary to the patient's immediate health. A nephrotomy, exploratory laparotomy, and a splenectomy would be completed because of a critical presentation in the animal. Bassert JM, Thomas JA, McCurnin's Clinical Textbook for Veterinary Technicians, ed 8, Elsevier, 2014, p. 1224.

369. b Taper-point needles do not leave small cuts associated with the cutting point; this is less traumatic for the patient and forms a sealed suture line. They would have difficulty passing through the skin and are no more expensive than cutting needles. They are able to pass easily through viscera. Tear M, Small Animal Surgical Nursing, ed 2, Elsevier, 2012, p. 32.

370. b The stem word thorac- refers to the chest; therefore, a thoracotomy would refer to an incision into the chest. Abdomin- refers to the abdominal cavity; crani- refers to the skull, and ot- refers to the ear. Colville T, Bassert JM, Clinical Anatomy and Physiology for Veterinary Technicians, ed 2, Mosby, 2008, p. 6.

371. a The suffix -ectomy means to remove surgically. Reduction is the replacement or realignment, exudate or aspiration refers to drainage, and -otomy refers to an incision. Sirois M, Principles and Practice of Veterinary Technology, ed 3, Mosby, 2011, p. 75.

372. d Often shortened to K-E, this apparatus has threaded cross-pins that are drilled into the bone and then attached to bars with clamps, nuts and bolts, or aluminum rings to make an external tension device. Rush pinning, Steinmann fixation, and stack pinning are all internal techniques that do not use bolts to hold in place. Tear M, Small Animal Surgical Nursing, ed 2, Elsevier, 2012, p. 186.

373. b The root arthro- refers to a joint and the suffix -otomy refers to making an incision. The root arteri- refers to an artery, my- refers to joint, and osteo- refers to bone. Sirois M, Principles and Practice of Veterinary Technology, ed 3, Mosby, 2011, p. 75.

374. c Hemostasis is the arrest of bleeding. Aspiration refers to removing air or liquid, fibrinolysis is the reduction or lysing of fibrin, and hemolysis refers to the breaking or lysing of blood cells. Sirois M, Principles and Practice of Veterinary Technology, ed 3, Mosby, 2011, p. 405.

375. b A thin membrane called the peritoneum lines the abdomen; when it becomes inflamed, it is known as peritonitis. Pericarditis is the inflammation of the pericardial space. Inflammation caused by parasites is termed *parasitosis*. Colville T, Bassert JM, Clinical Anatomy and Physiology for Veterinary Technicians, ed 2, Mosby, 2008, p. 6.

376. a If the testicle(s) have not descended into the scrotal sac, a cryptorchidectomy is performed. The procedure is not performed as a result of complications, nor is it similar to the vasectomy procedure done in humans. The only treatment of cryptorchidism is surgery and it is not related to cryptosporidiosis, which is a parasite. Sirois M, Principles and Practice of Veterinary Technology, ed 3, Mosby, 2011, p. 379.

377. b Fenestration is the creation of a window. Fenestrated drapes have a small window for the incision site; the surgeon fenestrates an intervertebral disk to remove disk material. Fossum TW, Small Animal Surgery, ed 3, Mosby, 2007, p. 1402.

378. b The primary indication for an OHE is to sterilize the animal. Contrary to common misconceptions, it does not reduce the activity level in animals. The procedure involves the removal of the ovaries and the uterus and therefore can only be performed on female patients. Having a litter is not a prerequisite for a spay/OHE procedure. Tear M, Small Animal Surgical Nursing, ed 2, Elsevier, 2012, p. 149.

379. b The prefix hepat- refers to the liver. Heme- refers to blood and gastro- refers to stomach. Heparin preparations refer to the use of heparin to preserve blood samples for later evaluation. Sirois M, Principles and Practice of Veterinary Technology, ed 3, Mosby, 2011, p. 76.

380. b Ligation can be used to occlude blood vessels and prevent bleeding. When vessels are ligated, they are not necessarily removed from the body and can be ligated via pressure, suture material, or cauterization. Ligation of vessels can occur in routine or emergency situations. Tobias KM, Johnston SA, Veterinary Surgery: Small Animal, Elsevier, 2012, p. 211.

381. c Slough of surrounding tissue may occur with the use of chemical cauterization and is therefore traumatic to adjacent tissues. Chemical cauterization is often used in veterinary medicine, especially when toenails have been clipped too short. Chemical cauterization does not release toxic fumes. Fossum TW, Small Animal Surgery, ed 3, Mosby, 2007, p. 512.

382. a "Moist tissues are happy tissues." If tissues are kept moist, the circulation is less compromised and tissue function remains intact. Moist tissue does not enhance bacterial regeneration. The use of 70% isopropyl alcohol would be tissue toxic and would not be done. Tear M, Small Animal Surgical Nursing, ed 2, Elsevier, 2012, p. 124.

383. c Bone plates are a type of internal orthopedic fixation device and can be used in many general practices. Insertion must be done with a skin incision. Tear M, Small Animal Surgical Nursing, ed 2, Elsevier, 2012, p. 182.

384. b Distal refers to the area farthest away from the trunk; proximal refers to the area of bone closest to the trunk. The inner portion of the bone is the medulla and the outer layer of the bone is the cortex. Sirois M, Principles and Practice of Veterinary Technology, ed 3, Mosby, 2011, p. 79.

385. d Torsion is the act of twisting or the state of being twisted. Studdert, VP, Gay CC, Blood DC, Saunders Comprehensive Veterinary Dictionary, ed 4, Saunders, 2012, p. 1114.

386. c Intramedullary pinning is performed on fractured long bones, such as the femur, and will not reduce complications to hip dysplasia. Triple pelvic osteotomy, a total hip replacement, and pectineal myotomy will help reduce complications associated with hip dysplasia. Tear M, Small Animal Surgical Nursing, ed 2, Elsevier, 2012, p. 183-186.

387. c Ear canal ablation is a surgical procedure in which the cartilaginous external ear canal is removed. Irrigation of the ear canal is simply known as flushing of the canal. An otoscope is used to examine the ear canal. Studdert, VP, Gay CC, Blood DC, Saunders Comprehensive Veterinary Dictionary, ed 4, Saunders, 2012, p. 3.

388. c Perioperative refers to the time immediately before and after a procedure. Studdert, VP, Gay CC, Blood DC, Saunders Comprehensive Veterinary Dictionary, ed 4, Saunders, 2012, p. 837.

389. b An onychectomy is also called a declaw procedure; the claw and associated third phalanx are removed. Onychectomies must be completed with anesthesia and analgesia and can be performed on both male and female cats. Castration removes a cat's testicles and spermatic cord. Tear M, Small Animal Surgical Nursing, ed 2, Elsevier, 2012, p. 163.

390. c There is always risk associated with surgery regardless of the surgeon's skill or the type of assistance provided in surgery. As a result, the client should be well informed of surgical risks and possible complications. Tear M, Small Animal Surgical Nursing, ed 2, Elsevier, 2012, p. 44-45.

391. b The purpose of any fracture fixation is to bring the opposing ends of the fracture and joints back into alignment, also known as reduction. Fracture reduction must be performed to ensure good healing and must be done with anesthesia and analgesia. Reduction does not always involve the trimming of bone adjacent to the fracture site. Tear M, Small Animal Surgical Nursing, ed 2, Elsevier, 2012, p. 182.

392. d Thoracic and abdominal radiographs are indicated for animals with major trauma to rule out the possibility of diaphragmatic hernias. Often the stomach and intestinal contents are displaced into the thoracic cavity, preventing the animal from breathing normally. These hernias can be repaired, but they can also be fatal if not repaired. Thomas JA, Lerche P, Anesthesia and Analgesia for Veterinary Technicians, ed 4, Mosby, 2011, p. 24.

393. b Part of the veterinary technician's job is to educate the client on how to care for their animal at home properly, post procedure. In addition to verbal direction given at the time of discharge, written home-care instructions should be provided to the client. Tear M, Small Animal Surgical Nursing, ed 2, Elsevier, 2012, p. 273.

394. a Gelatin sponges are placed directly into tissue defects to encourage hemostasis. The gelatin will slowly be absorbed and can be left in the body. They are not radiopaque and are available for veterinary surgery. Tear M, Small Animal Surgical Nursing, ed 2, Elsevier, 2012, p. 12.

395. a The exteriorizing of a contaminated part or organ reduces the likelihood of systemic infection. If done properly, it is not necessarily hazardous. Lavaging is still necessary. Care must be taken to keep the exteriorized part moist. Tear M, Small Animal Surgical Nursing, ed 2, Elsevier, 2012, p. 124.

396. c Intestinal resection and anastomosis is the excision of a segment of bowel followed by the reestablishment of the two remaining segments. Intussusception involves telescoping sections of the intestinal tract, enterotomy refers to incision into the intestines, and a celiotomy is incision into the abdomen. Tear M, Small Animal Surgical Nursing, ed 2, Elsevier, 2012, p. 142.

397. a Monofilament suture has less drag on the tissue and a taper-point needle should be selected when a sealed suture line is required. Nonabsorbable suture should be avoided in the urinary bladder or urethra because these sutures promote the formation of calculi. Fossum TW, Small Animal Surgery, ed 3, Mosby, 2007, p. 677.

398. d Increasing the fluid rate will increase the circulation volume, increasing overall blood pressure. Decreasing the anesthetic will result in a reversal of the cardiovascular depression caused by the anesthesia. Box 5-3, "Strategies to Prevent Hypotenstion," Thomas JA, Lerche P, Anesthesia and Analgesia for Veterinary Technicians, ed 4, Mosby, 2011, p. 153.

399. b Hypocarbia (decreased carbon dioxide levels) can be attributed to increased respiratory rate, too light a plane of anesthesia, pain, or overzealous artificial ventilation. Tear M, Small Animal Surgical Nursing, ed 2, Elsevier, 2012, p. 117.

400. c The most painful portion of the spay procedure is the plucking of the suspensory ligament. The patient may experience a temporary increase in heart rate and respiratory rate, which will resolve without intervention. Bassert JM, Thomas JA, McCurnin's Clinical Textbook for Veterinary Technicians, ed 8, Elsevier, 2014, p. 1233.

401. d Animals should be offered food as soon after recovery as possible. There is no nutritional reason to delay postoperative feeding. Delayed feeding can produce adverse effects on healing and recovery. Tear M, Small Animal Surgical Nursing, ed 2, Elsevier, 2012, p. 247.

402. a Vital signs are used primarily to determine patient safety and are only loosely correlated with the depth of anesthesia. Reflexes are more indicative of anesthetic depth. Bassert JM, Thomas JA, McCurnin's Clinical Textbook for Veterinary Technicians, ed 8, Elsevier, 2014, p. 1104.

403. d The corneal reflex should be present; its absence indicates that the anesthetic depth is too great. The other reflexes listed should be absent at a surgical plane of anesthesia. Table 29-8, "Interpretation of Reflexes and Other Indicators of Anesthetic Depth," Bassert JM, Thomas JA, McCurnin's Clinical Textbook for Veterinary Technicians, ed 8, Elsevier, 2014, p. 1107.

404. d Wound healing begins immediately after injury or incision. The four phases of wound healing are inflammation, debridement, repair, and maturation. Wound healing is dynamic; several phases occur simultaneously. The first 3 to 5 days are the lag phase of wound healing because inflammation and debridement predominate and wounds have not gained appreciable strength. Healing is influenced by host factors, wound characteristics, and other external factors. Fossum TW, Small Animal Surgery Textbook, ed 4, Mosby, 2013.

405. b An exudate composed of white blood cells, dead tissue, and wound fluid forms on wounds during the debridement phase. Fossum TW, Small Animal Surgery Textbook, ed 4, Mosby, 2013.

406. a A moist wound environment allows optimal healing. Wound fluid is allowed to remain on the wound, keeping it moist. In a moist environment, debridement is hastened and selective, granulation tissue formation is promoted, and epithelialization is faster. Allowing wound fluid to remain in contact with wounds fosters autolytic debridement by endogenous enzymes that break down necrotic, but not healthy, tissue. Moist wound healing does not promote bacterial contamination when treated appropriately. Fossum TW Small Animal Surgery Textbook, ed 4, Mosby, 2013.

407. d Corticosteroids depress all phases of wound healing and increase chances of infection. Some chemotherapeutic drugs (e.g., cyclophosphamide, methotrexate, and doxorubicin) inhibit wound healing. Radiation therapy can profoundly inhibit wound healing, depending on dose and time of exposure relative to the time of injury. It reduces the quantity of blood vessels, affects collagen maturation, and causes increased dermal fibrosis. Therefore, chemotherapeutic drugs and radiation therapy should be avoided for 2 weeks after surgery. Fossum TW, Small Animal Surgery Textbook, ed 4, Mosby, 2013.

408. d Healing is delayed if necrotic tissue is left in the wound. Devitalized tissue is removed from the wound by debridement. Debridement involves removal of dead or damaged tissue, foreign bodies, and microorganisms that compromise local defense mechanisms and delay healing. The goal of debridement is to obtain fresh clean wound margins and a wound bed for primary or delayed closure. Fossum TW, Small Animal Surgery Textbook, ed 4, Mosby, 2013.

409. b Surgical floors must be cleaned daily, whether used or not. In addition, they should be cleaned at night, allowing dust particles to settle overnight. Tear M, Small Animal Surgical Nursing, ed 2, Elsevier, 2012.

410. a Contact time refers to the amount of time a disinfectant must be in contact with a microorganism to kill or reduce levels. It is not the time required for the microorganism to develop resistance, nor is it a window of opportunity for the disinfectant to kill the microorganism. Tear M, Small Animal Surgical Nursing, ed 2, Elsevier, 2012.

411. b Ideally, the preparation area should be adjacent to the surgery room. The preparation room can be used for patient preparation and the storage of surgical supplies. AAHA also recommends placement of storage and cabinets in the preparation area, not the surgery room. The surgeon can use the preparation area to scrub and gown for surgery. Preparation should not occur within the surgical suite because this will increase the number of contaminants. It does not need to be separated by another room and it definitely does not need to be upstairs, above the surgical suite. Tear M, Small Animal Surgical Nursing, ed 2, Elsevier, 2012.

SECTION 7

1. a *Apical* is a directional term as it relates to the tooth. Apical is defined as toward the end portion or apex of the root. *Coronal* is the term that means toward the crown portion of the tooth. Cheeks and tongue are soft tissue structures related to the face and oral cavity. Mosby's Dental Dictionary, ed 2, Mosby, 2008, p. 45, 147.

2. c Gingival index 0: Clinically healthy gingiva; Gingival index 1: Mild gingivitis: slight reddening and swelling of the gingival margin; no bleeding on gentle probing of the gingival sulcus; Gingival index 2: Moderate gingivitis: the gingival margin is red and swollen; gentle probing of the gingival sulcus results in bleeding; Gingival index 3: Severe gingivitis: the gingival margin is very swollen with a red or bluish-red color; there is spontaneous hemorrhage and/or ulceration of the gingival margin. Gorrel C, "Oral examination and recording," Veterinary Dentistry for the General Practitioner, ed 2, Elsevier, 2013.
3. c Anodontia (total absence of teeth) and oligodontia (congenital absence of many but not all teeth) are associated with ectodermal dysplasia, are rare, and can occur in dogs with no apparent systemic problem or congenital syndrome. Hypodontia (absence of only a few teeth) is, however, a relatively common finding in dogs. Stomatitis is defined as inflammation of the mouth. Gorrel C, "Glossary," Veterinary Dentistry for the General Practitioner, ed 2, Elsevier, 2013, p. 215-221.
4. a UCF: Uncomplicated crown fracture; CCF: Complicated crown fracture; UCRF: Uncomplicated crown and root fracture; CCRF: Complicated crown and root fracture. Gorrel C, "Oral examination and recording," Veterinary Dentistry for the General Practitioner, ed 2, Elsevier, 2013, p. 56-66.
5. d Grade 0: No furcation involvement. Grade 1: Initial furcation involvement: the furcation can be felt with the probe/explorer, but horizontal tissue destruction is less than ⅓ of the horizontal width of the furcation. Grade 2: Partial furcation involvement: it is possible to explore the furcation but the probe/explorer cannot be passed through it; horizontal tissue destruction is >⅓ of the horizontal width of the furcation. Grade 3: Total furcation involvement: the probe/explorer can be passed through the furcation from buccal to palatal/lingual. Gorrel C, "Oral examination and recording," Veterinary Dentistry for the General Practitioner, ed 2, Elsevier, 2013, p. 56-66.
6. d Grade 0: No mobility. Grade 1: Horizontal movement of <1 mm. Grade 2: Horizontal movement of >1 mm. Note that multi-rooted teeth are scored more severely and a horizontal mobility in excess of 1 mm is usually considered a Grade 3 even in the absence of vertical movement. Grade 3: Vertical as well as horizontal movements are possible. Hence, for this question a multi-rooted tooth with >1 mm has Grade 3 mobility or a tooth with both horizontal and vertical movement can be assessed as Grade 3 mobility. Gorrel C, "Oral examination and recording," Veterinary Dentistry for the General Practitioner, ed 2, Elsevier, 2013, p. 56-66.
7. b The maxillary fourth premolar and the first and second molars have three roots. The maxillary third premolar has two roots, and there are no three-rooted teeth in the mandible. Teeth can, on occasion, develop extra or supernumerary roots; however, these are incidental findings and are only important if the tooth needs to be extracted or if it needs to have root canal therapy. Wiggs RB, Lobprise HB, Dental and oral radiology, in Veterinary Dentistry: Principles and Practices, Lippincott-Raven, 1997, p. 160.
8. b Permanent canines and premolars erupt at about 4–6 months. Adult incisors appear at 3–5 months. Adult molars appear at 5–7 months. Holzman G, The basics, in Perrone JR, ed, Small Animal Dental Procedures for Veterinary Technicians and Nurses, Wiley-Blackwell, 2013, p. 3-22.
9. a The Triadan system uses three numbers. The first number identifies one of the four quadrants of the mouth. The order is sequential, beginning with the upper right maxillary, which is assigned 1, 2 is the left maxillary, 3 the left mandibular, and 4 the right mandibular. The same format is followed for the deciduous teeth, starting with 5 for the deciduous maxillary right quadrant. The second and third numbers identify the teeth. There are always two numbers to represent the teeth. The tooth numbering begins in the front of the mouth with the central or first incisor being 01, the intermediate or second incisor 02, and the lateral or third incisor 03. The canine is always 04 and the first molar is always 09. Thus for 205, 2 refers to the left maxillary quadrant and 05 refers to the fifth tooth. 205 translates to the upper left first premolar anatomically. Holzman G, The basics, in Perrone JR, ed, Small Animal Dental Procedures for Veterinary Technicians and Nurses, Wiley-Blackwell, 2013, p. 3-22.
10. b 409 is the right mandibular first molar. 407 is the right mandibular third premolar. 408 is the right mandibular fourth premolar. 909 is the deciduous right maxillary second incisor. Cats have only three maxillary premolars and two mandibular premolars per side. The rule of 4 and 9 in the Triadan system helps standardize the nomenclature for species that have fewer teeth. The canine tooth is always designated as 04 and the first molar is always 09. The count begins backward from the first molar so that for the maxillary teeth, the fourth premolar is 08, the third premolar is 07, and the second premolar is 06, just as in the dog. The first lower right molar then is designated 409. Cats do not have a 105, 205, 305, 306, 405, or 406. These normally missing teeth are skipped in the numbering sequence. (Note: If the tooth is normally present and is not seen, it must be further investigated using dental radiographs.) Holzman G, The basics, in Perrone JR, ed, Small Animal Dental Procedures for Veterinary Technicians and Nurses, Wiley-Blackwell, 2013, p. 3-22.
11. d Collectively, these are all components of the pulp tissue that helps support odontoblastic cells that line the pulp chamber and root canal. Holzman G, The basics, in Perrone JR, ed, Small Animal Dental Procedures for Veterinary Technicians and Nurses, Wiley-Blackwell, 2013, p. 3-22.
12. c The odontoblasts that line the pulp chamber and root canal produce secondary dentin throughout life and fill in the canal, causing the dentin to widen within the parameters of the tooth body as the tooth ages. Enamel is the hardest surface in the body and it is made of an inorganic material. Pulp is within the pulp chamber/root canal of the tooth and is composed of blood vessels, nerves, and lymphatic vessels. The components of the pulp can be damaged but do not develop as the tooth ages. Gingiva surrounds the outside of the tooth as part of the tooth's support structure. Gingiva can also be damaged but does not develop as the tooth ages. Wiggs RB, Lobprise HB, Oral anatomy and physiology, in Veterinary Dentistry: Principles and Practices, Lippincott-Raven, 1997, p. 55-86.
13. d Enamel is relatively easy to clean and is slow to stain because it is acellular and is considered nonliving.

Cementum covers the root of the tooth, not enamel. Ameloblasts form enamel during tooth development, but enamel production (amelogenesis) stops just before tooth eruption and no more enamel is produced. Wiggs RB, Lobprise HB, Oral anatomy and physiology, in Veterinary Dentistry: Principles and Practices, Lippincott-Raven, 1997, p. 55-86.

14. c Dentin, which makes up the bulk of the tooth, is softer than enamel. It is a porous, organic structure. Dentin is covered by enamel on the crown surface and cementum over the root surface. The pulp is within the pulp chamber/root canal. The alveolar bone provides an anchor for the tooth root. The root is held in place by the periodontal ligament. The periodontal ligament spans from the surface of the cementum to the cribriform plate, which lines the alveolar sockets. Gorrel C, Derbyshire S, "Anatomy of the teeth and periodontium," Veterinary Dentistry for the Nurse and Technician, ed 1, Butterworth-Heinemann, 2005, p. 25-29.

15. b In a normal scissor bite, the upper fourth premolar should be buccal to the mandibular first molar. The maxillary incisors should slightly overlap the mandibular incisors. The mandibular canine teeth should fit comfortably in the diastema between the maxillary third incisor and maxillary canine with space between each tooth. The first tooth behind the upper canine is the first lower premolar. In the normal bite, each cusp points between the interdental spaces of the opposite premolar so that a zigzag or pinking-shear effect is seen. If the maxillary fourth premolar is level with or lingual to the mandibular teeth, this is called a caudal crossbite. If the maxillary fourth premolar is buccal to the mandibular fourth premolar, this is a Class 2 malocclusion where the mandibular arch occludes caudal to its normal position. Lobprise HB, "Malocclusions of teeth," Blackwell's Five-Minute Veterinary Consult Clinical Companion: Small Animal Dentistry, ed 2, Wiley-Blackwell, 2012, p. 195-203.

16. c 2 × {I 2/1:C 0/0:P 3/2:M 3/3} is the rabbit formula, 2 × {I 3/3:C 1/1:P 4/4:M 2/3} is the permanent formula for dogs, 2 × {I 3/3:C 1/1:P 3/2:M 1/1} is the permanent formula for cats. 2 × {I 3/3:C 1/1:P 3/3} is the primary formula for dogs. Gorrel C, "Anatomy of the teeth and periodontium," Veterinary Dentistry for the General Practitioner, ed 2, Elsevier, 2013, p. 36-41.

17. a Carnassial teeth in dogs are the maxillary fourth premolars and the mandibular first molars. The carnassial teeth are the largest shearing teeth in the dog and cat when compared with the other teeth. Carnassial means flesh cutting. Remember the subscript and superscript numbers tell you which side and jaw the tooth is on. The superscript means maxillary and subscript numbers mean mandibular. The number's location on the right or left of the letter tells you which side the tooth is on. Wiggs RB, Lobprise HB, "Oral anatomy and physiology," Veterinary Dentistry: Principles and Practices, Lippincott-Raven, 1997, p. 55-86.

18. c The free or marginal gingiva is the most coronal portion of the gingiva and in healthy patients lies closely around the tooth just slightly above the cementoenamel junction. This is also known as the free gingiva. The margin of the free gingiva is rounded so that a potential space is formed around the tooth called the sulcus. This sulcular depth can be measured with a periodontal probe and should normally be between 0.5 and 1.0 mm in cats and between 2.0 and 3.0 mm in dogs, depending on the tooth. The gingiva at the most apical portion is the attached gingiva. The cementum is the covering on the tooth root surface, which has no contact with the gingiva unless the support structures of the tooth recede because of periodontitis. Gorrel C, Derbyshire S, "Anatomy of the teeth and periodontium," Veterinary Dentistry for the Nurse and Technician, ed 1, Butterworth-Heinemann, 2005, p. 25-29.

19. d The periodontium is the supporting structure of the teeth and includes the periodontal ligament, gingiva, cementum, and the alveolar bone. The enamel covers the crown only. Like a shield, it protects the tooth from outside trauma. Gorrel C, Derbyshire S, "Anatomy of the teeth and periodontium," Veterinary Dentistry for the Nurse and Technician, ed 1, Butterworth-Heinemann, 2005, p. 25-29.

20. a Brachy means short and cephalic is head. Collies are described as being dolichocephalic (long head), whereas a retriever is a typical example of a mesaticephalic/mesocephalic breed (medium head). Prognacephalic is a made-up word. Bulldogs are considered brachycephalic Holzman G, "The basics," in Perrone JR, ed, Small Animal Dental Procedures for Veterinary Technicians and Nurses, Wiley-Blackwell, 2013, p. 3-22.

21. b Chlorhexidine has antibacterial properties. Cementoenamel erosion is a cavity-like lesion on the tooth. In dogs and cats this can occur from tooth resorption, which is caused by the sudden activity of odontoclasts. Normally, odontoclasts are responsible for the exfoliation of deciduous teeth. They start destroying tooth structure and replacing it with bone. On radiographs, one will see loss of root density and calcification of the periodontal ligament space. As the coronal tooth structure is destroyed, gingival tissue fills the holes until the tooth is treated or the crown falls off. At this point the patient is perceived to have a cavity. There is no way to prevent tooth resorption because it is an internal form of resorption. Chlorhexidine would have no effect on this condition. One of the side effects of prolonged use of chlorhexidine is a black staining of the teeth and tongue. Hence, chlorhexidine is not used to remove stains or to whiten teeth. Gingival hyperplasia is an overgrowth of gum tissue commonly seen in brachycephalic dogs. It causes an increase in gingival height, thus making a false pocket. Before treatment, chlorhexidine can be used to flush out the pockets to keep the bacterial levels at a minimum and to remove debris, but it does not change the condition. Treatment for this condition is to remove the excess tissue surgically, commonly called a gingivoplasty. Gorrel C, Derbyshire S, "Common oral and dental conditions," Veterinary Dentistry for the Nurse and Technician, ed 1, Butterworth-Heinemann, 2005, p. 87-107; Holmstrom SE, Frost P, Eisner ER, "Dental prophylaxis and periodontal disease stages," Veterinary Dental Techniques for the Small Animal Practitioner, ed 3, 2004, p. 175-232.

22. b A modified pen grasp should be used with overlapping pull strokes that are directed away from the gingival margin. Sickle scalers should not be used subgingivally and curettes should not be used supragingivally. Curettes are best used subgingivally. Bellows J, "Equipping your dental practice," The Practice of Veterinary Dentistry, Iowa State Press, 1999, p. 45-80.

23. b Periodontal pockets are diagnosed when the periodontal probe measures >3 mm in a dog and 0.5–1 mm in a cat. The pocket depth measurement is taken from the gingival margin to the bottom of the pocket. The normal location of the gingival margin is just slightly above the cementoenamel junction. If the gingiva has shrunk away from the normal location, two measurements are taken. The first measurement is from where the current gingival margin is to the cementoenamel junction. This measures the amount of recession or shrinkage. The second measurement is taken from where the current gingival margin is to the bottom of the pocket. This assesses whether or not there is an abnormal pocket depth. The probing depths along with dental radiographs determine the stage of periodontal disease. Wiggs RB, Lobprise HB, "Periodontology," Veterinary Dentistry: Principles and Practices, Lippincott-Raven, 1997, p. 186-231.

24. c The steps for cleaning and care of dental hand instruments are: (1) After the procedure, the instrument should be washed in disinfectant. (2) The instrument should be dried. (3) The instrument should be sharpened. (4) The instrument should be sterilized. Holmstrom SE, Frost P, Eisner ER, "Dental equipment and care," Veterinary Dental Techniques for the Small Animal Practitioner, ed 2, Saunders, 1998, p. 31-106.

25. d OSHA requires that veterinary employers provide hats, gloves, masks, and eye protection to members of staff who perform dental procedures. Dental procedures can aerosolize debris and oral bacteria, which could cause infection. Employees must take responsibility for their own safety by wearing said equipment. Holmstrom SE, Frost P, Eisner ER, "Personal safety and ergonomics," Veterinary Dental Techniques for the Small Animal Practitioner, ed 2, Saunders, 1998, p. 117-134; Cherry B, "Components of the dental operatory," in Perrone JR, ed, Small Animal Dental Procedures for Veterinary Technicians and Nurses, 2013, p. 29-44.

26. c Curettes have one or two sharp edges and a rounded toe; they are most effective for removing calculus, debris, and granulation tissue subgingivally. Curettes are designed so that each end is a mirror image of the opposite end to allow the user to treat different aspects of the tooth. The universal curette can reach all areas of the mouth. Other curettes, such as the Gracey, Columbia, and Barnhart, have variations in shank and blade length to reach specific areas of the mouth. The Morse and sickle scaler have two sharp sides and a pointed tip that allows it to be used supragingivally only. Holmstrom SE, Frost P, Eisner ER, "Dental equipment and care," Veterinary Dental Techniques for the Small Animal Practitioner, ed 2, Saunders, 1998, p. 31-106.

27. b A prophy angle used for polishing is used on low speed. Low-speed handpieces have a high torque and speeds of 5000 to 20,000 rpm. 5000 rpm is best for polishing teeth after a cleaning. 20,000 rpm is used for finishing and polishing tooth surfaces after a restoration. Holmstrom SE, Frost P, Eisner ER, "Dental equipment and care," Veterinary Dental Techniques for the Small Animal Practitioner, ed 2, Saunders, 1998, p. 31-106.

28. b When assessing jaw length, look at the word brachygnathism. Brachy- refers to short and gnath means jaw. In the word prognathism, pro refers to projecting forward. In mesaticephalic, mesati- refers to medium and cephalic means head. In dolichocephalic, dolico refers to long and narrow. Holzman G, "The basics," in Perrone JR, ed, Small Animal Dental Procedures for Veterinary Technicians and Nurses, Wiley-Blackwell, 2013, p. 3-22.

29. c Wry mouth (also known as wry bite) is a class IV malocclusion describing a discrepancy in jaw length between the right and left side of the mandible. One mandible appears longer than the maxilla whereas the opposite side is shorter. The upper and lower incisors do not align. Wry bite is a skeletal defect genetic condition in which the affected animal exhibits a nonsymmetrical head. Niemiec BA, "Pathology in the pediatric patient," Small Animal Dental, Oral and Maxillofacial Disease, Manson, 2010, p. 89-126.

30. a With posterior crossbite or caudal crossbite, the incisors are in the normal relationships, but the posterior teeth are not. The upper fourth premolars are either palatally displaced or the mandible is wider than the maxilla in the premolar area. This condition is common in dolichocephalic breeds. Bellows J, "Malocclusions of teeth," in Lobprise HB, ed, Blackwell's Five-Minute Veterinary Consult Clinical Companion: Small Animal Dentistry, ed 2, Wiley-Blackwell, 2012, p. 195-203.

31. b Base narrow mandibular canines is a class I malocclusion. The patient has a normal maxillary-to-mandible relationship, but the mandibular canines are lingually displaced. This is often seen in conjunction with retained lower deciduous teeth that push the mandibular canines inward. These base-narrow teeth then occlude with and cause trauma to the hard palate. Niemiec BA, "Pathology in the pediatric patient," Small Animal Dental, Oral and Maxillofacial Disease, Manson, 2010, p. 89-126.

32. d Rostral/anterior crossbite is a class I malocclusion and is the most common orthodontic abnormality. The premolar relationship is a normal scissor occlusion, but one or more of the incisors are misaligned. Bellows J, "Malocclusions of teeth," in Lobprise HB, ed, Blackwell's Five-Minute Veterinary Consult Clinical Companion: Small Animal Dentistry, ed 2, Wiley-Blackwell, 2012, p. 195-203.

33. d Extraction of teeth is a surgical procedure. Although it is not possible to achieve a sterile environment in the oral cavity, the mouth should be clean before extraction is performed. All teeth should be scaled and polished and the mouth should be rinsed with a chlorhexidine solution. Gorrel C, "Tooth extraction," Veterinary Dentistry for the General Practitioner, ed 2, Elsevier, 2013, p. 171-191.

34. d Dry socket or alveolar osteitis is a painful postoperative complication of extraction. It occurs mostly in humans but has occurred in dogs. It is thought to be a combination of trauma induced by the procedure, infection, loss of the primary clot, or a decreased blood supply to the alveolus. Palliative irrigation and pain management are used to treat this condition. Wiggs RB, Lobprise HB, "Oral surgery," in Veterinary Dentistry: Principles and Practices, Lippincott-Raven, 1997, p. 232-258.

35. c Gingivoplasty is the surgical contouring of the gingival tissues. This is performed to maintain tissue health and integrity. The suffix -plasty means formation or plastic repair. Gingival hyperplasia is treated using this method. Gingival hyperplasia is the excess growth of gingival tissue, causing a false pocket around the cementoenamel junction. Another condition for which gingivoplasty is performed is the suprabony pocket. The presence of a suprabony pocket means that the alveolar bone crest has decreased because of disease and will also cause a false pocket. The diseased gingiva is removed to eliminate suprabony pockets. The addition of more gingiva to a site is accomplished by performing flap surgery in which local gingiva is moved to cover a defect such as an oronasal fistula. If there are any exposed areas after the gingiva is removed, the tissue will granulate. The binding of loose teeth for stabilization is called periodontal splinting. Mosby's Dental Dictionary, ed 2, Mosby, 2008; Gorrel C, "Emergencies," Veterinary Dentistry for the General Practitioner, ed 1, 2004, Saunders, p. 131-155; Holmstrom SE, Frost P, Eisner ER, "Periodontal therapy and surgery," Veterinary Dental Techniques for the Small Animal Practitioner, ed 3, 2004, p. 233-290.

36. a When scaling the teeth, constant irrigation is essential to prevent overheating of the teeth. A water source is introduced into the scaling unit. The unit powers the water up into the scaling handpiece and out through the tip. The water acts to keep the scaler tip and the tooth from overheating. It is recommended that the tip be checked frequently for signs of wear and replaced according to the manufacturer's recommendations, but that has no bearing on the pulp tissue. The low-speed handpiece runs the prophy angle that delivers the paste and polishes the tooth surface after cleaning (and therefore does not apply to ultrasonic scaling). Low-speed handpieces that are used for polishing teeth should be run at a low speed. The rotational forces of the prophy cup holding the paste can cause thermal buildup if left longer than 3–5 seconds on a tooth. McMahon J, "The dental cleaning" in Perrone JR, ed, Small Animal Dental Procedures for Veterinary Technicians and Nurses, Wiley-Blackwell, 2013, p. 59-85.

37. c FORL is the acronym given to feline odontoclastic resorptive lesions. Although there are many names used to describe this, tooth resorption is caused by a sudden activity of cells called odontoclasts. Normally, odontoclasts are responsible for the exfoliation of deciduous teeth. They start destroying tooth structure and replacing it with bone. On radiographs, a loss of root density and a calcification of the periodontal ligament space can be seen. As the coronal tooth structure is destroyed, gingival tissue fills the holes until the tooth is treated or the crown falls off. At this point the patient is perceived to have a cavity. There is no way to prevent tooth resorption because it is an internal form of resorption. *Peripheral odontogenic fibroma* is the term used to describe fibromatous and ossifying epulides. Stomatitis is an inflammation of the soft tissues of the oral cavity caused by many different stimuli either localized or systemic. Enamel fracture is a fracture of the enamel layer of the crown. Gorrel C, Derbyshire S, "Common oral and dental conditions," Veterinary Dentistry for the Nurse and Technician, ed 1, Butterworth-Heinemann, 2005, p. 87-107; Baker L, "Stomatitis," in Lobprise HB, ed, Blackwell's Five-Minute Veterinary Consult Clinical Companion: Small Animal Dentistry, ed 2, Wiley-Blackwell, 2012, p. 237-248.

38. d Horses have teeth that can develop sharp points if they do not chew their food properly. Eating wears the teeth down, causing sharp edges to form. Floating is the filing or rasping of a horse's premolar and molar teeth to remove the sharp edges. This procedure should be performed on a regular basis to avoid oral pain. Quidding is the dropping of food while chewing, often a sign that the teeth need to be examined. Curettage, scaling, and dental radiographs are also available for equine patients. http://vetmedicine.about.com/od/equinehorseinformation/f/FloatingHorseTeeth.htm.

39. d Stoma is Greek for a mouth-like opening and -itis means inflammation. Stomatitis is the inflammation and infection of the tooth's supportive tissues. Halitosis is bad breath that will be noticed when periodontal disease is present. Tooth resorption results in the loss of tooth structure after activity of the odontoclasts in the tooth. Cheilitis is inflammation and infection of the lip. Baker L, "Stomatitis," in Lobprise HB, ed, Blackwell's Five-Minute Veterinary Consult Clinical Companion: Small Animal Dentistry, ed 2, Wiley-Blackwell, 2012, p. 237-242; Gorrel C, Derbyshire S, "Common oral and dental conditions," Veterinary Dentistry for the Nurse and Technician, Elsevier, 2005, p. 87-107.

40. c Dense rubber exercisers are the safest because they flex when the dog bites down. This flexibility will not in most cases allow the tooth to be fractured. Dried cow hooves and knucklebones are hard and could cause slab fractures and periodontal ankyloses (ligament shock-absorbing capacity that is lost because of calcification within the periodontal ligament space). Nylon ropes are abrasive and can cause gingival trauma and wear on the crowns of the teeth. If the rope fibers come loose, they can be swallowed and cause a linear foreign body. Roudebush P, Logan E, Hale FA, Evidence-based veterinary dentistry: a systemic review of homecare for prevention of periodontal disease in dogs and cats, J Vet Dent, 2005, p. 6-15.

41. c Size 4 dental film is the largest of the detail intraoral films. It is also referred to as occlusal film and is best used to ensure that the whole root is included on a large-breed dog. Size 0 dental film is for exotic breeds, toy-breed dogs, and cats. Size 2 is for small to medium dogs and cats. 8 in × 10 in screen film is used for skull x-rays or extraoral views of the jaws if dental radiographs are not available. Bellows J, "The why, when and how of small animal dental radiology," The Practice of Veterinary Dentistry, Iowa State Press, 1999, p. 81-105.

42. a Most dental radiographic film has a small raised dimple on one corner. The raised or convex side of the dimple will be on the side that should be facing up and toward the tube head and pointing rostrally. The back of the film has a tab that is used for opening the film during development. If the dimple is placed into the back of the mouth, there is an increased risk of the dimple showing up as an artifact on the tooth surface. If the backside of the film is placed toward the beam, the image will have a foil layer within the film. "The why, when and how of small animal dental radiology," Bellows J, The Practice of Veterinary Dentistry, Iowa State Press, 1999, p. 81-105.

43. c Most dental film packets have a tab in the back. The tab is used for opening the packet to remove the film for development. Within the film packet there is the film, lead foil, and black paper covering the film. The lead foil and black paper protect the film from radiation and light leaks. The lead foil sits just inside the flap side of the film, which should not face the tube head because it will cause an artifact. Bellows J, "The why, when and how of small animal dental radiology," The Practice of Veterinary Dentistry, Iowa State Press, 1999, p. 81-105.

44. c Two landmarks must be present to determine the bisecting angle—the plane of the film and the long axis of the tooth. An angle is formed where the tooth hinges to the film. That angle is bisected and the x-ray beam is at 90 degrees or perpendicular to that bisection line. If the beam is 90 degrees to the bisecting angle, minimal distortion will occur. Gorrel C, Derbyshire S, "Dental radiography," Veterinary Dentistry for the Nurse and Technician, ed 1, Butterworth-Heinemann, 2005, p. 55-67.

45. b If the x-ray beam is aimed more perpendicular to the tooth, causing too little vertical angulation, rather than to the bisecting angle, the tooth will appear more elongated. Foreshortening will occur if the beam is more perpendicular to the film, causing too much vertical angulation. The beam should be perpendicular to the bisecting angle to minimize distortion. If you think about the sun hitting an object at noon, the shadow will be very short (foreshortened). If you think about the sun hitting an object at sunset, the shadow will be very long (elongated). Bellows J, "The why, when and how of small animal dental radiology," The Practice of Veterinary Dentistry, Iowa State Press, 1999, p. 81-105.

46. d UCF: Uncomplicated crown fracture; CCF: Complicated crown fracture; UCRF: Uncomplicated crown and root fracture; CCRF: Complicated crown and root fracture. Gorrel C, "Oral examination and recording," Veterinary Dentistry for the General Practitioner, ed 2, Elsevier, 2013, p. 56-66.

47. c Hand scalers are used to remove calculus above the gum line or supragingivally. The scaler has a ridged back, two sharp sides, and a pointed tip. The tip of the scaler is used to remove debris in the developmental grooves along the crown surface. A dental explorer is used to check the tooth surface for any irregularities from an enamel fracture to pulp exposure in a fractured tooth. The working end of the explorer is a fine wire made to alert the handler that there is a defect by catching and making a pinging sound. The periodontal probe is an instrument that measures the gingival sulcus for any abnormal depths >3 mm in a dog and 0.5–1.0 mm in a cat. The periodontal probe is also used to measure how much gingival recession or gingival hyperplasia affects the tooth. The periodontal probe is marked in mm at varying intervals. Bellows J, "Equipping your dental practice," The Practice of Veterinary Dentistry, Iowa State Press, 1999, p. 45-80.

48. c Cementum is the mineralized layer that covers the root surface. The periodontal ligament arises from the cementum and attaches to the lining of the alveolar bone. Calculus is the presence of mineralized plaque bacteria on the tooth surface. Enamel is the hardest substance in the body and covers the crown of the tooth. Dentin is the mineralized layer beneath the enamel and the cementum. Perrone JR, "Common dental conditions and treatments: periodontal disease," in Perrone JR, ed, Small Animal Dental Procedures for Veterinary Technicians and Nurses, Wiley-Blackwell, 2013, p. 105-115. Gorrel C, Derbyshire S, "Anatomy of the teeth and periodontium, in Veterinary Dentistry for the Nurse and Technician, Elsevier, 2005, p. 25-29.

49. b The pulp cavity holds the blood vessels, lymphatic tissue, and nerves of the tooth. These structures exit through the apical delta at the tip of the root. In healthy patients, there is a portion of the gingiva that lies closely around the tooth just above the cementoenamel junction. This area is known as the free gingiva. The margin of the free gingiva is rounded so that a potential space is formed around the tooth called the sulcus. Teeth do not have marrow cavities; long bones do. Calculus is the presence of mineralized plaque bacteria on the tooth surface. Holzman G, "The basics," in Perrone JR, ed, Small Animal Dental Procedures for Veterinary Technicians and Nurses, Wiley-Blackwell, 2013, p. 3-22; Perrone JR, "Common dental conditions and treatments: periodontal disease," in Perrone JR, ed, Small Animal Dental Procedures for Veterinary Technicians and Nurses, Wiley-Blackwell, 2913, p. 105-114.

50. a The scaler removes plaque and calculus by making strokes across the tooth surface, taking care to scale away from the gums to avoid trauma. The scaler and all dental instruments are held using a modified pen grasp with a relaxed grip. This prevents repetitive motion injury of the hand, wrist, arm, and shoulder. There is no such thing as a screwdriver grasp. A scaler is used to remove gross calculus from the teeth, not a curette. Holmstrom SE, "Personal safety and ergonomics," Veterinary Dentistry: A Team Approach, ed 2, Saunders, 2013, p. 117-134.

51. d The spray from the ultrasonic scaler cools the tip to prevent burning the soft tissue and pulp tissue. Thermal damage to the tooth can happen if the scaler is kept on the tooth for longer than 10–15 seconds. Hand scaling should always be performed to access any surfaces that the ultrasonic scaler cannot reach. McMahon J, "The dental cleaning," in Perrone JR, ed, Small Animal Dental Procedures for Veterinary Technicians and Nurses, Wiley-Blackwell, 2013, p. 59-85.

52. b The normal sulcus depth in a cat is 0.5 to 1 mm. A periodontal probing depth of 3 mm or more in a dog or a cat is abnormal and requires further assessment with dental x-rays for signs of attachment loss and to make a treatment plan. Bellows J, "Equipping your dental practice," The Practice of Veterinary Dentistry, Iowa State Press, 1999, p. 45-80.

53. c Stomatitis is not a complication of extraction. Extraction is performed as a treatment for stomatitis. Hemorrhage, jaw fracture, and oronasal fistulas are common complications. Clotting defects may not be apparent until after extraction. Advanced periodontal disease around the mandibular teeth will weaken the mandible itself. Advanced periodontal disease destroys the medial bony wall of the alveolus, resulting in an oral nasal fistula. Gorrel C, "Emergencies;" Veterinary Dentistry for the General Practitioner, ed 2, Elsevier, 2013, p. 141-170.

54. a Carnassial tooth root abscesses can often present as a draining tract just below the eye of the affected side. Teeth can become infected through trauma, endodontic, or periodontal causes. The bacteria from infection can travel through the pulp of the tooth or along the periodontal ligament space. An abscess is a localized infection formed by the disintegration of tissues and it can cause facial swelling or travel from the tooth root and open to the outside either at the mucogingival line or erupt through the skin. Anthony JMG, Tooth root abscesses (apical abscesses), in Lobprise HB, ed, Blackwell's Five-Minute Veterinary Consult Clinical Companion: Small Animal Dentistry, ed 2, Wiley-Blackwell, 2012, p. 288-294.

55. d The care of the dental patient begins at the front desk. The receptionist must have enough knowledge of dental disease to be able to schedule the appointment to provide a balanced oral surgery session. The patient may need an initial examination for assessment and the creation of a treatment plan. The patient may have already been seen and might need a surgical appointment for treatment. The veterinary technician initially might speak to the owner on the phone, triage the patient, and involve the receptionist to schedule the patient. The veterinary technician may perform the initial conscious patient oral examination and bring findings to the veterinarian's attention. The veterinarian assesses the patient and writes up the treatment plan. The veterinary technician and the front-desk staff then prepare the owner and the patient for the next step in the treatment process. Berg M, "The examination room and the dental patient," in Perrone JR, ed, Small Animal Dental Procedures for Veterinary Technicians and Nurses, Wiley-Blackwell, 2013, p. 23-28.

56. a Adequate cooling of the bur by water (whether used in a high- or slow-speed handpiece) is mandatory. Overheating of the bur will result in damage to both the soft tissue and bone. Thermal necrosis of bone usually results in the development of a bone sequestrum that needs to be retrieved surgically as a second procedure. Elevators and extractors do not produce heat. Gorrel C, "Tooth extraction," Veterinary Dentistry for the General Practitioner, ed 2, Elsevier, 2013, p. 171-190.

57. a Brachygnathism is a class II malocclusion in which the mandible is shorter than the maxilla, causing an overshot jaw. Common problems with this condition include traumatic occlusion of the mandibular canines into the hard palate. Rhodesian ridgebacks and Labrador retrievers are prone to this condition. A mandible that is longer than the maxilla is called prognathism. The lack of incisors is hypodontia, in which some teeth are missing, and dental radiographs must be obtained to confirm that the teeth are truly missing. Polydontia is defined as an excessive number of teeth. Niemiec BA, "Pathology in the pediatric patient," Small Animal Dental, Oral and Maxillofacial Disease, Manson, 2010, p. 89-126; Lobprise HB, "Eruption disruption/abnormalities," Blackwell's Five-Minute Veterinary Consult Clinical Companion: Small Animal Dentistry, Wiley-Blackwell, ed 2, 2012, p. 157-162.

58. a Prognathism, also called an undershot jaw, is commonly seen in breeds such as the boxer, the Pekingese, and bulldogs. Prognathism is a class III malocclusion in which the mandible is longer than the maxilla. The mandibular incisors will be either level with or rostral to the maxillary incisors. The mandibular and maxillary premolars and molars will be out of alignment, causing tooth-to-tooth trauma. Brachygnathism is a class II malocclusion where the mandible is shorter than the maxilla, causing an overshot jaw. Wry bite, or wry mouth, is a class IV malocclusion describing a discrepancy in jaw length between the right and left side of the mandible. Elongated soft palate is common in these same breeds. The soft palate overlaps the epiglottis to obstruct the airway partially. Niemiec BA, "Pathology in the pediatric patient," Small Animal Dental, Oral and Maxillofacial Disease, Manson, 2010, p. 89-126.

59. d Resorptive lesions, or tooth resorption, are aggressive feline carious-like lesions that result in tooth loss; however, these are not related to malocclusion pathology. Tooth resorption is caused by a sudden activity of cells called odontoclasts. Normally, odontoclasts are responsible for the exfoliation of deciduous teeth. They start destroying tooth structure and replacing it with bone. On radiographs, loss of root density and a calcification of the periodontal ligament space can be seen. As the coronal tooth structure is destroyed, gingival tissue fills the holes until the tooth is treated or the crown falls off. At this point the patient is perceived to have a cavity. There is no way to prevent tooth resorption because it is an internal form of resorption. Gorrel C, Derbyshire S, "Common oral and dental conditions," Veterinary Dentistry for the Nurse and Technician, ed 1, Butterworth-Heinemann, 2005, p. 87-107.

60. a Adult cats do not have maxillary PM1 and mandibular PM1 and PM2. These missing teeth are not present on the feline dental chart. Holzman G, "The basics," in Perrone JR, ed, Small Animal Dental Procedures for Veterinary Technicians and Nurses, Wiley-Blackwell, 2013, p. 3-22.

61. b Furcation grades are assigned to teeth in an effort to determine how much attachment loss is present in a tooth with periodontal disease. The furcation is the space between two roots in a multirooted tooth. When the furcation is exposed, attachment loss is present. The tissues of the periodontium provide attachment and support to the tooth. Those tissues are the gingiva, periodontal ligament, and alveolar bone. Furcation exposure is graded using a periodontal probe. An attempt is made to enter the furcation using the probe and to measure how far into the furcation it goes. In grade F1 the probe just enters the furcation. In grade F2 the probe goes halfway across the furcation, and in grade F3 the probe goes all the way across the furcation. All grades of furcation exposure require dental radiographs to be taken to assess whether bone destruction is present. If >50% of the root's length has no bone attachment, the tooth is normally extracted. The area between the cementum and the enamel is the cementoenamel junction. The space between the root and the alveolar bone is the periodontal ligament space. The space between two teeth is the interdental space. McMahon J, "The dental cleaning," in Perrone JR, ed, Small Animal Dental Procedures for Veterinary Technicians and Nurses, Wiley-Blackwell, 2013, p. 59-85; Holzman G, "The basics," in Perrone JR, ed, Small Animal Dental Procedures for Veterinary Technicians and Nurses, Wiley Blackwell, 2013, p. 3-22.

62. c Feline stomatitis is an inflammation of any structures of the oral cavity. Tooth resorption or resorptive lesions are the resorption of the hard dental tissues by cells called odontoclasts. There are two types: internal resorption and external resorption. Internal resorption is caused by trauma. The lesions affect the area around the pulp chamber. External resorption of the tooth or root can also be caused by trauma, periapical disease, or neoplasia. Chronic osteitis/alveolitis occurs with chronic periodontitis, causing a bony change to the alveolus. Pocket formation and mobility can occur. Because of the excess bone deposition, the maxillary canine teeth become super erupted. Indolent ulcers are one of the oral manifestations of eosinophilic granuloma complex. They may have a hypersensitivity and genetic cause. Baker L, "Stomatitis," in Lobprise HB, ed, Blackwell's Five-Minute Veterinary Consult Clinical Companion: Small Animal Dentistry, ed 2, Wiley-Blackwell, 2012, p. 237-242; Reiter AM, "Tooth resorption: feline," in Lobprise HB, ed, Blackwell's Five-Minute Veterinary Consult Clinical Companion: Small Animal Dentistry, ed 2, Wiley-Blackwell, 2012, p. 369-379.

63. c The definition of an oronasal fistula is the communication between the oral cavity and the nasal cavity. Maxillary canine tooth root abscessation resulting from periodontal disease often results in the development of an oronasal fistula. The root tip of the maxillary canine is adjacent to a very thin plate of bone. The pathogenic bacteria found in periodontal disease causes bone destruction that breaks through that thin plate of bone into the nasal cavity. An incisor root abscess, although in the same vicinity as the maxillary canine tooth, does not usually cause an oronasal fistula. Retained deciduous incisors will have root resorption and will fall out. Should the retained deciduous incisors be fractured, an abscess could occur, but a fistula does not usually occur. Mandibular canine teeth are in the lower jaw and there is therefore no chance of an oronasal fistula even if an abscess develops on those teeth. Niemiec BA, "Pathologies of the oral mucosa," Small Animal Dental, Oral and Maxillofacial Disease, Manson, 2010, p. 183-198.

64. a Dogs with chronic allergies that engage in chewing and self-excoriation in combination with malocclusions have impaction of hair between the incisor teeth. The subsequent infection causes periodontal disease. The bacteria from the periodontal disease travels apically down the root to the alveolar bone, resulting in chronic osteomyelitis. The animals often lose their teeth and experience pain secondary to the infection. Toy-breed dogs are commonly affected with malocclusions. There are many toy breeds that have a brachycephalic head shape that causes malocclusion. Toy breeds should have the same number of teeth as large-breed dogs. The toy-breed mouth is very small and the teeth fit in however they can, usually by rotating or crowding. This can cause a malocclusion and abnormal wear. Enamel hypoplasia is a developmental disorder of the enamel layer of the tooth. Ameloblasts are the cells responsible for the formation of the enamel during the development of the deciduous and adult teeth. Illness in the animal during the development of the tooth can disrupt the normal function of the ameloblasts. The crowns of the affected teeth have areas of normal enamel and areas of missing or inadequate enamel. Anthony JMG, "Tooth root abscesses (apical abscesses)," in Lobprise HB, ed, Blackwell's Five-Minute Veterinary Consult Clinical Companion: Small Animal Dentistry, ed 2, Wiley-Blackwell, 2012, p. 288-294; Niemiec, "Pathology in the pediatric patient," Small Animal Dental, Oral, and Maxillofacial Disease, CRC Press, 2010, p. 89-126.

65. a The term *epulis* is primarily a descriptive term for any swelling in the oral cavity. Epulides are the fourth most common oral mass in dogs and they are rare in cats. Epulides arise from the periodontal connective tissue. There are three classifications: fibromatous epulis, ossifying epulis, and acanthomatous epulis. Fibromatous and ossifying epulides are now categorized as peripheral odontogenic fibromas. Acanthomatous epulides or acanthomatous ameloblastoma are nonmalignant, meaning they do not spread to other organs of the body. They are unique from other epulides in that they are locally invasive into the surrounding bone and therefore require wider margins around the tumor for complete removal. Lobprise HB, "Epulis," Blackwell's Five-Minute Veterinary Consult Clinical Companion: Small Animal Dentistry, ed 2, Wiley-Blackwell, 2012, p. 303-309.

66. c Eosinophilic granulomas and indolent ulcers are allergy-related lesions that occur in cats. The inciting cause has not been well defined. They resolve without treatment but are often responsive to corticosteroid administration. They often recur. Eosinophilic granulomas appear in the oral cavity as ulcerations on the tongue, palate, and palatine arches. Indolent ulcers are among the oral manifestations of the eosinophilic granuloma complex. They appear as raised ulcerated lesions confined to the lip margin adjacent to the philtrum. Feline resorptive lesions are resorptions of the hard dental tissues by cells called odontoclasts. There are two types: the internal resorption and the external resorption. Internal resorption is caused by trauma. The lesions affect the area around the pulp chamber. External resorption of the tooth or root can also be caused by trauma, periapical disease, or neoplasia. To rule out whether a lesion is caused by trauma or is a tumor, examination of a biopsy sample by a pathologist is recommended. Werner AH, Helton Rhodes K, "Eosinophilic granuloma complex," in Lobprise HB, ed, Blackwell's Five-Minute Veterinary Consult Clinical Companion: Small Animal Dentistry, ed 2, Wiley-Blackwell, 2012, p. 420-426; Reiter AM, "Tooth resorption: feline," in Lobprise HB, Blackwell's Five Minute Veterinary Consult clinical Companion: Small Animal Dentistry, ed 2, Wiley-Blackwell, 2012, p. 369-379.

67. c Feline resorptive lesions affect the hard tissue of the tooth. This is a progressive disease caused by the activity of cells that are called odontoclasts. Corticosteroid therapy has no effect on stopping the progression of the disease. Corticosteroid therapy in the oral cavity is used to treat inflammation and pain or to suppress the immune system. Reiter AM, "Tooth resorption: feline," in Lobprise HB, ed, Blackwell's Five-Minute Veterinary Consult Clinical Companion: Small Animal Dentistry, ed 2, Wiley-Blackwell, 2012, p. 369-379.

68. b The permanent lower canines usually erupt lingual to the deciduous canines. If the deciduous canines are still present when the dog or cat is 6 months of age, the deciduous teeth need to be extracted so that the mandibular canines can move into the proper position and avoid traumatic occlusion with the hard palate. Brannon R, "Persistent retained deciduous teeth," in Lobprise HB, ed, Blackwell's Five-Minute Veterinary Consult Clinical Companion: Small Animal Dentistry, ed 2, Wiley-Blackwell, 2012, p. 143-147.

69. c The pulp of the tooth is located in the center cavity of a tooth. It contains blood vessels (nutritive function) and nerves (providing sensation). Odontoblasts line the wall of the chamber and produce dentin. The periodontal ligament anchors the tooth to the alveolar bone. The enamel provides the crown with a protective, hard surface. The dentin makes up the bulk of the tooth below the enamel and cementum. Holzman G, "The basics," in Perrone JR, ed, Small Animal Dental Procedures for Veterinary Technicians and Nurses, Wiley-Blackwell, 2013, p. 3-22.

70. a A tooth in which the pulp is exposed should be extracted or should have a root canal procedure performed. This is a tooth in which the nerves are exposed, causing discomfort to the animal. Exposed pulp will become infected and the tooth will become abscessed as the pulp tissue becomes necrosed. Therefore, providing no treatment will leave the patient with a painful infected tooth. Crown amputation is used in cases in which tooth resorption has been diagnosed. To perform a crown amputation, the periodontal ligament space between the root and the alveolar bone must be ankylosed or fused. Any remaining crown or root structure is extracted, the area is smoothed to prevent trauma from sharp edges, and it is sutured closed. Reducing plaque and calculus may slow the progression of bacterial growth, but it does not stop it, and the exposed pulp can still become infected. Plaque bacteria build up on the tooth surface within 24 hours of cleaning. Gorrel C, "Tooth fracture," in Lobprise HB, ed, Blackwell's Five-Minute Veterinary Consult Clinical Companion: Small Animal Dentistry, ed 2, Wiley-Blackwell, 2012, p. 279-287; Dupont G, "Pathologies of the dental hard tissues," Niemiec BA, Small Animal Dental, Oral, and Maxillofacial Disease, Manson, 2010, p. 128-159.

71. b For chronic and severe periodontal disease, patients can be given antimicrobials for a week before the periodontal treatment and then for 7–10 days postoperatively. Corticosteroids are commonly used for the treatment of stomatitis. The clinical signs of stomatitis are severe inflammation and oral ulcerations that cause pain to the point of inappetence in some patients. Corticosteroids help to decrease the pain and inflammation for only a limited time. Surgical intervention with extractions of the teeth in the areas of the inflammation has shown the most promising results. Nonsteroidal anti-inflammatories are mostly used postoperatively in patients with severe periodontal disease. Immunostimulating drugs such as interferon have been used to treat stomatitis with poor results. Bellows J, "Periodontal disease: periodontitis," in Lobprise HB, ed, Blackwell's Five-Minute Veterinary Consult Clinical Companion: Small Animal Dentistry, ed 2, Wiley-Blackwell, 2012, p. 216-223; Bonello D, "Feline inflammatory, infectious and other oral conditions," in Tutt, C, Deeprose, J, Crossley, D, BSAVA Manual of Canine and Feline Dentistry, ed 3, British Small Animal Veterinary Association, 2007, p. 126-147.

72. a Oral masses do not usually present until after the patient is in adulthood. The oral tumor that arises at the earliest age is the fibrosarcoma. The fibrosarcoma or FSA is the third most common malignancy in dogs and the second most common malignancy in cats. It is important when doing an oral examination to count the teeth. Missing teeth in pediatric patients could mean the tooth has embedded at a location where an operculum, which is a tough fibrous gingival covering, has covered the tooth. The tooth could be impacted, making it unable to erupt because of bone or an adjacent tooth or deciduous tooth. The tooth could also never have erupted. Missing teeth should always be radiographed to assess whether the tooth is present or not. Extra teeth or supernumerary teeth can cause crowding or rotation of adjacent teeth and this could have an effect on periodontal health. Dental radiographs are taken to determine whether any of the supernumerary teeth are abnormal. This will help to prioritize extraction to alleviate the crowding. A class II malocclusion is present when the mandible is shorter than the maxilla. When the mandible is longer than the maxilla, it is considered a class III malocclusion or an undershot jaw. Dennis BD, "Fibrosarcoma," in Lobprise HB, ed, Blackwell's Five-Minute Veterinary Consult Clinical Companion: Small Animal Dentistry, ed 2, Wiley-Blackwell, 2012, p. 314-317; Lobprise HB, "Abnormal number of teeth," in Lobprise HB, ed, Blackwell's Five-Minute Veterinary Consult Clinical Companion: Small Animal Dentistry, ed 2, Wiley-Blackwell, 2012, p. 168-172.

73. b Perioceutics are drugs compounded so that they can be directly placed in the mouth, where the disease is occurring, and they can release the medication over time. Periodontal pockets that are 3–6 mm in a dog warrant placement of this locally applied antibiotic gel directly into the pocket. The placement of the gel allows more direct treatment of the infection and avoids any systemic or gastrointestinal side effects. In advanced periodontal disease, the support structure of the tooth or periodontium is destroyed. The periodontal ligament is one of the structures that make up the periodontium. Unfortunately, after the periodontal ligament is destroyed, it cannot be restored. Use of antibiotics in advance of a periodontal treatment can improve the patient's condition. The problem with systemic antibiotics is possible side-effect resistance. The procedure that caps the pulp cavity of a tooth is an endodontic therapy, which is the innermost structure of the tooth that carries the blood vessel and nerves. Common endodontic procedures are root canal therapy and vital pulp therapy. DeBowes L, "Periodontitis," Niemiec BA, Small Animal Dental, Oral and Maxillofacial Disease, Manson, 2010, p. 164-169.

74. a Correct bisecting angle technique is performed by directing the beam perpendicular to the bisection of the angle formed where the plane of the film meets the long axis of the tooth. If the beam is directed parallel to the bisection line, the beam will not strike the film or sensor and no image will appear. If the beam is directed perpendicular to the tooth root, the image will be elongated and nondiagnostic. If the beam is directed perpendicular to the film or sensor, the image will be foreshortened and nondiagnostic. Gorrel C, Derbyshire S, "Dental radiography," Veterinary Dentistry for the Nurse and Technician, ed 1, Butterworth-Heinemann, 2005, p. 55-67.

75. d Curettes are used to remove calculus, debris, and granulation tissue below the gum line or subgingivally. The curette is made with a rounded tip and a rounded back to facilitate insertion below the gum line without causing trauma. A dental explorer is used to check the tooth surface for any irregularities, from an enamel fracture to pulp exposure in a fractured tooth. The working end of the explorer is a fine wire made to alert the handler of any defect by catching and making a pinging sound. The periodontal probe is an instrument that measures the gingival sulcus for any abnormal depths >3 mm in a dog and 0.5–1.0 mm in a cat. The periodontal probe is also used to measure how much gingival recession or gingival hyperplasia is affecting the tooth. The periodontal probe is marked in mm at varying intervals. Scalers are used to remove calculus above the gum line or supragingivally. The scaler has a ridged back, two sharp sides, and a pointed tip. The tip of the scaler is used to remove debris in the developmental grooves along the crown surface. Bellows J, "Equipping your dental practice," The Practice of Veterinary Dentistry, Iowa State Press, 1999, p. 45-80.

76. d Ultrasonic scaling or power scaling can be used for both supragingival and subgingival scaling. Thanks to improvements in technology, there are subgingival tips and handpiece inserts available. The subgingival tip or insert is finer and thinner for insertion below the gum line. When using the subgingival tip, you will need to reduce the power to avoid any damage to the soft tissue. If visualization is difficult, hand instrumentation using a curette is recommended. Cherry B, "Components of the dental operatory," in Perrone JR, ed, Small Animal Dental Procedures for Veterinary Technicians and Nurses, Wiley-Blackwell, 2013, p. 29-44; McMahon J, "The dental cleaning," in Perrone JR, ed, Small Animal Dental Procedures for Veterinary Technicians and Nurses, Wiley-Blackwell, 2013, p. 59-86.

77. b It is advisable to use a cuffed endotracheal tube to prevent fluid and debris that are aerosolized during the procedure from gaining access to the lungs around the endotracheal tube. It is also a common practice to keep the endotracheal tube partially inflated when extubating to ensure that accumulated debris do not progress down the trachea. Mills A, "Anesthesia and the dental patient," in Perrone JR, ed, Small Animal Dental Procedures for Veterinary Technicians and Nurses, Wiley-Blackwell, 2013, p. 45-57; McMahon J, "The dental cleaning," in Perrone JR, ed, Small Animal Dental Procedures for Veterinary Technicians and Nurses, Wiley-Blackwell, 2013, p. 59-86.

78. c Distemper virus can result in abnormal formation of enamel (reduced deposition or absence of enamel). Enamel hypoplasia is a developmental disorder of the enamel layer of the tooth. Ameloblasts are the cells responsible for the formation of the enamel during the development of the deciduous and adult teeth. Illness during the development of the tooth can disrupt the normal function of the ameloblasts. The crowns of the affected teeth will have areas of normal enamel and areas of missing or inadequate enamel. Enamel staining or intrinsic staining usually occurs secondary to tetracycline exposure of animals at a young age. Tetracycline binds to enamel and dentin, causing a dark yellow discoloration. Adontia or missing teeth in pediatric patients could mean the tooth is embedded and covered with an operculum, a tough fibrous gingival covering. The tooth could be impacted where the tooth is unable to erupt because of bone or an adjacent tooth or deciduous tooth. The tooth could also have never erupted. Missing teeth should always be radiographed to assess whether the tooth is present or not. Extra teeth, supernumerary teeth, or polydontia can cause crowding or rotation of adjacent teeth, which could have an effect on periodontal health. Dental radiographs are obtained to determine whether any of the supernumerary teeth are abnormal. This will help prioritize extraction to alleviate crowding. Lobprise HB, "American veterinary dental college nomenclature," Blackwell's Five-Minute Veterinary Consult Clinical Companion: Small Animal Dentistry, ed 2, Wiley-Blackwell, 2012, p. 442-461; Dupont G, "Pathologies of the dental hard tissues," in Niemiec, BA Small Animal Dental, Orasl and Maxillofacial Disease, Manson, 2010, p. 128-159.

79. b There is no way to sterilize the oral cavity in any patient. Flushing with a dilute chlorhexidine solution may reduce the bacterial load that may potentially become aerosolized during the procedure. Veterinary technicians should wear surgical masks, shields or goggles, and gloves when performing a dental prophylaxis to decrease further their exposure to harmful pathogens. Chlorhexidine solution is a topical application and therefore does not provide any systemic or long-term treatment. Chlorhexidine is categorized as an antibacterial and does not have any anesthetic properties. McMahon J, "The dental cleaning," in Perrone JR, ed, Small Animal Dental Procedures for Veterinary Technicians and Nurses, Wiley-Blackwell, 2013, p. 59-85.

80. d Polishing is not a means for removing plaque; rather it is an effort to smooth the tooth surface to eliminate any etches on the tooth surface from the scaling process. These etches would potentially allow plaque and calculus to gain purchase on the tooth surface. You must be cautious not to overheat the tooth with the instrument by using too much pressure or by leaving it on the tooth longer than 3–5 seconds. McMahon J, "The dental cleaning," in Perrone JR, ed, Small Animal Dental Procedures for Veterinary Technicians and Nurses, Wiley-Blackwell, 2013, p. 59-85.

81. a The Triadan system is a charting system in which each tooth is identified with a specific number describing the quadrant in which it is located and the type of tooth it is. The Triadan system uses a series of three numbers. The first number identifies the quadrant. The mouth is divided into four quadrants: 1 = right maxillary; 2 = left maxillary; 3 = left mandibular; and 4 = right mandibular. The second and third numbers identify the tooth. The numbering starts with the central incisors with 01 and ends with the second or third molar with 10 or 11, respectively. When you put the numbers together, you will know the location of the tooth. In cats, the maxillary first premolar and the mandibular first and second premolar are missing. Using the Triadan system, those tooth numbers are skipped. A complete system that includes a power scaler and polisher is a dental unit. The method for radiographing molars is called the bisecting angle technique. Home care systems are products sent home with the client to maintain oral health. They can include toothbrushes, toothpaste, oral rinses, dental diets, and chews. Holzman G, The basics," in Perrone JR, ed, Small Animal Dental Procedures for Veterinary Technicians and Nurses, Wiley-Blackwell, 2013, p. 3-22; Cherry B, "Components of the dental operatory," in Perrone JR, ed, Small Animal Dental Procedures for Veterinary Technicians and Nurses, Wiley-Blackwell, 2013, p. 29-44.

82. a Anodontia (total absence of teeth) and oligodontia (congenital absence of many but not all teeth) are associated with ectodermal dysplasia, are rare and can occur in dogs with no apparent systemic problem or congenital syndrome. Hypodontia (absence of only a few teeth) is, however, a relatively common finding in dogs. Dysphagia means difficulty in eating. Gorrel C, "Glossary," Veterinary Dentistry for the General Practitioner, ed 2, Elsevier, 2013, p. 215-221.

83. a The canine tooth is long and pointed to grasp and tear with great pressure. The canine tooth also provides protection. For that reason, only ⅓ of the tooth's length is above the gum line. The other ⅔ are below the gum line. Bellows J, "Anatomy and nomenclature," The Practice of Veterinary Dentistry, Iowa State Press, 1999, p. 15-22.

84. c The upper fourth premolar communicates directly with the maxillary sinus. Mandibular refers to the lower jaw or mandible where no sinus is present. Occipital is the area of the skull at the back of the head. Orbital is the bony recess that holds the eye. Holzman G, "The basics," in Perrone JR, ed, Small Animal Dental Procedures for Veterinary Technicians and Nurses, Wiley-Blackwell, 2013, p. 3-22; Dyce KM, Sack WO, Wensing CJG, "The head and ventral neck of carnivores," Textbook of Veterinary Anatomy, ed 2, Saunders, 1996, p. 367-392.

85. a The crown of the teeth is the portion above the gum line and it is covered with enamel. The enamel is the hardest surface in the body and protects the tooth from most trauma. The most terminal portion of the root or the tip of the root is called the apex or apical portion. The portion below the gum line is the root. The layer of bony tissue that is attached to the alveolar bone by the periodontal ligament is the cementum. Holzman G, "The basics," in Perrone JR, ed, Small Animal Dental Procedures for Veterinary Technicians and Nurses, Wiley-Blackwell, 2013, p. 3-22.

86. b The normal sulcus depth in a cat is 0.5–1.0 mm. The normal sulcus depth in a dog is 1–3 mm. McMahon J, "The dental cleaning," in Perrone JR, ed, Small Animal Dental Procedures for Veterinary Technicians and Nurses, Wiley-Blackwell, 2013, p. 59-85.

87. c When the endotracheal tube cuff is overinflated, it can cause tracheal trauma to the point of rupture when the patient is turned from one side to the other without disconnecting the breathing circuit. To avoid tracheal trauma, properly inflate the endotracheal tube. The pop-off valve is closed to pressurize the system. The rebreathing bag is squeezed to a point where the seal will allow bagging at ≤20 cm of water. Packing the gauze too tightly in the pharyngeal area can impede venous return, causing the tongue to swell. Carpenter RE, Manfra Marretta S, "Dental patients," in Tranquilli WJ, Thurmon JC, Grimm KA, eds., Lumb and Jones' Veterinary Anesthesia and Analgesia, ed 4, Wiley-Blackwell, 2007, p. 993-995; Mills A, "Anesthesia and the dental patient," in Perrone JR, ed, Small Animal Dental Procedures for Veterinary Technicians and Nurses, Wiley-Blackwell, 2013, p. 45-57.

88. a Stage I periodontal disease shows no change to the alveolar height or architecture, but mild gingival inflammation is present. Stage II shows gingival inflammation and sometimes bleeding on probing. There is <25% bone loss or stage I furcation exposure. Stage III shows all of the signs of stage II but with 25%–50% bone loss, stage II furcation exposure, and possibly stage 1 mobility. Stage IV shows all the signs of stage III but with >50% bone loss, stage 3 furcation exposure, and stage II–III mobility. Perrone JR, "Common dental conditions and treatments: periodontal disease," Small Animal Dental Procedures for Veterinary Technicians and Nurses, Wiley-Blackwell, 2013, p. 105-115.

89. a Gingival index 0: Clinically healthy gingiva. Gingival index 1: Mild gingivitis: slight reddening and swelling of the gingival margin; no bleeding on gentle probing of the gingival sulcus. Gingival index 2: Moderate gingivitis: the gingival margin is red and swollen; gentle probing of the gingival sulcus results in bleeding. Gingival index 3: Severe gingivitis: the gingival margin is very swollen with a red or bluish-red color; there is spontaneous hemorrhage and/or ulceration of the gingival margin. Gorrel C, "Oral examination and recording" in Veterinary Dentistry for the General Practitioner, ed 2, Elsevier, 2013, p. 56-66.

90. b Enamel staining or intrinsic staining usually occurs secondary to tetracycline exposure of animals at a young age. Tetracycline binds to enamel and dentin, causing a dark yellow discoloration. Amoxicillin is a common antimicrobial given to dental patients either before or before and after periodontal therapy. Chloramphenicol, also an antimicrobial, is used mostly for tickborne illnesses such as Rocky Mountain spotted fever. Penicillin, although still used in veterinary medicine, is usually less preferred than amoxicillin because amoxicillin has fewer side effects. Dupont G, "Pathologies of the dental hard tissues," Niemiec BA, Small Animal Dental, Oral and Maxillofacial Disease, CRC Press, 2010, p. 127-157. http://www.petplace.com/article/drug-library/library/prescription/chloramphenicol-chloromycetin. Accessed 3/6.

91. c The occlusal surface of the tooth is the chewing surface. Dogs have flat surfaces on the cusps of the molars. The molars are used for grinding food into a form that can be swallowed. The surface of the tooth facing the hard palate is called palatal. The surface of the tooth facing the cheek is called buccal. The surface of the tooth facing the tongue is called lingual. Holzman G, "The basics," in Perrone JR, ed, Small Animal Dental Procedures for

Veterinary Technicians and Nurses, Wiley-Blackwell, 2013, p. 3-22.

92. b Dogs normally have 42 teeth. Holzman G, "The basics," in Perrone JR, ed, Small Animal Dental Procedures for Veterinary Technicians and Nurses, Wiley-Blackwell, 2013, p. 3-22.

93. c Grade 0: No mobility. Grade 1: Horizontal movement of ≤1 mm. Grade 2: Horizontal movement of >1 mm. Note that multi-rooted teeth are scored more severely and a horizontal mobility in excess of 1 mm is usually considered a Grade 3 even in the absence of vertical movement. Grade 3: Vertical as well as horizontal movement is possible. Gorrel C, "Oral examination and recording" in Veterinary Dentistry for the General Practitioner, ed 2, Elsevier, 2013, p. 56-66.

94. b Excessive force using a dental curette may degrade the epithelial attachment. Another way to cause trauma to the gingival tissue is the improper sharpening of the instrument. It is important when sharpening a curette to sharpen the blade and to maintain the rounded toe. Finally, hold the instrument using the pen grasp and use proper angulation against the tooth surface so the instrument does not slide off the tooth, which could cause trauma. Overheating of the tooth is caused by excessive pressure on the tooth surface with a power scaler or prophy angle because these instruments generate heat. Dental patients need to be under general anesthesia for a dental procedure to allow the use of invasive instruments in the mouth without the risk of bites. McMahon J, "The dental cleaning," in Perrone JR, ed, Small Animal Dental Procedures for Veterinary Technicians and Nurses, Wiley-Blackwell, 2013, p. 59-85.

95. d The maxillary or upper fourth premolar has three roots: the mesial buccal root, the palatal root, and the distal root. The canine tooth has one root. The first premolar and the first molar have two roots. Teeth can develop an extra root, which is considered an anatomic abnormality. Extra roots are charted as supernumerary roots. Holzman G, "The basics," in Perrone JR, ed, Small Animal Dental Procedures for Veterinary Technicians and Nurses, Wiley-Blackwell, 2013, p. 3-22.

96. c Prolonged application and/or excessive downward pressure of the prophy angle longer than 3–5 seconds on a tooth can cause overheating of the pulp, which could lead to pulpal death. When using the prophy angle, use a soft prophy cup and gently flange the edges of the cup to allow it to reach just under the gum line. McMahon J, "The dental cleaning," in Perrone JR, ed, Small Animal Dental Procedures for Veterinary Technicians and Nurses, Wiley-Blackwell, 2013, p. 59-85.

97. b Attrition is the active or passive wear of the tooth surface either by chewing, by biting, or when there is close contact with another tooth. Plaque attaches to the biofilm on the tooth surface and is made up of bacteria, salivary glycoproteins, and extracellular polysaccharides. Calculus is mineralized dental plaque. Abrasion is wear to the tooth surface from an outside source such as a toy, cage door, or excessive grooming. Lobprise HB, "Glossary," Blackwell's Five-Minute Veterinary Consult Clinical Companion: Small Animal Dentistry, ed 2, Wiley-Blackwell, 2012, p. 467-482.

98. b Grade 0: No furcation involvement. Grade 1: Initial furcation involvement: the furcation can be felt with the probe/explorer, but horizontal tissue destruction is less than ⅓ of the horizontal width of the furcation. Grade 2: Partial furcation involvement: it is possible to explore the furcation but the probe/explorer cannot be passed through it; horizontal tissue destruction is >⅓ of the horizontal width of the furcation. Grade 3: Total furcation involvement: the probe/explorer can be passed through the furcation from buccal to palatal/lingual. Gorrel C, "Oral examination and recording," Veterinary Dentistry for the General Practitioner, ed 2, Elsevier, 2013, p. 56-66.

99. d Abrasion is wear to the tooth surface from an outside source such as a toy, cage door, or excessive grooming. Plaque attaches to the biofilm on the tooth surface and is made up of bacteria, salivary glycoproteins, and extracellular polysaccharides. Attrition is the active or passive wear of the tooth surface either by chewing, by biting, or when there is close contact with another tooth. Calculus is mineralized dental plaque. Lobprise HB, "Glossary," Blackwell's Five-Minute Veterinary Consult Clinical Companion: Small Animal Dentistry, ed 2, Wiley-Blackwell, 2012, p. 467-482.

100. a Plaque attaches to the biofilm on the tooth surface and is made up of bacteria, salivary glycoproteins, and extracellular polysaccharides. Attrition is the active or passive wear of the tooth surface either by chewing, by biting, or when there is close contact with another tooth. Calculus is mineralized dental plaque. Abrasion is wear to the tooth surface from an outside source such as a toy, cage door, or excessive grooming. Lobprise HB, "Glossary," Blackwell's Five-Minute Veterinary Consult Clinical Companion: Small Animal Dentistry, ed 2, Wiley-Blackwell, 2012, p. 467-482.

101. a In cats, complete eruption of permanent dentition can occur anywhere from 4 to 6 months. The permanent incisors erupt at 3–4 months. The permanent canines erupt at 4–5 months. The permanent premolars erupt at 4–6 months and the permanent molars erupt at 4–5 months. Tooth eruption varies with breed, gender, overall health, body size, and season of birth. Hence healthy larger-breed, summer-born females tend to erupt earlier. Holzman G, "The basics," in Perrone JR, ed, Small Animal Dental Procedures for Veterinary Technicians and Nurses, Wiley-Blackwell, 2013, p. 3-22.

102. b A modified pen grip is the preferred method of holding dental instruments. This technique involves holding the instrument as you would a pen or a pencil. The instrument should be grasped with a light grip to avoid stress to the hand or wrist. Hold the instrument with the thumb and index finger at the junction of the handle and the shank. The ring finger is allowed to rest on the patient. This creates a triangle of movement. The ring finger provides stability while the movement of the instrument is provided using the thumb and the index finger. Holmstrom SE, "The complete prophy," Veterinary Dentistry: A Team Approach, ed 2, Saunders, 2013, p. 167-193.

103. d Grade 1 periodontal disease is among the top 10 diagnoses in dogs and gingivitis is the top 10 diagnoses in cats. Banfield State of Pet Health 2011 Report http://www.banfield.com/getmedia/89cdf49c-67e7-41ba-865a-c2d6ab123720/State_of_Pet_Health_2011.pdf. Accessed 3.31.2015.

104. a Curettage is the removal of calculus and necrotic cementum from the root surface using a dental curette. A dental curette is an instrument that has a rounded back and a rounded toe to facilitate scaling subgingivally. Splinting is used as a treatment for periodontal disease. Splinting immobilizes a tooth that is mobile because of periodontal disease. Removal of all calculus and granulation tissue subgingivally treats the tooth using an open flap technique. The flap is then sutured closed and the tooth is immobilized during healing by splinting the treated tooth to a healthy tooth using dental acrylic. Gingivoplasty is the surgical recontouring of the gingival surface. This can also be called a gingivectomy, a treatment for gingival hyperplasia. Gingivoplasty is performed to treat gingival hyperplasia if there are no false pockets present. Scaling is the removal of plaque and calculus above the gum line or supragingivally. This procedure is undertaken using power equipment and/or hand instrumentation. Holmstrom SE, Frost P, Eisner ER, "Periodontal therapy and surgery," Veterinary Dental Techniques for the Small Animal Practitioner, ed 3, 2004, p. 233-290.

105. b Full-mouth extractions are performed to treat conditions in which patients are hypersensitized to the presence of plaque on the teeth such as stomatitis in dogs and cats. The condition causes inflammation and ulcerations that cause pain. Selective or full-mouth extractions are performed to remove the source of reaction. The only situations in which full-mouth extractions might be viewed as preventative medicine are patients with systemic diseases that make them a possible anesthetic risk. If these patients require extractions of most of their teeth, extractions of the remaining teeth can be performed to prevent the need for further anesthesia and further dental treatment. Lobprise HB, "Extraction technique," Blackwell's Five-Minute Veterinary Consult Clinical Companion: Small Animal Dentistry, ed 2, Wiley-Blackwell, 2012, p. 95-121; Peak M, "Chronic ulceration and chronic ulcerative paradental stomatitis," in Lobprise HB, Blackwell's Five-Minute Veterinary Consult Clinical Companion: Small Animal Dentistry, ed 2. Wiley-Blackwell, 2012, p. 243-250.

106. a Attrition is the normal or pathological wearing down of the tooth crown resulting from chewing, biting, and/or tooth on tooth. An intrusion occurs when the tooth is pushed apically into the alveolar bone. An extrusion occurs when a tooth is partially dislocated from the alveolar bone. An avulsion occurs when the tooth is completely luxated from the alveolus. Holmstrom SE, "The complete prophy," Veterinary Dentistry: A Team Approach, ed 2, Saunders, 2013, p. 167-193.

107. d When using a hand scaler, the blade angle ranges from 45 to 90 degrees depending on the job being performed and on the area of the tooth involved. When scaling developmental grooves where the tip of the instrument is used, a 45-degree angle is used. When scaling the interdental spaces, a 70–80-degree angle is used. When scaling the buccal or lingual/palatal aspects of the crown, the angle can go as high as 90 degrees. Miltex Veterinary Dental Prophylaxis and Periodontal Procedure for Routine Treatment. Package insert SH-6809C.

108. d 2 × {I 2/1:C 0/0:P 3/2:M 3/3} is the rabbit formula, 2 × {I 3/3:C 1/1:P 4/4:M 2/3} is the permanent formula for dogs, 2 × I 3/3:C 1/1:P 3/2:M 1/1} is the permanent formula for cats. 2 × {I 3/3:C 1/1:P 3/3} is the primary formula for puppies. Gorrel C, "Oral examination and recording" in Veterinary Dentistry for the General Practitioner, ed 2, Elsevier, 2013, p. 56-66.

109. c As part of the anesthesia protocol, injections are usually administered during dental procedures. Injections are not usually sent home after a routine dental cleaning where no periodontal therapy was necessary. McMahon J, "The dental cleaning," in Perrone JR, ed, Small Animal Dental Procedures for Veterinary Technicians and Nurses, Wiley-Blackwell, 2013, p. 59-85; Mills A, "Anesthesia and the dental patient," in Perrone JR, ed, Small Animal Dental Procedures for Veterinary Technicians and Nurses, Wiley-Blackwell, 2013, p. 45-58.

110. a A bacterial layer that forms on the tooth is called plaque. Those bacteria that are attached to the tooth absorb calcium from the saliva and become calcified. This is known as calculus. The pellicle is a glycoprotein component of saliva and attaches to the tooth surface within 20 minutes of cleaning. The pellicle provides a foundation for the plaque bacteria to adhere. The aerobic bacteria then colonize and arrange themselves in a biofilm and continue to multiply and consume oxygen. This creates an environment for anaerobic bacteria to start forming. These bacteria often contain endotoxins sometimes called lipopolysaccharides and enzymes, which are toxic to gingival tissues. Holmstrom SE, "Pathogenesis of periodontal disease," Veterinary Dentistry: A Team Approach, ed 2, Saunders, 2013, p. 165.

111. b Rodents have constantly growing teeth. Malocclusion is the most common dental problem in rodents. This condition causes overgrowth of the incisor and/or premolar and molar teeth. It can cause overgrown incisor teeth, secondary tongue entrapment, and soft tissue laceration. Malocclusion can result from traumatic injury to a tooth, which causes a loss of normal wear to the opposing tooth. Malocclusion can also result from a mandible that is too short or too long or from nutritional deficiencies as well. Tooth root abscess, scurvy, and impaction of the cheek pouch can also occur in rodents but not as frequently. Istace K, "Dentistry and the exotic patient," in Perrone JR, ed, Small Animal Dental Procedures for Veterinary Technicians and Nurses, Wiley-Blackwell, 2013, p. 161-186.

112. c The periodontium is the supporting structure of the teeth and includes the periodontal ligament, gingiva, cementum, and the alveolar bone. The root is the structure of the tooth that is supported by the periodontium. Gorrel C, Derbyshire S, "Anatomy of the teeth and periodontium," Veterinary Dentistry for the Nurse and Technician, ed 1, Butterworth-Heinemann, 2005, p. 25-29.

113. d Combined client education, continuous reinforcement, and client recalls will generate better client compliance than instructing the client alone. Clients must be reminded about the importance of home care to prevent disease, which can be accomplished through repeated visits to the hospital and periodic phone calls. Gorrel C, "Preventive dentistry," Veterinary Dentistry for the General Practitioner, ed 2, Elsevier, 2013, p. 121-128.

114. d Resorptive lesions (RLs) occur as a result of an external root resorption, where the hard tissues of the root surfaces are destroyed by the activity of multinucleated cells called odontoclasts. Macrocytes are abnormally large erythrocytes and do not have any involvement with teeth. Osteoclasts are the basal metabolic units of bone. Chondrocytes are involved in developing cartilage. Gorrel C, "Resorptive lesions," Veterinary Dentistry for the General Practitioner, ed 2, Elsevier, 2013, p. 128-140.

115. c The furcation is the space between two roots in a multi-rooted tooth. Apical is defined as toward the end portion or apex of the tooth. *Rostral* is the term meaning toward the front of the head. Buccal is the surface facing the cheek. Lobprise HB, Wiggs RB, "Glossary," The Veterinarian's Companion for Common Dental Procedures, AAHA Press, 2000, p. 177-196.

116. d Buccal is the surface facing the cheek. Rostral means toward the front of the head. The furcation is the space between two roots in a multirooted tooth. Apical means toward the end portion or apex of the tooth. Lobprise HB, Wiggs RB, "Glossary," The Veterinarian's Companion for Common Dental Procedures, AAHA Press, 2000, p. 177-196.

117. a Apical is defined as toward the end portion or apex of the tooth. *Rostral* is the term meaning toward the front of the head. The furcation is the space between two roots in a multi-rooted tooth. Buccal is the surface facing the cheek. Lobprise HB, Wiggs RB, "Glossary," The Veterinarian's Companion for Common Dental Procedures, AAHA Press, 2000, p. 177-196.

118. b *Rostral* is the term meaning toward the front of the head. Apical is defined as toward the end portion or apex of the tooth. The furcation is the space between two roots in a multi-rooted tooth. Buccal is the surface facing the cheek. Lobprise HB, Wiggs RB, "Glossary," The Veterinarian's Companion for Common Dental Procedures, AAHA Press, 2000, p. 177-196.

119. b Chlorhexidine binds to the pellicle and slowly releases antimicrobial agents. Polyphosphates are mineral chelators and inhibitors. These agents bind to salivary calcium and make it unavailable for incorporation into the plaque biofilm. In short, polyphosphates do not allow plaque to mineralize into calculus. Fluoride reduces sensitivity when applied over exposed dentinal tubules. Fluoride forms fluoroapatite, causing the tooth surface to be strengthened and more resistant to the cariogenic bacteria that dissolve enamel. Bleaching stained teeth is not a procedure performed in dogs and cats at this time. Roudebush P, Logan E, Hale FA, Evidence-based veterinary dentistry: a systemic review of homecare for prevention of periodontal disease in dogs and cats, J Vet Dent, 2005; 22:6-15; Bellows J, "Equipping your dental practice," The Practice of Veterinary Dentistry, Iowa State University Press, 1999, p. 45-80.

120. a *Scissor bite* is a descriptive term for normal occlusion in a dog or cat. The maxillary and mandibular teeth align to each other like the blades of a scissor when closed. The mandibular incisors are just behind the maxillary incisors. The mandibular canine fits in the diastema between the maxillary third incisor and the maxillary canine. The maxillary premolars lie buccally to the mandibular premolars with the tips of some of the premolars interdigitating with the mandibular premolars, which looks like the blades of a pinking shear. Berg M, "The examination room and the dental patient," in Perrone JR, ed, Small Animal Dental Procedures for Veterinary Technicians and Nurses, Wiley-Blackwell, 2013, p. 23-28.

121. c In studies, the addition of 0.2% chlorhexidine to a dental chew decreased plaque on the tooth surface after 3 weeks. Chlorhexidine adheres to the tooth surfaces and slowly provides antimicrobial activity. The common concentration for oral chlorhexidine is 0.2%. Using a prediluted product is preferred rather than making up the correct solution from stock chlorhexidine. Prepackaged chlorhexidine is flavored to make it more palatable. Roudebush P, Logan E, Hale FA, Evidence-based veterinary dentistry: a systemic review of homecare for prevention of periodontal disease in dogs and cats, J Vet Dent, 2005, 22:6-15.

122. b Fluoride reduces sensitivity when applied over exposed dentinal tubules. Fluoride forms fluoroapatite, causing the tooth surface to be strengthened and more resistant to the cariogenic bacteria that dissolve enamel. Fluoride benefits cats by desensitizing a tooth that may have tooth resorption, but only until the tooth can be extracted. Fluoride does not stop the activity of odontoclasts, which are the cells responsible for progression of tooth resorption. Disclosing solution is the material that causes any missed plaque and calculus during a cleaning procedure to turn red. Bellows J, "Equipping your dental practice," The Practice of Veterinary Dentistry, Iowa State Press, 1999, p. 45-80.

123. d Curettes are used to remove calculus, debris, and granulation tissue below the gum line or subgingivally. The curette is designed with a rounded tip and a rounded back to facilitate insertion below the gum line without causing trauma. A dental explorer is used to check the tooth surface for any irregularities, from an enamel fracture to pulp exposure in a fractured tooth. The working end of the explorer is a fine wire made to alert the handler that there is a defect by catching and making a pinging sound. Scalers are used to remove calculus above the gum line or supragingivally. The scaler has a ridged back, two sharp sides, and a pointed tip. The tip of the scaler is used to remove debris in the developmental grooves along the crown surface. The periodontal probes are instruments that measure the gingival sulcus for any abnormal depths >3 mm in dogs and 0.5–1.0 mm in cats. The periodontal probe is also used to measure how much gingival recession or gingival hyperplasia is affecting the tooth.

The periodontal probe is marked in mm at varying intervals. Bellows J, "Equipping your dental practice," The Practice of Veterinary Dentistry, Iowa State Press, 1999, p. 45-80.

124. b A dental explorer is used to check the tooth surface for any irregularities, from an enamel fracture to pulp exposure in a fractured tooth. The working end of the explorer is a fine wire made to alert the handler if there is a defect by catching and making a pinging sound. The periodontal probes are instruments that measure the gingival sulcus for any abnormal depths >3 mm in dogs and 0.5–1.0 mm in cats. The periodontal probe is also used to measure how much gingival recession or gingival hyperplasia is affecting the tooth. The periodontal probe is marked in mm at varying intervals. Curettes are used to remove calculus, debris, and granulation tissue below the gum line or subgingivally. The curette is made with a rounded tip and a rounded back to facilitate insertion below the gum line without causing trauma. Scalers are used to remove calculus above the gum line or supragingivally. The scaler has a ridged back, two sharp sides, and a pointed tip. The tip of the scaler is used to remove debris in the developmental grooves along the crown surface. "Equipping your dental practice," Bellows J, The Practice of Veterinary Dentistry, Iowa State Press, 1999, p. 45-80.

125. c Scalers are used to remove calculus above the gum line or supragingivally. The scaler has a ridged back, two sharp sides, and a pointed tip. The tip of the scaler is used to remove debris in the developmental grooves along the crown surface. The periodontal probes are instruments that measure the gingival sulcus for any abnormal depths >3 mm in dogs and 0.5–1.0 mm in cats. The periodontal probe is also used to measure how much gingival recession or gingival hyperplasia is affecting the tooth. The periodontal probe is marked in mm at varying intervals. A dental explorer is used to check the tooth surface for any irregularities, from an enamel fracture to pulp exposure in a fractured tooth. The working end of the explorer is a fine wire made to alert the handler that there is a defect by catching and making a pinging sound. Curettes are used to remove calculus, debris, and granulation tissue below the gum line or subgingivally. The curette is made with a rounded tip and a rounded back to facilitate insertion below the gum line without causing trauma. Bellows J, "Equipping your dental practice," The Practice of Veterinary Dentistry, Iowa State Press, 1999, p. 45-80.

126. b Wry bite, or wry mouth, is a class IV malocclusion describing a discrepancy in jaw length between the right and left side of the mandible. You can see one mandible longer than the maxilla and the other side is shorter. The upper and lower incisors do not align. Wry bite is a skeletal defect genetic condition in which the affected animal has a nonsymmetrical head. If we are assessing jaw length, we look at the word brachygnathism; brachy refers to short and gnath means jaw. In the term *prognathism*, pro- refers to projecting forward. Prognathism, also called an undershot jaw, is commonly seen in breeds such as the boxer, Pekingese, and bulldogs. Prognathism is a class III malocclusion in which the mandible is longer than the maxilla. The mandibular incisors are either level with or rostral to the maxillary incisors. The mandibular and maxillary premolars and molars will be out of alignment, causing tooth-to-tooth trauma. Brachygnathism is a class II malocclusion where the mandible is shorter than the maxilla, causing an overshot jaw. Anterior or rostral crossbite is a class I malocclusion and is the most common orthodontic abnormality. The premolar relationship is a normal scissor occlusion, but one or more of the incisors are misaligned. Niemiec BA, "Pathology in the pediatric patient," Small Animal Dental, Oral and Maxillofacial Disease, CRC Press, 2010, p. 89-126; Bellows J, "Malocclusions of teeth," in Lobprise HB, ed, Blackwell's Five-Minute Veterinary Consult Clinical Companion: Small Animal Dentistry, Wiley-Blackwell, 2012, p. 195-206.

127. c Dentin forms the main supporting structure of the tooth. It spans from crown tip to root tip. It is the layer below the enamel in the crown and the cementum in the root. The odontoblasts that line the pulp chamber and root canal produce secondary dentin throughout life and fill in the canal, causing the dentin to widen within the parameters of the tooth body as the tooth ages. Pulp is within the pulp chamber/root canal of the tooth. It is made of blood vessels, nerves, and lymphatic vessels. Enamel is the hardest surface in the body and is made of an inorganic material. The enamel surface changes color and wears with age. The cementum is the covering on the tooth root surface that provides an attachment point for the periodontal ligament fibers that run from the cementum to the alveolar bone. Harvey CE, Dubielzig RR, "Anatomy of the oral cavity in the dog and cat," in Harvey CE, Veterinary Dentistry, Saunders, 1985, p. 11-22; Wiggs RB, Lobprise HB, "Oral anatomy and physiology," in Veterinary Dentistry: Principles and Practices, Lippincott-Raven, 1997, p. 55-86.

128. b Periodontal therapy is any treatment to stop the progression of periodontitis. Periodontitis is the loss of the support structure or periodontium of the tooth. The periodontium is made up of the gingiva, periodontal ligament, and the alveolar bone. When there is a loss of any of these support structures, gingivitis becomes periodontitis. When plaque and calculus invade subgingivally, periodontal pockets and/or gingival recession can occur. Root planing, whether open where a gingival flap is made for visualization or closed where no gingival flap is needed, is a periodontal therapy procedure. Inadequate root planing is a common mistake in treating periodontal disease. When plaque and calculus are left subgingivally, it becomes a source of infection. The bacteria left behind are not disrupted and will continue to grow. Thus care must be taken that all gingival, periodontal pockets, and areas of gingival recession are thoroughly scaled using both power scaling and hand scaling. Supragingival calculus localized to the crown of the tooth just needs to be scaled off. This procedure is not considered periodontal therapy. Inadequate removal of supragingival calculus could lead to the presence of subgingival calculus if left unchecked. Polishing removes microetchants left on the tooth surface from scaling. Polishing is a step of the cleaning process, but it is not a periodontal therapy.

Inadequate polishing can lead to quicker formation of calculus as the bacteria have a roughened surface on which to adhere. Although iatrogenic trauma to subgingival tissues may be a problem, it would not be considered the most common mistake in the treatment of periodontal disease. McMahon J, "The dental cleaning," in Perrone JR, ed, Small Animal Dental Procedures for Veterinary Technicians and Nurses, Wiley-Blackwell, 2013, p. 59-85.

129. d Brushing the teeth is the gold standard for disrupting plaque on the tooth surface. The mechanical action of the brush against the tooth disrupts the plaque bacteria from adhering temporarily. Brushing needs to be repeated daily in dogs and cats to provide optimum results. A dentifrice or toothpaste provides two additional benefits to the brushing procedure. It is made with a pleasant flavor that makes brushing more acceptable to dogs and cats and it includes an abrasive or chemical compound that improves the mechanical and/or chemical activity that brushing provides. Supra- and subgingival scaling is the most thorough way to remove calculus from the tooth and root surface. Polishing the teeth after a professional dental cleaning removes microetchants caused by scaling. These procedures are best performed with the patient under anesthesia. Roudebush P, Logan E, Hale FA, Evidence-based veterinary dentistry: a systemic review of homecare for prevention of periodontal disease in dogs and cats, J Vet Dent, 2005; 22:6-15.

130. a When chlorhexidine and fluoride are applied at the same time, the binding activity of each product can cancel out the another. It is best to wait 30 minutes between the application of fluoride and the application of chlorhexidine. Bellows J, "Periodontal equipment, materials and techniques," Small Animal Dental Equipment, Materials and Techniques: A Primer, 2004, p. 115-173.

131. b Mandibular symphyseal laxity is a common finding in cats and small dogs. In many of these types of dogs, the incisor teeth might not be in individual bony sockets but suspended in connective tissue, which allows them to be quite mobile. Although these may be healthy teeth, periodontal probing is necessary to rule out potential attachment loss. Probing and dental radiographs are used to assess attachment loss. If alveolar bone loss is >50%, an indicator of advanced periodontal disease, or if the tooth structure has an abnormal structure, the tooth should be extracted. Calcium deficiency is not a condition that is described in the veterinary dentistry literature. Hall B, "Maxillary and mandibular fractures," in Lobprise HB, ed, Blackwell's Five-Minute Veterinary Consult Clinical Companion: Small Animal Dentistry, ed 2, Wiley-Blackwell, 2012, p. 347-357; "Periodontal disease", in Perrone, JR, ed, Small Animal Dental Procedures for Veterinary Technicians and Nurses, Wiley-Blackwell, 2013, p. 106-115.

132. d The permanent tooth bud lies close to the deciduous tooth and could become infected if the deciduous tooth is fractured and left in place. As with an adult tooth with pulpal exposure, a deciduous tooth should be treated. The deciduous tooth has a pulp canal just like an adult tooth. If the deciduous tooth is fractured and the pulp is exposed, with time necrosis can occur, which can affect the health of the adult tooth bud. Fractured deciduous teeth should be carefully extracted to avoid disturbing the adult tooth bud. Repairing the deciduous tooth with endodontic therapy such as a root canal is not feasible, as the pulp canal is too narrow to access properly. Hale FA, "Juvenile veterinary dentistry," in Veterinary Clinics of North America Small Animal Practice: Dentistry, 35(4), p. 789-818.

133. d The patient should undergo its first dental examination when it comes in for its first vaccinations and it should have a dental examination every visit after that. At the first visit, usually at about 8 weeks of age, the primary/deciduous teeth should be in place. The occlusion should present as a normal scissor bite unless it is a breed that normally has an abnormal occlusion such as a brachycephalic breed. In a puppy or kitten with a significant jaw-length discrepancy, an abnormal dental interlock can occur. As the mandible continues to grow, the interlock holds it back and affects the jaw length. In this situation, the sharp deciduous canines can dig into the hard palate and the incisors can become trapped behind the incisive papilla. This trauma to the soft tissue is painful. Hale FA, "Juvenile veterinary dentistry," Veterinary Clinics of North America Small Animal Practice: Dentistry, 35 (4), p. 789-818.

134. b Deciduous incisors have long, thin, and fragile roots. They erupt at 3½ to 4 weeks of age in puppies and 2–3 weeks of age in kittens. Deciduous canine teeth also have long, thin, fragile roots. They are the most frequently retained teeth and are shed when the adult teeth erupt at 6 months of age. Hale FA, "Juvenile veterinary dentistry," Veterinary Clinics of North America Small Animal Practice: Dentistry, 35 (4), p. 789-818.

135. a The nerves and blood vessels that are found in the tooth enter through the apical delta. The apical delta is located at the bottommost portion of the root and it has multiple openings through which the nerves, blood vessels, and other structures pass into the tooth. Pulp is within the pulp chamber/root canal of the tooth. It is made of blood vessels, nerves, and lymphatic vessels. The crown of the tooth is the portion that is visible above the gum line. The crown is covered with enamel for protection. The most coronal portion of the gingiva in healthy patients lies closely around the tooth just slightly above the cementoenamel junction. This is also known as the free gingiva. The margin of the free gingiva is rounded so that a potential space is formed around the tooth, which is called the sulcus. Lobprise HB, Wiggs RB, "Glossary," The Veterinarian's Companion for Common Dental Procedures, AAHA Press, 2000, p. 177-196.

136. c Rostral crossbite is a class I malocclusion and is the most common orthodontic abnormality. The premolar relationship is a normal scissor occlusion, but one or more of the incisors are misaligned. A milder form of a rostral crossbite is a level bite. Level bite is when the mandibular and the maxillary incisors meet cusp tip to cusp tip. This is abnormal contact and it can cause wear to the tooth surface. Wry bite, or wry mouth, is a class IV malocclusion describing a discrepancy in jaw length between the right and left sides of the mandible. One mandible is visibly longer than the maxilla and the other side is shorter. The upper and lower incisors do not align. Wry bite is a skeletal defect genetic condition in which the affected animal has a nonsymmetrical head. Anodontia is the absence of one or all of the teeth because of developmental disorders rather than tooth extraction. Bellows J, "Malocclusions of teeth," in Lobprise HB, ed, Blackwell's Five-Minute Veterinary Consult Clinical Companion: Small Animal Dentistry, ed 2, Wiley-Blackwell, 2012, p. 195-203; Lobprise HB, "Malocclusions of teeth," Blackwell's Five-Minute Veterinary Consult Clinical Companion: Small Animal Dentistry ed 2, Wiley-Blackwell, 2012, p. 195-206.

137. b Polydontia is also known as supernumerary or extra teeth in addition to the normal number. A supernumerary tooth is usually an adult tooth. Retained deciduous teeth are deciduous or baby teeth that have not fallen out in their normal time frame. It is possible to observe supernumerary and retained deciduous teeth at the same time. Tooth loss resulting from periodontal disease occurs when the support structures of the tooth or periodontium are destroyed because of plaque bacteria. Lobprise HB, "Abnormal number of teeth (increased)," Blackwell's Five-Minute Veterinary Consult Clinical Companion: Small Animal Dentistry, ed 2, Wiley-Blackwell, 2012, p. 168-172.

138. a The sulcus depth should normally be between 2.0 and 3.0 mm in dogs, depending on the teeth. Lobprise HB, "Periodontal disease: gingivitis," Blackwell's Five-Minute Veterinary Consult Clinical Companion: Small Animal Dentistry, ed 2, Wiley-Blackwell, 2012, p. 211-215.

139. b Excessive growth on gingival tissue is termed *gingival hyperplasia*. Gingiva or gum tissue surrounds the base of the tooth and the alveolar bone. Gingivitis is the inflammation of the gingiva as a reaction to the presence of plaque bacteria. Gingival recession is the apical movement of the gum tissue from the gingival crest in response to the presence of plaque bacteria or calculus. Gingivectomy is the removal of unsupported gum tissue. Gingivectomy is the treatment for gingival hyperplasia. Mosby's Dental Dictionary, ed 2, Mosby, 2008.

140. d Gingival recession is the apical movement of the gum tissue from the gingival crest in response to the presence of plaque bacteria or calculus. Gingival hyperplasia is the excess growth of gingival tissue, causing a false pocket around the cementoenamel junction. Periodontitis is the loss of the support structure or periodontium of the tooth. The periodontium is made up of the gingiva, periodontal ligament, and the alveolar bone. When there is a loss of any of these support structures, gingivitis becomes periodontitis. Gingivectomy is the removal of unsupported gum tissue. Gingivectomy is the treatment for gingival hyperplasia. Mosby's Dental Dictionary, ed 2, Mosby, 2008.

141. b Fusion tooth is when two separate-forming tooth structures join to form a single structure, which can sometimes occur at the root. When this occurs, there will be one less tooth than normal. Gemini tooth is an incomplete separation of two teeth usually resulting in two crowns sharing one root system. Polydontia is more teeth than the normal number (also known as supernumerary teeth). Oligodontia is a decreased number of teeth, also known as hypodontia. Lobprise HB, "Glossary," Blackwell's Five-Minute Veterinary Consult Clinical Companion: Small Animal Dentistry, ed 2, Wiley-Blackwell, 2012, p. 467-482.

142. b Furcation is the location where the roots diverge into a multirooted tooth. The most terminal portion of the root, or the tip of the root, is called the apex or the apical portion. A fissure is an abnormal deep groove or a cleft in either the enamel or the gingiva. Mosby's Dental Dictionary, ed 2, Mosby, 2008.

143. a Gemini tooth is an incomplete separation of two teeth usually resulting in two crowns sharing one root system. Fusion tooth is when two separate-forming tooth structures join to form a single structure. You will sometimes see this fusion at the root. There will be one less tooth than normal. Polydontia is a greater number of teeth than normal (also known as supernumerary teeth). Oligodontia is a decreased number of teeth, also known as hypodontia. Lobprise HB, "Glossary," Blackwell's Five-Minute Veterinary Consult Clinical Companion: Small Animal Dentistry, ed 2, Wiley-Blackwell, 2012, p. 467-482.

144. b The most rostral surface is known as the labial aspect, or toward the lips. The occlusal surface is the flat surface found on the crowns of molars. The flat surface allows food to be ground to a form that can be swallowed. The buccal surface is the side of the tooth that comes into contact with the cheek mucosa. The mesial surface is the part closest to the midline of the arch. The midline is the interdental space between the right and left maxillary and mandibular first incisors. Holzman G, "The basics," in Perrone JR, ed, Small Animal Dental Procedures for Veterinary Technicians and Nurses, Wiley-Blackwell, 2013, p. 3-22.

145. b Oligodontia is a decreased number of teeth, which is also known as hypodontia. Polydontia is a greater number of teeth than normal, which are often referred to as supernumerary teeth. Fusion tooth is when two separate-forming tooth structures join to form a single structure. Wry bite, or wry mouth, is a class IV malocclusion describing a discrepancy in jaw length between the right and left sides of the mandible. One mandible will appear longer than the maxilla, whereas the other side appears shorter. The upper and lower incisors will not align. Wry bite is a skeletal defect genetic condition in which the affected animal has a nonsymmetrical head. Lobprise HB, "Glossary," Blackwell's Five-Minute Veterinary Consult Clinical Companion: Small Animal Dentistry, ed 2, Wiley-Blackwell, 2012, p. 467-482; Niemiec BA, "Pathology in the pediatric patient," Small Animal Dental, Oral and Maxillofacial Disease, Manson, 2010, p. 90-127.

146. c The buccal surface is the side of the tooth that comes into contact with the cheek mucosa. The occlusal surface is the flat surface found on the crowns of molars. The flat surface allows food to be ground to a form that can be swallowed. The most rostral surface is known as the labial aspect, or toward the lips. The mesial surface is the part closest to the midline of the arch. The midline is the interdental space between the right and left maxillary and mandibular first incisors. Holzman G, "The basics," in Perrone JR, ed, Small Animal Dental Procedures for Veterinary Technicians and Nurses, Wiley-Blackwell, 2013, p. 3-22.

147. c During the conscious feline patient oral examination, tooth resorption lesions are commonly seen at the cementoenamel junction. As the coronal tooth structure is destroyed, gingival tissue fills the holes until the tooth is treated or until the crown falls off. Gorrel C, Derbyshire S, "Common oral and dental conditions," Veterinary Dentistry for the Nurse and Technician, ed 1, Butterworth-Heinemann, 2005, p. 87-107.

148. b Fluoride reduces sensitivity when applied over exposed dentinal tubules. Fluoride forms fluoroapatite, causing the tooth surface to be strengthened and more resistant to the cariogenic bacteria that dissolve enamel. When polishing teeth, the use of the appropriate amount of prophy paste prevents heat buildup resulting from the spinning motion of the prophy angle on the tooth surface. The prophy paste also provides lubrication so that the prophy angle spins more freely. Constant irrigation helps prevent heat buildup in the tooth when power scaling. Power scalers use water to keep the tip cool. It is important to ensure that the water flow has a fine mist. The fine mist will keep the tip cool enough and will provide irrigation but not cause the patient's head to become drenched, which can lower the body temperature. Bellows J, "Equipping your dental practice," The Practice of Veterinary Dentistry, Iowa State Press, 1999, p. 45-80; McMahon J, "The dental cleaning," in Perrone JR, ed, Small Animal Dental Procedures for Veterinary Technicians and Nurses, Wiley-Blackwell, 2013, p. 59-86

149. b Enamel hypoplasia or enamel hypocalcification is an inadequate deposition of enamel on the crown. It can affect one or many teeth and can affect all of the crown or part of the crown. It occurs because of a disruption in enamel formation such as distemper virus or any fever during the development of the tooth. Prognathism, also called an undershot jaw, is commonly seen in breeds such as the boxer, Pekingese, and bulldogs. Prognathism is a class III malocclusion in which the mandible is longer than the maxilla. The mandibular incisors will be either level with or rostral to the maxillary incisors. The mandibular and maxillary premolars and molars will be out of alignment, causing tooth-to-tooth trauma. Abrasion is wear to the tooth surface from an outside source such as a toy, cage door, or excessive grooming. Attrition is the active or passive wear of the tooth surface either by chewing, biting, or when there is close contact with another tooth. Lobprise HB, "Enamel hypocalcification," Blackwell's Five-Minute Veterinary Consult Clinical Companion: Small Animal Dentistry, ed 2, Wiley-Blackwell, 2012, p. 152-156; Niemiec BA, "Pathology in the pediatric patient," Small Animal Dental, Oral and Maxillofacial Disease, Manson, 2010, p. 90-127.

150. b Class 2 malocclusion or mandibular distoclusion is an abnormal rostral–caudal relationship of the maxillary and mandibular arches. The mandibular arch occludes caudal (distal) to its normal position relative to the maxillary arch. Class 3 malocclusion or mandibular mesioclusion is an abnormal rostral–caudal relationship of the maxillary and mandibular arches. The mandibular arch is rostral (mesial) to its normal position relative to the maxillary arch. Class 1 malocclusion or neutroclusion is a normal rostral–caudal relationship of the maxillary and mandibular arches with malposition of one or more individual teeth. Dental malocclusion is a malocclusion caused by the abnormal positioning of one or more teeth. Lobprise HB, "Appendix B: American veterinary dental college nomenclature," Blackwell's Five-Minute Veterinary Consult Clinical Companion: Small Animal Dentistry, ed 2, Wiley-Blackwell, 2012, p. 442-461.

151. a Class 3 malocclusion or mandibular mesioclusion is an abnormal rostral–caudal relationship of the maxillary and mandibular arches. The mandibular arch is rostral (mesial) to its normal position relative to the maxillary arch. Class 2 malocclusion or mandibular distoclusion is an abnormal rostral–caudal relationship of the maxillary and mandibular arches. The mandibular arch occludes caudal (distal) to its normal position relative to the maxillary arch. Class 1 malocclusion or neutroclusion is a normal rostral–caudal relationship of the maxillary and mandibular arches with malposition of one or more individual teeth. Dental malocclusion is a malocclusion caused by the abnormal positioning of one or more teeth. Lobprise HB, "Appendix B: American veterinary dental college nomenclature," Blackwell's Five-Minute Veterinary Consult Clinical Companion: Small Animal Dentistry, ed 2, Wiley-Blackwell, 2012, p. 442-461.

152. c The carnassial teeth are the large caudal chewing teeth in dogs and cats. The maxillary carnassial tooth is the fourth and last premolar and the mandibular carnassial tooth is the first molar. The maxillary fourth premolar occludes buccal to the mandibular first molar. Their occlusion allows the dog or cat to shear meat from bones. Holzman G, "The basics," in Perrone JR, ed, Small Animal Dental Procedures for Veterinary Technicians and Nurses, Wiley-Blackwell, 2013, p. 3-22.

153. a The Triadan system uses three numbers. The first number identifies one of the four quadrants of the mouth. The order is sequential, beginning with the upper right maxillary that is assigned 1; 2 is the left maxillary, 3 the left mandibular, and 4 the right mandibular. The same format is followed for the deciduous teeth, starting with 5 for the deciduous maxillary right quadrant. The second and third numbers identify the teeth. There are always two numbers to represent a tooth. The tooth numbering begins in the front of the mouth with the central or first incisor being 01, the intermediate or second incisor 02, and the lateral or third incisor 03. The canine is always 04, and the first molar is always 09. Thus 205 refers to the left maxillary quadrant and the fifth tooth, which is the first premolar. Holzman G, "The basics," in Perrone JR, ed, Small Animal Dental Procedures for

Veterinary Technicians and Nurses, Wiley-Blackwell, 2013, p. 3-22.

154. a To radiograph the maxillary incisors, the rostral maxillary position is used. The film or sensor is placed below the incisors and canine teeth. The tube head or cone is angled between 50 and 60 degrees to the hard palate. To radiograph the mandibular premolars and molars, the parallel mandibular view is used. The film or sensor is placed between the tongue and the mandible parallel to the long axis of the teeth. The tube head is positioned perpendicular to the film at an approximate angle of 60 degrees to the horizontal plane. To radiograph the mandibular incisors and canine, the rostral mandibular view is used. The film or sensor is placed below the incisors and canine teeth. The tube head or cone is angled at about 60 degrees to the mandible. To radiograph the maxillary canine tooth, the lateral oblique view is used. The film or sensor is placed below the canine tooth to the second premolar. The tube head or cone is angled 45 degrees to the hard palate and 80–90 degrees oblique to the right or left, depending on which canine tooth is being radiographed. Mulligan TW, "Intraoral imaging techniques," Atlas of Canine and Feline Dental Radiography, Veterinary Learning Systems, 1998, p. 27-44.

155. c To radiograph the mandibular incisors and canine, the rostral mandibular view is used. The film or sensor is placed below the incisors and canine teeth. The tube head or cone is angled at about 60 degrees to the mandible. To radiograph the maxillary incisors, the rostral maxillary position is used. The film or sensor is placed below the incisors and canine teeth. The tube head or cone is angled between 50 and 60 degrees to the hard palate. To radiograph the mandibular premolars and molars, the parallel mandibular view is used. The film or sensor is placed between the tongue and the mandible parallel to the long axis of the teeth. The tube head is positioned perpendicular to the film at an approximate angle of 60 degrees to the horizontal plane. To radiograph the maxillary canine tooth, the lateral oblique view is used. The film or sensor is placed below the canine tooth to the second premolar. The tube head or cone is angled 45 degrees to the hard palate and 80–90 degrees oblique to the right or left, depending on which canine tooth is being radiographed. Mulligan TW, "Intraoral imaging techniques," Atlas of Canine and Feline Dental Radiography, Veterinary Learning Systems, 1998, p. 27-44.

156. b To radiograph the mandibular premolars and molars, the parallel mandibular view is used. The film or sensor is placed between the tongue and the mandible parallel to the long axis of the teeth. The tube head is positioned perpendicular to the film at an approximate angle of 60 degrees to the horizontal plane. To radiograph the maxillary incisors, the rostral maxillary position is used. The film or sensor is placed below the incisors and canine teeth. The tube head or cone is angled between 50 and 60 degrees to the hard palate. To radiograph the mandibular incisors and canine, the rostral mandibular view is used. The film or sensor is placed below the incisors and canine teeth. The tube head or cone is angled at about 60 degrees to the mandible. To radiograph the maxillary canine tooth, the lateral oblique view is used. The film or sensor is placed below the canine tooth to the second premolar. The tube head or cone is angled 45 degrees to the hard palate and 80–90 degrees oblique to the right or left, depending on which canine tooth is being radiographed. Mulligan TW, "Intraoral imaging techniques," Atlas of Canine and Feline Dental Radiography, Veterinary Learning Systems, 1998, p. 27-44.

157. b A tooth abscess will appear radiographically as a radiolucent area around the apex of the tooth. The area is radiolucent because the bacteria from the infection eat away the support structure that holds the tooth to the bone. A radiopaque area around the tooth root is a normal finding because bone and tooth are radiopaque. A radiopaque area inside the tooth pulp is a pulp stone. A radiolucent area inside the pulp is normal because the pulp is soft tissue that radiographs as radiolucent. Bellows J, "The why, when, and how of small animal dental radiography," The Practice of Veterinary Dentistry, Iowa State Press, 1999, p. 81-105.

158. c Pedodontics is the study of both genetic and acquired dental conditions of puppies and kittens. Exodontics is the extraction of teeth. Orthodontics is guidance and correction of malocclusion. Prosthodontics is the construction of an appliance designed to replace missing or other adjacent structures. Holmstrom SE, "The oral examination and disease recognition," Veterinary Dentistry: A Team Approach, ed 2, Saunders, 2013, p. 26-77.

159. a The periodontal probe is a hand instrument used to measure sulcus depth to rule out the presence of a periodontal pocket. A periodontal pocket is a deeper-than-normal measurement. Gorrel C, "Oral examination and charting," Small Animal Dentistry, Saunders, 2008, p. 13-21: Gorrel C, "Radiography," Small Animal Dentistry, Saunders, 2008, p. 22-28.

160. c In Class 5 tooth resorption there is no clinical crown but root tips remain, which are seen on dental radiographs. An acutely fractured tooth resulting from trauma will have a portion of the crown fractured off with the exposed pulp appearing as a pink dot in the middle of the fractured area. A normal-looking tooth with inflamed gums is considered gingivitis. An uncomplicated crown fracture is a fracture that does not involve the pulp. These teeth only require restoration for treatment. Bellows J, "Oral surgical equipment, materials and techniques," Small Animal Dental Equipment, Materials and Techniques: A Primer, Blackwell, 2004, p. 297-361.

161. c Internal resorption arises from the pulp. Trauma or death of the pulp can be contributing factors. It is diagnosed on dental radiography as an abnormally shaped pulp chamber. Bellows J, "Dental radiography," Small Animal Dental Equipment, Materials and Techniques: A Primer, Blackwell, 2004, p. 63-103.

162. a Periodontal disease is a bacterial infiltration that adheres to the biofilm that forms on the crown between brushings or cleanings. As the bacteria continue to multiply, they change from aerobic to anaerobic becoming more destructive. The bacterial growth moves apically down the tooth surface. The bacteria start destroying the support structures or periodontium (gingiva, periodontal ligament, alveolar bone). When this destruction affects multiple teeth and extends into the alveolar bone, this can be seen radiographically as horizontal bone loss. Fractured teeth only affect the crown or the root. Orthodontic disease is caused by malocclusion. Teeth affected with malocclusion need to be moved into proper position or extracted to provide a comfortable bite. Bellows J, "Dental radiography," Small Animal Dental Equipment, Materials and Techniques: A Primer, Blackwell, 2004, p. 63-103.

163. a If a tooth becomes fractured in a patient younger than 1 year of age and/or if the fracture is less than 48 hours old, the tooth can be treated with a vital pulp therapy procedure. This procedure stimulates apexogenesis in younger patients to allow the tooth apex to close. In patients with an acute fracture, the vital pulp therapy removes a small amount of the exposed pulp and then a liquid material is placed over the exposed pulp. This material irritates the exposed pulp, causing a dentinal bridge to form. A composite restoration is placed over the material to protect the area during healing. Root canal therapy is performed if the pulp is already dead or has a high chance of dying. Root canal therapy removes the entire tooth, the pulp chamber is cleaned, and a material is placed in the empty pulp chamber to remove the dead space and to prevent bacterial infiltration. After the procedure it is still a functional tooth but it is clinically dead. Bellows J, "Endodontic equipment, materials and techniques," Small Animal Dental Equipment, Materials and Techniques: A Primer, Blackwell, 2004, p. 175-229.

164. b A gray or black-colored pulp is an indication of necrotic or dead pulp. Root canal therapy or extractions are the only treatment options. In the case of a tooth that has been worn, the black discoloration is shiny and the pulp chamber will not be accessible using a dental explorer. In these cases regular probing and dental radiographs are needed for evaluation. A tooth with an open pulp chamber should never be left untreated. Bellows J, "Endodontic equipment, materials and techniques," Small Animal Dental Equipment, Materials and Techniques: A Primer, Blackwell, 2004, p. 175-229.

165. c The maxillary nerve block desensitizes the entire maxillary quadrant on both the palatal and lingua aspects. The location is the most caudal aspect of the hard palate. This is just caudal to the maxillary second molar of a dog or the maxillary first molar of a cat. The infraorbital block desensitizes all of the maxillary teeth rostral to the injection site. The infraorbital foramen is located dorsal to the roots of the maxillary third premolar. The middle mental block desensitizes the mandibular incisors and canines and the lower lip of the injected side. The foramen is located below the mesial root of the mandibular second premolar in the dog and mandibular third premolar in the cat. The mandibular or inferior alveolar nerve block desensitizes all the mandibular teeth on the injected side. The foramen is located on the lingual surface of the caudal mandible where the ventral cortex curves dorsally. Lewis JR, Miller BR, "Veterinary dentistry," in Bassett JM, Thomas JA, McCurnin's Clinical Textbook for Veterinary Technicians, ed 8, Elsevier, 2014, p. 1297-1354.

166. d In some cases malocclusion can be uncomfortable and in some cases it is painful. If the malocclusion causes the patient to experience difficulty or pain when chewing, it must be treated. The definition of orthodontics is the correction of malposition and malocclusion. In patients that are registered with the American Kennel Club (AKC) as show animals, orthodontic treatment can only be performed if the malocclusion or malposition causes harm to the animal. Movement of teeth to make a show animal more successful in the ring is illegal in the AKC. The goal with orthodontic treatment is to return a functional, comfortable bite to the patient. Bellows J, "Orthodontic equipment, materials, and treatment," Small Animal Dental Equipment, Materials and Techniques: A Primer, Blackwell, 2004, p. 263-296; "Rules dismissals," in Rules, Policies and Guidelines for Conformation Dog Show Judges REJ 999 https://images.akc.org/pdf/rulebooks/REJ999.pdf. Accessed September 9, 2020.

167. a Extraction forceps should only be used after the tooth has become mobile by elevation. The periodontium is initially incised using a surgical blade to allow a purchase point for the dental elevator to be inserted. The dental elevator is inserted between the tooth root and the alveolar bone. This is where the periodontal ligament fibers are located. After insertion, the dental elevator cuts and fatigues the periodontal ligament using downward and small twisting movements. The instrument is held using a short finger stop to avoid slippage, which could cause trauma to the patient or to the surgeon. This technique is repeated around the entire tooth until the tooth becomes mobile. The extraction forceps grasp the tooth as low as possible. A small twisting motion is used to release the tooth from the alveolus. Using the extraction forceps too early in the extraction process can result in a fractured root. Extracting the tooth without the extraction forceps is difficult because the tooth surface is slippery with blood and water. Bellows J, "Oral surgical equipment, materials, and techniques," Small Animal Dental Equipment, Materials and Techniques: A Primer, Blackwell, 2004, p. 297-361.

168. c Placement of an esophagostomy feeding tube benefits the dental patient after any major oral surgery that has necessitated the removal of large areas of jaw bone or after full-mouth extractions. The purpose of the esophagostomy feeding tube is to provide nutrition to the patient while bypassing the oral cavity during healing. Medications that are prepared to pass through the tube can also be administered. Routine cleanings, extractions, and small tumor removals do not require the placement of an esophagostomy tube because patients with proper pain management are able to eat comfortably the same day. Lewis JR, Miller BR, "Veterinary dentistry," in Bassett JM, Thomas JA, McCurnin's Clinical Textbook for Veterinary Technicians, ed 8, Elsevier, 2014, p. 1297-1354.

169. b Seal-point Siamese, greyhounds, collies, and borzois are breeds that are considered dolichocephalic.

Dolichocephalic heads are long and narrow. German shepherds and corgis are considered mesaticephalic and have medium heads. Persian cats are considered brachycephalic and have short, wide heads. Holmstrom SE, "Introduction to veterinary dentistry," Veterinary Dentistry: A Team Approach, ed 2, Saunders, 2013, p. 1-25.

170. d A lingually displaced mandibular canine is a condition in which the mandibular canine occludes directly into the hard palate. Normally the mandibular canine should occlude between and buccal to the maxillary third incisors and canine. The condition causes pain and potential communication with the nasal cavity. One option aside from orthodontic movement of the misplaced tooth into proper position is a crown reduction. A crown reduction involves cutting off the crown to the level of the incisors. The exposed pulp is treated and restored with a vital pulpotomy procedure, which allows the tooth to remain vital, and the crown tip can no longer enter the hard palate. Teeth affected by near pulpal exposure can be treated with a vital pulpotomy procedure if they are within the treatment parameters of either a patient younger than 12 months of age or a fracture that has occurred less than 48 hours previously. If the tooth does not fall into the parameters mentioned here, then root canal therapy or extraction is recommended. On a tooth with Stage 3 periodontal disease there is >50% bone loss. At this stage the only treatment option is extraction. Bellows J, "Orthodontic equipment, materials and techniques," Small Animal Dental Equipment, Materials and Techniques: A Primer, Blackwell, 2004, p. 263-296.

171. a Lip-fold dermatitis is a skin infection. The condition affects breeds with prominent lower lip folds and large pendulous upper lips. The combination of moisture from excess saliva, trapped food, and hair can cause increased bacterial growth, which, in turn, can lead to irritation, erythema, and a foul odor. Bulldogs, setters, spaniels, and bassets are the most commonly affected breeds. Summers AD, "Dogs and cats: diseases of the digestive system," Common Diseases of Companion Animals, ed 2, Mosby, 2007, p. 38-92.

172. b Periodontal probes come in various mm increments. The important point is to familiarize yourself with the probe before you begin measuring. 1, 2, 3, 4, 5, 6, 7, 8, 9, 10, 11, 12, 13, 14, 15 are the markings of a UNC 15 probe. The difference between the UNC and the Williams probe is that the Williams probe makes a jump. This was done to avoid confusion when measuring. 3, 6, 8 are the markings for the Michigan O probe. 1, 2, 3, 5, 7, 8, 9, 10 are the markings for the Goldman Fox probe. One of the unique traits of the Goldman Fox probe is that the probe can be either rounded or flat. The flat probe makes it easier to fit into a tight sulcus of pocket. Lewis JR, Miller BR, "Veterinary dentistry," in Bassett JM, Thomas JA, McCurnin's Clinical Textbook for Veterinary Technicians, ed 8, Elsevier, 2014, p. 1297-1354.

173. d It is critical that the owner is notified of any changes to the treatment plan. The oral examination is performed in two parts. The first part is in the examination room with the patient awake. The initial treatment plan can be presented at this point. The second part of the examination is performed after the patient is anesthetized. Radiographs are performed of each tooth, the oral cavity, and the full-mouth. After this is accomplished, the owner should be contacted and be told whether the treatment plan will remain the same or will change in any way. This is also a good opportunity to update the owner on the patient's condition under anesthesia and to provide a tentative completion time. Bellows J, "Dental radiography," Small Animal Dental Equipment, Materials and Techniques: A Primer, Blackwell, 2004, p. 63-103.

174. c Antibiotics can be administered into a periodontal pocket after root planing and/or gingival debridement. These antibiotics come in a gel form and are slowly released. This provides local control of the bacteria that causes periodontal disease, as well as reduces pocket depth, increases attachment levels, and decreases inflammation. Injectable antibiotics can be long acting or short acting and can treat systemic bacteria, which can be introduced into the blood stream before, during, or after the dental procedure. Systemic antibiotics are given IV, IL, or SC. Medications that are injected into a foramen are usually nerve block drugs. Holmstrom SE, "Periodontal therapy," Veterinary Dentistry: A Team Approach, ed 2, Saunders, 2013, p. 216-226.

175. a The vasoconstriction caused by the addition of epinephrine to a nerve block drug such as bupivacaine or lidocaine prolongs the effect of the nerve block drug and also provides some hemostasis. Epinephrine should not be used in patients that have uncontrolled hyperthyroidism, cardiac dysrhythmias, or asthma. Woodward TM, Local anesthesia in oral surgery, http://www.dentalaireproducts.com/local-anesthesia-in-oral-surgery/ Accessed 7 30 2015.

176. d Although all of the diseases mentioned cause a cat to paw at its face and cry out in pain, orofacial pain syndrome differentiates itself from the others by the aggression of the cat to make the pain stop. It is a pain disorder that presents with behavioral signs rather than a clinical presentation. In cases like these, a thorough oral examination with dental radiography is crucial to rule out an oral disease or trauma. It is thought that this condition is caused by damage to the nerves of the peripheral nervous system. The patient will proceed from very painful to pain-free intervals that will lessen with time. Mouth movements will usually trigger a reaction. The patient can become resistant to traditional pain-management treatments. The condition does, however, respond to an anticonvulsant with an analgesic effect. If the condition does not improve, testing for small intestinal lymphoma and/or inflammatory bowel disorder is recommended. Holmstrom SE, "Feline dentistry," Veterinary Dentistry: A Team Approach, ed 2, Saunders, 2013, p. 227-234.

177. a Gutta percha is used during a root canal procedure. After the pulp chamber has been debrided and flushed, a CE end or paste is used to seal the walls of the pulp chamber, preventing any bacteria from entering the dentinal tubules. Gutta percha fills in the remaining space in the pulp chamber. The gutta percha is packed into the pulp chamber using a plugger and a spreader. The spreader moves the gutta percha to the walls to allow more to be fitted in. Calcium hydroxide is an endodontic material used for a vital pulpotomy procedure. This material is placed on the exposed pulp and the tooth is restored. The material acts as an irritant to the tooth and causes it to form a dentist bridge over the exposed pulp, sealing it from any possible bacteria. The restoration is made from an acrylic resin. It acts as a permanent covering over any exposed tooth. The material comes in a paste or liquid form and is hardened and shaped to the tooth surface either by chemical curing or light bonding. Bellows J, "Endodontic equipment, materials, and techniques," Small Animal Dental Equipment, Materials and Techniques: A Primer, Blackwell, 2004, p. 175-229; Holmstrom SE, "Advanced veterinary dental procedures: periodontal surgery, endodontics, restorations and orthodontics," Veterinary Dentistry: A Team Approach, ed 2, Saunders, 2013, p. 307-342.

178. c The rostral maxillary, rostral caudal, and caudal mandibular blocks are known as regional blocks because they block sensation to entire quadrants of the oral cavity. Infiltration or splash blocks are least effective because they only block the area immediately around the injection point. Care is still taken to avoid hitting a blood vessel by aspirating before injecting. Infiltration blocks are usually performed after a dental procedure has been performed to reduce postoperative pain. Holmstrom SE, "Local anesthesia," Veterinary Dentistry: A Team Approach, ed 2, Saunders, 2013, p. 135-149; Woodward TM, Local anesthesia in oral surgery, http://www.dentalaireproducts.com/local-anesthesia-in-oral-surgery/ Accessed 7 30 2015.

179. a The most common cause of dental malocclusions is retained deciduous teeth. When these teeth do not fall out and the adult teeth start appearing, the adult teeth will erupt in the wrong position. Bad breeding can cause many malocclusion issues such as skeletal issues and overbites. In some breeds, overbites are normal occlusions as seen in brachycephalic breeds. Bellows J, "Orthodontic equipment, materials and techniques," Small Animal Dental Equipment, Materials and Techniques: A Primer, Blackwell, 2004, p. 263-296.

180. b West Highland white terriers can inherit a condition called cranial mandibular osteodystrophy. This condition presents as a non-neoplastic excess bone formation in the area of the temporomandibular joint (TMJ) and it can extend into the mandible. These patients experience pain, which lessens as the patient ages. Mandibular periostitis ossificans is found in immature large-breed dogs. This condition causes a unilateral bony swelling of the ventral mandible and is diagnosed radiographically by the presence of double-layered ventral cortex. It is considered an inflammatory reaction that will spontaneously disappear. An odontoma presents in the mandible as an oral swelling. Radiographically, that swelling is a mass of cells made up of enamel, dentin, cementum, and other toothpick structures. The mass can be extensive and invasive, but excisable. Osteomyelitis is inflammation of the bone and bone marrow secondary to a bacterial infection. Treatment with antibiotics is usually recommended. Holmstrom SE, "The oral examination and disease recognition," Veterinary Dentistry: A Team Approach, ed 2, Saunders, 2013, p. 26-77.

181. a Staging is a way to classify oral tumors. It is performed by the veterinarian and uses the system set up by the World Health Organization (WHO) for classifying cancerous tumors in humans. This system uses three features for assessment. T characterizes the tumor by its clinical features. N assesses the involvement of regional lymph nodes. M assesses whether the tumor has metastasized to other sites of the body. The system further assesses the tumor with quantitative measurements and the stage is further characterized with a number after each feature, such as T1, N1, and M1, depending on the results. Tumors are measured for size and recorded. Periodontal care and oral tumor surgery are assessed and a treatment plan is created. The treatment plan is discussed and agreed on with the owner of the patient. Komurek K, "Small animal medical nursing," in Bassett JM, Thomas JA, McCurnin's Clinical Textbook for Veterinary Technicians, ed 8, Elsevier, 2014, p. 672-719; Bellows J, "Oral surgical equipment, materials, and techniques," Small Animal Dental Equipment, Materials and Techniques: A Primer, Blackwell, 2004, p. 297-362.

182. a In horses, premolars 2–4 (Triadan 06–08) and the three molars (Triadan 09–11) can be collectively termed *cheek teeth.* Each type of tooth has certain morphological characteristics and specific functions. Incisor teeth are specialized for the prehension and cutting of food and the canine teeth are for defense and offence (for capture of prey in carnivores). Equine cheek teeth function as grinders for mastication. Dixon, PM, duToit, N "Dental anatomy," in Easley J, Padraic Dixon P, Schumacher J, Equine Dentistry, ed 3, Elsevier Health Sciences, 2011, p. 51-76.

183. c Coronal refers to the crown. The area furthest away from the occlusal surface is the apical surface. The area closest to the tongue is the lingual surface and the tooth closest to the incisors is the premolar. Easley J, Padraic Dixon P, Schumacher J, Equine Dentistry, ed 3, Elsevier Health Sciences, 2011, p. 51-76.

184. a Brachydont teeth (permanent dentition) fully erupt before maturity and are normally long and hard enough to survive for the life of the individual because they are not subjected to the prolonged and high levels of dietary abrasive forces with which herbivore teeth must contend. In contrast, hypsodont teeth slowly erupt during most of a horse's life at a rate of 2–3 mm/year, which is similar to the rate of attrition (wear) on the occlusal surface of the tooth, provided that the horse is on a grass diet (or some alternative fibrous diet, e.g., hay or silage) rather than being fed high levels of concentrate food. The latter type of diet reduces the rate of occlusal wear and also restricts the range of lateral chewing actions and thus dental overgrowths can occur. Both brachydont and hypsodont teeth have a limited growth period (although this period is very prolonged in the latter group) and thus are termed *anelodont teeth*. Dixon, PM, duToit, N, "Dental anatomy," in Easley J, Padraic Dixon P, Schumacher J, Equine Dentistry, ed 3, Elsevier Health Sciences, 2011, p. 51-76.

185. d Elodont teeth grow continually throughout all of an animal's life. Brachydont and hypsodont teeth are considered anelodont and have a period of growth. Dixon, PM, duToit, N, "Dental anatomy," in Easley J, Padraic Dixon P, Schumacher J, Equine Dentistry, ed 3, Elsevier Health Sciences, 2011, p. 51-76.

186. b Horses have 24 deciduous teeth 2(Di 3 / 3, Dc 0 / 0, Dm 3 / 3). Dixon, PM, duToit, N, "Dental anatomy," in Easley J, Padraic Dixon P, Schumacher J, Equine Dentistry, ed 3, Elsevier Health Sciences, 2011, p. 51-76.

187. b Adult horses also have 12 incisors in total, 6 in each arcade. The upper incisor teeth are embedded in the premaxillary (incisive) bone and the lower incisors in the rostral mandible, with the reserve crowns and apices of incisors converging toward each other. Dixon, PM, duToit, N, "Dental anatomy," in Easley J, Padraic Dixon P, Schumacher J, Equine Dentistry, ed 3, Elsevier Health Sciences, 2011, p. 51-76.

188. c Male horses normally have four permanent canine teeth: two maxillary and two mandibular. Canine teeth are usually absent or rudimentary in female horses, with a reported prevalence of 7.8%–28% in horses and 17.3%–30% in donkeys. Dixon, PM, duToit, N, "Dental anatomy," in Easley J, Padraic Dixon P, Schumacher J, Equine Dentistry, ed 3, Elsevier Health Sciences, 2011, p. 51-76.

189. b The 12 temporary premolars (506–508, 606–608, 706–708, and 806–808) erupt at birth or do so within a week. Dixon, PM, duToit, N, "Dental anatomy," in Easley J, Padraic Dixon P, Schumacher J, Equine Dentistry, ed 3, Elsevier Health Sciences, 2011, p. 51-76.

190. c An adult equine mouth normally contains 24 cheek teeth (06s–11s, i.e., 2nd–4th premolars and 1st–3rd molars), forming four rows of six teeth that are accommodated in the maxillary and mandibular bones. The molars erupt at approximately 1, 2, and 3.5 years of age, respectively. Dixon, PM, duToit, N, "Dental anatomy," in Easley J, Padraic Dixon P, Schumacher J, Equine Dentistry, ed 3, Elsevier Health Sciences, 2011, p. 51-76.

191. a The most appropriate teeth for aging horses are the (lower) incisors. The premolars and molars can be used with considerable accuracy to determine the horse's age, but their distal position has limited their use. Research has shown that cheek teeth morphology data can be used to predict age in horses that possess all permanent dentition. Radiographic assessment of cheek teeth root morphology can also help in determining age, especially in young horses. Because contact between upper and lower canines is seldom made, the canines do not wear down in a regular way and have no age-related occlusal surface. Dixon, PM, duToit, N "Dental anatomy," in Easley J, Padraic Dixon P, Schumacher J, Equine Dentistry, ed 3, Elsevier Health Sciences, 2011, p. 51-76.

192. b A variety of factors such as nature and quality of food, environmental conditions, heredity, injury, and disease can influence dental wear. It is, therefore, important that equine clinicians do not claim levels of accuracy that are unjustifiable. As it is impossible to assign specific ages to each dental feature, accuracy of age estimation in certain individuals can be very low. Dixon, PM, duToit, N "Dental anatomy," in Easley J, Padraic Dixon P, Schumacher J, Equine Dentistry, ed 3, Elsevier Health Sciences, 2011, p. 51-76.

193. b Foals develop a number of growth abnormalities, one being parrot mouth or an overbite. Overjet is known as overshot jaw, which will result in an overbite when not treated. Underjet is also known as undershot jaw and it is rare. Easley J, Padraic Dixon P, Schumacher J, Equine Dentistry, ed 3, Elsevier Health Sciences, 2011, p. 51-76.

194. c Dysplasia or abnormal development of teeth can involve the crown, roots, or the entire tooth. Commonly recorded disturbances in the gross form of teeth include dilacerations (abnormal bending of teeth), double teeth, abnormalities of size, and concrescence (roots of adjacent teeth joined by cementum) of teeth. Disturbances in the structure of teeth, including dysplasia (disturbances of development) of the individual calcified dental tissues or pulp, are well described. Dixon, PM, duToit, N "Dental anatomy," in Easley J, Padraic Dixon P, Schumacher J, Equine Dentistry, ed 3, Elsevier Health Sciences, 2011, p. 51-76.

195. d SCC, sarcoid, and ossifying fibroids are all soft tissue neoplasms, whereas an osteoma is an osteogenic neoplasm. Knottenbelt, DC, Kelly, DF, "Oral and dental tumors," in Easley J, Padraic Dixon P, Schumacher J, Equine Dentistry, ed 3, Elsevier Health Sciences, 2011, p. 149-184.

196. d Polyps, papillomas, and epulides are all non-neoplastic masses, whereas a cementoma is an odontogenic neoplasm. Knottenbelt, DC, Kelly, DF, "Oral and dental tumors," in Easley J, Padraic Dixon P, Schumacher J, Equine Dentistry, ed 3, Elsevier Health Sciences, 2011, p. 149-184.

197. a Chlorhexidine gluconate 0.05% (1:40 dilution of the 2% concentration) is the antiseptic of choice for oral rinses and has replaced chlorhexidine acetate because it is less likely to irritate mucous membranes. Dilute Betadine should not be used and glutaraldehyde can cause tissue necrosis. Galloway, SS, Galloway, MS, "Dental materials," in Easley J, Padraic Dixon P, Schumacher J, Equine Dentistry, ed 3, Elsevier Health Sciences, 2011, p. 345-368.

198. b If used improperly, all motorized floats can overheat teeth to the point of pulp damage. Lower speeds in the 2000 to 3000 rpm range are preferred because higher-speed rotation produces heat faster. (Note: Use light pressure on the float and keep it moving.) Easley J, Rucker, BA, "Equine dental equipment, supplies and instrumentation," in Easley J, Padraic Dixon P, Schumacher J, Equine Dentistry, ed 3, Elsevier Health Sciences, 2011, p. 245-260.

199. d Safety of the operator, the assistant(s), and the equine patient during motorized instrument use can be optimized in several ways. Protective eyewear and an air filter mask reduce the chance of debris and tooth dust entering the eyes and/or being inhaled. Ear protection should be considered if loud electric motors are used close to the operator's head or noisy air compressors are in operation nearby. Easley, J, Rucker, BA, "Equine dental equipment, supplies, and instrumentation," in Easley J, Padraic Dixon P, Schumacher J, Equine Dentistry, ed 3, Elsevier Health Sciences, 2011, p. 245-260

200. c Gelpi retractors are used in abdominal surgery to expose the abdominal cavity. Various forceps, elevators, and dental picks should be available to remove retained, displaced, or broken deciduous cheek tooth remnants (caps). Easley, J, Rucker, BA, "Equine dental equipment, supplies, and instrumentation," in Easley J, Padraic Dixon P, Schumacher J, Equine Dentistry, ed 3, Elsevier Health Sciences, 2011, p. 245-260.

201. c Nippers and cutters should not be used on canine teeth because these instruments offer minimal to no control during tooth fracturing. Opening the pulp or dentinal tubules can lead to pulpitis and tooth death years after the reduction. To avoid over-reduction of the canines, small files or diamond disc grinders (at low speed) should be used only for smoothening or to blunt the top of the canine. Elevators are not used to smooth tooth surfaces. Easley, J, Rucker, BA, "Equine dental equipment, supplies, and instrumentation," in Easley J, Padraic Dixon P, Schumacher J, Equine Dentistry, ed 3, Elsevier Health Sciences, 2011, p. 245-260.

202. b The objective of prophylactic antibiotics is to prevent treatment-induced bacteremia. Geriatric, debilitated, or immunocompromised individuals should receive antibiotics. In addition, those with preexisting heart conditions, gross infection, or chronic stomatitis should receive antibiotics. King Charles spaniels are more likely to have a preexisting heart condition, especially when they are over 10 years of age. Gorrel C, Antibiotics and antiseptics," Veterinary Dentistry for the General Practitioner, ed 2, Elsevier, 2013, p. 30-36.

203. b Numerous chemical agents have been evaluated for the supplementation of mechanical plaque control. Clinically effective antiplaque agents are characterized by a combination of intrinsic antibacterial activity and good oral retention properties. Agents that have been evaluated include chlorhexidine, essential oils, triclosan, sanguinarine, fluorides, oxygenating agents, quaternary ammonium compounds, substituted amino-alcohols and enzymes. Of these, the greatest effect on the reduction of plaque and gingivitis can be expected from chlorhexidine. Chlorhexidine is the gold standard and is the agent against which all antiplaque agents are tested. A diluted ampicillin solution is not available. The goal of a chlorhexidine flush in advance of the procedure is to reduce the number of bacteria in the oral cavity, to reduce the number of bacteria aerosolized during the procedure, and to supplement mechanical plaque control. Gorrel C, "Antibiotics and antiseptics," Veterinary Dentistry for the General Practitioner, ed 2, Elsevier, 2013, p. 30-35.

204. a Malocclusion is common and causes pain/discomfort and severe oral pathology. Malocclusions lead to periodontal disease, stomatitis, and gingival recession. Malocclusions should be diagnosed early in an attempt to prevent dental disease later in life. Gorrel C, "Occlusion and malocclusion," Veterinary Dentistry for the General Practitioner, ed 2, Elsevier, 2013, p. 42-55.

205. c Examination involves not only assessing the oral cavity but also palpation of the face (facial bones and zygomatic arch), the temporomandibular joint, the salivary glands (mandibular/sublingual; the parotids are usually only palpable if enlarged), and the lymph nodes (mandibular, cervical chain). The popliteal lymph nodes are not part of an oral assessment. Gorrel C, "Oral examination and recording," Veterinary Dentistry for the General Practitioner, ed 2, Elsevier, 2013, p. 56-66.

206. a Most animals allow at least a cursory inspection of the oral cavity after the jaws have been opened. The mucous membranes of the oral cavity should be examined in addition to the teeth. Apart from the color and texture of the mucous membranes, look for evidence of a potential bleeding problem (petechiation, purpura, ecchymoses). In addition, look for vesicle formation and ulceration, which could indicate a vesiculobullous disorder, for example, pemphigus and/or pemphigoid. Gingival recession falls into the pathology assessment category, and tonsillar crypts and fauces fall into the assessment of the oropharynx. Gorrel C, "Oral examination and recording," Veterinary Dentistry for the General Practitioner, ed 2, Elsevier, 2013, p. 56-66.

207. b Most animals allow at least a cursory inspection of the oral cavity after the jaws have been opened. The mucous membranes of the oral cavity should be examined, in which vesicle formation and ulceration should be observed, which could indicate a vesiculobullous disorder, for example, pemphigus and/or pemphigoid. Obvious pathology (tooth fracture, gingival recession, advanced furcation exposure) relating to the teeth can be identified. Tonsillar crypts, tonsils, and fauces would fall into the assessment of the oropharynx. Gorrel C, "Oral examination and recording," Veterinary Dentistry for the General Practitioner, ed 2, Elsevier, 2013, p. 56-66.

208. c Gingival index 0: Clinically healthy gingiva. Gingival index 1: Mild gingivitis: slight reddening and swelling of the gingival margin; no bleeding on gentle probing of the gingival sulcus. Gingival index 2: Moderate gingivitis: the gingival margin is red and swollen; gentle probing of the gingival sulcus results in bleeding. Gingival index 3: Severe gingivitis: the gingival margin is very swollen with a red or bluish-red color; there is spontaneous hemorrhage and/or ulceration of the gingival margin. Gorrel C, "Oral examination and recording," Veterinary Dentistry for the General Practitioner, ed 2, Elsevier, 2013, p. 56-66.

209. d The mesial surface is the part closest to the midline of the arch, whereas distal is the part farthest away from the midline. The midline is the interdental space between the right and left maxillary and mandibular first incisors. Holzman G, "The basics," in Perrone JR, ed, Small Animal Dental Procedures for Veterinary Technicians and Nurses, Wiley-Blackwell, 2013, p. 3-22.

210. b The curette can be used supra- and subgingivally on the tooth surface. It is not recommended for use in cleaning out the developmental grooves because the tips are not fine enough. Polishing removes the microetchants on the teeth by combining the fine-to-medium grit prophy paste with the spinning action of the prophy angle on the tooth surface. McMahon J, "The dental cleaning," in Perrone JR, ed, Small Animal Dental Procedures for Veterinary Technicians and Nurses, Wiley-Blackwell, 2013, p. 59-85.

211. c Grade 0: No furcation involvement. Grade 1: Initial furcation involvement: the furcation can be felt with the probe/explorer, but horizontal tissue destruction is <⅓ of the horizontal width of the furcation. Grade 2: Partial furcation involvement: it is possible to explore the furcation, but the probe/explorer cannot be passed through it; horizontal tissue destruction is >⅓ of the horizontal width of the furcation. Grade 3: Total furcation involvement: the probe/explorer can be passed through the furcation from buccal to palatal/lingual. Gorrel C, "Oral examination and recording," Veterinary Dentistry for the General Practitioner, ed 2, Elsevier, 2013, p. 56-66.

212. c Adult dogs have a total of 42 teeth, with each mandibular and maxillary side having 4 premolars. There are 2 maxillary and 3 mandibular molars per side. Holzman G, "The basics," in Perrone JR, ed, Small Animal Dental Procedures for Veterinary Technicians and Nurses, Wiley-Blackwell, 2013, p. 3-22.

213. c Calculus is mineralized dental plaque. Plaque attaches to the biofilm on the tooth surface and is made up of bacteria, salivary glycoproteins, and extracellular polysaccharides. Attrition is the active or passive wear of the tooth surface either by chewing, biting, or when there is close contact with another tooth. Abrasion is wear to the tooth surface from an outside source, such as a toy, cage door, or excessive grooming. Lobprise HB, "Glossary," Blackwell's Five-Minute Veterinary Consult Clinical Companion: Small Animal Dentistry, ed 2, Wiley-Blackwell, 2012, p. 467-482.

214. b Grade 0: No mobility. Grade 1: Horizontal movement of <1 mm. Grade 2: Horizontal movement of >1 mm. Note that multirooted teeth are scored more severely, and a horizontal mobility in excess of 1 mm is usually considered a Grade 3 even in the absence of vertical movement. Grade 3: Vertical as well as horizontal movement is possible. Gorrel C, "Oral examination and recording," Veterinary Dentistry for the General Practitioner, ed 2, Elsevier, 2013, p. 56-66.

215. b The premolars function to hold and carry food, as well as to break food down into smaller pieces. The canine teeth are used for holding and tearing and the incisors are for gnawing and grooming. The molars are used for grinding. Wiggs RB, Lobprise HB, "Oral anatomy and physiology," in Veterinary Dentistry: Principles and Practices, Lippincott-Raven, 1997, p. 55-86.

216. d The periodontal probe is an instrument that measures the gingival sulcus for any abnormal depths >3 mm in dogs and 0.5–1.0 mm in cats. The periodontal probe is also used to measure how much gingival recession or gingival hyperplasia is affecting the tooth. The periodontal probe is marked in mm at 1 mm or 3 mm intervals. Curettes are used to remove calculus, debris, and granulation tissue below the gum line or subgingivally. The curette is made with a rounded tip and a rounded back to facilitate insertion below the gum line without causing trauma. A dental explorer is used to check the tooth surface for any irregularities from an enamel fracture to pulp exposure in a fractured tooth. The working end of the explorer is a fine wire made to alert the handler that there is a defect by catching and making a pinging sound. Scalers are used to remove calculus above the gum line or supragingivally. The scaler has a ridged back, two sharp sides, and a pointed tip. The tip of the scaler is used to remove debris in the developmental grooves along the crown surface. Bellows J, "Equipping your dental practice," The Practice of Veterinary Dentistry, Iowa State Press, 1999, p. 45-80.

217. b UCF: Uncomplicated crown fracture; CCF: Complicated crown fracture; UCRF: Uncomplicated crown and root fracture; CCRF: Complicated crown and root fracture. Gorrel C, "Emergencies," Veterinary Dentistry for the General Practitioner, ed 2, Elsevier, 2013, p. 141-170.

218. d Buccal is the surface facing the cheek, whereas palatal is toward the upper palate. Lingual is the surface facing the tongue and is used in reference to the mandibular teeth. Labial means toward the lips. *Rostral* is the term meaning toward the front of the head and caudal is toward the back of the head. Holzman G, "The basics," in Perrone JR, ed, Small Animal Dental Procedures for Veterinary Technicians and Nurses, Wiley-Blackwell, 2013, p. 3-22.

219. d Fluoride reduces sensitivity when applied over exposed dentinal tubules. Fluoride forms fluoroapatite, causing the tooth surface to be more strengthened and resistant to cariogenic bacteria, which dissolve enamel. Fluoride does not have any effect on the structures of the periodontium such as the periodontal ligament. Bellows J, "Equipping your dental practice," The Practice of Veterinary Dentistry, Iowa State Press, 1999, p. 45-80.

220. b Full oral examination is only possible under general anesthesia. Oral examination should proceed in an orderly and structured fashion, using appropriate instrumentation. Adequate recording should occur at all stages, preferably on published or adapted dental charting systems. Several indices and measurements should be obtained to complement visual assessments, for example, gingival index, periodontal probing depth, and periodontal/clinical attachment level. Gorrel C, "Oral examination and recording," Veterinary Dentistry for the General Practitioner, ed 2, Elsevier, 2013, p. 56-66.

221. d Full-mouth radiographs (8–10 views) are strongly advocated in cats to detect odontoclastic resorptive lesions. All remaining statements are true. Gorrel C, "Dental radiography," Veterinary Dentistry for the General Practitioner, ed 2, Elsevier, 2013, p. 67-80.

222. b Anodontia (total absence of teeth) and oligodontia (congenital absence of many but not all teeth) are associated with ectodermal dysplasia, are rare, and can occur in dogs with no apparent systemic problem or congenital syndrome. Hypodontia (the absence of only a few teeth) is, however, a relatively common finding in dogs. Palatoschisis is known as a cleft palate. Gorrel C, "Glossary," Veterinary Dentistry for the General Practitioner, ed 2, Elsevier, 2013, p. 215-221.

223. a Cats have three maxillary premolars and two mandibular premolars per side. Holzman G, "The basics," in Perrone JR, ed, Small Animal Dental Procedures for Veterinary Technicians and Nurses, Wiley-Blackwell, 2013, p. 3-22.

224. d Cats, dogs, and horses have teeth that stop growing after the permanent teeth have erupted fully. The term for this is *anelodont*. Anelodont teeth have a limited growth period while the roots are developing. Rabbits and rats have elodont teeth. Elodont teeth grow throughout life and never develop roots. Equine patients are unique because they are hypsodonts, which means that much of the crown is subgingival and erupts about ⅛ inch per year until there is no more crown to erupt. Although equine patients are also anelodont, as are dogs and cats, the premolars and molars continue to erupt as the grinding surfaces are worn down through chewing. Verstraete FJM, "Question 42," in Self-Assessment Color Review of Veterinary Dentistry, CRC Press, 1999, p. 43-44.

225. d Radiographic evaluation allows differentiation between primary and permanent teeth. Primary teeth are smaller than their permanent counterparts, with long, slender roots. Compared with permanent teeth, the roots of primary teeth are relatively long in relation to the crown. Gorrel C, "Dental radiography," Veterinary Dentistry for the General Practitioner, ed 2, Elsevier, 2013, p. 67-80.

226. a Enamel hypoplasia (dysplasia) may be defined as an incomplete or defective formation of the organic enamel matrix of teeth. Anodontia (total absence of teeth) and oligodontia (congenital absence of many but not all teeth) are associated with ectodermal dysplasia, are rare, and can occur in dogs with no apparent systemic problem or congenital syndrome. Odontalgia is painful teeth. Gorrel C, "Common oral conditions," Veterinary Dentistry for the General Practitioner, ed 2, Elsevier, 2013, p. 81-96.

227. d Systemic factors include nutritional deficiencies, febrile disorders, hypocalcemia, and excessive intake of fluoride during the period of enamel formation. Gorrel C, "Common oral conditions," Veterinary Dentistry for the General Practitioner, ed 2, Elsevier, 2013, p. 81-96.

228. d Trauma (including a bite injury) and infection are examples of local factors that could affect enamel development. Hypocalcemia is a systemic factor resulting from a nutritional deficiency or endocrine disorder. Gorrel C, "Common oral conditions," Veterinary Dentistry for the General Practitioner, ed 2, Elsevier, 2013, p. 81-96.

229. c Dental decay is often referred to as caries. Enamel hypoplasia is also referred to as dysplasia, which can result from trauma. Furcation refers to a situation in which the bone between the roots of multirooted teeth is destroyed. Gorrel C, "Preventive dentistry," Veterinary Dentistry for the General Practitioner, ed 2, Elsevier, 2013, p. 121-127.

230. c Most epulides are non-neoplastic. The remaining statements are true. Gorrel C, "Common oral conditions," Veterinary Dentistry for the General Practitioner, ed 2, Elsevier, 2013, p. 81-96.

231. a Periodontal disease is the result of the inflammatory response to dental oral bacteria and it is limited to the periodontium. It is the most common oral disease in dogs. It is also common in cats. In fact, periodontal disease is probably the most common disease in small animal practice with the great majority of dogs and cats older than 3 years having a degree of disease that warrants intervention. Periodontal disease is unrelated to lupus and it may coexist with many conditions including lupus. Chronic stomatitis is not the result of the inflammatory process, but it is defined as inflammation of the oral mucosa. Gorrel C, "Periodontal disease," Veterinary Dentistry for the General Practitioner, ed 2, Elsevier, 2013, p. 97-120.

232. d The inflammatory reactions in periodontitis result in the destruction of the periodontal ligament and the alveolar bone. The result of untreated periodontitis is ultimately exfoliation of the affected tooth. Thus gingivitis is inflammation that is not associated with destruction (loss) of supporting tissue. Tooth enamel is not destroyed in the periodontitis inflammatory process. Gorrel C, "Periodontal disease," Veterinary Dentistry for the General Practitioner, ed 2, Elsevier, 2013, p. 97-120.

233. a Plaque accumulation starts within minutes on a clean tooth surface. The initial accumulation of plaque occurs supragingivally but will extend into the sulcus and will populate the subgingival region if left undisturbed. Gorrel C, "Periodontal disease," Veterinary Dentistry for the General Practitioner, ed 2, Elsevier, 2013, p. 97-120.

234. c Halitosis is common and is often the first sign that the pet owner notices. Individuals with untreated gingivitis may develop periodontitis. Gorrel C, "Periodontal disease," Veterinary Dentistry for the General Practitioner, ed 2, Elsevier, 2013, p. 97-120.

235. c The hyperplastic gingiva alters the position of the gingival margin and results in a false or pseudopocket. It is called a pseudopocket because the increased periodontal probing depth is not a result of the destruction of the periodontal ligament and the alveolar bone with apical migration of the junctional epithelium, as in periodontitis. Gorrel C, "Periodontal disease," Veterinary Dentistry for the General Practitioner, ed 2, Elsevier, 2013, p. 97-120.

236. d Veterinary technicians cannot perform surgery; however, they can perform all of the other techniques listed, in addition to root planing and tooth polishing. Gorrel C, "Periodontal disease," Veterinary Dentistry for the General Practitioner, ed 2, Elsevier, 2013, p. 97-120.

237. c Professional periodontal therapy (supra- and subgingival scaling and polishing) under general anesthesia to remove dental deposits (plaque and calculus) is required to reduce the incidence of dental disease. Gorrel C, "Periodontal disease," Veterinary Dentistry for the General Practitioner, Saunders, 2004, p. 87-110.

238. a Supragingival scaling is the removal of plaque and calculus above the gingival margin. It can be performed using hand instruments alone or with a combination of hand instruments and powered scalers. The recommended procedure is as follows: (1) Remove gross dental deposits (plaque-covered calculus) using rongeurs, extraction forceps, or calculus-removing forceps. (2) Remove residual supragingival dental deposits with sharp hand instruments (either a sickle-shaped scaler or a curette). (3) A powered scaler (either an ultrasonic or a sonic scaler) is then used to remove residual dental deposits. Powered scalers generate heat and have the potential to cause iatrogenic damage if not used properly. Overheating a tooth will cause desiccation of the dentine and consequent damage to the underlying pulp tissue. Pulp damage may be a reversible pulpitis but it can become severe enough to cause pulp necrosis, which would necessitate endodontic treatment of the affected tooth. Gorrel C, "Equipment and instrumentation," Veterinary Dentistry for the General Practitioner, ed 2, Elsevier, 2013, p. 1-13.

239. b A rough surface will facilitate plaque retention, not impede it. The remaining statements are true. Gorrel C, "Equipment and instrumentation," Veterinary Dentistry for the General Practitioner, ed 2, Elsevier, 2013, p. 1-13.

240. d Sulcular lavage involves gently flushing the gingival sulcus and pathologic pockets with saline or dilute chlorhexidine to remove any free-floating debris. This step is particularly important in a deep periodontal pocket because free-floating debris may occlude the orifice of the pocket and lead to the formation of a lateral periodontal abscess. The stream of fluid is directed subgingivally using a blunt-ended needle, a lachrymal catheter, or a Waterpik device. Gorrel C, "Periodontal disease," Veterinary Dentistry for the General Practitioner, ed 2, Elsevier, 2013, p. 97-120.

241. b Prevention is always preferable to treatment and many oral and dental conditions are readily amenable to preventive measures. Common conditions that can be prevented (totally or partially) include periodontal disease, caries, excessive wear, tooth fracture, and certain types of malocclusion. Gorrel C, "Preventive dentistry," Veterinary Dentistry for the General Practitioner, ed 2, Elsevier, 2013, p. 121-127.

242. b The owner is responsible for home care, which includes brushing the teeth to reduce the accumulation of plaque. The veterinary team will scale and lavage the patient's teeth while the patient is under general anesthesia. The benefit of any professional periodontal therapy is short-lived unless maintained by effective home care. In fact, if no home care is instituted after professional periodontal therapy, plaque will rapidly reform and disease will progress. It has been shown that, if no home care is instituted by 3 months after periodontal therapy, gingivitis scores are equivalent to those recorded before therapy. Gorrel C, "Preventive dentistry," Veterinary Dentistry for the General Practitioner, ed 2, Elsevier, 2013, p. 121-127.

243. a Tooth brushing is known to be the single most effective means of removing plaque. Studies have shown that in dogs with both experimentally induced gingivitis and naturally occurring gingivitis, daily tooth brushing is effective in returning the gingivae to health. In a 4-year study using beagle dogs, with no oral hygiene it was shown that plaque accumulated rapidly along the gingival margin, with gingivitis developing within a few weeks. Dogs that were fed an identical diet under identical conditions but that were subjected to daily tooth brushing developed no clinical signs of gingivitis. In the group that was not receiving daily tooth brushing, gingivitis progressed to periodontitis in most individuals. The type of toothpaste does not matter, except that is should be a pet-approved toothpaste. Dental diets are not as effective as tooth brushing. Gorrel C, "Preventive dentistry," Veterinary Dentistry for the General Practitioner, ed 2, Elsevier, 2013, p. 121-127.

244. c The use of a human toothpaste is not recommended, mainly because of the high fluoride (not salt) content, which may lead to acute, but more likely chronic, toxicity problems as pets do not rinse and spit but they swallow the toothpaste. Nonfoaming toothpaste is recommended, but it is not critical. A flavor pets like is recommended because it will allow owners to brush the teeth for a longer period. Gorrel C, "Preventive dentistry," Veterinary Dentistry for the General Practitioner, ed 2, Elsevier, 2013, p. 121-127.

245. c The brush is angled at 45-degrees to the tooth surfaces so that the bristles enter the gingival sulcus. A circling motion should ensure that all cracks and crevices in and around the teeth are cleaned. Preventive dentistry," Gorrel C, "Preventive dentistry," Veterinary Dentistry for the General Practitioner, ed 2, Elsevier, 2013, p. 121-127.

246. d All of the listed examples can lead to abrasion in veterinary patients. Excessive abrasion can occur under certain circumstances and stone chewing is a common cause. Another common cause is playing with a ball on a sandy surface. The ball becomes wet and covered with sand or grit and, as the animal bites on the ball, the teeth are worn excessively. Prevention in such circumstances is restricting access to stones and only playing with a ball in an environment where the ball does not become covered with abrasive material. Loss of teeth (because of disease or trauma) and malocclusion may also predispose to excessive attrition. If extensive extractions are required, the resultant occlusion must be evaluated and preventive measures instituted as appropriate. Gorrel C, "Preventive dentistry," Veterinary Dentistry for the General Practitioner, ed 2, Elsevier, 2013, p. 121-127.

247. c Veterinarians would remove primary teeth, not permanent teeth, to prevent malocclusion, and this should be performed before 12–14 weeks of age. Gorrel C, "Occlusion and malocclusion," Veterinary Dentistry for the General Practitioner, ed 2, Elsevier, 2013, p. 42-55.

248. a 2 × {I 2/1:C 0/0:P 3/2:M 3/3} is the rabbit formula; 2 × {I 3/3:C 1/1:P 4/4:M 2/3} is the permanent formula for dogs; 2 × {I 3/3:C 1/1:P 3/2:M 1/1} is the permanent formula for cats; 2 × {I 3/3:C 1/1:P 3/3} is the primary formula for dogs. Gorrel C, "Anatomy of the teeth and periodontium," Veterinary Dentistry for the General Practitioner, ed 2, Elsevier, 2013, p. 36-41.

249. d The heaviest calculus is usually found on the buccal surface of the upper check teeth because of the adjacent parotid salivary duct opening. The opening or parotid papilla is located in the mucosa above the distal root of the maxillary fourth premolar. The lower canine and incisor teeth are not adjacent to any salivary glands. There are two molar salivary glands in cats, which are the lingual molar salivary gland and the buccal molar salivary gland. These are not present in dogs. Wiggs RB, Lobprise HB, "Oral anatomy and physiology," in Veterinary Dentistry: Principles and Practices, Lippincott-Raven, 1997, p. 55-86.

250. a Lingual is the surface facing the tongue and is used in reference to the mandibular teeth. The most rostral surface is known as the labial aspect or toward the lips. The buccal surface is the side of the tooth that comes into contact with the cheek mucosa. The mesial surface is the part closest to the midline of the arch. The midline is the interdental space between the right and left maxillary and mandibular first incisors. Holzman G, "The basics," in Perrone JR, ed, Small Animal Dental Procedures for Veterinary Technicians and Nurses, Wiley-Blackwell, 2013, p. 3-22.

251. d Dental conditions in rabbits and rodents are generally a result of husbandry, diet intake, and lack of environmental enrichment, all of which should be addressed during examination procedures. Gorrel C, Verhaert, L, "Dental diseases in lagomorphs and rodents," Veterinary Dentistry for the General Practitioner, ed 2, Elsevier, 2013, p. 191-211.

252. b Scaling the teeth causes microetchants on the surface of the enamel, therefore polishing paste is applied to smooth the surface of the tooth and to remove any remaining plaque left behind by the cleaning. The polishing cup runs only over the surface of the teeth, not the gums. The polish does not disinfect and fluoride is not applied after polishing. Bellows J, "Equipping your dental practice," The Practice of Veterinary Dentistry, Iowa State Press, 1999, p. 45-80.

253. a Epulides are the fourth most common oral mass in dogs, but they are rare in cats. Epulides arise from the periodontal connective tissue, originating in the gingiva. There are three classifications of epulides: fibromatous epulis, ossifying epulis, and acanthomatous epulis. Fibromatous and ossifying epulides are now categorized as peripheral odontogenic fibromas. Acanthomatous epulides are unique. They are locally invasive and require wider margins around the tumor for complete removal. Fibrosarcoma, squamous cell carcinoma, and malignant melanoma are all malignant oral tumors. Lobprise HB, "Epulis," Blackwell's Five-Minute Veterinary Consult Clinical Companion: Small Animal Dentistry, ed 2, Wiley-Blackwell, 2012, p. 303-309; Dahliwal RS, "Malignant oral neoplasia," in Niemiec BA, Small Animal Dental, Oral and Maxillofacial Disease, Manson, 2010, p. 226-237.

254. c Normally, adult dogs have 6 incisors, 2 canines, 8 premolars, and 5 molars per side, which equals 42 teeth. Holzman G, "The basics," in Perrone JR, ed, Small Animal Dental Procedures for Veterinary Technicians and Nurses, Wiley-Blackwell, 2013, p. 3-22.

255. a Normally, adult cats have 6 incisors, 2 canines, 5 premolars, and 2 molars per side, which equals 30 teeth. Holzman G, "The basics," in Perrone JR, ed, Small Animal Dental Procedures for Veterinary Technicians and Nurses, Wiley-Blackwell, 2013, p. 3-22.

SECTION 8

1. a The *Vibrio* spp. morphology is a rod. The bacillus is also a rod. Coccus, spirochetes, and coccobacillus are not rods. Coccus is an arrangement of cocci bacteria, spirochetes are spiral in their morphology, and a coccobacillus has an oval morphology, intermediate between the coccus and the bacillus forms. Studdert VP, Gay CC, Blood DC, Saunders Comprehensive Veterinary Dictionary, ed 4, Elsevier Saunders, 2007.

2. a Fimbriae bind bacteria to cell surfaces. Locomotion, ion transport, and antibiotic resistance are the most important jobs of bacterial fimbriae. Tizard I, Veterinary Immunology, ed 9, Elsevier Saunders, 2013, p. 85.

3. a Bacterial endospores are resistant to heat, desiccation, chemicals, and radiation. Bacterial endospores are survival capsules that allow the organisms to survive harsh environments, but they are not a form of reproduction. Hendrix C, Sirois M, Laboratory Procedures for Veterinary Technicians, ed 5, Mosby Elsevier, 2007, p. 238.

4. d Bilirubin is assayed to determine the cause of jaundice, to evaluate liver function, and to check the patency of bile ducts. Blood levels of bilirubin are elevated with hepatocellular damage or with bile duct injury or obstruction. Blood levels of bilirubin are elevated with excessive erythrocyte destruction or defects in the transport mechanism that allows bilirubin to enter the hepatocytes for conjugation. Elevated lipase and amylase would be significant findings for a patient with acute pancreatitis. Hendrix C, Sirois M, Laboratory Procedures for Veterinary Technicians, ed 5, Mosby Elsevier, 2007, p. 200.

5. d A bacterial genus belongs to a species, versus being composed of one or more species, classes, or families. Suspected pathogens on the incubated plate should be further identified regarding their genus or species with the use of the flow chart. Determining the genus of a pathogenic organism is often possible by using just the staining and culture characteristics. Hendrix C, Sirois M, Laboratory Procedures for Veterinary Technicians, ed 5, Mosby Elsevier, 2007, p. 256.

6. a Antisepsis is the prevention of sepsis by antiseptic means, which is the result of the application of iodine on the skin. Asepsis (absence of pathogenic microorganisms that cause infection) makes the environment surgically clean, but not sterile (absence of all living microorganisms, including spores). Disinfection and sterilization are used on inanimate objects and fumigation is associated with disinfecting fumes. Tear M, Small Animal Surgical Nursing, ed 2, Mosby Elsevier, 2012, p. 102.

7. a Parenteral routes of medication administration include any of the injectable modalities. Of the options presented, transfusion is the only choice that includes an injectable modality. Studdert VP, Gay CC, Blood DC, Saunders Comprehensive Veterinary Dictionary, ed 4, Elsevier Saunders, 2007.

8. d The majority of bacteria grow in a neutral pH (6.5–7.0); however, there are some that thrive in acidic environments with a pH as low as 1.0 and there are very few that can thrive in a more alkaline environment. Sirois

M, Principles and Practice of Veterinary Technology, ed 3, Mosby Elsevier, 2011, p. 180.

9. b Bacterial flagella are long filaments used for bacterial movement. Attachment is the job of bacterial fimbriae. Bacterial cells contain a single DNA strand and reproduce primarily by binary fission. Ion transport is dependent on ATP (~65%). Tizard I, Veterinary Immunology, ed 9, Elsevier Saunders, 2013.

10. a As definitive hosts, most cats with *Toxoplasma gondii* will be asymptomatic. Humans and other mammals are the hosts of *Giardia lamblia*. Canines, felines, and swine can be definitive hosts of *Isospora rivolta*. Swine are the definitive hosts of *Balantidium coli*. Bassert J, Thomas J, McCurnin's Clinical Textbook for Veterinary Technicians, ed 8, Elsevier Saunders, 2014, p. 471.

11. b Exposure to saturated steam at 12°C for 13 minutes is considered a safe, minimum standard. Autoclave tape is activated is activated at 118°C, therefore 110°C would not be an acceptable temperature to achieve sterilization. Emergency sterilization can be achieved by reaching a temperature of 131°C for 3 minutes. Bassert J, Thomas J, McCurnin's Clinical Textbook for Veterinary Technicians, ed 8, Elsevier Saunders, 2014, p. 1164.

12. b B cells, also known as B lymphocytes, produce antibodies and are involved in humoral immunity. Monocytes are the largest of the leukocytes; they are phagocytic cells that migrate to the tissues and as they mature they become known as macrophages. Erythrocytes are red blood cells, which transport oxygen and a small proportion of carbon dioxide throughout the body. Tighe MM, Brown M, Mosby's Comprehensive Review for Veterinary Technicians, ed 4, Mosby Elsevier, 2015, p. 676.

13. b FIV is a common lentivirus infection in cats. Coronavirus can cause FIP in cats. Herpes virus causes nasal and ocular ulcers in cats. Parvovirus causes panleukopenia and cerebellar hypoplasia. Studdert VP, Gay CC, Blood DC, Saunders Comprehensive Veterinary Dictionary, ed 4, Elsevier Saunders, 2007, p. 424.

14. c Viruses only grow in living cells, which in the laboratory are provided by embryonated hen eggs, cell culture, or laboratory animals (rabbits, mice, etc.) All of the other options listed are a method of culturing animal viruses. Studdert VP, Gay CC, Blood DC, Saunders Comprehensive Veterinary Dictionary, ed 4, Elsevier Saunders, 2007, p. 1179.

15. d The antibody isotype IgG is the most common antibody and is found in the highest concentration in the blood. IgA is of primary importance for mucosal immunity and comprises approximately 20% of the circulating antibody. IgD is a monomer that, when present, is in very low abundance. IgE is the primary immunoglobulin associated with Type-1 hypersensitivity reactions and it is usually present in very small amounts. Sirois M, Principles and Practice of Veterinary Technology, ed 3, Mosby Elsevier, 2011, p. 282.

16. b Total bilirubin is used to evaluate liver function. Elevated lipase and amylase would be significant findings for a patient with pancreatitis. Kidney function is evaluated by BUN, creatinine, and phosphorus. Bile duct obstruction can cause an elevation in total bilirubin but a total bilirubin test would not be used primarily to determine bile duct health. If a possible obstruction is suspected, an abdominal ultrasound or other imaging is the primary diagnostic. Tighe MM, Brown M, Mosby's Comprehensive Review for Veterinary Technicians, ed 4, Mosby Elsevier, 2015, p. 82.

17. b A phagocyte refers to leukocytes that ingest foreign organisms and particles. A leukocyte is a white blood cell, not a red blood cell. A platelet functions to coagulate blood, not to phagocytize organisms and particles. An antibody's job is to coat bacteria and to bind them to receptors on the phagocytes cells and then to trigger them for ingestion. Christenson DE, Veterinary Medical Terminology, ed 2, Elsevier Saunders, 1997, p. 50.

18. b Nosocomial is defined as pertaining to or originating in a hospital. Endemic disease presents in a predictable and continuous pattern in a community. Iatrogenic disease results from the activity of the veterinarian or from any adverse condition in a patient that results from treatment by a veterinarian. Studdert VP, Gay CC, Blood DC, Saunders Comprehensive Veterinary Dictionary, ed 4, Elsevier Saunders, 2007, p. 768.

19. a Leukopenia clinically refers to a deficiency of white blood cells (leuko means white, and penia means deficiency). An increase in white blood cells is called leukocytosis. A clinical sign of bone marrow disease can be a leukopenia (along with other blood irregularities). Blood cancer is a form of cancer that attacks the blood, bone marrow, or lymphatic system, in which leukopenia might be a clinical sign. Saunders Veterinary Terminology Flash Cards, ed 1, Elsevier Saunders, 2009, p. 102.

20. d Blood urea nitrogen (BUN) is a laboratory test that evaluates kidney function and is a breakdown product of protein that healthy, functioning kidneys remove. High-protein diets and strenuous exercise may cause an elevated BUN level because of increased amino acid breakdown. Glucose is a test that measures the amount of sugar circulating in the blood and SGTP is a liver function test. Creatinine is also an evaluator for kidney function; however, it is a breakdown product of muscle creatine. Hendrix C, Sirois M, Laboratory Procedures for Veterinary Technicians, ed 5, Mosby Elsevier, 2007, p. 88.

21. c Hemolysins have the specific action of destroying red blood cells. Coagulated blood or clotting is the process by which blood changes from liquid to gel. The enzyme plasmin digests fibrin threads and other clotting products to cause clot lysis. The breakdown of red blood cells can occur from a virus, as well as from autoimmune disease, among other reasons. It is not by itself an indicator of a viral infection. Studdert VP, Gay CC, Blood DC, Saunders Comprehensive Veterinary Dictionary, ed 4, Elsevier Saunders, 2007, p. 527.

22. b High-protein diets and strenuous exercise may cause an elevated BUN level because of increased amino acid breakdown. Carbohydrate intake does not affect BUN levels (as it is not a protein that must be broken down). Insufficient insulin may result from a pancreas malfunction, whereas insufficient ADH is secreted from the pituitary gland. Hendrix C, Sirois M, Laboratory Procedures for Veterinary Technicians, ed 5, Mosby Elsevier, 2007, p. 88.

23. c Hypoalbuminemia may result as a loss of protein either through the kidneys or through the gastrointestinal tract. Decreased albumin can be seen in liver failure but is not usually seen in chronic liver disease. Decreased albumin is not associated with a carnivore or vegetarian diet. Bassert J, Thomas J, McCurnin's Clinical Textbook for Veterinary Technicians, ed 8, Elsevier Saunders, 2014, p. 425.

24. a An icteric or yellow sample may occur with liver disease or hemolytic anemia. A red serum sample indicates hemolysis, samples from dark brown to black can indicate digested hemoglobin from bacterial growth, and green blood is occasionally seen in birds suffering from intestinal parasites, such as coccidian. Sirois M, Principles and Practice of Veterinary Technology, ed 3, Mosby Elsevier, 2011, p. 132.

25. b Green top tubes contain heparin. Purple top tubes contain EDTA, blue top tubes contain citrate, and gray tubes contain sodium fluoride. Bassert J, Thomas J, McCurnin's Clinical Textbook for Veterinary Technicians, ed 8, Elsevier Saunders, 2014, p. 399.

26. a The kidneys excrete urea and ≤40% is reabsorbed by the tubules for re-excretion. Rate of reabsorption is inversely proportional to the amount of urine output; therefore, urea evaluates both filtration and function. Creatinine, glucose, and sodium can be altered in the face of kidney disease but they do not evaluate filtration and function. Tighe MM, Brown M, Mosby's Comprehensive Review for Veterinary Technicians, ed 4, Mosby Elsevier, 2015, p. 87.

27. a Dehydration results in increased urine specific gravity (SG) and increased PCV. With loss of fluid, both the urine and the plasma will become more concentrated. Bassert J, Thomas J, McCurnin's Clinical Textbook for Veterinary Technicians, ed 8, Elsevier Saunders, 2014, p. 875.

28. c Water deprivation and modified water deprivation tests are contraindicated in the presence of dehydration and azotemia. The patient is already stressed because of a preexisting condition, and the body may have already begun to produce ADH; therefore, it is not a good scientific baseline. Water deprivation in the presence of suspected tubular disease can lead to rapid dehydration. Tubular malfunction can affect the body's ability to reabsorb water; without the ability to replenish the body with water, the animal will quickly dehydrate. A sign of dehydration can be an elevated MCV. Depriving or restricting water from an animal that is already dehydrated is contraindicated. Hendrix C, Sirois M, Laboratory Procedures for Veterinary Technicians, ed 5, Mosby Elsevier, 2007, p. 92.

29. a The presence of glucose in the urine may indicate diabetes mellitus. When levels of glucose in the filtrate exceed the renal threshold, excess is excreted in the urine. Aspinall V, Cappello M, Introduction to Veterinary Anatomy and Physiology Textbook, ed 2, Elsevier, 2009, p. 121.

30. a A horse has higher normal AST values than other species. Test methods should be specific to the species being tested or the horse specimen can be diluted before beginning the test. ALP, ALT, and GGT have values similar to other species. Tighe MM, Brown M, Mosby's Comprehensive Review for Veterinary Technicians, ed 4, Mosby Elsevier, 2015, p. 118.

31. d GGT levels increase when there has been damage to cholangiocytes. ALKP may indicate obstruction of bile flow. ALT is an enzyme that, when elevated, might indicate hepatocyte injury. AST may be elevated in response to hepatocyte injury, but it can also be increased after injury to other tissues, including the heart. H Hendrix C, Sirois M, Laboratory Procedures for Veterinary Technicians, ed 5, Mosby Elsevier, 2007, p. 81.

32. a Electrochemical and ion-specific methods are most often used for the evaluation of electrolytes and other ionic components A popular electrolyte analyzer, the IDEXX VetLyte, uses ion-specific electrodes to measure sodium, potassium, and chloride. Adsorption is the action of a substance in attracting and holding other materials or particles to its surface and it has no relation to electrolyte measurement. Enzymatic digestion uses enzymes to break down materials and it has nothing to do with measuring electrolytes. Hendrix C, Sirois M, Laboratory Procedures for Veterinary Technicians, ed 5, Mosby Elsevier, 2007, p. 193.

33. d Elevated T4 concentration confirms the diagnosis of hyperthyroidism in most patients. T4, thyroxine, is typically elevated in hyperthyroidism, which may be seen in older cats. Luteinizing hormone (LH) is measured for reproductive studies, cortisol for Cushing's disease, and bile acids for liver abnormalities. Bassert J, Thomas J, McCurnin's Clinical Textbook for Veterinary Technicians, ed 8, Elsevier Saunders, 2014, p. 698.

34. c Ideally, samples should be analyzed within 30 minutes of collection to avoid postcollection artifacts and degenerative changes. Refrigeration preserves most urine constituents for an additional 6–12 hours. Hendrix C, Sirois M, Laboratory Procedures for Veterinary Technicians, ed 5, Mosby Elsevier, 2007, p. 157.

35. b Cells tend to break down rapidly in urine and therefore the urine should be centrifuged immediately after collection if cytologic evaluation is to be performed. This is necessary to concentrate any cells present; they are then removed from the supernatant. If the specimen cannot be centrifuged immediately, it should be refrigerated and not be allowed to sit at room temperature (bacteria can proliferate and cells will continue to degrade). Urine should never be frozen for cytological evaluation. Hendrix C, Sirois M, Laboratory Procedures for Veterinary Technicians, ed 5, Mosby Elsevier, 2007, p. 157.

36. a The minimum specific gravity (SG) in a healthy dog is 1.030. Higher SG levels may indicate various levels of dehydration and lower levels may be suggestive of kidneys or diabetes mellitus if glucose is present. Bassert J, Thomas J, McCurnin's Clinical Textbook for Veterinary Technicians, ed 8, Elsevier Saunders, 2014, p. 431.

37. b The minimum specific gravity (SG) in a healthy cat is 1.035. Higher SG levels may indicate various levels of dehydration and lower levels may be suggestive of kidneys or diabetes mellitus if glucose is present. Bassert J, Thomas J, McCurnin's Clinical Textbook for Veterinary Technicians, ed 8, Elsevier Saunders, 2014, p. 431.

38. d Counting the reticulocytes requires new methylene blue, which will result in an RBC's absorbing stain. A reticulocyte count can be done manually if indicated by the CBC. Total WBC count, differential WBC count, and total protein are all tests that are expected on a routine CBC. Sirois M, Principles and Practice of Veterinary Technology, ed 3, Mosby Elsevier, 2011, p. 148.
39. d Ketones are produced as a result of the breakdown of fatty acids. Because diabetic patients cannot normally utilize glucose, they get their energy from the breakdown of fatty acids. Liver disease, urinary tract infections, and renal failure are not associated with ketonuria. Hendrix C, Sirois M, Laboratory Procedures for Veterinary Technicians, ed 5, Mosby Elsevier, 2007, p. 167.
40. c Cystocentesis is the preferred method for obtaining a urine sample for bacterial culture. Catheterization, free catch samples, and manual expressions increase the potential for sample contamination. Bassert J, Thomas J, McCurnin's Clinical Textbook for Veterinary Technicians, ed 8, Elsevier Saunders, 2014, p. 430.
41. d Urine with an increased number of leukocytes should be cultured for bacteria. UTIs with nitrate-reducing bacteria cause nitrite formation. However, this test does not seem as sensitive in dogs and cats as it is in humans; therefore, it is important to look for bacteria in the sediment. Leukocytes are not commonly observed in cases of neoplasia, diabetes, or renal failure (unless multiple diseases processes are occurring). Hendrix C, Sirois M, Laboratory Procedures for Veterinary Technicians, ed 5, Mosby Elsevier, 2007, p. 174.
42. d The urine should be protected from exposure to UV light because this would result in the deterioration of constituents such as bilirubin. Ketones, protein, and glucose will not deteriorate as a result of UV light. Bassert J, Thomas J, McCurnin's Clinical Textbook for Veterinary Technicians, ed 8, Elsevier Saunders, 2014, p. 430.
43. a An early morning sample tends to be the most concentrated because the animal has likely not urinated all night. Throughout the day, frequent urination and water intake can affect the concentration of the urine. Hendrix C, Sirois M, Laboratory Procedures for Veterinary Technicians, ed 5, Mosby Elsevier, 2007, p. 157.
44. b Hematuria is the presence of intact red blood cells in the urine. During centrifugation, only intact red blood cells settle out, changing the color of the supernatant from red to clear. When hemoglobin concentration is sufficiently high in the urine to impart red discoloration, the urine remains red after centrifugation. Urine that is brown when voided may contain myoglobin (referred to as myoglobinuria) and is excreted during conditions that cause muscle cell lysis. Uroglobinuria does not exist. Hendrix C, Sirois M, Laboratory Procedures for Veterinary Technicians, ed 5, Mosby Elsevier, 2007, p. 163.
45. d If the pH of the urine is too acidic or too alkaline, specific crystals or uroliths can form, but crystal presence alone does not change the pH of urine, rather certain types of crystals are more likely to form if the urine is acidic or basic. Factors that may decrease the pH include fever, starvation, a high-protein diet, acidosis, excessive muscular activity, and the administration of certain drugs. Alkalosis, high-fiber diets, infection of the urinary tract with urease bacteria, and the use of certain drugs may cause increased pH. Hendrix C, Sirois M, Laboratory Procedures for Veterinary Technicians, ed 5, Mosby Elsevier, 2007, p. 165.
46. d Squamous epithelial cells are derived from the lower urinary passageways. Cystocentesis bypasses these tissues and therefore there is virtually no possibility of retrieving these cells when performing a cystocentesis. Squamous cells are frequently seen in catheterization, manual expression, and free catch samples. Hendrix C, Sirois M, Laboratory Procedures for Veterinary Technicians, ed 5, Mosby Elsevier, 2007, p. 170.
47. c Common interferences in clinical chemistries include bilirubin, hemolysis, and lipemia. Most samples need to be separated via centrifugation or preserved with EDTA or heparin for analysis. Dilution and concentration do not interfere with evaluation. Bassert J, Thomas J, McCurnin's Clinical Textbook for Veterinary Technicians, ed 8, Elsevier Saunders, 2014, p. 427.
48. a BUN and creatinine are biochemical tests of the renal profile and they may indicate azotemia. Cholestatic enzymes, hepatocellular leakage enzymes, and total protein and albumin are all associated with hepatic function. Bassert J, Thomas J, McCurnin's Clinical Textbook for Veterinary Technicians, ed 8, Elsevier Saunders, 2014, p. 425.
49. c Steatorrhea is excess fat in the feces because of a malabsorption syndrome caused by disease of the intestinal mucosa or by pancreatic enzyme deficiency. Dyschezia is difficult or painful evacuation of feces from the rectum. Dysentery is defined as a number of disorders marked by inflammation of the intestine, especially of the colon with abdominal pain, tenesmus, and frequent stools often containing blood and mucus. Tenesmus is ineffectual and painful straining at defecation or urination. Studdert VP, Gay CC, Blood DC, Saunders Comprehensive Veterinary Dictionary, ed 4, Elsevier Saunders, 2007, p. 1046.
50. d Paired serum samples are performed after 12 hours of fasting, food is then ingested, and 2 postprandial hours are needed to perform this test. Postprandial serum bile acid concentrations are higher than fasting concentrations, and the serum bile acid level is normally elevated after a meal because the gallbladder has contracted and released increased amounts of bile into the duodenum. The difference between the prefasted blood and the postprandial blood is what is reported. Inadequate fasting or spontaneous gallbladder contraction can increase fasting bile acid level. The exception to this is horses, which do not store bile in the gallbladder; only one sample is needed. Hendrix C, Sirois M, Laboratory Procedures for Veterinary Technicians, ed 5, Mosby Elsevier, 2007, p. 84.
51. b All tests listed evaluate liver function; however, bile acids (preprandial and postprandial) are considered the function test of choice. The great advantage of bile acids is that they evaluate the major anatomic component of the hepatobiliary system. Hendrix C, Sirois M, Laboratory Procedures for Veterinary Technicians, ed 5, Mosby Elsevier, 2007, p. 84.
52. c In dehydrated patients, fluid leaves the blood to enter the dehydrated tissues, leaving the blood more

concentrated. Therefore, total protein levels will be significantly increased. Hendrix C, Sirois M, Laboratory Procedures for Veterinary Technicians, ed 5, Mosby Elsevier, 2007, p. 32.

53. d The presence of calcium oxalate crystals suggests ethylene glycol toxicity. Ammonium biurate crystals are most common in animals with severe liver disease and are found in slightly acidic, neutral, or alkaline urine. Tyrosine crystals are not common findings and are mostly seen in animals that have liver disease. Triple phosphate crystals (also known as struvite crystals) are usually seen in urine that is alkaline to slightly acidic. Battaglia A, Small Animal Emergency and Critical Care for Veterinary Technicians, ed 2, Saunders, 2007, p. 316.

54. c Cats, unlike other species, have two forms of reticulocytes. The aggregate form contains large clumps of reticulum and is similar to reticulocytes in other species. The punctate form, unique to cats, contains from two to eight small, singular, basophilic granules. Hendrix C, Sirois M, Laboratory Procedures for Veterinary Technicians, ed 5, Mosby Elsevier, 2007, p. 56.

55. a *Borrelia burgdorferi* is Lyme disease. Lentivirus and coronavirus are both viruses and are not diseases. *Pasteurella multocida* is associated with cat bites and abscesses in cats. Bassert J, Thomas J, McCurnin's Clinical Textbook for Veterinary Technicians, ed 8, Elsevier Saunders, 2014, p. 430.

56. d Red top tubes should be left in a rack to clot; they should not be rocked to prevent coagulation. Blue, green, and purple top tubes all contain an anticoagulant and therefore should be rocked gently in the rocker until they can be read. Tighe MM, Brown M, Mosby's Comprehensive Review for Veterinary Technicians, ed 4, Mosby Elsevier, 2015, p. 421.

57. c Ideally, blood samples should be collected from an animal that has fasted for 12 hours. Lipemic, icteric, and hemolyzed serum may interfere with chemistry testing. Sirois M, Principles and Practice of Veterinary Technology, ed 3, Mosby Elsevier, 2011, p. 157.

58. c The differential count is performed in the smear monolayer by using oil immersion. The monolayer is selected because the cells are barely touching one another but are not so far apart that you would not be able to count 100 WBCs. The feathered edge area is the thinnest layer and contains cells that are usually distorted and erratically distributed. The thickest area is not diagnostic because it contains multilayers of cells, which increases the difficulty in evaluating cell size, color, and count. Hendrix C, Sirois M, Laboratory Procedures for Veterinary Technicians, ed 5, Mosby Elsevier, 2007, p. 59.

59. c Rouleaux cells appear to be stacked on top of one another and are considered normal in horses and abnormal in dogs, rats, and pigs. Sirois M, Principles and Practice of Veterinary Technology, ed 3, Mosby Elsevier, 2011, p. 141.

60. a Although amylase, lipase, and trypsin are produced and secreted by the pancreas, only amylase and lipase are measured in the serum. Trypsin can be qualitatively measured in the feces as an assessment of chronic pancreatitis. Hendrix C, Sirois M, Laboratory Procedures for Veterinary Technicians, ed 5, Mosby Elsevier, 2007, p. 210.

61. a Pollakiuria is the abnormally frequent passage of urine. Pollakiuria is commonly seen in blocked cats, which squat frequently to urinate but void small amounts only. Complete lack of urine is known as anuria; excessive urination at night is called enuresis. Excessive urinating and drinking is called polyuria and polydipsia, respectively. Studdert VP, Gay CC, Blood DC, Saunders Comprehensive Veterinary Dictionary, ed 4, Elsevier Saunders, 2007, p. 876.

62. c In dehydrated animals, hemoconcentration results in a smaller ratio of fluid to cells. An elevated hematocrit usually indicates that dehydration is present. A low hematocrit indicates that anemia is present. Leukocytosis does not change with dehydration. Hendrix C, Sirois M, Laboratory Procedures for Veterinary Technicians, ed 5, Mosby Elsevier, 2007, p. 32.

63. d An increased number of circulating band neutrophils is called a left shift and indicates that the bone marrow is releasing less-mature cells to meet demand. If the number of band neutrophils exceeds the number of segmented neutrophils, it is a called a degenerative left shift. Leukocytosis is seen in a regenerative left shift. The leukocyte count is normal or depressed and the immature neutrophils outnumber the mature neutrophils in a degenerative left shift. Bassert J, Thomas J, McCurnin's Clinical Textbook for Veterinary Technicians, ed 8, Elsevier Saunders, 2014, p. 413.

64. a Jaundice is also known as icterus and is characterized by the yellowness of skin, sclera, mucous membranes, and excretions because of hyperbilirubinemia and deposition of bile pigments. Xanthochromia is also associated with yellow discoloration but usually indicates hemorrhage into the central nervous system and is caused by the presence of xanthematin. Hemoglobinuria is the presence of hemoglobin in the urine and can cause discolored urine; ketonuria is the result of ketones in the urine and does not usually cause discoloration. Studdert VP, Gay CC, Blood DC, Saunders Comprehensive Veterinary Dictionary, ed 4, Elsevier Saunders, 2007.

65. c Bile acids convert fats and fatty acids into maltose. Proteins and carbohydrates have other functions but do not aid in digestion. Globulins are a form of protein produced in the liver. Aspinall V, Cappello M, Introduction to Veterinary Anatomy and Physiology Textbook, ed 2, Elsevier, 2009, p. 108.

66. d Samples should be inspected grossly for small clots before a sample is processed for a CBC; if a clot is present, a new sample should be collected. Clots in an EDTA tube are never acceptable because they can cause several false abnormalities such as decreased PCV and low platelet counts among others. Bassert J, Thomas J, McCurnin's Clinical Textbook for Veterinary Technicians, ed 8, Elsevier Saunders, 2014, p. 399.

67. c Only about 10%–30% of dogs with food allergies have GI problems. Most signs are cutaneous skin reactions that include skin rashes, ear infections, and pruritus. Tizard I, Veterinary Immunology, ed 9, Elsevier Saunders, 2013.

68. c A large buffy coat would be expected in a patient with an infection because the buffy coat is composed of leukocytes. Neutrophilia, leukocytosis, and a left shift are all expected in a patient with an infection. Hendrix C, Sirois M, Laboratory Procedures for

Veterinary Technicians, ed 5, Mosby Elsevier, 2007, p. 53.

69. a If the blood sample is from an anemic patient, increase the pusher slide angle to about 45 degrees. Anemic blood is thinner in consistency and using the normal angle creates too long a smear. Increasing the angle shortens the smear. Sirois M, Principles and Practice of Veterinary Technology, ed 3, Mosby Elsevier, 2011, p. 135.

70. c MCV (mean cell volume) indicates cell size. MCH (mean cell hemoglobin) is the quantity of hemoglobin in an average erythrocyte. MCHC (mean cell hemoglobin concentration) is an expression of the average concentration of hemoglobin per average erythrocyte. MPV (mean platelet volume) is the average size of circulating platelets. Studdert VP, Gay CC, Blood DC, Saunders Comprehensive Veterinary Dictionary, ed 4, Elsevier Saunders, 2007.

71. b NRBCs may be erroneously counted as WBCs by manual methods and by some automated hematology analyzers, resulting in a falsely increased WBC count. Bassert J, Thomas J, McCurnin's Clinical Textbook for Veterinary Technicians, ed 8, Elsevier Saunders, 2014, p. 412.

72. c An acanthocyte is an erythrocyte with protoplasmic projections giving it a thorny appearance. Acanthocytes have a few projections and may be of uneven length. Crenated cells have shorter projections that are evenly spaced around the cell. Schistocytes are pieces of RBCs and anisocytes are RBCs that show varying sizes (anisocytosis). Studdert VP, Gay CC, Blood DC, Saunders Comprehensive Veterinary Dictionary, ed 4, Elsevier Saunders, 2007, p. 6.

73. a When reticulocytes are stained with a vital stain, their RNA is visible as blue granules or aggregates. These cells correspond to the larger, blue-gray polychromatic RBCs seen in Wright-stained smears. Polychromasia is a slight bluish tinge caused by RNA that has not completely gone from the RBC. A hypochromic RBC is a cell that has insufficient hemoglobin and more central pallor than normal. Hyperchromasia is a condition that does not really exist, but spherocytes look hyperchromic; they appear darker than normal. Crenated RBCs have evenly spaced, short projections all around the cells, which are artifacts. Sirois M, Principles and Practice of Veterinary Technology, ed 3, Mosby Elsevier, 2011, p. 146.

74. c The WBC differential should be interpreted based on absolute numbers of each cell type. Absolute numbers are based on the total WBC count; percentages are based on 100 cells counted on the differential. Relative numbers and decimal numbers do not pertain to WBC differential results. Bassert J, Thomas J, McCurnin's Clinical Textbook for Veterinary Technicians, ed 8, Elsevier Saunders, 2014, p. 413.

75. d Fibrinogen rises in inflammatory processes and its detection is useful, especially in ruminants. Hematocrit, RBCs, and TP can be indicators of other processes if elevated but are not specific to dehydration. Hendrix C, Sirois M, Laboratory Procedures for Veterinary Technicians, ed 5, Mosby Elsevier, 2007, p. 80.

76. b The buffy coat is a pale layer consisting mainly of white blood cells overlaid by a thin layer of platelets. If the WBCs and/or platelets are elevated, you can see the larger, white layer on top of the RBC column in a spun-down hematocrit tube. NRBCs are found in the layer below the buffy coat known as the packed red blood cells. Studdert VP, Gay CC, Blood DC, Saunders Comprehensive Veterinary Dictionary, ed 4, Elsevier Saunders, 2007, p. 159.

77. b Postrenal azotemia is associated with urinary tract obstruction or perforation. Pathologic conditions occurring after the kidney, in the bladder and urethra, result in anuria or oliguria. An increase in BUN from severe renal disease is defined as azotemia. A decrease in BUN is associated with liver disease and an increase in BUN from dehydration is prerenal azotemia. Sirois M, Principles and Practice of Veterinary Technology, ed 3, Mosby Elsevier, 2011, p. 466.

78. c A phagocyte refers to leukocytes that ingest foreign organisms and particles. Neutrophils and macrophages (called monocytes in the blood) are phagocytes. Granulocytes include basophils and eosinophils and have other primary functions. Lymphocytes are responsible for antibody production. Christenson DE, Veterinary Medical Terminology, ed 2, Elsevier Saunders, 1997, p. 50.

79. c Monocyte nuclei are not segmented and are usually multilobed. Colville TP, Bassert JM, Clinical Anatomy and Physiology for Veterinary Technicians, ed 2, Mosby Elsevier, 2008, p. 233.

80. c The hemocytometer, with coverslip applied, is loaded with the diluted solution and placed on the microscope and the counting grid is found by using the 40× or 43× objective lens. For WBC counts, cells are counted in the nine primary squares with the 10× objective. The same numbers of cells are counted, no matter which objective lens is used. Poor positioning of the condenser obscures the WBCs. Too much time on the hemocytometer dries the diluted blood and could affect the count. Mini clots trap WBCs and would affect the count. Hendrix C, Sirois M, Laboratory Procedures for Veterinary Technicians, ed 5, Mosby Elsevier, 2007, p. 35.

81. c Spherocytes lack a central pallor and appear slightly smaller and denser than normal RBCs. Spherocytes result from the binding of antibodies to the RBC surface and the removal of a portion of the cell membrane by macrophages in the spleen. This occurs most commonly in immune-mediated hemolytic anemia. Spherocytes are seen with immune-mediated hemolytic anemia and will cause RBC degradation. All other responses are signs of regeneration. Bassert J, Thomas J, McCurnin's Clinical Textbook for Veterinary Technicians, ed 8, Elsevier Saunders, 2014, p. 1425.

82. a Left shift typically refers to increased numbers of immature neutrophils that may include any stage, from bands to more immature forms. Because a left shift applies to neutrophils, RBCs, platelets, and lymphocytes are incorrect responses. Sirois M, Principles and Practice of Veterinary Technology, ed 3, Mosby Elsevier, 2011, p. 148.

83. b Reticulocytes are evaluated when assessing anemia and counts can be performed using a blood film stained with new methylene blue. Lactophenol cotton blue is used for the identification of fungal elements. Gram stain is used to identify bacteria and acridine orange is a special stain used in a hematology analyzer. Sirois M, Principles and Practice of Veterinary Technology, ed 3, Mosby Elsevier, 2011, p. 146.

84. c A rubriblast is the earliest cell recognized in the erythroid maturation process. Any cell name ending in blast is the most immature cell that can be visually identified on a bone marrow or blood smear. Studdert VP, Gay CC, Blood DC, Saunders Comprehensive Veterinary Dictionary, ed 4, Elsevier Saunders, 2007, p. 971.

85. c The intermediate host for canine heartworms is mosquitoes. Fleas are the intermediate host for flea tapeworms, rodents are the intermediate host for cyclophyllid tapeworms, and snails are the intermediate host for flukes. Bassert J, Thomas J, McCurnin's Clinical Textbook for Veterinary Technicians, ed 8, Elsevier Saunders, 2014, p. 462.

86. d The prepatent period for canine heartworm is approximately 6 months and the detection antibody in the serology kit is directed at adult heartworms. Therefore, it is not possible to detect heartworm infection immediately. Hendrix C, Sirois M, Laboratory Procedures for Veterinary Technicians, ed 5, Mosby Elsevier, 2007, p. 297.

87. a Both cysts and trophozoites on direct fecal smear are diagnostic of *Giardia*. *Giardia* cysts are the infective form and are passed in formed feces; the trophozoite form is more apt to be seen in watery feces. *Isospora* is diagnosed with a mucosal scraping and examining for schizonts and merozoites. Sarcocystis are oocysts that contain two sporocysts and ova and L3 larvae are associated with canine heartworms. Bassert J, Thomas J, McCurnin's Clinical Textbook for Veterinary Technicians, ed 8, Elsevier Saunders, 2014, p. 470.

88. a Coccidia ova are unembryonated and spherical with a deeply pigmented center and a rough/pitted outer shell. They are slightly smaller than the ova of *Toxocara canis* (roundworm). Oocyst size for *Isospora canis* is 32 to 53 by 26 to 43 microns, compared with *Toxocara canis* ova, which are 90 by 75 microns. Hendrix C, Robinson E, Diagnostic Parasitology for Veterinary Technicians, ed 4, Elsevier, 2012, p. 31.

89. a Increased urine specific gravity is seen with decreased water intake. The kidneys would preserve water but still remove the wastes, resulting in more concentrated urine. Hendrix C, Sirois M, Laboratory Procedures for Veterinary Technicians, ed 5, Mosby Elsevier, 2007, p. 158.

90. d Fat droplets, artifacts, and contaminants may be seen in a urine sediment slide. If more than a few erythrocytes, leukocytes, hyperplastic, and/or neoplastic cells are identified in urine sediment, it is considered abnormal and further diagnostic tests should be performed. The presence of WBCs indicates inflammation somewhere in the urogenital tract and the presence of RBCs indicates bleeding in the urogenital tract. Squamous epithelial cells are normally seen in sediment. Hendrix C, Sirois M, Laboratory Procedures for Veterinary Technicians, ed 5, Mosby Elsevier, 2007, p. 167.

91. c Struvite crystals are commonly referred to as triple phosphate crystals and occasionally as ammonium-magnesium-phosphates. Hendrix C, Sirois M, Laboratory Procedures for Veterinary Technicians, ed 5, Mosby Elsevier, 2007, p. 174.

92. b Crystalluria is often of no clinical significance. Often, crystal formation is temperature dependent. If urine is allowed to cool, dissolved substances come out of solution. Occasionally there is a correlation between crystalluria and the presence of uroliths and other factors must be considered (pH, specific gravity, etc.). Bassert J, Thomas J, McCurnin's Clinical Textbook for Veterinary Technicians, ed 8, Elsevier Saunders, 2014, p. 435.

93. d The urine dipstick tests the levels of leukocytes, nitrates, protein, pH, blood, specific gravity, ketones, glucose, and bilirubin. Blood urea nitrogen (BUN) is a chemical analyzed in the blood whose increase is associated with kidney disease. Hendrix C, Sirois M, Laboratory Procedures for Veterinary Technicians, ed 5, Mosby Elsevier, 2007, p. 159.

94. c The presence of casts in the urine sediment (formed in the renal tubules) may offer evidence needed to warrant further diagnostics. Urinary casts may be made up of white blood cells, red blood cells, kidney cells, or substances such as protein or fat. Casts can be significant; however, they may be considered normal in such cases as granular and hyaline casts. Casts are cylinders composed of protein that is secreted by the renal tubules and may contain cells of various stages of disintegration. Christenson DE, Veterinary Medical Terminology, ed 2, Elsevier Saunders, 1997, p. 287.

95. c A trace amount of protein may be significant in a patient with chronic renal failure. In kidney disease, excessive amounts of protein enter the glomerular filtrate and are not reabsorbed, resulting in protein in the urine. Diabetes cases may have glucosuria and ketonuria. Hemolytic anemia cases have hematuria and bilirubinuria. If a patient is experiencing an acid-base imbalance, there will be a change in the pH of the urine. Hendrix C, Sirois M, Laboratory Procedures for Veterinary Technicians, ed 5, Mosby Elsevier, 2007, p. 161.

96. d Ketonuria occurs with metabolic diseases involving increased lipid or impaired carbohydrate metabolism, such as diabetic ketoacidosis in dogs and cats and starvation and ketosis in cattle. When carbohydrates are not metabolized in the normal way (such as in diabetes mellitus and starvation) or if there is a lack of sufficient carbohydrates, the animal's body uses fat as its energy source. Breakdown of fat results in ketones in the urine. Ketosis is also seen in dairy cattle in the first 6 weeks following parturition. Bassert J, Thomas J, McCurnin's Clinical Textbook for Veterinary Technicians, ed 8, Elsevier Saunders, 2014, p. 433.

97. b Horses have a large number of mucous glands located within the renal pelvis; therefore, normal equine urine may appear thick and mucoid. Mucus threads may be seen occasionally in other species. They are easily overlooked because of their faint appearance in the background. Bassert J, Thomas J, McCurnin's Clinical Textbook for Veterinary Technicians, ed 8, Elsevier Saunders, 2014, p. 746.

98. d Calcium oxalate dihydrate crystals generally appear as small squares, containing an X across the crystal that resembles the back of an envelope. Cystine crystals are hexagonal, and tyrosine crystals are dark, needle-like rods. Ammonium biurate crystals are brown spheres with long spicules. Hendrix C, Sirois M, Laboratory Procedures for Veterinary Technicians, ed 5, Mosby Elsevier, 2007, p. 174.

99. c Trypsin activity is more readily detectable in feces than in blood. Trypsin analyses are performed on fecal samples. Amylase, lipase, and bilirubin can be tested on serum blood chemistry, not feces. Hendrix C, Sirois M, Laboratory Procedures for Veterinary Technicians, ed 5, Mosby Elsevier, 2007, p. 210.

100. b Fat in the urine, called lipuria, is seen to some degree in most cats. Feline renal epithelial cells have a high fat content and fat droplets are released when these cells disintegrate. Hendrix C, Sirois M, Laboratory Procedures for Veterinary Technicians, ed 5, Mosby Elsevier, 2007, p. 180.

101. d Gram-positive organisms retain crystal violet stain and appear purple, whereas gram-negative organisms do not retain crystal violet, but counterstain with safranin, and they appear pink. The iodine in Gram stain fixes the crystal violet to the bacterial cell wall of the gram-positive bacteria. Decolorizer removes the crystal violet (primary stain) from gram-negative bacteria. Bassert J, Thomas J, McCurnin's Clinical Textbook for Veterinary Technicians, ed 8, Elsevier Saunders, 2014, p. 491.

102. c *Proteus* sp. is often seen swarming without distinct colonies on a blood agar plate. *Pseudomonas* sp. appears as an irregular spreading with grayish colonies. This species has variable hemolysis and may show a metallic sheen on a blood agar plate. *Staphylococcus* sp. appears smooth and glistening, with pigmented colonies that are white to yellow on a blood agar plate. *Escherichia coli* will appear large and gray, with smooth mucoid colonies. Hemolysis will be variable on a blood agar plate. Hendrix C, Sirois M, Laboratory Procedures for Veterinary Technicians, ed 5, Mosby Elsevier, 2007, p. 134.

103. d *Malassezia pachydermatis* is frequently found in patients with otitis externa, but it can also be seen in dermatitis. *Candida* is an opportunistic fungal organism mostly associated with avian respiratory and gastrointestinal tracts in veterinary medicine. *Cryptococcus* is a fungus mostly associated with feline nasal disease. *Microsporum* is feline ringworm and is not found in a dog's ear. Bassert J, Thomas J, McCurnin's Clinical Textbook for Veterinary Technicians, ed 8, Elsevier Saunders, 2014, p. 510.

104. a *Microsporum canis* accounts for a large percentage of canine and feline ringworm cases; two species of *Trichophyton* also cause the infection in dogs and cats. *Mycobacterium* is a genus of actinobacteria, which is given its own family called the *Mycobacteriaceae*. The genus includes pathogens known to cause serious diseases in mammals and is not associated with ringworm. *Micrococcus* is a gram-positive acid-fast bacteria that is known to cause serious disease in mammals. *Moraxella* is the causative agent of pink eye. Studdert VP, Gay CC, Blood DC, Saunders Comprehensive Veterinary Dictionary, ed 4, Elsevier Saunders, 2007, p. 712.

105. c *Bacillus* spp. are among the most common laboratory contaminants, but *Bacillus anthracis* is a pathogen of many mammals. *Bacillus anthracis* is the causative agent of anthrax in animals and human beings. *Corynebacterium pseudotuberculosis* is an important veterinary pathogen that causes caseous lymphadenitis in sheep and goats and both abscesses and ulcerative lymphangitis in horses. *Escherichia* (abbreviated as *E. coli*) are bacteria found in the environment, foods, and intestines of humans and animals. Hendrix C, Sirois M, Laboratory Procedures for Veterinary Technicians, ed 5, Mosby Elsevier, 2007, p. 115.

106. d *Staphylococcus* spp. are both normal resident cutaneous microflora and opportunistic pathogens frequently associated with pyoderma in dogs and cats. This organism can wall itself off from treatment but can still produce toxins that might kill the host. *Proteus* spp. are a common cause of urinary tract infections. *Escherichia coli* usually affects the GI tract and produces watery diarrhea. *Streptococcus* spp. are commonly linked to mastitis. Bonagura J, Twedt D, Kirk's Current Veterinary Therapy, XV, Elsevier Saunders, 2014, p. 435.

107. d Cats are particularly prone to stress-induced hyperglycemia. BUN is filtered by the kidneys and is often elevated in the presence of kidney disease or kidney injury, total protein can be elevated in a dehydrated patient, and elevated ALT reflects injury or disease of the liver. Bassert J, Thomas J, McCurnin's Clinical Textbook for Veterinary Technicians, ed 8, Elsevier Saunders, 2014, p. 699.

108. c Uric acid is increased in the blood of both birds and Dalmatians with kidney disease. In Dalmatians, a gene is responsible for elevated uric acid and the formation of uroliths. In birds, excessive amounts of uric acid and urates in tissue occur in visceral gout. Elevated BUN and creatinine is seen in all patients experiencing all kidney disease, not just birds and Dalmatians. Elevated AST can be seen in liver disease. Studdert VP, Gay CC, Blood DC, Saunders Comprehensive Veterinary Dictionary, ed 4, Elsevier Saunders, 2007, p. 1154.

109. b Cholesterol levels are frequently elevated in animals with hypothyroidism. Measuring cholesterol is useful, because the thyroid hormone controls the synthesis and destruction of cholesterol. ALT is usually assessed to determine liver health. Creatinine kinase is an enzyme that is usually elevated in association with muscle damage; however, it can also be elevated in instances of brain or heart damage. Total protein can be assessed to determine the amount of protein (albumin and globulin) in the blood; this is important for other diseases but is not assessed for hypothyroidism. Sirois M, Principles and Practice of Veterinary Technology, ed 3, Mosby Elsevier, 2011, p. 163.

110. b Prolonged hyperglycemia and glucosuria are consistent with diabetes mellitus. If adequate insulin is released and its target cells have healthy receptors, the artificially elevated blood glucose level peaks at 30 minutes after ingestion and begins to drop, reaching normal value within 2 hours, and no glucose appears in the urine. Hendrix C, Sirois M, Laboratory Procedures for Veterinary Technicians, ed 5, Mosby Elsevier, 2007, p. 213.

111. a The kidneys play a major role in maintaining homeostasis in animals. Their primary functions are to conserve water and electrolytes in times of a negative balance and to increase water and electrolyte elimination in times of a positive balance; to excrete or to conserve hydrogen ions to maintain blood pH within normal limits; to conserve nutrients (e.g., glucose, proteins); and to remove the end products of nitrogen metabolism. The liver and spleen also play a role in filtration of waste, but they do not conserve nutrients or control blood pressure. The pancreas has exocrine and endocrine functions and helps to regulate enzymes and hormones in the body. Hendrix C, Sirois M, Laboratory Procedures for Veterinary Technicians, ed 5, Mosby Elsevier, 2007, p. 203.

112. b The exocrine portion of the pancreas, also referred to as the acinar pancreas, comprises the greatest portion of the organ. This portion secretes an enzyme-rich juice that contains the enzymes necessary for digestion into the small intestine. The liver, spleen, and kidney all play an important role in homeostasis, but they do not secrete digestive enzymes. Hendrix C, Sirois M, Laboratory Procedures for Veterinary Technicians, ed 5, Mosby Elsevier, 2007, p. 93.

113. c Bile acids are a group of compounds synthesized by hepatocytes from cholesterol that aid in fat absorption. There are various digestive enzymes secreted throughout the digestive tract to help in the digestion of proteins (globulins are proteins) and carbohydrates. Sirois M, Principles and Practice of Veterinary Technology, ed 3, Mosby Elsevier, 2011, p. 162.

114. c Fibrinogen is a protein produced by the liver and is involved in blood coagulation. The pancreas produces hormones and enzymes. The spleen and bone marrow produce blood cells. Sirois M, Principles and Practice of Veterinary Technology, ed 3, Mosby Elsevier, 2011, p. 153.

115. c Some tests require serum to be frozen before running diagnostics. In addition, any prolonged delays in testing require the serum to be removed from the SST and placed in a sterile tube. The tube can then be frozen. Feces must be fresh or refrigerated to complete a float test. Freezing whole blood for a CBC will damage cells and alter results. Hendrix C, Sirois M, Laboratory Procedures for Veterinary Technicians, ed 5, Mosby Elsevier, 2007, p. 76.

116. d If little serum has separated after centrifuging, "rimming" the tube with a wooden applicator stick to loosen the clot may help. Rimming or ringing the clot means loosening the clotted blood from the tube, which may help release serum trapped in the clot. Inverting the tube will remix the blood if there is not a serum separator, but it will not produce more serum after being mixed again. Dehydration can be a reason for a low amount of serum being produced; however, it is not the only reason and it does not mean techniques cannot be used to try to get more serum if needed. Spinning blood longer and faster can result in hemolysis and is not recommended. Hendrix C, Sirois M, Laboratory Procedures for Veterinary Technicians, ed 5, Mosby Elsevier, 2007, p. 124.

117. b An arterial blood gas sample is the best source to evaluate blood CO_2 levels. Venous blood is generally used for hematology, chemistry, and organ function tests. Tear M, Small Animal Surgical Nursing, ed 2, Mosby Elsevier, 2012, p. 117.

118. b The chief function of bone marrow is to manufacture erythrocytes, leukocytes, and platelets. Lymphocytes are produced in lymphoid organs and peripheral lymphoid tissue (thymus, lymph nodes, spleen, tonsils). They are produced only secondarily in the bone marrow. Studdert VP, Gay CC, Blood DC, Saunders Comprehensive Veterinary Dictionary, ed 4, Elsevier Saunders, 2007, p. 142.

119. c In llamas, the predominant cell type is the erythrocyte. Hemoglobin pigment may appear evenly disbursed throughout the cell or concentrated at each end of the oval, lacking a central pallor. Bird and reptile erythrocytes are usually oval in shape and are nucleated. Horse erythrocytes are round and anucleated. Only red blood cells of llamas are ovoid and devoid of a nucleus. Hendrix C, Sirois M, Laboratory Procedures for Veterinary Technicians, ed 5, Mosby Elsevier, 2007, p. 54.

120. b Feline eosinophilic granules are rod shaped and small. Dog, horse, and cow eosinophils have round to globoid granules. Hendrix C, Sirois M, Laboratory Manual for Laboratory Procedures for Veterinary Technicians, ed 5, Mosby Elsevier, 2007.

121. c Spherocytes are significant in that they suggest immune-mediated destruction of RBCs, resulting in IMHA. Heinz bodies are usually a toxic reaction or are related to onion ingestion. Howell-Jolly bodies can be seen with markedly decreased splenic function. Target cells are commonly seen in association with liver disease. Hendrix C, Sirois M, Laboratory Procedures for Veterinary Technicians, ed 5, Mosby Elsevier, 2007, p. 54.

122. c The kidney plays a major role in maintaining homeostasis in animals. Their primary functions are to conserve water and electrolytes in times of a negative balance and to increase water and electrolyte elimination in times of a positive balance. When evaluating liver function, values for ALT, AST, and Alk Phos should be obtained. When evaluating pancreatic function, amylase and lipase should be evaluated. BNP (a cardiac enzyme) is a test that evaluates heart health. Hendrix C, Sirois M, Laboratory Procedures for Veterinary Technicians, ed 5, Mosby Elsevier, 2007, p. 203.

123. c Elevated levels of nitrogenous waste products accumulate in the blood, especially urea nitrogen, also known as azotemia. Hypernatremia is an increase in sodium levels in the blood; hypernaturia is an increase in sodium levels in the urine. Azoturia is an elevated level of nitrogenous compounds in the urine. Tighe MM, Brown M, Mosby's Comprehensive Review for Veterinary Technicians, ed 4, Mosby Elsevier, 2015, p. 28.

124. d Platelets are the smallest elements found in a peripheral blood smear and thus a higher magnification is necessary to view them adequately. 10× objective lenses should always be used to scan the feathered edge for the presence of rouleaux, RBC agglutination, and platelet clumping. Bassert J, Thomas J, McCurnin's Clinical Textbook for Veterinary Technicians, ed 8, Elsevier Saunders, 2014, p. 407.

125. a A toxic neutrophil is a neutrophil characterized by the presence of cytoplasmic basophilia, Döhle bodies, vacuoles, heavy granulation, and/or giantism. Howell-Jolly bodies are remnants of nuclear material found in erythrocytes, not leukocytes. Sirois M, Principles and Practice of Veterinary Technology, ed 3, Mosby Elsevier, 2011, p. 816.

126. c Buccal mucosal bleeding time is a primary assay for the detection of abnormalities in platelet function. ACT, APPT, and one-step PT are evaluators for secondary hemostasis. Sirois M, Principles and Practice of Veterinary Technology, ed 3, Mosby Elsevier, 2011, p. 152.

127. a Formation of the initial platelet plug is termed *primary hemostasis*. At the same time, tissue factors are released that activate the coagulation cascade or secondary hemostasis. Vascular spasm and platelet plug formation occur during primary hemostasis. Clot lysis occurs after the traumatized tissue has healed. Bassert J, Thomas J, McCurnin's Clinical Textbook for Veterinary Technicians, ed 8, Elsevier Saunders, 2014, p. 417.

128. b A buccal mucosal bleeding time should be evaluated in breeds with a high risk for von Willebrand disease. Because von Willebrand disease is a disorder of primary hemostasis, i.e., the coagulation cascade is normal, buccal mucosal bleeding time (BMBT) is the best screening test of those listed. ACT and APPT are evaluators of secondary hemostasis. Battaglia A, Small Animal Emergency and Critical Care for Veterinary Technicians, ed 2, Saunders, 2007, p. 142.

129. d Blood should be collected via a single venipuncture to avoid cell damage and excessive activation of coagulation factors. Trauma during venipuncture interferes with the results of a coagulation profile by increasing the blood's coagulability. Samples are collected in a blue citrate-containing Vacutainer. It is not necessary to test the sample immediately. Sirois M, Principles and Practice of Veterinary Technology, ed 3, Mosby Elsevier, 2011, p. 444.

130. d Thromboembolism occurs when blood clots form in the heart and lodge in the aortic trifurcation, disrupting the blood supply to the hind limbs. Petechiae, epistaxis, and hematuria are all symptoms of a bleeding disorder. Bassert J, Thomas J, McCurnin's Clinical Textbook for Veterinary Technicians, ed 8, Elsevier Saunders, 2014, p. 688.

131. c Eosinophilic bronchopneumopathy is a disease that can be caused by heartworm infection. Eosinophils are often found in greater numbers in the blood of animals that are allergic or that have parasitic infections. Bonagura J, Twedt D, Kirk's Current Veterinary Therapy, XV, Elsevier Saunders, 2014, p. 689.

132. b Bone marrow smears are much thicker than blood smears and a longer period of staining time is therefore necessary to identify adequately the various cells present. Bone marrow smears must be rapidly air dried and stained. Staining time must be increased in accordance with the cellularity and thickness of the sample. Hendrix C, Sirois M, Laboratory Procedures for Veterinary Technicians, ed 5, Mosby Elsevier, 2007, p. 80.

133. c Specific gravity is indicative of the concentration of dissolved materials in the urine and provides an indication of kidney function. The pH is an indicator of hydrogen ion concentration. Volume is only the amount of urine produced. Examinations of the sediment can answer questions regarding bacteria and white and red blood cells, but not the ability to concentrate urine. Sirois M, Principles and Practice of Veterinary Technology, ed 3, Mosby Elsevier, 2011, p. 204.

134. a Squamous epithelial cells are a common finding in urine samples and are the largest of the three types of epithelial cells. Transitional and renal cells are also epithelial cells but are not the largest. The term *caudate epithelial cells* refers to the shape of the cell, not the type. Sirois M, Principles and Practice of Veterinary Technology, ed 3, Mosby Elsevier, 2011, p. 207.

135. a The most frequently observed urolith is struvite. Calcium oxalate uroliths are seen in small numbers in horses and dogs. Cystine uroliths can be associated with renal tubular dysfunction and are not a common finding. Urate uroliths are mostly found in dalmatians. Tear M, Small Animal Surgical Nursing, ed 2, Mosby Elsevier, 2012, p. 161.

136. a Catheterization is the preferred method to assess patency of the urethra. If the urethra is not patent, it will not be possible to pass a urinary catheter. If there is a partial obstruction, it is still possible to express the bladder manually or to collect a sample by free catch. Cystocentesis involves direct puncture of the bladder, entirely bypassing the urethra. Sirois M, Principles and Practice of Veterinary Technology, ed 3, Mosby Elsevier, 2011, p. 202.

137. c Casts dissolve in alkaline urine. Casts generally dissolve in basic urine, i.e., urine that has been standing for some time before being examined. The remaining statements are true. Sirois M, Principles and Practice of Veterinary Technology, ed 3, Mosby Elsevier, 2011, p. 208.

138. d If a dehydrated patient has normally functioning kidneys, increases in BUN and serum creatinine should be accompanied by high urine SG, indicating that the kidneys are capable of concentrating urine to conserve as much water as possible. A state of dehydration causes the kidneys to conserve body water, thereby decreasing the amount of urine produced and increasing the concentration of urine excreted. Bassert J, Thomas J, McCurnin's Clinical Textbook for Veterinary Technicians, ed 8, Elsevier Saunders, 2014, p. 425.

139. a Small amounts of bilirubin are considered a normal finding in dogs. Because the renal threshold for bilirubin is low in dogs, bilirubinuria might be detected. Bilirubin should not be detected in the urine of a healthy cat, horse, or sheep; therefore, bilirubinuria in these species indicates disease. Bassert J, Thomas J, McCurnin's Clinical Textbook for Veterinary Technicians, ed 8, Elsevier Saunders, 2014, p. 433.

140. a Animals with chronic renal failure frequently produce isosthenuric urine. In animals with kidney disease, the closer the specific gravity is to isosthenuric, the greater the amount of kidney function that has been lost. Isosthenuria is when the specific gravity approaches that of glomerular filtrate (1.008–1.012). Hendrix C, Sirois M, Laboratory Procedures for Veterinary Technicians, ed 5, Mosby Elsevier, 2007, p. 162.

141. c Only the free-catch method involves no iatrogenic traumatization of the patient's urinary tract. Higher numbers of RBCs can be seen with manual expression, traumatic catheterization, or with cystocentesis if traumatic hemorrhage has occurred. Bassert J, Thomas J, McCurnin's Clinical Textbook for Veterinary Technicians, ed 8, Elsevier Saunders, 2014, p. 434.

142. a A healthy kidney should be able to concentrate urine in the face of dehydration or dilute urine to prevent overhydration. SG <1.008 indicates that the kidneys are functioning and are able to dilute urine actively. An overhydrated patient's body would need to excrete the excessive fluids, thereby increasing the amount of urine produced, diluting it, and thus lowering its specific gravity. Bassert J, Thomas J, McCurnin's Clinical Textbook for Veterinary Technicians, ed 8, Elsevier Saunders, 2014, p. 431.

143. c Treatment of patients with diabetes mellitus is achieved through subcutaneous insulin injections, generally administered once or twice daily, dietary changes, and maintenance of a healthy body condition score. As with many other hormone therapies, the dose of insulin must be titrated to effectiveness. This is achieved by monitoring glucose levels. Potassium and sodium can be affected by a diabetic crisis, such as diabetic ketoacidosis; however, they are not used to monitor insulin levels. Insulin is a hormone that is produced by the pancreas, which, among other things, controls the blood glucose in the body. Bassert J, Thomas J, McCurnin's Clinical Textbook for Veterinary Technicians, ed 8, Elsevier Saunders, 2014, p. 699.

144. d The condition of increased numbers of leukocytes is called pyuria and indicates inflammation in the urinary tract. UTIs with nitrate-reducing bacteria cause nitrite formation; however, this test does not seem as sensitive in dogs and cats as it is in humans. Therefore, it is important to look for bacteria in the sediment. Neoplasia, diabetes, and renal failure can all cause changes in the urine such as hematuria, glucosuria, ketonuria, and isosthenuria, but none of these would be associated with pyuria. Bassert J, Thomas J, McCurnin's Clinical Textbook for Veterinary Technicians, ed 8, Elsevier Saunders, 2014, p. 430.

145. d The adrenal glands are regulated by the anterior pituitary gland and during times of stress they release corticosteroids. The pancreas produces somatostatin, glucagon, and insulin. The thyroid gland produces T4, T3, and calcitonin. The pituitary gland produces TSH and growth hormone, ACTH, prolactin, FSH, and ADH. Aspinall V, Cappello M, Introduction to Veterinary Anatomy and Physiology Textbook, ed 2, Elsevier, 2009, p. 75.

146. a The calcium:phosphate ratio in the blood is altered by impaired kidney function. This leads to increased output of parathormone and consequently to increased resorption of bone in an effort to maintain blood calcium levels. Calcium plays a role in bone development, transmission of nerve impulses, and muscle contraction. Calcium concentrations are usually inversely related to phosphorus concentrations. Urea, nitrogen, and creatinine are measured by chemistry analysis to determine kidney health and to monitor kidney disease. Kidney disease can cause a calcium and phosphorus imbalance, which can lead to bone resorption and convulsions, but the calcium and phosphorus need to be measured to assess that, not the urea, nitrogen, and creatinine. Aspartate aminotransferase and alanine transaminase are monitored in liver disease. Sodium and potassium are electrolytes and can be disrupted by various diseases, but they are not associated with bone resorption or convulsions. Aspinall V, Cappello M, Introduction to Veterinary Anatomy and Physiology Textbook, ed 2, Elsevier, 2009, p. 74.

147. d The ACTH stimulation test evaluates the degree of adrenal gland response to the administration of exogenous ACTH. The liver, pancreas, and thyroid glands are all secreting glands that also produce hormones, but they are not the glands involved in the measurement of blood cortisol levels. Hendrix C, Sirois M, Laboratory Procedures for Veterinary Technicians, ed 5, Mosby Elsevier, 2007, p. 100.

148. b Struvite crystals are commonly referred to as magnesium ammonium phosphate crystals. Calcium carbonate and calcium oxalate calculi can be seen on radiographs of the urethra in small ruminants. Urates are composed mostly of uric acid. Hendrix C, Sirois M, Laboratory Procedures for Veterinary Technicians, ed 5, Mosby Elsevier, 2007, p. 174.

149. a The thyroid gland produces T3 and T4. The pancreas, the pituitary gland, and the thymus are secreting glands as well; however, they are not involved in the measurement of T3 and T4. The pancreas secretes glucagon and insulin. The pituitary gland produces TSH and growth hormone, ACTH, prolactin, FSH, and ADH. The thymus is part of the lymphatic system; it is active in late fetal and early postnatal life and is responsible for the production of T lymphocytes that give rise to the cell-mediated immune response. Aspinall V, Cappello M, Introduction to Veterinary Anatomy and Physiology Textbook, ed 2, Elsevier, 2009, p. 72.

150. c TSH and ACTH are both secreted by the anterior pituitary (adenohypophysis) gland, which is under the control of the hypothalamus. Blood levels of these hormones may be used to evaluate pituitary gland function. The pancreas produces somatostatin, glucagon, and insulin. The thyroid gland produces T4, T3, and calcitonin. The adrenal gland produces corticosteroids. Aspinall V, Cappello M, Introduction to Veterinary Anatomy and Physiology Textbook, ed 2, Elsevier, 2009, p. 72.

151. a Hypothyroidism is a disease that primarily affects dogs, although a rare congenital form can be seen in kittens. Patients with this disease have an underactive thyroid, resulting in subnormal circulating levels of thyroid hormones; this causes a subsequent decrease in metabolic rate. In dogs, the most common cause of hypothyroidism is immune-mediated destruction of the gland. Clinical signs are varied and many. The most common signs are weight gain, exercise intolerance, altered mentation, and lethargy caused by the decreased metabolic rate. On physical examination, hypothermia, bradycardia, truncal alopecia, and seborrhea may be noted. Diagnostic confirmation includes documenting low serum T4 and free T4 levels and elevated thyroid-stimulating hormone (TSH) levels, as well as evaluating the complete blood count and full chemistry. The pancreas produces somatostatin, glucagon, and insulin, whereas the adrenal gland produces corticosteroids. Neither the pancreas nor the adrenal glands is associated with all of the aforementioned clinical signs. The thymus is part of the lymphatic system, it is active in late fetal and early postnatal life and is responsible for the production of T lymphocytes that give rise to the cell-mediated immune response. Bassert J, Thomas J, McCurnin's Clinical Textbook for Veterinary Technicians, ed 8, Elsevier Saunders, 2014, p. 699.

152. c The primary indicator for IRIS staging of CKD is the concentration of creatinine in plasma or serum because currently this is the most useful and readily available test of kidney function in veterinary practice. The rest of the statements regarding creatinine are true. Bonagura J, Twedt D, Kirk's Current Veterinary Therapy, XV, Elsevier Saunders, 2014, p. 858.

153. d Urine cortisol/creatinine ratios have been used as screening tests for adrenal function. Only the cortisol/creatinine ratio is a test of urine. Endogenous ACTH, low-dose dexamethasone, and ACTH stimulation use blood, not urine, for testing. Hendrix C, Sirois M, Laboratory Procedures for Veterinary Technicians, ed 5, Mosby Elsevier, 2007, p. 223.

154. b Common tests for kidney function include blood urea nitrogen and creatinine. Aspartate aminotransferase and alanine transaminase can be used to evaluate the liver. Bilirubin and urobilinogen are associated with biliary disease, gallbladder disease, and liver disease. Ammonia and pyruvic acid are evaluated by a whole blood sample on serum chemistry. Hendrix C, Sirois M, Laboratory Procedures for Veterinary Technicians, ed 5, Mosby Elsevier, 2007.

155. c The commonly performed tests to evaluate the acinar functions of the pancreas include amylase and lipase. Kidney function can be measured by creatinine and BUN. ALT, AST, and Alk Phos can measure liver function. Adrenal glands can be assessed by a baseline cortisol test. Hendrix C, Sirois M, Laboratory Procedures for Veterinary Technicians, ed 6, Mosby Elsevier, 2015, p. 210.

156. d The liver converts ammonia to a nontoxic molecule called urea. Phosphorus and creatine are measured to evaluate kidney function but they are not byproducts of ammonia. Aspartate aminotransferase is measured to evaluate liver function. Colville TP, Bassert JM, Clinical Anatomy and Physiology for Veterinary Technicians, ed 2, Mosby Elsevier, 2008, p. 313.

157. d Bicarbonate is an electrolyte in plasma that maintains the blood pH in equilibrium. The other listed functions are influenced by electrolytes but not bicarbonate. Hendrix C, Sirois M, Laboratory Procedures for Veterinary Technicians, ed 5, Mosby Elsevier, 2007, p. 421.

158. a Azotemia is an excess of urea, creatinine, and other nitrogenous end products of protein and amino acid metabolism in the blood. Bilirubinemia is an increase of bilirubin in the blood. Hypernatremia is an increase of sodium in the blood. Hyperkalemia is an increase of potassium in the blood. Studdert VP, Gay CC, Blood DC, Saunders Comprehensive Veterinary Dictionary, ed 4, Elsevier Saunders, 2007, p. 1150.

159. c Prerenal azotemia is an increase in BUN values because of a pathologic condition that occurs prerenally, resulting from decreased blood flow, shock, and heart disease, and it is often secondary to dehydration. BUN may be high in patients with severe renal disease, not liver disease. BUN may be low in dogs with chronic liver disease, not renal disease. An increase in BUN resulting from the inability to urinate is termed *postrenal azotemia*. Bassert J, Thomas J, McCurnin's Clinical Textbook for Veterinary Technicians, ed 8, Elsevier Saunders, 2014, p. 912.

160. d Glucose tolerance tests directly challenge the pancreas with a glucose load, and they measure insulin's effect by evaluating blood or urine glucose concentration. Prolonged hyperglycemia and glucosuria are consistent with diabetes mellitus. Healthy animals have sufficient insulin to drop the increased glucose load to normal levels in approximately 2 hours. Animals with diabetes mellitus still typically show hyperglycemia and glucosuria in this same period. Cushing's disease, hypothyroidism, and Addison's disease are all diseases of the endocrine system, but they are diagnosed with different types of blood testing. Hendrix C, Sirois M, Laboratory Procedures for Veterinary Technicians, ed 5, Mosby Elsevier, 2007, p. 97.

161. d The neutrophils may be considered a first line of defense, converging rapidly on invading organisms and destroying them promptly, but they are incapable of a sustained effort. The neutrophil is the white cell that responds most quickly to the presence of microorganisms. It leaves the circulation, enters tissue, and becomes phagocytic. The eosinophil is a specialized cell of the immune system. Lymphocytes are the cells that determine the specificity of the immune response. Monocytes are a type of white blood cell, which fights off bacteria, viruses, and fungi, and they are the biggest type of white blood cell in the immune system (but they are not the first line of defense). Tizard I, Veterinary Immunology, ed 9, Elsevier Saunders, 2013, p. 40.

162. b The red top Vacutainer should be placed upright and allowed to clot for 15–30 minutes at room temperature. 0 and 5 minutes will not allow enough time for the clot to form. 1 hour will create changes in the test results that could falsely elevate glucose or decrease ketone levels. Bassert J, Thomas J, McCurnin's Clinical Textbook for Veterinary Technicians, ed 8, Elsevier Saunders, 2014, p. 426.

163. a Dioctophyma renale is the "giant kidney worm" of dogs. This largest parasitic nematodes frequently infects the right kidney of dogs and gradually ingests the renal parenchyma, leaving only the capsule of the kidney. Hendri C, Sirois M, Laboratory Procedures for Veterinary Technicians, ed 6, Mosby Elsevier, 2015, p. 210.

164. d Hematology testing primarily uses whole blood and samples that are not tested within 1 hour should be refrigerated for cell preservation. The sample should be allowed to warm to room temperature before analysis. Freezing the sample and adding formalin will destroy the cells. Spinning would separate the cells from the plasma and would render the cytology reading impossible. Hendrix C, Sirois M, Laboratory Procedures for Veterinary Technicians, ed 5, Mosby Elsevier, 2007, p. 31.

165. a The synovial fluid mucin forms a clot when added to acetic acid. The nature of the resultant clot reflects the quality and concentration of hyaluronic acid. This test is only performed with joint fluid. Hendrix C, Sirois M, Laboratory Procedures for Veterinary Technicians, ed 5, Mosby Elsevier, 2007, p. 111.

166. c Thrombocytopenia is a decrease in the number of platelets circulating in the blood and the function of platelets is related to clotting of blood. Anemia is a decrease in red blood cells and can be caused by a clotting problem, but it is not associated with a clotting disorder. Leukopenia is a decrease in white blood cells. Reticulocytosis is an excess of reticulocytes in the peripheral blood and is frequently associated with a regenerative anemia. Studdert VP, Gay CC, Blood DC, Saunders Comprehensive Veterinary Dictionary, ed 4, Elsevier Saunders, 2007, p. 1103.

167. b Line smears, starfish smears, and squash preps are compression smears. The compression prep method has been widely used for many years for cytology specimens and the squash preparation yields excellent cytologic smears. Wet prep is used to test the motility of a bacterial sample. A modified knot prep and Willis prep do not exist. Hendrix C, Sirois M, Laboratory Procedures for Veterinary Technicians, ed 5, Mosby Elsevier, 2007, p. 63.

168. c *Malassezia pachydermatis* is a common cause of otitis externa. Cerumen, epithelial cells, and debris are commonly found on an external ear canal cytology. Bassert J, Thomas J, McCurnin's Clinical Textbook for Veterinary Technicians, ed 8, Elsevier Saunders, 2014, p. 510.

169. a The primary function of neutrophils is phagocytosis. Eosinophils respond to allergic reactions and lymphocytes respond to immune issues. Hendrix C, Sirois M, Laboratory Procedures for Veterinary Technicians, ed 5, Mosby Elsevier, 2007, p. 62.

170. c The eosinophil's primary function is in the modulation of the immune system. Increased numbers of eosinophils are commonly seen in patients with allergic reactions and parasite infections or infestations. Neutrophils phagocytize invading pathogens and lymphocytes respond to immune issues. Hendrix C, Sirois M, Laboratory Procedures for Veterinary Technicians, ed 5, Mosby Elsevier, 2007, p. 63.

171. b A blood-filled capillary tube is centrifuged for 2–5 minutes. 1 minute is not enough time for the serum to separate and the buffy coat to form properly and it is not necessary to centrifuge the sample longer than 5 minutes. Sirois M, Principles and Practice of Veterinary Technology, ed 3, Mosby Elsevier, 2011, p. 132.

172. a Mean corpuscular volume measures the average size of red blood cells. PCV is the percentage of red blood cells in circulation. MCHC is the average concentration of hemoglobin in a volume of blood. Mean corpuscular hemoglobin and mean corpuscular volume are the same as MCHC. Bassert J, Thomas J, McCurnin's Clinical Textbook for Veterinary Technicians, ed 8, Elsevier Saunders, 2014, p. 437.

173. b Döhle bodies represent toxic changes to the neutrophil; feline neutrophils appear to form Döhle bodies easily, but they are also seen in canine neutrophils. Döhle bodies are found on WBCs, not erythrocytes, nor platelets, nor nRBCs. Sirois M, Principles and Practice of Veterinary Technology, ed 3, Mosby Elsevier, 2011, p. 148.

174. d Platelets, especially in cats, may be larger than erythrocytes. This can lead to inaccurate electronic blood cell counts when the cells are not differentiated by size. Platelets in the other species have a smaller appearance in comparison with the red blood cells. Hendrix C, Sirois M, Laboratory Procedures for Veterinary Technicians, ed 5, Mosby Elsevier, 2007, p. 59.

175. b Erythropoiesis is a formation of erythrocytes (red blood cells). Erythropoietin is a glycoprotein secreted by the kidneys, which acts on the bone marrow to stimulate erythropoiesis. Hematopoietin is also known as erythropoietin. Leukopoiesis is a formation of leukocytes. Studdert VP, Gay CC, Blood DC, Saunders Comprehensive Veterinary Dictionary, ed 4, Elsevier Saunders, 2007, p. 397.

176. c The order from least mature to most mature is rubriblast, rubricyte, reticulocyte, erythrocyte. Hendrix C, Sirois M, Laboratory Procedures for Veterinary Technicians, ed 5, Mosby Elsevier, 2007, p. 64.

177. c A positive direct Coombs test provides evidence of immune-mediated hemolytic disease. The red cell fragility test can add useful information in the differentiation among some forms of anemia, but it is not used to diagnose hemolytic anemia. The modified Knott test is used for the detection of circulating microfilariae. The Coggins test is a method used to detect antibodies against equine infectious anemia virus in horse serum. Hendrix C, Sirois M, Laboratory Procedures for Veterinary Technicians, ed 5, Mosby Elsevier, 2007, p. 279.

178. a Lymphocytosis in an increased number of circulating lymphocytes. Leukosis refers to a virus. Lymphocytopenia is a decrease in the number of circulating lymphocytes. *Lymphosarcoma* is a general term applied to a malignant neoplastic disorder of lymphoid tissue. Tighe MM, Brown M, Mosby's Comprehensive Review for Veterinary Technicians, ed 4, Mosby Elsevier, 2015, p. 52.

179. c Unstained smears should be stored away from formalin fumes and should be shipped separately from surgical biopsies that have been placed in formalin because formalin vapors inhibit optimal staining. Ether is not used in most labs or hospitals because it is not safe. Saline can be packed alongside unstained slides without any risk of harm to the slide. Acetone is used as a decol orizer when staining the slide. Bassert J, Thomas J, McCurnin's Clinical Textbook for Veterinary Technicians, ed 8, Elsevier Saunders, 2014, p. 405.

180. c A primary concern regarding ticks is the transmission of tickborne disease, which includes ehrlichiosis. Ticks do not spread toxoplasmosis, coccidiosis, or cryptosporidiosis. Bassert J, Thomas J, McCurnin's Clinical Textbook for Veterinary Technicians, ed 8, Elsevier Saunders, 2014, p. 274.

181. d Lice infestation is also called pediculosis. Myiasis is fly larvae penetration of living tissue (maggots). Acariasis is a mite or tick infestation. Paraphimosis is the inability to retract the penis because of a swollen state or constriction of the preputial orifice. Studdert VP, Gay CC, Blood DC, Saunders Comprehensive Veterinary Dictionary, ed 4, Elsevier Saunders, 2007, p. 660.

182. b Skin scraping is indicated whenever an ectoparasite infestation is suspected such as Notoedres. Bovicola is a louse and Otodectes is an ear mite. Ctenocephalides is a flea. Ford R, Mazzaferro E, Kirk and Bistner's Handbook of Veterinary Procedures and Emergency Treatments, ed 9, Saunders, 2012, p. 484.

183. b The hydatid cyst is the largest intermediate form of a tapeworm. Cysticercus, coenurus, and cysticercoid are all smaller intermediate forms of tapeworms. Bassert J, Thomas J, McCurnin's Clinical Textbook for Veterinary Technicians, ed 8, Elsevier Saunders, 2014, p. 448.

184. c *Spirocerca lupi* (the esophageal worm) is a nematode that often forms nodules in the esophagus. *Physaloptera* is the canine stomach worm. *Filaroides* is also known as the canine lungworm. *Neosporum* is a protozoan that causes neurologic disease in pups. Hendrix C, Sirois M, Laboratory Procedures for Veterinary Technicians, ed 5, Mosby Elsevier, 2007, p. 295.

185. b *Echinococcus* is not zoonotic. *Giardia*, *Toxoplasma*, and *Dipylidium* are all zoonotic conditions. Bonagura J, Twedt D, Kirk's Current Veterinary Therapy, XV, Elsevier Saunders, 2014, p. 1247.

186. c In fresh feces, *Tritrichomonas* move actively with jerky movements. *Giardia trophozoites*, on the other hand, have what is called a falling leaf movement. *Mycoplasma* and *E. canis* are not found in the feces. Hendrix C, Robinson E, Diagnostic Parasitology for Veterinary Technicians, ed 4, Elsevier, 2012, p. 169.

187. d Hookworms are voracious blood feeders. Pale mucous membranes and hydremia may be seen, signaling anemia, particularly in young puppies. Roundworms and tapeworms can cause, among other signs, vomiting and weight loss. Heartworms are usually associated with coughing and respiratory signs. None of the other listed parasites is associated with anemia. Bassert J, Thomas J, McCurnin's Clinical Textbook for Veterinary Technicians, ed 8, Elsevier Saunders, 2014, p. 456.

188. b *Sarcoptic ascariasis* is extremely pruritic. Patients with *Cheyletiella* can either present asymptomatic or with slight pruritus. *Demodex* presents as scaly lesions (usually on the face) but not necessarily pruritic. *Dermacentor* is a tick that can cause localized irritation at the site of the bite but will not cause generalized and/or extreme pruritus. Hendrix C, Robinson E, Diagnostic Parasitology for Veterinary Technicians, ed 4, Elsevier, 2012, p. 232.

189. c False negative occult heartworm tests are usually a result of immature infections, infections with low numbers of female worms or all-male infections. Antigen tests detect a glycoprotein found predominantly in the reproductive tract of the female worm. Bonagura J, Twedt D, Kirk's Current Veterinary Therapy, XV, Elsevier Saunders, 2014, p. 832.

190. a In the cat heartworm, infections generally consist of one to three worms that survive 3 years. In dogs, large numbers of adult heartworms can be present in the pulmonary arteries, right atrium and ventricle, and the caudal vena cava, and they can live up to 7 years. Bassert J, Thomas J, McCurnin's Clinical Textbook for Veterinary Technicians, ed 8, Elsevier Saunders, 2014, p. 689 .

191. c Known as the giant cell of bone marrow, a megakaryocyte is a large cell with a greatly lobulated nucleus that gives rise to blood platelets. Phagocytosis is the engulfing of microorganisms or other cells and foreign particles by neutrophils. Granulocytes are produced by stem cells within the bone marrow. Plasma cells are also produced within the bone marrow but they are not produced by the megakaryocyte. Studdert VP, Gay CC, Blood DC, Saunders Comprehensive Veterinary Dictionary, ed 4, Elsevier Saunders, 2007, p. 689.

192. a Poikilocytosis, which is a variation in the red cell shape, is not associated with a responsive anemia. Anisocytosis, reticulocytosis, and polychromasia are all seen in responsive anemias. Hendrix C, Sirois M, Laboratory Procedures for Veterinary Technicians, ed 5, Mosby Elsevier, 2007, p. 53.

193. b The mean corpuscular volume (MCV) represents the average size of the RBC. The mean corpuscular hemoglobin concentration (MCHC) provides an indication of the average amount of hemoglobin in a red blood cell. The reticulocyte count can indicate the regenerative ability of anemia (if it is present). The M/E ratio is the ratio of myeloid to erythroid precursors in bone marrow. Battaglia A, Small Animal Emergency and Critical Care for Veterinary Technicians, ed 2, Saunders, 2007, p. 232.

194. c A myeloblast is an immature cell in the bone marrow; it is the most primitive precursor in the granulocytic series. The megakaryoblast is the most immature cell in the thrombocyte series. A leukoblast is an immature granular leukocyte. Studdert VP, Gay CC, Blood DC, Saunders Comprehensive Veterinary Dictionary, ed 4, Elsevier Saunders, 2007, p. 737.

195. a The osteoclast is a large multinuclear cell frequently found in bone marrow. The megakaryocyte is similar, except that the nuclei are all attached and are not separate. The osteoblast and monoblast are also large cells, but they have a single nucleus. Studdert VP, Gay CC, Blood DC, Saunders Comprehensive Veterinary Dictionary, ed 4, Elsevier Saunders, 2007, p. 793.

196. b In responsive anemia, the majority of the bone marrow samples show erythroid hyperplasia (increased red cell production in the marrow). Erythroid hypoplasia is consistent with nonregeneration anemia. Myeloid metaplasia is associated with anemia, but it is not consistent with responsive anemia. Myeloid metaplasia is the occurrence of myeloid tissue in extramedullary sites; specifically, it is a syndrome characterized by splenomegaly, anemia, nucleated erythrocytes, and immature granulocytes in the circulating blood, and by extramedullary hematopoiesis in the liver and spleen. It is frequently associated with cancer and is not a form of responsive anemia. Bonagura J, Twedt D, Kirk's Current Veterinary Therapy, XV, Elsevier Saunders, 2014, p. 316.

197. c Warfarin toxicity leads to prolonged clotting times, which are commonly measured by one stage prothrombin time. Thrombocyte count is part of primary hemostasis, which is not affected by warfarin toxicity. Calcium levels are not part of the diagnosis for rodenticide toxicity. Warfarin affects factors 2, 7, 9, and 10, which are on the PT side of the coagulation cascade. PTT can be affected because these factors become depleted; however, this is a secondary response. PTT is not directly affected by warfarin toxicity. Bonagura J, Twedt D, Kirk's Current Veterinary Therapy, XV, Elsevier Saunders, 2014, p. 133.

198. a DIC often manifests as diffuse hemorrhage resulting from the ultimate consumption of coagulation factors and platelets. Icterus is not seen in disseminated intravascular coagulation (DIC). Because this is an abnormal activation of all of the coagulation pathways, hemorrhage, thrombocytopenia, and a prolonged activated clotting time (ACT) are all observed. Battaglia A, Small Animal Emergency and Critical Care for Veterinary Technicians, ed 2, Saunders, 2007, p. 224.

199. b Hypothyroidism can stimulate von Willebrand disease if the dog is already predisposed to von Willebrand disease. A deficiency in von Willebrand factor does not occur secondary to hypothyroidism in dogs without concurrent congenital von Willebrand disease. Hemophilia A, DIC, and coumarin toxicity are not stimulated by hypothyroidism. Bonagura J, Twedt D, Kirk's Current Veterinary Therapy, XV, Elsevier Saunders, 2014, p. e87.

200. d Ketosis is common and is considered normal in lactating cows. Ketonuria is an abnormal finding in canines, felines, and equines. Hendrix C, Sirois M, Laboratory Procedures for Veterinary Technicians, ed 5, Mosby Elsevier, 2007, p. 162.

201. c Renal epithelial cells are the smallest epithelial cells seen in the urine. A leukocyte is smaller, but it is not an epithelial cell. Squamous cells are the largest of the three types of epithelial cells. Transitional cells are larger than renal cells. Sirois M, Principles and Practice of Veterinary Technology, ed 3, Mosby Elsevier, 2011, p. 207.

202. b Insulin is necessary to transport glucose into body cells, and a deficiency causes hyperglycemia and the spilling of glucose into the urine (glucosuria). Uremia and azoturia can be associated with renal disease and do not cause glucosuria. Ketonemia is associated with diabetes and is often present when hyperglycemia is extreme. However, hyperglycemia and glucosuria occur before there is ketonemia. Hendrix C, Sirois M, Laboratory Procedures for Veterinary Technicians, ed 5, Mosby Elsevier, 2007, p. 167.

203. a Calcium oxalate urolithiasis is a condition affecting cats that has become more common during the last several decades. Silica, urate, and cystine crystals are not commonly seen in cats. Bonagura J, Twedt D, Kirk's Current Veterinary Therapy, XV, Elsevier Saunders, 2014, p. 897.

204. b Unlike in humans, a significantly increased urobilinogen level with the chemistry dipstick has not been observed in most patients; therefore, the usefulness of the test in animals is questionable. Glucose, protein, and ketones are tested reliably on urine dipsticks. Tighe MM, Brown M, Mosby's Comprehensive Review for Veterinary Technicians, ed 4, Mosby Elsevier, 2015, p. 32.

205. d Microalbumin levels can be an indicator of early glomerular renal disease. Protein often increases in the urine in glomerular disease because of the leakage of the large protein molecules through the glomerular filter. Bilirubin, ketones, and glucose can all be found in the urine for various other diseases. Tighe MM, Brown M, Mosby's Comprehensive Review for Veterinary Technicians, ed 4, Mosby Elsevier, 2015, p. 31.

206. c Uric acid stones appear yellow-brownish in color and are not commonly found in the dog and cat except in Dalmatian dogs. Basenji, German shepherd, and Shetland sheepdogs can form stones as well, but they are unlikely to form uric acid stones. Dalmatians have the most problems with uric acid stones because they lack the enzyme uricase to break down the uric acid. Sirois M, Principles and Practice of Veterinary Technology, ed 3, Mosby Elsevier, 2011, p. 165.

207. a Inducing dissolution can treat struvite uroliths. Providing a diet that reduces urine pH to 6–6.3 and is low in magnesium causes struvite uroliths to dissolve. The crystals that dissolve will not dissolve in basic, isosthenuric, or dilute urine. Summers A, Common Diseases of Companion Animals, ed 2, Mosby Elsevier, p. 302.

208. d The primary advantages of ELISA are that it is relatively rapid and easy to perform and can be quite sensitive and specific. The sensitivity and specificity of the assay can also be manipulated by selection of antigens and use of secondary antibodies selective for either immunoglobulin G (IgG) or immunoglobulin M (IgM). One of the major disadvantages of ELISA is that the results are often simply reported as positive or negative and not quantitatively to detect changes in titer. Sellon, D, Long, M. Equine Infectious Diseases, ed 2, W.B. Saunders, 2007.

209. a Acetaminophen, aflatoxin, benzimidazole anthelmintics, halogenated hydrocarbons (e.g., halothane, chloroform) hydrocarbon solvents, iron, melaleuca oil, mushrooms (*Amanita* spp.), phosphides, sago palm, xylitol, and zinc will all cause an increase in ALT. An increase in ammonia may be caused by the ingestions of ammonium-based fertilizers. Blood pH may change as a result of the ingestion of alcohols, bread dough, and ethylene glycol (among others). Calcium may increase as a result of the ingestion of Calcipotriene, cholecalciferol rodenticide, diuretics, grapes/raisins, hops, or xylitol. Willard M, Tvedten, H. Small Animal Clinical Diagnosis by Laboratory Methods, ed 5, W.B. Saunders, 2012.

210. d Chemical neutropenia and/or pancytopenia is generally a result of inhibition or destruction of stem cells after prolonged use of all of the drugs listed. Willard M, Tvedten, H. Small Animal Clinical Diagnosis by Laboratory Methods, ed 5, W.B. Saunders, 2012.

211. d Xylitol is reported to cause either hyperphosphatemia or hypophosphatemia. Willard M, Tvedten, H. Small Animal Clinical Diagnosis by Laboratory Methods, ed 5, W.B. Saunders, 2012.

212. a Blood or plasma is the major vehicle for body transport of toxicants. Whole blood should be collected in anticoagulant (ethylenediaminetetraacetic acid [EDTA] or heparin unless otherwise specified).

Vomitus or feces may provide evidence of recent oral exposure, biliary excretion, or both. Many organic toxicants are excreted in urine by direct secretion from renal tubule transport systems. Hair may document chronic accumulation of a toxicant (especially for metals or sulfur-containing compounds), showing prior exposure even when gastrointestinal and organ concentrations are no longer elevated or detectable. However, hair values must be interpreted carefully because assay may be influenced by external contamination rather than systemic accumulation. Willard M, Tvedten, H. Small Animal Clinical Diagnosis by Laboratory Methods, ed 5, W.B. Saunders, 2012.

213. b Plasma (from EDTA or heparin-preserved blood) or serum and urine are the preferred antemortem samples. Blood concentrations usually peak 4 to 6 hours after ingestion. Samples should be refrigerated if analyzed within 24 hours or frozen if longer delays are expected. A blood smear should be examined for Heinz bodies. Liver biopsies would not show immediate ingestion to aid in the treatment of the toxicant. Willard M, Tvedten, H. Small Animal Clinical Diagnosis by Laboratory Methods, ed 5, W.B. Saunders, 2012.

214. c Struvites are largely made up of magnesium ammonium phosphate, also called triple phosphate uroliths. Calcium carbonate and calcium oxalates are primarily composed of calcium, whereas silica crystals are mostly made up of 100% silica. Tighe MM, Brown M, Mosby's Comprehensive Review for Veterinary Technicians, ed 4, Mosby Elsevier, 2015, p. 38.

215. a Calcium is considered a mineral, not an electrolyte. Sodium, potassium, and chloride are all considered electrolytes. Tighe MM, Brown M, Mosby's Comprehensive Review for Veterinary Technicians, ed 4, Mosby Elsevier, 2015, p. 6.

216. d Hyperkalemia is commonly associated with hypoadrenocorticism, also known as Addison's disease. Hyperparathyroidism is associated with hypercalcemia. Hyperthyroidism results in elevated thyroid hormone. Diabetes insipidus usually results in decreased levels of potassium and calcium. Tighe MM, Brown M, Mosby's Comprehensive Review for Veterinary Technicians, ed 4, Mosby Elsevier, 2015, p. 517.

217. b A false positive test is one in which the animal is not affected and the test is positive. A false negative is when the animal is affected and the test is negative. Studdert VP, Gay CC, Blood DC, Saunders Comprehensive Veterinary Dictionary, ed 4, Elsevier Saunders, 2007, p. 941.

218. c Many animals will show no clinical signs of primary hyperparathyroidism; it is usually diagnosed on a routine serum chemistry examination. Therefore, polydipsia/polyuria (PU/PD) is not commonly seen in hyperparathyroidism. In hyperadrenocorticism, diabetes insipidus, and diabetes mellitus, PU/PD is a common clinical sign. Summers A, Common Diseases of Companion Animals, ed 2, Mosby Elsevier, p. 109.

219. d There is no universal cat blood donor, because cats have isoantibodies against other blood types. The good news is that most cats in the United States have the same blood type, which is A. Bassert J, Thomas J, McCurnin's Clinical Textbook for Veterinary Technicians, ed 8, Elsevier Saunders, 2014, p. 898.

220. a Cats have naturally occurring circulating alloantibodies to the blood type they do not have. Type B cats have high levels of type A antibodies and type A cats have a high number of type B antibodies. Therefore, transfusion of type A blood into a type B cat could result in severe, potentially fatal hemolytic transfusion reaction. Although rare, transfusion reactions in cats are much more severe than those in dogs and may occur with the first transfusion, which does not occur in dogs. Bassert J, Thomas J, McCurnin's Clinical Textbook for Veterinary Technicians, ed 8, Elsevier Saunders, 2014, p. 898.

221. c The spun hematocrit allows the evaluation of plasma color, PCV, buffy coat, and total protein. Hendrix C, Sirois M, Laboratory Procedures for Veterinary Technicians, ed 5, Mosby Elsevier, 2007, p. 53.

222. b A monolayer (mono means one) is the area on the blood film where the cells are evenly and randomly distributed and are not distorted. The feathered edge is the outer edge of a smear, and it may include a monolayer of cells; however, they may be slightly distorted in this area. The body of the blood smear is often multilayered and difficult to assess. Hendrix C, Sirois M, Laboratory Procedures for Veterinary Technicians, ed 5, Mosby Elsevier, 2007, p. 41.

223. c Capillary action, or capillarity, occurs when a liquid pushes against a solid and is caused to rise, such as blood entering a capillary tube. Therefore, blood will be drawn up into the tube by capillary action. Perfusion of mucous membranes provides information about proper oxygenation and blood pressure. Blood coursing through smaller veins is not an example of capillary action but is rather a normal physiological function for blood to course through all veins and is representative of blood pressure, heart function, and health. Removing serum from a clot with a pipette is sometimes necessary for certain testing and has nothing to do with capillary action. Aspinall V, Clinical Procedures in Veterinary Nursing, ed 2, Butterworth Heinemann Elsevier, 2008, p. 257.

224. c Anisocytosis is the presence in the blood of erythrocytes of varying sizes. Anisocytosis is the only selection that would be an abnormality of the substance being evaluated. All of the other answers are mechanical properties of the instrumentation and any inconsistencies with these will cause laboratory error. Studdert VP, Gay CC, Blood DC, Saunders Comprehensive Veterinary Dictionary, ed 4, Elsevier Saunders, 2007, p. 61.

225. b Remove serum or plasma from the cells as soon as possible to avoid increased serum phosphorus. Glucose will decrease, enzyme activity may be decreased, and potassium, not sodium, will increase. Tighe MM, Brown M, Mosby's Comprehensive Review for Veterinary Technicians, ed 4, Mosby Elsevier, 2015, p. 120.

226. b Lymphocytes are produced by the lymphatic system and act in the body's immune system. Neutrophils, monocytes, and macrophages phagocytize. Tighe

MM, Brown M, Mosby's Comprehensive Review for Veterinary Technicians, ed 4, Mosby Elsevier, 2015, p. 16.

227. b A complete urinalysis has the following parts in the following order: (1) Gross examination; (2) Specific gravity; (3) Biochemical analysis; (4) Sediment examination. Gross examination, looking at the sample in its presenting form, is required for all samples, including urine, blood, and feces, before beginning diagnostics. Sirois M, Principles and Practice of Veterinary Technology, ed 3, Mosby Elsevier, 2011, p. 203.

228. d The trematode lung fluke is *Paragonimus kellicotti*. The tapeworm is known as *Dipylidium caninum*. Mites, along with ticks, are small arthropods belonging to the subclass *Acari* and the class *Arachnida*. Bonagura J, Twedt D, Kirk's Current Veterinary Therapy, XV, Elsevier Saunders, 2014, p. 271.

229. b Leukocyte production occurs in bone marrow. The lymphatic system returns excessive tissue fluid that has leaked out of the capillaries to the circulating blood; it also removes bacteria and other foreign particles from the lymph in specialized filtering stations known as lymph nodes. The lymphatic system does not produce lymphocytes. Aspinall V, Cappello M, Introduction to Veterinary Anatomy and Physiology Textbook, ed 2, Elsevier, 2009, p. 77.

230. a The spleen is a fairly large organ that has both lymphatic and hematologic functions. The pancreas has endocrine and exocrine functions. The tonsils are similar to lymph nodes and the role of both of these structures is to fight infection. The liver is an extremely important organ in the body and is responsible for protein, fat, and carbohydrate metabolism; vitamin and mineral storage; digestion of food; and detoxification of waste. Aspinall V, Cappello M, Introduction to Veterinary Anatomy and Physiology Textbook, ed 2, Elsevier, 2009, p. 241.

231. a The spleen acts as a reservoir for blood when the animal is at rest and does not need a large amount of oxygen and other substances to be delivered to the muscles. The job of the pancreas is twofold: it has an endocrine function and an exocrine function releasing hormones such as insulin and digestive enzymes. The key role of the pancreas is not to store blood. The liver is an extremely important organ in the body. It is responsible for protein, fat, and carbohydrate metabolism; vitamin and mineral storage; digestion of food; and detoxification of waste. The parathyroid gland is responsible for secreting parathormone hormone, which is dependent on the calcium levels in the body. Aspinall V, Cappello M, Introduction to Veterinary Anatomy and Physiology Textbook, ed 2, Elsevier, 2009, p. 241.

232. b T cells mature within the thymus and are then released. The thyroid controls the metabolism of the body, and it has nothing to do with the T cells. Tonsils are part of the lymphatic system and help in the prevention of infection; they do not release T cells. The splenic trabeculae are small fibrous bands located within the spleen and do not release T cells. Tizard I, Veterinary Immunology, ed 9, Elsevier Saunders, 2013, p. 113.

233. c B cells migrate to the gut-associated lymphoid tissue (GALT), where they greatly increase their numbers as well as achieve the diversification of their B-cell receptor. GLNB, GALB, and GLAN are not associated with processing B cells. Tizard I, Veterinary Immunology, ed 9, Elsevier Saunders, 2013, p. 186.

234. d Human error is perhaps the most difficult testing parameter to control. New and/or outdated reagents may cause shifts, along with the recalibration of instruments. Hendrix C, Sirois M, Laboratory Procedures for Veterinary Technicians, ed 5, Mosby Elsevier, 2007, p. 22.

235. a Human error is perhaps the most difficult testing parameter to control. It is not possible to tell, through the use of quality-control measures, whether the samples are of acceptable quality. Example: A red top tube may have not been handled properly before separating, but the instrument may still produce a value; however, the value might not be accurate. Hendrix C, Sirois M, Laboratory Procedures for Veterinary Technicians, ed 5, Mosby Elsevier, 2007, p. 22.

236. b Refractometers should be checked daily with distilled water to ensure that the specific gravity is 1.000. Tap water, plasma, and urine will always read >1.000 and cannot be used to calibrate the refractometer. Hendrix C, Sirois M, Laboratory Procedures for Veterinary Technicians, ed 6, Mosby Elsevier, 2015, p. 13.

237. d Blood tubes are counterbalanced and centrifuged for 10 minutes at 2000–3000 rpm. Centrifuging a sample at too high a speed or for an extended period may cause hemolysis. Centrifuging a sample too slowly or for less than the proper time may not completely separate the specimen or concentrate the sediment. Tighe MM, Brown M, Mosby's Comprehensive Review for Veterinary Technicians, ed 4, Mosby Elsevier, 2015, p. 113.

238. b The centrifuge should never be operated with the lid unlatched. The centrifuge should always have balanced tubes, a timer should be set, and the tube holders should be checked to ensure contents have not leaked. Hendrix C, Sirois M, Laboratory Procedures for Veterinary Technicians, ed 5, Mosby Elsevier, 2007, p. 11.

239. c Enough blood should be collected to yield enough serum, plasma, or whole blood to run all planned assays three times. This allows for technician error, instrument failure, or the need to dilute a sample without having to collect another sample from the animal. Transcription errors are clerical errors and do not require extra use of a sample. Hendrix C, Sirois M, Laboratory Procedures for Veterinary Technicians, ed 5, Mosby Elsevier, 2007, p. 32.

240. a Prolonged contact of serum with RBCs will cause a false decrease in glucose. The other options offered would not decrease serum glucose levels. Ford R, Mazzaferro E, Kirk and Bistner's Handbook of Veterinary Procedures and Emergency Treatments, ed 9, Saunders, 2012.

241. b Dogs and cats should fast for 12 hours before sampling to avoid lipemia that may occur following a meal. Ingestion of food does not affect hemolysis, nor will the sample appear icteric or anemic because of food. Bassert J, Thomas J, McCurnin's Clinical Textbook for

Veterinary Technicians, ed 8, Elsevier Saunders, 2014, p. 426.

242. c Centrifuging a sample at too high a speed or for an extended period may cause hemolysis. Centrifuging that is run too slowly or for less than the proper time may not completely separate the specimen or concentrate the sediment. Tighe MM, Brown M, Mosby's Comprehensive Review for Veterinary Technicians, ed 4, Mosby Elsevier, 2015, p. 113.

243. c A hemolytic, or red, sample can occur from improper sample collection and handling. Icterus is caused by an increase in the total bilirubin in the blood; icteric (or yellow) serum or plasma is frequently seen in animals with liver disease or hemolytic anemia. Leukocytosis is an increase in white blood cells that would not be affected by mishandling. Lipemia is common in an unfasted animal. Sirois M, Principles and Practice of Veterinary Technology, ed 3, Mosby Elsevier, 2011, p. 132.

244. b Icterus is also called jaundice and is caused by elevated bilirubin. Elevated lipids will cause a white color in the serum. Changes in electrolytes and/or glucose will not change the color of serum. Studdert VP, Gay CC, Blood DC, Saunders Comprehensive Veterinary Dictionary, ed 4, Elsevier Saunders, 2007, p. 610.

245. d Plasma that appears deep yellow is described as icteric and can be seen in animals with liver disease or hemolytic anemia. Red is the proper color of blood; green and brown blood are not common findings. Hendrix C, Sirois M, Laboratory Procedures for Veterinary Technicians, ed 5, Mosby Elsevier, 2007, p. 36.

246. c Anticoagulants are required when whole blood or plasma samples are needed. Hendrix C, Sirois M, Laboratory Procedures for Veterinary Technicians, ed 5, Mosby Elsevier, 2007, p. 31.

247. b Hyperbilirubinemia can cause jaundice in the patient and icterus in the sample. Icterus is a condition that cannot be corrected or prevented by proper sample collection or handling. It is frequently seen in animals with liver disease or hemolytic anemia. Hemolysis is most commonly attributed to technician error, although hemolysis may occur in some anemias. Lipemia can usually be prevented or minimized by making the animal fast before collection. Tighe MM, Brown M, Mosby's Comprehensive Review for Veterinary Technicians, ed 4, Mosby Elsevier, 2015, p. 89.

248. d An immediate hypersensitivity reaction is systemic and life-threatening; it is known as an allergic anaphylaxis or anaphylactic shock. Agglutination, hemolysis, and DIC are all life-threatening hematological ailments; however, they are not triggered by allergy. Tizard I, Veterinary Immunology, ed 9, Elsevier Saunders, 2013, p. 327.

249. a In the United States, 99% of domestic short-hair and long-hair cats are type A. A total of 5% to 25% are B positive and <1% are AB. Tizard I, Veterinary Immunology, ed 9, Elsevier Saunders, 2013, p. 353.

250. d DEA is an acronym for dog erythrocyte antigen. Tighe MM, Brown M, Mosby's Comprehensive Review for Veterinary Technicians, ed 4, Mosby Elsevier, 2015, p. 563.

251. a Anticoagulant rodenticide poisoning initially prolongs the prothrombin time and factor VII is the first to be depleted. All the other clotting factors continue to be depleted. Coagulation tests would not be used to confirm adrenal or thyroid function or to confirm ethylene glycol poisoning. Hendrix C, Sirois M, Laboratory Procedures for Veterinary Technicians, ed 6, Mosby Elsevier, 2015, p. 230.

252. b Volumetric pipettes were designed to deliver microliter volumes. Graduated pipettes may contain a single volume designation or may have multiple gradations. Flasks and cylinders are not used to deliver microliter volumes of patient samples. A cuvette is a piece of laboratory glassware that is intended to hold samples for spectroscopic analysis. Hendrix C, Sirois M, Laboratory Procedures for Veterinary Technicians, ed 6, Mosby Elsevier, 2015, p. 14.

253. a Laser-flow technology is used to determine blood cell concentrations, white blood cell differential, and other hematology parameters. Laser flow technology is not applicable to chemistries, coagulation, or electrolyte analyzers. Hendrix C, Sirois M, Laboratory Procedures for Veterinary Technicians, ed 6, Mosby Elsevier, 2015, p. e4.

254. a ALT and AST are enzymes found in hepatocytes and are elevated when liver damage or disease is present. GGT and SDH are primarily measured to evaluate liver function in horses. Electrolytes, BUN, amylase, and lipase do not evaluate liver function. Tighe MM, Brown M, Mosby's Comprehensive Review for Veterinary Technicians, ed 4, Mosby Elsevier, 2015.

255. c GGT and SDH are primarily measured to evaluate liver function in horses. ALT and AST are enzymes found in hepatocytes and are elevated when liver damage or disease is present in dogs or cats. Electrolytes, BUN, amylase, and lipase do not evaluate liver function. Bassert J, Thomas J, McCurnin's Clinical Textbook for Veterinary Technicians, ed 8, Elsevier Saunders, 2014, p. 745.

256. d Liver function tests include AST, ALT, AP, bile acids, total bilirubin, serum albumin, and dye excretion. Kidney testing focuses on BUN, creatinine, and phosphorus among others, but not necessarily AST, ALT, AP, bile acids, total bilirubin, serum albumin, and dye excretion. Pancreatic testing may include the analysis of amylase and lipase, but it should mainly use ultrasound to evaluate the function. Heart disease testing may include BNP (B-type natriuretic peptide) and echocardiograms. Hendrix C, Sirois M, Laboratory Procedures for Veterinary Technicians, ed 6, Mosby Elsevier, 2015, p. 202.

257. b Impedance is the obstruction or opposition to passage or flow, as of an electric current or other form of energy. Impedance is commonly used to test blood samples in an instrument that passes a current of light or electricity through the sample. The change in current is measured as impedance. Studdert VP, Gay CC, Blood DC, Saunders Comprehensive Veterinary Dictionary, ed 4, Elsevier Saunders, 2007, p. 588.

258. d The key advantages of PCR assays are speed, cost, sensitivity, ability to detect nonviable virus, and in some cases, safety. The main disadvantages of PCR are false-positive reactions, the lack of a viable virus isolate, detection of virus that may not be clinically relevant, and the inability to detect new or poorly characterized viruses. Sellon, D, Long, M. Equine Infectious Diseases, ed 2, W.B. Saunders, 2007.

259. d *Gasterophilus* is a genus of flies called the horse botflies, the larvae of which develop in the gastrointestinal tract of horses and may sometimes infect humans. The larvae of *Gasterophilus* are known as bots and are equine parasites. The fly deposits eggs on the host's hair. The eggs hatch and the emerging larvae enter the mouth and migrate to the stomach, where they attach to the inner lining. They are members of the family *Gasterophilidae. Capillaria* is a genus of parasitic nematodes of the subfamily *Capillariinae* and is most commonly parasitic in birds; they cause capillariasis. *Otobius* is a genus of soft-bodied ticks in the family *Argasidae*. Thelazia is a genus of spiruroid worms in the family *Thelaziidae* and they are parasites of the lacrimal duct or conjunctival sac of mammals and birds. The larvae are deposited in the conjunctival sac by the intermediate host. Studdert VP, Gay CC, Blood DC, Saunders Comprehensive Veterinary Dictionary, ed 4, Elsevier Saunders, 2007, p. 472.

260. b Gasterophilus is a genus of flies, known as the horse botflies, the larvae of which develop in the gastrointestinal tract of horses and sometimes infect humans. Flea feces are referred to as flea dirt. A lice egg is called a nit and seed ticks are the six-legged larval stages of ticks. Studdert VP, Gay CC, Blood DC, Saunders Comprehensive Veterinary Dictionary, ed 4, Elsevier Saunders, 2007, p. 472.

261. a Nits are lice eggs; seed ticks are the six-legged larval stages of ticks; flea feces are referred to as flea dirt; and fly larvae are referred to as bots. Studdert VP, Gay CC, Blood DC, Saunders Comprehensive Veterinary Dictionary, ed 4, Elsevier Saunders, 2007, p. 762.

262. a *Strongylus vulgaris* sucks blood and also causes verminous arteritis, thromboembolic colic, anemia, and debility. The small strongyles can cause severe enteritis and diarrhea and are also known as redworm infestation. *Parascaris equorum* is an ascarid, *Anoplocephala perfoliata* is a tapeworm, and *Dictyocaulus arnfieldi* is a lungworm. Studdert VP, Gay CC, Blood DC, Saunders Comprehensive Veterinary Dictionary, ed 4, Elsevier Saunders, 2007, p. 1056.

263. b Sudan III or IV is used to stain fat. Fat droplets will float in and out of planes of focus, usually vary in size, and will stain shades of iridescent orange. New methylene blue provides excellent nuclear and nucleolar detail. Diff-Quik can be applied rapidly to smears of aspirated cells or exudate. Giemsa stain is used to detect spirochetes and rickettsiae as well as to demonstrate the capsule of *Bacillus anthracis* and the morphology of *Dermatophilus congolensis*. Tighe MM, Brown M, Mosby's Comprehensive Review for Veterinary Technicians, ed 4, Mosby Elsevier, 2015, p. 34.

264. a When stained with a supravital stain (e.g., new methylene blue), early reticulocytes demonstrate a network or reticulum that appears as aggregated material. Supravital stains contain no fixatives; Camco Quik, Eosin, and Sudan all have fixatives. Hendrix C, Sirois M, Laboratory Procedures for Veterinary Technicians, ed 6, Mosby Elsevier, 2015.

265. b An eosinophilia or raised number of eosinophils occurs in response to parasitic infestation. Bacterial and viral infections usually show an elevated white count, not just an increase in eosinophils. Eosinophilia is not a known marker for hormonal disorders. Aspinall V, Cappello M, Introduction to Veterinary Anatomy and Physiology Textbook, ed 2, Elsevier, 2009, p. 80.

266. b Jaundice or icterus is a result of excess bilirubin in the blood. Hyperhemoglobinemia is an excess of hemoglobin in the blood and does not cause discoloration. Ketonuria does not cause jaundice; however, hyperbilirubinemia can discolor urine. Anemia is not the cause of jaundice, but jaundice can appear in an anemic patient because of cellular degeneration. Tighe MM, Brown M, Mosby's Comprehensive Review for Veterinary Technicians, ed 4, Mosby Elsevier, 2015, p. 124.

267. a Basophilic stippling is the presence of small, dark-blue bodies within the erythrocyte that is observed in Wright-stained cells and represents residual RNA. It is common in immature RBCs of ruminants and occasionally in those of cats during a response to anemia. It is also characteristic of lead poisoning. Howell-Jolly bodies are one form of morphology that is usually seen in response to anemia. Immune-mediated diseases are frequently associated with spherocytes and neoplasia is frequently associated with keratocytes. Hendrix C, Sirois M, Laboratory Procedures for Veterinary Technicians, ed 6, Mosby Elsevier, 2015, p. 74.

268. c Spherocytes are significant in that they suggest the immune-mediated destruction of RBCs, resulting in hemolytic anemia. Basophilic stippling is associated with lead poisoning, whereas lymphocytosis is commonly linked to tickborne illness. Erythrocytes and smudge cells are linked to leukemia. Hendrix C, Sirois M, Laboratory Procedures for Veterinary Technicians, ed 6, Mosby Elsevier, 2015, p. 73.

269. a Heinz bodies are round structures that represent denatured hemoglobin and are caused by certain oxidant drugs or chemicals. A Howell-Jolly body is a small, round or oval body observed in erythrocytes when stains are added to fresh blood. H-J bodies may be found in various anemias and after splenectomy or reduced splenic function. *Anaplasma marginale* is a bacterium that lives within bovine red cells. A spherocyte is an intensely stained erythrocyte that has reduced or no central pallor. Hendrix C, Sirois M, Laboratory Procedures for Veterinary Technicians, ed 6, Mosby Elsevier, 2015, p. 74.

270. b Fresh frozen plasma (FFP) will retain its coagulation factor efficacy for 12 months, provided it is maintained at the appropriate temperature. After 1 year, it has to be relabeled as frozen plasma (FP). Battaglia A, Small Animal Emergency and Critical Care for Veterinary Technicians, ed 2, Saunders, 2007, p. 70.

271. b Plasma cells produce antibodies; hepatocytes, thymocytes, and T cells do not. Hendrix C, Sirois M, Laboratory Procedures for Veterinary Technicians, ed 6, Mosby Elsevier, 2015, p. 119.

272. b Howell-Jolly bodies are basophilic nuclear remnants seen in young erythrocytes during the response to anemia. Heinz bodies are round structures representing denatured hemoglobin. Reticulocytes are immature erythrocytes that contain organelles (ribosomes) that are lost as the cell matures. These organelles account for the diffuse blue-gray or polychromatophilic staining of immature cells with Wright stain. An increased membrane surface area relative to the cell volume characterizes a leptocyte. Hendrix C, Sirois M, Laboratory Procedures for Veterinary Technicians, ed 5, Mosby Elsevier, 2007, p. 55.

273. b To maintain adequate levels of all factors, plasma must be harvested from a unit of WB and frozen at -18°C or colder within 8 hours from the time of initial collection. After 8 hours, the product is labeled frozen plasma. Battaglia A, Small Animal Emergency and Critical Care for Veterinary Technicians, ed 2, Saunders, 2007, p. 70.

274. b When an antigen is injected into an animal, antibodies will be produced (by the patient) that can bind to that antigen and ensure its destruction. Immunoglobulin plays a role as a receptor in the body's defense system. T cells are responsible for mounting immune-mediated responses. Plasma cells produce antibodies when stimulated. Tizard I, Veterinary Immunology, ed 9, Elsevier Saunders, 2013, p. 7.

275. d A degenerative left shift occurs when the number of immature neutrophils exceeds the number of mature neutrophils and the total WBC is decreasing. A regenerative left shift is when the number of mature neutrophils exceeds the number of immature neutrophils and the total WBC is normal to increasing. Leukocytosis is an elevated number of white blood cells. Leukopenia is a decreased number of white blood cells. Tighe MM, Brown M, Mosby's Comprehensive Review for Veterinary Technicians, ed 4, Mosby Elsevier, 2015, p. 50.

276. b Anisocytosis clinically refers to size variations of the red blood cell. Polycytosis or polycythemia and erythrocytosis are both known as a condition in which there is a net increase in the total circulating erythrocyte (red blood cell) mass of the body. There are several types of polycythemia. *Poikilocytosis* is a general term denoting nondescript variations in shapes of erythrocytes that are scattered throughout the blood film. Christenson DE, Veterinary Medical Terminology, ed 2, Elsevier Saunders, 1997.

277. a Reticulocytes are immature erythrocytes that contain organelles (ribosomes) that are lost as the cell matures. Metarubricytes, rubriblasts, and rubricytes are all different phases of a developing red blood cell. The reticulocyte is the youngest of these phases. Hendrix C, Sirois M, Laboratory Procedures for Veterinary Technicians, ed 5, Mosby Elsevier, 2007, p. 56.

278. c The complete blood count includes total red blood cell and white blood cell counts, packed cell volume, hemoglobin concentration, erythrocyte indices, and the differential blood cell count. Whole blood is needed to test hemoglobin; serum and plasma are not whole blood. Whole blood is used to make a blood smear but it evaluates the blood cells, not the hemoglobin concentration. Hendrix C, Sirois M, Laboratory Procedures for Veterinary Technicians, ed 5, Mosby Elsevier, 2007, p. 27.

279. d The precision of a PCV is approximately 1%, making it a very accurate test. The erythrocyte count, Hgb determination, and leukocyte count are all part of the CBC; however, they have less accuracy. Sirois M, Principles and Practice of Veterinary Technology, ed 3, Mosby Elsevier, 2011, p. 132.

280. a Counting erythrocytes and leukocytes is a routine part of the CBC. Cell counts can be performed by manual or automated methods. The total WBC (leukocyte) is one of the most useful values determined in a CBC and is more accurate with a manual count. Total RBC (erythrocyte) and platelet (thrombocyte) counts may also be performed manually, although they are more difficult and less accurate. Manually spinning down hematocrit tubes and reading the values on a chart obtains PCV. Hendrix C, Sirois M, Laboratory Procedures for Veterinary Technicians, ed 5, Mosby Elsevier, 2007, p. 33.

281. d If stained with a vital stain (e.g., NMB or Diff-Quik), the reticular structure would be seen and the cell would be noted as a reticulocyte. This sign of regeneration is indicative of an active bone marrow. Schistocytosis is a common finding on a CBC for a patient with IMHA but is not representative of a regenerative anemia. Reticulocytosis is associated with regeneration but Diff-Quik is not needed for staining. Eosinophilia is not associated with regeneration. Tighe MM, Brown M, Mosby's Comprehensive Review for Veterinary Technicians, ed 4, Mosby Elsevier, 2015, p. 45.

282. b Target cells are leptocytes with a central area of pigment surrounded by a clear area and then a dense ring of peripheral cytoplasm. Plasma cells have an eccentric, round nucleus with condensed/clumped chromatin, deep-blue staining cytoplasm, perinuclear to juxtanuclear (next to) clear zone (Golgi apparatus) and they have a smaller nucleus in relation to cytoplasm compared with the typical lymphocyte. Spherocytes have a dark red staining appearance, are smaller than average size, are round, and lack a central pallor. Reticulocytes stained with Wright causes a polychromatophilic staining, or diffuse, blue-gray color. Hendrix C, Sirois M, Laboratory Procedures for Veterinary Technicians, ed 5, Mosby Elsevier, 2007, p. 54.

283. d The refractometer is a piece of equipment that can be used to approximate the total protein concentration in serum or plasma. The buffy coat layer is found between the packed red cells and plasma in a spun microhematocrit tube. Bassert J, Thomas J, McCurnin's Clinical Textbook for Veterinary Technicians, ed 8, Elsevier Saunders, 2014, p. 1425.

284. a Plasma has not been allowed to clot; therefore, it still contains the plasma protein fibrinogen (therefore has higher protein levels). Serum and plasma can both be used to measure electrolytes. Plasma and serum have the same color, and serum does not clot. Hendrix C, Sirois M, Laboratory Procedures for Veterinary Technicians, ed 5, Mosby Elsevier, 2007, p. 31.

285. b Lipemia is characterized by increased turbidity of the sample, ranging from haziness to an overtly milky appearance. Chylemia is the presence of chyle in blood and can result in lipemia but it is not a term to describe milky or white plasma. Leukemia and lactemia do not affect the color of serum or plasma. Bassert J, Thomas J, McCurnin's Clinical Textbook for Veterinary Technicians, ed 8, Elsevier Saunders, 2014, p. 426.

286. c The term *polychromasia* is used when there are varying degrees of bluish staining of the erythrocyte cytoplasm. Anemia is the decrease in the number of erythrocytes or red blood cells. *Anisocytosis* is a general term denoting variation of erythrocyte size. *Poikilocytosis* is a term denoting nondescript variations in the shapes of erythrocytes that are scattered throughout the blood film. Tighe MM, Brown M, Mosby's Comprehensive Review for Veterinary Technicians, ed 4, Mosby Elsevier, 2015, p. 45.

287. a Bilirubin is an insoluble molecule derived from the breakdown of hemoglobin. Urea results as a breakdown of protein. Carotene is yellow or red pigment (from carrots among other foods), which is converted into Vitamin A in the body. Erythropoietin is a hormone produced by the kidney and is used to stimulate red cell production. Hendrix C, Sirois M, Laboratory Procedures for Veterinary Technicians, ed 6, Mosby Elsevier, 2015, p. 199.

288. c Liver disease and/or hemolytic anemia is suspected when jaundice is present. A responsive and nonresponsive anemia can still be a hemolytic anemia; the responsiveness or nonresponsiveness characterizes the response to treatment, not the type of anemia. Megaloblastic anemia is described as megaloblasts in the bone marrow and macrocytic erythrocytes. There is no primary destruction of the red blood cells leading to a buildup of bilirubin in the circulating blood, which leads to icterus. Studdert VP, Gay CC, Blood DC, Saunders Comprehensive Veterinary Dictionary, ed 4, Elsevier Saunders, 2007, p. 522.

289. b The most immature erythrocyte is the rubriblast. Prorubricyte is the next step in maturity after the rubriblast. Multipotent stem cells means that they are stem cells that can divide into copies of themselves. Erythrocytoblast is a nucleated cell in bone marrow that develops into an erythrocyte. Tighe MM, Brown M, Mosby's Comprehensive Review for Veterinary Technicians, ed 4, Mosby Elsevier, 2015, p. 51.

290. a Rouleaux is most common in horses, although it is also seen in cats. In dogs and other animals, rouleaux may be an indication of inflammation and is considered abnormal. Bassert J, Thomas J, McCurnin's Clinical Textbook for Veterinary Technicians, ed 8, Elsevier Saunders, 2014, p. 406.

291. d Microcytosis is decreased MCV. Macrocytosis is an increased MCV. Hyperchromasia is an increased central pallor of red blood cells, and hypochromasia is a decreased central pallor of red blood cells. Tighe MM, Brown M, Mosby's Comprehensive Review for Veterinary Technicians, ed 4, Mosby Elsevier, 2015, p. 48.

292. b Forty is 4% of 1000. Tighe MM, Brown M, Mosby's Comprehensive Review for Veterinary Technicians, ed 4, Mosby Elsevier, 2015.

293. c A hypersegmented neutrophil implies an older neutrophil. Normal cells are not hypersegmented. Female animals and toxemia are not reasons for hypersegmented neutrophils, although toxemia can produce toxic changes such as Döhle bodies. Tighe MM, Brown M, Mosby's Comprehensive Review for Veterinary Technicians, ed 4, Mosby Elsevier, 2015, p. 50.

294. d Döhle bodies are considered toxic changes in the neutrophil. Leukemia, parasitic infection, and immaturity can cause changes in neutrophils such as a decreased or increased amount of neutrophils in the circulating blood or a left shift, but they do not include Döhle bodies. Hendrix C, Sirois M, Laboratory Procedures for Veterinary Technicians, ed 5, Mosby Elsevier, 2007, p. 48.

295. a Monocytes are very large WBCs that are found in the circulating blood. Neutrophils, eosinophils, and lymphocytes are also white blood cells and are commonly seen in peripheral blood, but they are smaller than monocytes. Sirois M, Principles and Practice of Veterinary Technology, ed 3, Mosby Elsevier, 2011, p. 145.

296. c Hydrogen peroxide is not a liquid that can be used to prepare direct fecal smears. A direct smear on fresh feces is prepared with isotonic saline; however, the type of liquid added depends on what you hope to accomplish with the technique. If you are examining a liquid fecal sample for the presence of protozoan trophozoites (live-active protozoa), use saline (if any extra liquid is needed). If you are looking for helminth eggs and protozoan cysts in a small sample (bird droppings, rectal smear, etc.), use either water or iodine. Sirois M, Principles and Practice of Veterinary Technology, ed 3, Mosby Elsevier, 2011.

297. a The total blood volume makes up 6%–8% (average 7%) of an animal's lean body weight. Colville TP, Bassert JM, Clinical Anatomy and Physiology for Veterinary Technicians, ed 2, Mosby Elsevier, 2008, p. 226.

298. c A minor crossmatch determines the compatibility of the donor's serum with the recipient's red cells. A major crossmatch determines the compatibility of the donor's red cells with the recipient's serum. A blood transfusion crossmatch does not use urine. T-cell growth can be stimulated by blood transfusions, but they are not involved in the crossmatch process. Bonagura J, Twedt D, Kirk's Current Veterinary Therapy, XV, Elsevier Saunders, 2014, p. 312.

299. c Ethylenediamine tetraacetic acid (EDTA) is the preferred anticoagulant for hematologic studies because it does not alter cell morphology when it is used in the proper ratio for samples to be analyzed soon after collection. EDTA is available as sodium or potassium salt and it prevents clotting by forming an insoluble complex with calcium, which is necessary for clot formation. EDTA tubes are available in either liquid or powder forms, but the liquid form is more commonly used. Heparin is a suitable anticoagulant for most tests that require plasma samples. Sodium citrates are also commonly used, especially in transfusion medicine, as an anticoagulant. Potassium oxalate cannot be used with blood samples to be assayed for potassium. Sodium citrates similarly interfere with sodium assays, as well as many of the commonly performed blood chemistry tests. Sodium heparin causes cell morphology. Hendrix C, Sirois M, Laboratory Procedures for Veterinary Technicians, ed 6, Mosby Elsevier, 2015, p. 42.

300. b The preferred anticoagulant for coagulation testing is citrate, whereas the preferred anticoagulant for hematology testing is ethylenediamine tetraacetic acid (EDTA). Heparin is a good choice when plasma is needed for a specific diagnostic test, but not APPT. Sodium fluoride, best known as a glucose preservative, also has anticoagulant properties, but it is not used to determine activated partial thromboplastin time and one-stage prothrombin time. Hendrix C, Sirois M, Laboratory Procedures for Veterinary Technicians, ed 5, Mosby Elsevier, 2007, p. 27.

301. a Myeloblasts are larger than rubriblasts and have a round-to-oval nucleus, a prominent nucleolus, and pale gray-blue cytoplasm. A Golgi apparatus acts to package proteins into membrane-bound vesicles inside the cell before the vesicles are sent to their destination. Heinz bodies and Döhle bodies are commonly seen when there are toxic changes in the blood. Hendrix C, Sirois M, Laboratory Procedures for Veterinary Technicians, ed 6, Mosby Elsevier, 2015.

302. d Heinz bodies are round structures representing denatured hemoglobin caused by certain oxidant drugs or chemicals. Howell-Jolly bodies are basophilic nuclear remnants seen in young erythrocytes during the response to anemia. Cells that have inclusions that contain immunoglobulin are commonly referred to as Russell bodies. Döhle bodies appear as small, gray-blue cytoplasmic inclusions, are indicative of mild toxemia, and are most abundant in cats and horses. Hendrix C, Sirois M, Laboratory Procedures for Veterinary Technicians, ed 5, Mosby Elsevier, 2007, p. 55.

303. b Hypochromia is a decrease in hemoglobin in erythrocytes so that they are abnormally pale, which is measured in calculation by the means of corpuscular hemoglobin concentration (MCHC). Low MCHC is often seen in iron-deficiency anemias, usually in association with microcytosis, and sometimes in dogs with congenital portosystemic shunts. Iron toxicity and increased erythrocyte production can also lead to decreased MCHC, but these are not the most common causes. Studdert VP, Gay CC, Blood DC, Saunders Comprehensive Veterinary Dictionary, ed 4, Elsevier Saunders, 2007, p. 568.

304. c Hemostasis (or blood clotting) requires interaction between blood vessel, platelets, and coagulation factors. Thrombin converts fibrinogen to fibrin. A meshwork of fibrin forms in and around the platelet plug, stabilizing the plug and preventing it from being washed away by the flow of blood. If the fibrin clot does not form, a patient may initially stop bleeding as the platelet plug forms, but may begin to bleed again as the primary platelet plug is dislodged. Phagocytosis and antibody production are not part of the clotting cascade. They play vital roles in the defense mechanisms of the body and the immune system. The complement fixation test is used to detect antibodies. Bassert J, Thomas J, McCurnin's Clinical Textbook for Veterinary Technicians, ed 8, Elsevier Saunders, 2014, p. 417.

305. a *Haemobartonella felis* is a fairly common parasite of feline erythrocytes. The disease is referred to as hemobartonellosis or feline infectious anemia. *Haemobartonella canis* infection is rare in dogs. There are strands of *Haemobartonella* that can affect horses and cattle, but they are very uncommon. Hendrix C, Sirois M, Laboratory Procedures for Veterinary Technicians, ed 5, Mosby Elsevier, 2007, p. 57.

306. c A left shift is an increased number of immature neutrophils in the peripheral blood. Neutropenia is a decreased number of neutrophils in the peripheral blood, whereas leukemia is a malignant condition that causes a decrease in leukocytes in the peripheral blood. Autoimmune hemolytic anemia (AIHA) is a condition in which the body attacks its own red blood cells. If the AIHA is a regeneration, an increased number of reticulocytes can be seen in the peripheral blood. Tighe MM, Brown M, Mosby's Comprehensive Review for Veterinary Technicians, ed 4, Mosby Elsevier, 2015, p. 50.

307. d The first line of defense against foreign invaders involves the protective barrier of the skin. Hair, neutrophils, and primary lymphoid tissue are also defense mechanisms and are part of nonspecific immunity, but they are not the first line of defense. Colville TP, Bassert JM, Clinical Anatomy and Physiology for Veterinary Technicians, ed 2, Mosby Elsevier, 2008, p. 243.

308. c Monocytes are phagocytic cells and when they migrate to the tissues they mature and become known as macrophages. Eosinophils play a major role in controlling parasitic infestation. An eosinophilia or raised numbers of eosinophils occur in response to parasitic infestation. Lymphocytes and neutrophils are both in charge of eliminating invading bacteria and antigens. Aspinall V, Cappello M, Introduction to Veterinary Anatomy and Physiology Textbook, ed 2, Elsevier, 2009, p. 80.

309. a IgG is the most abundant of the five classes (IgG, IgM, IgA, IgD, and IgE) of immunoglobulins, representing about 80% of serum immunoglobulin protein. IgM is the first antibody produced in the primary immune response. It represents about 20% of serum antibodies. IgD is found in trace quantities in the serum in humans and chickens. IgA is present in low concentrations in the serum. Studdert VP, Gay CC, Blood DC, Saunders Comprehensive Veterinary Dictionary, ed 4, Elsevier Saunders, 2007, p. 580.

310. b Production of substances in the body such as antibodies and interferon render the animal immune from disease. Active immunity can occur via immunization, as an immune response caused by natural exposure to the antigen, or as a sequela of the disease. Passive immunity is when antibodies were donated and therefore the individual's immune system was not stimulated to produce the antibodies (nor any memory cells). Colostral transfer of immunity is essential for the survival of young mammals. Bassert J, Thomas J, McCurnin's Clinical Textbook for Veterinary Technicians, ed 8, Elsevier Saunders, 2014, p. 1400.

311. a The placenta allows maternal IgG to transfer to the fetus, but not IgM, IgA, or IgE. Maternal IgG can enter the fetal bloodstream and the newborn human infant has circulating IgG levels comparable to those of its mother. IgG is the only immunoglobulin that can cross the placenta. Tizard I, Veterinary Immunology, ed 9, Elsevier Saunders, 2013, p. 231.

312. c Although a continuous process, phagocytosis can be divided into discrete stages: activation, chemotaxis, adherence, ingestion, and destruction. Tizard I, Veterinary Immunology, ed 9, Elsevier Saunders, 2013, p. 36.

313. b In an attenuated vaccine, specific genes are removed from the pathogen; it becomes harmless and can produce a safe vaccine that elicits strong immunity. When microorganisms are killed, the organisms used to produce the vaccines are also killed; therefore no microorganisms are found. A microorganism that is 100% virulent is prepared from live, usually attenuated, microorganisms. Tighe MM, Brown M, Mosby's Comprehensive Review for Veterinary Technicians, ed 4, Mosby Elsevier, 2015, p. 141.

314. d In passive immunity, the antibodies were donated and therefore the individual's immune system was not stimulated to produce the antibodies by exposure (nor by any memory cells). This involves short-term immunity because these antibodies will be quickly catabolized and cleared from the body and no replacements will be synthesized. Acquired immunity is developed after being exposed to pathogens. Tighe MM, Brown M, Mosby's Comprehensive Review for Veterinary Technicians, ed 4, Mosby Elsevier, 2015, p. 190.

315. d Myasthenia gravis is a disease that results in the esophageal muscle losing its normal muscle tone. Because it has little or no muscle tone, the esophagus relaxes and becomes more of a relaxed bag than a tight, muscular tube. This dilated esophagus is called a megaesophagus. The risk with the megaesophagus, and the principal reason that many animals die from it, is that the animal often breathes in some of the frequently regurgitated food, resulting in a lung condition called aspiration pneumonia. Generalized MG also causes exercise-related generalized muscle weakness that worsens after exercise and improves with rest. Colville TP, Bassert JM, Clinical Anatomy and Physiology for Veterinary Technicians, ed 2, Mosby Elsevier, 2008, p. 271; Bonagura J, Twedt D, Kirk's Current Veterinary Therapy, XV, Elsevier Saunders, 2014.

316. c Antigens that stimulate allergies can be called allergens. If an immediate hypersensitivity reaction is systemic and life-threatening, it is called allergic anaphylaxis or anaphylactic shock. Anaphylactic shock is not mild or moderate; it is a life-threatening emergency that stems from an allergy. It is not something that is caused by loss of blood flow or fluids. Tizard I, Veterinary Immunology, ed 9, Elsevier Saunders, 2013, p. 327.

317. d A condition called combined immunodeficiency affects animals in early life, after serum levels of maternally derived antibodies have declined. Arabian foals with this disease often die from opportunistic infection resulting from an absence or deficiency of immunoglobulins. Combined immunodeficiency occurs in approximately 2%–3% of Arabian foals. The foals fail to produce functional T or B cells. They may receive maternal immunoglobulins as they suckle successfully, but when the maternal immunoglobulins have been used, the foal cannot produce its own antibodies. All foals stricken usually die within 4–6 months as a result of infection. Hendrix C, Sirois M, Laboratory Procedures for Veterinary Technicians, ed 5, Mosby Elsevier, 2007, p. 269.

318. d Vaccination schedules are based on the age of the animal, anticipated exposure to infectious organisms, and the duration of immunity provided by the vaccine. Allergies, immunodeficiencies, and autoimmune disease are considered abnormal reactions of the immune system. Allergies are a hypersensitivity reaction, immunodeficiency is a lack of immune response, and protection and autoimmune disease is the immune system attacking itself. Bassert J, Thomas J, McCurnin's Clinical Textbook for Veterinary Technicians, ed 8, Elsevier Saunders, 2014, p. 276.

319. a Lymphocytes are central to the adaptive immune system and the defense of the body. There are three major types of lymphocyte. These are natural killer (NK) cells that play a role in innate immunity; T cells that regulate adaptive immunity and are responsible for cell-mediated immune responses; and B cells that are responsible for antibody production. The function of a neutrophil is to destroy and remove foreign substances. Monocytes are a type of white blood cell that fights off bacteria, viruses, and fungi. Monocytes are the biggest type of white blood cell in the immune system. Bassert J, Thomas J, McCurnin's Clinical Textbook for Veterinary Technicians, ed 8, Elsevier Saunders, 2014, p. 127.

320. c Memory B cells function as lymphocytes and therefore initiate a secondary immune response. Memory B cells are produced during the initial exposure and remain to produce antibodies more quickly in case there is a second exposure to the antigen. Thymocytes are present in the thymus and their main function is the production of T cells, which do not initiate a secondary immune response. Monocytes and neutrophils are a type of white blood cell that fights off bacteria, viruses, and fungi, and does not initiate a secondary immune response. Tizard I, Veterinary Immunology, ed 9, Elsevier Saunders, 2013, p. 10.

321. c Serology is the detection of antibody–antigen reactions. Endoparasites and ectoparasites are under the parasitology branch of science. The study of viruses or prions is called microbiology, whereas the study of fungi is called mycology. Studdert VP, Gay CC, Blood DC, Saunders Comprehensive Veterinary Dictionary, ed 4, Elsevier Saunders, 2007, p. 1004.

322. b Serological tests were used to identify the presence of viruses within tissues. The tests commonly used for this purpose included fluorescent antibody tests, enzyme-linked immunosorbent assay (ELISA), hemagglutination inhibition, virus neutralization, complement fixation, and gel precipitation. Tizard I, Veterinary Immunology, ed 9, Elsevier Saunders, 2013, p. 310.

323. b To perform this assay, microwells in polystyrene plates are first filled with an antigen solution. Proteins bind firmly to polystyrene surfaces, so that after unbound antigen is removed by vigorous washing, the wells remain coated with a layer of antigen. These coated plates can be stored until required. The serum under test is added to the wells. Any antibodies in the serum will bind to the antigen layer. After incubation and washing to remove unbound antibody, the presence of any bound antibodies can be detected by adding a solution containing an antiglobulin chemically linked to an enzyme. Complete washing of test wells used in ELISA is the critical step to ensure accurate results. Follow the manufacturer's instructions explicitly regarding washing procedures. Tizard I, Veterinary Immunology, ed 9, Elsevier Saunders, 2013, p. 498.

324. a A positive direct Coombs test provides evidence of immune-mediated hemolytic disease. Coombs tests are used to detect certain antigen–antibody reactions, one of which is used for the diagnosis of autoimmune hemolytic anemia. The Coggins test is a gel diffusion method used to detect antibodies against equine infectious anemia virus in horse serum. The latex agglutination test can be used for diagnosis and monitoring of *Cryptococcus* therapy. Intradermal skin testing using very dilute aqueous solutions of allergens has been widely used for the diagnosis of allergies, especially canine atopic dermatitis. Hendrix C, Sirois M, Laboratory Procedures for Veterinary Technicians, ed 5, Mosby Elsevier, 2007, p. 279.

325. d The adult *Ctenocephalides felis* (the cat flea) has piercing/sucking (siphon-like) mouth parts that are used to suck the blood of their host. *Macracanthorhynchus hirudinaceus* is the thorny-head worm of the small intestine of swine. Thorny head describes the spiny proboscis, which it embeds as an anchor into the small intestinal mucosa of the host. The unsheathed microfilariae of *Onchocerca cervicalis* have been incriminated as causing periodic ophthalmia and blindness in horses. These may be detected by ophthalmic examination. *Metastrongylus apri*, the swine lungworm, is found within the bronchi and bronchioles of pigs. Of the options listed, only *Ctenocephalides felis* is blood sucking. Hendrix C, Sirois M, Laboratory Procedures for Veterinary Technicians, ed 5, Mosby Elsevier, 2007, p. 246.

326. a *Trichinella spiralis* occurs in the small intestine of many hosts, most notably the pig. Swine become infected with *T. spiralis* when they ingest infective larval stages (juveniles) in undercooked meat. The larvae mature into adults in the host's small intestine in a few weeks and the female worms give birth to larvae. The males die after fertilizing the females and the females die after producing larvae. The larvae enter the bloodstream of the host and eventually end up in the pig's musculature. *Oesophagostomum* species are found in bovine stomachs. The *Eimeria* in pigs are considered to be fairly inconsequential as parasites in most instances; however, there have been cases both in natural infections and following experimental inoculation in which pigs have developed diarrhea as a result of *Eimeria* infections. *Fasciola hepatica* is the adult liver fluke. Hendrix C, Sirois M, Internal Parasites, Laboratory Procedures for Veterinary Technicians, ed 5, Mosby Elsevier, 2007, p. 256.

327. d Intraperitoneal injections are not used for vaccines because they would not be effective and can be dangerous. Vaccination by subcutaneous or intramuscular injection is the simplest and most common method of vaccine administration. Intranasal vaccines are available for infectious bovine rhinotracheitis of cattle; for *Streptococcus equi* infections in horses; for feline rhinotracheitis, *Bordetella bronchiseptica*, coronavirus, and calicivirus infections; for canine parainfluenza and *Bordetella* infection; and for infectious bronchitis and Newcastle disease in poultry. Tizard I, Veterinary Immunology, ed 9, Elsevier Saunders, 2013, p. 274.

328. b In a healthy animal, anesthesia will not affect the efficacy of the vaccine. The most common reason for vaccine failure is improper administration. Occasionally a vaccine may actually be ineffective. The method of production may have destroyed the protective epitopes or there may simply be insufficient antigen in the vaccine. Problems of this type are uncommon and can generally be avoided by using only vaccines from reputable manufacturers. In addition, an animal may simply fail to mount an immune response. Tizard I, Veterinary Immunology, ed 9, Elsevier Saunders, 2013, p. 277.

329. b *Paranoplocephala mamillana* is the Dwarf tapeworm. *Strongyloides westeri* is often referred to as the intestinal threadworm of horses. *Parascaris equorum* is often called the equine ascarid or equine roundworm. *Oxyuris equi* is the pinworm of horses. Hendrix C, Sirois M, Internal Parasites, Laboratory Procedures for Veterinary Technicians, ed 5, Mosby Elsevier, 2007.

330. a The coccidian *Cryptosporidium muris* is found in the stomach. *Bunostomum phlebotomum* is the hookworm of ruminants, and it produces trichostrongyle-type eggs. *Moniezia benedeni* are grain mites and *Haemonchus contortus* is known as barber's pole or wire worm. Sirois M, Laboratory Animal Medicine: Principles and Procedures, Elsevier Mosby, 2005.

331. b Pemphigus is classified as an autoimmune skin disease that attacks the skin and mucosa. Other autoimmune diseases may affect the blood and lymph systems, eyes, hooves, and claws, but they would not be classified as pemphigus. Tizard I, Veterinary Immunology, ed 9, Elsevier Saunders, 2013, p. 415.

332. c Patients with a low platelet count, known as thrombocytopenia, experience bleeding when adequate numbers of platelets are not available to form a platelet plug. With a lack of platelets, petechiae, ecchymoses, and anemia would be expected. Thrombocytosis is an elevated number of platelets, which would not be seen in ITP. Battaglia A, Small Animal Emergency and Critical Care for Veterinary Technicians, ed 2, Saunders, 2007, p. 221.

333. c The sequence of maturation for RBCs is rubriblast, prorubricyte, rubricyte, metarubricyte, reticulocyte, and mature RBC. Hendrix C, Sirois M, Laboratory Procedures for Veterinary Technicians, ed 5, Mosby Elsevier, 2007, p. 65.

334. a Histological results of spleen biopsies show both extramedullary hematopoiesis and areas of infarct and necrosis. One of the jobs of the spleen is blood storage. The kidneys filter blood but would not be associated with extramedullary hematopoiesis. Bone cortex helps facilitate the bones' main functions of supporting the whole body, protecting organs, providing levers for movement, and storing and releasing chemical elements (mainly calcium). The umbilicus is where the umbilical cord attaches to the fetus during pregnancy. Colville J, Oien S, Clinical Veterinary Language, Mosby Elsevier, 2014.

335. c *Baylisascaris procyonis* produces a condition called neurologic larva migrans, in which the larval stage of this ascarid migrates through neural tissues (e.g., brain and spinal cord). *Baylisascaris procyonis* is not associated with pneumonia, hemolytic anemia, or bloody diarrhea. Bassert J, Thomas J, McCurnin's Clinical Textbook for Veterinary Technicians, ed 8, Elsevier Saunders, 2014, p. 455.

336. a Hemagglutination is the aggregation of separate particles into clumps or masses; especially the clumping of bacteria, blood cells, or latex beads by antibodies specific to, or directed against, surface antigenic determinants. Lysing, crenation and swelling, and agglutination can be seen in the erythrocytes with a lot of the same disease, but each one is distinctly different. Lysing is the destruction of cells, crenation is the malformation of cells, and swelling is the condition of being swollen. Studdert VP, Gay CC, Blood DC, Saunders Comprehensive Veterinary Dictionary, ed 4, Elsevier Saunders, 2007, p. 27.

337. b The Coggins test is used to diagnose EIA. The indirect fluorescent antibody tests are for specific antibodies in a sample and these tests are commonly used to verify a tentative diagnosis. The direct Coombs test looks for antibodies bound to the surface of red blood cells and this test is associated with autoimmune diseases. A hemoglobin electrophoresis test checks the different types of hemoglobin in the blood. Hemoglobin is the substance in red blood cells that carries oxygen. Tighe MM, Brown M, Mosby's Comprehensive Review for Veterinary Technicians, ed 4, Mosby Elsevier, 2015, p. 464.

338. b Hypochromasia is defined as lacking the typical color of the erythrocyte for the species. These erythrocytes also have an increased central pallor. Polychromasia is a varying degree of bluish staining of the erythrocyte cytoplasm. These cells are usually also macrocytic. Basophilia is blue cytoplasm, usually with vacuoles. Hyperchromasia appears as an increase in color intensity. Tighe MM, Brown M, Mosby's Comprehensive Review for Veterinary Technicians, ed 4, Mosby Elsevier, 2015, p. 43.

339. c The presence of three to five nuclear lobes is characteristic of mammalian neutrophils. Band neutrophils are immature neutrophils with a horseshoe- or S-shaped nucleus. Normally the number of segments in the nucleus of a neutrophil increases as it matures and ages, after being released into the blood from the bone marrow. Whereas normal neutrophils only contain three or four nuclear lobes (the segments), hypersegmented neutrophils contain six or more lobes. Hendrix C, Sirois M, Laboratory Procedures for Veterinary Technicians, ed 5, Mosby Elsevier, 2007, p. 45.

340. b Sensitized cells release histamine through allergic or inflammatory mechanisms. Histamine combines with H1 receptors on smooth muscle fibers to cause bronchoconstriction. Histamine also increases the inflammatory response in the airways. Antihistamines are frequently provided to combat histamine release. Toxins build up in the blood in the event of severe disease or poisoning, but they are not a response to allergens. Lysin is an antibody or other substance able to cause lysis of cells and it is not released in the presence of an allergic response. Hendrix C, Sirois M, Laboratory Procedures for Veterinary Technicians, ed 5, Mosby Elsevier, 2007, p. 107.

341. a Gram-positive bacteria stain dark blue to purple, whereas Gram-negative bacteria stain red. Orange and lavender are not colors associated with a Gram stain. Hendrix C, Sirois M, Laboratory Procedures for Veterinary Technicians, ed 5, Mosby Elsevier, 2007, p. 229.

342. d In addition to the Gram stain, another commonly used stain is the acid-fast stain, which is used to identify organisms such as *Mycobacterium* spp., which have significant amounts of mycolic acid content in the cell wall. A modified acid fast is used to identify coccidia. Gram staining can be used to identify yeast. DTM and/or Sabouraud agar are commonly used to identify fungi. A Woods lamp may prove helpful and cellophane tape may also be used to collect certain types of samples for fungal analysis. Bassert J, Thomas J, McCurnin's Clinical Textbook for Veterinary Technicians, ed 8, Elsevier Saunders, 2014, p. 490.

343. a Immediate (type I) hypersensitivity reaction is the most common serious adverse event following vaccination in dogs. This reaction is mediated by immunoglobulin E (IgE), the principal cellular component is the mast cell or basophil, and the reaction is amplified or modified by eosinophils, neutrophils, and platelets. A type I hypersensitivity reaction triggers the release of histamine. Mast cells and basophils normally produce a small quantity of histamine, but when IgE sensitizes them, they react abnormally, producing large quantities of histamines and other chemicals. These chemicals cause allergic attacks (such as runny noses and swollen tissues). Bonagura J, Twedt D, Kirk's Current Veterinary Therapy, XV, Elsevier Saunders, 2014, p. 1250.

344. b T killer cells function to recognize cancer cells as abnormal cells and eliminate them. Mast cells and basophils are associated with releasing histamine. The antibody isotype IgG is the most common antibody and is found in the highest concentration in the blood. It helps defend tissues by coating the outer surface of pathogens, a process called opsonization, which allows them to be more easily phagocytized by macrophages. Endorphins are released from the body by chemical stimulation (opioids), exercise, or stress, and are not a function of T killer cells. Colville TP, Bassert JM, Clinical Anatomy and Physiology for Veterinary Technicians, ed 2, Mosby Elsevier, 2008, p. 238.

345. d Cats infected with FeLV can harbor the virus for long periods without clinical consequence. Battaglia A, Small Animal Emergency and Critical Care for Veterinary Technicians, ed 2, Saunders, 2007, p. 171.

346. c Acid-fast organisms stain bright pink to red. For non–acid-fast organisms, the background should stain green. Yellow, blue, and brown are not seen with acid-fast staining. Bassert J, Thomas J, McCurnin's Clinical Textbook for Veterinary Technicians, ed 8, Elsevier Saunders, 2014, p. 492.

347. b Because FIV is found in saliva, bite wounds serve as a means of transmission. FIV transmission in households with a stable social cat environment is rare, because FIV is transmitted mainly through biting and fighting; if no fights occur, FIV is not likely to be transmitted. Bonagura J, Twedt D, Kirk's Current Veterinary Therapy XV, Elsevier Saunders, 2014, p. 1276.

348. c Titer is a measure of antibody units per unit volume of serum. Titer testing is performed immediately after infection (acute phase) and 2 to 6 weeks after collection of the first serum sample (convalescent phase). IgG and IgM titers are typically reported individually. A titer >1:256 for IgM is consistent with active infection in patients with clinical signs (e.g., pneumonia in cats, myositis in dogs). It is recommended that two samples for IgG titer be submitted; samples should be collected 2 to 3 weeks apart. A fourfold or greater rise in titer within 2 to 3 weeks is supportive of the diagnosis of active infection. Ford R, Mazzaferro E, Kirk and Bistner's Handbook of Veterinary Procedures and Emergency Treatments, ed 9, Saunders, 2012, p. 632.

349. d Viruses are very small organisms that can only grow inside living cells. They are thus obligate intracellular parasites. Algae, fungi, and bacteria are free-living organisms and they do not depend on host cells to reproduce. Tizard I, Veterinary Immunology, ed 9, Elsevier Saunders, 2013, p. 87.

350. d The genus name is capitalized and both genus and species names are italicized in print or are underlined. Bowman DD, Georgis Parasitology for Veterinarians, ed 10, Elsevier Saunders, 2014, p. 1.

351. d *Mycobacterium* is diagnosed by acid-fast staining. Animals infected with *Mycobacterium tuberculosis, M. bovis*, and *M. avium* bacteria develop characteristic delayed hypersensitivity reactions when exposed to purified derivatives of the organism called tuberculin. Anaplasmosis, colibacillosis, and ringworm are not of the *Mycobacterium* sp. Sirois M, Principles and Practice of Veterinary Technology, ed 3, Mosby Elsevier, 2011, p. 175.

352. b Gram-negative organisms do not retain crystal violet, but they counterstain with safranin and appear pink. Gram-positive organisms retain crystal violet stain and appear purple. Stain procedures, such as acid-fast staining, are required to determine the identity of organisms such as *Mycobacterium* spp. and *Nocardia* spp. Non–acid-fast organisms and the background should stain green. If staining is used, then clear is not an option. Bassert J, Thomas J, McCurnin's Clinical Textbook for Veterinary Technicians, ed 8, Elsevier Saunders, 2014, p. 491.

353. c Viruses are very small organisms that can only grow inside living cells. They are thus obligate, non–free-living, intracellular parasites. Tizard I, Veterinary Immunology, ed 9, Elsevier Saunders, 2013, p. 86.

354. c The catalase test is performed on gram-positive cocci and small gram-positive bacilli. It tests for the enzyme catalase, which acts on hydrogen peroxide to produce water and oxygen. A small amount of a colony from a blood agar plate is placed on a microscope slide and a drop of catalase reagent (3% hydrogen peroxide) is added. If the colony is catalase positive, gas bubbles are produced. No bubble production indicates a negative result. Hendrix C, Sirois M, Laboratory Procedures for Veterinary Technicians, ed 5, Mosby Elsevier, 2007, p. 137.

355. b A nosocomial infection is an infection that was not present previously and develops during the course of medical care. An infection that is caused by medical personnel is called iatrogenic. An infection that is acquired during surgery is classed under nosocomial because it would occur during hospitalization and it is not limited just to surgery. Tighe MM, Brown M, Mosby's Comprehensive Review for Veterinary Technicians, ed 4, Mosby Elsevier, 2015, p. 314.

356. b As a general rule, Gram-negative bacteria contain endotoxins (substances that cause disease) in their cell walls, whereas Gram-positive bacteria contain preformed exotoxins, which they secrete into the surrounding medium. Viruses are extremely small infectious agents, ranging from 30 to 450 nm in diameter, which can cause disease in a wide variety of animals. Fungi are heterotrophs and are parasitic or saprophytic. Most are multicellular, except yeasts. They contain eukaryotic cells with cell walls composed of chitin. Fungal organisms consist largely of webs of slender tubes called hyphae. Sirois M, Principles and Practice of Veterinary Technology, ed 3, Mosby Elsevier, 2011, p. 280.

357. d Mannitol salt agar is not routinely used but is a highly selective medium for staphylococci and could be used to isolate *Staphylococcus aureus* from contaminated specimens. The medium has a high salt content (7.5%), and the pH indicator phenol red. Staphylococci are salt tolerant. *Streptococcus pyogenes, Bacillus subtilis*, and *Clostridium perfringens* are not salt tolerant and do not have the same reactions as a result. Hendrix C, Sirois M, Laboratory Procedures for Veterinary Technicians, ed 5, Mosby Elsevier, 2007, p. 125.

358. a The common wart is composed of epithelial and connective tissue and is caused by species-specific papillomaviruses. Variola (also known as smallpox) is a viral disease of humans and primates characterized by fever, rash, and scab formation. Feline herpes is associated with respiratory disease, whereas other forms of herpes produce genital warts, fevers, and rash. Studdert VP, Gay CC, Blood DC, Saunders Comprehensive Veterinary Dictionary, ed 4, Elsevier Saunders, 2007, p. 433.

359. c Hairs infected with some species of *Microsporum* may fluoresce a clear apple-green under the Woods lamp in a darkened room. Approximately 60% of positive cases involving *Microsporum canis* fluoresce, depending on whether the fungus has reached the right growth stage to produce fluorescence. *Microsporum gypseum, trichophyton mentagrophytes*, and *Epidermophyton floccosum* do not fluoresce under ultraviolet light. Hendrix C, Sirois M, Laboratory Procedures for Veterinary Technicians, ed 5, Mosby Elsevier, 2007, p. 145.

360. b *Moraxella bovis* is a Gram-negative diplococcus that causes pinkeye in cattle. *Haemophilus aegyptius* has six subspecies, which are known to cause pinkeye and flu-like symptoms in humans. *Streptococcus* spp. are opportunistic pathogens that normally reside in the upper respiratory, intestinal, lower urinary, and genital tracts, but they can cause localized infection or septicemia in dogs of all ages. *S. aureus* is dangerous because of its deleterious effects on animal health and its potential for transmission from animals to humans and vice versa. It thus has a huge impact on animal health and welfare and causes major economic losses in livestock production. Tighe MM, Brown M, Mosby's Comprehensive Review for Veterinary Technicians, ed 4, Mosby Elsevier, 2015, p. 128.

361. b Alpha is incomplete hemolysis, beta is complete hemolysis, and gamma is no hemolysis. Delta is not a classification. Sirois M, Principles and Practice of Veterinary Technology, ed 3, Mosby Elsevier, 2011, p. 184.

362. d Fleas (*Ctenocephalides felis*) are the most important vector of *D. caninum*, a common cestode of dogs and cats. The trematodes (flukes) are flatworms that, like cestodes, lack a body cavity. A nematode is a worm of the large phylum *Nematoda*, such as a roundworm or threadworm. An arthropod is an invertebrate animal of the large phylum *Arthropoda*, such as an insect, spider, or crustacean. Bowman DD, Georgis Parasitology for Veterinarians, ed 10, Elsevier Saunders, 2014, p. 259.

363. c Examples of digenetic trematodes of domestic animals are *Fasciola hepatica*. Trematodes refer to the class *Trematoda*, the flukes. A nematode is a worm of the large phylum *Nematoda*, such as a roundworm or a threadworm. Cestodes are multicellular organisms that lack a body cavity. Their organs are embedded in loose cellular tissue. Protozoa are single-celled organisms with one or more membrane-bound nuclei containing DNA and specialized cytoplasmic organelles; one example is *Giardia*. Sirois M, Principles and Practice of Veterinary Technology, ed 3, Mosby Elsevier, 2011, p. 218.

364. b *Dirofilaria immitis* is also referred to as the canine heartworm. The prepatent period in dogs is approximately 6 months and it takes 6–7 months for the heartworm to mature and to produce microfilariae. Hendrix C, Sirois M, Laboratory Procedures for Veterinary Technicians, ed 5, Mosby Elsevier, 2007, p. 196.

365. b The antigens are only released by female heartworms; therefore, the test can only detect the adult females. The tests can be used to identify an occult heartworm infection, that is, when microfilariae are not found to be circulating in the peripheral blood. ELISA antigen tests have been of somewhat limited use in cats because of their inability to detect all-male, immature, and low worm burden mature female infections (zero to one). Hendrix C, Sirois M, Laboratory Procedures for Veterinary Technicians, ed 5, Mosby Elsevier, 2007, p. 229; Bonagura J, Twedt D, Kirk's Current Veterinary Therapy, XV, Elsevier Saunders, 2014, p. 827.

366. c Nematodes are colloquially referred to as roundworms because of a unique feature—they are round when observed on cross-section. Some common species of canine nematodes are *Toxocara canis, Ancylostoma caninum, Trichuris vulpis*, and *Dirofilaria immitis*. Fleas (*Ctenocephalides felis*) are the most important vector of *D. caninum*, a common cestode in dogs and cats. An arthropod is an invertebrate animal of the large phylum *Arthropoda*, such as an insect, spider, or crustacean. The trematodes (flukes) are flatworms that, like cestodes, lack a body cavity. Bassert J, Thomas J, McCurnin's Clinical Textbook for Veterinary Technicians, ed 8, Elsevier Saunders, 2014, p. 452.

367. b *Otodectes cynotis* (ear mite) is an arthropod. The trematodes (flukes) are flatworms that, like cestodes, lack a body cavity. The cestodes are fleas and nematodes are colloquially referred to as roundworms. Bowman DD, Georgis Parasitology for Veterinarians, ed 10, Elsevier Saunders, 2014, p. 267.

368. d Dogs and cats become infected with *Dipylidium caninum* by ingesting intermediate or paratenic hosts such as fleas, lice, rodents, and ruminants containing larval cestodes. The infective stage of *Dipylidium caninum* is found in fleas. Rabbits are hosts for *Taenia pisiformis*, another tapeworm of dogs and cats. Hookworms and roundworms can be transmitted through feces and saliva. Bonagura J, Twedt D, Kirk's Current Veterinary Therapy, XV, Elsevier Saunders, 2014, p. 1247.

369. d *Taenia pisiformis* is commonly found in hunting dogs because the intermediate host is usually a rabbit. Flies can be the intermediate host for *Stephanofilaria stilesi* and *Habronema muscae*. Fleas are intermediate hosts for *Dipylidium caninum*. *Taenia hydatigena* and *Taenia ovis* involve ruminant intermediate hosts. Bassert J, Thomas J, McCurnin's Clinical Textbook for Veterinary Technicians, ed 8, Elsevier Saunders, 2014, p. 448.

370. b *Trichuris ovis* is commonly called the whipworm, infecting the cecum and colon of ruminants. It has a thick, yellow-brown, symmetric shell with plugs at both ends. *Strongyloides stercoralis* (threadworm) are seen in the male and female species and both genders possess a tiny buccal capsule and cylindrical esophagus without a posterior bulb. In the free-living stage, the esophagi of both sexes are rhabditiform. Males can be distinguished from females by two structures: the spicules and gubernaculum. Examples of roundworms are *Toxocara canis* and *Toxascaris leonine*. The adult *T. canis* has a round body with spiky cranial and caudal parts, covered by yellow cuticula. Hendrix C, Sirois M, Laboratory Procedures for Veterinary Technicians, ed 5, Mosby Elsevier, 2007, p. 202.

371. d Plague caused by *Yersinia pestis* is transmitted between animals and to humans via fleas; infection with *Y. pestis* is rare in North America, but a natural focus of transmission is maintained in a cycle involving fleas and prairie dogs in the western United States. Beavers are a reservoir for the plague organism but they are not prevalent in the western United States, which is where the plague is most prevalent. Dogs and cats cannot be reservoirs for the plague. They can have fleas that are part of the life cycle, but they themselves are not a reservoir. Bowman DD, Georgis Parasitology for Veterinarians, ed 10, Elsevier Saunders, 2014, p. 254.

372. d *Bordetella bronchiseptica* is a bacterial infection that is most commonly associated with infectious tracheobronchitis (kennel cough) in dogs. Fowl cholera is caused by *Pasteurella multocida*. *Staphylococcus aureus* is the leading cause of skin and soft tissue infections such as abscesses (boils), furuncles, and cellulitis. *Corynebacterium diphtheriae* is associated with diphtheria. Bassert J, Thomas J, McCurnin's Clinical Textbook for Veterinary Technicians, ed 8, Elsevier Saunders, 2014, p. 271.

373. d Leptospirosis is caused by the bacterium *Leptospira*, which is a spirochete. Common serovars are *Leptospira pomona*, *Leptospira hardjo*, and *Leptospira grippotyphosa*. *Corynebacterium pyogenes* is a Gram-positive, irregularly shaped rod. *Streptococcus pyogenes* are Gram-positive cocci. *Mycobacterium tuberculosis* is a rod-shaped bacterium. Holtgrew-Bohling K, Large Animal Clinical Procedures for Veterinary Technicians, ed 2, Elsevier Saunders, 2012, p. 386.

374. b *Streptococcus equi* is the organism that causes equine strangles. *Staphylococcus aureus* is the leading cause of skin and soft tissue infections such as abscesses (boils), furuncles, and cellulitis. *Corynebacterium equi* are Gram-positive rods of varying lengths, which cause corynebacterial pneumonia and abscesses in foals. Severe infections with *Strongylus vulgaris* can cause colic, gangrenous enteritis, torsion or rupture of the intestines, and death. Tighe MM, Brown M, Mosby's Comprehensive Review for Veterinary Technicians, ed 4, Mosby Elsevier, 2015, p. 563.

375. d Pathogenic mycobacteria have evolved to survive within host macrophages. *Mycobacterium* is not a spore former and antibiotics do not kill it easily. It is aerobic, not anaerobic. Tizard I, Veterinary Immunology, ed 9, Elsevier Saunders, 2013, p. 292.

376. d Gram stain procedure requires a primary stain, a mordant, a decolorizer, and a counterstain, and is therefore not considered a simple stain. Gram staining is used to categorize bacteria as gram positive or gram negative based on cell-wall structure. The Gram stain is a differential stain, whereas safranin is a counter stain. Simple stains, such as crystal violet or methylene blue, are typically used for yeasts. Hendrix C, Sirois M, Laboratory Procedures for Veterinary Technicians, ed 5, Mosby Elsevier, 2007, p. 253.

377. a Active immunity occurs in the body when the immune system develops antibodies to antigens such as viruses, yeast, or bacteria. The animal can be exposed to the antigen via natural exposure from the environment or by injection with a noninfectious form of the antigen in a vaccine. Antitoxin administration, ingestion of colostrum, and the administration of gamma globulin are examples of acquired passive immunity. Bassert J, Thomas J, McCurnin's Clinical Textbook for Veterinary Technicians, ed 8, Elsevier Saunders, 2014, p. 262.

378. b *Escherichia coli* organisms are among the normal flora of the intestines. Species that are typically found in a dog's small intestine primarily include streptococci, lactobacilli, and *Bifidobacterium* spp. Several species of anaerobic bacteria are found in the duodenum and jejunum, whereas *Escherichia coli* is present in the ileum. Bassert J, Thomas J, McCurnin's Clinical Textbook for Veterinary Technicians, ed 8, Elsevier Saunders, 2014, p. 263.

379. c Pediculosis is an infestation by lice. There are not specific alternative names for tick, flea, and mite infestations. Tighe MM, Brown M, Mosby's Comprehensive Review for Veterinary Technicians, ed 4, Mosby Elsevier, 2015, p. 676.

380. d Adult *Toxocara canis* and *Toxocara cati* are found in the small intestine of dogs and cats. When humans act as paratenic hosts, the conditions that result from this infection are known as visceral larva migrans (VLM). Visceral larva migrans is caused by ingestion of *Toxocara* eggs that hatch and develop into larvae that migrate through the abdominal viscera; creeping eruption is caused by skin penetration by *Ancylostoma* larvae; the sarcoptic mange mite causes scabies; hydatidosis is infection with the hydatid cyst of *Echinococcus*. Bassert J, Thomas J, McCurnin's Clinical Textbook for Veterinary Technicians, ed 8, Elsevier Saunders, 2014, p. 452.

381. a *Balantidium* species are found commonly in the feces of swine, but they are not considered pathogenic. *Giardia* and *Trichomonas* are flagellates. *Histomonas* species is a protozoan, but it is not found in swine feces. Tighe MM, Brown M, Mosby's Comprehensive Review for Veterinary Technicians, ed 4, Mosby Elsevier, 2015, p. 62.

382. a *Tritrichomonas foetus* is a flagellated protozoan parasite of the reproductive tract of cattle, which causes early-term abortions and repeat breeding. The organism can be found in fluid from the abomasum of aborted fetuses, uterine discharges, and vaginal and preputial washes. *Dioctophyma* species is the giant kidney worm and it is diagnosed through the patient's urine. It is difficult to obtain a definitive diagnosis for *Anaplasma*; basic blood work and a detailed history will help provide clues that the doctor can use to make decisions on treatment. *Anaplasma* is a genus of *Rickettsiales* bacteria. Hendrix C, Sirois M, Laboratory Procedures for Veterinary Technicians, ed 5, Mosby Elsevier, 2007, p. 354; Tighe MM, Brown M, Mosby's Comprehensive Review for Veterinary Technicians, ed 4, Mosby Elsevier, 2015.

383. b Respiratory roundworms include the lungworms of cattle and sheep (*Dictyocaulus* species and *Muellerius capillaris*). Diagnosis is made by finding the larvae on standard fecal flotation or flotation of the sputum–mucus discharge. *Dioctophyma* species is the giant kidney worm and is diagnosed by urine sediment exam. *Anaplasma* is a genus of *Rickettsiales* bacteria and is difficult to diagnose, but basic blood work provides clues to the clinician. *Tritrichomonas* is a genus of single-celled flagellated protozoan parasites, some of whose species are known to be pathogens of the bovine reproductive tract as well as the intestinal tract of felines; it is diagnosed by vaginal washing. Bowman DD, Georgis Parasitology for Veterinarians, ed 10, Elsevier Saunders, 2014.

384. c *Dioctophyma renale* is the giant kidney worm and it inhabits the walls of portions of the urinary system of both dogs and cats. The primary method of examining for parasites is by microscopic examination of the urine sediment. If a parasite egg is observed at low magnification, higher-power objective lenses may be used to examine it more closely. *Tritrichomonas foetus* is a flagellated protozoan parasite of the reproductive tract of cattle, which causes early-term abortions and repeat breeding. The organism can be found in fluid from the abomasum of aborted fetuses, uterine discharges, and vaginal and preputial washes. Respiratory roundworms include the lungworms of cattle and sheep (*Dictyocaulus* species and *Muellerius capillaris*). Diagnosis is made by finding the larvae on standard fecal flotation or flotation of the sputum–mucus discharge. *Anaplasma* is a genus of *Rickettsiales* bacteria and is difficult to diagnose, but basic blood work supplies clues for the clinician. Hendrix C, Robinson E, Diagnostic Parasitology for Veterinary Technicians, ed 4, Elsevier, 2012, p. 336.

385. d *Anaplasma* is diagnosed by examining blood sample. The disease may result in neutropenia, thrombocytopenia, and anemia. Chronically affected animals may be severely anemic, with marked leukopenia and thrombocytopenia, but sometimes the only hematologic abnormality is lymphocytosis. The total plasma protein level is usually increased. The organisms are best demonstrated during the acute phase but usually are present in small numbers. Blood films made from the buffy coat may aid in diagnosis. However, in most cases organisms are not seen and immunologic testing makes the diagnosis. *Tritrichomonas* species is diagnosed by vaginal washing. *Dictyocaulus* species diagnosis is made by finding the larvae on standard fecal flotation or flotation of the sputum-mucus discharge. *Dioctophyma* species is diagnosed by urine exam. Hendrix C, Sirois M, Laboratory Procedures for Veterinary Technicians, ed 5, Mosby Elsevier, 2007, p. 59.

386. a *Rhipicephalus sanguineus* is known as the brown dog tick. *Ixodes dammini* is known as the deer tick. *Dermacentor variabilis* is known as the American dog tick or wood tick. *Dermacentor albipictus* is known as the winter tick. Tighe MM, Brown M, Mosby's Comprehensive Review for Veterinary Technicians, ed 4, Mosby Elsevier, 2015, p. 78.

387. d *Dermacentor albipictus* is known as the winter tick. *Rhipicephalus sanguineus* is known as the brown dog tick. *Ixodes dammini* is known as the deer tick. *Dermacentor variabilis* is known as the American dog tick or the wood tick. Bowman DD, Georgis Parasitology for Veterinarians, ed 10, Elsevier Saunders, 2014, p. 61.

388. c *Dermacentor variabilis* is the American dog tick. *Rhipicephalus sanguineus* is known as the brown dog tick. *Ixodes dammini* is known as the deer tick. *Dermacentor albipictus* is the winter tick. Bassert J, Thomas J, McCurnin's Clinical Textbook for Veterinary Technicians, ed 8, Elsevier Saunders, 2014, p. 466.

389. b *Ixodes dammini* is the deer tick. *Rhipicephalus sanguineus* is known as the brown dog tick. *Dermacentor albipictus* is the winter tick. *Dermacentor variabilis* is the American dog tick. Summers A, Common Diseases of Companion Animals, ed 2, Mosby Elsevier, p. 246.

390. d *Otodectes cynotis* lives in the external ear canal of dogs and cats. *Sarcoptes* burrow into the skin. *Chorioptes* live on the skin's surface. *Demodex* live in the hair follicles. Sirois M, Principles and Practice of Veterinary Technology, ed 3, Mosby Elsevier, 2011, p. 235.

391. c *Chorioptes* species reside on the surface of the skin. *Demodex* live in the hair follicles. *Sarcoptes* burrow into the skin. *Otodectes cynotis* lives in the external ear canal of dogs and cats. Hendrix C, Robinson E, Diagnostic Parasitology for Veterinary Technicians, ed 4, Elsevier, 2012, p. 232.

392. a Sarcoptic mites burrow or tunnel within the epidermis of the infested definitive host. The *Otodectes cynotis* lives in the external ear canal of dogs and cats. *Demodex* live in the hair follicles. *Chorioptes* species reside on the surface of the skin. Hendrix C, Sirois M, Laboratory Procedures for Veterinary Technicians, ed 5, Mosby Elsevier, 2007, p. 248.

393. b *Demodex* species live in hair follicles. *Sarcoptes* burrow into the skin. *Chorioptes* live on the skin's surface. The *Otodectes cynotis* lives in the external ear canal of dogs and cats. Hendrix C, Sirois M, Laboratory Procedures for Veterinary Technicians, ed 5, Mosby Elsevier, 2007, p. 232.

394. a *Boophilus annulatus* is considered a single host tick, whereas *Otobius megnini*, *Ixodid* sp., and *Argasidae* are multi host ticks. Bassert J, Thomas J, McCurnin's Clinical Textbook for Veterinary Technicians, ed 8, Elsevier Saunders, 2014, p. 466.

395. a *Cheyletiella* spp. are highly contagious mites affecting dogs (*Cheyletiella yasguri*), cats (*Cheyletiella blakei*), and rabbits (*Cheyletiella parasitovorax*). *Cheyletiella* mites do not use birds or rodents as hosts. Bonagura J, Twedt D, Kirk's Current Veterinary Therapy, XV, Elsevier Saunders, 2014, p. 431.

396. d *Strongyloides stercoralis* larvae go through a free-living stage in the environment before becoming infective third-stage larvae that can penetrate the skin and cause migratory damage in the host. *Trichuris vulpis* is whipworm that lives in the large intestine of canines in its adult stages. *Taenia pisiformis*, commonly called the rabbit tapeworm, is an endoparasite that causes infection in lagomorphs, rodents, and carnivores. *Dipylidium caninum*, also called the flea tapeworm, double-pore tapeworm, or cucumber tapeworm, is a cyclophyllid cestode that infects organisms afflicted with fleas and canine chewing lice. Hendrix C, Robinson E, Diagnostic Parasitology for Veterinary Technicians, ed 4, Elsevier, 2012, p. 35.

397. a *Echinococcus granulosus* produces larvae that form hydatid cysts in the intermediate hosts, such as humans. *Anoplocephala magna*, *Taenia pisiformis*, and *Moniezia benedeni* do not use humans as an intermediate host. Hendrix C, Robinson E, Diagnostic Parasitology for Veterinary Technicians, ed 4, Elsevier, 2012, p. 288.

398. d The eggs of *Moniezia benedeni* for the most part seem to have fairly thin shells that distort in various flotation media (and also clear to some extent). In almost all cases, careful inspection of the egg allows visualization of the piriform apparatus containing the larva with its six hooklets (three pairs). The *Trichuris, Taenia*, and *Alaria* species do not have three pair of hooklets. B Bowman DD, Georgis Parasitology for Veterinarians, ed 10, Elsevier Saunders, 2014, p. 361.

399. a The egg of the whipworm is described as trichinelloid or trichuroid. It has a thick, yellow-brown, symmetric shell with plugs at both ends. *Taeni, Alaria*, and *Moniezia* species do not have bipolar plugs. Hendrix C, Sirois M, Laboratory Procedures for Veterinary Technicians, ed 5, Mosby Elsevier, 2007, p. 202.

400. c *Dipylidium caninum* is the double-pore tapeworm. *Paragonimus kellicotti* is a lung fluke. *Moniezia expansa* has hooklets. *Echinococcus granulosus* and *Echinococcus multilocularis* are tapeworms that are associated with unilocular and multilocular hydatid disease. It contains a single oncosphere with three pairs of hooks. Hendrix C, Sirois M, Laboratory Procedures for Veterinary Technicians, ed 5, Mosby Elsevier, 2007, p. 184.

401. d *Fasciola* species includes the liver fluke. *Diphyllobothrium* species and *Hymenolepis* species are both tapeworms and are not found in the liver. *Paragonimus* species is the lungworm. Hendrix C, Sirois M, Laboratory Procedures for Veterinary Technicians, ed 6, Mosby Elsevier, 2015, p. 310.

402. d *Cuterebra* species infect rabbits, squirrels, chipmunks, mice, cats, dogs, and occasionally humans (Baird, Podgore, and Sabrosky, 1982). Female *Cuterebra* flies lay their eggs along rabbit runs and near rodent burrows. As the host brushes past, the first-stage larvae hatch instantaneously and crawl immediately into the host's fur. These larvae enter the host through its natural body openings and migrate through the body of their host before reaching their final subcutaneous location. *Gasterophilus* species includes the horse botfly. *Hypoderma* species includes the warble fly where the eggs are laid on the forelegs of large animals. *Oestrus* species includes the nasal botfly found in the nostril and nares. Bowman DD, Georgis Parasitology for Veterinarians, ed 10, Elsevier Saunders, 2014, p. 36.

403. a *Gasterophilus* species (horse bots or stomach bots) adult females fly around the fetlocks of the forelegs and the chin and shoulders of the horse to oviposit eggs on the hairs in these regions. The *Hypoderma* species includes the warble fly where the eggs are laid on the forelegs of large animals. The *Oestrus* species includes the nasal botfly and is found in the nostril and nares. *Cuterebra* species are usually found in the skin of dogs and cats, wandering aberrantly into the brain of a dog. Hendrix C, Robinson E, Diagnostic Parasitology for Veterinary Technicians, ed 4, Elsevier, 2012, p. 225.

404. b *Hypoderma* species or warbles are found in subcutaneous tissue along the backs of cattle. *Oestrus species* includes the nasal botfly found in the nostril and nares. *Cuterebra* species are usually found in the skin of dogs and cats, wandering aberrantly into the brain of a dog. *Gasterophilus* species (horse bots or stomach bots) adult females fly around the fetlocks of the forelegs and the chin and shoulders of the horse to oviposit eggs on the hairs in these regions. Hendrix C, Robinson E, Diagnostic Parasitology for Veterinary Technicians, ed 4, Elsevier, 2012, p. 223.

405. c *Oestrus* species is the nasal botfly. *Gasterophilus* species (horse bots or stomach bots) adult females fly around the fetlocks of the forelegs and the chin and shoulders of the horse to oviposit eggs on the hairs in these regions. *Cuterebra* species are usually found in the skin of dogs and cats, wandering aberrantly into the brain of a dog. *Hypoderma* species includes the warble fly where the eggs are laid on the forelegs of large animals. Hendrix C, Robinson E, Diagnostic Parasitology for Veterinary Technicians, ed 4, Elsevier, 2012, p. 226.

406. b *Otodectes cynotis*, the ear mite, is an obligate parasite of the host but is not host specific. The life cycle is typically completed in about 3 weeks. *Ctenocephalides, Hypoderma*, and *Dermacentor* are not obligate parasites. Bonagura J, Twedt D, Kirk's Current Veterinary Therapy, XV, Elsevier Saunders, 2014, p. 431.

407. d *Cheyletiella* species is known as walking dandruff. *Sarcoptes* species and *Demodex* species both cause forms of mange. *Trombicula* is a genus of harvest mites (also known as red bugs, scrub-itch mites, berry bugs, or, in their larval stage, chiggers or chigoe). Tighe MM, Brown M, Mosby's Comprehensive Review for Veterinary Technicians, ed 4, Mosby Elsevier, 2015, p. 61.

408. d The disease caused by *Sarcoptes scabei* is called scabies. *Trombicula* is a genus of harvest mites (also known as red bugs, scrub-itch mites, berry bugs or, in their larval stage, chiggers or chigoe). *Oestrus* species includes the nasal botfly found in the nostril and nares. *Melophagus* species is a blood-sucking stable fly. Hendrix C, Robinson E, Diagnostic Parasitology for Veterinary Technicians, ed 4, Elsevier, 2012, p. 232.

409. b The larval stage has six legs. All of the other stages have eight legs. Bassert J, Thomas J, McCurnin's Clinical Textbook for Veterinary Technicians, ed 8, Elsevier Saunders, 2014, p. 466.

410. b Hematopoiesis is the production of blood cells and platelets. Fibrinogen is associated with the clotting cascade but not with hematopoiesis. Hendrix C, Sirois M, Laboratory Procedures for Veterinary Technicians, ed 6, Mosby Elsevier, 2015, p. 421.

411. b Uroliths are infection-induced. In dogs, in which 50% of nephroliths are struvite (infection-induced) uroliths, antibiotics may need to be administered for as long as 2 to 3 months before there is complete dissolution. Calcium oxalate, calcium carbonate, and cystine crystals are not associated with infection. Birchard S, Sherding R, Saunders Manual of Small Animal Practice, ed. 3, Saunders Elsevier, 2006, p. 901.

412. a Decreased glucose and bilirubin concentrations, increased pH resulting from bacterial breakdown of urea to ammonia, crystal formation with increased sample turbidity, breakdown of casts and RBCs (especially in dilute or alkaline urine), and bacterial proliferation may occur in samples allowed to stand for long periods at room temperature. Bacterial numbers continue to increase if the sample is left at room temperature. The number of epithelial cells will remain unchanged. Hendrix C, Sirois M, Laboratory Procedures for Veterinary Technicians, ed 5, Mosby Elsevier, 2007, p. 154.

413. a *Alaria* species is known as the intestinal fluke. *Metastrongylus* species is known as the lungworm. *Stephanurus* species is known as the kidney worm. *Fascioloides* species is known as the large American liver fluke. Bowman DD, Georgis Parasitology for Veterinarians, ed 10, Elsevier Saunders, 2014, p. 309.

414. d *Metastrongylus* species is known as the lungworm. *Alaria* species is known as the intestinal fluke. *Stephanurus* species is known as the kidney worm. *Fascioloides* species is known as the large American liver fluke. Hendrix C, Sirois M, Laboratory Procedures for Veterinary Technicians, ed 5, Mosby Elsevier, 2007, p. 210.

415. c *Stephanurus* species is known as the kidney worm. *Fascioloides* species is known as the large American liver fluke. *Alaria* species is known as the intestinal fluke. *Metastrongylus* species is known as the lungworm. Hendrix C, Sirois M, Laboratory Procedures for Veterinary Technicians, ed 6, Mosby Elsevier, 2015, p. 297.

416. b *Fascioloides* species is known as the large American liver fluke. *Stephanurus* species is known as the kidney worm. *Alaria* species is known as the intestinal fluke. *Metastrongylus* species is known as the lungworm. Hendrix C, Robinson E, Diagnostic Parasitology for Veterinary Technicians, ed 4, Elsevier, 2012, p. 134.

417. d Flea eggs resemble tiny, smooth pearls; they are nonsticky. Hendrix C, Sirois M, Laboratory Procedures for Veterinary Technicians, ed 5, Mosby Elsevier, 2007, p. 247.

418. b Hippoboscidae or sheep keds (*Melophagus ovinus*) are dorsoventrally flattened, wingless flies that resemble ticks. They suck blood and spend their entire lives on the host (sheep). They cause pruritus and damage the wool. *Ancylostoma* species is associated with hookworms and causes anemia. *Notoedres* is associated with the feline scabies mite. The *Echinococcus* species is associated with tapeworms, in which the eggs hatch and become larvae in the intermediate hosts; the larvae migrate throughout the intermediate host and form hydatids or cysts in various organs. Hendrix C, Sirois M, Laboratory Procedures for Veterinary Technicians, ed 6, Mosby Elsevier, 2015, p. 333.

419. a Red or reddish-brown urine indicates hematuria. It is cloudy because of the presence of intact red blood cell membranes. Brown and cloudy urine could be an indication of disease such as bilirubin from IMHA. Hemoglobin in the urine would cause red and clear blood. Brown and clear urine may be seen in the case of liver disease. Tighe MM, Brown M, Mosby's Comprehensive Review for Veterinary Technicians, ed 4, Mosby Elsevier, 2015, p. 28.

420. b Calcium carbonate crystals are commonly found in the urine of normal horses. These crystals are an abnormal finding in dogs and cats. Cattle do have these crystals but they are more often seen in horses. Sirois M, Principles and Practice of Veterinary Technology, ed 3, Mosby Elsevier, 2011, p. 210.

421. d Struvite crystals have a characteristic coffin-lid appearance. This type of crystal was formerly referred to as triple phosphate. Cystine crystals form a hexagonal shape. Calcium oxalate monohydrate crystals vary in shape and can be shaped like dumbbells, spindles, ovals, or picket fences, the last of which is most commonly seen as a result of ethylene glycol poisoning. Bilirubin crystals appear to have thorny edges. Sirois M, Elsevier's Veterinary Assisting Textbook, Elsevier Saunders 2013, p. 358.

422. c Ammonium biurate crystals are seen in slightly acidic, neutral, or alkaline urine. These crystals are brown in color and round, with long, irregular spicules (i.e., they have a "thorn apple" shape). Struvite crystals are colorless crystals shaped like a square envelope (also described as having a coffin-lid appearance). Calcium carbonate crystals look like a bicycle wheel. Calcium oxalate crystals look like a pyramid. Hendrix C, Sirois M, Laboratory Procedures for Veterinary Technicians, ed 6, Mosby Elsevier, 2015.

423. d Morning samples tend to be the most concentrated and least affected by dietary factors, thereby increasing the chances of finding formed elements. The urine from an early morning sample is concentrated, which allows for detection of substances that may not be present in a more dilute sample. Hendrix C, Sirois M, Laboratory Procedures for Veterinary Technicians, ed 6, Mosby Elsevier, 2015, p. 154.

424. b Morning samples tend to be the most concentrated and least affected by dietary factors, thereby increasing the chances of finding formed elements. The urine from an early morning sample is concentrated, which allows detection of substances that may not be present in a more dilute sample. Hendrix C, Sirois M, Laboratory Procedures for Veterinary Technicians, ed 6, Mosby Elsevier, 2015, p. 154.

425. c Cystocentesis and catheterization provide good samples for urinalysis that are free of contamination from the distal genital tract and external areas. Voiding and expressing the bladder to collect samples contaminates as the urine leaves the body and are therefore not considered sufficient for culture. Hendrix C, Sirois M, Laboratory Procedures for Veterinary Technicians, ed 6, Mosby Elsevier, 2015, p. 155.

426. b Polyuria is defined as the formation and excretion of large volumes of urine. Lack of urine is known as oliguria. *Proteinuria* is the term used to describe excessive protein in the urine. *Hypodipsia* is the term for low water intake. Tighe MM, Brown M, Mosby's Comprehensive Review for Veterinary Technicians, ed 4, Mosby Elsevier, 2015, p. 28.

427. d Oliguria is a decrease in the volume of urine produced. Polyphagia is excessive eating. Hyperbilirubinuria is excessive bilirubin in the urine (this can sometimes appear as green urine). Hendrix C, Sirois M, Laboratory Procedures for Veterinary Technicians, ed 6, Mosby Elsevier, 2015, p. 421.

428. c Anuria is the absence of urine. Oliguria is a decrease in the volume of urine produced. Hypodipsia is known as low water intake. Polydipsia is excessive drinking. Hendrix C, Sirois M, Laboratory Procedures for Veterinary Technicians, ed 6, Mosby Elsevier, 2015, p. 421.

429. a Alkalosis, high-fiber diets (plants), infection of the urinary tract with urease bacteria, the use of certain drugs, or urine retention, such as that which occurs with urethral obstruction or bladder paralysis, may cause increased pH (alkalinity). Diabetes, prolonged diarrhea, and starvation would be associated with acidic urine. Hendrix C, Sirois M, Laboratory Procedures for Veterinary Technicians, ed 6, Mosby Elsevier, 2015, p. 165.

430. b Red or red-brown urine indicates the presence of red blood cells (hematuria). Dysuria is painful urination. An excessive number of WBCs is referred to as pyuria or leukocyturia. Proteinuria is protein in the urine. Hendrix C, Sirois M, Laboratory Procedures for Veterinary Technicians, ed 6, Mosby Elsevier, 2015, p. 160.

431. c An excessive number of WBCs is referred to as pyuria or leukocyturia. Hematuria is blood in the urine. Dysuria is painful urination. Proteinuria is protein in the urine. Tighe MM, Brown M, Mosby's Comprehensive Review for Veterinary Technicians, ed 4, Mosby Elsevier, 2015, p. 34.

432. a Dysuria is difficulty or painful urination. Proteinuria is protein in the urine. Hematuria is blood in the urine. An excessive number of WBCs is referred to as pyuria or leukocyturia. Tighe MM, Brown M, Mosby's Comprehensive Review for Veterinary Technicians, ed 4, Mosby Elsevier, 2015, p. 27.

433. b Pancytopenia is the decrease in red blood cells, white blood cells, and platelet lines. Decreased numbers of white blood cells only is called leukopenia. Decreased numbers of red blood cells only is called anemia. Decreased numbers of granulocytes and monocytes is called neutropenia. Tighe MM, Brown M, Mosby's Comprehensive Review for Veterinary Technicians, ed 4, Mosby Elsevier, 2015, p. 676.

434. b Erythropoietin is a growth hormone produced by the kidneys that stimulates red blood cell production. Bone marrow produces red blood cells. The pituitary gland produces adrenocorticotropic hormone, which stimulates the adrenal glands to secrete steroid hormones, principally cortisol. The liver produces proteins that are important to blood clotting. Tighe MM, Brown M, Mosby's Comprehensive Review for Veterinary Technicians, ed 4, Mosby Elsevier, 2015, p. 390.

435. c In dogs, in which 50% of nephroliths are struvite (infection-induced) uroliths, antibiotic administration may be needed for as long as 2 to 3 months before there is complete dissolution. Bonagura J, Twedt D, Kirk's Current Veterinary Therapy, XV, Elsevier Saunders, 2014, p. 894.

436. a BUN and SC must be interpreted in conjunction with patient hydration status and a concurrent urine specific gravity (SG) to distinguish dehydration (prerenal azotemia) from impaired kidney function (renal azotemia). If a dehydrated patient has normally functioning kidneys, increases in BUN and SC should be accompanied by high urine SG, indicating that the kidneys are capable of concentrating urine to conserve as much water as possible. In patients with renal azotemia, the kidneys fail to concentrate urine adequately and SG is lower than expected to compensate for dehydration. Dehydration with true impaired kidney function is renal azotemia. Stage 1 renal disease and urinary tract infections are not associated with how prerenal azotemia and renal azotemia are characterized. Bassert J, Thomas J, McCurnin's Clinical Textbook for Veterinary Technicians, ed 8, Elsevier Saunders, 2014, p. 425.

437. c Coaxing: warming the food and feeding by hand are examples of enteral nutrition. ITP given through an IV catheter is an example of parental nutrition. Fasting, NPO, and water only are not nutrition options. Tighe MM, Brown M, Mosby's Comprehensive Review for Veterinary Technicians, ed 4, Mosby Elsevier, 2015, p. 257.

438. b Anticholinergics are sympatholytic drugs that exert their effects by blocking the actions of the parasympathetic neurotransmitter acetylcholine at the muscarinic receptors. Two examples are atropine and glycopyrrolate. Propofol, ketamine, cyclosporine, mycophenolate, dexdomitor, and antisedan are not anticholinergics. Tighe MM, Brown M, Mosby's Comprehensive Review for Veterinary Technicians, ed 4, Mosby Elsevier, 2015, p. 336.

439. c Expressed as MAC, this is the minimum alveolar concentration of an induction that produces no response in 50% of patients exposed to a painful stimulus. The lower the MAC, the more potent the anesthetic. A lower concentration is thus required to maintain a similar anesthetic depth. The remaining options have nothing to do with MAC or anesthesia depth. Tighe MM, Brown M, Mosby's Comprehensive Review for Veterinary Technicians, ed 4, Mosby Elsevier, 2015, p. 344.

440. a Iohexol clearance can be used to estimate GFR in dogs and cats. Iohexol is a radiographic agent that is administered as a single intravenous dose after a 12-hour fast, during which time the patient has free access to water. Serum samples are taken at 2, 3, and 4 hours after administration and are sent to a reference laboratory. Liver function, blood glucose, and food sensitivities are not associated with an iohexol clearance test. Hendrix C, Sirois M, Laboratory Procedures for Veterinary Technicians, ed 6, Mosby Elsevier, 2015, p. 33.

441. d Glucose can bind a variety of structures, including proteins. Fructosamine represents the irreversible reaction of glucose bound to protein, particularly albumin. When glucose concentrations are persistently elevated in blood, as occurs in patients with diabetes mellitus, the increased binding of glucose to serum proteins occurs. Fructosamine is a serum test that helps indicate whether a diabetic patient is controlled (long-term) or not. Hendrix C, Sirois M, Laboratory Procedures for Veterinary Technicians, ed 6, Mosby Elsevier, 2015, p. 213.

442. b Because the half-life of albumin in dogs and cats is 1 to 2 weeks, fructosamine provides an indication of the average serum glucose throughout that period. Hendrix C, Sirois M, Laboratory Procedures for Veterinary Technicians, ed 6, Mosby Elsevier, 2015, p. 213.

443. a Bone marrow cytology samples must be made immediately if they are not mixed with EDTA at the time of collection. If EDTA has been used, smears must be made within 1 hour of collection. Bone marrow can clot in seconds if not prepared with EDTA. Hendrix C, Sirois M, Laboratory Procedures for Veterinary Technicians, ed 6, Mosby Elsevier, 2015, p. 80.
444. a The buccal mucosa bleeding time (BMBT) is a primary assay for the detection of abnormalities in platelet function. PT, PTT, and fibrinogen all play a part in assessing clotting factors and the clotting cascade, but only the BMBT test can test for true platelet function. Hendrix C, Sirois M, Laboratory Procedures for Veterinary Technicians, ed 6, Mosby Elsevier, 2015, p. 80.
445. a High triglycerides indicate hyperlipidemia, resulting in a milky white serum. Serum may be yellow because of bilirubin; red serum would be a result of hemolysis of red blood cells; and clear serum would be obtained from a normal healthy dog or cat. Bassert J, Thomas J, McCurnin's Clinical Textbook for Veterinary Technicians, ed 8, Elsevier Saunders, 2014.
446. d A specific gravity of 1.040 would be expected in a healthy hydrated patient. 1.000 is the specific gravity of water (which would be used to calibrate a refractometer). 1.005 and 1.010 would indicate the kidneys are not concentrating the urine. Bassert J, Thomas J, McCurnin's Clinical Textbook for Veterinary Technicians, ed 8, Elsevier Saunders, 2014.
447. d Patients should fast for a minimum of 12 hours to avoid serum lipemia. Bassert J, Thomas J, McCurnin's Clinical Textbook for Veterinary Technicians, ed 8, Elsevier Saunders, 2014.

SECTION 9

1. a Ferrets are strict carnivores, requiring 30% protein and 25% fat in their diets. Dogs are omnivores. Prairie dogs and rabbits are herbivores. Bassert JM, Thomas JA, McCurnin's Clinical Textbook for Veterinary Technicians, ed 8, Elsevier, 2014.
2. c Pain in a patient can produce a catabolic state leading to wasting and suppressing the immune system, making the patient more prone to infections. In addition, pain promotes inflammation, which slows the healing process, increases anesthetic risk by increasing dosage required, and causes patient suffering. Goldberg ME, Shaffran N, Pain Management for Veterinary Technicians and Nurses, Wiley, 2014.
3. a The veterinary technician who is capable of obtaining a complete and accurate history can play a critical role in a busy veterinary practice. Obtaining information from clients is often time-consuming, and veterinary technicians who can do this well free veterinarians to complete other work. Using historical information, as well as other parts of the database, the veterinary technician should be able to generate technician evaluations and to formulate appropriate technician interventions to support the patient. Patient examinations are important every time a patient visits the hospital, even during wellness exams. Bassert JM, Thomas JA, "History and Physical Examination," McCurnin's Clinical Textbook for Veterinary Technicians, ed 8, Elsevier, St. Louis, 2014.
4. c Prairie dogs are herbivores, and ferrets are strict carnivores, requiring 30% protein and 25% fat in their diets. Dogs and iguanas are omnivores. Bassert JM, Thomas JA, McCurnin's Clinical Textbook for Veterinary Technicians, ed 8, Elsevier, St. Louis, 2014.
5. a Icterus manifests as yellow-to-orange serum caused by increased bilirubin levels in serum. Hemolyzed serum is red because of increased hemoglobin levels in serum. Hyperproteinemia results in increased total protein readings and when severe, presents yellow fluid with high viscosity, such as with feline infectious peritonitis. Lipemia manifests as turbid, white serum from an increased triglyceride level. Battaglia AM, Steele AM, Small Animal Emergency and Critical Care for Veterinary Technicians, ed 3, Elsevier, 2016.
6. d USDA: the United States Department of Agriculture regulates pet food labels and research facilities. AAFCO: the Association of American Feed Control Officials sets standards for substantiation claims and nutritional profiles for pet food; however, it has no regulatory authority. Government agencies often mandate AAFCO regulations into law. FDA: the Food and Drug Administration provides approval for new ingredients. FTC: the Federal Trade Commission regulates trade and the advertising of pet foods. Case LP, Daristotle L, Hayek MG, Raasch MF, "History and Regulation of Pet Foods," Canine and Feline Nutrition: A Resource for Companion Animal Professionals, ed 3, Mosby, 2011.
7. d AU refers to each ear (aures unitas). OD indicates right eye (oculus dexter). OS indicates left eye (oculus sinister). OU indicates both eyes (oculi unitas). Wanamaker BP, Massey KL, "Appendix A, Common Abbreviations Used in Veterinary Medicine," Applied Pharmacology for Veterinary Technicians, ed 5, Elsevier Saunders, 2015.
8. a Rabbits practice coprophagy, which means eating their night stools for nutrition. Dystrophic calcification is caused by a diet high in calcium or vitamin D, it results in chalky-white or cream-colored urine, and it can lead to urinary lithiasis. Dysbiosis occurs when antibiotic-impregnated feed is ingested, disrupting the intestinal flora. Vitamin A deficiency results in infertility, central nervous system defects, and increased neonatal mortality. Bassert JM, Thomas JA, McCurnin's Clinical Textbook for Veterinary Technicians, ed 8, Elsevier, St. Louis, 2014.
9. c The ASA score, or the American Society of Anesthesiologists scoring system, assesses anesthetic risk. The Glasgow Coma Scale assesses a patient's neurologic status. The Colorado Pain Scale is a systematic method of scoring a patient's pain. Shock index is a calculated value estimating the degree of shock that a patient is experiencing. Goldberg ME, Shaffran N, Pain Management for Veterinary Technicians and Nurses, Wiley, 2014.
10. b It is also important to ask open-ended questions, rather than leading questions. An open-ended question is one that requires clients to complete the information themselves, whereas a leading question is one that

potentially guides clients to an answer. When leading questions are asked, clients sense which response the interviewer prefers and are likely to give it; pet owners are anxious to help resolve their animal's problems. Asking leading questions can generate inaccurate historical information. Some owners have medical training and can be spoken to using medical jargon; however, most owners do not understand medical terminology and the veterinary technician must be careful to use simple language without belittling the client. Bassert JM, Thomas JA, "History and Physical Examination," McCurnin's Clinical Textbook for Veterinary Technicians, ed 8, Elsevier, St. Louis, 2014.

11. d The physical examination is the main component of the technician's observation of a patient, both during the initial presentation and when monitoring changes in a hospitalized patient. The key to a good physical examination is careful completion of all parts of the examination every time it is performed. You should perform all aspects of the physical examination in the same sequence for every patient. Developing this sort of routine will prevent you from forgetting to evaluate one area because you are overly focused on another. The routine you develop may have to vary slightly from patient to patient. Bassert JM, Thomas JA, "History and Physical Examination," McCurnin's Clinical Textbook for Veterinary Technicians, ed 8, Elsevier, St. Louis, 2014.

12. b Dysbiosis occurs when antibiotic-impregnated feed is ingested, disrupting the intestinal flora. Dystrophic calcification is caused by a diet high in calcium or vitamin D, it results in chalky-white or cream-colored urine, and it can lead to urinary lithiasis. Rabbits practice coprophagy, eating their night stools for nutrition. Vitamin A deficiency results in infertility, central nervous system defects, and increased neonatal mortality. Bassert JM, Thomas JA, McCurnin's Clinical Textbook for Veterinary Technicians, ed 8, Elsevier, St. Louis, 2014.

13. a Transduction occurs when sensing receptors called nociceptors sense a noxious stimulus. Transmission sends this signal to the spinal cord. Modulation occurs at the spinal cord to determine whether reflexes should be triggered, the signal amplified, or the signal dampened. Perception occurs when the stimulus is finally received by the brain and processed. Goldberg ME, Shaffran N, Pain Management for Veterinary Technicians and Nurses, Wiley, 2014.

14. d Vitamin A deficiency results in infertility, central nervous system defects, and increased neonatal mortality. Dystrophic calcification is caused by a diet high in calcium or vitamin D, it results in chalky-white or cream-colored urine, and it can lead to urinary lithiasis. Rabbits practice coprophagy, eating their night stools for nutrition. Dysbiosis occurs when antibiotic-impregnated feed is ingested, disrupting the intestinal flora. Bassert JM, Thomas JA, McCurnin's Clinical Textbook for Veterinary Technicians, ed 8, Elsevier, St. Louis, 2014.

15. b Dilated cardiomyopathy is a common cardiovascular disease of the dog, primarily seen in older males of large breed dogs. Boxer right ventricular cardiomyopathy is seen commonly in boxers; however, it is not commonly seen in other breeds. Hypertrophic cardiomyopathy is seen commonly in cats. Ventricular septal defects are not biased toward dogs or cats. Summers A, Common Diseases of Companion Animals, ed 3, Elsevier, 2014.

16. b Hallmarks of hypoadrenocorticism are hyponatremia and hyperkalemia. Clinical signs associated with hyperadrenocorticism include weight gain, muscle weakness, polyuria, polydipsia, skin and hair coat abnormalities, and a potbellied appearance. Hyperthyroidism is typically seen in cats, causing weight loss and a ravenous appetite among other signs. Hypothyroidism typically causes weight gain, bradycardia, exercise intolerance, and lethargy. Bassert JM, Thomas JA, McCurnin's Clinical Textbook for Veterinary Technicians, ed 8, Elsevier, St. Louis, 2014.

17. b Halitosis is malodorous breath, which is an indication of issues with either the oral cavity or the gastrointestinal tract. There are specific endocrine diseases that can lead to uniquely smelling breaths, although the choice is not on the list. The cardiovascular system involves the heart and the blood vessels creating blood flow. The nervous system consists of the brain, spinal cord, and nerves. The hematologic system involves blood cells and bone marrow. Summers A, Common Diseases of Companion Animals, ed 3, Elsevier, 2014.

18. a Peripheral arterial pulses should be palpated to determine pulse rate and pulse quality in every patient. Pulses generally are palpated by way of the femoral artery, which is located high on the medial thigh of the animal. Digital pressure should be applied over the femoral artery by using the tips of the fingers. It is essential to auscultate the heart while palpating pulses. Heart rate and pulse rate should be identical and a pulse of approximately equal quality should be produced by each heartbeat. Absence of a palpable pulse (or a significant change in pulse quality) with an audible heartbeat is called a pulse deficit. Pulse deficits usually indicate an abnormal heart rhythm and warrant further evaluation, such as electrocardiography. Palpating the pulse while taking the patient's temperature would serve no purpose. Bassert JM, Thomas JA, "History and Physical Examination," McCurnin's Clinical Textbook for Veterinary Technicians, ed 8, Elsevier, St. Louis, 2014.

19. b It is important to determine the pulse quality when palpating peripheral arterial pulses. The pressure you feel when palpating a pulse is called the pulse pressure. Pulse pressure represents the difference between systolic and diastolic arterial pressures. The intensity of the palpated pulse varies depending on the body condition of the animal, appearing stronger in thin animals and weaker in obese or heavily muscled animals. Pulse quality is a subjective measurement that is likely to vary from technician to technician, according to the level of experience and comfort attained in palpating peripheral pulses. Pulses may be described as slow to rise if the peak of intensity comes late in the pulse wave. This can be seen with obstruction to cardiac output, as occurs with aortic stenosis. A pulse that feels stronger than normal may also indicate a problem. Such pulses may be described as bounding, tall, or hyperkinetic. Bounding pulses may be palpated in hyperdynamic states (early septic shock, anemia) or when a rapid drop-off in diastolic pressure occurs (patent ductus arteriosus). Whenever pulse quality is abnormal, evaluation of blood pressure using direct or indirect means is warranted. The age of the patient should have no bearing on the pulse quality. Bassert JM, Thomas JA, "History and Physical Examination," McCurnin's Clinical Textbook for Veterinary Technicians, ed 8, Elsevier, St. Louis, 2014.

20. c Hyperthyroidism is typically seen in cats, causing weight loss and a ravenous appetite among other signs. Hallmarks of hypoadrenocorticism are hyponatremia and hyperkalemia. Clinical signs associated with hyperadrenocorticism include weight gain, muscle weakness, polyuria, polydipsia, skin and hair coat abnormalities, and a potbellied appearance. Hypothyroidism typically causes weight gain, bradycardia, exercise intolerance, and lethargy. Bassert JM, Thomas JA, McCurnin's Clinical Textbook for Veterinary Technicians, ed 8, Elsevier, St. Louis, 2014.

21. b The medial saphenous vein is located on the medial side (inside) of the pelvic limbs. To access this vein, the patient should be restrained in lateral recumbency (on its side) to expose the medial aspect of the pelvic limb. Dorsal recumbency means the patient is held on its back. Sternal recumbency means the patient is allowed to lie on its sternum. Medial recumbency is not a type of recumbency. Sheldon CC, Sonsthagen T, Topel JA, Animal Restraint for Veterinary Professionals, ed 1, Mosby Elsevier, 2006.

22. c An attempt should be made to describe the intensity of the pulse using terms such as *weak*, *moderate*, or *strong*. In general, a weak peripheral pulse is indicative of poor perfusion and might be caused by decreased cardiac output (as in congestive heart failure or hypovolemia) or increased peripheral resistance (as in shock). Pulses may be described as slow to rise if the peak of intensity comes late in the pulse wave. This can be seen with obstruction to cardiac output, as occurs with aortic stenosis. A pulse that feels stronger than normal may also indicate a problem. Such pulses may be described as bounding, tall, or hyperkinetic. Bounding pulses may be palpated in hyperdynamic states (early septic shock, anemia) or when a rapid drop-off in diastolic pressure occurs (patent ductus arteriosus). Whenever pulse quality is abnormal, evaluation of blood pressure using direct or indirect means is warranted. Patient attitude is generally described as bright, alert, and responsive, or a similar term that indicates how the patient is acting. Respiration is generally noted with terms such as increased inspiratory or expiratory effort. Bassert JM, Thomas JA, "History and Physical Examination," McCurnin's Clinical Textbook for Veterinary Technicians, ed 8, Elsevier, St. Louis, 2014.

23. d The cornea is the transparent covering of the front of the eye; it should be clear. The iris, lens, and anterior chamber are internal structures of the eye. The iris is the colored part of the eye. Bassert JM, Thomas JA, "History and Physical Examination," McCurnin's Clinical Textbook for Veterinary Technicians, ed 8, Elsevier, St. Louis, 2014.

24. d Hypothyroidism typically causes weight gain, bradycardia, exercise intolerance, and lethargy. Hallmarks of hypoadrenocorticism are hyponatremia and hyperkalemia. Clinical signs associated with hyperadrenocorticism include weight gain, muscle weakness, polyuria, polydipsia, skin and hair coat abnormalities, and a potbellied appearance. Hyperthyroidism is typically seen in cats, causing weight loss and a ravenous appetite, among other signs. Bassert JM, Thomas JA, McCurnin's Clinical Textbook for Veterinary Technicians, ed 8, Elsevier, St. Louis, 2014.

25. a A patient in right lateral recumbency will be lying with its right side down. This allows easy access to the lateral side of the left leg, facing the topmost aspect of the patient, where the lateral saphenous vein is located. The left medial saphenous, the left lateral saphenous, and the right jugular veins will all be on the underside of the patient. Sheldon CC, Sonsthagen T, Topel JA, Animal Restraint for Veterinary Professionals, ed 1, Elsevier, 2006.

26. b Hypoxemia is defined as low blood-oxygen levels. Hypovolemia is defined as a decrease in circulating blood volume. Hypoxia is defined as low tissue-oxygen levels. Hypervolemia is an increase in circulating fluid in the body. JM, Thomas JA, "Small Animal Medical Nursing," McCurnin's Clinical Textbook for Veterinary Technicians, ed 8, Elsevier, St. Louis, 2014.

27. c Dyspneic patients are in critical condition and the demonstration of a patent airway and the provision of oxygen are required immediately. If pleural effusion or pneumothorax is present, a thoracocentesis is performed as quickly as possible to help stabilize the patient. Additional stress can result in death of a dyspneic patient; therefore, thorough examination and diagnostic tests begin after the patient's condition has stabilized. Bassert JM, Thomas JA, "Small Animal Medical Nursing," McCurnin's Clinical Textbook for Veterinary Technicians, ed 8, Elsevier, St. Louis, 2014.

28. a The normal temperature for a horse is 99°F–101.5°F Bassert JM, Thomas JA, McCurnin's Clinical Textbook for Veterinary Technicians, ed 8, Elsevier, St. Louis, 2014.

29. d When proper restraint of a patient is not possible with gentle handling, the use of chemical restraint should be considered to alleviate risk of injury to all parties involved, and to ensure the highest chances of success in completing the procedure. Forcing a patient down and proceeding without full control will increase the chances of injury, is inhumane, and makes the chances of a successful outcome less likely. Recruiting help from the owner will expose him or her to potential injury and this would be a liability for the practice. Running the patient around until exhausted is inhumane and harmful to the patient that is presenting with illness. Sheldon CC, Sonsthagen T, Topel JA, Animal Restraint for Veterinary Professionals, ed 1, Elsevier, 2006.

30. c The normal temperature for a dog is 100°F–102.2°F Bassert JM, Thomas JA, McCurnin's Clinical Textbook for Veterinary Technicians, ed 8, Elsevier, St. Louis, 2014.

31. a Veterinarians, veterinary technicians, and veterinary assistants should be trained in restraining patients for various procedures. The person required to restrain might vary depending on the procedure performed.

Owners should never be asked to help restrain pets as they have not received proper training to minimize chances of injury and this can result in lawsuits filed against the practice should they become injured. Sheldon CC, Sonsthagen T, Topel JA, Animal Restraint for Veterinary Professionals, ed 1, Elsevier, 2006.

32. c The normal temperature for a cat is 100°F–102.2°F Bassert JM, Thomas JA, McCurnin's Clinical Textbook for Veterinary Technicians, ed 8, Elsevier, St. Louis, 2014.

33. a A patient with heart failure has clinical signs referable to the perfusion deficit: tachypnea, exercise intolerance (dogs), syncope, weakness, prolonged capillary refill time (CRT), and pale mucous membranes. A decreased respiratory rate (bradypnea) is most commonly associated with elevated intracranial pressure secondary to swelling of the brain, as can occur with traumatic brain injury. An abnormally rapid heart rate, called tachycardia, can indicate compensation for a shock state, pain, fear, anxiety, or any combination of those factors. An inappropriately slow heart rate, termed *bradycardia*, can indicate a life-threatening arrhythmia or, in animals with urethral obstruction, an extremely elevated potassium level. Bassert JM, Thomas JA, "Small Animal Medical Nursing," McCurnin's Clinical Textbook for Veterinary Technicians, ed 8, Elsevier, St. Louis, 2014.

34. c The most common presenting sign in a patient with undiagnosed severe hypertension is acute blindness caused by retinal detachment. After hypertension has been diagnosed, treatment with antihypertensive medication (calcium channel blockers, ACE inhibitors) is begun immediately. The goal is to lower blood pressure gradually into the normal range, avoiding a dramatic drop. Hypertension is not commonly seen with anorexia, cardiomyopathy, or hypothyroidism. Bassert JM, Thomas JA, "Small Animal Medical Nursing," McCurnin's Clinical Textbook for Veterinary Technicians, ed 8, Elsevier, St. Louis, 2014.

35. b Precautions for restraining cats include using the minimal restraint required, making sure all doors, windows, and cabinets are closed, clearing the table of any equipment that can be knocked down, treating each patient as an individual case and reading its body language, and distracting patients with gentle techniques such as tapping its forehead. Sheldon CC, Sonsthagen T, Topel JA, Animal Restraint for Veterinary Professionals, ed 1, Elsevier, 2006.

36. d The normal heart rate for a cat is 140–220 beats per minute. Bassert JM, Thomas JA, McCurnin's Clinical Textbook for Veterinary Technicians, ed 8, Elsevier, St. Louis, 2014.

37. a Regurgitation is the passive expulsion of material from the mouth, pharynx, or esophagus. Nausea and abdominal contractions are not typically seen. Patients can exhibit difficulty eating (dysphagia), hypersalivation, and gagging. Regurgitated material typically consists of undigested or partially digested food. Patients are at risk of aspiration of stomach contents and development of pneumonia. Vomiting is defined as the forceful expulsion of contents from the stomach and the upper small intestine; it is an active process that requires abdominal contraction (retching). Nausea often precedes vomiting, with patients exhibiting anxiety, hypersalivation, vocalization, and lip smacking. Vomitus can comprise any combination of undigested or digested food, hair, mucus, bile, and gastric secretions. If the patient is vomiting fresh or digested blood, it is termed *hematemesis*. B Bassert JM, Thomas JA, "Small Animal Medical Nursing," McCurnin's Clinical Textbook for Veterinary Technicians, ed 8, Elsevier, St. Louis, 2014.

38. a Puppies and kittens are unable to maintain their body temperatures during the first few days of life and the shiver reflex does not develop until after the first week of life. Body temperature at birth (94.5°F–97.3°F [34.5°C–36.3°C]) is lower than in adults and rises to 34.8°C–38.3°C during the first week of life. Normal temperature range for adult dogs and cats is 100.0°F–102.2°F, and for a horse it is 99.0°F–101.5°F. Bassert JM, Thomas JA, "Chapter 21, Neonatal Care of the Puppy, Kitten, and Foal," McCurnin's Clinical Textbook for Veterinary Technicians, ed 8, Elsevier, St. Louis, 2014.

39. b The best approach to a nervous patient in the cage is to try to lure the patient out with quiet, gentle urgings, standing clear of the door. This lets the patient walk out on its own, into an unfamiliar environment, and keeps them calm. Any excessive force, such as pulling it out with a leash, is stressful and provokes unpredictable reactions. Reaching into the cage, or quick, jerky movements, will often threaten the patient and these should be avoided. Sheldon CC, Sonsthagen T, Topel JA, Animal Restraint for Veterinary Professionals, ed 1, Elsevier, 2006.

40. c The normal heart rate for a dog is 60–160 beats per minute. Bassert JM, Thomas JA, McCurnin's Clinical Textbook for Veterinary Technicians, ed 8, Elsevier, St. Louis, 2014.

41. a An IV fluid that has the same solute concentration as the one to which it is being compared is considered an isotonic solution. Isotonic fluids have the same solute concentration as the intracellular space. Hypotonic solutions have lower solute concentrations than that of extracellular fluid. Hypertonic solutions have a higher solute concentration than that of extracellular fluid. 0.45% sodium chloride is a hypotonic solution. Donohoe C, "Body Water," Fluid Therapy for Veterinary Technicians and Nurses, Wiley-Blackwell, 2012.

42. d Contrary to popular belief, a bitch should not receive a greater amount of food immediately after she is bred. An increase of food at this time is unnecessary and could lead to excessive weight gain during pregnancy. After the fifth or sixth week of pregnancy, the bitch's food intake should be increased gradually so that at the time of whelping her daily intake is approximately 25% to 50% higher than her normal maintenance needs, depending on the size of the litter and the size of the bitch. Case LP, Daristotle L, Hayek MG, Raasch MF, "Pregnancy and Lactation," Canine and Feline Nutrition: A Resource for Companion Animal Professionals, ed 3, Mosby, 2011.

43. d A tourniquet is used to apply pressure around a limb to occlude the flow in a vein, making it stand out. An Elizabethan collar is a restraint device preventing chewing or tugging at areas on the body. A muzzle is a restraint device that prevents opening of the mouth.

A capture pole is used to restrain aggressive animals to prevent the patient from getting close enough to the personnel to bite. Sheldon CC, Sonsthagen T, Topel JA, Animal Restraint for Veterinary Professionals, ed 1, Elsevier, 2006.

44. b The normal pulse for a horse is 28–44 beats per minute. Bassert JM, Thomas JA, McCurnin's Clinical Textbook for Veterinary Technicians, ed 8, Elsevier, St. Louis, 2014.

45. a Fat and lactose are the primary sources of energy in milk; puppies and kittens have high intestinal lactase activity and are capable of digesting milk fat very early in life. Case LP, Daristotle L, Hayek MG, Raasch MF, "Nutritional Care of Neonatal Puppies and Kittens," Canine and Feline Nutrition: A Resource for Companion Animal Professionals, ed 3, Mosby, 2011.

46. a Many disease processes such as vomiting, anorexia, diarrhea, and hemorrhagic shock cause isotonic dehydration. Body water that has a solute concentration equal to that remaining in the compartment is defined as isotonic dehydration. Hypovolemia refers to a deficit in fluid volume that is circulating throughout the body. Hypotonic dehydration describes loss of body water that has a low concentration of dissolved particles. Hypertonic dehydration involves the loss of fluid that has a high solute concentration. Donohoe C, "Patient Assessment," Fluid Therapy for Veterinary Technicians and Nurses, Wiley-Blackwell, 2012.

47. d When two people are involved in lifting a large dog, the person at the front should wrap one arm around the dog's neck and the other arm under and around the dog's chest, behind the front legs. The second person wraps one arm around the abdomen in front of the rear limbs. Lifting by the head can cause harm to the patient and hugging the neck should control the head. Sheldon CC, Sonsthagen T, Topel JA, Animal Restraint for Veterinary Professionals, ed 1, Elsevier, 2006.

48. a The normal respiratory rate for a horse is 6–16 breaths per minute. Bassert JM, Thomas JA, McCurnin's Clinical Textbook for Veterinary Technicians, ed 8, Elsevier, St. Louis, 2014.

49. b An increase in PCV in conjunction with elevated TS often indicates dehydration. An increase in PCV in conjunction with a decrease in TS is likely an indication of protein loss. Decreased PCV and TS indicate anemia. This can also be seen in patients receiving fluid therapy. Donohoe C, "Patient Assessment," Fluid Therapy for Veterinary Technicians and Nurses, Wiley-Blackwell, 2012.

50. d 1 microgram (µg) = 0.000001 gram (g) (µg) 1 milligram (mg) = 0.001 g = 1000 µg 1 gram (g) = 1.0 g = 1000 mg 1 kilogram (kg) = 1000.0 g. Wanamaker BP, Massey KL, "Appendix B, Weights and Measures," Applied Pharmacology for Veterinary Technicians, ed 5, Elsevier Saunders, 2015.

51. a A gait is defined as the series of joint, segment, and whole body movements used for locomotion. It is made up of repeated strides, which cycles through a stance and swing phase. A gallop is a type of gait, much like a walk, trot, or pace. Millis DL, Levine D, Canine Rehabilitation and Physical Therapy, ed 2, Elsevier, 2014.

52. c The normal respiratory rate for a cat is 20–42 breaths per minute. Bassert JM, Thomas JA, McCurnin's Clinical Textbook for Veterinary Technicians, ed 8, Elsevier, St. Louis, 2014.

53. c Mixtures consist of aqueous solutions (i.e., water) and suspensions for oral administration. A suspension usually separates after long periods of shelf life and must be shaken well before it is used so that a uniform dose is provided. Syrups contain the drug and a flavoring in a concentrated solution of sugar water or other aqueous liquid. In veterinary medicine, an antibiotic (e.g., doxycycline) may be mixed with a liquid vitamin (e.g., Lixotinic) to ensure a more palatable taste for the patient. Elixirs usually consist of a hydroalcoholic liquid that contains sweeteners, flavoring, and a medicinal agent. Emulsions consist of oily substances dispersed in an aqueous medium with an additive that stabilizes the mixture. Wanamaker BP, Massey KL, "Routes and Techniques of Drug Administration," Applied Pharmacology for Veterinary Technicians, ed 5, Elsevier Saunders, 2015.

54. a Cleaning the rubber diaphragm of the medication vial with an alcohol swab is important to reduce the likelihood of foreign material or bacteria from being introduced into the vial and its contents. Wiping the diaphragm after inserting the needle serves no purpose. Inspecting the diaphragm for foreign material does not in itself prevent that material from entering the vial. The rubber diaphragm should not be removed from multidose vials because this would cause a greater risk of contaminating the contents of the vial. Wanamaker BP, Massey KL, "Routes and Techniques of Drug Administration," Applied Pharmacology for Veterinary Technicians, ed 5, Elsevier Saunders, 2015.

55. a Wound healing goes through the inflammatory phase, proliferation phase, and then the maturation phase. The inflammatory phase involves an acute vascular response and cellular infiltration. The proliferative phase can also be called the reparative or fibroblastic phase when the fibroblasts proliferate to repair damaged tissue. Granulation occurs during this phase. The maturation phase involves collagen fibers forming crosslinks to become stable. Millis DL, Levine D, Canine Rehabilitation and Physical Therapy, ed 2, Elsevier, 2014.

56. b The normal respiratory rate for a dog is 16–32 breaths per minute. Bassert JM, Thomas JA, McCurnin's Clinical Textbook for Veterinary Technicians, ed 8, Elsevier, St. Louis, 2014.

57. a 16 gauge is the largest needle size. Needles are available in various sizes and styles, but all needles have the following three parts: hub, shaft, and bevel. Needle sizes vary by gauge and by length. The gauge refers to the inside diameter of the shaft. There is an inverse relationship between the gauge number and the size of the inside diameter of the needle. In other words, the larger the gauge number, the smaller the diameter. Wanamaker BP, Massey KL, "Routes and Techniques of Drug Administration," Applied Pharmacology for Veterinary Technicians, ed 5, Elsevier Saunders, 2015.

58. a AD indicates right ear (auris dextra). AS refers to left ear (auris sinistra). AU refers to each ear (auris utraque). OD refers to right eye (oculus dexter). Standard Abbreviations for Veterinary Medical Records. ed. 3, AAHA Press, 2010.

59. b Passive range of motion involves manually creating motion in the joint, without muscle contraction occurring, using external forces. It is used to reduce joint pain and scar tissue formation. Active range of motion involves active muscle contraction to achieve the range of motion of a joint. Proprioception is the body's ability to sense balance. Stretching is a sustained maneuver on a joint used to help elongate tissues that have undergone shortening resulting from immobility. Millis DL, Levine D, Canine Rehabilitation and Physical Therapy, ed 2, Elsevier, 2014.

60. a The normal systolic blood pressure for a cat is 120–160 mmHg. Bassert JM, Thomas JA, McCurnin's Clinical Textbook for Veterinary Technicians, ed 8, Elsevier, St. Louis, 2014.

61. a q.i.d. = four times a day. q.o.d. = every other day. s.i.d. = once a day. t.i.d. = three times a day. Wanamaker BP, Massey KL, "Appendix A, Common Abbreviations Used in Veterinary Medicine," Applied Pharmacology for Veterinary Technicians, ed 5, Elsevier Saunders, 2015.

62. b μg = microgram. mEq = milliequivalent. mg = milligram. mm = millimeter. Wanamaker BP, Massey KL, "Appendix A, Common Abbreviations Used in Veterinary Medicine," Applied Pharmacology for Veterinary Technicians, ed 5, Elsevier Saunders, 2015.

63. b Bladder expression is the act of manually applying pressure to the bladder and expressing urine. Neurologic conditions can lead to the development of an atonic bladder or a bladder that has lost muscle tone to make the patient urinate, in which bladder expression would be required. Bladder palpation is the act of feeling the bladder through the abdominal walls. Distension urination occurs when the bladder is overdistended with urine, causing involuntary urination. Millis DL, Levine D, Canine Rehabilitation and Physical Therapy, ed 2, Elsevier, 2014.

64. b The normal systolic blood pressure for a dog is 130–160 mmHg. Bassert JM, Thomas JA, McCurnin's Clinical Textbook for Veterinary Technicians, ed 8, Elsevier, St. Louis, 2014.

65. c 15 mL = 1 tbsp. 5 mL = 1 tsp. 30 mL = 1 oz. 240 mL = 1 cup. Wanamaker BP, Massey KL, "Practical Calculation," Applied Pharmacology for Veterinary Technicians, ed 5, Elsevier Saunders, 2015.

66. a The cerebrum is responsible for higher functions of the brain, such as learning, memory, and interpretation of sensory input (e.g., vision and pain recognition). The thalamus serves as a relay center for sensory impulses from the spinal cord, brainstem, and cerebellum to the cerebrum. The thalamus may also be involved in pain interpretation. The hypothalamus serves as the primary mediator between the nervous system and the endocrine system through its control of the pituitary gland. The hypothalamus also controls and regulates the ANS. The medulla carries both sensory and motor impulses between the spinal cord and the brain. It contains centers that control vital physiologic activities, such as breathing, heartbeat, blood pressure, vomiting, swallowing, coughing, body temperature, hunger, and thirst. The reticular formation is a network of nerve cells scattered through bundles of fibers that begin in the medulla and extend upward through the brainstem. The reticular activating system is a part of the reticular formation, which functions to arouse the cerebral cortex and is responsible for consciousness, sleep, and wakefulness. Wanamaker BP, Massey KL, "Drugs Used in Nervous System Disorders," Applied Pharmacology for Veterinary Technicians, ed 5, Elsevier Saunders, 2015.

67. b Nosocomial infections are one of the most common complications with urinary catheterization. Because of this, the catheter is disinfected periodically after placement, the prepuce or vulva is disinfected before placement, and strict aseptic technique is required when handling any part of the urinary catheter and collection set. Periodic checking for continued proper placement is also required because dislodgment of the catheter is not uncommon. Millis DL, Levine D, Canine Rehabilitation and Physical Therapy, ed 2, Elsevier, 2014.

68. b Permanent canines and premolars erupt at about 4 to 6 months of age. Adult incisors appear at 3 to 5 months. Adult molars appear at 5 to 7 months. Holzman G, "The basics," in Perrone JR, ed, Small Animal Dental Procedures for Veterinary Technicians and Nurses, Wiley-Blackwell, 2013, p. 3-22.

69. a The wall of each alveolus is composed of the thinnest epithelium in the body—simple squamous epithelium. The capillaries that surround the alveoli are also composed of simple squamous epithelium, Therefore, the main physical barriers between the air in the alveoli and the blood in the capillaries are the thin epithelium of the alveolus and the adjacent, equally thin epithelium of the capillaries. These two thin layers allow oxygen and carbon dioxide to diffuse freely back and forth between the air and the blood. Colville T, Bassert JM, Clinical Anatomy and Physiology for Veterinary Technicians ed 3, Elsevier , 2015.

70. b Physiologic pain is a protective sensation of pain that allows individuals to move away from potential tissue damage. Physiologic pain can be beneficial in that it can allow the animal to avoid damaging stimuli. Pathologic pain results from tissue or nerve damage and may be further classified according to its origin, severity, or duration. Visceral pain arises from hollow abdominal organs, peritoneum, heart, liver, and lungs, whereas somatic pain arises from the musculoskeletal system. Somatic pain may be further described as superficial (arising from the skin) or deep (arising from periosteum, tendon, or joint tissues). Neuropathic pain can arise as a result of injury to the peripheral or central nervous system and it is described in humans as burning or shooting. Pain can have varying degrees of severity (none, mild, moderate, or severe) and may be acute or chronic. Wanamaker BP, Massey KL, "Drugs Used to Relieve Pain and Inflammation," Applied Pharmacology for Veterinary Technicians, ed 5, Elsevier Saunders, 2015.

71. a The nursing process is the act of collecting patient data, identifying and prioritizing patient problems to be addressed, developing a nursing plan, implementing interventions, and assessing the treatment's effectiveness. This cycle is repeated as the veterinary technician continues to work with a patient. Physical examination is only the initial portion of this process. Patient treatment is the intervention for problems. Diagnosis is a veterinarian task that involves determining the ailment the patient is experiencing. Bassert JM, Thomas JA, McCurnin's Clinical Textbook for Veterinary Technicians, ed 8, Elsevier, St. Louis, 2014.

72. a Brachy means short and cephalic means relating to the head. Collies are described as being dolichocephalic (long head), whereas a retriever is a typical example of a mesaticephalic/mesocephalic breed (medium head). Prognacephalic is a made-up word. Holzman G, "The basics," in Perrone JR, ed, Small Animal Dental Procedures for Veterinary Technicians and Nurses, Wiley-Blackwell, 2013, p. 3-22.

73. b Colloid solutions are used for expansion of the plasma volume in the treatment of patients with hypovolemia not caused by dehydration, septic shock, or hypoalbuminemia. Colloids are useful in treating patients prone to edema because smaller fluid volumes are required for effective treatment. Hetastarch (hydroxyethyl starch) is a large molecular weight starch and a colloid solution. Dextrose 5% in water, lactated Ringer solution, and Normosol R are all examples of crystalloid solutions. Wanamaker BP, Massey KL, "Therapeutic Nutritional, Fluid, and Electrolyte Replacements," Applied Pharmacology for Veterinary Technicians, ed 5, Elsevier Saunders, 2015.

74. d Sodium bicarbonate is an alkalizing agent that may be added to correct metabolic acidosis and certain other conditions. Because lactate or acetate in fluid preparations often cannot correct severe metabolic acidosis, supplementation becomes necessary. Potassium chloride is a solution that is used to supplement hypokalemia. Calcium gluconate or calcium chloride is given as an intravenous infusion to correct hypocalcemia. Wanamaker BP, Massey KL, "Therapeutic Nutritional, Fluid, and Electrolyte Replacements," Applied Pharmacology for Veterinary Technicians, ed 5, Elsevier Saunders, 2015.

75. b Azotemia is defined as an increase in serum creatinine and blood urea nitrogen, seen with kidney disease. Anemia is a reduction of red blood cell mass. Hypoproteinemia is a reduction of total protein. Isosthenuria is when the urine specific gravity is neither high nor low. Bassert JM, Thomas JA, McCurnin's Clinical Textbook for Veterinary Technicians, ed 8, Elsevier, St. Louis, 2014.

76. b When assessing jaw length, we should understand the meaning of the word brachygnathism. Brachy refers to short and gnath means jaw. Prognathism: pro refers to projecting forward. Mesaticephalic: mesati refers to medium, and cephalic means relating to the head. Dolichocephalic–dolico refers to long and narrow. Holzman G, "The basics," in Perrone JR, ed, Small Animal Dental Procedures for Veterinary Technicians and Nurses, Wiley-Blackwell, 2013, p. 3-22.

77. c The green electrode is attached to the right hind limb, the white electrode is attached to the right forelimb, the black electrode is attached to the left forelimb, and the red electrode is attached to the left hind limb. Summers A, "Diseases of the Cardiovascular System," Common Diseases of Companion Animals, ed 3, Elsevier, 2014.

78. b Clinical signs of saddle thrombus in cats include acute onset of rear leg pain and paresis, cold, bluish footpads resulting from decreased circulation, and a lack of palpable pulses in the rear limbs. Thrombus formation is a common and serious complication of myocardial disease in cats. Thrombi develop in the left side of the heart, which may dislodge and become trapped elsewhere in the arterial system. Approximately 90% of these emboli lodge as saddle thrombi in the distal aortic trifurcation, resulting in hind-limb pain and paresis. Summers A, "Diseases of the Cardiovascular System," Common Diseases of Companion Animals, ed 3, Elsevier, 2014.

79. c Colostrum is rich in immunoglobulins and absorption of immunoglobulins through the gastrointestinal system of the neonate is required before gut closure occurs, which prevents absorption of whole proteins beyond this initial stage. Bassert JM, Thomas JA, McCurnin's Clinical Textbook for Veterinary Technicians, ed 8, Elsevier, St. Louis, 2014.

80. b Stoma is Greek for a mouth-like opening and -itis means inflammation. Halitosis is bad breath that can be noticed when periodontal disease is present. Tooth resorption results in the loss of tooth structure after activity of the odontoclasts in the tooth. Inflammation and infection of the periodontal support tissues indicate periodontal disease. Baker L, "Stomatitis," in Blackwell's Five-Minute Veterinary Consult Clinical Companion: Small Animal Dentistry, ed 2, Wiley-Blackwell, 2012, p. 237-242; Gorrel C, Derbyshire S, Common oral and dental conditions," in Veterinary Dentistry for the Nurse and Technician, Butterworth-Heinemann, 2009, p. 87-107.

81. b The duodenum is the first portion of the small intestine that exits the stomach and leads to the jejunum. The pylorus is the opening between the stomach and the duodenum. The serosa is the third layer of the stomach wall. The cecum is located at the beginning of the large intestine. Summers A, "Diseases of the Digestive System," Common Diseases of Companion Animals, ed 3, Elsevier, 2014.

82. d Some animals with liver disease may develop bleeding tendencies because of vitamin K malabsorption. Vitamin K requires bile acids for absorption. Jaundice may develop as the disease progresses and is common in chronic liver damage. Common clinical signs of heart disease include coughing, pulmonary edema, and ascites. Common clinical signs of intestinal disease include vomiting and/or diarrhea. Common clinical signs of kidney disease include oliguria, polyuria, anorexia, and dehydration. Summers A, "Diseases of the Digestive System," Common Diseases of Companion Animals, ed 3, Elsevier, 2014.

83. b Gut closure, or closing of absorptive pores, allowing immunoglobulin G and immunoglobulin A molecules through the gastrointestinal system occurs within 16 hours in kittens and 24 hours in puppies. Consumption of colostrum before gut closure is very important to augment the immune system neonatally. Bassert JM, Thomas JA, McCurnin's Clinical Textbook for Veterinary Technicians, ed 8, Elsevier, St. Louis, 2014.

84. a D5W is a hypotonic fluid that is the least useful. It is oxidized to CO_2 and H_2O, providing free water and it should be used in the face of a free-water deficit or hypernatremia. Plasma-Lyte 48 is an isotonic crystalloid and will provide rapid intravascular volume expansion. Hypertonic saline is a hypertonic crystalloid and Hetastarch is a colloid. Both will expand vascular volume and are useful in patients that will not tolerate a large volume of fluids (head trauma, heart failure). Bassert JM, Thomas JA, McCurnin's Clinical Textbook for Veterinary Technicians, ed 8, Elsevier, St. Louis, 2014, p. 883-885.

85. c Animals with leptospirosis might pose a health risk for humans and other animals. Infected animals should be isolated and anyone handling them should wear protective clothing and practice strict hygiene. Laboratory technicians should take care when handling fluids. The urine of animals with leptospirosis should be considered infectious. Cholangiohepatitis, infectious canine hepatitis, and toxin-induced liver disease are not known to be zoonotic. Summers A, "Diseases of the Digestive System," Common Diseases of Companion Animals, ed 3, Elsevier, 2014.

86. c The use of complicated terminology or jargon may be a hindrance in the communication process. A veterinary technician's role can be a vital bridge between a veterinary surgeon and the client. Often a client does not want to ask the vet to repeat what he or she has said, especially if the client does not understand the vet's use of a lot of specialized terminology. It is often the technician's role to interpret to the client what the vet has said. It is also important to avoid using complicated jargon; if it is necessary, take a moment to explain what the terms mean in plain English. Repeating what was said using the same terms does not help the client to understand. Having the client look up terms in a dictionary would not be good client service. The Internet is full of incorrect information; veterinary professionals should use great care in suggesting clients consult Dr. Google! Aspinall V, "The Art of Communication," The Complete Textbook of Veterinary Nursing, ed 2, Saunders Elsevier, 2011.

87. a All of these choices are true in neonates. However, the only point that affects consideration for drug dosing is the liver. Neonates have reduced hepatic metabolism of drugs and less albumin production, both relating to a necessity to reduce the drug dosage. Bassert JM, Thomas JA, McCurnin's Clinical Textbook for Veterinary Technicians, ed 8, Elsevier, St. Louis, 2014.

88. a Diazepam is a benzodiazepine and is considered the drug of choice for treating seizures in both dogs and cats. It is considered a first-line drug, whereas pentobarbital is a second-line drug, and propofol is a third. Potassium bromide is a maintenance drug and is not used as an emergency treatment for status epilepticus. Silverstein D, Hopper K, Small Animal Critical Care Medicine, ed 1, Elsevier, p. 417-418, 794.

89. c A cathode is a negatively charged electrode that produces electrons in the x-ray tube. Anodes are positively charged electrodes within the x-ray tube that consist of a tungsten target that produce x-rays when hit with electrons from the cathode. An artifact is a structure or feature not normally present, but visible, that diminishes the quality of a radiograph. A collimator is a device on an x-ray machine that is used to restrict the x-ray beam to reduce scatter. Sirois M, "Diagnostic Imaging," Principles and Practice of Veterinary Technology, ed 3, Elsevier, 2011.

90. a The mAs is a product of the milliamperage and the exposure time. The milliamperage controls the number of electrons in the electron cloud generated at the filament of the cathode. Controlling the temperature of the cathode filament does this. The kilovoltage peak (kVp) is the voltage applied between the cathode and the anode. It is used to accelerate electrons flowing from the cathode toward the anode side. Increasing the kVp increases the positive charge on the anode. This causes the electrons to move faster, increasing the force of the collision with the target. Source image distance (SID) is the distance from the target to the recording surface (film). For most radiographic procedures, this distance is held constant, around 36 to 40 inches. The object-image distance (OID) is the distance from the object being imaged to the recording surface (film or digital recording plate). This distance should be as short as possible to minimize the penumbra effect and the magnification that occurs with a long OID. Sirois M, "Diagnostic Imaging," Principles and Practice of Veterinary Technology, ed 3, Elsevier, 2011.

91. a Blood type for cats is governed by the AB system and an individual can be of type A, B, or AB. A secondary antigen called Mik has also been described. DEA 1 is a canine blood type, Q is an equine blood type, and Tr is a canine blood type of nonstandard nomenclature. Bassert JM, Thomas JA, McCurnin's Clinical Textbook for Veterinary Technicians, ed 8, Elsevier, 2014.

92. d Palpation is the act of using one's hands and fingers to feel anatomical features to determine the presence of any abnormalities. Centrifugation is a process of using centrifugal force to separate dense from less dense matter in fluid. Mentation is the assessment of a patient's alertness to assess nervous system function. Auscultation is the act of using a stethoscope to listen to organs of the body. Battaglia AM, Steele AM, Small Animal Emergency and Critical Care for Veterinary Technicians, ed 3, Elsevier, 2016.

93. c A tension pneumothorax occurs when air is able to enter the pleural space but is unable to escape (it has been compared to a one-way valve that allows air in but it is not able to allow air to exit). Pressure builds up in the pleural space and after that pressure becomes greater than atmospheric pressure, the patient is unable to expand the lungs. A tension pneumothorax will not resolve without a thoracocentesis to remove air from the pleural space. Battaglia AM, Small Animal Emergency and Critical Care for Veterinary Medicine, ed 2, Elsevier, 2007, p. 266.

94. b Hydrocarbons, such as fuels, solvents, etc., are life-threatening because of the possibility of aspiration pneumonia. Aspiration can occur when the substance is ingested or when the patient vomits. Because of this risk, inducing emesis is contraindicated. The less viscous (thinner) a hydrocarbon is, the more likely it is to be aspirated. The lungs are very vulnerable to hydrocarbons and aspiration of less than 1 mL can lead to death. Emesis is beneficial when a patient has ingested organophosphates (pesticides, insecticides), salicylates (aspirin), and anticholinergics (commonly found in medications). Peterson ME, Talcott PA, Small Animal Toxicology, ed 2, Elsevier, 2006, p. 128-129.

95. b Septic shock occurs when there is a circulatory failure secondary to sepsis. Early in septic shock, there is a hyperdynamic response (tachycardia, vasodilation, fever, and bounding pulses) causing hyperemic (red) mucous membranes. Icteric (yellow) mucous membranes are caused by an excessive amount of bilirubin in the blood. Bilirubin increases with liver disease or the breakdown of RBCs. Pale mucous membranes are seen when there is vasoconstriction or a decrease in perfusion (both of which decrease blood flow to the membranes) or anemia. Cyanosis (blue mucous membranes) is seen when hemoglobin is not carrying oxygen. This deoxygenated hemoglobin causes the blood to be blue. To detect cyanosis, there must be more than 5 g/dL of deoxygenated hemoglobin present in the blood (5 g/dL is equivalent to a PCV of 15%). Cyanosis is not detectable in a patient that is severely anemic and cannot be relied on to indicate hypoxemia. Bassert JM, Thomas JA, McCurnin's Clinical Textbook for Veterinary Technicians, ed 8, Elsevier, 2014, p. 675; Bonagura JD, Twedt DC, Kirk's Current Veterinary Therapy XV, Elsevier, 2014, p. 52.

96. b A patient with diarrhea of unknown causes should always be treated as a possible source of infection. Always suspect an infectious disease if no diagnosis has been made or while diagnostic tests are being performed. It is likely that the kennel occupied by a patient with diarrhea will require regular cleaning and disinfection and management of this task should therefore be considered. Infectious diseases that may have diarrhea as a clinical sign include canine parvovirus and feline infectious enteritis. Diseases that are also zoonotic include campylobacteriosis and salmonellosis. If an infectious disease is suspected, barrier nursing should be maintained throughout the patient's stay. Aspinall V, "Medical Nursing Procedures," Clinical Procedures in Veterinary Nursing, ed 3, Butterworth-Heinemann, 2014.

97. d When liquids must be administered with a syringe or dropper, the muzzle should be held at a neutral angle and not elevated. Hyperextension of the neck or movement by the patient during administration may result in fluid aspiration into the trachea. If the patient struggles or coughs or if fluid spills out of the mouth, the patient should be allowed to rest before further administration attempts are made. Holding the patient's neck at a downward angle would easily allow the liquid to spill out of the mouth. Aspinall V, "Medical Nursing Procedures," Clinical Procedures in Veterinary Nursing, ed 3, Butterworth-Heinemann, 2014.

98. c Propofol does not cross the placental barrier, therefore it is the safest induction agent in regard to fetuses. Etomidate crosses the placental barrier, but it is eliminated quickly and it might therefore be a good second choice if the bitch cannot tolerate propofol. Diazepam and thiopental cross the placental barrier and have adverse effects on neonates. Thomas JA, Lerche P, Anesthesia and Analgesia for Veterinary Technicians, ed 4, Mosby Elsevier, 2011, p. 73, 83.

99. a The most common cause of feline aortic thromboembolism is cardiomyopathy. The turbulent blood flow seen with cardiomyopathy causes the formation of thrombi. This clot (or pieces of a clot) breaks free, travels through the circulatory system, and becomes lodged in the distal aorta where it causes an aortic thromboembolism. This is commonly known as a saddle thrombosis and causes loss of the use of one, or both, hind limbs. Common clinical signs include acute loss of motor in the hind legs, loss of femoral and/or dorsal pedal pulses, and cyanotic pads or toenail beds. Because it is cardiac in origin, the liver, renal, and respiratory systems do not apply. Bass Bassert JM, Thomas JA, McCurnin's Clinical Textbook for Veterinary Technicians, ed 8, Elsevier, 2014, p. 688; Battaglia AM, Small Animal Emergency and Critical Care for Veterinary Medicine, ed 2, Elsevier, 2007, p. 257-259.

100. d Gathering patient data starts with taking immediate history and description of the patient's complaint from the owner. The past medical history should be consulted to learn of any preexisting conditions or past illnesses. The physical examination should be performed thoroughly, evaluating the patient in a systematic manner each time. The veterinarians should be consulted to ask questions that might not be answered by the medical record. Bassert JM, Thomas JA, McCurnin's Clinical Textbook for Veterinary Technicians, ed 8, Elsevier, 2014.

101. d Mannitol is an osmotic diuretic that decreases intracranial pressure by reducing blood viscosity. This allows an increase in blood flow (and thus an increase in oxygen delivery) to the brain as well as causing a decrease in the water content of the brain. Atropine is an anticholinergic used to treat bradycardia, as a preanesthetic, or as an antidote for organophosphate toxicity. Diazepam is a benzodiazepine used for sedation, muscle relaxation, or treatment of seizure activity. Dexamethasone is a glucocorticoid that is often used to decrease inflammation. However, it is contraindicated in head trauma and should never be administered as often as every 4–6 hours. Silverstein D, Hopper K, Small Animal Critical Care Medicine, ed 1, Elsevier, p. 427-428.

102. c Tubes should be measured to the 13th rib to pass into the stomach. The thoracic inlet is the landmark for endotracheal intubation. The 8th rib is the landmark if the tube is to end in the distal esophagus. The medial canthus is the landmark used when placing a nasal oxygen cannula. Bassert JM, Thomas JA, "Chapter 18, Diagnostic Sampling and Therapeutic Techniques," McCurnin's Clinical Textbook for Veterinary Technicians, ed 8, Elsevier, 2014.

103. c Transdermal drugs are delivered via absorption through the skin, such as in a patch or cream. A diuretic is a drug (not a delivery method) that increases the rate of urine output. Emetics are agents (not a delivery method) used to induce vomiting. Viscus is defined as any large internal organ (i.e., the intestines) in any of the body cavities and has nothing to do with drug delivery. Bassert JM, Thomas JA, "Chapter 18, Diagnostic Sampling and Therapeutic Techniques," McCurnin's Clinical Textbook for Veterinary Technicians, ed 8, Elsevier, 2014.

104. a The most life-threatening problem should be treated first. In this scenario, the dyspneic patient should be seen first. Respiratory distress or dyspnea can quickly worsen and may even turn into respiratory arrest. It is always treated first. Proptosis, laceration, and dystocia can be serious emergencies but are not immediately life-threatening conditions. Bassert JM, Thomas JA, McCurnin's Clinical Textbook for Veterinary Technicians, ed 8, Elsevier, 2014, p. 908-911.

105. c First-intention healing occurs when the edges of a wound are brought together and closed with sutures or staples. This can be done with a laceration. A degloving wound is usually too extensive to close without performing daily bandage changes for several days until the tissue has developed a bed of granulation tissue. After this has occurred, the wound can be closed. This is referred to as third-intention healing. An abscess or puncture wound can be cleaned, flushed, and then left to heal with no closure, or second-intention healing. Aspinall V, "Table 8.1," Clinical Procedures in Veterinary Nursing, ed 3, Butterworth-Heinemann, 2014; Sirois M, Principles and Practice of Veterinary Technology, ed 3, Elsevier, 2011, p. 312.

106. c Intravenous administration is the most effective route of delivery, with a catheter in the jugular vein being most desirable. Intracardiac delivery should be avoided because of the possibility of causing cardiac arrhythmias or damage to the heart and lungs. Administering medications through the e-tube (intratracheal) is appropriate, but it is not as effective as intravenous administration. It is important to keep in mind that sodium bicarbonate cannot be administered via the trachea. Intraosseous is another possibility in small animals; however, this route will be inaccessible in larger animals and is contraindicated in those with sepsis or if there is an infection present in the area of the insertion site. Silverstein D, Hopper K, Small Animal Critical Care Medicine, ed 1, Elsevier, p. 16-18.

107. d The subcutaneous (SC) injection is easily and frequently performed and is the most common route for administering vaccines, isotonic fluids, and some types of antibiotics. With the exception of delayed absorption in obese animals, the SC route for injection offers relatively rapid absorption rates for most injectables; however, it is the slowest absorbed route of those listed previously. The SC route is not recommended in severely dehydrated or critically ill patients when immediate absorption is required. In an emergency situation, the IV or intraosseous route provides much faster absorption. The IV route is preferred when large volumes of fluid must be administered. If an extremely rapid onset of action is required, the intravenous or intraosseous route is chosen. Medications administered by intramuscular injection are not absorbed as quickly as those given via the intravenous or intraosseous route. Bassert JM, Thomas JA, "Chapter 18, Diagnostic Sampling and Therapeutic Techniques," McCurnin's Clinical Textbook for Veterinary Technicians, ed 8, Elsevier, 2014.

108. c Current recommendations from RECOVER (Reassessment Campaign on Veterinary Resuscitation) are for chest compressions to be performed at a rate of 100–120 (compressions per minute) on any size, age, or species. Recover web site: http://onlinelibrary.wiley.com/doi/10.1111/vec.2012.22.issue-s1/issuetoc.

109. d Lipemia manifests as turbid, white serum from increased triglyceride level. Icterus manifests as yellow-to-orange serum caused by increased bilirubin levels in serum. Hemolyzed serum manifests is red because of increased hemoglobin levels in serum. Hyperproteinemia results in increased total protein readings and when severe, presents as yellow fluid with high viscosity, such as with feline infectious peritonitis. Battaglia AM, Steele AM, Small Animal Emergency and Critical Care for Veterinary Technicians, ed 3, Elsevier, 2016.

110. b Both packed cell volume and total protein increase with dehydration because it leads to loss of intravascular plasma volume and concentration of red cells and proteins. A low packed cell volume indicates anemia. Patients suffering from hemorrhaging can exhibit normal-to-decreased packed cell volume and total protein depending on the chronicity. Packed cell volume and total protein is often used as a measure of effectiveness of blood transfusions. Battaglia AM, Steele AM, Small Animal Emergency and Critical Care for Veterinary Technicians, ed 3, Elsevier, 2016.

111. c Pressure applied at the area adjacent and ventral to the mandible will allow control of maxillary blood flow and hemorrhage to the head. The temporomandibular joint is the area where the jaw hinges and applying pressure to this area will not stop hemorrhage to the head. By applying pressure to one or both jugular grooves, you will prevent venous drainage from the head and may actually cause an increase in hemorrhage. This may also increase intracranial pressure, which should be avoided in any patient with possible head trauma. Battaglia AM, Small Animal Emergency and Critical Care for Veterinary Medicine, ed 2, Elsevier, 2007, p. 206.

112. d Only veterinarians may legally prescribe medications. Technicians do not prescribe medications. Technician assessment is defined as the clinical judgment that the veterinary technician makes regarding the physiologic needs and psychological problems of a patient. Technician evaluations are conclusions drawn from patient assessment and analysis of the database related to the animal's (or the owner's) physical and psychological response to a veterinary medical condition. Technician intervention is the third phase of the veterinary technician practice model and is an action planned and implemented by the veterinary technician using independent critical thinking to address a patient's reaction to illness and risk of future problems, as well as owner knowledge deficits. Typically, a technician intervention is performed to address each of the technician's evaluations. Bassert JM, Thomas JA, "Chapter 19, Small Animal Medical Nursing," McCurnin's Clinical Textbook for Veterinary Technicians, ed 8, Elsevier, 2014.

113. c A calorie is a very small unit, which is not of practical use in the science of animal nutrition. The kilocalorie (kcal) is a commonly used unit of measure. One kcal is equal to 1000 calories. Case LP, Daristotle L, Hayek MG, Raasch MF, "Energy and Water," Canine and Feline Nutrition: A Resource for Companion Animal Professionals, ed 3, Mosby, 2011.

114. b In cases in which large volumes of fluids are contraindicated (head trauma, congestive heart failure), hypertonic saline will provide intravascular volume expansion with a small volume. Hypertonic saline will pull fluid from the interstitial space into the vascular space. Because dehydrated patients are already deficient in fluid in the interstitial space and hypertonic saline pulls fluid from here, it will worsen dehydration and should not be used in these patients. DiBartola SP, Fluid, Electrolyte, and Acid-Base Disorders in Small Animal Practice, ed 4, Elsevier, p. 568.

115. b Petechiae, or pinpoint bruising of the tissue surfaces, and ecchymoses, or wide bruised areas on the tissue surfaces, indicate dysfunction of coagulation mechanisms. Anemia can result from bleeding disorders, although not always present with the two signs. Dehydration is related to fluid balance and is unrelated to petechiae and ecchymoses. Hypertension is an elevation of the blood pressure, which is also unrelated. Battaglia AM, Steele AM, Small Animal Emergency and Critical Care for Veterinary Technicians, ed 3, Elsevier, 2016.

116. c Cranial nerve X is the vagus nerve. Stimulation of this nerve will increase vagal tone, causing bradycardia. Cranial nerve I is the olfactory nerve, which transmits smell. Cranial nerve XII is the hypoglossal nerve, which controls the tongue and geniohyoid muscles. Cranial nerve IV is the trochlear nerve, which controls the dorsal oblique muscles of the eye. Stimulation of these last three nerves will not cause bradycardia. Colville TP, Bassert JM, Clinical Anatomy and Physiology for Veterinary Technicians, ed 2, Elsevier, p. 327-328.

117. a Arginine is an essential amino acid. Alanine, asparagine, and aspartate are nonessential amino acids. Case LP, Daristotle L, Hayek MG, Raasch MF, “Protein and Amino Acids,” Canine and Feline Nutrition: A Resource for Companion Animal Professionals, ed 3, Mosby, 2011.

118. d Tyrosine is a nonessential amino acid. Histidine, isoleucine, and methionine are essential amino acids. Case LP, Daristotle L, Hayek MG, Raasch MF, “Protein and Amino Acids,” Canine and Feline Nutrition: A Resource for Companion Animal Professionals, ed 3, Mosby, 2011.

119. b Epistaxis (blood coming from the nose) can indicate head trauma or hemorrhage in the respiratory tract. If this occurs, the patient should be allowed to breathe through his mouth or to pant. Tying the mouth shut will prevent this. The good Samaritan should be told to watch for aggression, apply pressure to any wounds (if possible), and transport the dog on a board (again, if possible). Battaglia AM, Small Animal Emergency and Critical Care for Veterinary Medicine, ed 2, Elsevier, 2007, p. 350.

120. b The most common reason for peripheral edema is hypoproteinemia, and specifically reduction of albumin, which reduces the colloid osmotic pressure of plasma, leading to effusion of fluid into the tissues. Coagulation disorders can occur because of a loss of coagulation proteins, but they do not cause edema readily. Hypotension can occur as a result of reduced colloid osmotic pressure but is not directly related to edema. Hypoxia can result from hypotension, but it is not directly related to edema. Battaglia AM, Steele AM, Small Animal Emergency and Critical Care for Veterinary Technicians, ed 3, Elsevier, 2016.

121. a The CVP measures the heart’s ability to pump the blood that returns from the body. The higher the CVP, the less able the heart is to pump the blood forward. Although the normal CVP varies depending on the patient’s condition, a healthy, normally hydrated patient has a CVP between 0 and 5 cm H_2O. A CVP of 5–10 cm H_2O indicates borderline hypervolemia, whereas a CVP >10 cm H_2O indicates fluid overload. Ford RB, Mazzaferro EM, Kirk and Bistner’s Handbook of Veterinary Procedures and Emergency Treatment, ed 9, Elsevier, 2011, p. 30-31.

122. c Vitamin C is a water-soluble vitamin. Vitamins A, E, and K are fat-soluble vitamins. Case LP, Daristotle L, Hayek MG, Raasch MF, “Vitamins,” Canine and Feline Nutrition: A Resource for Companion Animal Professionals, ed 3, Mosby, 2011.

123. b Deficiency in vitamin D causes rickets. Deficiency in vitamin A and E may cause reproductive failure. Deficiency in vitamin K is a cause of increased clotting time. Case LP, Daristotle L, Hayek MG, Raasch MF, “Vitamins,” Canine and Feline Nutrition: A Resource for Companion Animal Professionals, ed 3, Mosby, 2011.

124. b Normal urine output of a patient on intravenous fluids is 1–2 mL/kg/h. Urine output <0.5 mL/kg/h is considered anuria. Urine output between 0.5 mL/kg/h and 1 mL/kg/h is considered oliguria. Urine output >2 mL/kg/h is considered polyuria. Silverstein D, Hopper K, Small Animal Critical Care Medicine, ed 1, Elsevier, p. 31; Sirois M, Principles and Practice of Veterinary Technology, ed 3, Elsevier, 2011, p. 417.

125. a Auscultation of the ventral side of the abdomen should indicate borborygmus or gurgling made by fluid and gas moving along the gastrointestinal tract. A lack of these sounds indicates gastric motility impairment. Crackles are abnormal lung sounds heard when pulmonary edema is present. Stertor is a snorting sort of breathing noise often heard with brachycephalic animals. Battaglia AM, Steele AM, Small Animal Emergency and Critical Care for Veterinary Technicians, ed 3, Elsevier, 2016.

126. a The CVP measures the right ventricular end diastolic pressure and the heart’s ability to pump blood forward. Anything that decreases this ability will also increase the CVP. Cardiogenic shock occurs when there is a decrease in the contractility of the heart. This decrease in contractility prevents the heart from pumping blood forward. In this type of shock, the CVP will be elevated. Hypovolemic shock is supported by a decrease in the CVP because the decrease in vascular volume will decrease the right ventricular end diastolic pressure. Distributive shock is a result of an inability of the body to cause vasoconstriction in response to a decrease in blood volume or tissue perfusion. In this case, the CVP may be normal (if the blood volume is normal) or decreased (if the blood volume is low). Septic shock also causes vasodilation and the CVP will be normal because the heart is still able to pump blood forward. DiBartola SP, Fluid, Electrolyte, and

Acid-Base Disorders in Small Animal Practice, ed 4, Elsevier, p. 559-561.

127. c Vitamin C is the one vitamin that can be synthesized from glucose by dogs and cats; humans, however, must receive vitamin C from dietary sources. Dogs and cats must receive vitamins A, B6, and K in their diets and they are not able to synthesize these vitamins. Case LP, Daristotle L, Hayek MG, Raasch MF, "Vitamins," Canine and Feline Nutrition: A Resource for Companion Animal Professionals, ed 3, Mosby, 2011.

128. b Ergocalciferol is vitamin D2. Thiamin is also referred to as vitamin B1. Pyridoxine vitamin is B6. Cobalamin is vitamin B12. Case LP, Daristotle L, Hayek MG, Raasch MF, "Vitamins," Canine and Feline Nutrition: A Resource for Companion Animal Professionals, ed 3, Mosby, 2011.

129. d Septic shock occurs when sepsis has caused hypotension that is unresponsive to fluid therapy. Hypoglycemia occurs because inflammatory mediators, hypotension, and hypovolemia all combine to cause a decreased intake, decreased production, and increased use of glucose. Hypoglycemia is rarely seen with anaphylactic, cardiogenic, or neurogenic shock unless there is an underlying cause. Silverstein D, Hopper K, Small Animal Critical Care Medicine, ed 1, Elsevier, p. 298, 459.

130. c An esophageal stethoscope is most useful when monitoring anesthetized patients, allowing the passage of the device into the esophagus. While it is inserted into the esophagus, it has very little use in evaluating esophageal abnormalities such as megaesophagus. Detection of ileus is performed by abdominal auscultation, which an esophageal stethoscope will not accomplish. Routine physical examinations involve alert and awake patients, which make esophageal stethoscopes difficult to use without harm. Battaglia AM, Steele AM, Small Animal Emergency and Critical Care for Veterinary Technicians, ed 3, Elsevier, 2016.

131. b Total bilirubin is used to evaluate liver function. Elevated lipase and amylase would be significant findings for a patient with pancreatitis. Kidney function is evaluated by BUN, creatinine, and phosphorus. Bile duct obstruction can cause an elevation in total bilirubin, but a total bilirubin test would not be used primarily to determine bile duct health. If a possible obstruction is suspected, an abdominal ultrasound or other imaging technique is the primary diagnostic. Tighe MM, Brown M, Mosby's Comprehensive Review for Veterinary Technicians, ed 4, Mosby Elsevier, 2015, p. 82.

132. c Copper deficiency is known to cause anemia. Deficiencies in calcium or phosphorus may cause rickets. Deficiencies in zinc are known to cause dermatoses. Case LP, Daristotle L, Hayek MG, Raasch MF, "Minerals," Canine and Feline Nutrition: A Resource for Companion Animal Professionals, ed 3, Mosby, 2011.

133. d Zinc is a trace mineral. Macrominerals include calcium, phosphorus, magnesium, sulfur, iron, and the electrolytes sodium, potassium, and chloride. Case LP, Daristotle L, Hayek MG, Raasch MF, "Minerals," Canine and Feline Nutrition: A Resource for Companion Animal Professionals, ed 3, Mosby, 2011.

134. b Nosocomial is defined as pertaining to or originating in a hospital. Endemic disease presents in a predictable and continuous pattern in a community. Iatrogenic disease results from the activity of the veterinarian, or from any adverse condition in a patient that results from treatment by a veterinarian. Studdert VP, Gay CC, Blood DC, Saunders Comprehensive Veterinary Dictionary, ed 4, Elsevier Saunders, 2007, p. 768.

135. a Dogs are sensitive to and show preferences for sweet foods. Studies have shown that one of the two receptor genes known to encode for the sweet taste receptors in taste buds is not expressed in cats. This is one of the reasons that theobromine toxicity, as a result of chocolate ingestion, is a more commonly seen in dogs than in cats. Case LP, Daristotle L, Hayek MG, Raasch MF, "Digestion and Absorbtion," Canine and Feline Nutrition: A Resource for Companion Animal Professionals, ed 3, Mosby, 2011.

136. c Hypoalbuminemia may result as a loss of protein either through the kidneys or the gastrointestinal tract. Decreased albumin can be seen in liver failure but is not usually seen in chronic liver disease. Decreased albumin is not associated with a carnivore or vegetarian diet. Bassert JM, Thomas JA, McCurnin's Clinical Textbook for Veterinary Technicians, ed 8, Elsevier, 2014, p. 425.

137. c A fever is hyperthermia resulting from inflammatory processes in the body. Responses a and b are hypothermic and normothermic, respectively. The patient in d is experiencing hyperthermia from mechanical and environmental heat accumulation. Answer c is the only patient with hyperthermia with inflammation/infection. Battaglia AM, Steele AM, Small Animal Emergency and Critical Care for Veterinary Technicians, ed 3, Elsevier, 2016.

138. c The pulse pressure is the difference between systolic and diastolic pressure. When bounding pulses are present, it indicates a large difference between the systolic and diastolic pressure. This can occur whether the mean arterial pressure is high or low and it is more likely to occur when diastolic pressure is low. Bounding pulse in itself does not indicate one way or another regarding cardiovascular function. Battaglia AM, Steele AM, Small Animal Emergency and Critical Care for Veterinary Technicians, ed 3, Elsevier, 2016.

139. a Dehydration results in increased urine specific gravity (SG) and increased PCV. With loss of fluid, both the urine and the plasma become more concentrated. Bassert JM, Thomas JA, McCurnin's Clinical Textbook for Veterinary Technicians, ed 8, Elsevier, 2014, p. 875.

140. d In contrast to the small intestine, the primary function of the large intestine (colon) in dogs and cats is the absorption of water and certain electrolytes, especially sodium. Food passes from the mouth to the stomach through the esophagus. The stomach acts as a reservoir for the body, allowing food to be ingested as a meal rather than continuously throughout the day. Before reaching the small intestine, most of the digestive processes that occur in dogs and cats are mechanical in nature. In dogs and cats, the chemical digestion of food is completed in the small intestine. Case LP, Daristotle L, Hayek MG, Raasch MF, "Digestion and Absorbtion," Canine and Feline Nutrition: A Resource for Companion Animal Professionals, ed 3, Mosby, 2011.

141. a Vitamin C is the one vitamin that can be synthesized from glucose by dogs and cats. The domestic cat's requirements include high protein, arachidonic acid, preformed vitamin A, and taurine. Case LP, Daristotle L, Hayek MG, Raasch MF, "Nutritional Idiosyncrasies of the Cat," Canine and Feline Nutrition: A Resource for Companion Animal Professionals, ed 3, Mosby, 2011.

142. d Ketones are produced as a result of the breakdown of fatty acids. Because diabetic patients cannot normally use glucose, they obtain their energy from the breakdown of fatty acids. Liver disease, urinary tract infections, and renal failure are not associated with ketonuria. Sirois M, Hendrix CM, Laboratory Procedures for Veterinary Technicians, ed 6, Mosby Elsevier, 2015, p. 167.

143. c The oscillometric device is a machine that senses pressure oscillations on a cuff and uses an algorithm to calculate the blood pressure. A Doppler ultrasound can be used to detect arterial pulses for manual blood pressure measurement. Direct blood pressure measurement is performed through an arterial catheter with a pressure transducer. Stethoscopes are used to auscultate pulses in human medicine. Battaglia AM, Steele AM, Small Animal Emergency and Critical Care for Veterinary Technicians, ed 3, Elsevier, 2016.

144. a Catheter sites are observed at least once a day and they should look clean, with no signs of inflammation or discharge. When redness, swelling, or purulent discharge is noted, it indicates inflammation and infection. Presence of fluid exiting the insertion site or a subcutaneous pocket of fluids indicates catheter leakage. Occluded catheters cannot be flushed. Battaglia AM, Steele AM, Small Animal Emergency and Critical Care for Veterinary Technicians, ed 3, Elsevier, 2016.

145. c In dehydrated patients, fluid leaves the blood to enter the dehydrated tissues, leaving the blood more concentrated. Therefore, total protein levels will be significantly increased. Sirois M, Hendrix CM, Laboratory Procedures for Veterinary Technicians, ed 5, Mosby Elsevier, 2007, p. 32.

146. c Only about 10%–30% of dogs with food allergies have GI problems. Signs are usually cutaneous skin reactions, including skin rashes, ear infections, and pruritus. Tizard I, Veterinary Immunology, ed 9, Elsevier Saunders, 2013.

147. a Current recommendations for feeding critically ill patients are to begin feeding equal to the patient's estimated resting energy requirement. Adding food for additional stress or illness factors, which was often done in the past, is no longer recommended. Wortinger A, Burns K, Nutrition and Disease Management for Veterinary Technicians and Nurses, ed 2, Wiley Blackwell, 2015.

148. c A trace amount of protein may be significant in a patient with chronic renal failure. In kidney disease, excessive amounts of protein enter the glomerular filtrate and are not reabsorbed, resulting in protein in the urine. Diabetes cases may have glucosuria and ketonuria. Hemolytic anemia cases have hematuria and bilirubinuria. If a patient is experiencing an acid-base imbalance, there will be a change in the pH of the urine. Sirois M, Hendrix CM, Laboratory Procedures for Veterinary Technicians, ed 5, Mosby Elsevier, 2007, p. 161.

149. b An arterial blood gas sample is the best source to evaluate blood CO_2 levels. Venous blood is generally used for hematology, chemistry, and organ function tests. Tear M, Small Animal Surgical Nursing, ed 2, Mosby Elsevier, 2012, p. 117.

150. a Factors affecting basal metabolic rate include gender, reproductive status, hormonal status, autonomic nervous system function, body composition, body surface area, nutritional stage, and age. Factors affecting voluntary muscular activity involve exercise, size, and weight of the animal. Factors affecting meal-induced thermogenesis include caloric and nutrient composition of the meal. Factors affecting adaptive thermogenesis include ambient temperature and emotional stress. Case LP, Daristotle L, Hayek MG, Raasch MF, "Energy Balance," Canine and Feline Nutrition: A Resource for Companion Animal Professionals, ed 3, Mosby, 2011.

151. a AAFCO: the Association of American Feed Control Officials sets standards for substantiation claims and nutritional profiles for pet food; however, it has no regulatory authority. Government agencies often mandate AAFCO regulations into law. FDA: the Food and Drug Administration has approval over new ingredients. FTC: the Federal Trade Commission regulates trade and advertising of pet foods. USDA: the United States Department of Agriculture regulates pet food labels and research facilities. Case LP, Daristotle L, Hayek MG, Raasch MF, "History and Regulation of Pet Foods," Canine and Feline Nutrition: A Resource for Companion Animal Professionals, ed 3, Mosby, 2011.

152. b Hypothyroidism can stimulate von Willebrand disease if the dog is already predisposed to von Willebrand disease. A deficiency in von Willebrand factor does not occur secondary to hypothyroidism in dogs without concurrent congenital von Willebrand disease. Hemophilia A, DIC, and coumarin toxicity are not stimulated by hypothyroidism. Bonagura JD, Twedt DC, Kirk's Current Veterinary Therapy XV, Elsevier, 2014, p. 87.

153. c Infected catheters should be removed and an IV catheter replaced in another site. Blood stream infections from catheters can cause fevers, but they should be removed regardless of the presence of fever. The catheter insertion site should be disinfected after the catheter is removed to prevent further bacterial growth, but disinfection should not be considered adequate for continued use. Catheter-related blood stream infections are a serious complication of IV catheters and intervention is required. Battaglia AM, Steele AM, Small Animal Emergency and Critical Care for Veterinary Technicians, ed 3, Elsevier, 2016.

154. c The presence of subcutaneous fluids indicates a catheter that is no longer in the vein or a case in which there is significant leaking out of the vessels. Continuing to use the catheter at the same or reduced rate and checking later will likely lead to more subcutaneously injected fluids. Removing the catheter is most appropriate as the catheter is not useful as an intravenous delivery device. Battaglia AM, Steele AM, Small Animal Emergency and Critical Care for Veterinary Technicians, ed 3, Elsevier, 2016.

155. d Hyperkalemia is commonly associated with hypoadrenocorticism, also known as Addison's disease. Hyperparathyroidism is associated with hypercalcemia. Hyperthyroidism will result in elevated thyroid hormone. Diabetes insipidus usually results in decreased levels of potassium and calcium. Tighe MM, Brown M, Mosby's Comprehensive Review for Veterinary Technicians, ed 4, Mosby Elsevier, 2015, p. 517.

156. d Vomiting is defined as the forceful expulsion of contents from the stomach and the upper small intestine; it is an active process that requires abdominal contraction (retching). Regurgitation is the passive expulsion of material from the mouth, pharynx, or esophagus. Nausea and abdominal contractions are not typically seen. Patients can exhibit difficulty eating (dysphagia), hypersalivation, and gagging. Regurgitated material typically consists of undigested or partially digested food. Patients are at risk for aspiration of stomach contents and development of pneumonia. Cachexia is weight loss, loss of muscle mass, and general debilitation that may accompany chronic disease. Cathartics are medications that through their chemical effects serve to promote the clearing of intestinal contents. Bassert JM, Thomas JA, "Chapter 19, Small Animal Medical Nursing," McCurnin's Clinical Textbook for Veterinary Technicians, ed 8, Elsevier, 2014.

157. a Vomiting fresh or digested blood is termed *hematemesis*. Frank, red blood in feces is hematochezia. Blood in the urine is hematuria. Hemoabdomen is the abnormal accumulation of blood in the abdomen. Bassert JM, Thomas JA, "Chapter 19, Small Animal Medical Nursing," McCurnin's Clinical Textbook for Veterinary Technicians, ed 8, Elsevier, 2014.

158. c Many animals will show no clinical signs of primary hyperparathyroidism; it is usually diagnosed on a routine serum chemistry examination. Therefore, polydipsia/polyuria (PU/PD) is not commonly seen in hyperparathyroidism. In hyperadrenocorticism, diabetes insipidus, and diabetes mellitus, PU/PD is a common clinical sign. Summers A, Common Diseases of Companion Animals, ed 2, Elsevier, 2007, p. 109.

159. a Cats have naturally occurring circulating alloantibodies to the blood type they do not have. Type B cats have high levels of type A antibodies and type A cats have a high number of type B antibodies. Therefore, transfusion of type A blood into a type B cat could result in severe, potentially fatal hemolytic transfusion reaction. Although rare, transfusion reactions in cats are much more severe than those in dogs and may occur with the first transfusion, which does not occur in dogs. Bassert JM, Thomas JA, McCurnin's Clinical Textbook for Veterinary Technicians, ed 8, Elsevier, 2014, p. 898.

160. d Central and peripheral veins and intraosseous routes of administration all directly allow fluids to enter the intravascular space and are effective routes in fluid resuscitation for a 12% dehydrated animal (severe dehydration). Subcutaneous fluids will not swiftly enter the intravascular space, especially because of a lack of intravascular volume and blood flow to the tissues. Battaglia AM, Steele AM, Small Animal Emergency and Critical Care for Veterinary Technicians, ed 3, Elsevier, 2016.

161. d Dehydration causes a loss of volume in the orbit and surrounding tissues, leading to the orbit being sunken into the eye socket. Pinpoint pupils indicate a neurologic issue. Eyes are typically rotated ventrally during heavy sedation or anesthesia. Lateral nystagmus can result in the patient suffering from a nervous system–related ataxia. Battaglia AM, Steele AM, Small Animal Emergency and Critical Care for Veterinary Technicians, ed 3, Elsevier, 2016.

162. d An immediate hypersensitivity reaction is systemic and life-threatening and it is known as an allergic anaphylaxis or anaphylactic shock. Agglutination, hemolysis, and DIC are all life-threatening hematological ailments; however, they are not triggered by an allergy. Tizard I, Veterinary Immunology, ed 9, Elsevier Saunders, 2013, p. 327.

163. d DEA is an acronym for dog erythrocyte antigen. Tighe MM, Brown M, Mosby's Comprehensive Review for Veterinary Technicians, ed 4, Mosby Elsevier, 2015, p. 563.

164. c Hard labor for 30 to 60 minutes with no new young is a form of dystocia. Eclampsia is a condition of hypocalcemia arising from lactation, resulting in muscle spasms, fever, tachycardia, and seizures. Mastitis results in a hard and painful nipple and galactostasis (loss of milk production). Vaginal discharge, vomiting, diarrhea, dehydration, anorexia, polyuria, and polydipsia are all signs of pyometra. Battaglia AM, Steele AM, Small Animal Emergency and Critical Care for Veterinary Technicians, ed 3, Elsevier, 2016.

165. c Passive range of motion is used to keep from joints becoming stiff. Warm compressing is a technique used to increase blood flow to an area to increase draining and healing of the area, such as with mastitis. Coupage is a technique used to help loosen purulent material within the pulmonary parenchyma with pneumonia. Cold compress is used to minimize inflammation. Battaglia AM, Steele AM, Small Animal Emergency and Critical Care for Veterinary Technicians, ed 3, Elsevier, 2016.

166. a Anticoagulant rodenticide poisoning initially prolongs the prothrombin time and factor VII is the first to be depleted. All the other clotting factors continue to be depleted. Coagulation tests would not be used to confirm adrenal or thyroid function or ethylene glycol poisoning. Sirois M, Hendrix CM, Laboratory Procedures for Veterinary Technicians, ed 6, Mosby Elsevier, 2015, p. 230.

167. c Normal frequency of bowel movements is commonly seen in patients with small bowel diarrhea; increased frequency of bowel movements is a common sign of large bowel diarrhea. Decreased volume of feces, mucus in feces, and tenesmus are all common indicators of large bowel diarrhea. Bassert JM, Thomas JA, "Chapter 19, Small Animal Medical Nursing," McCurnin's Clinical Textbook for Veterinary Technicians, ed 8, Elsevier, 2014.

168. d Tenesmus is defined as painful straining at urination or defecation. A thorough medical history and physical examination must be completed to determine the body system that is involved. Tenesmus of GI origin is usually a result of colonic disease, often accompanying diarrhea or constipation. Hematochezia is the presence of blood in the feces. It can be seen with diarrhea or as streaks of blood on the outside of a normally formed stool. Hematochezia usually indicates a problem with the colon or the rectum. Hematuria is blood in the urine. Melena is defined as the presence of digested blood in the feces. The stool is characteristically a tarry black color. Melena may be seen in patients with upper GI bleeding, caused by, for example, endoparasites, ulcerations, neoplasms, or coagulopathies. Bassert JM, Thomas JA, "Chapter 19, Small Animal Medical Nursing," McCurnin's Clinical Textbook for Veterinary Technicians, ed 8, Elsevier, 2014.

169. b Jaundice or icterus is a result of excess bilirubin in the blood. Hyperhemoglobinemia is an excess of hemoglobin in the blood and does not cause discoloration. Ketonuria does not cause jaundice; however, hyperbilirubinemia can discolor urine. Anemia is not the cause of jaundice, but jaundice can appear in an anemic patient because of cellular degeneration. Tighe MM, Brown M, Mosby's Comprehensive Review for Veterinary Technicians, ed 4, Mosby Elsevier, 2015, p. 124.

170. b Fresh frozen plasma (FFP) will retain its coagulation factor efficacy for 12 months, provided it is maintained at the appropriate temperature. After 1 year, it has to be relabeled as frozen plasma (FP). Battaglia AM, Small Animal Emergency and Critical Care for Veterinary Medicine, ed 2, Elsevier, 2007, p. 70.

171. c Pancreatitis may be acute or chronic in nature. Acute pancreatitis is seen more commonly in dogs. Chronic pancreatitis is more common in cats. Acute pancreatitis is often caused by dietary indiscretion. In most cases, the cause of chronic pancreatitis is unknown. Bassert JM, Thomas JA, "Chapter 19, Small Animal Medical Nursing," McCurnin's Clinical Textbook for Veterinary Technicians, ed 8, Elsevier, 2014.

172. b A bland, low-fat diet is recommended for patients suffering from acute pancreatitis. A common risk factor for developing acute pancreatitis is ingestion of a high-fat meal. Feeding any high-fat diet is contraindicated. Bassert JM, Thomas JA, "Chapter 19, Small Animal Medical Nursing," McCurnin's Clinical Textbook for Veterinary Technicians, ed 8, Elsevier, 2014.

173. b To maintain adequate levels of all factors, plasma must be harvested from a unit of WB and frozen at −18°C or colder within 8 hours from the time of initial collection. After 8 hours, the product is labeled frozen plasma. Battaglia AM, Small Animal Emergency and Critical Care for Veterinary Medicine, ed 2, Elsevier, 2007, p. 70.

174. a Skin turgor, or the speed at which the skin returns to normal position after being pinched and pulled away from the body, is prolonged in dehydrated animals. Shortened skin turgor indicates overhydration. Skin turgor is a commonly used method for determining hydration status. Battaglia AM, Steele AM, Small Animal Emergency and Critical Care for Veterinary Technicians, ed 3, Elsevier, 2016.

175. c Liver disease and/or hemolytic anemia is suspected when jaundice is present. A responsive and nonresponsive anemia can still be a hemolytic anemia; the words responsive or nonresponsive characterize the response to treatment, not the type of anemia. Megaloblastic anemia is the presence of megaloblasts in the bone marrow and macrocytic erythrocytes. There is not a primary destruction of the red blood cells leading to a buildup of bilirubin in the circulating blood, leading to icterus. Studdert, V.P, Gay, C.C, Blood, D.C. Saunders Comprehensive Veterinary Dictionary, 4th Edition. Elsevier Saunders, 2007, p. 522.

176. a The total blood volume makes up an average of 6% to 8% (average 7%) of an animal's lean body weight. Colville TP, Bassert JM, Clinical Anatomy and Physiology for Veterinary Technicians, ed 2, Elsevier, 2008, p. 226.

177. a The pulse rate increases in patients that are moderately dehydrated because their intravascular volume will be depleted, leading to compensatory tachycardia. The pulse rate can decrease with overhydration and increased intravascular volume or with very severe shock. The pulse rate can be inconsistent with cardiac disease or severe shock. Pulses that are not palpable indicate severe shock or vasoconstriction. Battaglia AM, Steele AM, Small Animal Emergency and Critical Care for Veterinary Technicians, ed 3, Elsevier, 2016.

178. a Mucous membrane (MM) is pale and capillary refill time (CRT) is prolonged in a patient experiencing hypovolemic shock resulting from vasoconstriction reducing blood flow to the periphery. MM is normally pink, with a normal CRT (1–2 seconds). Red mucous membranes indicate vasodilation that can occur with systemic inflammation or hyperthermia. In these cases, the CRT is often very rapid. Yellow MM indicates elevated bilirubin (liver disease, hemolytic anemia) in which the CRT is often not affected. Battaglia AM, Steele AM, Small Animal Emergency and Critical Care for Veterinary Technicians, ed 3, Elsevier, 2016.

179. d Myasthenia gravis is a disease that results in the esophageal muscle losing its normal muscle tone. Because it has little or no muscle tone, the esophagus relaxes and becomes more of a relaxed bag than a tight, muscular tube. This dilated esophagus is called a megaesophagus. The risk with megaesophagus, and the principal reason many animals die from it, is that the animal often breathes in some of the frequently regurgitated food, resulting in a lung condition called aspiration pneumonia. Generalized MG also causes exercise-related generalized muscle weakness that worsens after exercise and improves with rest. Colville TP, Bassert JM, Clinical Anatomy and Physiology for Veterinary Technicians, ed 2, Elsevier, 2008, p. 271;

Bonagura JD, Twedt DC, Kirk's Current Veterinary Therapy XV, Elsevier, 2014.

180. d Chronic kidney disease (CKD) is characterized by an irreversible, progressive loss of functioning renal tissue. Treatment focuses on slowing the progression of the disease because restoring function to the damaged kidneys is not possible. Renal transplantation is the only possible curative treatment. Medical management of chronic kidney disease focuses on slowing progression of the disease, treating concurrent disease, correcting electrolyte imbalances, ameliorating clinical signs, and providing nutritional support. Bassert JM, Thomas JA, "Chapter 19, Small Animal Medical Nursing," McCurnin's Clinical Textbook for Veterinary Technicians, ed 8, Elsevier, 2014.

181. a Eclampsia is a postpartum complication caused by a deficiency of blood calcium (hypocalcemia). Galactostasis is stasis of milk in the mammary glands, resulting in enlarged, painful mammary glands. Mastitis refers to inflammation of one or more of the mammary glands. Metritis is a bacterial infection of the uterus. Bassert JM, Thomas JA, "Chapter 19, Small Animal Medical Nursing," McCurnin's Clinical Textbook for Veterinary Technicians, ed 8, Elsevier, 2014.

182. d Intraperitoneal injections are not used for vaccines because they would not be effective and could be dangerous. Vaccination by subcutaneous or intramuscular injection is the simplest and most common method of vaccine administration. Intranasal vaccines are available for infectious bovine rhinotracheitis of cattle; for *Streptococcus equi* infections in horses; for feline rhinotracheitis, *Bordetella bronchiseptica*, coronavirus, and calicivirus infections; for canine parainfluenza and *Bordetella* infection; and for infectious bronchitis and Newcastle disease in poultry. Tizard I, Veterinary Immunology, ed 9, Elsevier Saunders, 2013, p. 274.

183. b Pemphigus is classified as an autoimmune skin disease that attacks the skin and mucosa. Other autoimmune diseases may affect the blood and lymph systems, eyes, hooves, and claws, but they would not be classified as pemphigus. Tizard I, Veterinary Immunology, ed 9, Elsevier Saunders, 2013, p. 415.

184. c Patients with a low platelet count, known as thrombocytopenia, experience bleeding when inadequate numbers of platelets are available to form a platelet plug. With a lack of platelets, petechiae, ecchymoses, and anemia would be expected. Thrombocytosis is an elevated number of platelets, which would not be seen in ITP. Battaglia AM, Small Animal Emergency and Critical Care for Veterinary Medicine, ed 2, Elsevier, 2007, p. 221.

185. b Mucus in feces is a common indication of large bowel diarrhea. Normal or decreased volume of feces, normal frequency of bowel movements, and weight loss are commonly seen in patients with small bowel diarrhea. Bassert JM, Thomas JA, "Chapter 19, Small Animal Medical Nursing," McCurnin's Clinical Textbook for Veterinary Technicians, ed 8, Elsevier, 2014.

186. d NE tubes should never be used in unconscious or semiconscious patients. These patients would be at risk of aspiration. Donohoe C, "Routes of Administration," Fluid Therapy for Veterinary Technicians and Nurses, Wiley-Blackwell, 2012.

187. a Auscultation is the act of using a stethoscope to listen to the organs of the body. Palpation is the act of using one's hands and fingers to feel anatomical features to determine the presence of any abnormalities. Centrifugation is a process of using centrifugal force to separate dense from less-dense matter in fluids. Mentation is the assessment of a patient's alertness to evaluate nervous system function. Battaglia AM, Steele AM, Small Animal Emergency and Critical Care for Veterinary Technicians, ed 3, Elsevier, 2016.

188. b Maintaining the chamber at approximately half its capacity prevents large volumes of air from passing into the line and subsequently into the patient. If filled to the top, the veterinary technician will be unable to count the number of drops being delivered per minute. Leaving the chamber empty will allow air to flow into the line. The chamber will not fill by gravity. Donohoe C, "Fluid Pumps and Tools of Administration," Fluid Therapy for Veterinary Technicians and Nurses, Wiley-Blackwell, 2012.

189. b Only the veterinarian may legally prescribe (order) the type of fluids the patient will receive. The veterinary technician is responsible for calculating fluid rate as ordered by the veterinarian, for initiating fluid therapy, and for monitoring the infusion. Donohoe C, "Calculating Rates of Administration," Fluid Therapy for Veterinary Technicians and Nurses, Wiley-Blackwell, 2012.

190. d Cats infected with FeLV can harbor the virus without clinical consequence for long periods. Battaglia AM, Small Animal Emergency and Critical Care for Veterinary Medicine, ed 2, Elsevier, 2007, p. 171.

191. b Isotonic crystalloids are used primarily to replace intravascular volume, mimicking the osmolarity of plasma. Hypertonic crystalloids and synthetic colloids are used to increase colloid osmotic pressure. Whole blood is used primarily to supplement red blood cells and, in some cases, plasma proteins. Battaglia AM, Steele AM, Small Animal Emergency and Critical Care for Veterinary Technicians, ed 3, Elsevier, 2016.

192. b Because FIV is found in saliva, bite wounds serve as a means of transmission. FIV transmission in household cats with a stable social environment is rare because FIV is transmitted mainly through biting and fighting; if no fights occur, FIV is not likely to be transmitted. Bonagura JD, Twedt DC, Kirk's Current Veterinary Therapy XV, Elsevier, 2014, p. 1276.

193. b *Moraxella bovis* is a Gram-negative diplococcus that causes pinkeye in cattle. *Haemophilus aegypti* has six subspecies; they are known to cause pinkeye in humans and flu-like symptoms. *Streptococcus* spp. are opportunistic pathogens that normally reside in the upper respiratory, intestinal, lower urinary, and genital tracts, but which can cause localized infection or septicemia in dogs of all ages. *S. aureus* is dangerous because of its deleterious effects on animal health and its potential for transmission from animals to humans and vice versa. It thus has a huge impact on animal health and welfare and causes major economic losses in livestock production. Tighe MM, Brown M, Mosby's Comprehensive Review for Veterinary Technicians, ed 4, Mosby Elsevier, 2015, p. 128.

194. b Rate (drops/min) = Rate (mL/h) × drops/mL ÷ 60 min/h. Using the specified rate and drip set mentioned earlier, the rate in drops/min would equal: 20 mL/h × 60 drops/mL ÷ 60 min/h = 20 drops/min. This would be equivalent to 1 drop every 3 seconds. Battaglia AM, Steele AM, Small Animal Emergency and Critical Care for Veterinary Technicians, ed 3, Elsevier, 2016.

195. c Placing a patient in the oxygen cage is the least stressful method of oxygen supplementation in most scenarios because it allows oxygen delivery without handling the patient. Mask oxygen delivery often requires someone to place the mask on the patient, which can cause stress by holding an object to the face. A nasal cannula requires significant physical or chemical restraint. Transtracheal catheters are the most invasive of the options mentioned. Battaglia AM, Steele AM, Small Animal Emergency and Critical Care for Veterinary Technicians, ed 3, Elsevier, 2016.

196. c Pyrexia (fever or febrile condition) can result from a reaction to blood products. Pyrexic patients have an elevated body temperature resulting from causes that exist within the patient's own body. Common causes of pyrexia include inflammation, infection, sepsis, neoplasia, and reaction to the transfusion of blood products. *Hyperthermia* is the term that describes a patient whose body temperature is increased because of external causes. *Hypothermia* is the term that describes a patient with a low body temperature. Pyridoxine is one of the forms of vitamin B6 and has nothing to do with inflammation, infection, sepsis, neoplasia, or reactions. Donohoe C, "Patient Monitoring," Fluid Therapy for Veterinary Technicians and Nurses, Wiley-Blackwell, 2012.

197. d Common causes of bradycardia include hyperkalemia, hypocalcemia, toxin ingestion, and increased intracranial pressure. Common causes of tachycardia include hypovolemia, hypoxia, and hypokalemia. Donohoe C, "Patient Monitoring," Fluid Therapy for Veterinary Technicians and Nurses, Wiley-Blackwell, 2012.

198. b Polyuria is defined as the formation and excretion of large volumes of urine. Lack of urine is known as oliguria. *Proteinuria* is the term used to describe excessive protein in the urine. *Hypodipsia* is the term for low water intake. Tighe MM, Brown M, Mosby's Comprehensive Review for Veterinary Technicians, ed 4, Mosby Elsevier, 2015, p. 28.

199. d Formation of uroliths is dependent on urine pH, urine concentration, and urine saturation. Protein in the urine has not been shown to have any effect on the formation of uroliths. Bassert JM, Thomas JA, "Chapter 19, Small Animal Medical Nursing," McCurnin's Clinical Textbook for Veterinary Technicians, ed 8, Elsevier, 2014.

200. a Bacterial infections of the bladder are common in dogs and are rare in healthy cats. Female dogs are more prone to infection than male dogs. Treatment consists of appropriate antimicrobial therapy for 1 to 2 weeks. Seven to 10 days after completion of the antibiotic course, a urine culture is performed to confirm resolution of the UTI. If the UTI is still present, it is important to ascertain from the owner whether failure to give the patient the entire course of antibiotics occurred. In truly resistant or recurrent cases, a 4-week course of antibiotics is required. Bassert JM, Thomas JA, "Chapter 19, Small Animal Medical Nursing," McCurnin's Clinical Textbook for Veterinary Technicians, ed 8, Elsevier, 2014.

201. d Oliguria is a decrease in the volume of urine produced. Polyphagia is excessive eating. Hyperbilirubinuria is excessive bilirubin in the urine (this can sometimes appear as green urine). Sirois M, Hendrix CM, Laboratory Procedures for Veterinary Technicians, ed 6, Mosby Elsevier, 2015, p. 421.

202. b UTI is a common secondary complication in cats and dogs with diabetes mellitus, chronic kidney disease, or hyperadrenocorticism, and it also occurs in patients with indwelling urinary catheters. A UTI is not a common secondary complication in patients experiencing congestive heart failure, hepatic lipidosis, or hyperthyroidism. Bassert JM, Thomas JA, "Chapter 19, Small Animal Medical Nursing," McCurnin's Clinical Textbook for Veterinary Technicians, ed 8, Elsevier, 2014.

203. c Dysuria (painful urination) is a very common clinical sign resulting from inflammation of the urethra and bladder. Azotemia is a condition in which the blood contains increased concentrations of nitrogenous wastes such as urea nitrogen (BUN) and it is more commonly seen with obstruction of the urinary tract. An elevated BUN is more commonly seen when an animal is on a high-protein diet, is dehydrated, or exhibits renal insufficiency. Dehydration is not a common indication of UTI but might be seen in an extremely severe case or if the patient has other concurrent disease. Bassert JM, Thomas JA, "Chapter 19, Small Animal Medical Nursing," McCurnin's Clinical Textbook for Veterinary Technicians, ed 8, Elsevier, 2014.

204. c Anuria is the absence of urine. Oliguria is a decrease in the volume of urine produced. Hypodipsia is known as low water intake. Polydipsia is excessive drinking. Sirois M, Hendrix CM, Laboratory Procedures for Veterinary Technicians, ed 6, Mosby Elsevier, 2015, p. 421.

205. a Dysuria is difficulty or painful urination. Proteinuria is protein in the urine. Hematuria is blood in the urine. An excessive number of WBCs is referred to as pyuria or leukocyturia. Tighe MM, Brown M, Mosby's Comprehensive Review for Veterinary Technicians, ed 4, Mosby Elsevier, 2015, p. 27.

206. b Patients can show signs similar to pain with boredom, thirst, anxiety, and the need to urinate and defecate. Patient positioning is important for patient comfort. Each patient has unique needs and a technician can help by understanding each patient as an individual. All of these points cannot be ignored, even when pharmacologic interventions are used, because they affect patient comfort. Battaglia AM, Steele AM, Small Animal Emergency and Critical Care for Veterinary Technicians, ed 3, Elsevier, 2016.

207. c Eyes are typically rotated ventrally during heavy sedation or anesthesia. Pinpoint pupils indicate a neurologic issue. Dehydration causes a loss of volume in the orbit and surrounding tissues, leading to the orbit being sunken into the eye socket. Lateral nystagmus can result from the patient suffering from a nervous system–related ataxia. Battaglia AM, Steele AM, Small Animal Emergency and Critical Care for Veterinary Technicians, ed 3, Elsevier, 2016.

208. a Hemolytic anemia is characterized by erythrocyte (red blood cell) destruction. Leukocytes, lymphocytes, and monocytes are white blood cells. Bassert JM, Thomas JA, "Chapter 19, Small Animal Medical Nursing," McCurnin's Clinical Textbook for Veterinary Technicians, ed 8, Elsevier, 2014.

209. d Fructosamine levels are often used to help diagnose and monitor diabetes mellitus. Diagnosis of IMHA is based on CBC findings consistent with hemolytic anemia and evidence of autoimmunity via autoagglutination and a positive Coombs test. Bassert JM, Thomas JA, "Chapter 19, Small Animal Medical Nursing," McCurnin's Clinical Textbook for Veterinary Technicians, ed 8, Elsevier, 2014.

210. c Communicating directly with the clinician about particular concerns shows the veterinarian that the technician is aware of pain and assessment. It also provides the clinician with information if medication changes are necessary. Although monitoring urine and fecal output is important, unless it has direct bearing on a particular case, it would not be the best answer to this question. Veterinary technicians cannot change medication when it is not effective without input from the attending clinician. It is important that the veterinary technician sees the animal receiving the medication directly and that should therefore not be passed off to another person. Goldberg ME, "Pain Management," in Tighe MM, Brown M, Mosby's Comprehensive Review for Veterinary Technicians, ed 4, Mosby Elsevier, 2015, p. 474.

211. d Regurgitation is food substances being expelled by the esophagus without digestion. Forceful contraction of the abdomen and diaphragm is seen with vomiting. Restlessness and salivation are signs of nausea that are not seen with regurgitation. Battaglia AM, Steele AM, Small Animal Emergency and Critical Care for Veterinary Technicians, ed 3, Elsevier, 2016.

212. c Green fluid in the vomitus indicates the involvement of fresh bile in the duodenum. Gastric or esophageal disorders commonly manifest as white, frothy vomitus. Gastrointestinal ulceration results in frank blood if the bleeding from ulceration is fresh, whereas dark, black flecks resembling coffee grounds indicate blood digested in the stomach. Pyloric outflow obstruction results in projectile vomiting. Battaglia AM, Steele AM, Small Animal Emergency and Critical Care for Veterinary Technicians, ed 3, Elsevier, 2016.

213. b Resentment of being handled, aggression, and abnormal posture are three characteristics of pain in cats. Sleeping continuously, overeating, and attention-seeking behaviors are not indicative of pain. Hyperactivity, pupillary enlargement, and tail swishing combined would not necessarily indicate pain. Hypotension, hypocapnia, hypopnea, and bradycardia are not signs of pain; signs to be expected are increased heart rate, increased respiratory rate, and dilated pupils instead. Goldberg ME, "Pain Management," Tighe MM, Brown M, Mosby's Comprehensive Review for Veterinary Technicians, ed 4, Mosby Elsevier, 2015, p. 475.

214. a A pain assessment should be completed every 4–6 hours. It is unnecessary to assess every 30 minutes to 1 hour unless the time period is within the immediate postoperative period. Assessing every 8 hours and 12–24 hours is not often enough. Goldberg ME, "Pain Management," Tighe MM, Brown M, Mosby's Comprehensive Review for Veterinary Technicians, ed 4, Mosby Elsevier, 2015, p. 476.

215. b Phenothiazine tranquilizers, such as acepromazine (PromAce), chlorpromazine (Thorazine), and prochlorperazine (Compazine, Darbazine), are commonly used antiemetics. Apomorphine quickly causes emesis in dogs; however, it is a less effective emetic in cats. An effective emetic for cats is the sedative xylazine, which produces emesis within minutes of injection. Hydrogen peroxide is a commonly used emetic at home; however, it does not work consistently. Sirois M, "Pharmacology and Pharmacy," Principles and Practice of Veterinary Technology, ed 3, Elsevier, 2011.

216. b Aspiration is the act of inhaling vomitus or mucus into the respiratory tract. Patients with myasthenia gravis, a disorder of neuromuscular transmission that causes muscle weakness, may also suffer from megaesophagus (large, dilated esophagus). This muscle weakness increases the risk of aspiration in these patients. *Acephalus* is a term used to describe a headless fetus. Asteatosis refers to a skin disease with dry scaling. Astrocytoma is a common tumor of the brain or spinal cord. Bassert JM, Thomas JA, "Chapter 19, Small Animal Medical Nursing," McCurnin's Clinical Textbook for Veterinary Technicians, ed 8, Elsevier, 2014.

217. d Yellow mucous membrane (MM) indicates elevated bilirubin (liver disease, hemolytic anemia), in which the CRT is often not affected. MM is pale and capillary refill time (CRT) is prolonged in a patient experiencing hypovolemic shock resulting from vasoconstriction reducing blood flow to the periphery. MM is normally pink, with a normal CRT (1–2 seconds). Red mucous membranes indicate vasodilation that can occur with systemic inflammation or hyperthermia. In these cases the CRT is often rapid. Battaglia AM, Steele AM, Small Animal Emergency and Critical Care for Veterinary Technicians, ed 3, Elsevier, 2016.

218. b Gastrointestinal ulceration results in frank blood if the bleeding from ulceration is fresh, whereas dark, black flecks resembling coffee grounds indicate blood digested in the stomach. Green fluid in the vomitus indicates involvement of fresh bile in the duodenum. Gastric or esophageal disorders commonly manifest as white, frothy vomitus. Pyloric outflow obstruction results in projectile vomiting. Battaglia AM, Steele AM, Small Animal Emergency and Critical Care for Veterinary Technicians, ed 3, Elsevier, 2016.

219. b Speaking in low tones and interacting with the animal makes the patient feel better, but behaviors will resume when the interaction stops (this will show that the patient has pain and is not dysphoric). Placing the patient on comfortable blankets will not relieve an animal with dysphoria; it would be comforting, but it will not stop dysphoric behavior. Moving the animal to a different ward would make it better; again this shows that the patient can be comforted, but it will not stop dysphoric behavior. Automatically reversing the analgesic medication is reserved for those patients that typically do not seem to recognize that a human is with them, do not make eye contact, and do not necessarily respond to light palpation of painful sites. Goldberg ME, "Pain Management," Tighe MM, Brown M, Mosby's Comprehensive Review for Veterinary Technicians, ed 4, Mosby Elsevier, 2015, p. 476.

220. d Fleas spread *Yersinia pestis*, which is commonly known as the plague. *Borrelia burgdorferi* (Lyme disease), *Rickettsia rickettsii* (Rocky Mountain spotted fever), *Ehrlichia* spp. (canine ehrlichiosis) are all vector-borne pathogens that are spread by ticks. Bassert JM, Thomas JA, "Chapter 19, Small Animal Medical Nursing," McCurnin's Clinical Textbook for Veterinary Technicians, ed 8, Elsevier, 2014.

221. b Sarcomas arise from mesenchymal tissue, such as cartilage, connective tissue, or bone. Lymphoma is commonly found in the liver and spleen. Adenocarcinoma is found in glandular tissue, such as mammary glands. Carcinoma is found in the skin and is common in the sublingual tissue. Bassert JM, Thomas JA, "Chapter 19, Small Animal Medical Nursing," McCurnin's Clinical Textbook for Veterinary Technicians, ed 8, Elsevier, 2014.

222. a Massage is an example of manual therapy. Effleurage technique is a type of massage and physical modalities involve the use of light, heat, sound, water, and electrotherapies. Therapeutic exercise is not a form of massage because massage does not involve the use of the animal's movement. Goldberg ME, "Pain Management," Tighe MM, Brown M, Mosby's Comprehensive Review for Veterinary Technicians, ed 4, Mosby Elsevier, 2015, p. 496.

223. c Diarrhea originating in the large intestine results in high-frequency diarrhea, often accompanied with straining and mucus. Involvement of the stomach causes no distinct change to diarrhea and it is most associated with vomiting. Diarrhea and bleeding that originates in the jejunum and ileum presents as melena. Colitis results in frank blood mixed in the diarrhea. Battaglia AM, Steele AM, Small Animal Emergency and Critical Care for Veterinary Technicians, ed 3, Elsevier, 2016.

224. d Vaginal discharge, vomiting, diarrhea, dehydration, anorexia, polyuria, and polydipsia are all signs of pyometra. Eclampsia is a condition of hypocalcemia arising from lactation, resulting in muscle spasms, fever, tachycardia, and seizures. Mastitis results in hard, painful nipples, and galactostasis (loss of milk production). Hard labor for 30 to 60 minutes with no new young is a form of dystocia. Battaglia AM, Steele AM, Small Animal Emergency and Critical Care for Veterinary Technicians, ed 3, Elsevier, 2016.

225. d Viscera are defined as any internal organ within the body that is enclosed within a cavity. Osteosarcoma is not part of the viscera, whereas the pancreas and intestinal tract are. Therefore, pancreatitis, gastroenteritis, and bowel ischemia are examples of visceral pain. Goldberg ME, "Pain Management," Tighe MM, Brown M, Mosby's Comprehensive Review for Veterinary Technicians, ed 4, Mosby Elsevier, 2015, p. 482.

226. c Speaking can temporarily soothe most animals experiencing mild to moderate pain. Animals that are dysphoric or delirious because of opioid overdose rarely respond to soothing interaction or to light palpation of the painful area. Thrashing and yowling alone do not prove dysphoria because many times the pained animal will calm down when spoken to or touched, until it is alone again. The claustrophobic animal generally weaves in the cage or tries to escape by digging or chewing on bars. Shaffran, N, "Pain Management: The Veterinary Technician's Perspective," in Mathews KA, ed, The Veterinary Clinics of North America: Small Animal Practice: Update on Pain Management, 2008, 38(6), p. 1423.

227. b Some intravascular (IV) chemotherapy agents are potent vesicants and irritants, which, if accidentally administered perivascularly, can cause local tissue necrosis potentially severe enough to require limb amputation. It is important when administering IV chemotherapy drugs that the IV catheter is confidently and properly placed and secured. If, despite all precautions, the chemotherapy agent is provided perivascularly, do not remove the IV catheter. Irrigate the area with sterile saline both through the catheter and subcutaneously to dilute the drug. Subcutaneous administration of dexamethasone in the area is often recommended. Apply cold compresses to the area for the next 72 hours. Close monitoring for redness, swelling, pain, and skin sloughing is necessary. The veterinarian may need to intervene and debride the necrotic tissue. Bassert JM, Thomas JA, "Chapter 19, Small Animal Medical Nursing," McCurnin's Clinical Textbook for Veterinary Technicians, ed 8, Elsevier, 2014.

228. b The jugular vein is generally recommended for obtaining a blood sample from neonatal puppies and kittens because of its larger size compared with other vessels. Blood collection from the cephalic, lateral saphenous, or medial saphenous veins can prove very challenging for even the most experience technician because of their small size in these patients. Bassert JM, Thomas JA, "Chapter 21, Neonatal Care of the Puppy, Kitten, and Foal," McCurnin's Clinical Textbook for Veterinary Technicians, ed 8, Elsevier, 2014.

229. b The small intestine is divided into three parts, the duodenum, jejunum, and ileum. The duodenum is the first and shortest portion of the small intestine and is where the pancreatic and bile ducts enter the intestine. The jejunum and ileum form the main portion of the small intestine; there is not a clear division between the different parts of the small intestine. The cecum is part of the large intestine. Wortinger A, "Digestion and Absorption," in Nutrition for Veterinary Technicians and Nurses, Blackwell, 2007.

230. c Panting, anorexia, and depression are very common behaviors seen in dogs experiencing pain. Although vocalization is seen in dogs in pain, increased appetite is not (decreased appetite is seen more commonly). Playful actions, excessive licking, and increased attention to activities occurring in the environment are behavioral signs of a dog not experiencing pain. Muir WW, Gaynor JS, "Pain Behaviors," Handbook of Veterinary Pain Management, Mosby, 2009, p. 64-65.

231. a A Doppler ultrasound can detect arterial pulses for manual blood pressure measurement by using ultrasound to create an audible signal from blood flow. The oscillometric device is a machine sensing pressure oscillations on a cuff and using an algorithm to calculate the blood pressure. Direct blood pressure measurement is performed through an arterial catheter with a pressure transducer. Stethoscopes are used to auscultate pulses in human medicine. Battaglia AM, Steele AM, Small Animal Emergency and Critical Care for Veterinary Technicians, ed 3, Elsevier, 2016.

232. d Colitis results in frank blood mixed in the diarrhea. Involvement of the stomach causes no distinct change to diarrhea and is the condition most associated with vomiting. Diarrhea and bleeding that originates in the jejunum and ileum presents as melena. Diarrhea of the large intestinal origin results in high-frequency diarrhea, often accompanied with straining and mucus. Battaglia AM, Steele AM, Small Animal Emergency and Critical Care for Veterinary Technicians, ed 3, Elsevier, 2016.

233. b The large intestine begins at the ileocecocolic valve and continues as the cecum, ascending, transverse, and descending colon, rectum, and anus. Wortinger A, "Digestion and Absorption," Nutrition for Veterinary Technicians and Nurses, Blackwell, 2007.

234. a Basal energy requirement is defined as the energy required for a normal animal in a thermoneutral environment, awake but resting, in a fasting state. Resting energy requirement is defined as the energy required for a normal animal in a thermoneutral environment, awake but not fasted. Maintenance energy requirement is the energy required for a moderately active adult animal in a thermoneutral environment. Daily energy requirement is the energy required for average daily activity of any animal, dependent on lifestyle and activity. Wortinger A, "Energy Balance," Nutrition for Veterinary Technicians and Nurses, Blackwell, 2007.

235. c Dogs and cats that willingly stretch their abdominal muscles are not in pain. Dogs experiencing pain show a decreased appetite, are more aggressive, and have less social interaction. Muir WW, Gaynor JS, "Pain Behaviors," Handbook of Veterinary Pain Management, Mosby, 2009, p. 63-6528.

236. b Enteral feeding has been observed as more effective at preventing gastrointestinal ulcerations than traditional medications. Drugs aimed at reducing acidity of the gastric content (such as famotidine) are helpful in preventing ulceration, but they are not as effective as feeding. Antibiotic administration is helpful only when microbial causes are present. Withholding food is the most harmful to gastrointestinal healing. Battaglia AM, Steele AM, Small Animal Emergency and Critical Care for Veterinary Technicians, ed 3, Elsevier, 2016.

237. d Warm-water blankets are helpful in warming a patient, although prevention of hypothermia is best achieved when combined with other measures of warming and prevention of heat loss. When in use, providing insulation between the device and the patient is recommended because instances of heat injury are possible for all of these devices. Warming should be directed at the core as opposed to the periphery to prevent peripheral vasodilation and impaired heat exchange. Battaglia AM, Steele AM, Small Animal Emergency and Critical Care for Veterinary Technicians, ed 3, Elsevier, 2016.

238. c Joint mobility treatment consists of ROM and stretching exercises. Muir WW, Gaynor JS, Handbook of Veterinary Pain Management, Mosby, 2009, p. 514.

239. b A pet food with "chicken dinner" as part of its name must contain >10% chicken. A pet food named "chicken" must contain >70% chicken. A pet food named "chicken flavor" may contain <3% chicken. Wortinger A, "Pet Food Labels," in Nutrition for Veterinary Technicians and Nurses, Blackwell, 2007.

240. d Nutritional claim is optional on the PDP. The manufacturer's name, brand name, product name, designator or statement of intent, and net weight are all required for inclusion on the PDP. Wortinger A, "Pet Food Labels," in Nutrition for Veterinary Technicians and Nurses, Blackwell, 2007.

241. c The most common types of pain in the horse are orthopedic pain and abdominal/colic pain. Orthopedic pain typically presents as lameness and can include pain of the joints, tendons/ligaments, long bones, and back. Lameness is a result of the horse trying to avoid the painful area by compensating on the other limbs. Sometimes the behaviors associated with pain can be nonspecific or can correlate with a specific location such as the abdomen, limb, foot, head, mouth, or castration site. Goldberg ME, Shaffran N, Pain Management for Veterinary Technicians and Nurses, Wiley, 2014, p. 22.

242. b The Universal Product Code, batch information, and freshness date are all optional and are not required to appear on the information panel. The ingredient statement, guaranteed analysis, nutritional adequacy statement, feeding guidelines, and manufacturer or distributor are all required to appear on the information panel. Wortinger A, "Pet Food Labels," in Nutrition for Veterinary Technicians and Nurses, Blackwell, 2007.

243. d Minimum percentage of crude protein, minimum percentage of crude fat, maximum percentage of moisture, and maximum percentage of crude fiber are required to be listed on the guaranteed analysis panel of all pet foods. The minimum percentage of taurine is optional. Case LP, Daristotle L, Hayek MG, Raasch MF, "Pet Food Labels," Canine and Feline Nutrition: A Resource for Companion Animal Professionals, ed 3, Mosby, 2011.

244. c Hypothermia interferes with normal metabolic functions by decreasing the metabolic rate: it leads to decreased peripheral perfusion, it causes cardiac dysfunction, and it increases coagulation time by interfering with the coagulation cascade. Battaglia AM, Steele AM, Small Animal Emergency and Critical Care for Veterinary Technicians, ed 3, Elsevier, 2016.

245. d A cow may experience depression and appear dull. In addition, grinding teeth, lack of appetite, and standing with one foot behind the other may be exhibited. Goldberg ME, Shaffran N, Pain Management for Veterinary Technicians and Nurses, Wiley, 2014, p. 26.

246. c Obesity can be defined as an increase in fat-tissue mass sufficient to contribute to disease; therefore, 10% or 20% is negligible. Goldberg ME, Shaffran N, Pain Management for Veterinary Technicians and Nurses, Wiley, 2014, p. 286.

247. b Apomorphine quickly causes emesis in dogs when administered by IV or IM injection, or when an apomorphine tablet is placed in the conjunctival sac of the eye. Apomorphine is a less-effective emetic in cats. Acepromazine (PromAce), chlorpromazine (Thorazine), and prochlorperazine (Compazine, Darbazine) are commonly used antiemetics that combat vomiting caused by motion sickness. Sirois M, "Pharmacology and Pharmacy," Principles and Practice of Veterinary Technology, ed 3, Elsevier, 2011.

248. b Lactulose is another laxative that increases osmotic pressure by drawing water into the colon and causing the fecal material to contain more liquid. It also has an acidifying aspect, which is used in the treatment of hepatic encephalopathy because it traps ammonia in the form of ammonium. It is used most commonly in small animals with chronic constipation problems. Antidiarrheals are drugs used to combat various types of diarrhea and include diphenoxylate (Lomotil), paregoric (tincture of opium), and loperamide (Imodium). Sirois M, "Pharmacology and Pharmacy," Principles and Practice of Veterinary Technology, ed 3, Elsevier, 2011.

249. a Obesity is a risk factor for OA and the most common traumatic cause of OA in dogs is ruptured cruciate ligaments. Overweight/obese dogs are two to three times more likely to rupture cruciate ligaments compared with normal-weight dogs. Understanding the correlation between maintaining their dog at a healthy weight and decreasing the risk of disease may be a powerful motivator for many owners. Torn Achilles, hip dysplasia, and phalangeal fractures are not the most common traumatic causes of OA in dogs. Goldberg ME, Shaffran N, Pain Management for Veterinary Technicians and Nurses, Wiley, 2014, p. 287.

250. c In a patient with limited mobility, passive range of motion prevents muscle atrophy and stiffening of joints and sling walking will help a patient to go outside when necessary. The neck and head should be slightly elevated, especially to prevent aspiration in patients at risk of vomiting or regurgitation. These patients should also be turned every 2–4 hours to prevent consolidation of lungs, creation of pressure sores, and pooling of fluid in tissues. Battaglia AM, Steele AM, Small Animal Emergency and Critical Care for Veterinary Technicians, ed 3, Elsevier, 2016.

251. c Porphyrin staining in rodents is red-colored hematoporphyrin exudate, which may encircle the eye. Therefore, the answer is not the hair standing on end or the color of cage litter resulting from urine. Goldberg ME, Shaffran N, Pain Management for Veterinary Technicians and Nurses, Wiley, 2014, p. 217.

252. a Pain in rabbits is usually characterized by a reduction in food and water intake (and thus increasing weight loss and dehydration) and limited movement. Teeth grinding (bruxism) can be a sign of pain but is not the most common. Squinted eyes can be a sign of pain but not closed eyes. Lateral recumbency would indicate a severely ill rabbit. Goldberg ME, Shaffran N, Pain Management for Veterinary Technicians and Nurses, Wiley, 2014, p. 223.

253. d Sucralfate (Carafate) is an antiulcer drug used to treat ulcers of the stomach and upper small intestine. Systemic antacids decrease acid production in the stomach. Systemic antacids include cimetidine (Tagamet), ranitidine (Zantac), and famotidine (Pepcid). Sirois M, "Pharmacology and Pharmacy," Principles and Practice of Veterinary Technology, ed 3, Elsevier, 2011.

254. d The white lead is attached to the right foreleg, the red lead is attached to the left rear leg, the green lead is attached to the right rear leg, and the black lead is attached to the left front leg. "Green and white is always right; newspaper (white and black) comes in the morning (front), Christmas comes at the end of the year (back legs)." Sirois M, "Pharmacology and Pharmacy," Principles and Practice of Veterinary Technology, ed 3, Elsevier, 2011, p. 609.

255. c An insulin overdose results in hypoglycemia, which can lead to weakness, lethargy, and hypoglycemic seizures. Muscle wasting is a sign of uncontrolled diabetes. Diabetics with hyperglycemia often exhibit polyuria. Vomiting and halitosis can occur with diabetic ketoacidosis, a condition that develops in cases of diabetics when insulin therapy is not maintained. Battaglia AM, Steele AM, Small Animal Emergency and Critical Care for Veterinary Technicians, ed 3, Elsevier, 2016.

256. c First-intention wound healing occurs with no infection or suppuration (pus formation). First-intention wound healing occurs with skin edges held together and with minimal scar formation. Sirois M, "Table 13-1," Principles and Practice of Veterinary Technology, ed 3, Elsevier, 2011.

257. b FDA: the Food and Drug Administration provides approval for new ingredients. AAFCO: the Association of American Feed Control Officials sets standards for substantiation claims and nutritional profiles for pet food; however, it has no regulatory authority. Government agencies often mandate AAFCO regulations into law. FTC: the Federal Trade Commission regulates trade and advertising of pet foods. USDA: the United States Department of Agriculture regulates pet food labels and research facilities. Case LP, Daristotle L, Hayek MG, Raasch MF, "History and Regulation of Pet Foods," Canine and

Feline Nutrition: A Resource for Companion Animal Professionals, ed 3, Mosby, 2011.

258. a Common causes of tachycardia include hypovolemia, hypoxia, and hypokalemia. Common causes of bradycardia include hyperkalemia, hypocalcemia, toxin ingestion, and increased intracranial pressure. Donohoe C, "Patient Monitoring," Fluid Therapy for Veterinary Technicians and Nurses, Wiley-Blackwell, 2012.

259. b Not all bandages need to be removed 24 hours after application. A bandage should be checked three or four times a day for signs of swelling, slippage, moisture, or soiling. If any of these scenarios occurs, the bandage should be changed. Tear M, Small Animal Surgical Nursing, ed 2, Mosby Elsevier, 2012, p. 178.

260. b Eclampsia is a condition of hypocalcemia arising from lactation, resulting in muscle spasms, fever, tachycardia, and seizures. Mastitis results in hard, painful nipples and galactostasis (loss of milk production). Hard labor for 30 to 60 minutes with no new young is a form of dystocia. Vaginal discharge, vomiting, diarrhea, dehydration, anorexia, polyuria, and polydipsia are all signs of pyometra. Battaglia AM, Steele AM, Small Animal Emergency and Critical Care for Veterinary Technicians, ed 3, Elsevier, 2016.

261. b Immediately after feeding the patient with a gruel-type meal, the tube should be slowly flushed with water. The technician should never rapidly inject food or fluids because this could induce immediate vomiting. In addition, the tube should never be flushed with air. Patients should gradually be introduced to larger volumes of food after the initial placement; never administer the total caloric amount on the first postoperative day. Tear M, Small Animal Surgical Nursing, ed 2, Mosby Elsevier, 2012, p. 248.

262. a Nonsystemic antacids, in liquid or tablet form, are composed of calcium, magnesium, or aluminum and they directly neutralize acid molecules in the stomach or rumen. Over-the-counter (OTC) products such as Tums and Rolaids are nonsystemic antacids made primarily of calcium. Other nonsystemic antacids include magnesium products (Riopan, Carmilax), aluminum products (Amphojel), and combinations of magnesium and aluminum products (Maalox). Sucralfate is an antiulcer drug used to treat ulcers of the stomach and upper small intestine. Omeprazole is a gastric acid pump inhibitor that binds irreversibly to the secretory surface of cells in the stomach. It therefore decreases acid secretion (antacid) and helps to support the stomach lining (antiulcer). Misoprostol is a synthetic prostaglandin that helps decrease acid secretion in the stomach and increases production of the stomach lining (mucosa). Misoprostol is primarily used to combat insults to the stomach caused by nonsteroidal anti-inflammatory agents. Sirois M, "Pharmacology and Pharmacy," Principles and Practice of Veterinary Technology, ed 3, Elsevier, 2011.

263. d Feeding tubes are not placed through the mouth. The patient would chew through a tube placed through the mouth, rendering it useless. Nasogastric, pharyngostomy, and gastrostomy tubes all bypass the mouth. Bassert JM, Thomas JA, McCurnin's Clinical Textbook for Veterinary Technicians, ed 8, Elsevier, 2014, p. 330-331.

264. b The two small pterygoid bones support part of the lateral walls of the pharynx (throat). The turbinates are also called the nasal conchae. They are four, thin, scroll-like bones that fill most of the space in the nasal cavity. Each side has a dorsal and a ventral turbinate. The moist, very vascular soft tissue lining of the nasal passages covers the turbinates. The scroll-like shape of the turbinates forces air inhaled through the nose around many twists and turns as it passes through the nasal cavity. This helps warm and humidify the air and also helps trap any tiny particles of inhaled foreign material in the moist surface of the nasal epithelium. This process helps condition the inhaled air before it reaches the delicate lungs. The two palatine bones make up the caudal portion of the hard palate (the bony part of the roof of the mouth), which separates the mouth from the nasal cavity. The rest of the hard palate (the rostral portion) is made up of part of the maxillary bones. The single vomer bone is located on the midline of the skull and forms part of the nasal septum, which is the central wall between the left and right nasal passages. Colville TP, Bassert JM, Clinical Anatomy and Physiology for Veterinary Technicians, ed 3, Elsevier, 2016.

265. c Appropriate analgesic therapy is necessary for patient comfort; however, it will not prevent decubital ulcers. Repositioning the patient, adequate padding, and massage will all reduce pressure and/or increase circulation to the pressure points, decreasing the likelihood of decubital ulcer formation. Sirois M, "Pharmacology and Pharmacy," Principles and Practice of Veterinary Technology, ed 3, Elsevier, p. 638-639.

266. d Warm compressing is a technique used to increase blood flow to an area to increase draining and healing of the area, such as with mastitis. Coupage is a technique used to help loosen purulent material within the pulmonary parenchyma with pneumonia. Passive range of motion is used to keep joints from becoming stiff. Cold compress is used to minimize inflammation. Battaglia AM, Steele AM, Small Animal Emergency and Critical Care for Veterinary Technicians, ed 3, Elsevier, 2016.

267. a Brachycephalic breeds of cats and dogs run the risk of proptosis (dislocation of the eye globe from the socket) when held too tightly around the neck. Proptosed eyes are always an emergency and are never the result of conjunctivitis. Dolichocephalic breeds rarely experience proptosed globes. Morgan RV, Small Animal Practice Client Handouts, Saunders, 2011.

268. a The metabolic alterations that occur after nutritional support is started in a severely malnourished, underweight, and/or starved patient are known as refeeding syndrome. When the body is in a starved state, the body maintains extracellular concentrations of electrolytes at the expense of intracellular concentrations. This may result in inward restricting when glucose and insulin are introduced to the patient with refeeding. The result of this shift is critical decreases in vital serum electrolyte concentrations, which may be life-threatening. Refeeding syndrome may result from starvation; however, starvation and simple starvation refer to an extreme lack of nutrition and not metabolic alterations. Wortinger A, Burns K, Nutrition and Disease Management for Veterinary Technicians and Nurses, ed 2, Wiley Blackwell, 2015.

269. a It is important to keep a splint or bandage clean and dry; it should therefore not be washed at any time. Clients should inspect the bandage daily for any swelling, shifting, or moisture collection. Tighe MM, Brown M, Mosby's Comprehensive Review for Veterinary Technicians, ed 3, Mosby, p. 445.

270. c Icterus manifests as yellow-to-orange serum because of increased bilirubin levels in serum. Hemolyzed serum is red because of increased hemoglobin levels in serum. Hyperproteinemia results in increased total protein readings and, when severe, presents as yellow fluid with high viscosity, such as with feline infectious peritonitis. Lipemia manifests as turbid, white serum from an increased triglyceride level. Battaglia AM, Steele AM, Small Animal Emergency and Critical Care for Veterinary Technicians, ed 3, Elsevier, 2016.

271. d Pneumothorax is when air has been trapped in the chest cavity between the lungs and the chest wall and the lungs collapse because of increased pressure within the chest cavity. A chest tube can help evacuate the air and allow the lungs to expand. Pulmonary edema is fluid within the lungs (chest tubes are never placed within lungs). Ascites is fluid within the abdominal cavity. Subcutaneous emphysema is air trapped under the skin, and a chest tube does not treat emphysema. Fossum TW, Small Animal Surgery, ed 3, Mosby, 2007, p. 899.

272. d Refeeding syndrome occurs in disease conditions such as starvation from feline hepatic lipidosis, overall malnutrition, and prolonged diuresis as ensues in uncontrolled diabetes renal failure. Wortinger A, Burns K, Nutrition and Disease Management for Veterinary Technicians and Nurses, ed 2, Wiley Blackwell, 2015.

273. b The coccygeal vertebrae are the bones of the tail. The cervical vertebrae are in the neck region. The lumbar vertebrae are dorsal to the abdominal region. The thoracic vertebrae are located dorsal to the thorax. The sacral vertebrae are unique in that they fuse to form a single, solid structure called the sacrum. Colville TP, Bassert JM, Clinical Anatomy and Physiology for Veterinary Technicians, ed 3, Elsevier, 2016.

274. d Hexachlorophene is a phenolic surgical scrub that has decreased in popularity because of its suspected neurotoxicity (damage to the nervous system) and teratogenic effects (birth defects) in pregnant nurses who performed hexachlorophene scrubs on a regular basis. Chlorhexidine, povidone, and quaternary compounds remain safe to use in cats. Sirois M, "Pharmacology and Pharmacy," Principles and Practice of Veterinary Technology, ed 3, Elsevier, 2011, p. 273.

275. b Direct blood pressure measurement is performed through an arterial catheter with a pressure transducer. The oscillometric device is a machine sensing pressure oscillations on a cuff and using an algorithm to calculate the blood pressure. Ultrasound can create an audible signal from blood flow and a Doppler ultrasound can detect arterial pulses for manual blood pressure measurement. Stethoscopes are used to auscultate pulses in human medicine. Battaglia AM, Steele AM, Small Animal Emergency and Critical Care for Veterinary Technicians, ed 3, Elsevier, 2016.

276. b Anterior drawer movement is used to detect cranial cruciate ligament (CCL) damage/rupture in the stifle joint. The anterior drawer movement test is not used with elbows, stifles, or hocks. Colville TP, Bassert JM, Clinical Anatomy and Physiology for Veterinary Technicians, ed 2, Elsevier, 2008, p. 186.

277. b Nutrients in excess of the patient's needs will not be used in a critically ill patient as they would be in a healthy patient. Overfed patients are at increased risk of developing hepatic lipidosis, hypercapnia, and a multitude of metabolic abnormalities. Literature shows that metabolic disturbances of any type are less likely to occur if estimates of caloric needs are conservative. Current recommendations are to begin feeding critically ill patients their resting energy requirement (RER). Wortinger A, Burns K, Nutrition and Disease Management for Veterinary Technicians and Nurses, ed 2, Wiley Blackwell, 2015.

278. b Catheter sites are observed at least once a day and they should look clean, with no signs of inflammation or discharge. The presence of fluid exiting the insertion site or a subcutaneous pocket of fluids indicates catheter leakage. Redness, swelling, or purulent discharge are indications of inflammation and infection. Catheters that are occluded cannot be flushed. Battaglia AM, Steele AM, Small Animal Emergency and Critical Care for Veterinary Technicians, ed 3, Elsevier, 2016.

279. a Pleural effusion is the accumulation of fluid in the thoracic cavity. Treatment includes oxygen supplementation and thoracocentesis. Pulmonary edema is fluid in the lungs, ascites is fluid in the abdomen, and a pyothorax is defined as pus in the thoracic cavity. Bassert JM, Thomas JA, McCurnin's Clinical Textbook for Veterinary Technicians, ed 8, Elsevier, 2014, p. 684.

280. c Shortened skin turgor indicates overhydration. Skin turgor, or the speed at which the skin returns to normal position after being pinched and pulled away from the body, is prolonged in dehydrated animals. Skin turgor is a commonly used method of determining hydration status. Battaglia AM, Steele AM, Small Animal Emergency and Critical Care for Veterinary Technicians, ed 3, Elsevier, 2016.

281. b Second intention healing is indicated for heavily contaminated wounds. Primary intention is used for surgically induced incisions. Healing of a wound that has already formed granulation tissue undergoes secondary closure. Fourth intention does not exist. Bassert JM, Thomas JA, McCurnin's Clinical Textbook for Veterinary Technicians, ed 8, Elsevier, 2014, p. 1433.

282. d Chronic mitral valvular disease is the more commonly acquired cardiac abnormality in dogs, affecting more than ⅓ of patients older than 10 years of age. Chronic mitral valvular disease is not commonly seen in younger dogs. Wortinger A, Burns K, Nutrition and Disease Management for Veterinary Technicians and Nurses, ed 2, Wiley Blackwell, 2015.

283. b Taurine is an essential amino acid in cats; deficiencies have been shown to be the leading cause of dilated cardiomyopathy in cats. The minimum recommended allowance of taurine in cat food is 0.04% DM. Deficiency in glutamine, arginine, and copper has not been linked to dilated cardiomyopathy in cats. Wortinger A, Burns K, Nutrition and Disease Management for Veterinary Technicians and Nurses, ed 2, Wiley Blackwell, 2015.

284. b Isotonic saline is a sterile solution that can be used to flush wounds, abdominal cavities, or instruments that have been soaking in a cold sterile solution. Tap water could be contaminated and should not be used. Povidone and hydrogen peroxide can be irritating to tissues and cannot be used in internal cavities. Bassert JM, Thomas JA, McCurnin's Clinical Textbook for Veterinary Technicians, ed 8, Elsevier, 2014.

285. b Pinpoint pupils indicate a neurologic issue. Dehydration causes a loss of volume in the orbit and surrounding tissues, leading to the orbit being sunken into the eye socket. Eyes are typically rotated ventrally during heavy sedation or anesthesia. Lateral nystagmus can result when the patient suffers from a nervous system–related ataxia. Battaglia AM, Steele AM, Small Animal Emergency and Critical Care for Veterinary Technicians, ed 3, Elsevier, 2016.

286. c Red mucous membranes indicate vasodilation that can occur with systemic inflammation or hyperthermia. In these cases the CRT is often very rapid. Mucous membrane (MM) is pale and capillary refill time (CRT) is prolonged in a patient experiencing hypovolemic shock as a result of the vasoconstriction reducing blood flow to the periphery. MM is normally pink, with a normal CRT (1–2 seconds). Yellow MM indicates elevated bilirubin (liver disease, hemolytic anemia) in which the CRT is often not affected. Battaglia AM, Steele AM, Small Animal Emergency and Critical Care for Veterinary Technicians, ed 3, Elsevier, 2016.

287. d Redistribution of blood flow results in pale mucous membranes, poor capillary refill, and cold extremities, which are all symptoms seen in an animal experiencing shock. Acidosis, alkalosis, and cell death are not attributable to excessive blood loss. Bassert JM, Thomas JA, McCurnin's Clinical Textbook for Veterinary Technicians, ed 8, Elsevier, 2014, p. 912.

288. a Within a few hours of ingesting high levels of sodium, normal dogs and cats easily excrete the excess in their urine. However, patients in the early stages of cardiac disease may lose their ability to excrete excess sodium. Retention for longer periods has been implicated in the pathogenesis of congestive heart failure (CHF) and some forms of hypertension. Wortinger A, Burns K, Nutrition and Disease Management for Veterinary Technicians and Nurses, ed 2, Wiley Blackwell, 2015.

289. b Potassium or magnesium homeostasis abnormalities may cause cardiac dysrhythmias, may decrease myocardial contractility, might produce profound muscle weakness, and might potentiate adverse effects from cardiac glycosides and other cardiac drugs. Potassium or magnesium homeostasis abnormalities may decrease, not increase, myocardial contractility. Wortinger A, Burns K, Nutrition and Disease Management for Veterinary Technicians and Nurses, ed 2, Wiley Blackwell, 2015.

290. a Omega-3 fatty acids have been shown to have a significant effect on survival times when used in dogs diagnosed with dilated cardiomyopathy (DCM) or chronic valvular disease (CVD). The effects of omega-3 fatty acids may be attributed to anti-inflammatory effects, cachexia prevention, improved appetite, or antiarrhythmic effects. Omega-6 and omega-9 fatty acids have not been shown to elicit positive effects for patients with cardiac disease. Wortinger A, Burns K, Nutrition and Disease Management for Veterinary Technicians and Nurses, ed 2, Wiley Blackwell, 2015.

291. c Horses with respiratory disease may have increased respiratory rate (tachypnea) and effort (dyspnea), nasal discharge, and cough, as well as decreased performance, fever, and lymphadenopathy. Horses with problems in the upper respiratory tract, larynx, pharynx, guttural pouches, nasal passages, and sinuses may have unilateral or bilateral nasal discharge or decreased airflow from one or both nostrils and they may make a noise when breathing (stridor or stertor). Bassert JM, Thomas JA, McCurnin's Clinical Textbook for Veterinary Technicians, ed 8, Elsevier, 2014.

292. b Horses with problems in the lower respiratory tract (lungs and trachea) may have bilateral nasal discharge, but abnormal lung sounds are often audible during rebreathing examination. Abnormal sounds may include crackles, wheezes, decreased airflow, and prolonged recovery from the rebreathing examination. Stridor and stertor refer to making noise while breathing and are seen with upper respiratory complications. Bassert JM, Thomas JA, McCurnin's Clinical Textbook for Veterinary Technicians, ed 8, Elsevier, 2014.

293. d Pyloric outflow obstruction results in projectile vomiting, in which the cause can be mechanical (e.g., foreign body) or functional (e.g., pyloric thickening). Green fluid in the vomitus indicates involvement of fresh bile in the duodenum. Gastric or esophageal disorders commonly manifest as white, frothy vomitus. Gastrointestinal ulceration results in frank blood if the bleeding from ulceration is fresh, whereas dark, black flecks resembling coffee grounds indicate blood digested in the stomach. Battaglia AM, Steele AM, Small Animal Emergency and Critical Care for Veterinary Technicians, ed 3, Elsevier, 2016.

294. c An MRI can be used to assess the upper airway of a horse. BAL (bronchoalveolar lavage), TTW (transtracheal wash), and pulmonary function testing are all used to assess the lower airway of horses. Bassert JM, Thomas JA, McCurnin's Clinical Textbook for Veterinary Technicians, ed 8, Elsevier, 2014.

295. a Typical clinical signs of advanced arthritis in dogs include difficulty in rising from rest, stiffness, lameness, reluctance to walk, run, climb stairs, jump, or play. Reduced appetite is not a usual sign of advanced arthritis provided that food is available in areas that are easily accessible to the dog. Wortinger A, Burns K, Nutrition and Disease Management for Veterinary Technicians and Nurses, ed 2, Wiley Blackwell, 2015.

296. a Strangles causes the submandibular and retropharyngeal lymph nodes to swell and abscess. Common clinical signs seen with equine influenza, herpes, and viral arteritis include coughing, nasal discharge, and pyrexia. Bassert JM, Thomas JA, McCurnin's Clinical Textbook for Veterinary Technicians, ed 8, Elsevier, 2014.

297. b Diarrhea and bleeding that originate in the jejunum and ileum present as melena. Diarrhea of large intestinal origin will result in high-frequency diarrhea, often accompanied with straining and mucus. Involvement of the stomach causes no distinct change to diarrhea and it is most associated with vomiting. Colitis results in frank blood mixed in the diarrhea. Battaglia AM, Steele AM, Small Animal Emergency and Critical Care for Veterinary Technicians, ed 3, Elsevier, 2016.

298. b Equine herpes virus is the causative agent of rhinopneumonitis in horses. Streptococcus equi is the causative agent of strangles, in which *Aspergillus* spp. is the agent of guttural pouch mycosis. Bassert JM, Thomas JA, McCurnin's Clinical Textbook for Veterinary Technicians, ed 8, Elsevier, 2014.

299. d Risk factors, in dogs, for developing osteoarthritis include: age, large or giant breeds, genetics, developmental orthopedic disease, trauma, and obesity. Spayed or neutered pets are at increased risk for obesity because of their reduced energy needs. However, being spayed or neutered is not a risk factor for the development of osteoarthritis. Wortinger A, Burns K, Nutrition and Disease Management for Veterinary Technicians and Nurses, ed 2, Wiley Blackwell, 2015.

300. d Hyperthyroidism is very rare in dogs and is commonly seen in cats older than 10 years of age. Hypothyroidism is rare in cats and is common in dogs 6–10 years of age. Hyperadrenocorticalism, also known as Cushing's disease, is common in dogs and rare in cats. Hypoadrenocorticism, also known as Addison's disease, mainly affects dogs. Aspinall V, The Complete Textbook of Veterinary Nursing, ed 2, Saunders Elsevier, 2011.

301. d Common symptoms of osteoarthritis in cats include: mobility changes such as reluctance to jump or to jump as high, changes in activity level such as decreased playing or hunting, and changes in grooming habits, as the cat may not be able to reach certain areas easily. Changes in eating habits are not a normal symptom of osteoarthritis in cats, provided that the food is located in an area that the cats are able to access easily. Wortinger A, Burns K, Nutrition and Disease Management for Veterinary Technicians and Nurses, ed 2, Wiley Blackwell, 2015.

302. c Absence seizures are brain seizure activities that result in a loss of consciousness with or without external signs. Focal seizures can be referred to as petit mal seizures, resulting in partial seizures with or without loss of consciousness. Generalized seizures can be referred to as grand mal seizures and can involve loss of consciousness with tonic–clonic whole body movements and are often accompanied by salivation, urination, and defecation. Myoclonus refers to brief twitches of a muscle or muscle groups. Battaglia AM, Steele AM, Small Animal Emergency and Critical Care for Veterinary Technicians, ed 3, Elsevier, 2016.

303. c Equine herpesvirus (the causative agent of rhinopneumonitis) is a contagious virus that produces respiratory disease, abortion, and neonatal and neurologic disease (ascending paralysis) in horses and it is a reportable disease in some states. Abortion is not associated with strangles, influenza, or EIA. Thomas JA, McCurnin's Clinical Textbook for Veterinary Technicians, ed 8, Elsevier, 2014.

304. d In avian patients, nutritional deficiencies and excesses in avians may result in immune dysfunction, increased susceptibility to infectious diseases, and metabolic and biochemical derangements. Clinically, veterinary teams may see nutritional secondary hyperparathyroidism, thyroid hyperplasia (dysplasia), hemochromatosis, and potentially many other issues. Wortinger A, Burns K, Nutrition and Disease Management for Veterinary Technicians and Nurses, ed 2, Wiley Blackwell, 2015.

305. b Absence seizures are brain seizure activities that result in a loss of consciousness with or without external signs. Focal seizures can be referred to as petit mal seizures, resulting in partial seizures with or without loss of consciousness. Generalized seizures can be referred to as grand mal seizures and they involve loss of consciousness with tonic–clonic whole body movements and are often accompanied by salivation, urination, and defecation. Myoclonus refers to brief twitches of a muscle or muscle groups. Battaglia AM, Steele AM, Small Animal Emergency and Critical Care for Veterinary Technicians, ed 3, Elsevier, 2016.

306. a Absence seizures are brain seizure activities that result in a loss of consciousness with or without external signs. Focal seizures can be referred to as petit mal seizures, resulting in partial seizures with or without loss of consciousness. Generalized seizures can be referred to as grand mal seizures and involve loss of consciousness with tonic–clonic whole body movements, and are often accompanied by salivation, urination, and defecation. Myoclonus refers to brief twitches of a muscle or muscle groups. Battaglia AM, Steele AM, Small Animal Emergency and Critical Care for Veterinary Technicians, ed 3, Elsevier, 2016.

307. a Heaves, or recurrent airway obstruction (RAO), is an allergic airway disease caused by airway inflammation, narrowing of small airways (bronchoconstriction), and excessive production of mucus. Heaves typically affects horses 15 years of age and older. Viral arteritis, IAD, and EIPH are not associated with allergic airway disease. Bassert JM, Thomas JA, McCurnin's Clinical Textbook for Veterinary Technicians, ed 8, Elsevier, 2014.

308. d Brachycephalic syndrome is a collection of anatomical features that a brachycephalic is predisposed to having, which impedes proper breathing (stenotic nares, hypoplastic trachea, elongated soft palate, and acquired everted laryngeal saccules). Horner syndrome is described as miosis, ptosis (drooping eyelid), enophthalmos (posterior displacement of eye because of muscle dysfunction), and protruding nictitans. Wobbler syndrome is ataxia and paresis that occurs from vertebral malformations (spondylosis). Vestibular syndrome is characterized by head tilt, facial paresis, nystagmus, positional strabismus, and ataxia. Battaglia AM, Steele AM, Small Animal Emergency and Critical Care for Veterinary Technicians, ed 3, Elsevier, 2016.

309. a Ferrets are strict carnivores that have a short, simple gastrointestinal (GI) tract. GI tracts of ferrets lack a cecum and ileocolic valve. Because of their shorter GI tract, ferrets' GI transit time is rapid—approximately 3–6 hours. Highly digestible foods containing large amounts of protein and fat, from animal-based ingredients, should be offered. Also the nutritional makeup includes minimal digestible (soluble) carbohydrate and fiber. Herbivores eat only, or primarily, plant material. Omnivore refers to an animal that eats plants and animal tissue. Granivores is not a word. Wortinger A, Burns K, Nutrition and Disease Management for Veterinary Technicians and Nurses, ed 2, Wiley Blackwell, 2015.

310. d When bacterial infection spreads from lung tissue to the pleural space, called pleuropneumonia, pleural effusion can occur. Bassert JM, Thomas JA, McCurnin's Clinical Textbook for Veterinary Technicians, ed 8, Elsevier, 2014.

311. b Brachycephalic syndrome is a collection of anatomical features that a brachycephalic is predisposed to having, which impedes proper breathing (stenotic nares, hypoplastic trachea, elongated soft palate, and acquired everted laryngeal saccules). Horner syndrome is described as miosis, ptosis (drooping eyelid), enophthalmos (posterior displacement of eye because of muscle dysfunction), and protruding nictitans. Wobbler syndrome is ataxia and paresis that occurs from vertebral malformations (spondylosis). Vestibular syndrome is characterized by head tilt, facial paresis, nystagmus, positional strabismus, and ataxia. Battaglia AM, Steele AM, Small Animal Emergency and Critical Care for Veterinary Technicians, ed 3, Elsevier, 2016.

312. b Equine viral arteritis is a contagious viral disease that produces limb swelling, conjunctivitis, abortion, and respiratory disease in horses. Limb swelling is painful and results from vasculitis (inflammation of blood vessels). Bassert JM, Thomas JA, McCurnin's Clinical Textbook for Veterinary Technicians, ed 8, Elsevier, 2014.

313. c Lagomorphs have a rapid gut transit time resulting in starch and simple sugars not being completely digested in the small intestine. These are then directed into the cecum, where they may be used for fermentation by the cecal microorganisms. The GI tract of rabbits consists of a simple (noncompartmentalized) stomach and a large cecum. Wortinger A, Burns K, Nutrition and Disease Management for Veterinary Technicians and Nurses, ed 2, Wiley Blackwell, 2015.

314. a Hamsters, gerbils, mice, and rats naturally hoard food items. Therefore it is difficult to determine exactly how much food is being ingested. Rabbits, guinea pigs, and ferrets are not food hoarders. Wortinger A, Burns K, Nutrition and Disease Management for Veterinary Technicians and Nurses, ed 2, Wiley Blackwell, 2015.

315. c Brachycephalic syndrome is a collection of anatomical features that a brachycephalic is predisposed to having, which impedes proper breathing (stenotic nares, hypoplastic trachea, elongated soft palate, and acquired everted laryngeal saccules). Horner syndrome is described as miosis, ptosis (drooping eyelid), enophthalmos (posterior displacement of eye because of muscle dysfunction), and protruding nictitans. Wobbler syndrome is ataxia and paresis that occurs from vertebral malformations (spondylosis). Vestibular syndrome is characterized by head tilt, facial paresis, nystagmus, positional strabismus, and ataxia. Battaglia AM, Steele AM, Small Animal Emergency and Critical Care for Veterinary Technicians, ed 3, Elsevier, 2016.

316. c Anaplasmosis, also known as equine granulocytic ehrlichiosis, is caused by infection with the bacteria *Anaplasma phagocytophilum*, formerly called *Ehrlichia equi*. Biting ticks of the genus *Ixodes* transmit these bacteria. Clinical signs include fever, anemia, icterus, lethargy, stiffness, and limb edema. Bassert JM, Thomas JA, McCurnin's Clinical Textbook for Veterinary Technicians, ed 8, Elsevier, 2014.

317. a Gastric ulcers are common in performance horses of all disciplines. Clinical signs of gastric ulceration include bruxism (grinding of teeth), hypersalivation, abdominal pain after eating, and anorexia. Bassert JM, Thomas JA, McCurnin's Clinical Textbook for Veterinary Technicians, ed 8, Elsevier, 2014.

318. c Guinea pigs require a dietary source of vitamin C because they lack the enzyme L-gulonolactone involved in synthesizing glucose to ascorbic acid. Guinea pigs do not require dietary sources of vitamins B or K. Wortinger A, Burns K, Nutrition and Disease Management for Veterinary Technicians and Nurses, ed 2, Wiley Blackwell, 2015.

319. b Ferrets are strict carnivores that have a short, simple gastrointestinal (GI) tract. The GI tract of ferrets lacks a cecum and an ileocolic valve. Because of their shorter GI tract, ferrets' GI transit time is rapid—approximately 3–6 hours. Highly digestible foods containing large amounts of protein and fat, from animal-based ingredients, should be offered. Being strict carnivores, ferrets do not require plant-based ingredients, nor do they use them well. It is believed that ferrets do not have dietary requirements for carbohydrates, including fiber, as seen in other obligate carnivores. Wortinger A, Burns K, Nutrition and Disease Management for Veterinary Technicians and Nurses, ed 2, Wiley Blackwell, 2015.

320. b Bathing the patient with mild dishwashing detergent alleviates exposure to dermal or topical toxins. Applying chemical solvents can be just as harmful or more harmful to the patient. Induction of emesis (vomiting) is indicated when there is recent ingestion of toxin and is not required for dermal/topical decontamination. Wiping off the chemical with a dry towel removes some of the chemical but will not adequately decontaminate the fur compared with bathing. Battaglia AM, Steele AM, Small Animal Emergency and Critical Care for Veterinary Technicians, ed 3, Elsevier, 2016.

321. b Phenylbutazone (NSAID) toxicosis in horses can produce renal insufficiency and oral, gastric, and colonic ulceration in horses. Colonic ulcers occur in the right dorsal colon and are difficult to treat. Colonic ulcers secondary to phenylbutazone toxicity can produce abdominal pain, marked protein loss, melena (blood in manure), peritonitis, colonic stricture, or colonic rupture—a syndrome known as right dorsal colitis. Phenylbutazone toxicosis does not cause limb edema. Bassert JM, Thomas JA, McCurnin's Clinical Textbook for Veterinary Technicians, ed 8, Elsevier, 2014.

322. d A prescription for a controlled substance must be signed and dated at the time of issue. The prescription must include the patient's (owner's) full name and address, the practitioner's full name and address, and the practitioner's DEA number. It must be written in ink, in indelible pencil, or printed, and the practitioner must manually sign it on the date issued. A designated individual may be assigned to prepare prescriptions for the practitioner's signature. The prescription must also include the drug name, drug strength, dosage form, quantity prescribed, directions for use, and number of refills authorized. The name and address of the drug manufacturer is not required. Wanamaker BP, Massey KL, Applied Pharmacology for Veterinary Technicians, ed 5, Elsevier Saunders, 2015.

323. c Colitis in horses can result in rapid, life-threatening fluid loss (hypovolemia), shock, endotoxemia, electrolyte loss, and acid-base imbalance as a result of diarrhea. Some horses may develop hypovolemic shock and electrolyte imbalance before the appearance of diarrhea. Bassert JM, Thomas JA, McCurnin's Clinical Textbook for Veterinary Technicians, ed 8, Elsevier, 2014.

324. d Each of these choices is a valid venipuncture point for a bird. However, the jugular veins are the largest of the vessels and the right jugular is anatomically larger than the left jugular vein. Battaglia AM, Steele AM, Small Animal Emergency and Critical Care for Veterinary Technicians, ed 3, Elsevier, 2016.

325. d To determine how many tablets to give to this patient, divide the dose you are to administer (250 mg) by the concentration of the tablet (100 mg). 250÷100 = 2.5. Each tablet is 100 mg; therefore, ½ tablet is 50 mg. You must provide 2.5 tablets. 1½ tablets = 150 mg, 2 tablets = 200 mg, 2¼ tablets = 225 mg. Lake T, Green N, Essential Calculations for Veterinary Nurses and Technicians, ed 2, Butterworth-Heinemann, 2009.

326. a Complications of colitis include laminitis (founder), cardiovascular collapse, cardiac arrhythmias, and thrombophlebitis. Stertor/stridor are noises made while breathing and bruxism is grinding of the teeth (although this is a clinical symptom of colitis, it is not a complication). Bassert JM, Thomas JA, McCurnin's Clinical Textbook for Veterinary Technicians, ed 8, Elsevier, 2014.

327. a Lymphosarcoma is the most common neoplasia in horses and most commonly affects the gastrointestinal tract. Infiltration of the intestine may result in chronic weight loss, diarrhea, and hypoalbuminemia. A presumptive diagnosis is supported by the exclusion of other causes of weight loss, the thickening of the intestinal wall on ultrasound, and the palpation of enlarged mesenteric lymph nodes on rectal examination. Definitive diagnosis is made by biopsy of the intestine (via gastroscopy, rectal mucosal biopsy, laparoscopy, or laparotomy) or identification of neoplastic cells in abdominal fluid. The liver, spleen, and kidney may also be affected. Bassert JM, Thomas JA, McCurnin's Clinical Textbook for Veterinary Technicians, ed 8, Elsevier, 2014.

328. b Blood weighs approximately 1 g/mL. 1% of 450 g = 4.5 g. 4.5 g of blood is approximately 4.5 mL. 450 g × 0.01 × 1 mL/g = 4.5 mL. Battaglia AM, Steele AM, Small Animal Emergency and Critical Care for Veterinary Technicians, ed 3, Elsevier, 2016.

329. c Eastern, Western, Venezuelan, and West Nile are the four main types of viral equine encephalitis. Bassert JM, Thomas JA, McCurnin's Clinical Textbook for Veterinary Technicians, ed 8, Elsevier, 2014.

330. c 1 lb = 2.2 kg. To convert the patient's weight from pounds to kilograms, divide 88 by 2.2 = 40. 20 kg = 44 lb, 24 kg = 52.8 lb, 44 kg = 96.8 kg. Lake T, Green N, Essential Calculations for Veterinary Nurses and Technicians, ed 2, Butterworth-Heinemann, 2009.

331. c Clinical signs of West Nile encephalitis include weakness, ataxia, muscle fasciculations, and cranial nerve deficits (such as droopy lip). Hyperesthesia (extreme sensitivity to touch) around the head and neck is a common clinical sign. Bassert JM, Thomas JA, McCurnin's Clinical Textbook for Veterinary Technicians, ed 8, Elsevier, 2014.

332. d The blood feather should be pulled and pressure applied at the follicle to stop the bleeding. Applying pressure to the broken edge is ineffective in stopping the bleeding because there is no tissue that can be occluded in the area, making clotting difficult. Applying styptic powder to the blood feather is also unlikely to stop the bleeding. Cutting the feather at the base will only relocate the bleeding edge to the base, without providing any measures for the blood to stop. Battaglia AM, Steele AM, Small Animal Emergency and Critical Care for Veterinary Technicians, ed 3, Elsevier, 2016.

333. c Vaccines for Eastern, Western, and West Nile equine encephalitis are highly efficacious and clinical disease in vaccinated horses is rare. Horses in the United States should be vaccinated against Eastern and Western equine and West Nile encephalomyelitis viruses before the mosquito season begins in the spring. Horses living in southern states with a year-round mosquito season should be vaccinated 2 to 3 times per year. Broodmares should receive a booster of their vaccination in the 10th month of gestation (use only killed-virus vaccines in pregnant animals) to ensure adequate colostral antibody protection for the foal. Vaccination against Venezuelan equine encephalomyelitis is not routinely recommended because the disease has not been reported recently in the United States and it does not currently pose a threat to the US horse population, except those near the Mexican border. Bassert JM, Thomas JA, McCurnin's Clinical Textbook for Veterinary Technicians, ed 8, Elsevier, 2014.

334. b 1 mL is equal to 120 mg. To determine how much to give (60 mg), divide the number of mg you wish to give (60) by the concentration of the liquid medication (120). 60÷120 = 0.5. You would administer 0.5 mL of this medication to the patient. 2.0 mL of this medication = 240 mg, which is four times the dose the patient is prescribed. 0.2 mL of this medication = 24 mg, which is much less than the prescribed dose. 5.0 mL of this medication = 600 mL, which is 10 times the dose prescribed for this patient. Lake T, Green N, Essential Calculations for Veterinary Nurses and Technicians, ed 2, Butterworth-Heinemann, 2009

335. b Tetanus is a highly fatal neurologic disease in horses characterized by a stiff, stilted gait, hyperexcitability, seizure, and coma. Bassert JM, Thomas JA, McCurnin's Clinical Textbook for Veterinary Technicians, ed 8, Elsevier, 2014.

336. b The caudal tail vein and the heart are two common locations of blood sampling from a reptile. The basilic vein can be used in an avian, but, along with the cephalic and jugular, these veins are all very difficult to access or are nonexistent. Battaglia AM, Steele AM, Small Animal Emergency and Critical Care for Veterinary Technicians, ed 3, Elsevier, 2016.

337. a Botulism is a rapidly progressive, often fatal neurologic disease in horses, which is characterized by profound weakness, muscle fasciculations, and dysphagia (inability to swallow). The causal organism produces a neurotoxin that may gain entry to the body by colonizing the intestinal tract (foals) through infected wounds or by contaminated feedstuff. Bassert JM, Thomas JA, McCurnin's Clinical Textbook for Veterinary Technicians, ed 8, Elsevier, 2014.

338. b To determine how many mL the patient has received, multiply the amount initially in the bag of fluids (1000 mL) by the percent the patient received (25%). 1000 mL × 25% is equal to 1000 mL × 0.25 = 250 mL. The patient has received 250 mL of fluid. 100 mL = 10% of the 1000 mL bag, 350 mL = 35% of the 1000 mL bag, 500 mL = 50% of the 1000 mL bag. Lake T, Green N, Essential Calculations for Veterinary Nurses and Technicians, ed 2, Butterworth-Heinemann, 2009.

339. b To determine how many mL of fluid per kg of body weight the patient has received, divide the total amount of fluid the patient has received (250 mL) by the patient's weight in kg (25 kg). 250 ÷ 25 = 10 mL of fluid per kg. At 5 mL/kg of body weight, the patient would have only received 125 mL of fluid; at 15 mL/kg, the patient would have received 375 mL of fluid; at 25 mL/kg, the patient would have received 625 mL of fluid. Lake T, Green N, Essential Calculations for Veterinary Nurses and Technicians, ed 2, Butterworth-Heinemann, 2009.

340. b Acute renal failure in horses is most often the result of toxic causes. Aminoglycoside antibiotics (gentamicin, amikacin), oxytetracycline, polymyxin B, an antibiotic used in the treatment of endotoxemia, and NSAIDs are commonly implicated. Dehydration exacerbates renal damage caused by these drugs. Age and hereditary factors do not contribute to renal failure in horses. Colic is a gastrointestinal emergency and although renal failure may result from drugs administered (sometimes at toxic levels) to treat colic, it is not a direct result. Bassert JM, Thomas JA, McCurnin's Clinical Textbook for Veterinary Technicians, ed 8, Elsevier, 2014.

341. b Chronic kidney disease is an irreversible, progressive loss of functioning renal tissue leading to azotemia and reduced urine specific gravity. Acute kidney injury is a quick onset renal dysfunction that can be reversible, depending on the cause. Acute or chronic liver disease applies to the hepatic tissues and thus not to the renal tissue. Bassert JM, Thomas JA, McCurnin's Clinical Textbook for Veterinary Technicians, ed 8, Elsevier, 2014.

342. c Surgical removal of worms from the right atrium is necessary as a life-saving procedure for patients with a heavy worm load and caval syndrome. Adulticide therapy is used for lighter worm load and is thought to be sufficient. Microfilaricide is used as a preventative measure against the development of adult worms. Heavy heartworm load is not transient and requires treatment. Bassert JM, Thomas JA, McCurnin's Clinical Textbook for Veterinary Technicians, ed 8, Elsevier, 2014.

343. c Horses normally drink between 4% and 6% of their body weight daily (20 to 30 L for a full-sized horse). Bassert JM, Thomas JA, McCurnin's Clinical Textbook for Veterinary Technicians, ed 8, Elsevier, 2014.

344. a To determine the quantity to feed, divide the total number of kcal in the can (360) by the number of kcal that the cat is to be fed (90); 360 ÷ 90 = 0.25. This cat should be fed 0.25 cans of this food at each meal. Feeding 0.2 cans, the cat would receive 72 kcal per meal; feeding 0.5 cans, the cat would receive 180 kcal; feeding 1 can, the cat would receive 360 kcal. Lake T, Green N, Essential Calculations for Veterinary Nurses and Technicians, ed 2, Butterworth-Heinemann, 2009.

345. c The cell is the basic unit of the body. All cells contain a nucleus, cell membrane, and cytoplasm. They also possess other features that are specific to their type and function. Neurons (or nerve cells) have slender arm-like processes that transmit electrical impulses through the nervous system to reach the whole body. Aspinall V, The Complete Textbook of Veterinary Nursing, ed 2, Saunders Elsevier, 2011.

346. c Horses normally urinate 1% to 3% of their body weight daily (5 to 15 L for a full-sized horse) because most water is lost via feces. Bassert JM, Thomas JA, McCurnin's Clinical Textbook for Veterinary Technicians, ed 8, Elsevier, 2014.

347. b Hemoptysis, dyspnea, and coughing are signs of pulmonary thromboembolism that can occur with adulticide treatment of heartworm. Ecchymoses and anemia are signs of coagulopathy and related red blood cell loss. Hematuria and stranguria are signs of irritation to the bladder. Melena and lethargy are signs of upper gastrointestinal ulceration and possibly anemia. Bassert JM, Thomas JA, McCurnin's Clinical Textbook for Veterinary Technicians, ed 8, Elsevier, 2014.

348. a The most common sign associated with severe hypertension is acute blindness resulting from retinal detachment. Syncope (fainting) and weakness are signs of hypotension. Tachycardia is often associated with hypotension rather than hypertension, which tends to cause bradycardia. Bassert JM, Thomas JA, McCurnin's Clinical Textbook for Veterinary Technicians, ed 8, Elsevier, 2014.

349. b Dietary indiscretion, especially with high-fat meals, is a common trigger for pancreatitis in dogs. Blunt force trauma, pancreatic hypoperfusion, and pancreotoxic drugs are all sources of pancreatitis for both dogs and cats. Bassert JM, Thomas JA, McCurnin's Clinical Textbook for Veterinary Technicians, ed 8, Elsevier, 2014.

350. d Erythrocytes, or red blood cells, are designed to hold the red pigment hemoglobin to convey oxygen around the body; they are among the few cells in the body that have no nucleus. Epithelial cells are found lining the surface of the body, the body cavities, and the organs within it. Glandular cells are responsible for producing some kind of secretion, for example, mucus to lubricate the tissues. Osteoblasts produce bone tissue. Aspinall V, The Complete Textbook of Veterinary Nursing, ed 2, Saunders Elsevier, 2011.

351. b The highly convoluted renal tubule extends from the glomerular capsule to the connection with the collecting duct. The urethra carries urine from the bladder to the outside. The two ureters are thin tubes, one leading from each renal pelvis to the bladder. The functional unit of the kidney is called a nephron. Aspinall, V, The Complete Textbook of Veterinary Nursing, ed 2, Butterworth-Heinemann, 2011.

352. c Objective observation relates to measurable factors such as heart rate, body temperature, capillary refill time, blood pressure, and blood biochemistry. Subjective relates to immeasurable observations that can be made, such as demeanor, behavior, degree of lameness, or head tilt. Aspinall V, The Complete Textbook of Veterinary Nursing, ed 2, Butterworth-Heinemann, 2011.

353. d Polyuria/polydipsia (PU/PD) can be the result of physiologic causes, including lactation, heat, exercise, diarrhea, and glucocorticoid administration. Certain diseases can also result in PU/PD. PU/PD is a common sign of equine pituitary pars intermedia syndrome (Cushing's disease) in older horses. PU/PD can also result from drinking psychogenic water, behavioral problems, diabetes, or chronic renal failure. A water deprivation test may be performed to help differentiate the causes. Bassert JM, Thomas JA, McCurnin's Clinical Textbook for Veterinary Technicians, ed 8, Elsevier, 2014.

354. b Coupage is a technique used to help loosen purulent material within the pulmonary parenchyma with pneumonia. Warm compressing is a technique used to increase blood flow to an area to increase draining and healing of the area, such as with mastitis. Passive range of motion is used to keep joints from becoming stiff. Cold compress is used to minimize inflammation. Battaglia AM, Steele AM, Small Animal Emergency and Critical Care for Veterinary Technicians, ed 3, Elsevier, 2016.

355. a Subjective: personal assessment of immeasurable observations, for example, patient's behavior, demeanor, and posture. Objective: factual assessment of measurable observations, for example, temperature, pulse, and respiration (TPR). Assessment: a comparative exercise to assess the progress of the patient; may include both subjective and objective observations. Planning: an outline of the plan for each patient for that day, whether it is a specific treatment protocol or a procedure to be performed. Aspinall V, The Complete Textbook of Veterinary Nursing, ed 2, Butterworth-Heinemann, 2011.

356. b Dermatophilosis is also known as rain rot or rain scold and is a common bacterial infection. Dermatophytosis is fungal infection and is referred to as ringworm, and *Culicoides* hypersensitivity is a syndrome characterized by mane and tail rubbing, whereby affected horses develop an allergic pruritic skin condition secondary to a bite of the *Culicoides* fly. Sarcoid is a benign, locally invasive tumor of the skin. Bassert JM, Thomas JA, McCurnin's Clinical Textbook for Veterinary Technicians, ed 8, Elsevier, 2014.

357. c Hyperthyroidism is an endocrine disorder seen almost exclusively in cats. Chronic kidney disease is commonly seen in cats, but the kidney is not a part of the endocrine system. Diabetes mellitus is endocrine in origin, but it is seen in both cats and dogs. Hypothyroidism is most commonly seen in dogs. Bassert JM, Thomas JA, McCurnin's Clinical Textbook for Veterinary Technicians, ed 8, Elsevier, 2014.

358. b Hematochezia is the production of fresh, bright red blood in the feces: evidence of blood loss in the lower gastrointestinal tract. Dyschezia is the difficult and painful passage of feces. Melena refers to the production of dark, tarry feces with or without mucus, which presents evidence of blood loss in the upper gastrointestinal tract. Tenesmus is the painful, ineffectual straining to pass feces, seen in cases of constipation. Aspinall V, The Complete Textbook of Veterinary Nursing, ed 2, Butterworth-Heinemann, 2011.

359. d Equine recurrent uveitis (moon blindness) is the most common cause of blindness in horses. It is an immune-mediated condition and many factors (heredity, parasites, leptospirosis) have been implicated in its development; however, the inciting cause is often unknown. Dermatophilosis is also known as rain rot or rain scold and it is a common bacterial infection. Dermatophytosis is a fungal infection and is referred to as ringworm. Corneal ulcerations commonly result from ocular trauma and do not have an alternate name. Bassert JM, Thomas JA, McCurnin's Clinical Textbook for Veterinary Technicians, ed 8, Elsevier, 2014.

360. a Clinical signs associated with hyperadrenocorticism include weight gain, muscle weakness, polyuria, polydipsia, skin and hair coat abnormalities, and a potbellied appearance. Hallmarks of hypoadrenocorticism are hyponatremia and hyperkalemia. Hyperthyroidism is typically seen in cats, causing weight loss and a ravenous appetite, among other signs. Hypothyroidism typically causes weight gain, bradycardia, exercise intolerance, and lethargy. Bassert JM, Thomas JA, McCurnin's Clinical Textbook for Veterinary Technicians, ed 8, Elsevier, 2014.

361. c Isolation wards should be designed with separation from other patients in mind. Equipment should be dedicated to the isolation area. A negative pressure air ventilation system is ideal to prevent particles from leaving the room and a single wall of cage banks prevents cross contamination across cages. A double-door entryway with an anteroom also serves as an appropriate barrier. Bassert JM, Thomas JA, McCurnin's Clinical Textbook for Veterinary Technicians, ed 8, Elsevier, 2014.

362. c Steatorrhea is the passage of large volumes of pale, fatty feces, usually associated with exocrine pancreatic insufficiency. Anuria is the complete cessation of urine production. Coprophagia is when an animal eats its own feces. Oliguria is a reduction in the daily production of urine. Aspinall V, The Complete Textbook of Veterinary Nursing, ed 2, Butterworth-Heinemann, 2011.

363. a Dysuria is when the passage of urine is difficult and uncomfortable. Poikuria is the irregular passage of urine. Polyuria is the passing of larger volumes of urine than normal. Stranguria is when the passage of urine is painful and uncomfortable. Aspinall V, The Complete Textbook of Veterinary Nursing, ed 2, Butterworth-Heinemann, 2011.

364. a Equine recurrent uveitis (moon blindness) is the most common cause of blindness in horses. It is an immune-mediated condition and many factors (heredity, parasites, leptospirosis) have been implicated in its development; however, the inciting cause is often unknown. Bassert JM, Thomas JA, McCurnin's Clinical Textbook for Veterinary Technicians, ed 8, Elsevier, 2014.

365. a Barrier nursing for isolation includes gloves, gown, and shoe covers as a standard set. Personnel may opt to wear a mask, although a filtered respirator mask is only required when airborne zoonotic diseases are involved. Bassert JM, Thomas JA, McCurnin's Clinical Textbook for Veterinary Technicians, ed 8, Elsevier, 2014.

366. c Nauseous patients often appear unusually depressed and may intermittently lick their lips. These patients will often turn their heads away from food when it is offered and they may attempt to hide or bury it if food is left with them. Nauseous patients will generally not eat willingly. Ability to urinate is not considered a sign of nausea. Aspinall V, The Complete Textbook of Veterinary Nursing, ed 2, Butterworth-Heinemann, 2011.

367. c Coughing is an expulsive mechanism transmitted by the vagus nerve to the thoracic muscles to expel mucus or foreign bodies. Conditions that can induce a coughing reflex include bronchitis/tracheitis/laryngitis, kennel cough or infectious rhinotracheitis, left-sided congestive heart failure, pneumonia, laryngeal spasm (in cats following endotracheal tube extubation), malformation (e.g., an overlong soft palate). A foreign body in the throat may cause coughing; however, an intestinal foreign body would not. Aspinall V, The Complete Textbook of Veterinary Nursing, ed 2, Butterworth-Heinemann, 2011.

368. a Coupage and nebulization may be used to help loosen secretions and to encourage a more productive cough. To perform coupage, cupped hands should be used to tap firmly on the chest wall, starting caudally and working forward. Working in this direction will encourage a more productive cough and the patient may potentially expel secretions. Caudally refers to the hind end of the patient, thus starting caudally and working backward would not be logical. Coupage involves percussion of the thorax; starting cranially and working forward would not involve the chest. Starting cranially and working backward may encourage loose secretions to move away from the patient's mouth and they may therefore not be as readily expelled. Aspinall V, The Complete Textbook of Veterinary Nursing, ed 2, Butterworth-Heinemann, 2011.

369. c Pica is cravings for unusual items of food, licking, and eating at foreign objects; it is usually seen in animals with nutritional deficiencies. Inappetence is a partial reduction in appetite. Anorexia is a loss of desire for food before calorific requirements have been met. Coprophagia is the ingestion of an animal's own feces. Aspinall V, The Complete Textbook of Veterinary Nursing, ed 2, Butterworth-Heinemann, 2011.

370. d Recumbent horses and foals quickly develop pressure sores (decubital ulcers) over the pelvis (tuber coxae), elbows, and head if not properly managed Bassert JM, Thomas JA, McCurnin's Clinical Textbook for Veterinary Technicians, ed 8, Elsevier, 2014.

371. b Ultraviolet light is required for cholecalciferol synthesis, promoting shell formation and repair, and it also stimulates appetite. Vitamin A deficiency occurs because of nutritional deficiencies. Vitamin D is cholecalciferol and the light helps increase levels, not decrease them. Sunlight is important in body temperature regulation, although the question is specific for ultraviolet light. Bassert JM, Thomas JA, McCurnin's Clinical Textbook for Veterinary Technicians, ed 8, Elsevier, 2014.

372. c Discharge in the pinna or ear might indicate an ear infection or other diseases of the ear canal; however, they are not an indication of the patient's hydration stratus. There are various measurements and observations used to determine a patient's hydration status, which include: capillary refill time (CRT)—the gum is blanched by finger pressure and the time taken for the gum to return to normal color is recorded; in a dehydrated patient, this may take longer than in a healthy CRT. Dry mucous membranes are indicative of a dehydrated patient and can also be assessed while carrying out the previously mentioned measurement. When observing eye position within the socket, retraction of the eye back into its socket indicates that the patient is dehydrated. Gently pinching or tenting the patient's skin is a test for dermal elasticity. In a healthy patient, the skin should resume its normal form almost immediately, but in cases of dehydration there will be less elasticity within the skin and it will take longer to resume a normal position. This assessment is objective and depends on the age, condition, and amount of subcutaneous fat in the patient. A packed cell volume (PCV) may be performed if a blood sample is available. This test is normally used to measure the amount of red blood cells in a given volume of blood, but the figure obtained can also be indicative of hydration status. The normal PCV for a cat or dog is 32%–45%. A higher PCV (>45%) would indicate dehydration because the top layer of the plasma sample, the fluid component of the blood, is reduced so that the relative proportion of red blood cells is greater. When assessing dehydration, the rule is that a 1% increase in PCV is equivalent to a water loss of 10 mL/kg. Aspinall V, The Complete Textbook of Veterinary Nursing, ed 2, Butterworth-Heinemann, 2011.

373. c Administering warmed sterile isotonic fluids subcutaneously can be particularly useful in patients where intravenous access would be difficult, for example, in neonates or in patients in which oral administration would be difficult. Absorption of fluids using this method is very slow and should be avoided in severely dehydrated animals. Small boluses should only be administered at any one time and different areas of skin should be used each time. Warmed sterile hypotonic or isotonic fluids may also be administered directly into the peritoneal cavity. Because of the high absorptive capacity of the peritoneum, it is a more efficient way of administering fluids than the subcutaneous route. This method must be undertaken in a strictly aseptic manner to avoid introducing infection into the peritoneal cavity. Intraosseous fluid administration allows the administration of fluids into the medullary cavity of a long bone, for example, the proximal femur or tibia in cats or dogs. It is especially useful in small exotic species, neonates, and trauma patients in which venous access is fragile or compromised. Absorption of fluids from this route is as rapid as the intravenous route. For intravenous fluid administration, access is gained using an intravenous catheter. Sterile warmed fluids are administered into the vein—commonly the cephalic or saphenous vein. This method is the most rapid and effective way of introducing fluids into a severely dehydrated patient and it can be used for continual fluid administration. Aspinall V, The Complete Textbook of Veterinary Nursing, ed 2, Butterworth-Heinemann, 2011.

374. b The position of the horse should be changed every 6 hours; multiple attendants are required to move an adult recumbent horse. A sling can be used only in horses that can partially support their own weight but are not able to stand on their own. Bassert JM, Thomas JA, McCurnin's Clinical Textbook for Veterinary Technicians, ed 8, Elsevier, 2014.

375. b Ferrets are strict carnivores, requiring 30% protein and 25% fat in their diets. Dogs are omnivores. Prairie dogs and rabbits are herbivores. Bassert JM, Thomas JA, McCurnin's Clinical Textbook for Veterinary Technicians, ed 8, Elsevier, 2014.

376. c The lumbar vertebrae are dorsal to the abdominal region. The cervical vertebrae are in the neck region. The thoracic vertebrae are located dorsal to the thorax. The sacral vertebrae are unique in that they fuse to form a single, solid structure called the sacrum. Colville TP, Bassert JM, Clinical Anatomy and Physiology for Veterinary Technicians, ed 3, Elsevier, 2016.

377. a Endotoxemia refers to the group of clinical signs caused by endotoxin circulating through the bloodstream. Clinical signs associated with endotoxemia include fever, tachycardia, hyperemic mucous membranes, leukopenia, laminitis, and depression. Bassert JM, Thomas JA, McCurnin's Clinical Textbook for Veterinary Technicians, ed 8, Elsevier, 2014.

378. c Dystrophic calcification is caused by a diet high in calcium or vitamin D, results in chalky-white or cream-colored urine, and can lead to urinary lithiasis. Rabbits practice coprophagy, eating their night stool for nutrition. Dysbiosis occurs when antibiotic-impregnated feed is ingested, disrupting the intestinal flora. Vitamin A deficiency results in infertility, central nervous system defects, and increased neonatal mortality. Bassert JM, Thomas JA, McCurnin's Clinical Textbook for Veterinary Technicians, ed 8, Elsevier, 2014.

379. b Thrombus: formation of a blood clot because of the flow of blood being impeded, for example, by the presence of a catheter within the lumen of the vein, which may lead to an embolism. Thrombophlebitis: inflammation of a vein usually associated with thrombus formation. Air embolism: sudden obstruction of a blood vessel because of the introduction of air into the lumen of a blood vessel. An embolism may also be caused by a blood clot or piece of tissue. Septicemia/bacteremia: introduction of microorganisms into the vein through poor catheter placement and management. Swelling, redness, pain, and discharge from the catheter site and surrounding area lead to systemic infection. Aspinall V, The Complete Textbook of Veterinary Nursing, ed 2, Butterworth-Heinemann, 2011.

380. c After medical resolution of colic, horses should be offered soft feed, such as bran mash, fresh grass, and small amounts of good-quality hay. Feed should be offered to horses with gastrointestinal tract disease frequently in small quantities rather than in two large daily meals. Bassert JM, Thomas JA, McCurnin's Clinical Textbook for Veterinary Technicians, ed 8, Elsevier, 2014.

381. c Female hamsters are known to hide their young in their check pouches when disturbed, which can lead to suffocation of the young. Female hamsters are the ones that attack newly introduced males. Hamsters live 18–24 months. The best method of restraint in hamsters is to hold the nape of the skin at the base of the neck or by cupping the hands under the hind limbs. Bassert JM, Thomas JA, McCurnin's Clinical Textbook for Veterinary Technicians, ed 8, Elsevier, 2014.

382. b Inappetent horses should be offered highly palatable, calorie-dense feed to increase energy intake. Bassert JM, Thomas JA, McCurnin's Clinical Textbook for Veterinary Technicians, ed 8, Elsevier, 2014.

383. b Hypostatic pneumonia can be a complication in laterally recumbent patients, especially those that are geriatric or are seriously ill. Pooling of blood and fluids can occur in the lower lung, that is, the lung closest to the floor, and it provides an ideal medium for the growth of bacterial microorganisms. This then reduces the viability of the lung, resulting in the development of pneumonia. Clinical signs include coughing, tachypnea, and a rapid shallow breathing pattern. Preventative treatment includes turning the patient every 4 hours, if not contraindicated, preventing the lower lung from becoming nonviable. The patient can also be repositioned into sternal recumbency, allowing both lungs to inflate fully. Coupage may also be performed to aid expulsion of secretions. Antibiotics may be needed to treat the pneumonia; however, they are not recommended as a method of prevention. Ensuring that the patient is fully awake and is able to protect its own airway in advance of extubation might prevent aspiration pneumonia. Aspinall V, The Complete Textbook of Veterinary Nursing, ed 2, Butterworth-Heinemann, 2011.

384. d Muscle atrophy may be a potential complication through reduced limb use and it can lead to joint adhesions and muscle spasms, which can be painful and can cause permanent damage. Physical therapy under instruction from the veterinarian, in the form of controlled passive limb movement and voluntary exercise, can help to reduce the risks of these complications occurring. Passive limb movement involves the nurse gently extending and flexing the joints in the limbs. Care should be taken not to overstretch the muscles and checks must be made to ensure that all limbs are fully functional and amenable to such activity. Hydrotherapy may be of benefit because the water provides much of the support for the patient. Massage has also been shown to increase circulation in immobile limbs, as well as increasing fluid exchange, flushing toxins out of the tissues via the pulmonary and lymphatic drainage system, and reducing the presence of edematous fluid formation. Massage can prevent fibrous adhesions from occurring between connective tissue in the limbs and can provide mental relaxation for the patient. In spinal cases, massage has been beneficial in alleviating painful spasms associated with spinal disease and trauma. Aspinall V, The Complete Textbook of Veterinary Nursing, ed 2, Butterworth-Heinemann, 2011.

385. d Physical therapy for companion animals presents multiple therapeutic benefits, improves the quality of life, and speeds functional recovery. It can be helpful in pain management, combating acute and chronic inflammatory processes, improving the range of motion of affected joints, improving blood perfusion and consequently tissue growth, reducing muscle contraction and tension, maintaining and strengthening muscles, stimulating the nervous system, encouraging proprioceptive rehabilitation and relearning of motor patterns, improving cardiorespiratory capacity, reducing edema, and managing weight in overweight patients. Successful veterinary physical therapy is directly related to the assessment of the patient and requires knowledge of functional anatomy and physiology, excellent communication skills, and the ability to observe and assess movement patterns. Aspinall V, The Complete Textbook of Veterinary Nursing, ed 2, Butterworth-Heinemann, 2011.

386. a Septic thrombophlebitis can be life-threatening in horses and is more likely to occur in horses with endotoxemia, systemic infection, and in those being treated with parenteral nutrition. Bassert JM, Thomas JA, McCurnin's Clinical Textbook for Veterinary Technicians, ed 8, Elsevier, 2014.

387. a Mastitis results in hard, painful nipples, and galactostasis (loss of milk production). Eclampsia is a condition of hypocalcemia arising from lactation, resulting in muscle spasms, fever, tachycardia, and seizures. Hard labor for 30 to 60 minutes with no new young is a form of dystocia. Vaginal discharge, vomiting, diarrhea, dehydration, anorexia, polyuria, and polydipsia are all signs of pyometra. Battaglia AM, Steele AM, Small Animal Emergency and Critical Care for Veterinary Technicians, ed 3, Elsevier, 2016.

388. b Petrissage: when performing petrissage, the therapist rolls, squeezes, compresses and kneads the skin and muscles to increase the circulation. This increases the supply of oxygen and nutrients to the tissues, while encouraging muscle relaxation. Petrissage is used to encourage the breakdown and mobilization of adhesions in damaged tissues, to soften fascia, and to prevent injury. It is very important for the therapist to observe the patient closely while performing petrissage to assess pain levels and tolerance. Effleurage: this is a gentle form of massage that should be used before other forms of physical therapy and it familiarizes the animal to being touched. The technique can be performed all over the body. The therapist makes gentle contact with the patient's skin using the palm of the hand and stroking toward the heart, which encourages lymphatic and venous return. When massaging the limbs, effleurage should be performed from the distal to the proximal limb. A session of effleurage should last for approximately 10 minutes. Percussion: this involves gently tapping the skin with the palm or the side of the hand and large areas of muscle can be treated in this way. Percussion increases blood supply to the surrounding tissues and also aids in relaxation of the muscles. Vibration: this is a useful technique in which a group of muscles is slowly moved in a to-and-fro movement or by holding the paw to stimulate the whole limb. Vibration is useful at the end of a massage session because it relaxes the muscles. Effleurage may also be used at the end of the massage session. Aspinall V, The Complete Textbook of Veterinary Nursing, ed 2, Butterworth-Heinemann, 2011.

389. b Penicillin has good efficacy against common Gram-positive pathogens in the horse (*Streptococcus zooepidemicus, S. equi equi*) and is relatively safe. It is frequently administered intramuscularly (procaine penicillin) and intravenously (potassium penicillin). Procaine penicillin should never be administered intravenously. Life-threatening anaphylactic reactions are reported with IV procaine penicillin administration and should be treated with epinephrine. Aminoglycosides can safely be administered IV and trimethoprim is administered orally. Metronidazole can be administered orally or rectally. Bassert JM, Thomas JA, McCurnin's Clinical Textbook for Veterinary Technicians, ed 8, Elsevier, 2014.

390. b Sheep are gregarious and stay together as a group, even during lambing. Rams have very little to do with rearing of their young and although lamb–lamb bonds may form, they are not as important a resource as the ewe is to a lamb. Bassert JM, Thomas JA, McCurnin's Clinical Textbook for Veterinary Technicians, ed 8, Elsevier, 2014, p. 749.

391. d Outpatients include those that visit the practice for examinations, vaccinations, lab work, or services that do not require hospitalization. Prendergast H, Front Office Management for the Veterinary Team, ed 2, Saunders, 2011, p. 2.

392. a A veterinary technologist can graduate from a 4-year Bachelor of Science program in veterinary technology accredited by the AVMA. A veterinary technologist may also hold an associate's degree in veterinary technology along with a bachelor's degree in another program, such as business, management, or health science. Technologists tend to work in positions that require a higher level of education and they may hold teaching positions within technology programs or veterinary schools. Prendergast H, Front Office Management for the Veterinary Team, ed 2, Saunders, 2011, p. 7.

393. c Receptionists are often the face of the veterinary practice. They play a significant role in the success of a practice and must appear professional, polite, and caring. They must listen to client stories, show empathy when needed, and be able to collect money from clients under difficult circumstances. Prendergast H, Front Office Management for the Veterinary Team, ed 2, Saunders, 2011, p. 8.

394. a The purpose of any safety program is to reduce or eliminate the possibility of injury or illness for any human being on the premises. Prevention of injury in the workplace does make OSHA happy, but it is not the motivator for implementing a safety program. Prendergast H, Front Office Management for the Veterinary Team, ed 2, Saunders, 2011, p. 8.

395. c Glutaraldehyde is a potent chemical used in the veterinary practice to sterilize hard instruments without the use of an autoclave. Because it is so effective at killing germs, glutaraldehyde can be harmful to other living organisms, including you when you are using this cold-sterilization solution. Be sure to follow all safe-handling rules put forth by the manufacturer, including washing your hands after handling instruments exposed to the solution and keeping trays covered to minimize evaporation. Ethylene oxide is used for gas sterilization. Formalin and formaldehyde are tissue preservatives. Bassert JM, Thomas JA, McCurnin's Clinical Textbook for Veterinary Technicians, ed 8, Elsevier, 2014, p. 123.

396. b Dogs in cages will inevitably bark and barking dogs can adversely affect hearing, especially if working in an indoor kennel. Noise levels in dog wards can reach as high as 110 dB. Although relatively short-duration exposure to these noise levels, such as going into the kennel just to retrieve a patient, poses no serious damage to your hearing, chronic or long-term exposure can contribute to hearing loss. Ear ablation is a type of ear surgery in which the ear canal is removed. Simple barking would not cause ear infections. Hyphema, or bleeding in the eyes, includes non-sound–related causes. Bassert JM, Thomas JA, McCurnin's Clinical Textbook for Veterinary Technicians, ed 8, Elsevier, 2014, p. 124.

397. c Dogs in cages will inevitably bark and barking dogs can adversely affect your hearing, especially if you work in an indoor kennel. Noise levels in dog wards can reach as high as 110 dB. Although relatively short-duration exposure to these noise levels, such as going into the kennel just to retrieve a patient, poses no serious damage to your hearing, chronic or long-term exposure can contribute to hearing loss. Bassert JM, Thomas JA, McCurnin's Clinical Textbook for Veterinary Technicians, ed 8, Elsevier, 2014, p. 124.

398. a Infectious diseases that can be passed from animals to humans are known as zoonotic diseases. Some zoonotic diseases are not easily transmitted from animals to humans, whereas others are easily spread. You can be exposed to the organisms that cause disease by several means: inhalation, contact with broken skin, ingestion, contact with eyes and mucous membranes, and via accidental inoculation by needle. A veterinary technician may be exposed to a wide variety of zoonotic agents. Bassert JM, Thomas JA, McCurnin's Clinical Textbook for Veterinary Technicians, ed 8, Elsevier, 2014, p. 124.

399. d Infectious diseases that can be passed from animals to humans are known as zoonotic diseases. Some zoonotic diseases are not easily transmitted from animals to humans, whereas others are easily spread. You can be exposed to the organisms that cause disease by several means: inhalation, contact with broken skin, ingestion, contact with eyes and mucous membranes, and via accidental inoculation by needle. A veterinary technician may be exposed to a wide variety of zoonotic agents. Bassert JM, Thomas JA, McCurnin's Clinical Textbook for Veterinary Technicians, ed 8, Elsevier, 2014, p. 124.

400. b Adverse effects of corticosteroid administration include immunosuppression, polyuria or polydipsia, poor hair coat, muscle wasting, poor wound healing, laminitis, and progression of degenerative joint disease. Therefore, corticosteroids are administered with caution and only when specifically indicated. Bassert JM, Thomas JA, McCurnin's Clinical Textbook for Veterinary Technicians, ed 8, Elsevier, 2014.

401. b Coupage is contraindicated in cases in which there are fractured ribs or other thoracic traumas. Coupage is important in recumbent animals and in those suffering from pulmonary disease because this type of patient is likely to suffer from reduced lung volume and pooling of pulmonary secretions. Coupage is used to maintain optimal respiratory function by loosening secretions and assisting airway clearance by encouraging coughing. Patients suffering from pulmonary disease are liable to have a reduced lung capacity and function and it is therefore important not to stress the patient before, during, or after the treatment. Aspinall V, The Complete Textbook of Veterinary Nursing, ed 2, Butterworth-Heinemann, 2011.

402. b Orally administered drugs travel through the gastrointestinal tract and most are absorbed in the small intestine. After absorption across the intestinal wall, orally administered drugs enter the hepatic portal circulation and are routed directly to the liver. One of the roles of the liver is to remove potentially toxic substances before they reach the systemic blood circulation and drugs may be partially or completely broken down because of this mechanism. This is known as the first-pass effect. The small intestine is located after the stomach and therefore drugs would not enter the stomach after the small intestine. Some toxins and drugs may be eliminated from the body in the urine or feces; however, the liver generally eliminates that which is absorbed in the wall of the small intestine and is not used in the body. Aspinall V, The Complete Textbook of Veterinary Nursing, ed 2, Butterworth-Heinemann, 2011.

403. c Specialized epithelial cells in the jejunum and ileum absorb antibodies by pinocytosis. Normal intestinal epithelial cells replace these cells soon after birth and absorption of antibodies terminates within 24 hours of birth. Bassert JM, Thomas JA, McCurnin's Clinical Textbook for Veterinary Technicians, ed 8, Elsevier, 2014.

404. b Diarrhea or scours, a common problem among young dairy and beef calves, is associated with multiple infectious and noninfectious causes. Muscle weakness in calves is known as white muscle disease. Diarrhea in calves can lead to hypoglycemia, not hyperglycemia. Calves experiencing scours may also exhibit hypothermia. Bassert JM, Thomas JA, McCurnin's Clinical Textbook for Veterinary Technicians, ed 8, Elsevier, 2014.

405. c The movement of a drug from the systemic circulation into the body tissues is known as distribution. Most drugs must reach a specific area or target tissue to produce their desired effect, known as the therapeutic effect. When a drug enters the systemic circulation, drug molecules attach themselves to a certain site on plasma proteins (notably to albumin). This is called protein binding. Tissue perfusion in the target organ or organs also affects distribution. Well-perfused organs receive the drug quickly. After a time, the drug also distributes into the poorly perfused areas and drug concentration levels will drop in the blood plasma. Because distribution of a drug occurs along a concentration gradient, it can cause the drug to leave the well-perfused organs and re-enter the circulation, then move into a less-perfused area until equilibrium is reached. This is called redistribution. Aspinall V, The Complete Textbook of Veterinary Nursing, ed 2, Butterworth-Heinemann, 2011.

406. c A noninfectious disease is a disease that is not caused by microorganisms but usually results from a disturbance in the normal metabolism of the animal, for example, diabetes mellitus, neoplasia, or poisoning. A contagious disease is a disease that can spread from one animal to another via direct or indirect contact. An infectious disease is a disease caused by microorganisms that can spread among individuals. A vector is an animate object that carries the microorganisms. Aspinall V, The Complete Textbook of Veterinary Nursing, ed 2, Butterworth-Heinemann, 2011.

407. c Glomerulonephritis is often immune-mediated and affects the renal glomerulus and thus renal filtration. Pyelonephritis is infection of the renal pelvis, usually resulting from an ascending bacterial infection from the lower urinary tract. Nephritis refers to any inflammatory condition of the kidney. Aspinall V, The Complete Textbook of Veterinary Nursing, ed 2, Butterworth-Heinemann, 2011.

408. a Struvite uroliths, also known as triple phosphate uroliths, are found in alkaline urine. Ammonium urate uroliths, also known as ammonium acid urate uroliths, are found in acidic urine. Calcium oxalate uroliths are found in acidic urine. Cystine uroliths are found in acidic urine. Aspinall V, The Complete Textbook of Veterinary Nursing, ed 2, Butterworth-Heinemann, 2011.

409. d White muscle disease (WMD), also known as nutritional myodegeneration, occurs in young calves, lambs, and kids born to dams receiving diets deficient in selenium during gestation. Dietary deficiency of selenium and/or vitamin E may cause degeneration of cardiac or skeletal muscle. If skeletal muscles are affected, muscular weakness or stiffness followed by eventual recumbency and death may occur. Diarrhea or scours is a common problem among calves and is often a result of a virus (bovine viral diarrhea) or bacteria (bacterial enteritis). Bassert JM, Thomas JA, McCurnin's Clinical Textbook for Veterinary Technicians, ed 8, Elsevier, 2014.

410. d Early cases of the skeletal form of WMD may respond to injections of vitamin E and selenium. Prevention includes ensuring that the dam's ration has adequate amounts of vitamin E and selenium and administering supplements of selenium to the dam before parturition in areas of the country where the soil is deficient in selenium. Selenium can be toxic and the manufacturer's recommendations must be followed carefully. High protein levels in alfalfa will not treat WMD. Bassert JM, Thomas JA, McCurnin's Clinical Textbook for Veterinary Technicians, ed 8, Elsevier, 2014.

411. d Causes of right-sided heart failure include tricuspid dysplasia, pulmonic stenosis, endocardiosis, congestive cardiomyopathy, pericardial effusions, neoplasia, and myocarditis. Causes of left-sided heart failure include aortic stenosis, mitral valve dysplasia, and dysrhythmias. Aspinall V, The Complete Textbook of Veterinary Nursing, ed 2, Butterworth-Heinemann, 2011.

412. b Hypoadrenocorticism, also known as Addison's disease, mainly affects dogs. Hyperadrenocorticalism is also known as Cushing's disease. It is common in dogs and rare in cats. Hypothyroidism is rare in cats and common in dogs 6–10 years of age. Hyperthyroidism is very rare in dogs and commonly seen in cats that are more than 10 years of age. Aspinall V, The Complete Textbook of Veterinary Nursing, ed 2, Butterworth-Heinemann, 2011.

413. b Enterotoxemia caused by *C. perfringens* is recognized worldwide as a common, frequently fatal disease of young sheep and goats. Aspects of enterotoxemia in small ruminants include severe enterocolitis, sudden death, diarrhea in goats, and neurologic signs in lambs. Small ruminants are considered highly susceptible to enterotoxemia and should be vaccinated every 6 months. In herds with a history of disease, 4-month vaccination intervals may be more appropriate. Initial vaccinations should be followed 3 to 4 weeks later by booster vaccinations; semiannual or triannual vaccinations should be followed 3 weeks before parturition by booster vaccinations for maximal benefit for the newborns. Kids should be vaccinated at 4 to 6 weeks of age and again at weaning. Vaccines with *C. perfringens* type C and D with or without tetanus are preferable to the polyvalent clostridial vaccines available for cattle. Bassert JM, Thomas JA, McCurnin's Clinical Textbook for Veterinary Technicians, ed 8, Elsevier, 2014.

414. b The pH of rumen fluid is normally 6.5 to 6.8 (5.5 to 6.5 with high-grain diets). Rumen fluid with pH <5.5 is suggestive of grain overload. Bassert JM, Thomas JA, McCurnin's Clinical Textbook for Veterinary Technicians, ed 8, Elsevier, 2014.

415. b Portosystemic shunt is a vascular abnormality in which the hepatic portal vein empties directly into the caudal vena cava, thus bypassing the liver. A portosystemic shunt may be either congenital (most common) or acquired. Analyzing blood liver enzymes, radiography, and ultrasound confirms diagnosis. Typically, affected animals have a small liver. Treatment is by surgical correction. Hepatic lipidosis is usually seen in overweight patients after a prolonged period of anorexia. Cardiomyopathy and aortic stenosis are both forms of heart disease. Aspinall V, The Complete Textbook of Veterinary Nursing, ed 2, Butterworth-Heinemann, 2011.

416. a Crackle (course or fine) is defined as a high-pitched, discontinuous inspiratory sound associated with the reopening of airways that closed during expiration. *Stertor* is the term used to describe noise generated from the nasal passages. *Stridor* is the term used to describe the high-pitched inspiratory sound generated from turbulent airflow in the extrathoracic airways. A wheeze is a high-pitched, continuous inspiratory or expiratory sound associated with narrowing of the airways. Aspinall V, The Complete Textbook of Veterinary Nursing, ed 2, Butterworth-Heinemann, 2011.

417. d In ruminants, the term *indigestion* describes the disruption of normal reticulorumen function; this condition is very common in ruminants. It results from a rapid feed change or the introduction of feed materials that rapidly change the rumen environment. Moldy or overheated feeds are typically implicated. Bassert JM, Thomas JA, McCurnin's Clinical Textbook for Veterinary Technicians, ed 8, Elsevier, 2014.

418. c Hyperemic (injected) membranes are a deep brick-red color and appear injected. This change is most commonly seen in hyperthermia, sepsis, and polycythemia. In hyperthermia, it occurs because of the massive vasodilation needed for heat loss hence there is a huge amount of blood present at locations such as the peripheral membranes. In a septic patient, there is pooling of blood because of the loss of vascular tone, yielding a dark, brick-colored appearance. Cyanotic membranes are generally recognized as bluish in tone, but the color can range from a deep red-purple to a pale or dusky blue caused by excessive amounts of desaturated hemoglobin in the capillary blood. In cases in which the mucous membranes are pigmented, it is necessary to look at other, nonpigmented areas, for example the vagina or the prepuce. There might also be a difference in the appearance of the mucous membranes under natural or artificial lights, especially under fluorescent lighting. If the animal is found with cyanosed mucous membranes, supply with oxygen before calling the veterinary surgeon. Icteric (jaundice) occurs when there is a buildup of bilirubin in the plasma and tissues (hyperbilirubinemia), which causes a yellow discoloration of the skin, mucous membranes, and also the sclera of the eye. Pale mucous membranes vary from a pale pink to gray/white. This may indicate that the animal has a low packed cell volume (PCV) or that the animal is exhibiting circulatory shutdown. Aspinall V, The Complete Textbook of Veterinary Nursing, ed 2, Butterworth-Heinemann, 2011.

419. d Sites for intraosseous catheter placement include the cranial aspect of the diaphysis of the ulna, the cranial aspect of the greater tubercle of the humerus, the trochanteric fossa of the proximal femur, and the flat medial aspect of the proximal tibia (at a site that is distal to the tibial tuberosity and the proximal tibial growth plate). The last two sites are the most common in dogs and cats. Aspinall V, The Complete Textbook of Veterinary Nursing, ed 2, Butterworth-Heinemann, 2011.

420. d Clinical signs include acute anorexia, reduced rumen motility, and potentially malodorous diarrhea. The disease is self-limiting and affected cattle return to normal. Bassert JM, Thomas JA, McCurnin's Clinical Textbook for Veterinary Technicians, ed 8, Elsevier, 2014.

421. c *Polyuria* is the term used to describe passing larger volumes of urine than normal. A fomite is a contaminated, inanimate (nonliving) object, such as a feeding bowl or a litter tray. Poikuria refers to the irregular passage of urine. Vector refers to an animate object that carries the microorganisms. Aspinall V, The Complete Textbook of Veterinary Nursing, ed 2, Butterworth-Heinemann, 2011.

422. d Ptyalism refers to excessive salivation. Borborygmus refers to the rumbling sound in the gut, caused by a moving gas–fluid interface, from the stomach through the intestines. Dyschezia refers to difficulty or painful passing of feces. Polyphagia refers to the excessive eating or ingestion of food. Merrill L, Small Animal Internal Medicine for Veterinary Technicians and Nurses, Wiley Blackwell, 2012.

423. a Grain overload in ruminants results from the consumption of excessive amounts of highly fermentable carbohydrate feed and subsequent production of large quantities of lactic acid in the rumen. Medical treatment involves rapid removal of rumen contents. In cattle, this may be achieved by lavaging the rumen with a large-bore stomach tube or by performing rumenotomy surgery. In small ruminants, rumen lavage is not possible with a large-bore tube and rumenotomy is required. In addition, animals are given oral antacids, antibiotics, anti-inflammatories when rehydrated, and thiamine, all of which help to prevent liver abscess, polioencephalomalacia, and laminitis. In more severe cases, IV fluids with sodium bicarbonate should be administered to correct dehydration and acidosis. Whether an animal is treated medically or surgically, rumen transfaunation is often helpful to reestablish normal rumen microflora and to improve appetite. Bassert JM, Thomas JA, McCurnin's Clinical Textbook for Veterinary Technicians, ed 8, Elsevier, 2014.

424. c Regurgitation refers to the passive, retrograde movement of ingested material to a level above the upper esophageal sphincter. Typically, regurgitation happens before the ingested material reaches the stomach and it is not an active process. Vomiting is the forceful discharge of ingested material from the stomach and sometimes from the proximal small intestines. Vomiting involves three stages: nausea, retching, and, subsequently, vomiting. Expectoration refers to the expulsion of material from the respiratory tract and is generally associated with coughing. However, some dogs that cough and gag excessively may stimulate themselves to vomit. Hematemesis refers to vomiting with the presence of blood in the vomitus and may involve the expulsion of digested blood or fresh blood. Merrill L, Small Animal Internal Medicine for Veterinary Technicians and Nurses, Wiley Blackwell, 2012.

425. b Transverse plane: a plane across the body that divides it into cranial (head-end) and caudal (tail-end) parts that are not necessarily equal. The sagittal plan runs the length of the body and divides it into left and right parts that are not necessarily equal halves. The median plane is a special kind of sagittal plane that runs down the center of the body lengthwise and divides it into equal left and right halves. It could also be called a midsagittal plane, but that term is not commonly used. The dorsal plane is a plane at right angles to the sagittal and transverse planes. It divides the body into dorsal (toward the animal's back) and ventral (toward the belly) parts that are not necessarily equal. If an animal stands in water with its body partially submerged, the surface of the water describes a dorsal plane. In humans this plane is called the frontal plane. Colville TP, Bassert JM, Clinical Anatomy and Physiology for Veterinary Technicians, ed 3, Elsevier, 2016.

426. c Gas production is a normal occurrence during rumen fermentation and healthy animals are capable of eructating the gas that the rumen produces. However, in some cases, abnormal distention of the rumen with gas may occur, resulting in bloat or rumen tympany. Lactic acidosis is known as grain overload. Tetany is a state of calcium deficiency and it can cause bloat. Rumenitis is inflammation of the rumen. Bassert JM, Thomas JA, McCurnin's Clinical Textbook for Veterinary Technicians, ed 8, Elsevier, 2014.

427. c *Rostral* is a special term used only to describe positions or directions on the head. The term *cranial* loses its meaning on the head because the cranium is part of the head. Caudal retains its normal meaning on the head because it still means toward the tail end of the animal. In humans, the term *nasal* means toward the nose. Cranial and caudal refer to the ends of the animal as it stands on four legs. Cranial means toward the head (cranium), and caudal means toward the tail (cauda). The caudal end of the sternum (breastbone) is called the xiphoid process. Dorsal and ventral refer to up and down directions or positions with the animal in a standing position. Dorsal means toward the back (top surface) of a standing animal and ventral means toward the belly (bottom surface) of a standing animal. Dorsal and ventral are easiest to visualize in a standing animal, but they retain their meanings regardless of the animal's position. Colville TP, Bassert JM, Clinical Anatomy and Physiology for Veterinary Technicians, ed 3, Elsevier, 2016.

428. a Medial and lateral refer to positions relative to the median plane. Medial means toward the median plane (toward the center line of the body) and lateral means away from the median plane. The medial surface of an animal's leg is the one closest to its body. The lateral surface of the leg is the outer surface. Proximal and distal are used to describe positions only on extremities, such as legs, ears, and tail, relative to the body. Proximal means toward the body and distal means away from the body. The proximal end of the tail attaches it to the body. The toes are located on the distal end of the leg. Colville TP, Bassert JM, Clinical Anatomy and Physiology for Veterinary Technicians, ed 3, Elsevier, 2016.

429. d Because scaling and polishing procedures are the most common dental procedures performed in practice, special attention is paid in this chapter to instrumentation and techniques of proper periodontal therapy. These procedures are often mistakenly referred to as prophylaxis, or prophy. Because of the variation in severity of disease at the time of treatment, the term *dental prophylaxis* is largely being replaced with the term *professional dental cleaning*. The technician who is involved in performing a professional dental cleaning should be capable of performing assessment, periodontal debridement (supragingival and subgingival scaling), polishing, home care education, and counseling about proper diet, treats, and toys as they relate to dentistry. Bassert JM, Thomas JA, McCurnin's Clinical Textbook for Veterinary Technicians, ed 8, Saunders, 2014.

430. a The American Veterinary Dental College (AVDC) published a position statement in 1998 regarding veterinary dental health care providers. This statement provides recommendations for the qualifications of persons who perform veterinary dental procedures. The AVDC considers it appropriate for the veterinarian to delegate certain dental tasks to veterinary technicians. Tasks appropriately performed by veterinary technicians include professional dental cleaning and certain procedures that do not result in alterations in the shape, structure, or positional location of teeth in the dental arch. Bassert JM, Thomas JA, McCurnin's Clinical Textbook for Veterinary Technicians, ed 8, Elsevier, 2014.

431. b Cheek teeth and incisors of rabbits and some rodents are aradicular hypsodont (also called elodont) teeth, indicating a lack of true root structure along with lifelong tooth growth, which compensates for occlusal wear. Dogs and cats have four types of teeth: incisors, canines, premolars, and molars. Incisor teeth are the most rostral teeth and are used for gnawing and grooming. Canine teeth are distal to the incisors. They are long and are used for prehending and holding. Premolars and molars (often referred to as cheek teeth) are used for shearing and grinding. Bassert JM, Thomas JA, McCurnin's Clinical Textbook for Veterinary Technicians, ed 8, Elsevier, 2014.

432. d *Vestibular* is a term that describes the tooth surface facing the lips or vestibule (acceptable alternatives are buccal and labial). *Rostral* is a term that, when used to describe cranial anatomy, refers to a structure that is closer to the front of the head in comparison with another structure. *Caudal* is a term that is used to describe a structure that is toward the back of the head when compared with another structure. *Facial* is a term that describes the vestibular surface of teeth visible from the front (incisors). Lingual refers to the surface of the mandibular teeth adjacent to the tongue. Bassert JM, Thomas JA, McCurnin's Clinical Textbook for Veterinary Technicians, ed 8, Elsevier, 2014.

433. a Causes of right-sided heart failure include pulmonic stenosis, neoplasia, and myocarditis. Causes of left-sided heart failure include mitral valve dysplasia, aortic stenosis, endocardiosis, cardiomyopathy, obstruction of aorta, and dysrhythmias. Aspinall V, The Complete Textbook of Veterinary Nursing, ed 2, Butterworth-Heinemann, 2011.

434. c Coronal refers to a structure with a location that is closer to the crown of the tooth in relation to another structure. Palatal refers to the surface of maxillary teeth adjacent to the palate. Mesial refers to the portion of the tooth in line with the dental arcade that is closest to the most rostral portion of the midline of the dental arch. Distal refers to the portion of the tooth that is closest to the most caudal portion of the dental arch. The concepts of mesial and distal surfaces are difficult to describe without referring to a diagram. It may help to remember that the terms *mesial* and *distal* are used to describe surfaces of the teeth where adjacent teeth touch or nearly touch. Apical refers to a portion of the tooth that is closer to the apex (tip of the root). Coronal refers to a structure with a location that is closer to the crown of the tooth in relation to another structure. Bassert JM, Thomas JA, McCurnin's Clinical Textbook for Veterinary Technicians, ed 8, Elsevier, 2014.

435. c Treatment of free gas bloat involves passing an orogastric tube. If hypocalcemia is the underlying problem, administration of calcium is therapeutic. Forced exercise stimulates rumen motility and eructation. In addition, rumen stimulants improve motility and normal belching. If an animal is critically bloated and the passing of a stomach tube is too stressful, an emergency procedure, called rumen trocharization, should be performed. Bassert JM, Thomas JA, McCurnin's Clinical Textbook for Veterinary Technicians, ed 8, Elsevier, 2014.

436. d Frothy bloat requires a different treatment because the froth must first be dissipated before gas can be expelled from the rumen. To reduce the surface tension of the froth, several products may be used, including poloxalene, household detergent, mineral oil, or dioctyl sodium sulfosuccinate (DSS). After the frothy bloat becomes a free gas bloat, it can be eructated or relieved via an orogastric tube. Bassert JM, Thomas JA, McCurnin's Clinical Textbook for Veterinary Technicians, ed 8, Elsevier, 2014.

437. c Most mammals are diphyodont, meaning that they have two sets of teeth. The first set of teeth is referred to as deciduous (also referred to as primary or baby teeth); these are replaced with permanent teeth (also referred to as secondary or adult teeth). Occlusion refers to the spatial relationship of teeth within the mouth. Malocclusion refers to the situation in which teeth or jaws are not correctly aligned. Although the cosmetic issues of misaligned teeth are not typically a concern in dogs and cats, malocclusions can result in discomfort from impingement of teeth on soft tissue structures of the opposing dental arcade. The cingulum is a smooth convex bulge located on the palatal side of the gingival third of the incisor teeth. Bassert JM, Thomas JA, McCurnin's Clinical Textbook for Veterinary Technicians, ed 8, Elsevier, 2014.

438. a A normal feline mouth contains 30 teeth and a normal canine mouth contains 42 teeth. Bassert JM, Thomas JA, McCurnin's Clinical Textbook for Veterinary Technicians, ed 8, Elsevier, 2014.

439. b Chronic valvular disease (CVD) resulting from thickening of the heart valves affects many older dogs, especially smaller breeds, but it occurs less commonly in cats. Larger-breed dogs, although also affected by CVD, may develop a different cardiac disease, such as dilated cardiomyopathy. Cats are more likely to develop hypertrophic cardiomyopathy (HCM), a condition in which the heart muscle becomes thickened. Hypertrophic cardiomyopathy can affect younger cats, but many are middle-aged at the time of initial presentation. Cardiac disease in pets can lead to arrhythmias, congestive heart failure, and other complications, such as renal damage secondary to reduced renal perfusion. Bassert JM, Thomas JA, McCurnin's Clinical Textbook for Veterinary Technicians, ed 8, Elsevier, 2014.

440. c Traumatic reticuloperitonitis (TRP), or hardware disease, results from penetration of the reticulum by a foreign body and is one of the most common gastrointestinal problems affecting the forestomach compartments of mature dairy cattle. Grain overload is also known as lactic acidosis. Rumen tympany is referred to as bloat. Polioencephalomalacia is also known as cerebrocortical necrosis and it is characterized by altered function of the central nervous system. Bassert JM, Thomas JA, McCurnin's Clinical Textbook for Veterinary Technicians, ed 8, Elsevier, 2014.

441. c Bovine viral diarrhea (BVD) is a common viral pathogen affecting all ages of cattle. BVD can manifest as sudden onset of fever, depression, anorexia, oral and GI ulcers and erosions, and diarrhea (sometimes with blood and mucus). The disease may progress rapidly through a group of animals. BVD also plays an important role in respiratory diseases in cattle by causing immunosuppression and susceptibility to secondary bacterial pathogens. The virus is responsible for abortions, in utero infections, and birth defects. Bassert JM, Thomas JA, McCurnin's Clinical Textbook for Veterinary Technicians, ed 8, Elsevier, 2014.

442. d Chronic renal disease is one of the diseases seen most commonly in geriatric patients, especially cats. In addition to causing increased urination (polyuria) and water intake (polydipsia), kidney disease can cause complications such as anemia, gastric upset, anorexia, weight loss, and muscle weakness. Routine screening for proteinuria, azotemia, and other abnormalities associated with kidney disease should be part of any diagnostic evaluation in a senior pet. With early detection, the implementation of diet changes, fluid support, and specific medications may be used to slow progression. Bassert JM, Thomas JA, McCurnin's Clinical Textbook for Veterinary Technicians, ed 8, Elsevier, 2014.

443. c Ivermectin is a microfilaricide treatment that is administered after an adulticide treatment. It is given as a single dose. Thiacetarsamide is an adulticide treatment that is no longer used because of serious side effects occurring with its use. Melarsomine dihydrochloride is an adulticide treatment that is given at 24-hour intervals. Injections should be made deep into the lumbar muscles. Summers A, Common Diseases of Companion Animals, ed 3, Elsevier, 2014.

444. c In healthy eyes, production of aqueous fluid is equal to the amount leaving the eye and the intraocular pressure (IOP) remains fairly constant. If more aqueous fluid is produced than that leaving the eye, IOP increases and glaucoma results. The term *pannus* is used to describe superficial corneal vascularization and infiltration of granulation tissue. Keratoconjunctivitis sicca (KCS): dogs and cats have two lacrimal glands, one located in the lateral superior orbit and one at the base of the third eyelid. Loss of both glands (atrophy) produces KCS. Summers A, Common Diseases of Companion Animals, ed 3, Elsevier, 2014.

445. d The sclera is composed of tough fibrous tissue, which helps maintain the shape of the eye. The sclera and the cornea make up the fibrous layer. The cornea is composed of four layers: the epithelium, the stroma, the descemet membrane, and the endothelium. The epithelium covering provides a barrier against microorganisms entering the eye. Summers A, Common Diseases of Companion Animals, ed 3, Elsevier, 2014.

446. d No treatment is available for BVD, but antimicrobials are often used to prevent secondary bacterial infection. Vaccination of dairy and beef animals is important to help prevent the disease. Killed-virus and modified live-virus vaccines are both available. Bassert JM, Thomas JA, McCurnin's Clinical Textbook for Veterinary Technicians, ed 8, Elsevier, 2014.

447. a Epiphora, an overflow of tears, may be the result of the overproduction of tears or of faulty drainage by the lacrimal system. Overproduction of tears is always the result of ocular pain or irritation. Faulty functioning of the lacrimal drainage system may occur for several reasons, including blockage of lacrimal duct by swelling or inflammatory cells, imperforate puncta, or trauma. Dogs and cats do not cry as humans do when feeling sad or frightened. Excessive dietary protein has not been linked to epiphora. Summers A, Common Diseases of Companion Animals, ed 3, Elsevier, 2014.

448. c *Progressive retina atrophy* is a term used to describe a group of hereditary diseases seen in many breeds of dogs. The disease is common in toy poodles, golden retrievers, and cocker spaniels, to name only a few. All of the other choices are also eye diseases; however, none has been shown to be a hereditary disease. Summers A, Common Diseases of Companion Animals, ed 3, Elsevier, 2014.

449. d Cattle with BRDS experience depression, standing with their heads lowered, anorexia, fever (104°F–107°F), mucopurulent ocular and nasal discharge, cough, and dyspnea. Bassert JM, Thomas JA, McCurnin's Clinical Textbook for Veterinary Technicians, ed 8, Elsevier, 2014.

450. a Metaphylaxis, which involves the mass treatment of animal populations before onset of overt disease, is commonly used by feedlots and involves the treatment of cattle with long-acting antimicrobial agents. Preconditioning refers to the castration, deworming, and so forth, of calves before transport and it may prevent or lessen the severity of the disease being prevented. Megascript is not used in veterinary medicine. Bassert JM, Thomas JA, McCurnin's Clinical Textbook for Veterinary Technicians, ed 8, Elsevier, 2014.

451. c Ear mites live on the surface of the skin in the external ear canal, feeding on epidermal debris. Treatment involves carefully cleaning the exudates from the ear canal and then applying a miticide into the ear canal. Flea, ticks, and mange mites may be treated with a number of products including shampoos and dips formulated to treat these parasites. Summers A, Common Diseases of Companion Animals, ed 3, Elsevier, 2014.

452. c Until the late 1980s, feline fibrosarcomas were unrecognized. During that time, a killed rabies vaccine and the feline leukemia vaccine became available to practitioners. These tumors are rapidly developing, highly invasive, and malignant. They occur at the site of the vaccination, usually 4 to 6 weeks after the vaccine has been given. By the time many owners act, it is too late to provide successful treatment for cats. In an effort to prevent or reduce the incidence of this disease, the Vaccine-Associated Sarcoma Task Force issued the following guidelines for vaccination: use single-dose vaccines, use intranasal vaccines when possible, and never vaccinate between the shoulder blades. Rabies vaccine should be given as low as possible on the right rear leg, leukemia vaccine low on the left rear leg, and distemper combinations on the right shoulder. Summers A, Common Diseases of Companion Animals, ed 3, Elsevier, 2014.

453. c The use of barrier nursing is to help prevent staff members from transmitting infection from the patients they are nursing to others of the same species or to those susceptible to infection such as immunologically challenged patients and pediatric or geriatric patients. Personal protective clothing such as disposable gloves, aprons, and foot covers should be worn. These should be placed in the clinical waste after use. Patients who are most likely to spread disease should be cleaned and treated after all other patients in the isolation facility.

This will also help to prevent disease being spread from the most infectious patients by the nursing staff. Patient care should always take priority; uniforms can be washed and/or replaced as needed. Aspinall V, "Medical Nursing Procedures," Clinical Procedures in Veterinary Nursing, ed 3, Butterworth-Heinemann, 2014.

454. a Diabetes insipidus results from the failure in production of antidiuretic hormone (ADH) from the posterior pituitary gland or a failure of the kidneys to respond to ADH. Hyperadrenocorticism, also known as Cushing's disease, is caused by excessive production of glucocorticoids, such as cortisol, released from the adrenal cortex. Elevations in blood glucocorticoid levels cause a variety of clinical signs, such as polyuria, polydipsia, muscle wasting, and increased appetite. Hypothyroidism is relatively common among middle-aged and older dogs, although younger dogs can also be affected. The condition is caused by inadequate production of thyroid hormone. Clinical signs include weight gain, lethargy, and muscle weakness—changes that pet owners may mistake for simple signs of aging or slowing down. Insulinoma: functional tumors of the beta cells of the pancreas secrete insulin or proinsulin independent of a negative feedback effect. Hyperinsulinemia results in the development of hypoglycemia. Aspinall V, The Complete Textbook of Veterinary Nursing, ed 2, Butterworth-Heinemann, 2011.

455. d BRDS, which primarily affects feedlot calves and dairy calves younger than 6 months of age, is caused by a complex interaction of respiratory viruses, bacteria, and stress. Bassert JM, Thomas JA, McCurnin's Clinical Textbook for Veterinary Technicians, ed 8, Elsevier, 2014.

456. d OPP manifests as progressive respiratory failure but also causes mastitis (hard bag), neurologic signs, and arthritis. The pulmonary form is predominant in the United States and clinical signs include exercise intolerance, open-mouth breathing, exaggerated expiratory effort, and an occasional dry cough. In the later stages of the disease, weight loss occurs despite a good appetite. The disease causes an interstitial pneumonia and affected animals usually die within 3 to 8 months of onset of clinical signs. Diagnosis is based on clinical signs, necropsy, and serology testing. Bassert JM, Thomas JA, McCurnin's Clinical Textbook for Veterinary Technicians, ed 8, Elsevier, 2014.

457. d Three types of cells that make up bone are osteoblasts, osteocytes, and osteoclasts. Osteoblasts are the cells that form bone. Colville TP, Bassert JM, Clinical Anatomy and Physiology for Veterinary Technicians, ed 3, Elsevier, 2016.

458. a The bones of the skeleton can be conveniently divided into two main groups: the bones of the head and trunk and the bones of the limbs. Because the bones of the head and trunk are located along the central axis of the body, they are referred to as the axial skeleton. The limbs are appendages of the trunk and their bones are collectively called the appendicular skeleton. Some animals may have a third category of bones called the visceral skeleton. These are bones formed in the viscera or soft organs. The metacarpal bones extend distally from the distal row of carpal bones to the proximal phalanges of the digits. Colville TP, Bassert JM, Clinical Anatomy and Physiology for Veterinary Technicians, ed 3, Elsevier, 2016.

459. b The occipital bone is a single bone that forms the caudoventral portion or base of the skull. It is the most caudal skull bone and is very important because it is where the spinal cord exits the skull; it is the skull bone that articulates (forms a joint) with the first cervical (neck) vertebra. The interparietal bones are two small bones located on the dorsal midline between the occipital bone and the parietal bones. They are usually clearly visible in young animals. In older animals, they may fuse together into one bone or they may fuse to the parietal bones and become indistinguishable. The two parietal bones form the dorsolateral walls of the cranium. They are large and well developed in dogs, cats, and humans, but they are relatively small in horses and cattle. The two temporal bones are located below or ventral to the parietal bones. The temporal bones are important for several reasons: they form the lateral walls of the cranium, they contain the middle and inner ear structures, and they are the skull bones that form the temporomandibular joints (TMJs) with the mandible (lower jaw). Colville TP, Bassert JM, Clinical Anatomy and Physiology for Veterinary Technicians, ed 3, Elsevier, 2016.

460. d The lacrimal bones are two small bones that form part of the medial portion of the orbit of the eye. The three tiny but very important pairs of ear bones are hidden away in the middle ear. Known as the ossicles, starting from the outside these bones are the malleus or hammer, the incus or anvil, and the stapes or stirrup. Colville TP, Bassert JM, Clinical Anatomy and Physiology for Veterinary Technicians, ed 3, Elsevier, 2016.

461. c Retained placenta is a common postpartum disease affecting dairy cattle. After calving, the placenta usually is passed within 2 to 4 hours and is considered retained if it has not been expelled by 12 hours. The cause is unknown, but it is more likely to occur after the birth of twins, after abortion during the last half of pregnancy, and in cases of dystocia. Selenium and vitamin A and E deficiencies have been suggested as the cause of an increased incidence of retained placenta. Bassert JM, Thomas JA, McCurnin's Clinical Textbook for Veterinary Technicians, ed 8, Elsevier, 2014.

462. b Metritis is known as a postpartum uterine infection and is common in dairy cattle. Retained placentas are also known as fetal membranes. Pseudopregnancy is a condition characterized by the accumulation of fluid in the uterus and in one or more corpus lutea in the ovaries. Milk fever is a metabolic disorder in which there is a severe decline in the serum calcium, usually occurring within 48 hours of calving. Bassert JM, Thomas JA, McCurnin's Clinical Textbook for Veterinary Technicians, ed 8, Elsevier, 2014.

463. a The two zygomatic bones are also known as the malar bones. They form a portion of the orbit of the eye and join with a process from the temporal bones to form the zygomatic arches on either side of the skull. The two maxillary bones make up most of the upper jaw. (The incisive bones make up the rest.) The maxillary bones house the upper canine teeth, all of the upper cheek teeth (premolars and molars), and the maxillary sinuses. The lacrimal bones are two small bones that form part of the medial portion of the orbit of the eye. A space within each lacrimal bone houses the lacrimal sac, which is part of the tear drainage system of the eye. The two nasal bones form the bridge of the nose, which is the dorsal or upper part of the nasal cavity. Considerable variety is seen in the relative size and shape of the nasal bones, depending on the species and breed of animal. The length of the animal's face is the main influence on the nasal bones. Colville TP, Bassert JM, Clinical Anatomy and Physiology for Veterinary Technicians, ed 3, Elsevier, 2016.

464. c The turbinates are also called the nasal conchae. They are four thin, scroll-like bones that fill most of the space in the nasal cavity. Each side has a dorsal and a ventral turbinate. The moist, very vascular soft tissue lining of the nasal passages covers the turbinates. The scroll-like shape of the turbinates forces air inhaled through the nose around many twists and turns as it passes through the nasal cavity. This helps warm and humidify the air and also helps trap any tiny particles of inhaled foreign material in the moist surface of the nasal epithelium. This process helps condition the inhaled air before it reaches the delicate lungs. The two palatine bones make up the caudal portion of the hard palate (the bony part of the roof of the mouth), which separates the mouth from the nasal cavity. The rest of the hard palate (the rostral portion) is made up of part of the maxillary bones. The two small pterygoid bones support part of the lateral walls of the pharynx (throat). The single vomer bone is located on the midline of the skull and forms part of the nasal septum, which is the central wall between the left and right nasal passages. Colville TP, Bassert JM, Clinical Anatomy and Physiology for Veterinary Technicians, ed 3, Elsevier, 2016.

465. c Pseudopregnancy is a condition characterized by the accumulation of fluid in the uterus and one or more corpus lutea in the ovaries. Metritis is known as a postpartum uterine infection and is common in dairy cattle. Retained placentas are also known as fetal membranes. Milk fever is a metabolic disorder in which there is a severe decline in the serum calcium, usually occurring within 48 hours of calving. Bassert JM, Thomas JA, McCurnin's Clinical Textbook for Veterinary Technicians, ed 8, Elsevier, 2014.

466. d The sacral vertebrae are unique in that they fuse to form a single, solid structure called the sacrum. The cervical vertebrae are in the neck region. The thoracic vertebrae are located dorsal to the thorax. The lumbar vertebrae are dorsal to the abdominal region. Colville TP, Bassert JM, Clinical Anatomy and Physiology for Veterinary Technicians, ed 3, Elsevier, 2016.

467. c The ingredient statement, a key portion of a pet food label, should be reviewed whenever a product is purchased or recommended. All ingredients are required to be listed in order by descending weight. Bassert JM, Thomas JA, McCurnin's Clinical Textbook for Veterinary Technicians, ed 9, Elsevier, 2018.

468. d Milk fever is a metabolic disorder in which there is a severe decline in the serum calcium, usually occurring within 48 hours of calving. Metritis is known as a postpartum uterine infection and is common in dairy cattle. Retained placentas are also known as fetal membranes. Pseudopregnancy is a condition characterized by the accumulation of fluid in the uterus and in one or more corpus lutea in the ovaries. Bassert JM, Thomas JA, McCurnin's Clinical Textbook for Veterinary Technicians, ed 8, Elsevier, 2014.

469. c The sternum, also called the breastbone, forms the floor of the thorax. It is made up of a series of rod-like bones called sternebrae. The last, most caudal sternebra is called the xiphoid or xiphoid process. Only the first and last sternebrae are named and used as landmarks. The others are numbered from cranial to caudal. The first, most cranial sternebra is called the manubrium or manubrium sterni. In dogs, the eleventh thoracic vertebra (T11) is called anticlinal because its spinous process, unlike those of the surrounding vertebrae, projects straight up. Colville TP, Bassert JM, Clinical Anatomy and Physiology for Veterinary Technicians, ed 3, Elsevier, 2016.

470. b The scapula is the most proximal bone of the thoracic limb. It is a flat, somewhat triangular bone with a prominent, longitudinal ridge on its lateral surface, which is referred to as the spine of the scapula. At its distal end, it forms the socket portion of the ball-and-socket shoulder joint. This fairly shallow, concave articular surface is called the glenoid cavity. It is connected with the main body of the scapula by a narrowed area known as the neck. The humerus is the long bone of the upper arm or brachium. The ball portion of the ball-and-socket shoulder joint is on its proximal end: the head of the humerus, which is joined to the shaft by the neck. Opposite the head on the proximal end are some large processes called tubercles, where the powerful shoulder muscles attach. The largest one is called the greater tubercle. Colville TP, Bassert JM, Clinical Anatomy and Physiology for Veterinary Technicians, ed 3, Elsevier, 2016.

471. c Two bones form the forearm or antebrachium: the ulna and the radius. The ulna forms a major portion of the elbow joint with the distal end of the humerus. The scapula is the most proximal bone of the thoracic limb. It is a flat, somewhat triangular bone with a prominent, longitudinal ridge on its lateral surface, which is referred to as the spine of the scapula. The humerus is the long bone of the upper arm or brachium. Colville TP, Bassert JM, Clinical Anatomy and Physiology for Veterinary Technicians, ed 3, Elsevier, 2016.

472. a The anatomical term for fibrous joints is *synarthroses*. Fibrous joints are immovable in that the bones are firmly united by fibrous tissue. The internal bones of the face are the palatine bones, the pterygoid bones, the vomer bone, and the turbinates. Colville TP, Bassert JM, Clinical Anatomy and Physiology for Veterinary Technicians, ed 3, Elsevier, 2016.

473. b Postpartum uterine infection, or metritis, is common in dairy cattle and is less common in beef cattle and small ruminants. Uterine infection in ruminants is associated with retained placenta, dystocia, delivery of twins, and unbalanced prepartum diets. Many bacterial species have been isolated from bovine uterine infections, but the organism most commonly associated with bovine metritis is *Arcanobacterium pyogenes*. Bassert JM, Thomas JA, McCurnin's Clinical Textbook for Veterinary Technicians, ed 8, Elsevier, 2014.

474. a Cows with hypocalcemia develop muscle tremors, weakness, and a staggering gait, eventually leading to recumbency. Cows with milk fever often lie in sternal recumbency with their heads turned into their flank. Affected cows have a dry nose, rumen atony with bloat, and no urine or feces production. Unless the cow is treated quickly, she may die from the effects of low serum calcium. Cows in the early stages of milk fever (before recumbency) often respond to the administration of oral calcium. For recumbent cows, slow administration of IV calcium gluconate is the treatment of choice. Cows often respond rapidly to calcium therapy and will begin to lacrimate, eructate, urinate, and defecate during treatment. Additional calcium gluconate should be administered subcutaneously for more prolonged calcium supplementation. Bassert JM, Thomas JA, McCurnin's Clinical Textbook for Veterinary Technicians, ed 8, Elsevier, 2014.

475. d Omega-3 fatty acids have been shown to have a significant effect on survival times when used in dogs diagnosed with dilated cardiomyopathy (DCM) or chronic valvular disease (CVD). Omega-3 fatty acids may be attributed to anti-inflammatory effects, cachexia prevention, improved appetite, or antiarrhythmic effects. Wortinger A, Burns K, Nutrition and Disease Management for Veterinary Technicians and Nurses, ed 2, Wiley Blackwell, 2015.

476. d The American Veterinary Dental College (AVDC) supports the advanced training of veterinary technicians to perform additional dental services, such as taking impressions, making models, charting veterinary dental lesions, taking and developing dental radiographs, and performing nonsurgical subgingival root planing. Bassert JM, Thomas JA, McCurnin's Clinical Textbook for Veterinary Technicians, ed 8, Elsevier, 2014.

477. b Prevention of milk fever is achieved by providing a well-balanced, low-calcium diet during the dry period. Total dietary intake of calcium should be restricted during the dry period. It is important to keep dry cows separated from the rest of the herd so that they can be fed appropriately. Administrating calcium IV is a treatment option, not a preventative. Oral administration of dextrose will neither treat nor prevent milk fever. Bassert JM, Thomas JA, McCurnin's Clinical Textbook for Veterinary Technicians, ed 8, Elsevier, 2014.

478. d Ball-and-socket joints are also called spheroidal joints. They allow the most extensive movements of all the joint types and allow all the synovial joint movements. Ball-and-socket joints permit flexion, extension, abduction, adduction, rotation, and circumduction. The shoulder and hip joints are ball-and-socket joints. Pivot joints are also known as trochoid joints. One bone pivots or rotates on another. The only movement possible is rotation. Only one true pivot joint is found in the bodies of most animals, that being the atlantoaxial joint, which is the joint between the first and second cervical vertebrae. The complicated name for gliding joints is arthrodial joints, but the term *rocking joints* would be more descriptive. The joint surfaces of a gliding joint are relatively flat. The movement between them is a rocking motion of one bone on the other. Colville TP, Bassert JM, Clinical Anatomy and Physiology for Veterinary Technicians, ed 3, Elsevier, 2016.

479. a Hyperadrenocorticalism is also known as Cushing's disease. It is common in dogs and is rare in cats. Hypoadrenocorticism, also known as Addison's disease, affects mainly dogs. Hypothyroidism is rare in cats and is common in dogs 6–10 years of age. Hyperthyroidism is very rare in dogs and is commonly seen in cats that are more than 10 years of age. Aspinall V, The Complete Textbook of Veterinary Nursing, ed 2, Butterworth-Heinemann, 2011.

480. d Ketosis occurs in high-producing dairy cows during the first few months of lactation if they are unable to meet the energy demands of lactation. To provide energy for milk production, the cow begins to mobilize fat, the breakdown of which results in the formation of ketone bodies that accumulate in the blood. Ketosis in dairy cows may result from a primary deficiency in energy intake or it may be secondary to a disease process that causes anorexia, such as abomasal displacement, mastitis, or metritis. Milk fever does not cause ketosis. Bassert JM, Thomas JA, McCurnin's Clinical Textbook for Veterinary Technicians, ed 8, Elsevier, 2014.

481. d Caseous lymphadenitis (CL) is the most common cause of lymph node abscess in small ruminants and is a major cause of carcass condemnation in sheep. This highly contagious disease is caused by *Corynebacterium pseudotuberculosis*. The disease is readily spread from animal to animal by contact with contaminated purulent material. The bacterium usually gains entry through broken skin, but the organism may also invade intact skin or enter the body via inhalation or ingestion. It then infects the lymphatic system, in which characteristic abscesses develop. The disease can become endemic in a herd or flock and it is difficult to eradicate because of its poor response to therapeutics and its ability to persist in the environment for long periods (up to 8 months in soil). Bassert JM, Thomas JA, McCurnin's Clinical Textbook for Veterinary Technicians, ed 8, Elsevier, 2014.

482. d Risk factors for overweight/obesity in dogs include age, certain breeds, being neutered, consuming semi-moist food, homemade diets, or canned food as the dog's major diet source, and consumption of other foods (meat or other food products, commercial treats, or table scraps). Feeding dry dog food is not a risk factor for overweight/obesity in dogs provided that the correct amount of food for the diet is fed. Wortinger A, Burns K, Nutrition and Disease Management for Veterinary Technicians and Nurses, ed 2, Wiley Blackwell, 2015.

483. c Osteoclasts are like the evil twins of osteoblasts; instead of forming bone, they eat it away. Actually, they are not evil at all. Bones are dynamic structures that must be remodeled constantly. Osteoclasts are necessary for remodeling to take place by removing bone from areas in which it is not needed; osteoblasts form new bone in areas where it is needed. Osteoclasts also allow the body to withdraw calcium from the bones when it is needed to raise the calcium level in the blood. Osteoblasts are the cells that form bone. They secrete the matrix of bone and then supply the minerals necessary to harden it. After the osteoblasts become trapped in the ossified matrix they have created, they are called osteocytes. Talk about painting yourself into a corner! Osteocytes are always ready to revert to their former lives as osteoblasts and they form new bone if an injury makes that necessary. Some of the bones serve as sites for blood cell formation in the bone marrow that fills their interiors, which is called hematopoiesis. Colville TP, Bassert JM, Clinical Anatomy and Physiology for Veterinary Technicians, ed 3, Elsevier, 2016.

484. a Sheep are more prone than goats to the development of copper toxicity. Sheep absorb copper from the diet in proportion to the amount offered rather than according to the body's need. Copper accumulates in the liver, causing liver damage that precedes the onset of clinical signs. Usually, stress, such as shipping, handling, traveling to shows, and feed changes, triggers the release of copper from the liver. Copper is not stored in the kidneys, gallbladder, or lymph nodes. Bassert JM, Thomas JA, McCurnin's Clinical Textbook for Veterinary Technicians, ed 8, Elsevier, 2014.

485. b Pinkeye, or infectious keratoconjunctivitis, usually caused by *Chlamydia psittaci* in sheep and *Mycoplasma conjunctivae* in goats, is often treated with tetracycline in both species. Cattle can be treated with subconjunctival injection of antibiotics, usually penicillin. Phenylbutazone is an anti-inflammatory, not an antibiotic, and it will not prevent the spread of infection. Aminoglycosides are not used to treat pinkeye. Bassert JM, Thomas JA, McCurnin's Clinical Textbook for Veterinary Technicians, ed 8, Elsevier, 2014.

486. a The interparietal bones are two small bones located on the dorsal midline between the occipital bone and the parietal bones. They are usually clearly visible in young animals. In older animals, they may fuse together into one bone or they may fuse to the parietal bones and become indistinguishable. The occipital bone is a single bone that forms the caudoventral portion or base of the skull. It is the most caudal skull bone and is very important because it is where the spinal cord exits the skull and it is the skull bone that articulates (forms a joint) with the first cervical (neck) vertebra. The two parietal bones form the dorsolateral walls of the cranium. They are large and well developed in dogs, cats, and humans, but they are relatively small in horses and cattle. The two temporal bones are located below or ventral to the parietal bones. The temporal bones are important for several reasons: they form the lateral walls of the cranium, they contain the middle and inner ear structures, and they are the skull bones that form the temporomandibular joints (TMJs) with the mandible (lower jaw). Colville TP, Bassert JM, Clinical Anatomy and Physiology for Veterinary Technicians, ed 3, Elsevier, 2016.

487. a Digestive upset can be limited by allowing a slow change and adjustment from one diet to another. A transition time of 5 to 7 days is recommended. Shorter transition times will often cause diarrhea. A longer transition time might be necessary in some specific cases, but these cases would be unusual. Sirois M, "Pharmacology and Pharmacy," Principles and Practice of Veterinary Technology, ed 3, Elsevier, 2011, p. 592.

488. b Fewer calories are required after growth is complete and fiber is beneficial for GI function. An increase in calories, feeding table scraps, and reduced fiber could lead to additional weight gain and could increase the possibility of obesity. Hand MS, et al, Small Animal Clinical Nutrition, ed 5, Mark Morris Institute, 2010.

489. a Vitamins A, E, C, and beta carotene are considered antioxidants. Vitamin K is a fat-soluble vitamin that is involved in the clotting process. The Krebs cycle is an important component of the oxygenation process. Fascetti AJ, Delaney SJ, Applied Veterinary Clinical Nutrition, Wiley-Blackwell, 2012, p. 149.

490. d The color or colors of foods may impact an owner's perception of the food; however, colors have no bearing in dog or cat acceptability. For patients, ingredients and their associated impact on palatability, along with texture (i.e., dry, wet, semi-moist) and macronutrient distribution (e.g., protein, fat, and carbohydrate percentages), play key roles in the foods they choose to consume when given a choice. Fascetti AJ, Delaney SJ, Applied Veterinary Clinical Nutrition, Wiley-Blackwell, 2012, p. 6.

491. b Interdigital necrobacillosis, or foot rot, is an infection of the interdigital skin and underlying tissues. Polioencephalomalacia is also known as cerebrocortical necrosis and is characterized by altered function of the central nervous system. Hardware disease is the ingestion of metal objects by ruminants. Hairy heel wart is also known as papillomatous digital dermatitis. Bassert JM, Thomas JA, McCurnin's Clinical Textbook for Veterinary Technicians, ed 8, Elsevier, 2014.

492. d Laminitis, or founder, is a diffuse, aseptic inflammation of the corium (sensitive lamina) of the feet. Acute laminitis occurs sporadically and may be a result of sudden excessive grain ingestion or it may occur secondary to other diseases that occur during the postparturient period. Chronic laminitis is more often associated with constant feeding of high-grain diets. The hoof grows from the coronary band. The wall is the convex, external portion of the hoof that is visible from the anterior, lateral, and medial views. It is divided into three regions: the toe, the quarters, and the heels. The coffin bone is the distal phalanx bone, which is the entire third phalanx of the skeletal foot of the horse. Bassert JM, Thomas JA, McCurnin's Clinical Textbook for Veterinary Technicians, ed 8, Elsevier, 2014.

493. c Horses are classified as a hindgut fermenter. The cecum of horses is a very large chamber stretching from the upper right flank to the xiphoid process of the sternum. Ruminants have a stomach with four compartments;

for example, a cow is a ruminant. An omnivore is an animal that eats meat and plant material; a dog is an omnivore. A carnivore is an animal that requires a diet of meat; a cat is a carnivore. Holtgrew-Bohling K, Large Animal Clinical Procedures for Veterinary Technicians, ed 2, Elsevier, 2012, p. 181.

494. a Higher protein is necessary for lactation and growth than for an adult maintenance diet to meet the additional energy requirements of lactating dams/queens and growing puppies and kittens. Higher fiber and lower-calorie diets are contraindicated and would not meet the dietary requirements of these patients. Vitamin supplementation is not required and, except in rare cases, is contraindicated. Hand MS, et al, Small Animal Clinical Nutrition, ed 5, Mark Morris Institute, 2010.

495. d Vitamin E, mixed tocopherols, and vitamin C are considered natural preservatives. Omega-3 oils are fatty acids. Sucrose and dextrose are forms of sugar. Lactated Ringer's solution is a type of IV fluid. Fascetti AJ, Delaney SJ, Applied Veterinary Clinical Nutrition, Wiley-Blackwell, 2012, p. 97.

496. a Trichophyton verrucosum is the organism responsible for ringworm in cattle. *Microsporum canis* and *Microsporum gypseum* are found in dogs and cats, whereas *Epidermophyton floccosum* is found in humans. Sykes J, Canine and Feline Infectious Diseases, Saunders, 2014, VitalBook file; Bassert JM, Thomas JA, McCurnin's Clinical Textbook for Veterinary Technicians, ed 8, Elsevier, 2014.

497. d Contagious ecthyma (sore mouth, orf), a common zoonotic viral disease of small ruminants, causes crusty, proliferative lesions around the mouth and nose of lambs and kids and causes similar lesions on the teats and udders of ewes and does. Sorf does not exist. Bassert JM, Thomas JA, McCurnin's Clinical Textbook for Veterinary Technicians, ed 8, Elsevier, 2014.

498. c Corticosteroids have potent anti-inflammatory properties and are administered for allergic airway disease, allergic skin conditions, immune-mediated disease, and joint inflammation. Corticosteroids are administered topically, orally, parenterally (intravenously or intramuscularly), and intra-articularly. Adverse effects of corticosteroid administration include immunosuppression, polyuria or polydipsia, poor hair coat, muscle wasting, poor wound healing, laminitis, and progression of degenerative joint disease. Therefore, corticosteroids are administered with caution and only when specifically indicated. Corticosteroids have not been shown to have any effect on tear production or hair coat. Bassert JM, Thomas JA, McCurnin's Clinical Textbook for Veterinary Technicians, ed 8, Elsevier, 2014, p. 744.

499. b Joint supplements and chondroprotective agents, such as nutraceuticals, chondroitin sulfate, hyaluronic acid, and glycosaminoglycans (GAGs), are used more commonly in horses than in any other species. These products generally are not truly analgesic agents, but they may help to improve joint health, thereby decreasing pain. Flavor enhancers are used to increase palatability of animal feeds. Dentifrice is a paste, liquid, or powder used to help maintain good oral hygiene. Parenteral medications are those that are administered intravenously. Bassert JM, Thomas JA, McCurnin's Clinical Textbook for Veterinary Technicians, ed 8, Elsevier, 2014, p. 1071.

500. d Processing of piglets raised in confinement includes iron dextran injections at 3 days of age and clipping needle teeth prevents injury to the dam's udder and to other piglets in the litter. Castration may also be performed and tails may be docked to prevent tail biting, which can result in an ascending infection. Dewclaws on piglets are not removed. Bassert JM, Thomas JA, McCurnin's Clinical Textbook for Veterinary Technicians, ed 8, Elsevier, 2014.

501. c The typical length of gestation for swine is 114 days (3 months, 3 weeks, 3 days). The average gestation period for ferrets is 42 days and for dogs is 63 days. For sheep the average is 147 days. Bassert JM, Thomas JA, McCurnin's Clinical Textbook for Veterinary Technicians, ed 8, Elsevier, 2014.

502. b Exertional myopathy causes cramping, fatigue, and muscle pain in horses and is most often associated with exercise. One common result of exertional myopathy, especially associated with exercise, is necrosis of the striated skeletal muscle. Necrosis of the striated skeletal muscle is also known as exertional rhabdomyolysis. Other terms for exertional rhabdomyolysis are *azoturia*, *cording up*, and *tying up*. Exertional rhabdomyolysis can be divided into two categories: sporadic exertional rhabdomyolysis and chronic rhabdomyolysis. Polydipsia is excessive thirst. Anorexia is the loss of appetite (not eating). Pyrexia is a fever or febrile condition. Holtgrew-Bohling K, Large Animal Clinical Procedures for Veterinary Technicians, ed 2, Elsevier, 2012, p. 319.

503. c Water-soluble vitamins include B complex and C. Vitamins A, D, E, and K are fat-soluble vitamins. Case LP, Daristotle L, Hayek MG, Raasch MF, "Vitamins," Canine and Feline Nutrition: A Resource for Companion Animal Professionals, ed 3, Mosby, 2011.

504. c An ideal diet for dogs with acute pancreatitis is highly digestible, low in fat, and palatable. The main goals to manage the patient with pancreatitis are to provide enough calories and nutrients to support recovery while decreasing pancreatic stimulation. Protein levels, appropriate for the patient's life stage, are appropriate for these patients provided the diet is low in fat. Fascetti AJ, Delaney SJ, Applied Veterinary Clinical Nutrition, Wiley-Blackwell, 2012, p. 224-226.

505. c L-carnitine is a water-soluble, vitamin-like compound synthesized from the amino acids lysine and methionine, which is critical for myocardial energy production. Although taurine is an essential nutrient for cats, dogs are thought to be able to synthesize adequate amounts of taurine endogenously, therefore it is not classified as an essential nutrient for dogs. Dilated cardiomyopathy in dog breeds that are at highest risk of the disease (e.g., Doberman pinschers, boxers) does not appear to be related to taurine deficiency, but taurine deficiency has been documented in some dogs with DCM of certain breeds, such as the American cocker spaniel, Newfoundland, Portuguese water dog, and golden retriever. Taurine deficiency may occur more commonly in certain breeds because of higher requirements or breed-specific metabolic abnormalities, but diet may also play a role. Taurine and L-carnitine have not been shown to play any role in inappetence, dysphagia, and temperament. Fascetti AJ, Delaney SJ, Applied Veterinary Clinical Nutrition, Wiley-Blackwell, 2012, p. 308-309.

506. a Intracellular cation is essential for smooth, skeletal, and cardiac muscle contraction. Dietary deficiencies of K lead to neurologic disease, especially ventroflexion of the head (similar to thiamin deficiency), along with weakness, poor growth, and cardiac abnormalities. Potassium deficiency has not been shown to cause weight gain; these patients are often anorexic and therefore are more prone to weight loss. Palatability is not affected by potassium deficiency. Poor growth, not improved growth, can be a result of potassium deficiency. Bassert JM, Thomas JA, McCurnin's Clinical Textbook for Veterinary Technicians, ed 8, Elsevier, 2014, p. 304.

507. b The typical length of gestation for dogs is 63 days, whereas swine average 114 days (3 months, 3 weeks, 3 days). An average ferret gestation period is 42 days, whereas sheep average 147 days. Bassert JM, Thomas JA, McCurnin's Clinical Textbook for Veterinary Technicians, ed 8, Elsevier, 2014.

508. a Technicians should know the physiology of the GI tract (in this instance the large intestine) and how the GI tract responds to VFA. The optimum pH for microbial activity that promotes volatile fatty acid (VFA) absorption in the equine large intestine is 6.5. A pH of 6.1 is lower than optimum and a pH of 6.7 and 7.1 are higher than optimum to promote absorption. Frape D, Equine Nutrition and Feeding, ed 4, Wiley-Blackwell, 2010, p. 18.

509. a AAFCO has established feeding trial guidelines for diets labeled as complete and balanced for adult maintenance, growth, and gestation/lactation. No feeding trial guidelines have been established for senior diets. Bassert JM, Thomas JA, McCurnin's Clinical Textbook for Veterinary Technicians, ed 8, Elsevier, 2014, p. 304.

510. b Porcine stress syndrome (PSS) is also known as malignant hyperthermia. A single autosomal recessive gene causes susceptibility to PSS and disease is manifested only in pigs that are homozygous recessive for this gene. Sodium ion toxicosis is known as salt poisoning and it results from the ingestion of excess salt or from water deprivation. Porcine parvovirus is not referred to by any other name. Bassert JM, Thomas JA, McCurnin's Clinical Textbook for Veterinary Technicians, ed 8, Elsevier, 2014.

511. a Unqualified use of the term *beef* in a product name requires that beef ingredients be at least 95% or more of the total weight of all ingredients, exclusive of water used in processing, but in no case <70% of the total product. The term *beef* with a qualifier, such as beef dinner, beef platter, or beef formula, requires at least 25% of the total weight of all the ingredients, exclusive of water used in processing, but in no case <10% of the total product. There are no label terms that require 40% or 50% of an ingredient to be included in a diet. Hand MS, et al, Small Animal Clinical Nutrition, ed 5, Mark Morris Institute, 2010, p. 195.

512. a Canning as a way to preserve food was invented in 1810 and it is an important method to destroy bacteria and to extend the shelf life of human and pet foods. As with dry foods, the ingredients are first ground and then mixed with water and steam to a consistent moisture content. At this point, instead of entering an extruder, they are processed in a cooker/mixer. A filler/seamer machine is used to fill cans and seal the lids. Cans are placed in a machine called a retort because the process of retorting canned food is necessary to achieve sterilization. This heating and cooling step is sufficient to kill *Clostridium botulinum*, a bacterial pathogen that causes botulism. Preservatives must be used in dry and semi-moist foods to inhibit the growth of mold and bacteria and to prevent spoilage and contamination. Bassert JM, Thomas JA, McCurnin's Clinical Textbook for Veterinary Technicians, ed 8, Elsevier, 2014, p. 313.

513. c PSS results in hyperthermia, not hypothermia. Bassert JM, Thomas JA, McCurnin's Clinical Textbook for Veterinary Technicians, ed 8, Elsevier, 2014.

514. a Cats are obligate carnivores and require a significantly higher amount of protein in their diets than dogs. Feeding a variety of different diets may cause gastrointestinal upset and is not recommended. Hairballs may cause vomiting or intestinal blockage; however, hairballs are not a sign of illness. Animal and fish liver contains high levels of vitamin A. Bassert JM, Thomas JA, McCurnin's Clinical Textbook for Veterinary Technicians, ed 8, Elsevier, 2014, p. 298.

515. a Veterinary therapeutic dietary products, although not strictly prescription items, such as pharmaceuticals, may in most areas be sold (dispensed) only at the veterinary clinic where the patient is seen. Often the label includes a phrase such as "Use under the direction of a veterinarian." To purchase therapeutic diets from other clinics, online pharmacies, or other suppliers, a veterinarian must prescribe or request the order. This is done to prevent dispensing or recommending an inappropriate product. Raw pet foods and ingredients are marketed to those consumers who believe that food in its natural, uncooked state is healthier than cooked, or to those who think that nutrients are destroyed during processing, leading to unhealthy products. Holistic is a more recent product claim seen on certain pet food labels. There is no official definition or general agreement on what the term *holistic* means. Over-the-counter (OTC) diets are those that may be purchased without the involvement of a veterinarian. Bassert JM, Thomas JA, McCurnin's Clinical Textbook for Veterinary Technicians, ed 8, Elsevier, 2014, p. 308.

516. b Pigs are sensitive to heat and wallow in mud to help them thermoregulate. Rooting is a normal foraging behavior for pigs; however, they do not wallow in mud to root. Pigs do not root in mud to remove parasites or to prevent sunburn. Bassert JM, Thomas JA, McCurnin's Clinical Textbook for Veterinary Technicians, ed 8, Elsevier, 2014.

517. a Adulthood in cats is reached by 10 to 12 months of age and cats should be fed growth formula until this time. During the postweaning period, kittens are usually active and playful. Energy requirements are two to three times that of adult cats based on body weight. Feeding kittens an adult formula at 6 months of age is not recommended because these diets are not formulated to meet their increased energy needs. Adult cats fed a growth formula may become overweight or obese because their energy requirements are generally less than those of a growing kitten. Bassert JM, Thomas JA, McCurnin's Clinical Textbook for Veterinary Technicians, ed 8, Elsevier, 2014, p. 325.

518. d The current recommendation is to feed >10% of a pet's daily caloric requirement in treats to avoid nutritional deficiencies and excesses. Treats are not required to be, and generally are not, complete and balanced. Pets fed >10% of their daily caloric requirements may become overweight or obese. Low-calorie treats are not complete and balanced. Wortinger A, Burns K, Nutrition and Disease Management for Veterinary Technicians and Nurses, ed 2, Wiley Blackwell, 2015, p. 121.

519. b The most common misconception held by owners of pet pigs is that their potbellied pig will weigh only 40 to 50 lb when fully grown. Although a few pigs remain small, most of them will weigh closer to 120 lb when mature and they do not reach full size until they are 2 to 3 years old. Bassert JM, Thomas JA, McCurnin's Clinical Textbook for Veterinary Technicians, ed 8, Elsevier, 2014.

520. c Taurine, an amino acid, is unique in that it is required in the diet for cats but not for dogs because healthy dogs are able to synthesize taurine from other amino acids. L-carnitine is a vitamin-like substance and is a natural compound found in all animal cells. Glutamine is a conditionally essential amino acid and may need to be supplemented in pets with certain disease conditions such as cancer. Lysine is an essential amino acid and is required in the diet of both dogs and cats. Bassert JM, Thomas JA, McCurnin's Clinical Textbook for Veterinary Technicians, ed 8, Elsevier, 2014, p. 297.

521. d Law requires ingredients to be listed in order by weight, with the heaviest first and the lightest last. Units cannot be used (e.g., it is illegal to state "chicken 40%, rice 20%," or "beef 90 grams"). The pet food label is not required to indicate dietary importance, nutrient bioavailability, and caloric percentage of ingredients. Bassert JM, Thomas JA, McCurnin's Clinical Textbook for Veterinary Technicians, ed 8, Elsevier, 2014, p. 312.

522. c The most common nutritional disease of potbellied pigs is obesity; however, many stunted and malnourished pigs are seen because of their owner's misguided attempts to keep them small. Several companies have developed diets specifically for miniature pigs. Miniature pigs should never be fed commercial swine feed; feed for miniature swine is lower in protein and fat and has a higher fiber content than commercial swine rations. Miniature pig feed is generally classified as starter, grower, breeder, or maintenance. Bassert JM, Thomas JA, McCurnin's Clinical Textbook for Veterinary Technicians, ed 8, Elsevier, 2014.

523. a The US Department of Agriculture (USDA) is broadly responsible for agricultural products, including ingredients used in pet foods. The USDA conducts inspections of farms and pet food manufacturers to ensure safety and proper handling. The Food and Drug Administration (FDA) and its division the Center for Veterinary Medicine (CVM) are the main regulators of the safety of pet foods. The FDA-CVM has authority regarding much of the information on pet food labels, including health and nutrition claims. The Association of American Feed Control Officials (AAFCO) is a private, nongovernmental organization that does not have regulatory or enforcement power. However, federal and state governments employ many members of AAFCO as feed control officials. The Federal Trade Commission (FTC) regulates business practices in the United States. False, misleading, or deceptive marketing practices in the manufacture, distribution, and sale of pet food may be subject to FTC enforcement. Bassert JM, Thomas JA, McCurnin's Clinical Textbook for Veterinary Technicians, ed 8, Elsevier, 2014, p. 309.

524. b During the first week postpartum, daily energy intake should be 25% to 50% higher than maintenance and by week 4 or 5 of lactation, energy needs may be 100% to 200% higher. Protein and fat requirements also increase during the last 4 to 5 weeks of gestation. To meet these additional needs, pregnant dogs should be offered more food per day, as has been described. Recommendations range from 20% to 100% more dietary protein and from 20% to 60% more dietary fat. During the final weeks of gestation, it is reasonable to switch gradually from a maintenance diet to one formulated for growth (puppy food) or reproduction (gestation and lactation). Similar to growing puppies, pregnant dogs have an increased need for energy and other nutrients. However, for the first 5 to 6 weeks of gestation, fetal growth is minimal, so the nutritional requirements are the same as for adult maintenance. Beginning in week 5, a pregnant dog's energy intake should increase by approximately 30% to 60% depending on breed, size, number of puppies, and stage of gestation. To prevent adverse health effects of loss of weight and lean body mass during lactation, weaning should begin when puppies are 3 to 4 weeks of age. Offering solid food to puppies at an early age provides the benefit of reducing stress on the mother by reducing milk demand. Bassert JM, Thomas JA, McCurnin's Clinical Textbook for Veterinary Technicians, ed 8, Elsevier, 2014, p. 323-324.

525. c A murmur is an atypical heart sound associated with a functional or structural valve abnormality. An arrhythmia is an abnormal heart rate or rhythm. Fibrillations are the rapid, irregular myocardial contractions resulting in loss of a simultaneous heartbeat and pulse. Infarct is a localized area of tissue that is dying or dead because of a lack of blood supply. Colville J, Sharon O, Clinical Veterinary Language, Mosby, 2014.

526. a Although patients requiring weight control and management of diabetes mellitus benefit from a consistent food dose, the higher sugar content and lower fiber content of semi-moist foods make them ill-suited for these feeding applications. Any food type, including semi-moist foods, labeled complete and balanced for all life stages, may be fed to healthy geriatric, growing, and lactating dogs and cats. Hand MS, et al, Small Animal Clinical Nutrition, ed 5, Mark Morris Institute, 2010, p. 160.

527. d The term *fish flavor* does not stipulate a minimum percentage and should be an amount that is detectable by the pet. The fish flavor designation usually indicates that fish is <3% of the total product. An ingredient that provides the characterizing flavor (e.g., fish digest, fish byproducts) may be <1% of the total product and may still appear in the product name as a flavor. The unqualified use of the term *fish* in a product name requires that fish ingredients be at least 95% or more of the total weight of all ingredients, exclusive of water used in processing, but in no case <70% of the total product. The use of the term *fish* with a qualifier, such as fish dinner, fish platter, fish entree, fish formula, or any similar designation, requires that fish ingredients be at least 25% of the total weight of all ingredients, exclusive of water used in processing, but in no case <10% of the total product. The term *with fish* is intended to highlight minor ingredients and requires that fish ingredients be at least 3% of the total product. Hand MS, et al, Small Animal Clinical Nutrition, ed 5, Mark Morris Institute, 2010, p. 194-195.

528. b The words dog food, for cats, or some similar terminology must appear conspicuously on the principal display panel of pet foods sold in the United States. These terms clearly identify the animal for which the product is intended and that the product is not for human consumption. The term *beef entrée* requires that beef ingredients be at least 25% of the total weight of all ingredients, exclusive of water used in processing, but in no case <10% of the total product. Nine Lives is an example of a product brand name. "Complete and balanced for adult dogs" is a nutrition adequacy statement. Hand MS, et al, Small Animal Clinical Nutrition, ed 5, Mark Morris Institute, 2010, p. 195.

529. a An equine that is around 1 year old is referred to as a yearling. Foaling is the process of giving birth to a colt or filly. A weanling is a young equine that has been weaned from its mother. A filly is an intact female younger than 4 years. Colville JL, Oien SA, Clinical Veterinary Language, ed 1, Elsevier Mosby, 2014, VitalBook file.

530. b The guaranteed analysis consists of four required diet components and amounts, along with several others that are optional but are found on many pet foods. Only the minimum crude protein and crude fat amounts are required, along with the maximum fiber and moisture amounts. The exact amounts of nutrients and moisture levels are not listed on pet food labels. Maximum levels of some nutrients are required to be listed on pet food labels. The minimum levels of some nutrients are required to be listed on pet food labels. Bassert JM, Thomas JA, McCurnin's Clinical Textbook for Veterinary Technicians, ed 8, Elsevier, 2014, p. 311.

531. c Digestibility provides a measure of the final diet's quality because it directly determines the proportion of nutrients in the food that are available for absorption into the body. Currently, AAFCO regulations do not require companies to determine or provide digestibility levels for their foods. Dry-matter basis refers to the amount of nutrient in a food after the moisture has been removed. Energy density is the percentage in the diet of a nutrient multiplied by the modified Atwater factor for that nutrient. Hydrolyzation refers to a process that reduces proteins to small peptides and amino acids. Wortinger A, Burns K, Nutrition and Disease Management for Veterinary Technicians and Nurses, ed 2, Wiley Blackwell, 2015, p. 66.

532. a Warming the food to between room and body temperature (70°F–100°F) increases the palatability of pet foods. Onions can be toxic to dogs and cats. Food should not be overheated to avoid the pet burning the tissue of its mouth and tongue. Milk is not easily digestible by adult dogs and cats and may cause diarrhea. Wortinger A, Burns K, Nutrition and Disease Management for Veterinary Technicians and Nurses, ed 2, Wiley Blackwell, 2015, p. 173.

533. c As described earlier, fats are composed of triglycerides, which include three fatty acids attached to a glycerol chain. Different types of fatty acids are found in dietary sources and in the body based on chain length, location and number of double bonds, and function. The first variable to consider is how many carbon molecules the fatty acid contains. These are divided into short-chain (2 to 6), medium-chain (8 to 12), and long-chain (14 to 24) varieties. Short-chain fatty acids are building blocks and are not an important part of diet or function in dogs and cats. Although only limited research has examined the effects and benefits of MCT compared with other triglycerides, it is thought that it is more easily broken down and absorbed in the intestinal tract. MCT oil is less palatable than long-chain triglycerides, therefore it cannot be used as the only dietary source of fat. Long-chain fatty acids are the most common types found in foods and include linoleic and alpha-linolenic acids (essential for dogs and cats) and arachidonic acid (essential for cats). Bassert JM, Thomas JA, McCurnin's Clinical Textbook for Veterinary Technicians, ed 8, Elsevier, 2014, p. 298.

534. c An intact male donkey is referred to as a jack, whereas a jenny is an intact female donkey. A dam is the female parent of her offspring and a sire is the male parent of his offspring. Colville JL, Oien SA, Clinical Veterinary Language, ed 1, Elsevier Mosby, 2014.

535. c Farrowing is the process of giving birth to pigs. Freshening is the process whereby dairy goats give birth to kids. A stag is a male that was castrated/neutered after sexual maturity. Kidding is the process of giving birth to kids. Colville JL, Oien SA, Clinical Veterinary Language, ed 1, Elsevier Mosby, 2014, VitalBook file.

536. c Specific-purpose products are intended for certain life stages, such as growth, or for certain medical conditions such as obesity, kidney disease, hairballs, etc. Most veterinary therapeutic diets fall into this category, which should be prescribed and monitored by animal health professionals. All-purpose pet foods are intended for feeding healthy animals of any age or life stage. They are complete and balanced, meaning that they contain all known nutrients in adequate amounts and that the nutrients are bioavailable. Ideally, these products have undergone feeding trials for growth of puppies or kittens, as well as reproduction (gestation and lactation), to ensure that they meet the increased nutritional demands. Premium products are sold on the basis that more expensive ingredients and foods are healthier than lower-priced value products. Some companies market certain pet foods as super-premium. Although no standard definition has been established, in general, premium products are sold at specialty retailers such as pet stores, kennels, and veterinary clinics. By making some products exclusive to certain retailers, pet food companies hope to attract more demanding owners or those consumers who equate high price with high quality. Value or low-priced products are aimed at consumers looking for bargains or who are feeding multiple animals. Many store brands, private labels, and generic pet foods are positioned as low-cost, high-value. These are often sold at discount and grocery stores, feed stores, and warehouse clubs, and sometimes at pet retailers as an alternative to higher-priced products. Value-oriented pet foods are typically complete and balanced and are acceptable for feeding healthy dogs and cats. Bassert JM, Thomas JA, McCurnin's Clinical Textbook for Veterinary Technicians, ed 8, Elsevier, 2014, p. 306.

537. a Organic pet foods generally include those that use food ingredients that are not exposed to insecticides, pesticides, or, in the case of animals, medications such as antibiotics or growth promotants. At present, no complete and balanced pet food can be considered 100% organic because of the need to add inorganic vitamins, minerals, and trace nutrients. Although organic products appeal to consumers who try to avoid artificial chemicals, no evidence currently suggests that organic foods are by definition healthier or more nutritious. Raw pet foods and ingredients are marketed to those consumers who believe that food in its natural, uncooked state is healthier than cooked, or to those who think that nutrients are destroyed during processing, leading to unhealthy products. Natural pet foods claim to avoid any chemically synthesized ingredients. This term most often applies to preservatives used in dry products (moist foods usually do not need added preservatives because the sealed cans prevent spoilage). Holistic is a more recent product claim seen on certain pet food labels. There is no official definition or general agreement on what the term *holistic* means. Bassert JM, Thomas JA, McCurnin's Clinical Textbook for Veterinary Technicians, ed 8, Elsevier, 2014, p. 307.

538. d Pet food recipes found in books and on the Internet are almost always incomplete and unbalanced. Several studies have attempted to evaluate the nutrient content of these generic diet recipes and have found missing or deficient nutrients in the vast majority of cases. Some people claim that home recipes will be balanced over time, meaning that nutrients not provided one day will be made up for in the future. However, this concept is difficult to understand, because a nutrient deficiency in the recipe cannot necessarily be corrected by an excessive amount at a different time. Although some proponents believe that human diets are not complete each day and become balanced over time, this is a false assumption. A majority of Americans, and probably people in other countries, do not eat complete, balanced diets daily or over time, which leads to many adverse effects later in life. On the other hand, pets that are provided at least 100% of their nutrient requirements daily are much more likely to live long, healthy lives than those with daily deficiencies. Bassert JM, Thomas JA, McCurnin's Clinical Textbook for Veterinary Technicians, ed 8, Elsevier, 2014, p. 316.

539. a Morbidity is the number of animals in a population that become sick. Mortality is the number of animals in a population that die from a disease. Chronic is the slow onset of an abnormal condition that lasts a long time. Acute is the sudden onset of an abnormal condition and lasts a short duration. Colville JL, Oien SA, Clinical Veterinary Language, ed 1, Elsevier Mosby, 2014.

540. c Hemothorax refers to a collection of blood in the cranial portion of the ventral cavity. Pneumothorax refers to a collapsed lung. Pneumonia refers to fluid within the lungs. Hemostasis refers to an interruption of blood flow to a part of the body. Colville JL, Oien SA, Clinical Veterinary Language, ed 1, Elsevier Mosby, 2014.

541. a Overweight and obese puppies are a common health concern seen in our veterinary hospitals today. This observation is a result of overfeeding as well as a common misconception that puppies should be allowed to eat as much as they want. It is unusual for owners to feed too little and it is unfortunately not uncommon for owners to feed in excess. Fortunately, most owners today understand that puppies do not need nor can easily digest milk and therefore this is generally no longer a problem. Bassert JM, Thomas JA, McCurnin's Clinical Textbook for Veterinary Technicians, ed 8, Elsevier, 2014, p. 319.

542. b Feeding cats meals twice a day is considered the most appropriate feeding plan for cats that tend to overeat. Spacing these two meals out to approximately 12 hours apart, as opposed to feeding once per day, often reduces the likelihood that these cats will act hungry. A common way of feeding cats in the past was to place dry food in a bowl and simply refill the bowl whenever empty. Cats would self-regulate their food intake and eat multiple small meals throughout the day and night. Because of the high prevalence of overweight and obese cats, this practice is no longer recommended. The current theory is that spayed and neutered cats lose some of their appetite inhibition. When presented with free-choice food, cats cannot stop themselves from eating more than their energy expenditure warrants. The result is excess body weight, especially fat mass. To reduce this risk, cats that act hungry and tend to overeat should be fed twice a day. Obviously, feeding a cat only once a week is not recommended! Bassert JM, Thomas JA, McCurnin's Clinical Textbook for Veterinary Technicians, ed 8, Elsevier, 2014, p. 328.

543. a The most common sign of malnutrition is lack of energy and protein intake because of a reluctance or inability to eat voluntarily. Proper nutrition is necessary in sick patients for immune system function, tissue synthesis to promote healing, proper GI function, and regulation of many physiologic processes. Assisted feeding of a complete and balanced diet containing the appropriate amount of protein might be necessary to address this problem. When the dietary protein needs are addressed, any lack of sugar, carbohydrates, or minerals is of little concern for most hospitalized patients. Bassert JM, Thomas JA, McCurnin's Clinical Textbook for Veterinary Technicians, ed 8, Elsevier, 2014, p. 329.

544. c Oral feeding is the most physiologic and often the safest route. However, force-feeding is contraindicated because it may cause food aversion and even aspiration pneumonia if the animal struggles. Parenteral nutrition, although an appropriate method of feeding in certain cases, is not without risk, and the body does not use this type of nutrition as readily. Intraosseous and subcutaneous feeding is never an option; however, these methods are appropriate options for fluid administration in certain cases. Bassert JM, Thomas JA, McCurnin's Clinical Textbook for Veterinary Technicians, ed 8, Elsevier, 2014, p. 330.

545. d NG and NE tubes are effective and inexpensive methods of providing short-term nutritional support to hospitalized patients that are unable or unwilling to eat. They are less expensive and easier to place than any of the other methods for supplying nutritional support to patients unwilling or unable to eat. NG and NE tubes are useful for short-term nutritional support, generally 7 days or less. Bassert JM, Thomas JA, McCurnin's Clinical Textbook for Veterinary Technicians, ed 8, Elsevier, 2014, p. 330.

546. d A keloid is an overgrowth of scar tissue at the site of injury. A papule is a small, solid, usually pointed elevated of the skin. A petechia is tiny bleeds or bruising within the dermal layer. A laceration is a rough or jagged skin tear. Colville JL, Oien SA, Clinical Veterinary Language, ed 1, Elsevier Mosby, 2014.

547. b Osteomalacia refers to softening of bones. Osteopetrosis refers to hardening of bone. Multiple myeloma refers to the collection of abnormal cells that accumulate within the bones. Pachydermia refers to thickened skin. Colville JL, Oien SA, Clinical Veterinary Language, ed 1, Elsevier Mosby, 2014.

548. d Foods inadequate in protein and energy can cause abnormalities in the hair coat including a dry, dull hair coat and hair loss. This may also lead to depigmentation of the hair coat, not excessive pigmentation. Protein and energy deficiencies have not been shown to cause skin depigmentation, crusting around the eyes, or pyoderma. Hand MS, et al, Small Animal Clinical Nutrition, ed 5, Mark Morris Institute, 2010, p. 643.

549. d Dogs and cats may develop an adverse reaction to virtually any pet food ingredient; however, adverse reactions to protein sources are the most common. Homemade diets containing only one protein source to which the patient has never been exposed are commonly used as elimination diets. Patients suffering from adverse reactions to diet often exhibit concurrent allergies to environmental allergens. Hand MS, et al, Small Animal Clinical Nutrition, ed 5, Mark Morris Institute, 2010, p. 619-622.

550. a Dogs and cats might develop an adverse reaction to virtually any pet food ingredient; however, adverse reactions to protein sources are the most common. High levels of protein in the diet are not recommended to manage adverse reactions. Adverse food reactions to a carbohydrate source is uncommon in dogs and cats. Preservatives have not been shown to cause adverse food reactions. Hand MS, et al, Small Animal Clinical Nutrition, ed 5, Mark Morris Institute, 2010, p. 619.

551. a The Veterinary Oral Health Council (VOHC) is a private, independent agency established in 1997. The purpose of the VOHC is to provide an independent, objective, and credible means of recognizing veterinary dental products that effectively control the accumulation of plaque and/or calculus. The VOHC system is similar to the American Dental Association Seal of Acceptance system and is recognized worldwide. The American Veterinary Dental Association, the Academy of Veterinary Oral Health, and the Veterinary Dental Society are all associations composed of veterinary professionals interested in veterinary oral health. None of the other listed organizations is an approval body. Hand MS, et al, Small Animal Clinical Nutrition, ed 5, Mark Morris Institute, 2010, p. 987.

552. b Tendons connect muscles to bones. Ligaments connect bones to bones. A foramen refers to an opening or perforation. A process is a natural overgrowth or projection. Colville JL, Oien SA, Clinical Veterinary Language, ed 1, Elsevier Mosby, 2014, VitalBook file.

553. b Acute diarrhea is most often caused by dietary indiscretion or by the ingestion of a high-fat diet. Malignancy, histoplasmosis, and pythiosis are associated with severe large bowel disease, and as such most often result in chronic diarrhea. Wortinger A, Burns K, Nutrition and Disease Management for Veterinary Technicians and Nurses, ed 2, Wiley Blackwell, 2015, p. 169.

554. c Clinical signs IBD in cats include vomiting, diarrhea, and weight loss. Weight gain in cats with IBD is highly unusual. Wortinger A, Burns K, Nutrition and Disease Management for Veterinary Technicians and Nurses, ed 2, Wiley Blackwell, 2015.

555. a Increased frequency of defecation resulting in larger than normal soft-to-watery stool is often seen in small bowel diarrhea. Signs of large bowel diarrhea include fecal mucus and marked tenesmus. Hematochezia (bright red blood) typically originates in the anus, rectum, or descending colon. Melena may originate in the stomach or upper small intestine. Wortinger A, Burns K, Nutrition and Disease Management for Veterinary Technicians and Nurses, ed 2, Wiley Blackwell, 2015.

556. d Dietary indiscretion or ingestion of a high-fat meal is the most common cause of acute diarrhea. Taking a detailed nutritional history is important to determine what may have caused the acute diarrhea. Wortinger A, Burns K, Nutrition and Disease Management for Veterinary Technicians and Nurses, ed 2, Wiley Blackwell, 2015.

557. a Panosteitis refers to inflammation of all bones or the inflammation of every part of one bone. Polypathia refers to the presence of many diseases at the same time. Pandemic refers to a widespread disease across a region, a continent, or worldwide. Osteoporosis refers to weak or brittle bones. Colville JL, Oien SA, Clinical Veterinary Language, ed 1, Elsevier Mosby, 2014.

558. a Amyoplasia refers to the lack of muscle formation or development. Myoplegia refers to the paralysis of muscles. Hemiparesis refers to muscular weakness or partial paralysis restricted to one side of the body. Myopathy refers to any disease of a muscle. Colville JL, Oien SA, Clinical Veterinary Language, ed 1, Elsevier Mosby, 2014.

559. b Patients suffering from SBS should be fed a low-fat, highly digestible diet on a long-term basis to reduce and manage the diarrhea that is a clinical sign in many of these patients because of decreased intestinal transit time. Diets high in fats and moderately digestible diets are more difficult for these patients to digest as a result of decreased intestinal transit time. Merrill L, Small Animal Internal Medicine for Veterinary Technicians and Nurses, Wiley Blackwell, 2012.

560. d Water losses due to vomiting, diarrhea, and reduced water consumption can quickly lead to dehydration, which can be become severe and life-threatening without supportive care. Wortinger A, Burns K, Nutrition and Disease Management for Veterinary Technicians and Nurses, ed 2, Wiley Blackwell, 2015.

561. c Alkalemia should be expected if vomiting patients lose hydrogen and chloride ions in excess of sodium and bicarbonate. Acidemia may occur in vomiting patients if the vomited gastric fluid is relatively low in hydrogen and chloride content (e.g., during fasting) or if concurrent loss of intestinal sodium and bicarbonate occurs. Wortinger A, Burns K, Nutrition and Disease Management for Veterinary Technicians and Nurses, ed 2, Wiley Blackwell, 2015.

562. b Hydremia refers to a disorder in which there is excess fluid in the blood. Ischemia refers to an inadequate supply of blood to a part of the body. Anemia refers to a low red blood cell count in the body. Apex refers to the narrow point at the bottom of the heart. Colville JL, Oien SA, Clinical Veterinary Language, ed 1, Elsevier Mosby, 2014.

563. c Ascites is the accumulation of fluid in the abdominal cavity. Auscultate means to evaluate by listening with the aid of a stethoscope. Infarct is a localized area of tissue that is dying or dead because of a lack of blood supply. Edema is the excess fluid accumulation around cells of connective tissue. Colville JL, Oien SA, Clinical Veterinary Language, ed 1, Elsevier Mosby, 2014.

564. a It is important to flush all enteral feeding tubes before feeding to ensure they are not clogged and have not become dislodged. Flushing after feeding is important to eliminate remaining food from the tube to prevent the tube from becoming clogged. Flushing only after use increases the risk of food being administered into areas other than the digestive tract. Flushing only before use can result in the tube becoming clogged, possibly requiring its replacement. Never flushing the tube can result in all of these complications. Bassert JM, Thomas JA, McCurnin's Clinical Textbook for Veterinary Technicians, ed 8, Elsevier, 2014, p. 333.

565. a Intravenous feeding is referred to as parenteral feeding and is an effective method of providing nutritional support to patients unable to receive or tolerate enteral feeding. Enteral and oral feeding are both methods of feeding via the digestive tract. Providing nutrition in a true emergency is not of primary concern. True lifesaving measures are only necessary in true emergency situations. Bassert JM, Thomas JA, McCurnin's Clinical Textbook for Veterinary Technicians, ed 8, Elsevier, 2014, p. 334.

566. a Cats are obligate carnivores and have a higher protein requirement than dogs, which are omnivores. Given this physiologic difference it is never recommended to feed dog food to a cat. Wortinger A, Burns K, Nutrition and Disease Management for Veterinary Technicians and Nurses, ed 2, Wiley Blackwell, 2015, p. 124, 139.

567. c Leukopenia refers to an abnormally low white blood cell count. *Normocytic* is a descriptive term applied to the size of a normal red blood cell. Leukocytosis refers to a high white blood cell count. Anemia refers to a low red blood cell count. Colville JL, Oien SA, Clinical Veterinary Language, ed 1, Elsevier Mosby, 2014.

568. b Apepsia refers to a lack of digestion. Bradypeptic pertains to slow digestion. Monogastric refers to having a single digestion system (also referred to as a simple-stomach). Anastomosis refers to a surgical connection of two hollow organs or the joining of blood vessels. Colville JL, Oien SA, Clinical Veterinary Language, ed 1, Elsevier Mosby, 2014.

569. c The American Animal Hospital Association recommends five vital assessments of patient health at every examination to ensure the highest standard of care. These five vital assessments are temperature, cardio function, respiratory health, pain, and nutrition. 2010 AAHA Nutritional Assessment Guidelines for Dogs and Cats. https://www.aaha.org/globalassets/02-guidelines/nutritional-assessment/nutritionalassessmentguidelines.pdf.

570. d Patients suffering from acute or chronic vomiting are at increased risk of becoming dehydrated; without water or fluid therapy, these patients can become severely dehydrated. Protein, vitamins, and minerals are all important nutrients; however, a lack of these items is not as immediately life-threatening as severe dehydration. Merrill L, Small Animal Internal Medicine for Veterinary Technicians and Nurses, Wiley Blackwell, 2012.

571. d Acute diarrhea is typically the result of diet, parasites, or infectious disease (e.g., parvovirus, coronavirus, etc.). Wortinger A, Burns K, Nutrition and Disease Management for Veterinary Technicians and Nurses, ed 2, Wiley Blackwell, 2015.

572. d The goals of nutritional management of hepatic disease include maintaining normal metabolic processes, correction of electrolyte disturbances, providing substrates to support hepatocellular repair and regeneration, avoiding toxic byproduct accumulation, and avoiding and managing hepatic encephalopathy. Wortinger A, Burns K, Nutrition and Disease Management for Veterinary Technicians and Nurses, ed 2, Wiley Blackwell, 2015.

573. a The term *melena* refers to the passing of dark, tarry feces containing blood that has been acted on by bacteria in the intestines. Chyme refers to a semi-fluid mass of partially digested food that enters the small intestine from the stomach. An enzyme is a protein produced by living cells that initiates a chemical reaction but is not affected by the reaction. Relapse refers to falling back into a diseased state after an apparent recovery. Colville JL, Oien SA, Clinical Veterinary Language, ed 1, Elsevier Mosby, 2014.

574. a Cold compress is used to minimize inflammation. Warm compressing is a technique used to increase blood flow to an area to increase draining and healing of the area, such as with mastitis. Coupage is a technique used to help loosen purulent material within the pulmonary parenchyma with pneumonia. Passive range of motion is used to keep from joints becoming stiff. Battaglia AM, Steele AM, Small Animal Emergency and Critical Care for Veterinary Technicians, ed 3, Elsevier, 2016.

575. a Dogs and cats weighing 10%–19% more than the optimal weight for their breed are considered overweight; those weighing 20% or more than the optimal weight for their breed are considered obese. Wortinger A, Burns K, Nutrition and Disease Management for Veterinary Technicians and Nurses, ed 2, Wiley Blackwell, 2015.

576. a Overweight and obese pets should be introduced gradually to an exercise plan. Excessive running or exercising may cause pets to tire easily, which can cause owners to become frustrated. Starting with moderate exercise will often produce a more successful result. Exercise promotes weight loss; in fact, some pets do not lose weight unless exercise is included in their weight-reduction plan. Wortinger A, Burns K, Nutrition and Disease Management for Veterinary Technicians and Nurses, ed 2, Wiley Blackwell, 2015.

577. c Sebaceous glands that deposit the cat's scent are located around the lips and chin, interdigitally, and in the perianal area. Cats leave olfactory signals by rubbing the sebaceous glands of the face on objects, on other cats, and on humans; scratching (to deposit scent from the interdigital glands); and spraying. Spraying is usually a normal olfactory communication among cats (although inter-cat conflict in a household can induce spraying). Additionally, some cats communicate through urination and middening (fecal marking). Little S, The Cat, Saunders, 2012.

578. b Before the late 1980s, feline DCM was one of the most frequent cardiac diseases reported in cats. After the association of the disease with taurine deficiency, additional taurine was added to commercial diets, and the incidence of the disease significantly decreased. The pathologic condition is similar to DCM in dogs. Evidence exists of a genetic predisposition to DCM in cats fed taurine-deficient diets. Summers A, Common Diseases of Companion Animals, ed 3, Elsevier, 2014.

579. c The formula RER kcal/day = 70 (ideal body weight in kg) 0.75 is widely considered the most accurate formula to calculate resting energy requirements (RER). None of the other options listed are correct and these would underestimate or overestimate RER. Wortinger A, Burns K, Nutrition and Disease Management for Veterinary Technicians and Nurses, ed 2, Wiley Blackwell, 2015.

580. d Recommendations for a successful weight-loss program include an emphasis on feeding consistency, feeding the pet from its designated dish only, ensuring the client is using an 8-oz measuring cup to measure food, and appropriate exercise for the pet. Wortinger A, Burns K, Nutrition and Disease Management for Veterinary Technicians and Nurses, ed 2, Wiley Blackwell, 2015.

581. b The most common cause of FLUTD in cats younger than 10 years of age is feline idiopathic cystitis (FIC). In cats more than 10 years old, urinary tract infection and/or struvite uroliths are the most common cause of FLUTD. From 1994 to 2002, approximately 55% of uroliths were calcium oxalate crystals. Wortinger A, Burns K, Nutrition and Disease Management for Veterinary Technicians and Nurses, ed 2, Wiley Blackwell, 2015.

582. b Clinical signs of a thromboembolism include acute onset of rear leg pain and paresis, cold, bluish footpads (decreased circulation), lack of palpable pulses in the rear limbs, and a history of clinical findings of myocardial disease. Summers A, Common Diseases of Companion Animals, ed 3, Elsevier, 2014.

583. b Causes of congenital heart disease include genetic, environmental, infectious, nutritional, and drug-related factors. More is understood of the genetic factors than the other causes. Studies suggest the defects are polygenetic in nature and that they might be difficult to eliminate entirely from a specific breed. Summers A, Common Diseases of Companion Animals, ed 3, Elsevier, 2014.

584. c Cat owners, especially those owning cats prone to FLUTD, should be encouraged to have one litter box per cat plus one additional litter box. Cats may have individual preferences to the type of litter and litter box; however, many cats prefer unscented litters. Many cats dislike covered litter boxes, which tend to keep odors trapped in the litter box. Some cats prefer clumping litter whereas others prefer nonclumping. Wortinger A, Burns K, Nutrition and Disease Management for Veterinary Technicians and Nurses, ed 2, Wiley Blackwell, 2015.

585. d Urinalysis, including microscopic sediment examination and diagnosis of the urinary tract, including the bladder, is recommended for cats with lower urinary tract disease. Thyroid screening is not necessary when diagnosing urinary tract disease. Wortinger A, Burns K, Nutrition and Disease Management for Veterinary Technicians and Nurses, ed 2, Wiley Blackwell, 2015.

586. a Urinalysis is best performed on fresh urine samples within 30 minutes of collection. Crystals may form in urine samples evaluated >30 minutes after collection. Samples may be refrigerated for up to 8 hours and then evaluated after returning to room temperature. However, this method is not best for evaluating crystalluria and should be avoided. Ultrasound is not useful for evaluating crystalluria. Wortinger A, Burns K, Nutrition and Disease Management for Veterinary Technicians and Nurses, ed 2, Wiley Blackwell, 2015.

587. d Clinical signs associated with FHD include: coughing, dyspnea, vomiting, anorexia, weight loss, lethargy, right-sided CHF, sudden death, or acute development of neurologic signs. Summers A, Common Diseases of Companion Animals, ed 3, Elsevier, 2014.

588. d Nowadays, the Center for Veterinary Medicine (CVM), within the FDA, regulates pet foods in cooperation with the individual states. The FDA is responsible for: (1) establishing certain animal food labeling regulations, (2) specifying certain permitted ingredients such as drugs and additives, (3) enforcing regulations about chemical and microbiologic contamination, and (4) describing acceptable manufacturing procedures. The FDA is not responsible for enforcing manufacturing procedures. Hand MS, et al, Small Animal Clinical Nutrition, ed 5, Mark Morris Institute, 2010, p. 193.

589. b An adverse reaction to food is an abnormal response to an ingested food or food additive. An ingested toxin or inhaled toxin is by definition a poison. Inhaled food is defined as aspiration. Hand MS, et al, Small Animal Clinical Nutrition, ed 5, Mark Morris Institute, 2010, p. 609.

590. b Protein malnutrition is seen in patients with hepatic disease, manifesting clinically as weight loss, muscle atrophy, and hypoalbuminemia. Zinc toxicity, vitamin K toxicity, and weight gain are not clinical signs of protein malnutrition resulting from hepatic disease. Liver disease can cause zinc accumulation and vitamin K accumulation. Wortinger A, Burns K, Nutrition and Disease Management for Veterinary Technicians and Nurses, ed 2, Wiley Blackwell, 2015.

591. d Small frequent meals are recommended for patients with hepatic disease to optimize blood flow through the liver, to manage fasting glucose, and to minimize hepatic encephalopathy. Wortinger A, Burns K, Nutrition and Disease Management for Veterinary Technicians and Nurses, ed 2, Wiley Blackwell, 2015.

592. b Cats with hepatic lipidosis often present with a history of anoxia and weight loss. The cause is not completely understood; however, potential causes include protein deficiency, excessive peripheral lipolysis, and excessive lipogenesis. Thyroid disease, lower urinary tract disease, and cardiac disease have not been shown to result in hepatic lipidosis. Wortinger A, Burns K, Nutrition and Disease Management for Veterinary Technicians and Nurses, ed 2, Wiley Blackwell, 2015.

593. a Chronic hepatitis may result from copper accumulation, from infectious diseases, from drugs, from breed-associated hepatitis, and possibly from autoimmune disease. Copper storage, not copper deficiency, is a type of liver disease. Zinc deficiency and vitamin K deficiency, although related to liver disease, are not common in chronic hepatitis. Wortinger A, Burns K, Nutrition and Disease Management for Veterinary Technicians and Nurses, ed 2, Wiley Blackwell, 2015.

594. b When administering oral medication to cats, ensure that the medication is washed down with water to prevent the tablet or capsule from sticking in the lower portion of the esophagus and causing irritation. Summers A, Common Diseases of Companion Animals, ed 3, Elsevier, 2014.

595. a Clinical signs of acute gastritis include anorexia, acute onset of vomiting, presence or absence of dehydration, painful abdomen, and a history of dietary change or toxin ingestions. Polyuria and anuria have to do with urination and have no relation to acute gastritis. Polydipsia (increased intake of water) is not a clinical sign of acute gastritis, because most cases present with acute vomiting. Summers A, Common Diseases of Companion Animals, ed 3, Elsevier, 2014.

596. c Immune-mediated inflammatory bowel disease (IBD) is the result of the accumulation of inflammatory cells within the lining of the small intestine, stomach, or the large bowel, and it is seen most commonly in cats, although it occurs in dogs as well. The etiology of the disease is unknown, but it is thought that a disruption of the immunologic tolerance to the normal bacterial flora of the small intestine, or to dietary substances, develops and results in an inflammatory response with cellular infiltration. Gastritis and colitis may be conditions that the patient experiences as a result of IBD. Summers A, Common Diseases of Companion Animals, ed 3, Elsevier, 2014.

597. b The microscopic examination of the urine sediment is the only way to identify hematuria accurately. The blood reagent pad on the urine dipstick is not specific for hematuria. In addition to red blood cells, it also becomes positive with hemoglobin and myoglobin. Hemoglobin may also cause the urine sample to appear red. Erythrocytes may or may not be present in the urine of a cat with FIC. Wortinger A, Burns K, Nutrition and Disease Management for Veterinary Technicians and Nurses, ed 2, Wiley Blackwell, 2015.

598. d Methods for increasing water intake in cats include placing ice cubes in water, adding broth to foods, and providing water fountains. Wortinger A, Burns K, Nutrition and Disease Management for Veterinary Technicians and Nurses, ed 2, Wiley Blackwell, 2015.

599. b Inflammation plays a role in many causes of FLUTD, especially FIC and urolithiasis. Therefore, a key nutritional factor to managing these cats includes omega-3 fatty acid, specifically EPA and DHA, which are known to have potent anti-inflammatory effects. Increasing the salt content of food is an effective method for causing urine dilution in cats, but the potential for adverse effects should be considered. Feeding schedule has not evidenced a positive effect in the management of FIC. Therapeutic veterinary diets and canned diets are recommended for cats prone to FIC. Varying the diet types has not resulted in a positive effect on cats with FIC and any diet changes should be made gradually, giving the cat adequate time to adapt and to avoid becoming stressed. Wortinger A, Burns K, Nutrition and Disease Management for Veterinary Technicians and Nurses, ed 2, Wiley Blackwell, 2015.

600. d Nutritional management, environmental enrichment, and stress reduction are all recommended treatments for cats with FIC. Wortinger A, Burns K, Nutrition and Disease Management for Veterinary Technicians and Nurses, ed 2, Wiley Blackwell, 2015.

601. c Pruritus is the most common sign in dogs and cats with allergic skin disease. Lethargy and reluctance to eat are not generally associated with allergic skin disease. Hyperpigmentation can be a result of chronic licking, rubbing, and chewing. Wortinger A, Burns K, Nutrition and Disease Management for Veterinary Technicians and Nurses, ed 2, Wiley Blackwell, 2015.

602. b Pets that are diagnosed with IBD require a special diet for life, in which table scraps and treats must be eliminated. The diagnosis of IBD requires a complete laboratory workup to rule out other causes of the clinical symptoms and a definitive diagnosis requires an intestinal biopsy. Therapy is required for the life of the animal and the immunosuppressive drugs used to treat this disease have side effects in animals. Polyuria, polydipsia, polyphagia, weight gain, and skin and urinary infections may occur. The veterinarian must closely monitor the animal and the lowest possible dose of anti-inflammatory drug must be used. Summers A, Common Diseases of Companion Animals, ed 3, Elsevier, 2014.

603. a Gastric ulceration and erosion is the common result of drug therapy in dogs and cats. Nonsteroidal anti-inflammatory drugs (NSAIDs) are the most commonly implicated drugs, which produce ulceration in humans as well as in dogs. These drugs, which include aspirin, ibuprofen, flunixin meglumine, and phenylbutazone, disrupt the normal gastric mucosal barrier, resulting in ulceration. Stress, as seen in severely traumatized animals or animals in strenuous training, can also result in gastric erosion. Renal failure, hepatic failure, and hypoadrenocorticism may also result in gastric erosion or ulceration. Antibiotics, parasiticides, and immunotherapy drugs are not implicated as causes of gastric ulceration. Summers A, Common Diseases of Companion Animals, ed 3, Elsevier, 2014.

604. d Miliary dermatitis, eosinophilic granuloma complex, and adverse reactions to food are among the most commonly diagnosed skin disorders in cats. Hyperthyroidism is not considered a skin disorder. Wortinger A, Burns K, Nutrition and Disease Management for Veterinary Technicians and Nurses, ed 2, Wiley Blackwell, 2015.

605. b An abnormal response to an ingested food is considered an adverse reaction to food. Inhaling food, liquid, or other foreign material is considered aspiration. Ingesting or inhaling a toxin is considered poisoning. Wortinger A, Burns K, Nutrition and Disease Management for Veterinary Technicians and Nurses, ed 2, Wiley Blackwell, 2015.

606. a Feline eosinophilic granuloma complex describes a skin disorder that involves several syndromes, including indolent ulcers, eosinophilic plaques, and linear granulomas. *Indolent ulcers* is a term used to describe raised, ulcerated lesions in cats, most commonly seen on the upper lip and in the mouth. An eosinophilic plaque describes reddened, raised, flat, and firm lesions commonly seen on the abdomen or inner thigh regions. A linear granuloma is a series of raised plaques in a linear configuration often seen on the caudal aspect of a cat's thighs. Wortinger A, Burns K, Nutrition and Disease Management for Veterinary Technicians and Nurses, ed 2, Wiley Blackwell, 2015.

607. d Intestinal lymphangiectasia is a chronic protein-losing intestinal disease of dogs that is characterized by impaired intestinal lymphatic drainage resulting from obstruction of normal lymphatic flow. The backup of lymph releases fluid into the intestinal lumen, causing a loss of lipids, plasma protein, and lymphocytes. Summers A, Common Diseases of Companion Animals, ed 3, Elsevier, 2014.

608. a A complete nutritional protocol in the management of inflammatory skin disorders includes an assessment of current foods being ingested, the method of feeding, the identification of an appropriate feeding plan, and a reassessment of the feeding plan. Corn, gluten, and carbohydrates are not generally associated with inflammatory skin disorders. To develop an appropriate feeding plan, it is extremely important to determine which food ingredients, if any, might be causing the adverse food reaction. Wortinger A, Burns K, Nutrition and Disease Management for Veterinary Technicians and Nurses, ed 2, Wiley Blackwell, 2015.

609. d For a dietary elimination trial to be successful, the patient's diet must be limited to one novel protein source or hydrolyzed protein. The patient must not ingest any other food or treats during the elimination process and all other concurrent allergic skin disorders must be addressed, especially atopy and flea allergy hypersensitivity. Wortinger A, Burns K, Nutrition and Disease Management for Veterinary Technicians and Nurses, ed 2, Wiley Blackwell, 2015.

610. b Although the literature reports megacolon as an uncommon condition, it is seen frequently in cats. Of the many reasons suggested for feline obstipation, approximately 62% of them are attributed to idiopathic megacolon. The typical affected cat is middle-aged to older and is obese; the presenting symptom is straining to defecate. Some cats are able to pass a liquid stool that contains blood, mucus, or both. Dogs can become constipated. Immune-mediated inflammatory bowel disease (IBD) is the result of the accumulation of inflammatory cells within the lining of the small intestine, stomach, or the large bowel, and it is seen most commonly in cats, although it occurs in dogs as well. Summers A, Common Diseases of Companion Animals, ed 3, Elsevier, 2014.

611. d Although toxicosis is not a frequent occurrence in dogs and cats, drugs that are most commonly implicated are acetaminophen, phenobarbital, thiacetarsamide sodium (Carparsolate), antifungals, diethylcarbamazine, anabolic steroids, and halothane or methoxyflurane (Metofane). Acute onset of hepatic disease usually results from an overdose of these medications, whereas chronic damage may occur with long-term use at clinical doses. Summers A, Common Diseases of Companion Animals, ed 3, Elsevier, 2014.

612. a Dogs with DM typically present to the veterinary hospital with the following signs: polydipsia, polyphagia, weight loss, and lethargy. Weight gain, especially in undiagnosed and/or poorly regulated DM, would be highly unusual in dogs. Although chronic kidney disease and DM might occur in some patients, CKD is not a typical presenting sign of DM. Wortinger A, Burns K, Nutrition and Disease Management for Veterinary Technicians and Nurses, ed 2, Wiley Blackwell, 2015.

613. b Nutritional management of feline hyperthyroidism has been evaluated since approximately the mid-2000s. The results of studies support the conclusion that feeding <0.32 ppm iodine on a dry-matter basis (DMB) provides safe and effect therapy for cats with naturally occurring hyperthyroidism.

Thyroidectomy, anti-thyroid drugs, and radioactive iodine therapy are also effective in the management of feline hyperthyroidism, which have been used more commonly for a number of years. All of these methods are considered appropriate; the veterinarian and pet owner must determine and select the best course of action. Wortinger A, Burns K, Nutrition and Disease Management for Veterinary Technicians and Nurses, ed 2, Wiley Blackwell, 2015.

614. c Multiple independent studies have shown 90% of hyperthyroid cats remained euthyroid when fed <0.32 ppm iodine DMB as the sole source of nutrition. All of the other options listed are lower than these studies showed. Wortinger A, Burns K, Nutrition and Disease Management for Veterinary Technicians and Nurses, ed 2, Wiley Blackwell, 2015.

615. a Signs of liver disease are usually vague in the early stages. These signs include anorexia, vomiting, diarrhea or constipation, weight loss, polyuria, polydipsia, pyrexia, melena, and hematuria. Cats often display hypersalivation. Some animals may experience the development of bleeding tendencies because of vitamin K malabsorption. (Vitamin K requires bile acids for absorption.) Jaundice may develop as the disease progresses. Liver diseases can be categorized as follows: drug- or toxin-induced liver disease, infectious liver disease, feline hepatic lipidosis, neoplastic liver disease, and congenital portosystemic shunts. Summers A, Common Diseases of Companion Animals, ed 3, Elsevier, 2014.

616. d The thyroid gland is located in the ventral cervical region along the lateral margins of the trachea. The gland is not usually palpable in a healthy animal. The gland is composed of follicles that produce the thyroid hormones triiodothyronine (T3) and tetraiodothyronine (T4). These hormones are produced by the follicular cells and are stored in the gland until the body needs them. A third hormone, calcitonin, is produced by the parafollicular cells in the thyroid gland. Calcitonin acts to increase calcium deposition within bone to decrease blood calcium concentration, whereas T3 and T4 function to control all of the body's metabolic processes. Summers A, Common Diseases of Companion Animals, ed 3, Elsevier, 2014.

617. a Patients that are 12%–15% dehydrated will show obvious signs of shock and death is imminent. Patients that are 6%–8% dehydrated will have a prolonged CRT and slightly dry mucous membrane. Patients that are 10%–12% dehydrated will have eyes that are sunken into the orbits. Sirois M, Mosby's Veterinary PDQ, ed 2, Mosby Elsevier, 2014.

618. c Surgery and radioactive iodine therapy are intended to provide long-term solutions to hyperthyroidism and both are required to provide a lifelong solution. Oral anti-thyroid medications are used to control hyperthyroidism and must be administered daily to achieve and maintain their effects. Wortinger A, Burns K, Nutrition and Disease Management for Veterinary Technicians and Nurses, ed 2, Wiley Blackwell, 2015.

619. b Hyperthyroidism is a clinical condition that results from excessive production and secretion of thyroxine (T4) and triiodothyronine (T3) by the thyroid gland. Malnutrition and diets containing high levels of protein have not been associated with hyperthyroidism. Excessive cortisol production can result from abnormalities in the pituitary gland that cause excessive hormone secretion by the adrenal glands and might cause Cushing's disease. Wortinger A, Burns K, Nutrition and Disease Management for Veterinary Technicians and Nurses, ed 2, Wiley Blackwell, 2015.

620. b Diabetic animals may have increased amino acid losses through their urine. Poorly controlled diabetic patients may experience muscle wasting as protein is catabolized to meet energy needs. It is important to provide protein quality and quantity that will meet the requirements of diabetic animals in the face of increased aminoaciduria while avoiding excess protein content. Fat and carbohydrates are not stored in the muscle tissue and therefore are not catabolized to provide energy for these patients. Wortinger A, Burns K, Nutrition and Disease Management for Veterinary Technicians and Nurses, ed 2, Wiley Blackwell, 2015.

621. a Hyperthyroidism is the most commonly seen endocrine disorder in cats; however, it is rarely seen in dogs except as a result of neoplasia. The excess of both T3 and T4 results in a multisystemic disease seen primarily in older cats. Clinical symptoms include weight loss, polyphagia, vomiting, increased appetite, tachycardia with or without murmurs, aggressive behavior, hyperactivity, increased systolic blood pressure, and blindness with retinal detachment. Summers A, Common Diseases of Companion Animals, ed 3, Elsevier, 2014.

622. b The endocrine portion consists of pancreatic islet cells (formerly called the islets of Langerhans). These islets are dispersed throughout the gland and produce several important hormones: beta cells (β2 cells), which produce insulin, the best-known hormone; alpha cells (α cells), which secrete glucagon; and delta cells, which produce somatostatin. F cells secrete pancreatic polypeptides. The hypothalamus produces oxytocin and the thyroid gland produces calcitonin. Excess glucose is stored in the liver and muscle as glycogen, which can be converted to fat. Summers A, Common Diseases of Companion Animals, ed 3, Elsevier, 2014.

623. c Key nutritional factors that help to maintain healthy skin and aid in the management of skin disorders are protein, energy, essential fatty acids, copper, zinc, and vitamins A, E, and B-complex. Calcium and carbohydrates should be included in all complete and balanced diets at the recommended levels for the life stage of the pet; however, they are not key nutritional factors in the management of skin disorders. Wortinger A, Burns K, Nutrition and Disease Management for Veterinary Technicians and Nurses, ed 2, Wiley Blackwell, 2015.

624. b Cancer cachexia is a paraneoplastic syndrome manifested by weight loss and a decrease in body condition despite adequate nutritional intake. Anorexia and inappetence refer to patients that are not willing to eat or are unable to eat. Wortinger A, Burns K, Nutrition and Disease Management for Veterinary Technicians and Nurses, ed 2, Wiley Blackwell, 2015.

625. a The key nutritional factors in animals with cancer include soluble carbohydrates, fiber, protein, fat, and omega-3 fatty acids. Soluble fibers may be poorly used by animals with cancer but are important to help maintain intestinal health, especially in animals undergoing chemotherapy, radiation therapy, or surgery, and they may help prevent and resolve abnormal stool quality. Insoluble fibers do not tend to absorb liquid and are not generally helpful in preventing or resolving soft stools. Polyphenols may help improve oral health. Arginine and calcium are not considered key nutritional factors for animals with cancer. Wortinger A, Burns K, Nutrition and Disease Management for Veterinary Technicians and Nurses, ed 2, Wiley Blackwell, 2015.

626. d Almost 100% of dogs and about 50% of cats will have insulin-dependent diabetes (type I) at examination. As many as 50% of presenting cats will have non-insulin dependent diabetes (type II), which does not require insulin therapy. Summers A, Common Diseases of Companion Animals, ed 3, Elsevier, 2014.

627. b At one time it was estimated that about 25% of Bedlington terriers were affected with copper storage disease and another 50% were carriers. In the breed, the incidence of the disease has been significantly reduced as a result of genetic testing and responsible breeding practices. Afghan hounds, Pekinese dogs, and cats are not associated with copper storage disease. Wortinger A, Burns K, Nutrition and Disease Management for Veterinary Technicians and Nurses, ed 2, Wiley Blackwell, 2015.

628. c The liver's main responsibility is maintaining homeostasis and removing waste products that have accumulated within the body. Wortinger A, Burns K, Nutrition and Disease Management for Veterinary Technicians and Nurses, ed 2, Wiley Blackwell, 2015.

629. d Dogs and cats presenting with vomiting and diarrhea may have abnormal serum potassium, chloride, and sodium concentrations. Mild hypokalemia, hypochloremia, and either hypernatremia or hyponatremia are the electrolyte abnormalities most commonly associated with acute vomiting and diarrhea. Wortinger A, Burns K, Nutrition and Disease Management for Veterinary Technicians and Nurses, ed 2, Wiley Blackwell, 2015.

630. d In clinical trials of dogs with spontaneous cancer, high levels of omega-3 fatty acids and arginine in food were shown to benefit dogs with lymphoma, nasal carcinomas, hemangiosarcomas, and osteosarcoma. Omega-3 fatty acids in conjunction with arginine were shown to influence clinical signs, to increase survival time, to provide longer remission time, and to improve quality of life. Wortinger A, Burns K, Nutrition and Disease Management for Veterinary Technicians and Nurses, ed 2, Wiley Blackwell, 2015.

631. d Almost 100% of dogs and about 50% of cats will have insulin-dependent diabetes (type I) at examination. As many as 50% of presenting cats will exhibit non-insulin dependent diabetes (type II), which does not require insulin therapy. Summers A, Common Diseases of Companion Animals, ed 3, Elsevier, 2014.

632. a The levels of vitamin E and other antioxidant nutrients should be appropriate as related to the levels of polyunsaturated fatty acids, trace minerals, and oxidants in the food. A complete and balance diet, including highly digestible protein, is the appropriate treatment for cachexia; supplementation with vitamin E has not been shown to have a positive effect on cachexia. Supplementation with mega doses of vitamins is not recommended, especially when feeding a commercial diet. Wortinger A, Burns K, Nutrition and Disease Management for Veterinary Technicians and Nurses, ed 2, Wiley Blackwell, 2015.

633. c Hypokalemia is the most commonly detected electrolyte disturbance when providing nutritional support to a patient suffering from refeeding syndrome. With refeeding syndrome, glucose is absorbed, insulin is secreted, and cells along with glucose take up potassium. Hyponatremia, hypochloremia, and hypomagnesemia are not commonly seen in refeeding syndrome patients. Hypomagnesemia is more commonly seen in starvation patients Wortinger A, Burns K, Nutrition and Disease Management for Veterinary Technicians and Nurses, ed 2, Wiley Blackwell, 2015.

634. b Common signs of diabetes include PU/PD, tachypnea, weight loss, depression, weakness, and vomiting. Bradycardic and pitting edema are not symptoms associated with diabetes. Summers A, Common Diseases of Companion Animals, ed 3, Elsevier, 2014.

635. b Hyperglycemia is never acutely fatal, whereas hypoglycemia can be life-threatening. PU/PD is not life-threatening and is often recognized early. Summers A, Common Diseases of Companion Animals, ed 3, Elsevier, 2014.

636. b Addison's disease and Cushing's syndrome are the two main diseases of the adrenal glands. Diabetes rises from the pancreas, IBD from the intestines, and eclampsia can be a thyroid disorder because the thyroid gland produces calcitonin. Summers A, Common Diseases of Companion Animals, ed 3, Elsevier, 2014.

637. c Increased stool volume is commonly associated with small intestine diarrhea. Mucus, hematochezia (fresh blood in feces), and dyschezia (inability to defecate) are all clinical signs of large intestine diarrhea. Cote, E. Clinical Veterinary Advisor: Dogs and Cats, Ed. 2. Mosby, 2011.

638. c Tenesmus (straining) is seen with large intestinal diarrhea. Halitosis (bad breath), borborygmus and steatorrhea (undigested fat in the feces) are all seen with small intestinal diarrhea. Cote E, Clinical Veterinary Advisor: Dogs and Cats, ed 2, Mosby, 2011.

639. a Oleander (Nerium oleander) causes vomiting and diarrhea, along with digitoxin-like effects with bradycardia, tachycardia, arrhythmias, and hyperkalemia. Marijuana (*Cannabis sativa*) causes CNS depression, while morning glory (*Ipomoea*) and tobacco plant (*Nicotiana*) cause CNS stimulation. Cote E, Clinical Veterinary Advisor: Dogs and Cats, ed 2, Mosby, 2011.

640. b Easter lily (*Lilium* spp.) plants will cause vomiting, lethargy and acute renal failure in cats. Apricot seeds affect the respiratory system, onions cause hemolysis, and mistletoe is cardiotoxic. Cote E, Clinical Veterinary Advisor: Dogs and Cats, ed 2, Mosby, 2011.

641. a Pomeranians most commonly experience PDA. Bull terriers are more likely to experience AS, and a variety of breeds, including boxers may experience ASD. English bulldogs and the English springer spaniel may experience VSD. Summers A, Common Diseases of Companion Animals, ed 3, Elsevier, 2014.

642. b Patients that are 5%–6% dehydrated will have a subtle loss of skin elasticity. Patients that are 6%–8% dehydrated will have prolonged CRT, and patients that are 10%–12% dehydrated will have eyes that are sunken into the orbits. Sirois M, Mosby's Veterinary PDQ, ed 2, Mosby Elsevier, 2014.

643. d All symptoms presented would describe an anemic patient. Sirois M, Mosby's Veterinary PDQ, ed 2, Mosby Elsevier, 2014.

644. a Iron deficiency would be the most common cause of anemia. Lethargy is a clinical sign, not a cause of a disease. Alopecia would be seen with atopy and calicivirus is a disease associated with a viral infection of the URT. Sirois M, Mosby's Veterinary PDQ, ed 2, Mosby Elsevier, 2014.

645. c Cataracts are often inherited or secondary to diabetes (among other diseases). Clinical signs include opaque pupillary opening and progressive vision loss. Patients with calicivirus would experience anorexia, lethargy, fever, ulcerative stomatitis, and/or nasal discharge. Patients with parvovirus experience bloody diarrhea, lethargy, vomiting, dehydration, and fever. Distemper patients experience fever, cough, mucopurulent ocular and nasal discharge, V/D, hyperkeratosis of foot pads, and ataxia. Sirois M, Mosby's Veterinary PDQ, ed 2, Mosby Elsevier, 2014.

646. d All of the organisms listed will contribute to ringworm, or dermatophytosis. Sirois M, Mosby's Veterinary PDQ, ed 2, Mosby Elsevier, 2014.

647. b FAD is caused by a hypersensitivity to a Ctenocephalides infestation. Environmental allergens and mite infestations may cause atopy, but do not contribute to FAD. *Blastomyces dermatitidis* is a fungal infection. Sirois M, Mosby's Veterinary PDQ, ed 2, Mosby Elsevier, 2014.

648. b Otitis media is the cause of GVS, with clinical signs such as head tilt, circling, disorientation, ataxia, nystagmus. Increased intraocular fluid production is seen with glaucoma. *Coccidioides immitis* and *Histoplasma capsulatum* are both fungal infections. Sirois M, Mosby's Veterinary PDQ, ed 2, Mosby Elsevier, 2014.

649. b The accumulation of triglycerides in the liver is hepatic lipidosis. Renal lipidosis does not exist. Hyperthyroidism is the overproduction of thyroid hormone, whereas hypothyroidism is the underproduction of thyroid hormone. Sirois M, Mosby's Veterinary PDQ, ed 2, Mosby Elsevier, 2014.

650. c Clinical signs of distemper include coughing, fever, and mucopurulent discharge. Kennel cough and ICT are the same and include a dry, hacking, paroxysmal cough. Clinical signs of canine parvovirus do not include a cough, but rather vomiting and diarrhea. Sirois M, Mosby's Veterinary PDQ, ed 2, Mosby Elsevier, 2014.

651. d *Borrelia burgdorferi* causes Lyme disease. *Rickettsia rickettsia* is a tick-borne disease, while *Scabies scabei* is sarcoptic mange. *Staphylococcus* is a bacteria that may cause pyometra. Sirois M, Mosby's Veterinary PDQ, ed 2, Mosby Elsevier, 2014.

652. c Herpesvirus infection causes viral rhinotracheitis. Canine distemper is a paramyxoviral infection and parvovirus is a viral infection if the GI tract. von Willebrand disease is a decreased or deficient production of von Willebrand factor. Sirois M, Mosby's Veterinary PDQ, ed 2, Mosby Elsevier, 2014.

653. d All listed are forms of viral enteritis, causing bloody diarrhea, lethargy, vomiting, dehydration, and fever. Sirois M, Mosby's Veterinary PDQ, ed 2, Mosby Elsevier, 2014.

654. a Petechial hemorrhage, ecchymosis, epistaxis, and lethargy are all clinical signs associated with thrombocytopenia. Clinical signs of urolithiasis include dysuria and hematuria and renal failure signs include oliguria, polyuria, anorexia, and dehydration (among others). Pyometra clinical signs include vulvular discharge, abdominal enlargement, PU/PD, and dehydration. Sirois M, Mosby's Veterinary PDQ, ed 2, Mosby Elsevier, 2014.

655. c A dog that consumes excess amounts of fat is at higher risk of experiencing pancreatitis. A patella luxation is generally a genetic predisposition but can also occur due to trauma. It is an orthopedic issue, not GI. Cushing's disease is an endocrine disease, not GI. Panosteitis is also an orthopedic issue and is usually caused by metabolic disease, allergic reactions, excess hormones, and could possibly be a viral infection. Sirois M, Mosby's Veterinary PDQ, ed 2, Mosby Elsevier, 2014.

656. b von Willebrand's disease is a decreased or deficient production of von Willebrand's factor and has nothing to do with orthopedics. Sirois M, Mosby's Veterinary PDQ, ed 2, Mosby Elsevier, 2014.

657. d All vaccines listed, except *Leptospira*, are considered core vaccines recommended in the United States. Sirois M, Mosby's Veterinary PDQ, ed 2, Mosby Elsevier, 2014.

658. c All vaccines listed, except leukemia are considered core vaccines in the United States. Sirois M, Mosby's Veterinary PDQ, ed 2, Mosby Elsevier, 2014.

659. b *Bordetella bronchiseptica* has a DOI of 1 year. Sirois M, Mosby's Veterinary PDQ, ed 2, Mosby Elsevier, 2014.

660. b The objective portion of the medical record contains physiologic data. The subjective portion contains the appearance of the patient, the assessment includes the current status and differential diagnosis, and the plan includes the next steps to be completed. Sirois M, Mosby's Veterinary PDQ, ed 2, Mosby Elsevier, 2014.

661. c A murmur that is graded 6/6 is significant and can be heard (and sometimes felt) very well. A 1/6 is barely audible and may be missed by some. Sirois M, Mosby's Veterinary PDQ, ed 2, Mosby Elsevier, 2014.

662. b As stated earlier, animals can be hurt and can become psychologically upset if restraint is overly harsh. Restraint techniques must be applied properly and in such a manner as to minimize any pain experienced by the animal. You must have a good working knowledge of animal anatomy, physiology, and behavior to decide which restraint technique to use for a particular procedure. Sheldon CC, Sonsthagen T, Topel JA, Animal Restraint for Veterinary Professionals, ed 1, Elsevier, 2006.

663. c Chemical restraint involves the use of drugs with effects ranging from sedation to complete immobilization. Sedation or tranquilization can remove fear and anxiety. However, the flight-or-fight response can override the effects, so do not rely heavily on chemical restraint to slow the animal's reactions. Sheldon CC, Sonsthagen T, Topel JA, Animal Restraint for Veterinary Professionals, ed 1, Elsevier, 2006.

664. a The square knot is used to secure the ends of two ropes together or to form a nonslipping noose. A nonslip knot is one that will not come untied or tighten if pressure is applied to both ends. It is most commonly used to secure surgical knots. The reefer knot allows you to tie a nonslipping, quick-release knot. The reefer knot is the same as the square knot, with one exception. You make the second throw by first forming a bight in the left-hand rope and tightening the knot with the bight in place. Sheldon CC, Sonsthagen T, Topel JA, Animal Restraint for Veterinary Professionals, ed 1, Elsevier, 2006.

665. b Use minimal restraint to start a procedure and tighten your hold as necessary. Applying medium or maximum restraint at the onset will often upset the cat and it will fight to escape. This does not mean that you should not maintain a secure hold; you can maintain control by holding gently but firmly and by being alert to the cat's changing temperament. Do not treat all cats the same. Read the cat's body language; if it is a gentle cat, handle it gently. Use towels, cat bags, gauntlets, and chemical restraint as necessary. Use distraction techniques. A cat's attention can be diverted while you perform unpleasant procedures. Timing is of the utmost importance. Begin the diversion just as you start the procedure. Otherwise, you may convey anxiety to the cat by increasing the strength of your diversion just as the injection is being given or as a painful procedure begins. Techniques that seem to work well include making a funny noise (be careful with this one; you do not want to scare the cat), scratching the cat's ears or under its chin, gently tapping its face, blowing on its nose, or wiggling its legs. Sheldon CC, Sonsthagen T, Topel JA, Animal Restraint for Veterinary Professionals, ed 1, Elsevier, 2006.

666. c A cat placed in sternal recumbency can have all of the listed procedures completed, except a cystocentesis, in which the patient would need to be placed in lateral recumbency with a shift to the more dorsal position. Sheldon CC, Sonsthagen T, Topel JA, Animal Restraint for Veterinary Professionals, ed 1, Elsevier, 2006.

667. a Signs of impending aggression include a head held low, either below or level with the dog's shoulders; a gaze that is averted to the side; raised hair along the back, ears down, and tail straight out; and an ominous growl or snarl. Dogs showing any of these signs should be handled with extreme caution and must always be considered dangerous. Sheldon CC, Sonsthagen T, Topel JA, Animal Restraint for Veterinary Professionals, ed 1, Elsevier, 2006.

668. c In addition to butting, another defensive mechanism of cattle is kicking. They are accurate with their feet and can kick out 6 to 8 feet from their bodies. The 6 to 8 feet is a kill zone because whatever happens to be kicked can die or be damaged. Most cattle do not usually kick straight backward as a horse does. Rather, they usually kick in a slight forward motion that then arcs backward. Sheldon CC, Sonsthagen T, Topel JA, Animal Restraint for Veterinary Professionals, ed 1, Elsevier, 2006.

669. c A chute is used to restrain beef cattle and bulls. The chute is usually at the end of an alleyway that allows one animal access to the chute at a time. Cattle are loaded into a chute or stanchion before applying a nose ring, nose lead, or halter (all of these are restraining devices for the head). Sheldon CC, Sonsthagen T, Topel JA, Animal Restraint for Veterinary Professionals, ed 1, Elsevier, 2006.

670. b Horses have keen eyesight for seeing movement at great distances, but they do not see well near themselves, nor do they see just below their noses or directly behind themselves. Never walk directly behind a horse unless you stay close and talk to the horse so that it knows you are there. Never walk under a horse's neck. The horse cannot see you there and may throw its head, raise a front leg and knock you down, or rear up and come down on you. Sheldon CC, Sonsthagen T, Topel JA, Animal Restraint for Veterinary Professionals, ed 1, Elsevier, 2006.

671. d Horses kick as a means of protection. They can kick with either back hoof directly behind themselves as well as out to the sides. They can kick with both back legs at once by rocking their weight onto their front legs. They can strike with one front leg at a time or rock all their weight onto their back legs and rear up and strike with both front legs. Sheldon CC, Sonsthagen T, Topel JA, Animal Restraint for Veterinary Professionals, ed 1, Elsevier, 2006.

672. c The tail also indicates a horse's attitude. A wringing or circling tail indicates nervousness. A tail held straight down indicates pain or sleeping. A tail that is clamped tight indicates fear. Sheldon CC, Sonsthagen T, Topel JA, Animal Restraint for Veterinary Professionals, ed 1, Elsevier, 2006.

673. d The halter and lead rope are the main tools of equine restraint and should always be used when leading or working on a horse. Check the halter and lead rope for splits or fraying because a horse can easily break a defective lead rope or halter with a sharp jerk of its head. Sheldon CC, Sonsthagen T, Topel JA, Animal Restraint for Veterinary Professionals, ed 1, Elsevier, 2006.

674. d Rocking the ear, grabbing skin on the shoulder, and hand twitching are all methods of distraction for horses. Tail jacking is a distraction technique used for cattle. Sheldon CC, Sonsthagen T, Topel JA, Animal Restraint for Veterinary Professionals, ed 1, Elsevier, 2006.

675. c The safest method of capturing a single pig from a herd is to move all of the pigs into a small pen using barriers or hurdles. Hurdles are flat, solid pieces of wood, plastic, or metal large enough to cover your legs. Some are equipped with handles or holes cut into them so you can easily carry them in front of you. Sheldon CC, Sonsthagen T, Topel JA, Animal Restraint for Veterinary Professionals, ed 1, Elsevier, 2006.

SECTION 10

1. b Ultrasound uses sound waves to produce images and after 30 years of study, it has proven to have no associated health risks. X-ray, fluoroscopy, and CT all use radiation as a source to produce images. Brown M, Brown L, Lavin's Radiography for Veterinary Technicians, ed 6, Saunders, 2018, p. 163.
2. d To obtain a view with both temporomandibular joint projections, the patient is placed in sternal recumbency. To obtain a radiograph of the right temporomandibular joint, the patient should be placed in right lateral recumbency, allowing the skull to oblique naturally down toward the table at approximately 10 degrees. To obtain an image of the left temporomandibular joint, the patient should be placed in left lateral recumbency, allowing the skull to be oblique and naturally down toward the table at approximately 10 degrees. To obtain a DV temporomandibular joint projection of both joints, the patient is placed in sternal recumbency. Ventral recumbency is typically not used to view the temporomandibular joint. Sirois M, Anthony E, Mauragis D, Handbook of Radiographic Positioning for Veterinary Technicians, ed 1, Delmar Cengage Learning, 2010, p. 130.
3. b To obtain a lateral projection of the skull, the beam should be centered at the lateral canthus of the eye socket. When obtaining either a VD or DV projection of the skull, the center should be midway between the tip of the nose to just caudal to the occipital protuberance at the base. To obtain a rostrocaudal foramen magnum projection, the center should be between the eyes. To obtain a rostrocaudal tympanic bullae open-mouth projection, the beam is centered just above the base of the tongue and just below the soft palate, approximately at the commissure of the mouth. Sirois M, Anthony E, Mauragis D, Handbook of Radiographic Positioning for Veterinary Technicians, ed 1, Delmar Cengage Learning, 2010, p. 110.
4. d Closed metacarpal and metatarsal physes describe a grade level 4. An open proximal 3rd metacarpal or metatarsal growth plate describes grade level 2. A closed proximal 3rd metacarpal or metatarsal growth plate describes a grade level 3. Farrow CS, Veterinary Diagnostic Imaging: The Horse, Mosby Elsevier, 2006, p. 15.
5. b The transducer of an ultrasound machine is the handheld unit that touches the patient. Within each transducer are piezoelectric ceramics that aid in creating and receiving the sound waves to produce images. A bucky is the tray that holds the film in place to obtain an x-ray. Magnets are not used in ultrasound but rather in MRI units. Brown M, Brown L, Lavin's Radiography for Veterinary Technicians, ed 6, Saunders, 2018, p. 164.
6. b To obtain a dorsoventral abdominal view of a rabbit, the beam should be centered over the liver. To obtain a view of the thorax of a rabbit, the center of the beam should be focused over the heart. To obtain a whole body view, the beam should be focused over the center of the body from cranial to caudal or at the thoracolumbar area. Han CM, Hurd CD, Practical Diagnostic Imaging for the Veterinary Technician, ed 3, Mosby, 2005, p. 162.
7. c When strong short electrical pulses strike the crystals within an ultrasound transducer, the crystals vibrate, creating a sound frequency that the sonographer can control. Brown M, Brown L, Lavin's Radiography for Veterinary Technicians, ed 6, Saunders, 2018, p. 164.
8. d Radioisotopes used in nuclear medicine studies may be administered by injection, inhalation or oral consumption. Brown M, Brown L, Lavin's Radiography for Veterinary Technicians, ed 6, Saunders, 2018, p. 29.
9. b Closure of the proximal growth plate of P2 occurs between 18 and 30 weeks. The first radiographic appearance of the crena occurs between 4 and 22 weeks. The closure of the proximal growth plate of P1 occurs between 22 and 38 weeks. The closure of the distal growth plate of MC3 occurs between 18 and 38 weeks. Farrow CS, Veterinary Diagnostic Imaging: The Horse, Mosby Elsevier, 2006, p. 4.
10. d A varus deformity is one in which the interior angle of the joint, viewed frontally, is less than 180 degrees. A valgus deformity is one in which the interior angle, viewed frontally, is greater than 180 degrees. The term *axial rotation* pertains to foals with angular limb deformities. The term *windswept* refers to the combination of valgus and varus deformity. Farrow CS, Veterinary Diagnostic Imaging: The Horse, Mosby Elsevier, 2006, p. 10.
11. a When obtaining a dorsomedial-palmarolateral oblique view, the cassette should be held against the palmarolateral aspect of the leg. When obtaining a lateromedial view of the carpus of a horse, the cassette should be held on the medial aspect of the leg. When obtaining a dorsopalmar view of the carpus, the cassette should be held on the palmar aspect of the carpus. When obtaining a dorsolateral-palmaromedial oblique view, the cassette should be held on the palmaromedial aspect of the leg. Han CM, Hurd CD, Practical Diagnostic Imaging for the Veterinary Technician, ed 3, Mosby, 2005, p. 190.
12. c Atrophy occurs as an effect of radiation overdose to lymphoid tissue. Cataracts can occur to the eyes as a result of radiation overdose. Ulcers occur to the gastrointestinal tract as a result of radiation overdose. Necrosis occurs to the brain as a result of radiation overdose. Brown M, Brown L, Lavin's Radiography for Veterinary Technicians, ed 6, Saunders, 2018, p. 29.
13. a The term *plantar* describes the caudal surface of the hind limb distal to the tarsus. The term *palmar* describes the caudal surface of the forelimb distal to the carpus. The term *dorsopalmar* describes the radiographic views distal to the carpus obtained by passing the primary x-ray beam from the dorsal direction to the palmar surface of the forelimb. The term *caudocranial* describes the radiographic projection obtained by passing the primary x-ray beam from the caudal surface to the cranial surface of a structure. Sirois M, Anthony E, Mauragis D, Handbook of Radiographic Positioning for Veterinary Technicians, ed 1, Delmar Cengage Learning, 2010, p. 3.
14. d There are approximately 256 shades of gray that are incorporated into the display of an ultrasound image. This creates a much superior level of contrast than that

with plain radiographs. The human eye can distinguish approximately 32–64 shades of gray. Brown M, Brown L, Lavin's Radiography for Veterinary Technicians, ed 6, Saunders, 2018, p. 165.

15. a The abbreviation B-mode in ultrasound stands for brightness. B-mode is what is displayed in gray scale on the image and the different shades of gray are assigned to create a range from bright to dark. Bits are the basic units of information used in computers. The binary system is a numerical system that represents values using two different symbols, 0 and 1, which interprets into a numeric value. Power mode in ultrasound is the use of Doppler to image low-velocity movements. Brown M, Brown L, Lavin's Radiography for Veterinary Technicians, ed 6, Saunders, 2018, p. 165.

16. b Doppler ultrasound is used to image the flow of blood and other liquids as well to measure their velocities. M-mode or motion mode is used simultaneously with B-mode to display the motion of the tissues over a two-dimensional scale. B-mode or brightness mode is used to display the different shades of gray. Brown M, Brown L, Lavin's Radiography for Veterinary Technicians, ed 6, Saunders, 2018, p. 166.

17. c Color-flow Doppler indicates the presence of blood flow. In standard imaging, when the color bar shows the red on top and blue on the bottom, blue indicates flow away and red indicates flow toward the transducer. The blue and red do not distinguish veins from arteries or the velocity of the flow. Brown M, Brown L, Lavin's Radiography for Veterinary Technicians, ed 6, Saunders, 2018, p. 166.

18. a The lateral view is best for evaluating major fracture dislocation and conformational abnormalities. The flexed lateral view has proven to be the most accurate in detecting carpal fractures and it shows fragment mobility. The dorsopalmar view is the least revealing in carpal fractures, but it is best to evaluate distal radial growth plate closures. The medial oblique view is best for detecting slab fractures. Farrow CS, Veterinary Diagnostic Imaging: The Horse, Mosby Elsevier, 2006, p. 159.

19. b Color Doppler indicates direction of blood flow, whereas power Doppler is sensitive to pick up slow blood flow but does not indicate direction. Neither color Doppler nor power Doppler provide a velocity of blood flow or indicate whether an image is an artery or a vein. Brown M, Brown L, Lavin's Radiography for Veterinary Technicians, ed 6, Saunders, 2018, p. 166.

20. c Pulse wave imaging can detect a maximum velocity of 1.4 m/s. Any velocity that exceeds 1.4 m/s starts to alias and cannot be measured accurately. Brown M, Brown L, Lavin's Radiography for Veterinary Technicians, ed 6, Saunders, 2018, p. 166.

21. a In ultrasound, the Nyquist point is the point at which the maximum blood velocity is reached; beyond that is when aliasing of color and pulse wave occurs. Ultrasound is limited to depth of penetration based on the medium in which the sound is traveling and it varies with the different frequencies used. Drop-out signal occurs in ultrasound for many reasons such that the sound frequency used has reached maximum depth and sound attenuation has occurred within the medium it has traveled. Brown M, Brown L, Lavin's Radiography for Veterinary Technicians, ed 6, Saunders, 2018, p. 166.

22. a Most dental radiographic film has a small raised dimple on one corner. The raised or convex side of the dimple will be on the side that should be facing up and toward the tube head, and pointing rostrally. The back of the film has a tab that is used for opening the film during development. If the dimple is placed into the back of the mouth, there is an increased risk of the dimple appearing as an artifact on the tooth surface. If the backside of the film is placed toward the beam, the image will have a foil layer within the film. Bellows J, "The why, when and how of small animal dental radiology," in The Practice of Veterinary Dentistry: A Team Effort, Iowa State Press, 1999, p. 81-105.

23. c Continuous wave (CW) Doppler measures very high blood flow velocities by using two different crystals working together. One crystal sends out a signal whereas the other receives a signal, at the same time allowing high-velocity reading. However, this type of ultrasound does not produce B-mode imaging; it only produces a pulse wave. Color Doppler only detects direction of blood flow. PW Doppler detects velocities but has a maximum limit of 1.4 m/s. Harmonics is a useful tool in decreasing artifacts with imaging. Brown M, Brown L, Lavin's Radiography for Veterinary Technicians, ed 6, Saunders, 2018, p. 167.

24. b The gain control knob controls the overall brightness of the image. The power output has its own knob, which changes the amount of power used to penetrate into the patient. The PRF scale in PW Doppler has its own knob and it changes the measurement scale for velocity purposes. The depth of the image is changed with the depth knob, allowing the viewing of shallow or deep images. Brown M, Brown L, Lavin's Radiography for Veterinary Technicians, ed 6, Saunders, 2018, p. 170.

25. c Time gain compensation knobs allow the gain to be adjusted at various depths of the image. The time it takes for sound to travel through different mediums cannot be changed. Frame time on ultrasound is adjusted in multiple ways either to slow it down or speed it up, such as in the use of too many or too few focal points. The faster the frame time, the more quickly the image will be produced. Brown M, Brown L, Lavin's Radiography for Veterinary Technicians, ed 6, Saunders, 2018, p. 170.

26. b A carpal hematoma usually results from a ruptured accessory cephalic vein in the horse. The buccal vein is located in the head of horses. The medial saphenous vein is located in the hind limbs of horses. The superficial thoracic vein is located at the thorax of horses. Farrow CS, Veterinary Diagnostic Imaging: The Horse, Mosby Elsevier, 2006, p. 172.

27. a Two is the maximum number of focal points recommended. Different manufacturers suggest varying maximum numbers of focal points; typically the maximum number is five. Anything beyond two focal points will slow the frame rate and will produce an unclear image. Brown M, Brown L, Lavin's Radiography for Veterinary Technicians, ed 6, Saunders, 2018, p. 170.

28. a The lower the frequency, the deeper the level of penetration that can be achieved, therefore the 4 MHz frequency allows the deepest level of penetration. The higher the frequency, the less penetration is achieved. The 12 MHz frequency provides the best resolution at shallow depths, and the 9 MHz will penetrate a little deeper than the 12 MHz. The 5 MHz penetrates deeper than the 9 and 12, but the 4 MHz provides the deepest penetration. Brown M, Brown L, Lavin's Radiography for Veterinary Technicians, ed 6, Saunders, 2018, p. 171.

29. b Lateral resolution is the ability to distinguish between two objects that are adjacent to one another yet perpendicular to the sound wave. Axial, longitudinal, and azimuthal resolutions are all synonymous terms. Axial resolution is the ability to differentiate between two structures along the beam's length and is equal to half of a pulse's length. Brown M, Brown L, Lavin's Radiography for Veterinary Technicians, ed 6, Saunders, 2018, p. 171.

30. d To obtain a lateromedial view of the femorotibial joint, the cassette should be placed on the medial aspect. The cassette should be placed on the cranial aspect when obtaining a caudocranial view of the femorotibial joint of the horse. The caudocranial and lateromedial views are the only two typical views of the femorotibial joint and therefore the lateral and medial aspects do not apply. Han CM, Hurd CD, Practical Diagnostic Imaging for the Veterinary Technician, ed 3, Mosby, 2005, p. 221.

31. c Wiping the transducer and cord with a glutaraldehyde-based disinfectant is the best method for cleaning the transducers. Autoclaving and gas sterilization should never be used because it can permanently damage the ceramic crystals inside. The transducers should never be immersed in an alcohol-based solution because it can damage the housing seals. Brown M, Brown L, Lavin's Radiography for Veterinary Technicians, ed 6, Saunders, 2018, p. 174.

32. b When a sound wave strikes a metal object or air, a comet-tail artifact will probably be produced. A comet-tail artifact appears as a series of closely interspaced and intense reverberations or reflections that resemble the tail of a comet. Edge shadowing occurs when the sound wave is redirected by an interface and a shadow is cast from the edge of an object. Mirror image artifact occurs when the sound wave strikes a strong reflective surface and is misinterpreted by the ultrasound machine, which writes the same image on the opposite side of the reflector to create a mirror image. Acoustic enhancement occurs when the sound wave accelerates through a fluid-filled medium and the intensity is stronger, which enhances the tissue behind it. Brown M, Brown L, Lavin's Radiography for Veterinary Technicians, ed 6, Saunders, 2018, p. 175.

33. a The correct abbreviation for caudocranial is CdCr. The abbreviation for craniocaudal is CrCd. The abbreviation for dorsopalmar is Dpa. The abbreviation for cranial is Cr. Sirois M, Anthony E, Mauragis D, Handbook of Radiographic Positioning for Veterinary Technicians, ed 1, Delmar Cengage Learning, 2010, p. 3.

34. b The term *hypoechoic* describes the pixels as being dark gray. Hyperechoic describes the pixels as bright gray. Anechoic describes the pixels as black. White is referred to a bright gray and is therefore called hyperechoic. Brown M, Brown L, Lavin's Radiography for Veterinary Technicians, ed 6, Saunders, 2018, p. 164.

35. d The most important components of an ultrasound machine are the elements in the transducer. These elements are predominantly made of piezoelectric ceramics. These materials have unique properties that allow them to change shape in the presence of an electrical current. When the ultrasound machine emits a desired frequency, strong but very short electrical pulses make the ceramics vibrate. This vibration causes the crystals within the ceramics to emit a mechanical vibration at a preset frequency. Each of the crystals is connected to an individual circuit, known as an element, allowing them to be directed independently. It is this individual control of the crystals that allows them to be steered and focused through timing delays. When mechanical energy from the returning sound waves makes contact with the transducer elements, they once again distort the shape of the individual ceramics, creating electrical energy that is released back to the machine to analyze. It is this electrical current that is digitized to create a diagnostic image. Brown M, Brown L, Lavin's Radiography for Veterinary Technicians, ed 6, Saunders, 2018, p. 164.

36. c To obtain a dorsolateral-palmaromedial oblique view, the cassette should be on the palmaromedial aspect of the metacarpus. To obtain a lateromedial view of the metacarpus of a horse, the cassette should be on the medial aspect of the limb. To obtain a dorsomedial-palmarolateral oblique view, the cassette should be on the palmarolateral aspect of the metacarpus. To obtain a dorsopalmar view of the metacarpus, the cassette should be on the palmar surface of the metacarpus. Han CM, Hurd CD, Practical Diagnostic Imaging for the Veterinary Technician, ed 3, Mosby, 2005, p. 203.

37. a The term *dorsoventral* describes a radiograph produced when the primary x-ray beam enters the dorsal surface and exits the ventral surface of the patient. The term *ventrodorsal* describes a radiograph produced when the primary x-ray beam enters the ventral surface and exits the dorsal surface of the patient. The term *craniocaudal* describes the radiographic projection obtained by passing the primary x-ray beam from the cranial surface to the caudal surface of a structure. The term *caudocranial* describes a radiographic projection obtained by passing the primary x-ray beam from the caudal surface to the cranial surface of a structure. Sirois M, Anthony E, Mauragis D, Handbook of Radiographic Positioning for Veterinary Technicians, ed 1, Delmar Cengage Learning, 2010, p. 3.

38. b Dorsal recumbency is used to obtain a craniocaudal view of the tibia. To obtain a caudocranial view of the tibia, the patient should be in the sternal recumbent position with the limb of interest extended caudally. Right or left lateral recumbent positions would be used to obtain a lateral view of the tibia. Han CM, Hurd CD, Practical Diagnostic Imaging for the Veterinary Technician, ed 3, Mosby, 2005, p. 118.

39. b A microconvex probe is the ideal probe when performing an examination through the intercostal view because of the smaller footprint size and the spread of the wide-angle view. The linear probe is appropriate for high resolution imaging for fine details. The phased array is useful in cardiac studies. Brown M, Brown L,

Lavin's Radiography for Veterinary Technicians, ed 6, Saunders, 2018, p. 174.

40. a When scanning in a sagittal plane, the cranial aspect of the patient's body is located on the left side of the monitor. The caudal portion of the patient's body is located on the right side of the monitor. The anterior portion of the patient's body is located at the top of the monitor and the posterior portion of the patient's body is located at the bottom of the monitor. Brown M, Brown L, Lavin's Radiography for Veterinary Technicians, ed 6, Saunders, 2018, p. 172.

41. b M-mode in ultrasound stands for motion. M mode simultaneously creates a B-mode imaged while displaying the motion of the tissues over a two-dimensional scale. B-mode stands for brightness. Harmonics is a mode which helps decrease artifacts. Multiplanar reconstruction involves reconstructing images from various planes to allow simultaneous visualization on the monitor. Brown M, Brown L, Lavin's Radiography for Veterinary Technicians, ed 6, Saunders, 2018, p. 167.

42. d A 3 MHz transducer frequency will allow imaging at a depth of 20 cm. 5 MHz allows imaging at a depth of 15 cm. 7.5 MHz allows imaging at a depth of 10 cm. 10MHz allows imaging at a dept of 7 cm. Brown M, Brown L, Lavin's Radiography for Veterinary Technicians, ed 6, Saunders, 2018, p. 171.

43. a Radiation units have recently been changed to follow an international naming code. REM has been changed to Siever (Sv), Roentgen has been changed to Coulomb/ kg (C/kg), RAD has been changed to Gray (Gy1), Curie has been changed to Becquerel (Bq). Brown M, Brown L, Lavin's Radiography for Veterinary Technicians, ed 6, Saunders, 2018, p. 33.

44. d Dental imaging uses film and small phosphor plates as image receptors. The phosphor plates are used both for direct digital imaging and for computerized imaging. Brown M, Brown L, Lavin's Radiography for Veterinary Technicians, ed 6, Saunders, 2018, p. 399.

45. b Slab fractures, also known as biarticular fractures, are considered the most destabilizing and most serious of all carpal fractures. Corner fractures are more serious than chip fractures, creating more bone, cartilage, and capsular damage. Chip fractures are the least serious of the carpal fractures in that small flakes or chunks of bone are sheared off. Farrow CS, Veterinary Diagnostic Imaging: The Horse, Mosby Elsevier, 2006, p. 156.

46. b A 110-V power outlet is required to operate a dental radiograph unit. The standard preset to operate a dental unit is 70 kV and 8 mA. 110 kV is incorrect for a power outlet. Brown M, Brown L, Lavin's Radiography for Veterinary Technicians, ed 6, Saunders, 2018, p. 395.

47. a The foil backing used on dental x-ray film is designed to absorb any exiting remnant radiation. The film and foil are encased in a waterproof plastic covering to protect them. The small phosphor plates used in digital and computerized imaging are able to bend to accommodate the dental architecture. Brown M, Brown L, Lavin's Radiography for Veterinary Technicians, ed 6, Saunders, 2018, p. 397.

48. c The correct order to process dental film is as follows: pass it through the developer, the wash, the fixer, and then the wash again. It is important to follow this order otherwise the film does not develop correctly. The intermediary wash tanks serve as a stop bath that arrests the activity of the developer and washes off some of the surface developer before entering the fixer. Brown M, Brown L, Lavin's Radiography for Veterinary Technicians, ed 6, Saunders, 2018, p. 399.

49. b The term *dorsopalmar* describes the radiographic views distal to the carpus obtained by passing the primary x-ray beam from the dorsal direction to the palmar surface of the forelimb. The term *plantar* describes the caudal surface of the hind limb distal to the tarsus. The term *palmar* describes the caudal surface of the forelimb distal to the carpus. The term *caudocranial* describes the radiographic projection obtained by passing the primary x-ray beam from the caudal surface to the cranial surface of a structure. Sirois M, Anthony E, Mauragis D, Handbook of Radiographic Positioning for Veterinary Technicians, ed 1, Delmar Cengage Learning, 2010, p. 3.

50. d The typical kilovoltage preset used for dental x-rays is 70 kV. A 110 kV power outlet is required to operate a dental unit. Kilovoltages of 25 kV and 50 kV do not provide enough kV to obtain a radiograph. Brown M, Brown L, Lavin's Radiography for Veterinary Technicians, ed 6, Saunders, 2018, p. 395.

51. e A CT image is a three-dimensional image or a matrix of voxels that includes the third dimension of depth. A radiograph is a two-dimensional image or a matrix of pixels or picture elements. Brown M, Brown L, Lavin's Radiography for Veterinary Technicians, ed 6, Saunders, 2018, p. 190.

52. c A computed tomography x-ray tube rotates 360 degrees around the patient. A dental x-ray unit can rotate in a range ≤270 degrees. A stationary x-ray machine does not rotate at all. Brown M, Brown L, Lavin's Radiography for Veterinary Technicians, ed 6, Saunders, 2018, p. 190.

53. c Blood is read at 80 HU in computed tomography. When using CT imaging, fat reads as –50 HU and calcium reads as 160 HU. Brown M, Brown L, Lavin's Radiography for Veterinary Technicians, ed 6, Saunders, 2018, p. 192.

54. b The scan field of view is the number of detectors that are covered by the x-ray beam. Scan data (also known as raw data) are collected from the detectors and are used to create the images. The image data are the data that are sent either to films or to a PACS system. Display field of view provides a resolution of the CT images, is either equal to or is smaller than the scan field of view, and can resolve structures. Brown M, Brown L, Lavin's Radiography for Veterinary Technicians, ed 6, Saunders, 2018, p. 194.

55. a Anything below –750 HU will be seen as black on the CT image. Anything that falls between –750 and 1250 will be visible as shades of gray. Brown M, Brown L, Lavin's Radiography for Veterinary Technicians, ed 6, Saunders, 2018, p. 192.

56. d Anything above 1250 HU in CT imaging appears as white on the image. Black colors appear at the –755 HU level. Different shades of gray appear between –750 and 1250 HU, therefore 120 HU and 1200 HU both appear as shades of gray. Brown M, Brown L, Lavin's Radiography for Veterinary Technicians, ed 6, Saunders, 2018, p. 192.

57. d Modern CT scanners use multi-slice technology and are able to acquire image slices that are thinner than 1 mm. The original CT scanner acquired images in 10 mm or 1 cm-thick slices. Ten cm slices are not used by CT imaging because they are too thick and can potentially miss minute details. Brown M, Brown L, Lavin's Radiography for Veterinary Technicians, ed 6, Saunders, 2018, p. 196.

58. b The term *pitch* in CT scanning refers to the ratio between the table movement in mm and the CT slice thickness. The calculation of an unknown value based on two known values on either side is termed *interpolation* algorithm. Helical scanning, also known as spiral scanning, allows the x-ray tube and detectors to rotate continuously. Brown M, Brown L, Lavin's Radiography for Veterinary Technicians, ed 6, Saunders, 2018, p. 195.

59. c IV contrast used in conjunction with CT imaging helps view arteries, veins, and other various organs throughout the body, as well as infections seen in the extremities. Contrast will not aid in viewing bone marrow. Brown M, Brown L, Lavin's Radiography for Veterinary Technicians, ed 6, Saunders, 2018, p. 195.

60. b When using the shaded-surface display with CT imaging, 160 HU and higher should be selected to view bone. A −200 HU would demonstrate the skin. A −750 HU or lower, including −800 HU, would display as black. Brown M, Brown L, Lavin's Radiography for Veterinary Technicians, ed 6, Saunders, 2018, p. 196.

61. a A fulcrum is best described as the point of interest. The fulcrum is typically the central point at which a lever rotates. In CT imaging, the fulcrum is the point of interest within the patient's body. In CT imaging, blur is the distortion of the resolution of anatomy above and below the region of interest. A matrix is a series of boxes or individual shades of information. Brown M, Brown L, Lavin's Radiography for Veterinary Technicians, ed 6, Saunders, 2018, p. 189.

62. a The word tomography is derived from the Greek word tomos, which means cut or section. A fulcrum is known as the point of interest. A matrix is a series of boxes or individual shades of information. Brown M, Brown L, Lavin's Radiography for Veterinary Technicians, ed 6, Saunders, 2018, p. 188.

63. c Fluoroscopy provides dynamic real-time imaging of anatomical structures using continuous radiation. If the skin of the patient is too close to the unit or remains in exposure for too long, it can cause radiation burns. CT imaging uses radiation; however, it provides static images and the exposure time is therefore short. MRI uses magnets, not radiation, to produce images. Ultrasound uses sound waves, not radiation, to produce images. Brown M, Brown L, Lavin's Radiography for Veterinary Technicians, ed 6, Saunders, 2018, p. 181.

64. a The acronym ALARA stands for "as low as reasonably achievable", which is a universal principle to limit the amount of radiation doses to patients or employees. Choices b and c do not pertain to radiography examinations. Brown M, Brown L, Lavin's Radiography for Veterinary Technicians, ed 6, Saunders, 2018, p. 28.

65. b Radionuclides are atoms that emit particles and energy to become stable. Photons are elementary particles of electromagnetic radiation. Radioactive decay is the process of radioactive disintegration. Isotopes are variants of atoms of particular chemical elements that have differing numbers of neutrons. Brown M, Brown L, Lavin's Radiography for Veterinary Technicians, ed 6, Saunders, 2018, p. 29.

66. c When an isotope becomes radioactive, it is termed a radioisotope. A photon is an elementary particle of electromagnetic radiation. A radionuclide is an atom that emits particles and energy to become stable. Brown M, Brown L, Lavin's Radiography for Veterinary Technicians, ed 6, Saunders, 2018, p. 29.

67. d Alpha and beta particles both have high linear energy transfer (LET) and low penetrability. The term *LET* describes the amount of energy imparted to the target. Gamma rays have low LET and high penetrability. Brown M, Brown L, Lavin's Radiography for Veterinary Technicians, ed 6, Saunders, 2018, p. 29.

68. a Bone is denser than soft tissue and fat; therefore, it efficiently absorbs more radiation and prevents the image receptor from exposure. This explains why bone appears white on x-ray. Brown M, Brown L, Lavin's Radiography for Veterinary Technicians, ed 6, Saunders, 2018, p. 29.

69. a A mediolateral view of the tarsal joint would require the cassette to be held on the lateral surface of the joint. To obtain a lateromedial view of the tarsal joint of a horse, the cassette should be placed on the medial surface of the joint. The dorsoplantar view would require the cassette to be held on the plantar surface of the joint. To obtain a dorsolateral-plantaromedial oblique view, the cassette should be held on the plantaromedial aspect of the tarsus. Han CM, Hurd CD, Practical Diagnostic Imaging for the Veterinary Technician, ed 3, Mosby, 2005, p. 196.

70. d The higher the kilovolts used, the higher the scatter and secondary radiation, which increases the risk to the patient and employee. The kilovoltage should be optimized to penetrate the body part and the mAs should be set according to the density of the film to provide the best image optimization and best kV amount. Brown M, Brown L, Lavin's Radiography for Veterinary Technicians, ed 6, Saunders, 2018, p. 29.

71. d Distance, time, and shielding are considered the three cardinal rules for radiation protection. Reducing the time of exposure, increasing the distance between the source of the radiation and the subject, and placing a shield or barrier between the subject and the source are the three primary methods of reducing exposure. Brown M, Brown L, Lavin's Radiography for Veterinary Technicians, ed 6, Saunders, 2018, p. 34.

72. d When obtaining a dorsopalmar view of the carpus, the cassette should be held on the palmar aspect of the carpus. When obtaining a dorsomedial-palmarolateral oblique view, the cassette should be held against the palmarolateral aspect of the leg. When obtaining a lateromedial view of the carpus of a horse, the cassette should be held on the medial aspect of the leg. When obtaining a dorsolateral-palmaromedial oblique view, the cassette should be held on the palmaromedial aspect of the leg. Han CM, Hurd CD, Practical Diagnostic Imaging for the Veterinary Technician, ed 3, Mosby, 2005, p. 188.

73. c It is extremely important to limit radiation exposure to pregnant workers at any gestation period because of the potential for causing birth defects. The time between weeks 2 and 10 is the most critical because this is the time of major organogenesis. Brown M, Brown L, Lavin's Radiography for Veterinary Technicians, ed 6, Saunders, 2018, p. 34.

74. b The medial oblique view is best for detecting slab fractures. The lateral view is best for evaluating major fracture dislocation and conformational abnormalities. The flexed lateral view is the most accurate in detecting carpal fractures and showing fragment mobility. The dorsopalmar view is the least revealing in carpal fractures but is best to evaluate distal radial growth plate closures. Farrow CS, Veterinary Diagnostic Imaging: The Horse, Mosby Elsevier, 2006, p. 159.

75. a A meter to measure the rate of exposure is known as a dosimeter. Fluoroscopy is a type of imaging modality that uses continuous radiation techniques. Collimation is the act of reducing the exposure size of the radiation beam. Shielding is the act of creating a barrier between the employee and the radiation exposure unit as well as between the patient and the exposure unit. Brown M, Brown L, Lavin's Radiography for Veterinary Technicians, ed 6, Saunders, 2018, p. 30.

76. b When lead x-ray gowns are not in use, they should be hung up by the shoulders so that the lead can freely hang, which helps avoid the risk of cracking. If the lead is folded or partially hung over the side of something, there is a risk of the lead cracking, which can lead to inadequate protection from radiation. Brown M, Brown L, Lavin's Radiography for Veterinary Technicians, ed 6, Saunders, 2018, p. 35.

77. d Dosimeter badges should be stored away from any exposure to radiation, away from heat, and away from natural light, and they should not be taken home. The best choice to store dosimeter badges is in a dry, cool place away from any radiation exposure. Brown M, Brown L, Lavin's Radiography for Veterinary Technicians, ed 6, Saunders, 2018, p. 31.

78. c Per OSHA guidelines, it is recommended that x-ray equipment in a veterinarian's office should be tested every 2 years. This testing includes the accuracy of kilovoltage, half-value layer, milliampere linearity, reproducibility, timer accuracy, and collimator accuracy. Brown M, Brown L, Lavin's Radiography for Veterinary Technicians, ed 6, Saunders, 2018, p. 32.

79. d Lead aprons are designed to be effective for $\leq$125 kV of radiation. The levels of 50 kV, 70 kV, and 90 kV are all typical x-ray exposure doses in which the use of a lead apron is needed for protection. Brown M, Brown L, Lavin's Radiography for Veterinary Technicians, ed 6, Saunders, 2018, p. 35.

80. d Dosimetry reports should be available for anyone who is exposed to radiation to view; individuals are only allowed to see their specific results, not those of other team members. However, OSHA inspectors and practice owners/managers can view all reports. OSHA often inspects these reports for any discrepancy and to ensure that proper exposure limits are maintained. Brown M, Brown L, Lavin's Radiography for Veterinary Technicians, ed 6, Saunders, 2018, p. 31.

81. d If the DNA is affected by radiation, all of the following may occur: the cell may display no immediate effects but damage may have occurred internally that will affect the individual later, when mitosis occurs cell damage may be obvious with portions of the DNA compromised, or cell death may occur. Brown M, Brown L, Lavin's Radiography for Veterinary Technicians, ed 6, Saunders, 2018, p. 28.

82. b MRI shows the concentration of free-floating hydrogen molecules in tissue, demonstrates better contrast than CT, and is considered superior in imaging the brain and spinal cord. Ultrasound uses sound waves to produce imaging; however, it has huge impedances with penetrating bone. X-ray does not provide good imaging of soft tissue, especially in the brain and spinal cord. Fluoroscopy is a form of continuous real-time x-ray that is effective for dense structures such as bones, but it also does not produce good imaging of soft tissue. Brown M, Brown L, Lavin's Radiography for Veterinary Technicians, ed 6, Saunders, 2018, p. 202.

83. c MRI machines use an extremely strong magnet, which poses danger to anyone in close proximity to the machine with metallic objects. People have been severely injured or killed when metallic objects have become projectiles because of the force of the magnet. MRI machines do not use radiation to obtain images. The intensity of the magnet on the patient is not a concern unless the patient has a metal object within or attached to them. MRI machines are safe; however, they still have safety concerns. Brown M, Brown L, Lavin's Radiography for Veterinary Technicians, ed 6, Saunders, 2018, p. 202.

84. b The most common measurement of magnetism and magnetic equivalency is the Tesla (T). Tesla is the unit that people use to describe the medical magnet's field strength. The imperial unit of measurement for magnetism is the gauss. Polarity is the separation of electric charge leading to a molecule or its chemical groups having an electric dipole or multipole moment. Precession is when the atom wobbles in space. Brown M, Brown L, Lavin's Radiography for Veterinary Technicians, ed 6, Saunders, 2018, p. 203.

85. a Permanent magnets consist of two slabs of magnetic material facing each other. Electromagnets, also known as resistive magnets, create an electrical charge applied through copper wire wrapped around a center. Superconducting magnets are electromagnets made of windings that are superconductive. Brown M, Brown L, Lavin's Radiography for Veterinary Technicians, ed 6, Saunders, 2018, p. 202.

86. b Superconducting magnets are the most common medical magnets used, which are electromagnets made of windings that are superconductive in very low temperatures. Liquid helium is used to keep this magnet alive. Resistive magnets, also known as electromagnets, are created by an electrical charge applied through copper wire wrapped around a center that creates 0.6 T. Permanent magnets consist of two slabs of magnetic material facing each other and they have a measurement of 0.3 T. Brown M, Brown L, Lavin's Radiography for Veterinary Technicians, ed 6, Saunders, 2018, p. 202.

87. a Shims are pieces or plates of metal used to correct the magnetic field within the magnet. Gradients are coils or assemblies within the magnetic bore that enable the machine to create images in any plane. Surface coils are devices that receive radio wave signals from a body part that is covered or is contained by them. Brown M, Brown L, Lavin's Radiography for Veterinary Technicians, ed 6, Saunders, 2018, p. 204.

88. c A lower repetition time of ≤699 ms shows the T1 decay response of the tissues. A higher repetition time of ≤1500 ms shows the T2 decay response and changes the contrast of the images. Brown M, Brown L, Lavin's Radiography for Veterinary Technicians, ed 6, Saunders, 2018, p. 206.

89. c Radio waves are used to manipulate hydrogen atoms in and out of an excited energy state. Helium is used to keep some magnets active. Water does not aid nor hinder the MRI unit. Oxygen does not aid nor hinder the MRI unit. Brown M, Brown L, Lavin's Radiography for Veterinary Technicians, ed 6, Saunders, 2018, p. 203.

90. b In MRI, the various shades of gray are referred to as signal intensities. Densities are factors in the different body tissues that can play a role in the different imaging modalities. Hypoechoic and hyperechoic refer to the different echogenicities of ultrasound. Brown M, Brown L, Lavin's Radiography for Veterinary Technicians, ed 6, Saunders, 2018, p. 206.

91. b Cerebrospinal fluid has a low signal intensity on a true T1-weighted image and appears black. Fat and skin have a high signal intensity and appear bright or white. Between the low and high signal intensities are different shades of gray. Brown M, Brown L, Lavin's Radiography for Veterinary Technicians, ed 6, Saunders, 2018, p. 206.

92. a MRI requires the use of a contrast agent known as gadolinium, a paramagnetic, to highlight injection, tumors, or vascular disease. Iodine and barium contrast are both used in CT imaging. Brown M, Brown L, Lavin's Radiography for Veterinary Technicians, ed 6, Saunders, 2018, p. 207.

93. b Gadolinium is a paramagnetic contrast used in MRI and is excreted by the kidneys. It is very important that the kidneys are functioning properly before administration. The liver plays a role in the metabolism of drugs but does not excrete drugs. The lungs excrete certain drugs through respiration. Gadolinium is administered intravenously. The GI tract aids in removing barium from the body but does not remove gadolinium. Brown M, Brown L, Lavin's Radiography for Veterinary Technicians, ed 6, Saunders, 2018, p. 207.

94. d The term *caudocranial* describes the radiographic projection obtained by passing the primary x-ray beam from the caudal surface to the cranial surface of a structure. The term *dorsopalmar* describes the radiographic views distal to the carpus obtained by passing the primary x-ray beam from the dorsal direction to the palmar surface of the forelimb. The term *plantar* describes the caudal surface of the hind limb distal to the tarsus. The term *palmar* describes the caudal surface of the forelimb distal to the carpus. Sirois M, Anthony E, Mauragis D, Handbook of Radiographic Positioning for Veterinary Technicians, ed 1, Delmar Cengage Learning, 2010, p. 3.

95. c MRI machines are acoustically very loud and reach noise levels between 60 dB and 90 dB. Ear shielding is necessary for patients and for anyone staying in the MRI room during a scan. Brown M, Brown L, Lavin's Radiography for Veterinary Technicians, ed 6, Saunders, 2018, p. 209.

96. e All personnel working in a facility that contains an MRI machine should be aware of the following: every patient/employee should be screened for safety purposes, no loose metallic objects can be near the machines, the MRI consists of a strong magnetic field, and the magnet is always on. Brown M, Brown L, Lavin's Radiography for Veterinary Technicians, ed 6, Saunders, 2018, p. 202.

97. b To obtain a dorsopalmar view of the metacarpus, the cassette should be on the palmar surface of the metacarpus. To obtain a dorsolateral-palmaromedial oblique view, the cassette should be on the palmaromedial aspect of the metacarpus. To obtain a lateromedial view of the metacarpus of a horse, the cassette should be on the medial aspect of the limb. To obtain a dorsomedial-palmarolateral oblique view, the cassette should be on the palmarolateral aspect of the metacarpus. Han CM, Hurd CD, Practical Diagnostic Imaging for the Veterinary Technician, ed 3, Mosby, 2005, p. 200.

98. c Technetium 99m is used for nuclear scintigraphy, also referred to as nuclear medicine. MRI uses magnetic fields. Ultrasound uses sound waves. Fluoroscopy uses continuous x-ray to obtain images. Brown M, Brown L, Lavin's Radiography for Veterinary Technicians, ed 6, Saunders, 2018, p. 214.

99. b The flexed lateral view of the carpal joint is the best view for detecting distal corner fractures. The lateral view is the best view for judging a major fracture dislocation and conformational abnormalities. The dorsopalmar view is the best view to evaluate distal radial growth-plate closure. The medial oblique view of the carpal joint is the best view for detecting slab fractures. Farrow CS, Veterinary Diagnostic Imaging: The Horse, Mosby Elsevier, 2006, p. 153.

100. c Radioisotopes used for each examination in a nuclear medicine study are measured in millicurie (mCi) units. X-rays are measured in units of kV and mA. Ultrasound is measured in MHz. Brown M, Brown L, Lavin's Radiography for Veterinary Technicians, ed 6, Saunders, 2018, p. 214.

101. b With nuclear medicine studies, an area that shows an indication of higher radiation emission is termed a *hot spot.* The term *cold spot* suggests an area of a less intense or smaller concentration of radiation. A gamma photon burst is an emission of radiation seen with the nuclear medicine camera. Brown M, Brown L, Lavin's Radiography for Veterinary Technicians, ed 6, Saunders, 2018, p. 215.

102. b A tooth abscess will appear radiographically as a radiolucent area around the apex of the tooth. The area is radiolucent because the bacteria from the infection eat away the support structure that holds the tooth to the bone. A radiopaque area around the tooth root is a normal finding because bone and tooth are radiopaque. A radiopaque area inside the tooth pulp is a pulp stone. A radiolucent area inside the pulp is normal because the pulp is soft tissue that shows on radiographs as radiolucent. Bellows J, "The why, when and how of small animal dental radiology," in The Practice of Veterinary Dentistry: A Team Effort, Iowa State Press, 1999, p. 81-105.

103. a The soft tissue phase occurs approximately 5–10 minutes post injection. This detects the pooling of the nuclide and demonstrates tendons and ligaments. The vascular phase can be seen immediately, with the injection used to look primarily for thrombosis. The bone phase is performed 2–3 hours after the injection to ensure the maximum amount of nucleide has gathered at the point of interest. The pet is usually hospitalized for 48 hours following the injection so that the isotope can decay. Brown M, Brown L, Lavin's Radiography for Veterinary Technicians, ed 6, Saunders, 2018, p. 215.

104. b The color blue seen on nuclear medicine studies indicates an area of low activity for emitted radiation bursts. The color red indicates high activity for radiation bursts. No activity on a nuclear medicine study could suggest areas of tissue necrosis. The normal anatomy of the patient is displayed along with the plotted series of dots to identify easily the area of interest, because these images only demonstrate function and not anatomy. Brown M, Brown L, Lavin's Radiography for Veterinary Technicians, ed 6, Saunders, 2018, p. 215.

105. b The correct abbreviation for dorsopalmar is Dpa. The abbreviation for craniocaudal is CrCd. The abbreviation for caudocranial is CdCr. The abbreviation for cranial is Cr. Sirois M, Anthony E, Mauragis D, Handbook of Radiographic Positioning for Veterinary Technicians, ed 1, Delmar Cengage Learning, 2010, p. 3.

106. b The half-life of a radioisotope means that the patient is emitting half of the original strength of the isotope. Technetium Tc99m is the most common radioisotope used in nuclear medicine and has a half-life of 6 hours. Typically it is recommended to keep the patient hospitalized for 24–48 hours to protect the surrounding people from radiation emissions. Brown M, Brown L, Lavin's Radiography for Veterinary Technicians, ed 6, Saunders, 2018, p. 216.

107. d After a patient has received the radioisotope, the entire body as well as the waste products are considered radioactive for at least 48 hours. Brown M, Brown L, Lavin's Radiography for Veterinary Technicians, ed 6, Saunders, 2018, p. 216.

108. d When handling a patient that is considered radioactive, all of the following must be worn: lab coat, gloves, disposable boots, and a dosimeter badge. Brown M, Brown L, Lavin's Radiography for Veterinary Technicians, ed 6, Saunders, 2018, p. 218.

109. a Radiographic projections are named according to the direction in which the central beam anatomically enters the body part, followed by the area of exit of the x-ray beam. This is a standard rule for naming the radiographic projection direction; therefore, the remaining options are incorrect in the naming of the direction. Scatter radiation bounces off objects. Brown M, Brown L, Lavin's Radiography for Veterinary Technicians, ed 6, Saunders, 2018, p. 225.

110. b The term *ventral recumbency* refers to a patient lying on its abdomen. Dorsal recumbency refers to the patient lying on its back. The term *left lateral recumbency* refers to the patient lying on its left side. The term *right lateral recumbency* refers to the patient lying on its right side. Brown M, Brown L, Lavin's Radiography for Veterinary Technicians, ed 6, Saunders, 2018, p. 225.

111. b The abbreviation Cd refers to caudal. The abbreviation Cr refers to cranial. The abbreviation V refers to ventral. The abbreviation PaP refers to palmar. Brown M, Brown L, Lavin's Radiography for Veterinary Technicians, ed 6, Saunders, 2018, p. 225.

112. b The term *proximal* is abbreviated as Pr. The term *palmar* is abbreviated as Pa. The term *plantar* is abbreviated as Pl. The term *distal* is abbreviated as Di. Brown M, Brown L, Lavin's Radiography for Veterinary Technicians, ed 6, Saunders, 2018, p. 226.

113. a The abbreviation CrCd refers to craniocaudal. The abbreviation ML refers to mediolateral. The abbreviation DP refers to dorsopalmar and dorsoplantar. Brown M, Brown L, Lavin's Radiography for Veterinary Technicians, ed 6, Saunders, 2018, p. 226.

114. c The term *craniocaudal* describes the radiographic projection obtained by passing the primary x-ray beam from the cranial surface to the caudal surface of a structure. The term *dorsoventral* describes a radiograph produced when the primary x-ray beam enters the dorsal surface and exits the ventral surface of the patient. The term *ventrodorsal* describes a radiograph produced when the primary x-ray beam enters the ventral surface and exits the dorsal surface of the patient. The term *caudocranial* describes a radiographic projection obtained by passing the primary x-ray beam from the caudal surface to the cranial surface of a structure. Sirois M, Anthony E, Mauragis D, Handbook of Radiographic Positioning for Veterinary Technicians, ed 1, Delmar Cengage Learning, 2010, p. 3.

115. c The term *oblique* is generally used in reference to the limbs. The abdomen, spine, and head views are usually taken parallel to the x-ray beam. Brown M, Brown L, Lavin's Radiography for Veterinary Technicians, ed 6, Saunders, 2018, p. 226.

116. b The term *rostral* refers to the direction toward the nose. The term *cranial* refers to the direction toward the head. The term *caudal* refers to the direction toward the tail. The term *medial* refers to the direction toward the middle or midline of the body. Brown M, Brown L, Lavin's Radiography for Veterinary Technicians, ed 6, Saunders, 2018, p. 226.

117. a The median plane divides the body into left and right portions. The dorsal plane divides the body in anterior/posterior portions. The transverse plane divides the body into cranial/caudal portions. Brown M, Brown L, Lavin's Radiography for Veterinary Technicians, ed 6, Saunders, 2018, p. 225.

118. b The x-ray marker should indicate the side that is down when obtaining a lateral recumbent x-ray. For right lateral recumbency, the right side is down and therefore the right marker should be used. In left lateral recumbency, the left side is down and therefore the left marker should be used. The front and hind markers should be used to denote the front side or hind side of any anatomical structure and these markers are especially useful when referring to equine x-rays when there are symmetrical anatomical areas. Brown M, Brown L, Lavin's Radiography for Veterinary Technicians, ed 6, Saunders, 2018, p. 233.

119. a When viewing a lateral radiograph, the cranial part of the animal is to the left on the illuminator. When reviewing a lateral or oblique radiograph of the limbs, the cranial or dorsal aspect of the limb is to the viewer's left. When viewing cranial/caudal or dorsal/plantar images of extremities, the proximal end should be at the top of the illuminator. Directions of viewing will always typically be to the left or to the top of the illuminator. Brown M, Brown L, Lavin's Radiography for Veterinary Technicians, ed 6, Saunders, 2018, p. 234.

120. c When obtaining an x-ray, the area of interest should be closest to the image receptor. This location provides the best imaging optimization of the x-ray beam. Any other location would not be as accurate. The restrainer should be as far away as possible from the x-ray beam for safety reasons. Brown M, Brown L, Lavin's Radiography for Veterinary Technicians, ed 6, Saunders, 2018, p. 235.

121. a To obtain a lateromedial view of the metacarpus of a horse, the cassette should be on the medial aspect of the limb. To obtain a dorsolateral-palmaromedial oblique view, the cassette should be on the palmaromedial aspect of the metacarpus. To obtain a dorsomedial-palmarolateral oblique view, the cassette should be on the palmarolateral aspect of the metacarpus. To obtain a dorsopalmar view of the metacarpus, the cassette should be on the palmar surface of the metacarpus. Han CM, Hurd CD, Practical Diagnostic Imaging for the Veterinary Technician, ed 3, Mosby, 2005, p. 202.

122. b To collimate the x-ray beam is to limit the beam exposure to just the area of interest within the film. For safety concerns, the lowest kV possible should be used when obtaining x-rays. The film should never have full exposure because of increased amounts of scatter radiation. Brown M, Brown L, Lavin's Radiography for Veterinary Technicians, ed 6, Saunders, 2018, p. 224.

123. b To help prevent motion artifacts, a high milliamperage should be used, which produces the shortest exposure time. Lower milliamperage creates longer exposure time and thus does not help with motion artifacts. The kVp is used to obtain the correct penetration to provide for the best gray scale of the area of interest. Brown M, Brown L, Lavin's Radiography for Veterinary Technicians, ed 6, Saunders, 2018, p. 238.

124. c The dorsoplantar view requires the cassette to be held on the plantar surface of the joint. A mediolateral view of the tarsal joint requires the cassette to be held on the lateral surface of the joint. To obtain a lateromedial view of the tarsal joint of a horse, the cassette should be placed on the medial surface of the joint. To obtain a dorsolateral-plantaromedial oblique view, the cassette should be held on the plantaromedial aspect of the tarsus. Han CM, Hurd CD, Practical Diagnostic Imaging for the Veterinary Technician, ed 3, Mosby, 2005, p. 194.

125. b When obtaining an x-ray of a vomiting patient, left lateral recumbency is ideal because gas is moved to the pyloric antrum and can potentially highlight a foreign body. Right lateral recumbency can also be used, but it is not ideal because overlying bowel gas moves to the anterior portion of the stomach. Dorsal/ventral or ventral/dorsal can be a challenge in a vomiting patient because of overlying bowel gas as well as the possible risk of aspiration of vomit. Brown M, Brown L, Lavin's Radiography for Veterinary Technicians, ed 6, Saunders, 2018, p. 239.

126. a To ensure the animal is properly positioned in the lateral view, the coxofemoral joints should be superimposed, intervertebral foramina should be the same size, rib heads should be superimposed, and transverse processes should be superimposed at the origin from the vertebral bodies. Brown M, Brown L, Lavin's Radiography for Veterinary Technicians, ed 6, Saunders, 2018, p. 239.

127. e The following are ways to help determine whether the animal is properly positioned in the ventrodorsal view: rib and abdominal symmetry, wings of the ilium are symmetrical, spinous processes are aligned in the center of the vertebral bodies, and obturator foramina is symmetrical. Superimposing the coxofemoral joints and superimposing the rib heads help to determine whether the animal is properly positioned in the lateral view. Brown M, Brown L, Lavin's Radiography for Veterinary Technicians, ed 6, Saunders, 2018, p. 239.

128. c To obtain a rostrocaudal foramen magnum projection, the center should be between the eyes. To obtain a lateral projection of the skull, the beam should be centered at the lateral canthus of the eye socket. When obtaining either a VD or a DV projection of the skull, the center should be midway between the tip of the nose to just caudal to the occipital protuberance at the base. To obtain a rostrocaudal tympanic bullae open-mouth projection, the beam is centered just above the base of the tongue and just below the soft palate, approximately at the commissure of the mouth. Sirois M, Anthony E, Mauragis D, Handbook of Radiographic Positioning for Veterinary Technicians, ed 1, Delmar Cengage Learning, 2010, p. 110.

129. c The liver, kidneys, bladder, stomach, small intestine, and large intestine are just a few organs normally seen on radiographs. The pancreas is not seen on radiographs. Brown M, Brown L, Lavin's Radiography for Veterinary Technicians, ed 6, Saunders, 2018, p. 246.

130. a The lungs are clearly seen on x-ray. The urethra, ureters, adrenal glands, pancreas, gallbladder, and mesenteric and rectal lymph nodes are not seen on ultrasound images. Brown M, Brown L, Lavin's Radiography for Veterinary Technicians, ed 6, Saunders, 2018, p. 174.

131. a The colon appears in the shape of a question mark on the dorsoventral view of an x-ray. The spleen appears as a small triangle shape caudal to the fundus of the stomach and the right kidney is a bean-shaped organ that is seen cranial to the left kidney. The diaphragm has a bumpy appearance in the dorsoventral view on an x-ray. Brown M, Brown L, Lavin's Radiography for Veterinary Technicians, ed 6, Saunders, 2018, p. 246.

132. c The liver lies in the cranial abdomen between the diaphragm and stomach and is the largest organ in the abdominal cavity. The adrenal glands are not generally visualized on a radiograph, but they are located in the retroperitoneal space craniomedial to each kidney. The normal pancreas is not visualized radiographically. The spleen is located in the craniodorsal abdomen and is dorsal and caudal to the stomach. Brown M, Brown L, Lavin's Radiography for Veterinary Technicians, ed 6, Saunders, 2018, p. 246.

133. e The right kidney is seen cranial to the left kidney in the left lateral view, right lateral view, ventrodorsal view and the dorsoventral view. Brown M, Brown L, Lavin's Radiography for Veterinary Technicians, ed 6, Saunders, 2018, p. 246.

134. c If pneumonia is suspected in small animals, both lateral views and a ventrodorsal view are recommended. If cardiac disease is suspected, either a right or left lateral view and a dorsoventral view are recommended. Brown M, Brown L, Lavin's Radiography for Veterinary Technicians, ed 6, Saunders, 2018, p. 254.

135. b A false diagnosis of pneumothorax obtained using x-ray can be caused by overexposure. Underexposure might lead to an incorrect diagnosis of interstitial opacification. Panting can lead to motion artifacts, making it difficult to obtain a good-quality x-ray. Patient movement can cause motion artifacts, which makes it more difficult to obtain a good quality x-ray. Increasing the mAs can minimize motion artifacts. Brown M, Brown L, Lavin's Radiography for Veterinary Technicians, ed 6, Saunders, 2018, p. 254.

136. c The VD view is recommended to view the lungs. Right lateral and left lateral views are good for imaging the lung fields; however, the VD view provides an image of both lung fields on the same image. The DV view is acceptable if the patient has difficulty breathing while in the VD position (however, this view is not ideal). A VD position is ideal to image the heart. Brown M, Brown L, Lavin's Radiography for Veterinary Technicians, ed 6, Saunders, 2018, p. 260.

137. d The maximum permissible dose for a person is 5000 millirems per year. Prendergast H, Front Office Management for the Veterinary Team, ed 3, Saunders, 2020, p. 81.

138. c Dosimetry reports should be kept for a minimum of 30 years in case any medical issues arise regarding team members who might have been exposed. Harmful effects of radiation can take several years to arise; therefore, dosimetry reports should be kept for ≥30 years. Prendergast H, Front Office Management for the Veterinary Team, ed 3, Saunders, 2020, p. 81.

139. b To obtain a thoracic radiograph, exposure should be taken at maximum inspiration to maximize lung contrast by increasing aeration of the lung field. With maximum expiration, the lungs are not fully expanded, which is not ideal for obtaining an x-ray. Panting causes motion artifact leading to poor-quality x-rays, making it difficult to obtain accurate diagnoses. Brown M, Brown L, Lavin's Radiography for Veterinary Technicians, ed 6, Saunders, 2018, p. 254.

140. b It is best to measure the patient in the position in which it is to be x-rayed to allow for the most accurate measurement. If the patient is standing, the measurement might not be completely accurate and may change after the patient is in the proper position for x-ray. When measuring the patient, the thickest part should be measured to allow for proper exposure rather than measuring the thinnest portion. Brown M, Brown L, Lavin's Radiography for Veterinary Technicians, ed 6, Saunders, 2018, p. 254.

141. a The central ray should be located at the center of the scapula when obtaining a caudocranial view of the scapula. This image includes the scapula, humerus, and shoulder joint. The borders should be the shoulder joint and the caudal border of the scapula (which is at the level of the eighth rib). The measurement should be taken at the level of the scapulohumeral articulation and should extend over the first thoracic vertebral body. Brown M, Brown L, Lavin's Radiography for Veterinary Technicians, ed 6, Saunders, 2018, p. 282.

142. b To radiograph the mandibular premolars and molars, the parallel mandibular view is used. The film or sensor is placed between the tongue and the mandible, parallel to the long axis of the teeth. The tube head is positioned perpendicular to the film at an approximate angle of 60 degrees to the horizontal plane. To radiograph the maxillary incisors, the rostral maxillary position is used. The film or sensor is placed below the incisors and canine teeth. The tube head or cone is angled between 50 and 60 degrees to the hard palate. To radiograph the mandibular incisors and canine, the rostral mandibular view is used. The film or sensor is placed below the incisors and canine teeth. The tube head or cone is angled at about 60 degrees to the mandible. To radiograph the maxillary canine tooth, the lateral oblique view is used. The film or sensor is placed below the canine tooth to the second premolar. The tube head or cone is angled at 45 degrees to the hard palate and 80–90 degrees oblique to the right or left, depending on which canine tooth is being radiographed. Mulligan TW, Aller MS, Williams CA, "Intraoral imaging techniques," Atlas of Canine and Feline Dental Radiography, Veterinary Learning Systems, 1998, p. 27-44.

143. c The patient should be placed in a dorsal recumbent position when obtaining a caudocranial view of the humerus. The ventral recumbent position is used to obtain a craniocaudal image of the humerus. The right or left lateral recumbent positions are used to obtain a lateral image of the forelimb, not a caudocranial view. Brown M, Brown L, Lavin's Radiography for Veterinary Technicians, ed 6, Saunders, 2018, p. 287.

144. b The film density will be doubled if the mA or exposure time is doubled. If the mA or exposure time is halved, the film density will also be halved. Both the mA and exposure time work together and have a linear effect on film density. Han CM, Hurd CD, Practical Diagnostic Imaging for the Veterinary Technician, ed 3, Mosby, 2005, p. 10.

145. d The milliamperage control on the machine affects the current to the cathode, which controls the amount of radiation that is produced. A step-down transformer controls the amount of incoming voltage. Han CM, Hurd CD, Practical Diagnostic Imaging for the Veterinary Technician, ed 3, Mosby, 2005, p. 4.

146. a The radiographic density is the degree of blackness on a radiograph. The radiographic contrast is defined as the differences in radiographic density between adjacent areas on a radiographic image. A focal-film distance is the distance from the target to the film. Radiographic fogging decreases the differences in densities between two adjacent shadows. Han CM, Hurd CD, Practical Diagnostic Imaging for the Veterinary Technician, ed 3, Mosby, 2005, p. 10.

147. c Foreshortening occurs when the object is not parallel to the recording surface. Distortion occurs when there is a misrepresentation of the size, shape, and location of anatomic structures. Penumbra causes blurring at the edges of the shadows cast by the x-ray exposure. Fogging decreases the differences in densities between two adjacent shadows. Han CM, Hurd CD, Practical Diagnostic Imaging for the Veterinary Technician, ed 3, Mosby, 2005, p. 15.

148. b When an x-ray photon strikes an object, one of three different things can occur: the photon penetrates the object, the photon is absorbed by the object, or the photon produces scatter radiation. Han CM, Hurd CD, Practical Diagnostic Imaging for the Veterinary Technician, ed 3, Mosby, 2005, p. 17.

149. b Scatter radiation has a longer wavelength than the primary beam and is projected in all directions. Because it has a longer wavelength, it is less energetic and is absorbed by the next object it strikes. The wavelength is the distance, not the width, that a wave can move in the time it takes to complete one cycle and it is measured in nanometers. Han CM, Hurd CD, Practical Diagnostic Imaging for the Veterinary Technician, ed 3, Mosby, 2005, p. 17.

150. c A wavelength of an x-ray is measured in nanometers (nm). A nanometer is equal to one millionth of a millimeter. The typical wavelength of a medical x-ray is 0.05–0.01 nanometers (nm). The choices millimeter, meter, and decimeter are the incorrect units. Han CM, Hurd CD, Practical Diagnostic Imaging for the Veterinary Technician, ed 3, Mosby, 2005, p. 3.

151. d Collimators are lead shutters installed in the tube head of the x-ray machine and are adjustable to increase or decrease the exposure size. Filters are thin sheets of aluminum and are placed over the tube window, which are used to absorb the less penetrating x-rays as they leave the tube head. Diaphragms are sheets of lead with rectangular, square, or circular openings that limit the size of the primary beam. Cones are lead cylinders of fixed size and are placed over the collimator on the x-ray tube head. Han CM, Hurd CD, Practical Diagnostic Imaging for the Veterinary Technician, ed 3, Mosby, 2005, p. 18.

152. d To obtain a rostrocaudal tympanic bullae open-mouth projection, the beam is centered just above the base of the tongue and just below the soft palate, approximately at the commissure of the mouth. To obtain a rostrocaudal foramen magnum projection, the center should be between the eyes. To obtain a lateral projection of the skull, the beam should be centered at the lateral canthus of the eye socket. When obtaining either a VD or DV projection of the skull, the center should be midway between the tip of the nose to just caudal to the occipital protuberance at the base. Sirois M, Anthony E, Mauragis D, Handbook of Radiographic Positioning for Veterinary Technicians, ed 1, Delmar Cengage Learning, 2010, p. 110.

153. a A grid is used to decrease scatter radiation and increase the contrast on the radiograph. Filters are used to absorb the less penetrating x-rays as they leave the tube head. Cones are used to restrict the primary beam to the size of the cone being used. Diaphragms are used to limit the size of the primary beam to the size of the diaphragm used. Han CM, Hurd CD, Practical Diagnostic Imaging for the Veterinary Technician, ed 3, Mosby, 2005, p. 18.

154. d When obtaining a dorsolateral-palmaromedial oblique view, the cassette should be held on the palmaromedial aspect of the leg. When obtaining a dorsomedial-palmarolateral oblique view, the cassette should be held against the palmarolateral aspect of the leg. When obtaining a lateromedial view of the carpus of a horse, the cassette should be held on the medial aspect of the leg. When obtaining a dorsopalmar view of the carpus, the cassette should be held on the palmar aspect of the carpus. Han CM, Hurd CD, Practical Diagnostic Imaging for the Veterinary Technician, ed 3, Mosby, 2005, p. 189.

155. c A grid is a series of thin, linear strips made of alternating radiodense and radiolucent material. The radiodense material is composed of lead. The radiolucent interspacers are plastic, aluminum, or fiber. Han CM, Hurd CD, Practical Diagnostic Imaging for the Veterinary Technician, ed 3, Mosby, 2005, p. 18.

156. b The grid is located between the patient and the cassette and is used to decrease scatter radiation and increase the contrast on the radiograph. Because the grid helps to increase the contrast on the radiograph, it cannot be located below the cassette, on top of the patient, or within the housing unit. Han CM, Hurd CD, Practical Diagnostic Imaging for the Veterinary Technician, ed 3, Mosby, 2005, p. 18.

157. c A black irregular border on one end of the film is caused by light exposure while still in the box before being processed. Film that has expired or has been exposed to radiation while still in storage will cause a fogged film. Rough handling of the film before exposure will cause black crescents or lines. Han CM, Hurd CD, Practical Diagnostic Imaging for the Veterinary Technician, ed 3, Mosby, 2005, p. 49.

158. c A fogged film can be caused by exposure to excessive scatter radiation. Chemical spills on the screen as well as foreign material between the film and the screen can cause white areas. Film exposure resulting from static electricity causes black crescents or lines. Han CM, Hurd CD, Practical Diagnostic Imaging for the Veterinary Technician, ed 3, Mosby, 2005, p. 49.

159. d Grid lines on the entire film appear as a result of the focal-film distance not being in the range of the grid's focus. Patient motion and poor film-screen contact results in a decrease in detail. When the grid is not centered with the primary beam, it causes grid lines that are more visible on one end of the film with an overall decrease in radiographic density. Han CM, Hurd CD, Practical Diagnostic Imaging for the Veterinary Technician, ed 3, Mosby, 2005, p. 51.

160. d The correct temperature for an automatic processor tank is 95°F (35°C). Manual tanks should be at 68°F (20°C). Han CM, Hurd CD, Practical Diagnostic Imaging for the Veterinary Technician, ed 3, Mosby, 2005, p. 52.

161. c Decreased radiographic density with poor contrast can result from an underexposed film. Increased radiographic density with poor contrast results from the film being overdeveloped or overexposed or developed in chemicals that were too hot. Han CM, Hurd CD, Practical Diagnostic Imaging for the Veterinary Technician, ed 3, Mosby, 2005, p. 52.

162. d To obtain a whole body view, the beam should be focused over the center of the body from cranial to caudal or at the thoracolumbar area. To obtain a dorsoventral abdominal view of the rabbit, the beam should be centered over the liver. To obtain a view of the thorax of a rabbit, the center of the beam should be focused over the heart. Han CM, Hurd CD, Practical Diagnostic Imaging for the Veterinary Technician, ed 3, Mosby, 2005, p. 167.

163. c The limb should be extended cranially to obtain a mediolateral view of the brachio-antebrachial joint. To obtain a craniocaudal view of the brachio-antebrachial joint, the limb of the horse should be abducted to separate the elbow from the thoracic musculature, which pulls the limb away from midline. To adduct the limb would be to move it toward the midline of the body, which would not be ideal for this image. To extend the limb caudally does not assist in obtaining a view of the brachio-antebrachial joint. Han CM, Hurd CD, Practical Diagnostic Imaging for the Veterinary Technician, ed 3, Mosby, 2005, p. 223.

164. d The right or left lateral recumbent position would be used to obtain a lateral view of the tibia. Dorsal recumbency would be used to obtain a craniocaudal view of the tibia. To obtain a caudocranial view of the tibia, the patient should be in the sternal recumbent position with the limb of interest extended caudally. Han CM, Hurd CD, Practical Diagnostic Imaging for the Veterinary Technician, ed 3, Mosby, 2005, p. 117.

165. c Closure of the distal growth plate of MC3 of a foal occurs between 18 and 38 weeks. The first radiographic appearance of the distal epiphyseal ossification in metacarpal 2 and metacarpal 4 occurs between 4 and 38 weeks. The first radiographic appearance of the crena occurs between 4 and 22 weeks. Closure of the proximal growth plate P1 occurs between 22 and 38 weeks. Farrow CS, Veterinary Diagnostic Imaging: The Horse, Mosby Elsevier, 2006, p. 4.

166. a Uneven development of film results from uneven chemical levels. Film that is developed in chemicals that are too cold or film that is underexposed results in decreased radiographic density with poor contrast. Good radiographic density with poor contrast results from a low-grade light leak in the darkroom. Han CM, Hurd CD, Practical Diagnostic Imaging for the Veterinary Technician, ed 3, Mosby, 2005, p. 53.

167. d When the entire film appears clear, it can be caused either from a lack of exposure or a case in which the film was processed in the fixer before the developer. When the final wash has been conducted improperly, it can result in the film turning brown. Han CM, Hurd CD, Practical Diagnostic Imaging for the Veterinary Technician, ed 3, Mosby, 2005, p. 54.

168. a When obtaining a lateral view of the cervical vertebrae of a small animal, it is important not to overextend the limbs caudally, which could result in rotation of the spine. A pad may be placed under the mandible to superimpose the wings of the atlas as well as under the neck to prevent sagging of the spine. The wings of the atlas and center of the spine of the scapula should be placed in the longitudinal center of the primary beam. Han CM, Hurd CD, Practical Diagnostic Imaging for the Veterinary Technician, ed 3, Mosby, 2005, p. 71.

169. b The topographic landmark for the caudal cervical vertebrae is the center of the spine of the scapula. The base of the skull is the landmark for the cranial cervical vertebrae. The level of C4 does include the full survey of the cervical vertebrae. The level of T4 is part of the thoracic vertebrae and it is not necessary to include it in a cervical vertebrae survey. Han CM, Hurd CD, Practical Diagnostic Imaging for the Veterinary Technician, ed 3, Mosby, 2005, p. 75.

170. c The spin of the scapula is the cranial landmark for a radiographic view of the thoracic vertebrae. The wings of the ilium are the caudal landmark for a radiographic view of the lumbar vertebrae. The base of the skull is the cranial landmark for a radiographic view of the cervical vertebrae. Halfway between the xiphoid process and the last rib is the caudal landmark for a radiographic view of the thoracic vertebrae. Han CM, Hurd CD, Practical Diagnostic Imaging for the Veterinary Technician, ed 3, Mosby, 2005, p. 82.

171. d When obtaining a radiograph of the thoracic vertebrae, the highest point of the thorax should be measured for the kVp setting. The lowest point does not account for the widest portion of the body and the film will be underexposed. The cranial or caudal end of the thoracic vertebrae is not an ideal measurement location for the kVp setting because it is not the widest portion of the animal and will result in underexposure of the film. Han CM, Hurd CD, Practical Diagnostic Imaging for the Veterinary Technician, ed 3, Mosby, 2005, p. 78.

172. d The correct abbreviation for cranial is Cr. The abbreviation for craniocaudal is CrCd. The abbreviation for caudocranial is CdCr. The abbreviation for dorsopalmar is Dpa. Sirois M, Anthony E, Mauragis D, Handbook of Radiographic Positioning for Veterinary Technicians, ed 1, Delmar Cengage Learning, 2010, p. 3.

173. b The kVp should be increased slightly to adjust for the thick density of the lumbosacral vertebrae. Decreasing the kVp may result in underexposure. Changing the mAs will account for motion artifact, which does not help the exposure for thicker densities. Han CM, Hurd CD, Practical Diagnostic Imaging for the Veterinary Technician, ed 3, Mosby, 2005, p. 88.

174. c The patient should be placed in the sternal recumbency position to obtain a dorsopalmar view of a limb. Right or left lateral recumbency will be needed to obtain a lateral or oblique view of the limb. Dorsal recumbency is not typical when obtaining an x-ray of the metacarpus and digits. Han CM, Hurd CD, Practical Diagnostic Imaging for the Veterinary Technician, ed 3, Mosby, 2005, p. 84.

175. b The cranial landmark for a ventrodorsal x-ray of the thorax is the manubrium. The caudal landmark for a ventrodorsal x-ray of the thorax is halfway between the xiphoid and the last rib. The base of the skull is the cranial landmark for a cervical vertebrae x-ray. The ilium wings are the caudal landmark for a lumbar vertebrae x-ray. Han CM, Hurd CD, Practical Diagnostic Imaging for the Veterinary Technician, ed 3, Mosby, 2005, p. 105.

176. b The greater trochanter of the femur is the caudal landmark for an abdominal x-ray in the lateral position. The cranial landmark for a lateral abdominal x-ray is three rib spaces cranial to the xiphoid. The ilium wings are used as landmarks for the lumbar vertebrae. The manubrium is the cranial landmark for a ventrodorsal x-ray of the thorax. Han CM, Hurd CD, Practical Diagnostic Imaging for the Veterinary Technician, ed 3, Mosby, 2005, p. 108.

177. b An abdominal x-ray should be obtained at peak expiration to avoid pressure on the abdominal contents from the diaphragm. Peak inspiration is best used during an x-ray of the thorax. Panting is never ideal during x-rays because of motion artifact. Han CM, Hurd CD, Practical Diagnostic Imaging for the Veterinary Technician, ed 3, Mosby, 2005, p. 108.

178. a The caudal landmark used in lateral pelvic x-ray is the border of the ischium. The cranial landmark is the wings of the ilium for a lateral pelvic x-ray. The xiphoid process is located at the base of the sternum and is used as a landmark for thoracic and abdominal x-rays. The greater trochanter of the femur is used as a caudal landmark for an abdominal x-ray. Han CM, Hurd CD, Practical Diagnostic Imaging for the Veterinary Technician, ed 3, Mosby, 2005, p. 109.

179. d The term *caudocranial* describes a radiographic projection obtained by passing the primary x-ray beam from the caudal surface to the cranial surface of a structure. The term *craniocaudal* describes the radiographic projection obtained by passing the primary x-ray beam from the cranial surface to the caudal surface of a structure. The term *dorsoventral* describes a radiograph produced when the primary x-ray beam enters the dorsal surface and exits the ventral surface of the patient. The term *ventrodorsal* describes a radiograph produced when the primary x-ray beam enters the ventral surface and exits the dorsal surface of the patient. Sirois M, Anthony E, Mauragis D, Handbook of Radiographic Positioning for Veterinary Technicians, ed 1, Delmar Cengage Learning, 2010, p. 3.

180. b Palpating the tibial tuberosity will help determine the amount of rotation necessary for an exact caudocranial projection of the stile joint. The location of the patella will vary in each patient and does not aid in this view. The greater trochanter of the femur is used as the caudal landmark for an abdominal x-ray. The manubrium is used as the cranial landmark for the ventrodorsal x-ray of the thorax. Han CM, Hurd CD, Practical Diagnostic Imaging for the Veterinary Technician, ed 3, Mosby, 2005, p. 116.

181. b Radiopaque areas appear white on x-ray images. Radiolucent areas appear as black on x-ray images. Hyperechoic describes bright echoes seen on ultrasound. Hypoechoic described dark echoes seen on ultrasound. Han CM, Hurd CD, Practical Diagnostic Imaging for the Veterinary Technician, ed 3, Mosby, 2005, p. 129.

182. b If the x-ray beam is aimed more perpendicular to the tooth rather than to the bisecting angle, causing too little vertical angulation, the tooth will appear more elongated. Foreshortening will occur if the beam is more perpendicular to the film, causing too much vertical angulation. The beam should be perpendicular to the bisecting angle to minimize distortion. If you think about the sun hitting an object at noon, the shadow will be very short (foreshortened). If you think about the sun hitting an object at sunset, the shadow will be very long (elongated). Bellows J, "The why, when and how of small animal dental radiology," in The Practice of Veterinary Dentistry: A Team Effort, Iowa State Press, 1999, p. 81-105.

183. a Barium sulfate is commonly used as a positive contrast for gastrointestinal studies only when perforation is not suspected. Meglumine diatrizoate and sodium diatrizoate are commonly used together as a water-soluble organic iodide solution used in GI studies when perforation is suspected. Betadine is not used as a contrast in radiographs. Han CM, Hurd CD, Practical Diagnostic Imaging for the Veterinary Technician, ed 3, Mosby, 2005, p. 130.

184. d It takes approximately 3 hours for barium sulfate to travel from the stomach to the colon. It may take longer than 3 hours to travel to the colon, but it is typically not any faster. Han CM, Hurd CD, Practical Diagnostic Imaging for the Veterinary Technician, ed 3, Mosby, 2005, p. 130.

185. d Barium sulfate preparations are manufactured in the form of powders, colloid suspension, and pastes, and they are for oral use only. The barium sulfate preparation is not injectable. Han CM, Hurd CD, Practical Diagnostic Imaging for the Veterinary Technician, ed 3, Mosby, 2005, p. 130.

186. d Negative-contrast agents used for radiography include air, oxygen, and carbon dioxide because they all have a low atomic number or low density and they appear as radiolucent on x-ray images. Han CM, Hurd CD, Practical Diagnostic Imaging for the Veterinary Technician, ed 3, Mosby, 2005, p. 130.

187. b Water-soluble organic iodides should be avoided in dehydrated patients because they draw excessive amounts of water to the bowel, causing the patient to become more dehydrated. Water-soluble iodide is recommended for use in patients with suspected bowel perforation and in well-hydrated patients. Contrast used in CT imaging should not be used in a patient with kidney failure. Han CM, Hurd CD, Practical Diagnostic Imaging for the Veterinary Technician, ed 3, Mosby, 2005, p. 133.

188. a Placing a reptile on a cool surface or chilling it briefly results in a temporary lethargy or immobility. Excitement, rapid breathing, or aggressiveness can all occur when handling reptiles. Han CM, Hurd

CD, Practical Diagnostic Imaging for the Veterinary Technician, ed 3, Mosby, 2005, p. 169.

189. d To obtain a dorsolateral-plantaromedial oblique view, the cassette should be held on the plantaromedial aspect of the tarsus. The dorsoplantar view would require the cassette to be held on the plantar surface of the joint. A mediolateral view of the tarsal joint would require the cassette to be held on the lateral surface of the joint. To obtain a lateromedial view of the tarsal joint of a horse, the cassette should be placed on the medial surface of the joint. Han CM, Hurd CD, Practical Diagnostic Imaging for the Veterinary Technician, ed 3, Mosby, 2005, p. 197.

190. b When positioning a lizard in the right lateral recumbent position for x-ray imaging, the left limbs are always caudal to the right limbs. In a left lateral recumbent position, the left limbs are always cranial to the right limbs. In a lateral recumbent position the limbs would be placed cranial/caudal to each other, not lateral/medial. Han CM, Hurd CD, Practical Diagnostic Imaging for the Veterinary Technician, ed 3, Mosby, 2005, p. 172.

191. c The tabletop technique is commonly used for all patients whose girth does not exceed 10–12 cm. If the girth exceeds 10–12 cm, a grid technique would be more effective. Han CM, Hurd CD, Practical Diagnostic Imaging for the Veterinary Technician, ed 3, Mosby, 2005, p. 172.

192. c When using a Plexiglas tube to assist in obtaining an x-ray, the kVp should be increased approximately 2–4 units to compensate for the thickness of the tube. The mAs can be left unchanged because this helps in motion artifact. Han CM, Hurd CD, Practical Diagnostic Imaging for the Veterinary Technician, ed 3, Mosby, 2005, p. 175.

193. c Gloved hands are considered a form of manual restraint when obtaining x-ray images. Physical restraints used to obtain x-ray images are tape, radiolucent Plexiglas, foam pads, wooden blocks, and cardboard boxes. Han CM, Hurd CD, Practical Diagnostic Imaging for the Veterinary Technician, ed 3, Mosby, 2005, p. 175.

194. b The cathode is the site of electron generation in the x-ray tube and contains a filament consisting of a tightly coiled tungsten wire. The anode is also the site of electron generation and contains a tungsten metal plate on which the electrons are focused. B-mode is known as brightness mode in ultrasound. A transducer is the handheld unit, which emits a series of pulses and then receives the returning echoes to produce an ultrasound image. Han CM, Hurd CD, Practical Diagnostic Imaging for the Veterinary Technician, ed 3, Mosby, 2005, p. 283.

195. a Roentgen equivalent man (REM) is the amount used to express the dose equivalent that results from exposure to ionizing radiation. The term *ALARA* means "as low as reasonably achievable" and refers to the duty to use the lowest amount of radiation possible to achieve what is necessary. The term *MPD* stands for "maximum permissible dose per person" and should not exceed 5 rem per year. The term *Sv* stands for Sievert, which is used to define a rem: 1 Sv = 100 rem. Han CM, Hurd CD, Practical Diagnostic Imaging for the Veterinary Technician, ed 3, Mosby, 2005, p. 40.

196. b The protective lead worn as required PPE is approximately 0.5 mm thick and only decreases the primary beam exposure by 25%. Han CM, Hurd CD, Practical Diagnostic Imaging for the Veterinary Technician, ed 3, Mosby, 2005, p. 41.

197. d The copper element within the monitoring badges measures the highest level of exposure to radiation. The open window measures the lowest level of exposure, whereas the plastic and aluminum elements measure the medium exposure ranges. Han CM, Hurd CD, Practical Diagnostic Imaging for the Veterinary Technician, ed 3, Mosby, 2005, p. 41.

198. b Film badges are the most common method of monitoring ionizing radiation and are typically worn on the thyroid collar of the team member being exposed. Thermoluminescent dosimeters, optically stimulated luminescence badges, and ion chambers are also used to monitor ionizing radiation exposure, but they are more complex and are not commonly used in practice. Han CM, Hurd CD, Practical Diagnostic Imaging for the Veterinary Technician, ed 3, Mosby, 2005, p. 42.

199. b Digital radiography, CT, MRI, and ultrasound all use the universally accepted format to store images known as DICOM (digital imaging and communication in medicine). CCD is known as a charge-coupled device and is a type of digital radiography. MOD is a magnetic optical disc and is a type of unit that stores DICOM images. PACS is a widely used picture archiving and communication system, which greatly reduces the amount of space needed for storage. Sirois M, Elsevier's Veterinary Assisting Textbook, ed 2, Mosby, 2017, p. 345.

200. b When obtaining a lateromedial view of the carpus of a horse, the cassette should be held on the medial aspect of the leg. When obtaining a dorsomedial-palmarolateral oblique view, the cassette should be held against the palmarolateral aspect of the leg. When obtaining a dorsopalmar view of the carpus, the cassette should be held on the palmar aspect of the carpus. When obtaining a dorsolateral-palmaromedial oblique view, the cassette should be held on the palmaromedial aspect of the leg. Han CM, Hurd CD, Practical Diagnostic Imaging for the Veterinary Technician, ed 3, Mosby, 2005, p. 191.

201. c The limb of a horse should be flexed approximately 60 degrees, keeping the metacarpus parallel and the radius perpendicular to the ground when obtaining an x-ray of the lateromedial view of the carpus. Han CM, Hurd CD, Practical Diagnostic Imaging for the Veterinary Technician, ed 3, Mosby, 2005, p. 192.

202. d For standard radiographs of the tarsus of a horse, the weight should be evenly distributed on all four legs. The limb should be positioned so that the metatarsus is perpendicular to the ground. Han CM, Hurd CD, Practical Diagnostic Imaging for the Veterinary Technician, ed 3, Mosby, 2005, p. 195.

203. b To obtain a lateromedial view of the tarsal joint of a horse, the cassette should be placed on the medial surface of the joint. A mediolateral view of the tarsal joint would require the cassette to be held on the lateral surface of the joint. The dorsoplantar view would require the cassette to be held on the plantar surface of the joint. To obtain a dorsolateral-plantaromedial oblique view, the cassette should be held on the plantaromedial aspect of the tarsus. Han CM, Hurd CD, Practical Diagnostic Imaging for the Veterinary Technician, ed 3, Mosby, 2005, p. 197.

204. c The primary beam projection should be at 60 degrees to obtain a flexed dorsoplantar radiographic view of the tarsal joint of a horse. The metatarsus should be parallel to the ground at a 90-degree angle. The angles of 15 and 45 degrees do not provide an accurate view of the tarsal bones for a flex view. Han CM, Hurd CD, Practical Diagnostic Imaging for the Veterinary Technician, ed 3, Mosby, 2005, p. 199.

205. b To obtain a standard x-ray of the metacarpus of a horse, the limb of interest should be perpendicular to the ground with an even weight distribution all on four limbs. The positions parallel, at 45 degrees, or at 60 degrees would be used for a flexed view. Han CM, Hurd CD, Practical Diagnostic Imaging for the Veterinary Technician, ed 3, Mosby, 2005, p. 199.

206. d To help reduce exposure to the staff, sandbags, sponges, tape, or other restraining devices should be used for positioning the patient rather than manual restraint. Thrall, D. Textbook of Veterinary Diagnostic Radiology, ed 6. W.B. Saunders, 2013, p. 8.

207. b The primary beam needs to be angled 20 degrees proximal to distal to obtain a dorsopalmar view of the fetlock joint. The cassette needs to be placed against the palmar surface of the limb. The natural angle of this joint requires the primary beam to be at 20 degrees proximal to distal. Han CM, Hurd CD, Practical Diagnostic Imaging for the Veterinary Technician, ed 3, Mosby, 2005, p. 208.

208. a The primary beam needs to be angled 15–20 degrees proximal to distal when obtaining a dorsopalmar view of the interphalangeal joint. All four limbs need to be equal in weight bearing and the limb needs to be in its natural position with the leg perpendicular to the ground, which requires the primary beam angle of 15–20 degrees. Han CM, Hurd CD, Practical Diagnostic Imaging for the Veterinary Technician, ed 3, Mosby, 2005, p. 211.

209. d Before imaging the coffin bone it is ideal to do the following in preparation: remove horseshoes, clean and trim the hoof to the new sole, and pack the sulcus with radiolucent material to prevent artifact. Han CM, Hurd CD, Practical Diagnostic Imaging for the Veterinary Technician, ed 3, Mosby, 2005, p. 213.

210. a The cassette should be placed on the cranial aspect when obtaining a caudocranial view of the femorotibial joint of the horse. To obtain a lateromedial view of the femorotibial joint, the cassette should be placed on the medial aspect. The caudocranial and lateromedial views are the only two typical views of the femorotibial joint; therefore, the lateral and medial aspects do not apply. Han CM, Hurd CD, Practical Diagnostic Imaging for the Veterinary Technician, ed 3, Mosby, 2005, p. 221.

211. b To obtain a craniocaudal view of the brachio-antebrachial joint, the limb of the horse should be abducted to separate the elbow from the thoracic musculature, which pulls the limb away from midline. To adduct the limb would mean moving it toward the midline of the body, which would not be ideal for this image. The limb should be extended cranially to obtain a mediolateral view of the brachio-antebrachial joint. To extend the limb caudally does not assist in obtaining a view of the brachio-antebrachial joint. Han CM, Hurd CD, Practical Diagnostic Imaging for the Veterinary Technician, ed 3, Mosby, 2005, p. 224.

212. a To obtain a caudocranial view of the tibia, the patient should be in the sternal recumbent position with the limb of interest extended caudally. Dorsal recumbency would be used to obtain a craniocaudal view of the tibia. The right or left lateral recumbent position would be used to obtain a lateral view of the tibia. Han CM, Hurd CD, Practical Diagnostic Imaging for the Veterinary Technician, ed 3, Mosby, 2005, p. 119.

213. a To obtain a dorsoventral view of the thorax of a rabbit, the center of the beam should be focused over the heart. To obtain an abdominal view of the rabbit, the beam should be centered over the liver. To obtain a whole body view, the beam should be focused over the center of the body from cranial to caudal or at the thoracolumbar area. Han CM, Hurd CD, Practical Diagnostic Imaging for the Veterinary Technician, ed 3, Mosby, 2005, p. 163.

214. c For avian radiography, chemical restraint is the most common form of restraint to avoid injury to the patient. Manual restraint consists of gloved hands to hold the patient, which is not possible in most cases (gloved hands should never enter the direct radiation beam). Physical restraint devices can be used, such as soft nylon ropes, paper tape, IV tubing, or cardboard, but these can only be used in combination with chemical restraints. Han CM, Hurd CD, Practical Diagnostic Imaging for the Veterinary Technician, ed 3, Mosby, 2005, p. 181.

215. a When restraining a bird, grasping the patient around the neck should be avoided because of the potential for tracheal collapse. The correct way to restrain a bird is to grasp it gently by the mandibular articulation and the feet and then to stretch out the bird gently. Han CM, Hurd CD, Practical Diagnostic Imaging for the Veterinary Technician, ed 3, Mosby, 2005, p. 181.

216. b For a lateral avian view, the left wings and limbs should be caudal to the right wings and limbs. For ventrodorsal views, the limbs should be symmetrically extended caudally and the wings abducted laterally. The wings and limbs should never be superimposed on any view; they should be viewed separately. Han CM, Hurd CD, Practical Diagnostic Imaging for the Veterinary Technician, ed 3, Mosby, 2005, p. 181.

217. a The keel is known as the sternum. In a ventrodorsal avian view, the keel should be superimposed over the spine. If the keel is lateral, cranial, or caudal, then the bird is not positioned correctly in the ventrodorsal view. Han CM, Hurd CD, Practical Diagnostic Imaging for the Veterinary Technician, ed 3, Mosby, 2005, p. 181.

218. d To obtain a craniocaudal appendicular skeletal radiograph in a larger species of bird, the limb can be taped directly on the cassette as well as a gloved hand can be placed directly behind the hock to restrain the limb for exposure. The limb should not be directly taped to a Plexiglas plate for larger species. Han CM, Hurd CD, Practical Diagnostic Imaging for the Veterinary Technician, ed 3, Mosby, 2005, p. 183.

219. b The wings should be taped across the humerus, close to the body, to avoid the possibility of a wing fracture if the patient awakens. Placing tape across the radius–ulna area or at the most distal end could result in fracturing the wings if the pet awakens from sedation. Han CM, Hurd CD, Practical Diagnostic Imaging for the Veterinary Technician, ed 3, Mosby, 2005, p. 183.

220. d For obtaining an avian lateral view, the dependent limb should be cranial to the contralateral limb. Moving the limbs in a lateral or medial position is not ideal in a lateral x-ray. Having the limbs superimposed makes it difficult to distinguish one from the other. Han CM, Hurd CD, Practical Diagnostic Imaging for the Veterinary Technician, ed 3, Mosby, 2005, p. 183.

221. c For small patients, a tabletop technique is preferred along with higher mA, shorter exposure time, and lower kVp. The use of a lower mA can result in motion artifact. The use of higher kVp is too much exposure for a small patient. Han CM, Hurd CD, Practical Diagnostic Imaging for the Veterinary Technician, ed 3, Mosby, 2005, p. 158.

222. b The front legs should be extended cranially when obtaining a dorsoventral radiograph of a rodent. The hind limbs should be extended caudally. The limbs should never be superimposed because superimposition makes it difficult to distinguish one from the other. It is not ideal to abduct the limbs away from the body for a dorsoventral view because this would result in the lack of collimation. Han CM, Hurd CD, Practical Diagnostic Imaging for the Veterinary Technician, ed 3, Mosby, 2005, p. 158.

223. b When using a nonscreen film to radiograph a snake, it is important that movement is minimal to prevent motion artifact. The length or size of girth of the snake does not alter the use of nonscreen film. Han CM, Hurd CD, Practical Diagnostic Imaging for the Veterinary Technician, ed 3, Mosby, 2005, p. 175.

224. d Postprocessing manipulation is a huge advantage of using digital x-ray because it allows magnification, rotation, and contrast adjustment. Thrall DE, Textbook of Veterinary Diagnostic Radiology, ed 6, Elsevier, 2013, p. 29.

225. c A digital x-ray includes numerous advantages over analog x-ray, such as elimination of the darkroom, image postprocessing capabilities, exposure latitude and contract optimization, and consolidated image storage. Digital x-ray still uses radiation to obtain an x-ray and all proper precautions should still be considered. Thrall DE, Textbook of Veterinary Diagnostic Radiology, ed 6, Elsevier, 2013, p. 29.

226. b Contrast optimization is a feature of digital radiography that is related to the bit depth of each pixel and the software that accompanies the digital-imaging system. Spatial resolution refers to how small a structure can actually be discriminated in the image. Dynamic range is the difference between the smallest and the largest usable signal through a transmission or processing chain. Exposure latitude refers to the relative independence of digital radiographic image quality on the magnitude of incident x-ray exposure. Thrall DE, Textbook of Veterinary Diagnostic Radiology, ed 6, Elsevier, 2013, p. 29.

227. b Exposure creep can occur in both analog and digital systems. It is concerning in digital systems because it is not as clearly recognized, creating a concern for unnecessary patient and personnel exposure to ionizing radiation. Exposure creep is recognized in an analog system by excessive film blackening. The films are overexposed and not underexposed. Thrall DE, Textbook of Veterinary Diagnostic Radiology, ed 6, Elsevier, 2013, p. 33.

228. d Horses have approximately seven carpal bones, each with its own unique shape, and they are arranged in two rows. The most distal row is composed of the 2nd, 3rd, and 4th carpal bones. The accessory carpal bone stands alone behind the ulnar carpal bone. The upper row comprises the radial, intermediate, and ulnar carpal bones. Farrow CS, Veterinary Diagnostic Imaging: The Horse, Mosby Elsevier, 2006, p. 150.

229. b The dorsopalmar view of the carpal joint provides the best view in which to judge the width of the cartilage spaces. The lateral view is the best view for judging a major fracture dislocation and conformational abnormalities. The medial oblique view of the carpal joint is the best view for detecting slab fractures. The flexed lateral view of the carpal joint is the best view for detecting distal corner fractures. Farrow CS, Veterinary Diagnostic Imaging: The Horse, Mosby Elsevier, 2006, p. 153.

230. d The dorsopalmar view is the best view to evaluate distal radial growth plate closure. The lateral view is the best view for judging a major fracture dislocation and conformational abnormalities. The flexed lateral view of the carpal joint is the best view for detecting distal corner fractures. The medial oblique view of the carpal joint is the best view for detecting slab fractures. Farrow CS, Veterinary Diagnostic Imaging: The Horse, Mosby Elsevier, 2006, p. 153.

231. c In the presence of fresh carpal chips in horses, the surrounding bone density appears normal on x-ray images. In old carpal chips, the adjacent bone density appears decreased. Farrow CS, Veterinary Diagnostic Imaging: The Horse, Mosby Elsevier, 2006, p. 155.

232. a Old carpal chip fractures in horses have all of the following radiographic characteristics: vague fragment margination, decreased adjacent bone density, presence of osteoarthritis, and normal or cool surrounding tissue. Sharp fragment margination is seen with fresh carpal chips in horses. Farrow CS, Veterinary Diagnostic Imaging: The Horse, Mosby Elsevier, 2006, p. 155.

233. b Slab fractures, also known as biarticular fractures, are considered the most destabilizing and most serious of all carpal fractures. Corner fractures are more serious than chip fractures, creating more bone, cartilage, and capsular damage. Chip fractures are the least serious of the carpal fractures, in that small flakes or chunks of bone are sheared off. Farrow CS, Veterinary Diagnostic Imaging: The Horse, Mosby Elsevier, 2006, p. 156.

234. c Radiographically, the flexed lateral view has been shown as the most accurate in detecting carpal fractures and it shows fragment mobility. The dorsopalmar view is the least revealing in carpal fractures but it is best for evaluating distal radial growth plate closures. The lateral view is best for evaluating major fracture dislocation and conformational abnormalities. The medial oblique view is best for detecting slab fractures. Farrow CS, Veterinary Diagnostic Imaging: The Horse, Mosby Elsevier, 2006, p. 159.

235. b The bones of foals radiographically appear as smoother, rounder, and smaller than those of the adult horse. They also are unfused and composed mostly of cartilage in which the spaces appear wider than those seen in adults. Farrow CS, Veterinary Diagnostic Imaging: The Horse, Mosby Elsevier, 2006, p. 1.

236. c The first radiographic appearance of the crena occurs between 4 and 22 weeks. The closure of the distal growth plate of MC3 occurs at 18–38 weeks. The closure of the proximal growth plate of P1 occurs between 22 and 38 weeks. Between 0 and 4 weeks, most growth plates are still visible. Farrow CS, Veterinary Diagnostic Imaging: The Horse, Mosby Elsevier, 2006, p. 4.

237. a The following are considered key radiographic features of carpal or tarsal bone immaturity: poor calcification, increased number of visible vascular canals causing increased porosity, abnormally tapered profile, and one or more fringed margins. Farrow CS, Veterinary Diagnostic Imaging: The Horse, Mosby Elsevier, 2006, p. 7.

238. c A valgus deformity is one in which the interior angle of the joint, viewed frontally, is greater than 180 degrees. A varus deformity is one in which the interior angle, viewed frontally, is less than 180 degrees. The term *axial rotation* pertains to foals with angular limb deformities. The term *windswept* refers to the combination of valgus and varus deformity. Farrow CS, Veterinary Diagnostic Imaging: The Horse, Mosby Elsevier, 2006, p. 10.

239. a A grade level 1 for the carpal and tarsal ossification index of newborn foals is described as an unossified carpal and tarsal bone. A grade 2 is described as the partial ossification of carpal and tarsal bones. A grade 3 describes all carpal or tarsal bones mineralized. A grade 4 describes the carpal and tarsal bones fully mineralized. Farrow CS, Veterinary Diagnostic Imaging: The Horse, Mosby Elsevier, 2006, p. 15.

240. c The correct abbreviation for craniocaudal is CrCd, which describes the projection obtained by passing the primary x-ray beam from the cranial surface to the caudal surface of a structure. The abbreviation for caudocranial is CdCr. The abbreviation for dorsopalmar is Dpa. The abbreviation for cranial is Cr. Sirois M, Anthony E, Mauragis D, Handbook of Radiographic Positioning for Veterinary Technicians, ed 1, Delmar Cengage Learning, 2010, p. 3.

241. c The term *palmar* describes the caudal surface of the forelimb distal to the carpus. The term *plantar* describes the caudal surface of the hind limb distal to the tarsus. The term *dorsopalmar* describes the radiographic views distal to the carpus obtained by passing the primary x-ray beam from the dorsal direction to the palmar surface of the forelimb. The term *caudocranial* describes the radiographic projection obtained by passing the primary x-ray beam from the caudal surface to the cranial surface of a structure. Sirois M, Anthony E, Mauragis D, Handbook of Radiographic Positioning for Veterinary Technicians, ed 1, Delmar Cengage Learning, 2010, p. 3.

242. b The term *ventrodorsal* describes a radiograph produced when the primary x-ray beam enters the ventral surface and exits the dorsal surface of the patient. The term *dorsoventral* describes a radiograph produced when the primary x-ray beam enters the dorsal surface and exits the ventral surface of the patient. The term *craniocaudal* describes the radiographic projection obtained by passing the primary x-ray beam from the cranial surface to the caudal surface of a structure. The term *caudocranial* describes a radiographic projection obtained by passing the primary x-ray beam from the caudal surface to the cranial surface of a structure. Sirois M, Anthony E, Mauragis D, Handbook of Radiographic Positioning for Veterinary Technicians, ed 1, Delmar Cengage Learning, 2010, p. 3.

243. c Radiographs of long bones should include both the proximal and distal joints. If the patient is too large to fit on one film, then multiple images might be necessary. Sirois M, Anthony E, Mauragis D, Handbook of Radiographic Positioning for Veterinary Technicians, ed 1, Delmar Cengage Learning, 2010, p. 6.

244. d Radiographs of joints must include ⅓ of the bones both proximal and distal to the joint. It is important to include bones on both sides of the joint in question to rule out any complications. Sirois M, Anthony E, Mauragis D, Handbook of Radiographic Positioning for Veterinary Technicians, ed 1, Delmar Cengage Learning, 2010, p. 6.

245. b The proper collimated radiograph appears as clear, unexposed areas of all four edges of the film of a finished radiograph. Black, fully exposed edges of the film demonstrate a fully exposed noncollimated radiograph. Collimation includes all four edges; any edge that has full exposure does not meet the collimation requirements. Sirois M, Anthony E, Mauragis D, Handbook of Radiographic Positioning for Veterinary Technicians, ed 1, Delmar Cengage Learning, 2010, p. 6.

246. d When using a V-trough, the correct measurement should include both the V-trough and the thickest portion of the body to be measured. The thinnest portion of the body is incorrect and does not accommodate for the correct kVp setting. The V-trough alone does not allow for the proper kVp setting to include the body being imaged. Sirois M, Anthony E, Mauragis D, Handbook of Radiographic Positioning for Veterinary Technicians, ed 1, Delmar Cengage Learning, 2010, p. 6.

247. b The thickest part of the area of interest should be placed toward the cathode end of the x-ray tube, which takes advantage of the heel effect. The thickest part of the area of interest being placed toward the anode end of the x-ray tube does not aid in the heel effect. The primary area of interest should be placed in the center of the x-ray beam, but it is not necessarily the thickest portion. Being placed close to the radiographer does not have any bearing on the creation of a better image. Sirois M, Anthony E, Mauragis D, Handbook of Radiographic Positioning for Veterinary Technicians, ed 1, Delmar Cengage Learning, 2010, p. 5.

248. a To decrease magnification of an x-ray, the patient should be positioned as close to the x-ray cassette as possible. To increase magnification of an x-ray there should be an increase in the amount of distance between the patient and the cassette. The amount of collimation does not change the amount of magnification of the x-ray; it only provides a clearer image and less scatter radiation. Sirois M, Anthony E, Mauragis D, Handbook of Radiographic Positioning for Veterinary Technicians, ed 1, Delmar Cengage Learning, 2010, p. 6.

249. b The term *splitting the plate* refers to using a lead shield on half of the film to prevent exposure and allowing for two views to be obtained on the same film. After the first side is exposed, the lead is switched and the desired view is obtained on the other side. If there is only a large cassette and film available, the beam should be collimated to accommodate the size of the patient. A large cassette cannot be split to create multiple smaller cassettes. Sirois M, Anthony E, Mauragis D, Handbook of Radiographic Positioning for Veterinary Technicians, ed 1, Delmar Cengage Learning, 2010, p. 6.

250. e To obtain images of the nasal passages of small animals, the following are required: lateral view, DV or VD, rostrocaudal view, and an open-mouth view. Sirois M, Anthony E, Mauragis D, Handbook of Radiographic Positioning for Veterinary Technicians, ed 1, Delmar Cengage Learning, 2010, p. 109.

251. c The correct area to obtain a measurement for radiographs of the nasal passages is slightly rostral to the widest area of the cranium to avoid overexposing the air-filled sinuses. The most rostral end of the cranium may be too thin and might not allow enough exposure to obtain quality images. The most caudal end of the cranium is typically wide and will cause overexposure of the nasal passages. Using the widest portion of the cranium will allow overexposure of the nasal passages. Sirois M, Anthony E, Mauragis D, Handbook of Radiographic Positioning for Veterinary Technicians, ed 1, Delmar Cengage Learning, 2010, p. 109.

252. a When obtaining either a VD or DV projection of the skull, the center should be midway between the tip of the nose to just caudal to the occipital protuberance at the base. To obtain a lateral projection of the skull, the beam should be centered at the lateral canthus of the eye socket. To obtain a rostrocaudal foramen magnum projection, the center should be between the eyes. To obtain a rostrocaudal tympanic bullae open-mouth projection, the beam is centered just above the base of the tongue and just below the soft palate, approximately at the commissure of the mouth. Sirois M, Anthony E, Mauragis D, Handbook of Radiographic Positioning for Veterinary Technicians, ed 1, Delmar Cengage Learning, 2010, p. 110.

253. c To obtain a radiograph of the right temporomandibular joint, the patient should be placed in right lateral recumbency, allowing the skull to be oblique toward the table at approximately 10 degrees. To obtain an image of the left temporomandibular joint, the patient should be placed in left lateral recumbency, allowing the skull to be oblique toward the table at approximately 10 degrees. To obtain a DV temporomandibular joint projection of both joints, the patient is placed in sternal recumbency. Typically, ventral recumbency is not used to view the temporomandibular joint. Sirois M, Anthony E, Mauragis D, Handbook of Radiographic Positioning for Veterinary Technicians, ed 1, Delmar Cengage Learning, 2010, p. 130.

254. b To obtain a radiograph of the VD extended hip projection, the beam is centered at a midline between the left and right ischial tuberosity. The lateral projection of the pelvis is centered at the greater trochanter of the femur. The level of the 7th vertebra is at the level of the beginning of the pelvis and is too high to center the beam for a VD extended hip projection. The level of the mid-femur is too low to obtain a full view of the VD extended hip projection. Sirois M, Anthony E, Mauragis D, Handbook of Radiographic Positioning for Veterinary Technicians, ed 1, Delmar Cengage Learning, 2010, p. 26.

255. a To obtain a lateral projection of the pelvis, the area that should be measured is at the highest level of the trochanter. To obtain a VD frog-leg projection or extended hip projection, the measurement should be taken at the thickest part of the pelvis. Measuring the thinnest part of the pelvis will create an underexposed film. Measuring at the level of the 7th vertebra does not account for the thickest part of the pelvis and will not provide proper technique and exposure of the film. Sirois M, Anthony E, Mauragis D, Handbook of Radiographic Positioning for Veterinary Technicians, ed 1, Delmar Cengage Learning, 2010, p. 30.

256. c To obtain a CdCr (caudocranial) projection of the scapula, the patient should be in a dorsal recumbent position with the forelimbs extended cranially and the hind limbs extended caudally. To obtain a lateral projection of the scapula, the patient should be in a lateral recumbent position. Sternal recumbency or standing positions are not typically used in imaging the scapula. Sirois M, Anthony E, Mauragis D, Handbook of Radiographic Positioning for Veterinary Technicians, ed 1, Delmar Cengage Learning, 2010, p. 38.

257. a To obtain a CdCr projection of the humerus, the measurement should be taken from the table to the midshaft humerus; this accounts for the distance from the humerus to the table because they are not in contact. The thickest part of the humerus does not account for the distance between the humerus and the table. Measuring from the dorsal side from the table to the height of the scapula is the technique used for the lateral projection of the scapula. Measuring the midshaft humerus does not account for the distance from the humerus to the table. Sirois M, Anthony E, Mauragis D, Handbook of Radiographic Positioning for Veterinary Technicians, ed 1, Delmar Cengage Learning, 2010, p. 42.

258. b To obtain a flexed lateral projection of the carpal joint, the measurement should be obtained at the thickest part of the flexed joint. Measuring caudal to the carpal joint does not account for the thickest part of the carpus. This view requires a flexed joint and should be measured in the flexed position. Measuring in the nonflexed position does not account for increasing thickness. Measuring cranial to the carpal joint does not account for the thickness of the joint. Sirois M, Anthony E, Mauragis D, Handbook of Radiographic Positioning for Veterinary Technicians, ed 1, Delmar Cengage Learning, 2010, p. 60.

259. c Two landmarks must be present to determine the bisecting angle—the plane of the film and the long axis of the tooth. An angle is formed where the tooth hinges to the film. That angle is bisected and the x-ray beam comes in 90 degrees or perpendicular to that bisection line. If the beam is 90 degrees to the bisecting angle, minimal distortion occurs. Gorrel C, Derbyshire S, "Dental radiography," Veterinary Dentistry for the Nurse and Technician, ed 1, Saunders, 2009, p. 55-67.

260. c The grid is located in or under the table. The cathode, anode, and tungsten filament are housed in the x-ray tube. Sirois M, Elsevier's Veterinary Assisting Textbook, ed 2, Mosby, 2017, p. 337.

261. d With film-based x-ray imaging there are three receptor components that include the cassette, the intensifying screen, and the film. Brown M, Brown L, Lavin's Radiography for Veterinary Technicians, ed 6, Saunders, 2018, p. 43.

SECTION 11

1. a Larger areas can be targeted by use of regional anesthesia, which refers to a loss of sensation in a limited area of the body produced by administration of a local anesthetic or other agent in proximity to sensory nerves. Local anesthesia refers to loss of sensation in a small area of the body produced by administration of a local anesthetic agent in proximity to the area of interest. Infiltration of local anesthetic into the tissues surrounding a small tumor to facilitate removal is an example of local anesthesia. Topical anesthesia is the loss of sensation of a localized area produced by administration of a local anesthetic directly to a body surface or to a surgical or traumatic wound. Hypnosis is a drug-induced sleep-like state that impairs the ability of the patient to respond appropriately to stimuli. Thomas J, Phillip L, Anesthesia and Analgesia for Veterinary Technicians, ed 5, Elsevier, 2017.

2. b If a ball is used instead of a bobbin to read oxygen flow rate through the system, the gas flow is read from the center of the ball. The top of the ball would give an erroneous reading that is too high, and the bottom would give a reading that is too low. Alibhai H, "The anaesthetic machine and vaporizers," in Duke-Novakovski T, de Vries M, Seymour C, BSAVA Manual of Canine and Feline Anaesthesia and Analgesia, ed 3, British Small Animal Veterinary Association, 2016.

3. b Balanced anesthesia is defined as the administration of multiple drugs concurrently in smaller quantities than would be required if each were given alone. Balanced anesthesia maximizes benefits, minimizes adverse effects, and gives the anesthetist the ability to produce anesthesia with the degree of CNS depression, muscle relaxation, analgesia, and immobilization appropriate for the patient and the procedure. General anesthesia does not always produce balanced anesthesia; the same applies when a local anesthesia is added. Thomas J, Phillip L, Anesthesia and Analgesia for Veterinary Technicians, ed 5, Elsevier, 2017.

4. d Local anesthesia is a loss of sensation in a small area of the body produced by administration of a local anesthetic. Sedation is a drug-induced CNS depression and drowsiness that vary in intensity from light to deep. Surgical anesthesia refers to the specific stage within general anesthesia in which there is a sufficient degree of analgesia and muscle relaxation to allow surgery to be performed without patient pain or movement. Thomas J, Phillip L, Anesthesia and Analgesia for Veterinary Technicians, ed 5, Elsevier, 2017.

5. a Most anesthetic agents have a very narrow therapeutic index and the consequences of a calculation or administration error may be serious. Therefore, care and attention to detail are critical when doses are calculated and rates of administration are adjusted. Thomas J, Phillip L, Anesthesia and Analgesia for Veterinary Technicians, ed 5, Elsevier, 2017.

6. b Methadone is the least likely to cause vomiting and may be preferred in the ophthalmology patient. Morphine is the opioid most likely to cause vomiting and should be avoided when possible in the patient undergoing an ophthalmic procedure because of the potential rise in IOP. Midazolam and diazepam are not opioids; they are benzodiazepines. Lockhead K, "Anesthesia for Ophthalmology Patients," in Bryant S, Anesthesia for Veterinary Technicians, ed 1, Blackwell, 2010, p. 196.

7. d Of the listed drugs, only butorphanol can be classified as an opioid. Carprofen is a nonsteroidal anti-inflammatory and amantadine and ketamine are NMDA receptor antagonists. Murrell JC, "Premedications and Sedation," in Seymour C, Duke-Novakovski T, BSAVA Manual of Canine and Feline Anesthesia and Analgesia, ed 2, British Small Animal Veterinary Association, 2007. Murrell JC, "Pre-anaesthetic medication and sedation," in Duke-Novakovski T, de Vries M, Seymour C, BSAVA Manual of Canine and Feline Anaesthesia and Analgesia, ed 3, British Small Animal Veterinary Association, 2016.

8. d The body condition score is important because changes in body weight influence patient management. Excessive thinness may indicate the presence of an underlying disorder such as hyperthyroidism or chronic parasitism, which may increase patient risk. Animals with little body fat are more sensitive to the effects of some anesthetics such as the ultra–short-acting barbiturates and are more prone to hypothermia than patients of normal body weight. Obesity also poses difficulties for the anesthetist. Obese animals may have compromised cardiovascular function and decreased functional lung volume. In addition, venipuncture and auscultation are more difficult in obese patients. When patients are significantly overweight, anesthetics should be dosed according to lean body weight (excluding body fat) instead of total body weight. This is because body fat increases the total body weight but not the volume or weight of the nervous tissue on which anesthetics exert their effect. Administration of a dose calculated by using total body weight results in an anesthetic overdose. Therefore, the anesthetist must use the body condition score along with the actual patient weight to estimate lean body weight. Dehydration, anemia, and bruising all increase the risk associated with anesthesia. Thomas J, Phillip L, Anesthesia and Analgesia for Veterinary Technicians, ed 5, Elsevier, 2017.

9. b When a capnometer is combined with a continuous graphical display, this monitoring device is referred to as a capnograph. A pulse oximeter provides information about the saturation of oxygen; however, it does not give information about carbon dioxide levels. There is not a device to measure CRT. Schauvliege S "Patient Monitoring and Monitoring Equipment," in Duke-Novakovski T, de Vries M, Seymour C, BSAVA Manual of Canine and Feline Anaesthesia and Analgesia, ed 3, British Small Animal Veterinary Association, 2016.

10. a The Doppler probe is placed over the artery with the blood pressure cuff placed proximal to it. The sphygmomanometer is used to inflate the cuff until the heartbeat is no longer audible. The cuff is slowly deflated until the heartbeats are audible again. The number on the sphygmomanometer correlating to the first audible heartbeat is the systolic blood pressure. This method is only used for systolic blood pressure. Reuss-Lamky, HL, "Monitoring Blood Pressure and End-Tidal CO2 in the Anesthetized Patient," in Muir WW, Hubbell JA, Bednarski RM, Lerche P, Handbook of Veterinary Anesthesia, ed 5, Elsevier, 2013.

11. a When activating the oxygen flush valve, oxygen is delivered into the system at a very high flow 30–70 L/min at a pressure of approximately 400 kPa. This can cause severe barotrauma and even death if a patient is attached to the system. This becomes even more dangerous if the oxygen flush valve is pushed while the patient is connected and the pop-off valve is closed. The oxygen supply needs to be connected for the flush valve to work. For this reason, a patient should be disconnected from the breathing circuit. Alibhai H, "The anaesthetic machine and vaporizers," in Duke-Novakovski T, de Vries M, Seymour C, BSAVA Manual of Canine and Feline Anaesthesia and Analgesia, ed 3, British Small Animal Veterinary Association, 2016.

12. c A stuporous patient (noun form stupor) is in a sleep-like state and can be aroused only with a painful stimulus. Patients with a mildly decreased LOC that can be aroused with minimal difficulty are said to be lethargic. The word lethargy is a noun describing this state. Patients that are more depressed and that cannot be fully aroused are referred to as obtunded (noun form obtundity). A comatose patient (noun form coma) cannot be aroused and is unresponsive to all stimuli including pain. Thomas J, Phillip L, Anesthesia and Analgesia for Veterinary Technicians, ed 5, Elsevier, 2017.

13. c Direct blood pressure monitoring is done by placing a catheter into an artery and hooking up a transducer to the monitor. This is the gold standard of blood pressure monitoring and is also referred to as invasive blood pressure monitoring. The other methods are indirect or noninvasive blood pressure methods. Reuss-Lamky HL, "Monitoring Blood Pressure and End-Tidal CO_2 in the Anesthetized Patient," in Bryant S, Anesthesia for Veterinary Technicians, ed 1, Wiley-Blackwell, 2010.

14. c Hetastarch is a colloid solution. Lactated Ringer's (LR), normal saline, and 5% dextrose are all considered crystalloid solutions. Thomas J, Phillip L, Anesthesia and Analgesia for Veterinary Technicians, ed 5, Elsevier, 2017.

15. b The vaporizer is a device that delivers clinically safe and effective concentrations of anesthetic vapors. Most anesthetic gases are liquids at room temperature and pressure and therefore need to be vaporized before being delivered to the patient. The vaporizer does not regulate the flow of oxygen; that is the function of the oxygen flowmeter. The vaporizer does not measure the pressure of gas in the system. Alibhai H, "The anaesthetic machine and vaporizers," in Duke-Novakovski T, de Vries M, Seymour C, BSAVA Manual of Canine and Feline Anaesthesia and Analgesia, ed 3, British Small Animal Veterinary Association, 2016.

16. c A patient that is moderately dehydrated or anemic would be classified as P3 and at moderate risk. A patient with mild dehydration or obese would be considered P2, low risk, whereas a patient suffering from internal hemorrhage would be classified as P4, high risk. Thomas J, Phillip L, Anesthesia and Analgesia for Veterinary Technicians, ed 5, Elsevier, 2017.

17. c Whole blood is considered a colloid. The LR, NR, and hypertonic saline are examples of crystalloids, which are solutions that contain electrolyte and nonelectrolyte solutes. Beiter C, "Fluid Therapy and Blood Products," in Bryant S, Anesthesia for Veterinary Technicians, ed 1, Wiley-Blackwell, 2010, p. 124.

18. a In healthy, calm patients, lung sounds should be very quiet. The presence of discontinuous lung sounds (crackles, rales, or rhonchi) or continuous sounds (wheezes) may indicate either pulmonary conditions (including pneumonia, bronchial disease, or asthma) or heart failure. An animal that appears lethargic is important to recognize but is not the most significant factor in the options provided. A body temperature of 104.1°F is also important but may be attributed to other factors. A sinus arrhythmia is a common finding in dogs. Thomas J, Phillip L, Anesthesia and Analgesia for Veterinary Technicians, ed 5, Elsevier, 2017.

19. b Desflurane has a very low boiling point (23°C) and therefore has to be contained within an electrically heated chamber that raises the temperature of desflurane to 39°C so that it can be used effectively by the vaporizer. Isoflurane and sevoflurane do not require a temperature-controlled vaporizer that needs to be heated. Halothane is sensitive to temperature; however, it does not come with a vaporizer that heats the gas. Alibhai H, "The anaesthetic machine and vaporizers," in Duke-Novakovski T, de Vries M, Seymour C, BSAVA Manual of Canine and Feline Anaesthesia and Analgesia, ed 3, British Small Animal Veterinary Association, 2016.

20. a Brachycephalic animals are difficult to intubate and must be watched closely to ensure a patent airway before, during, and after any anesthetic procedure. Members of these breeds often require use of smaller endotracheal tubes than most other breeds. Exotic breeds, cats, horses, and sighthounds have fewer sections and larger airways, therefore decreasing the risk associated with airway obstruction. Thomas J, Phillip L, Anesthesia and Analgesia for Veterinary Technicians, ed 5, Elsevier, 2017.

21. d Tidal volume is the volume of gas exhaled in one breath, with an approximate value of 10–20 mL/kg. Hughes L, "Breathing Systems and Ancillary Equipment," in Duke-Novakovski T, de Vries M, Seymour C, BSAVA Manual of Canine and Feline Anaesthesia and Analgesia, ed 3, British Small Animal Veterinary Association, 2016.

22. a Inappropriate cuff size is the leading cause of inaccurate blood pressure readings. The width of the cuff should be approximately 40% of the circumference of the leg in dogs. A circumference that is larger or smaller leads to inappropriate readings. Reuss-Lamky HL, "Monitoring Blood Pressure and End-Tidal CO_2 in the Anesthetized Patient," in Bryant S, Anesthesia for Veterinary Technicians, ed 1, Wiley-Blackwell, 2010.

23. c Minute volume refers to the sum of all gas volumes exhaled in one minute. It is calculated as a multiple of tidal volume and respiration rate. The volume of gas exhaled in one breath is the tidal volume. Hughes L, "Breathing Systems and Ancillary Equipment," in Duke-Novakovski T, de Vries M, Seymour C, BSAVA Manual of Canine and Feline Anaesthesia and Analgesia, ed 3, British Small Animal Veterinary Association, 2016.

24. d When possible, choose a large-diameter catheter in case rapid fluid administration is necessary, as would be the case with excessive blood loss or hypotension. Thomas J, Phillip L, Anesthesia and Analgesia for Veterinary Technicians, ed 5, Elsevier, 2017.

25. c Calcium hydroxide is the main component of soda lime and is the product used to absorb CO2 from the breathing system. Potassium hydroxide had previously been used as a component to absorb CO2, but it has been long discontinued. Baking soda cannot be used to absorb excess CO2 from the breathing system. Hughes L, "Breathing Systems and Ancillary Equipment," in Duke-Novakovski T, de Vries M, Seymour C, BSAVA Manual of Canine and Feline Anaesthesia and Analgesia, ed 3, British Small Animal Veterinary Association, 2016.

26. d The blood pressure cuff is most commonly placed on the forelimb, followed by the hind limb and then tail. The foot is not an acceptable area for cuff placement. Reuss-Lamky HL, "Monitoring Blood Pressure and End-Tidal CO_2 in the Anesthetized Patient," in Bryant S, Anesthesia for Veterinary Technicians, ed 1, Wiley-Blackwell, 2010.

27. c The Murphy eye is an oval hole opposite the bevel. This hole allows gas to flow through the tube if the bevel edge should become obstructed. Hughes L, "Breathing Systems and Ancillary Equipment," in Duke-Novakovski T, de Vries M, Seymour C, BSAVA Manual of Canine and Feline Anaesthesia and Analgesia, ed 3, British Small Animal Veterinary Association, 2016.

28. a Water is the most prevalent substance in the body. In adult animals, about 60% of the body weight is water. Thomas J, Phillip L, Anesthesia and Analgesia for Veterinary Technicians, ed 5, Elsevier, 2017.

29. c Isotonic, polyionic replacement crystalloids including lactated Ringer's and Normosol-R are the first choice for fluid therapy for healthy patients undergoing routine surgery as well as many sick patients (as long as the PCV is >20% and the plasma protein is >3.5 gm/dL). Consequently, these fluids are used in the vast majority of anesthetized patients. Hypertonic saline acts rapidly but temporarily and is often used in emergency settings. A 50% dextrose solution is not used to support dehydration. Thomas J, Phillip L, Anesthesia and Analgesia for Veterinary Technicians, ed 5, Elsevier, 2017.

30. d There are many disadvantages of using a chamber to induce anesthesia, which include but are not limited to the patient struggling causes increased catecholamines, an increased risk of cardiac arrhythmias, and staff exposure to harmful waste gases when the chamber is opened when the animal is retrieved. Hughes L, "Breathing Systems and Ancillary Equipment," in Duke-Novakovski T, de Vries M, Seymour C, BSAVA Manual of Canine and Feline Anaesthesia and Analgesia, ed 3, British Small Animal Veterinary Association, 2016.

31. d An intestinal foreign body would not call for the use of a controlled ventilator because the condition will most likely not involve the thoracic cavity. All of the remaining factors can be indicators for placing a patient on a controlled ventilator. If a patient has an inability to ventilate because of factors such as decreased ventilator drive resulting from anesthetic agents or the patient having a thoracotomy, the patient should be placed on a ventilator for controlled ventilation during the anesthetic event. Hammond R, Murison P, "Automatic ventilators," in Duke-Novakovski T, de Vries M, Seymour C, BSAVA Manual of Canine and Feline Anaesthesia and Analgesia, ed 3, British Small Animal Veterinary Association, 2016.

32. d Microdrip sets deliver fluids at a rate of 60 drops per milliliter and are used for infusion rates less than 100 mL/h. Thomas J, Phillip L, Anesthesia and Analgesia for Veterinary Technicians, ed 5, Elsevier, 2017.

33. b An ear pinch would not be a clinical sign used to evaluate the depth of anesthesia. Eye position, jaw tone, and presence of absence of palpebral reflex should be used to evaluate the patient's depth while under anesthesia. Schauvliege S, "Patient Monitoring and Monitoring Equipment," in Duke-Novakovski T, de Vries M, Seymour C, BSAVA Manual of Canine and Feline Anaesthesia and Analgesia, ed 3, British Small Animal Veterinary Association, 2016.

34. b Patients with perioperative hemorrhage may benefit from colloid solutions, which draw water into the vascular space and raise blood pressure. Standard shock doses of fluids can be up to 90 mL/h/kg in dogs, whereas routine surgery rates are approximately 10 mL/kg/h. Colloids are given at lower administration rates than crystalloids. Hypertonic saline is administered in small volumes to patients in shock. Thomas J, Phillip L, Anesthesia and Analgesia for Veterinary Technicians, ed 5, Elsevier, 2017.

35. a An esophageal stethoscope is an easy way for the technician anesthetist to auscultate the heart and lungs at times when placing a traditional stethoscope on a patient's chest would be contraindicated (as it is in surgical cases because of sterility). An esophageal stethoscope cannot measure central venous pressure, temperature, or end tidal carbon dioxide. Schauvliege S "Patient Monitoring and Monitoring Equipment," in Duke-Novakovski T, de Vries M, Seymour C, BSAVA Manual of Canine and Feline Anaesthesia and Analgesia, ed 3, British Small Animal Veterinary Association, 2016.

36. b Of the described terms, capnometry correctly describes the monitoring parameter used for the measurement and numerical display of the carbon dioxide concentration in the respiratory gas. An electrocardiogram gives information about the electrical activity through the heart. The pulse oximeter does give information about the saturation of oxygen; however, it does not give information about carbon dioxide levels. Carbon dioxide levels are not a monitoring parameter for capillary refill times. Schauvliege S "Patient Monitoring and Monitoring Equipment," in Duke-Novakovski T, de Vries M, Seymour C, BSAVA Manual of Canine and Feline Anaesthesia and Analgesia, ed 3, British Small Animal Veterinary Association, 2016.

37. b When monitoring any anesthetized patient that is receiving IV fluids, the anesthetist should be alert for signs of overhydration. These include ocular and nasal discharge, chemosis (edema and swelling of the conjunctiva), subcutaneous edema, increased lung sounds, increased respiratory rate, and dyspnea. Thomas J, Phillip L, Anesthesia and Analgesia for Veterinary Technicians, ed 5, Elsevier, 2017.

38. c A capnometer in which the measuring chambers are placed directly in the airway and the measurement signal is generated there is referred to as a mainstream capnometer. Sidestream capnometers are connected to the endotracheal tube via an end piece that contains a sampling line that continuously samples respiratory gases. The terms *endstream* and *invasive* are not used to describe capnometers. Schauvliege S, "Patient Monitoring and Monitoring Equipment," in Duke-Novakovski T, de Vries M, Seymour C, BSAVA Manual of Canine and Feline Anaesthesia and Analgesia, ed 3, British Small Animal Veterinary Association, 2016.

39. d All of the given locations can be used as placement for a pulse oximeter. A pulse oximeter uses a transmitter and receiver of red and infrared light and is positioned to transilluminate a pulsatile arteriolar bed. In small animal patients, it can be placed in any light-colored or nonpigmented area such as the tongue, toes, or prepuce. Schauvliege S, "Patient Monitoring and Monitoring Equipment," in Duke-Novakovski T, de Vries M, Seymour C, BSAVA Manual of Canine and Feline Anaesthesia and Analgesia, ed 3, British Small Animal Veterinary Association, 2016.

40. d Third-degree AV block is an abnormal rhythm in which the atrial and ventricular contractions occur independently. It is recognized by a complete loss of the normal relationship between the P waves and QRS complexes and is characterized by randomly irregular PR intervals. This rhythm indicates cardiac disease and is infrequently seen in anesthetized patients, but when present, it decreases cardiac output and requires treatment. NSR is a regular rhythm in which the HR is normal and the distance between each heartbeat (each QRS complex) is approximately equal. SA is a cyclic change in the HR coordinated with respirations, in which the HR decreases (recognized by an increased distance between QRS complexes) during expiration and increases (recognized by a decreased distance between QRS complexes) during inspiration. Second-degree AV block appears as occasional missing QRS complexes. Thomas J, Phillip L, Anesthesia and Analgesia for Veterinary Technicians, ed 5, Elsevier, 2017.

41. a Invasive blood pressure measurements via either CVP or direct arterial measurements are considered gold standard in terms of accurate measurements when it comes to blood pressure. Doppler and oscillometric methods are both considered noninvasive methods and are thought to be not as accurate as direct or invasive blood pressure monitoring. Schauvliege S, "Patient Monitoring and Monitoring Equipment," in Duke-Novakovski T, de Vries M, Seymour C, BSAVA Manual of Canine and Feline Anaesthesia and Analgesia, ed 3, British Small Animal Veterinary Association, 2016.

42. a Tidal volume is the volume of gas exhaled in one breath. An approximate value is 10–20 mL/kg. Hughes L, "Breathing Systems and Ancillary Equipment," in Duke-Novakovski T, de Vries M, Seymour C, BSAVA Manual of Canine and Feline Anaesthesia and Analgesia, ed 3, British Small Animal Veterinary Association, 2016.

43. c Neuroleptanalgesia is a state of profound sedation and analgesia induced by the simultaneous administration of an opioid and a tranquilizer. Thomas J, Phillip L, Anesthesia and Analgesia for Veterinary Technicians, ed 5, Elsevier, 2017.

44. a The classic approach to measurement of central venous pressures is to position a long intravenous catheter via the jugular vein in the thoracic portion of the vena cava. The catheter is not placed into the atrium or ventricles of the heart. Peripheral veins such as cephalic veins or saphenous veins are not used to obtain central venous pressures. Schauvliege S, "Patient Monitoring and Monitoring Equipment," in Duke-Novakovski T, de Vries M, Seymour C, BSAVA Manual of Canine and Feline Anaesthesia and Analgesia, ed 3, British Small Animal Veterinary Association, 2016.

45. a Of the listed drugs, only acepromazine is a phenothiazine tranquilizer. Diazepam and midazolam are benzodiazepines, and morphine is an opioid analgesic. Murrell JC, "Pre-anaesthetic medication and sedation," in Duke-Novakovski T, de Vries M, Seymour C, BSAVA Manual of Canine and Feline Anaesthesia and Analgesia, ed 3, British Small Animal Veterinary Association, 2016.

46. a Acetylcholine is the primary neurotransmitter in the parasympathetic nervous system responsible for parasympathetic effects (also referred to as cholinergic effects). The PNS has two types of receptors for acetylcholine: the nicotinic receptors and the muscarinic receptors. Anticholinergics competitively block binding of the neurotransmitter acetylcholine at the muscarinic receptors. Thomas J, Phillip L, Anesthesia and Analgesia for Veterinary Technicians, ed 5, Elsevier, 2017.

47. c Acepromazine is an antagonist at alpha-1 adrenoreceptors. This causes a peripheral vasodilation, which results in decrease in temperature and overall blood pressure. For this reason acepromazine should be avoided in patients with cardiovascular instability or in shock. Murrell JC, "Pre-anaesthetic medication and sedation," in Duke-Novakovski T, de Vries M, Seymour C, BSAVA Manual of Canine and Feline Anaesthesia and Analgesia, ed 3, British Small Animal Veterinary Association, 2016.

48. d All of the listed drugs are examples of alpha-2 adrenoreceptor agonists, which function as sedatives and analgesics. Murrell JC, "Pre-anaesthetic medication and sedation," in Duke-Novakovski T, de Vries M, Seymour C, BSAVA Manual of Canine and Feline Anaesthesia and Analgesia, ed 3, British Small Animal Veterinary Association, 2016.

49. d If bradycardia develops, the best treatment is administration of an appropriate reversal agent, and in this case, atipamezole. Atropine reverses the adverse effects caused by organophosphates and some nerve gases such as sarin, soman, tabun, and toxic ingestion of mushrooms containing muscarine. Naloxone reverses opioids. Epinephrine reverses anaphylaxis. Thomas J, Phillip L, Anesthesia and Analgesia for Veterinary Technicians, ed 5, Elsevier, 2017.

50. b The primary effect of naloxone is reversal of both the desirable and undesirable effects of an agonist, partial agonist, or agonist-antagonist, including sedation, dysphoria, panting, respiratory depression, hypotension, bradycardia, GI effects, and analgesia. Therefore, naloxone is the drug of choice to reverse the effects of opioids. Atipamezole reverses the effects of dexmedetomidine. Atropine reverses organophosphate poisonings. Yohimbine reverses xylazine. Thomas J, Phillip L, Anesthesia and Analgesia for Veterinary Technicians, ed 5, Elsevier, 2017.

51. b Benzodiazepines are commonly used to manage convulsions and are used not only as premedicants but also as a first-line intervention for animals presenting in status epilepticus. Opioids, antibiotics, and alpha-2 adrenoreceptor agonist drugs are not used in this manner. Murrell JC, "Pre-anaesthetic medication and sedation," in Duke-Novakovski T, de Vries M, Seymour C, BSAVA Manual of Canine and Feline Anaesthesia and Analgesia, ed 3, British Small Animal Veterinary Association, 2016.

52. d Benzodiazepines do not have analgesic properties; they reduce skeletal muscle spasm and produce sedation through depression of the limbic system. Dexmedetomidine, methadone, and morphine do provide analgesia. Murrell JC, "Pre-anaesthetic medication and sedation," in Duke-Novakovski T, de Vries M, Seymour C, BSAVA Manual of Canine and Feline Anaesthesia and Analgesia, ed 3, British Small Animal Veterinary Association, 2016.

53. a After a brief period of hypotension, etomidate has little effect on heart rate, rhythm, blood pressure, and cardiac output. It is therefore the induction agent of choice for animals with moderate to severe heart disease or shock. Propofol would be the drug of choice for renal patients. Orthopedic patients could have any induction, not just etomidate. Pediatric patients have a high metabolism rate. It is not recommended for these patients to fast for more than 1 to 2 hours before surgery. Permeability of the blood–brain barrier is increased in pediatric patients, therefore reducing the dosage of most drugs used in anesthesia. Low percentage of body fat in pediatric patients results in little adipose tissue for redistribution with the potential for delayed elimination of the drug. Thomas J, Phillip L, Anesthesia and Analgesia for Veterinary Technicians, ed 5, Elsevier, 2017.

54. a The most common way for a drug to be eliminated from the body is through urine excretion via the kidneys. Before a drug is excreted and eliminated, it is often metabolized (or biotransformed). This occurs most often in the liver. Drugs are not digested in the gastrointestinal system to be eliminated. Muir WW, "Physiology and Pathophysiology of Pain," in Gaynor JS, Muir WW (eds), Handbook of Veterinary Pain Management, ed 2, Elsevier, 2009.

55. c Methadone is the only one in the list that is an opioid agonist, which is a good choice for patients that are in moderate to severe pain. Naloxone is the opposite and considered an opioid antagonist, which means it has no analgesic activity. Butorphanol is one of the opioids known as opioid agonists–antagonists. This means they are mu receptor antagonists but also kappa receptor agonists. Because they are not full mu receptor agonists like morphine and methadone, they are considered weak analgesics. Muir WW, "Physiology and Pathophysiology of Pain," in Gaynor JS, Muir WW (eds), Handbook of Veterinary Pain Management, ed 2, Elsevier, 2009; McNerney T, "Surgical Pain Management," Shaffran ME, Goldberg N (eds), Pain Management for Veterinary Technicians and Nurses, ed 1, Wiley Blackwell, 2014.

56. c Ketamine hydrochloride is used alone to induce dissociative anesthesia in cats for minor procedures. It is also commonly used in combination with a variety of tranquilizers and opioids to induce general anesthesia in a wide variety of species and it is given in subanesthetic doses by CRI to provide analgesia. Thiopental sodium and pentobarbital sodium are barbiturates and propofol is an ultra–short-acting nonbarbiturate injectable anesthetic with a wide margin of safety. Thomas J, Phillip L, Anesthesia and Analgesia for Veterinary Technicians, ed 5, Elsevier, 2017.

57. c For any inhalation anesthetic, 1.5×MAC will maintain moderate surgical anesthesia. Thomas J, Phillip L, Anesthesia and Analgesia for Veterinary Technicians, ed 5, Elsevier, 2017.

58. b Naloxone hydrochloride is a pure mu opioid antagonist that reverses all opioid effects at all receptors. Oppositely, morphine and hydromorphone are opioid agonists and fully activate the mu receptors. Butorphanol is a mixed agonist antagonist; it functions to antagonize mu receptors, but it also acts as a kappa agonist eliciting full effect at those receptors. Albino M, "Analgesic Pharmacology," Shaffran ME, Goldberg N (eds), Pain Management for Veterinary Technicians and Nurses, ed 1, Wiley Blackwell, 2014.

59. b Local anesthetics reversibly bind sodium channels and block nerve conduction in nerve fibers. All other choices listed relate to the effect of nonsteroidal anti-inflammatory drugs. Duke-Novakovski T, "Pain management II: local and regional anaesthetic techniques," in Duke-Novakovski T, de Vries M, Seymour C, BSAVA Manual of Canine and Feline Anaesthesia and Analgesia, ed 3, British Small Animal Veterinary Association, 2016.

60. d Propofol is a potent respiratory depressant. High doses or rapid injection may cause significant respiratory depression, including apnea. To lessen the respiratory depression associated with the use of propofol, the anesthetist should give the initial bolus gradually during 1 to 2 minutes, carefully titrating the dose to effect, and monitoring respiratory rate and depth carefully during the first few minutes after injection. Propofol is given by infusion/injection intravenously, but this does not decrease the risk of transient apnea and neither does the addition of opioids to the premedication cocktail. Thomas J, Phillip L, Anesthesia and Analgesia for Veterinary Technicians, ed 5, Elsevier, 2017.

61. a One disadvantage of tiletamine-zolazepam is the long and difficult recovery seen in some animals. As with ketamine, ataxia and increased sensitivity to stimuli are commonly observed during the recovery period. Tremors, muscle rigidity, seizure activity, and hyperthermia can also be seen, especially in dogs given tiletamine-zolazepam at labeled doses by the IM route. IV diazepam administration may be helpful in affected animals. In cats, recovery may be prolonged (up to 5 hours after IM injection), particularly if high doses are administered. Because the drug is metabolized by the liver and excreted via the kidneys, prolonged recovery should be expected in animals with liver or kidney dysfunction. Bradycardia is not a recorded side effect with this drug. Hypotension is not seen because of the tiletamine effect. Laryngospasms are not an issue in dogs. Thomas J, Phillip L, Anesthesia and Analgesia for Veterinary Technicians, ed 5, Elsevier, 2017.

62. b *Regional anesthesia* is the correct term to describe the injection of a local anesthetic into the area around a peripheral nerve to block sensory and/or motor function. Although some regional anesthesia can be given by subcutaneous injection, this term does not adequately describe what is happening (blocking sensory and motor function). Other listed techniques describe various ways to deliver local anesthetics, either in the subarachnoid space with spinal anesthesia or to the skin or mucous membranes via topical anesthesia. Albino M, "Analgesic Pharmacology," Shaffran ME, Goldberg N (eds), Pain Management for Veterinary Technicians and Nurses, ed 1, Wiley Blackwell, 2014.

63. c NMDA receptor antagonists include the drugs ketamine, amantadine, and memantine. The opioid methadone is also thought to have activity at the NMDA receptor as well as being a mu opioid agonist. Morphine does not have activity at the NMDA receptor. Plumb DC, Veterinary Drug Handbook, ed 9, Wiley Blackwell, 2018.

64. c Isoflurane depresses the respiratory system. In patients anesthetized with isoflurane, the respiratory rate decreases with time. A concentration of two to three times the MAC causes respiratory arrest in common domestic species. Hepatic toxicity is mostly seen with halothane. Isoflurane does not accumulate in the body fat in the same way as injectable anesthetics. Seizures are not seen during recovery with isoflurane. Thomas J, Phillip L, Anesthesia and Analgesia for Veterinary Technicians, ed 5, Elsevier, 2017.

65. b Of the listed opioids, methadone has been shown to have the lowest likelihood of causing vomiting in cats. Thomas J, Phillip L, Anesthesia and Analgesia for Veterinary Technicians, ed 5, Elsevier, 2017.

66. a Maropitant has been shown to be useful at reducing not only opioid-related nausea and vomiting but also the MAC of anesthetic gases needed when given preoperatively. Carprofen is an anti-inflammatory and has not been shown to reduce nausea and vomiting. Morphine and hydromorphone are opioids and often a main side effect of their use is nausea and vomiting. Laird JMA, Olivar T, Roza C, De Felipe C, Hunt SP, Cervero F, "Deficits in Visceral Pain and Hyperalgesia of Mice with a Disruption of the Tachykinin NK1 Receptor Gene," Neuroscience, p. 98, 345-352, 2000.

67. c Pain can originate from organs, in which case it is visceral pain (e.g., pleuritis or colic), or from the musculoskeletal system, in which case it is somatic pain. Somatic pain can be divided into superficial (i.e., skin) and deep (i.e., joints, muscles, bones) pain. Some diseases or surgeries may result in more than one of these types of pain; for example, abdominal surgery has components of somatic pain (skin and abdominal wall incisions) and visceral pain (organ manipulation and surgery). Thomas J, Phillip L, Anesthesia and Analgesia for Veterinary Technicians, ed 5, Elsevier, 2017.

68. a Morphine is the opioid most commonly used for epidural analgesia. Buprenorphine can be used; however, it is less potent than morphine because it is a partial agonist. Lidocaine and bupivacaine are local anesthetics and although they are commonly used as epidural analgesics, they are not opioids. Thomas J, Phillip L, Anesthesia and Analgesia for Veterinary Technicians, ed 5, Elsevier, 2017.

69. b Morphine is commonly administered via either the subcutaneous or intramuscular route. Rapid administration IV can cause histamine release, causing vasodilation, decreased blood pressure, and urticaria. Testosterone and estrogen are not given intravenously. Endogenous opioids are natural opioids present in the body and are not injected. Kerr C, "Pain management I: systemic analgesics in in Duke-Novakovski T, de Vries M, Seymour C, BSAVA Manual of Canine and Feline Anaesthesia and Analgesia, ed 3, British Small Animal Veterinary Association, 2016.

70. c The first step is the transformation of noxious thermal, chemical, or mechanical stimuli into electrical signals called action potentials by peripheral A-delta and C nerve fibers, which is called transduction. During perception, impulses are transmitted to the brain, where they are processed and recognized. During modulation, the impulses can be altered by other neurons, which either amplify or suppress them. When sensory impulses are conducted to the spinal cord, the process known as transmission occurs. Thomas J, Phillip L, Anesthesia and Analgesia for Veterinary Technicians, ed 5, Elsevier, 2017.

71. b All of the listed opioids can cause vomiting; however, methadone has been shown to have the lowest likelihood of causing vomiting, which can lead to increased intracranial and intraocular pressures. Thomas J, Phillip

L, Anesthesia and Analgesia for Veterinary Technicians, ed 5, Elsevier, 2017.

72. c In young puppies and kittens, hypothermia and hypotension can be of concern when they are under anesthesia. However, hypoglycemia is of particular concern in young puppies and kittens that have been fasted because they may not have glucose reserves to make up for the fasting, therefore putting them at risk of hypoglycemia. Murrell JC, "Pre-anaesthetic medication and sedation," in Duke-Novakovski T, de Vries M, Seymour C, BSAVA Manual of Canine and Feline Anaesthesia and Analgesia, ed 3, British Small Animal Veterinary Association, 2016.

73. b The first step is the transformation of noxious thermal, chemical, or mechanical stimuli into electrical signals called action potentials by peripheral A-delta and C nerve fibers, which is called transduction. During perception, impulses are transmitted to the brain, where they are processed and recognized. During modulation, the impulses can be altered by other neurons, which either amplify or suppress them. When sensory impulses are conducted to the spinal cord, the process known as transmission occurs. Thomas J, Phillip L, Anesthesia and Analgesia for Veterinary Technicians, ed 5, Elsevier, 2017.

74. b Centrally, in the spinal cord, neurons that are stimulated by constant nociceptive input from the periphery become hyperexcitable and sensitive to low-intensity stimuli that would not normally elicit a pain response. This phenomenon is called central nervous system hypersensitivity and is also referred to as wind-up. Clinically this may manifest as an area of hypersensitivity that is farther away from the initial injury and is known as secondary hyperalgesia. A receptor that is activated in wind-up is the N-methyl-D-aspartate (NMDA) receptor. Drugs such as ketamine can block this receptor. The brain is where perception occurs, but not the actual event. Visceral and peripheral pain receptors do not exist. Thomas J, Phillip L, Anesthesia and Analgesia for Veterinary Technicians, ed 5, Elsevier, 2017.

75. a Of the side effects listed, vomiting is commonly associated with opioids given preoperatively. Decreased mucous membrane secretions, tachycardia, and hypertension are all side effects of anticholinergics. Murrell JC, "Pre-anaesthetic medication and sedation," in Duke-Novakovski T, de Vries M, Seymour C, BSAVA Manual of Canine and Feline Anaesthesia and Analgesia, ed 3, British Small Animal Veterinary Association, 2016.

76. c Propofol is not considered a barbiturate anesthetic. Barbiturate anesthetics exert their effect by depression of the central nervous system via enhanced exhibition and inhibited excitation at the level of synaptic neurotransmission. Pentobarbital, methohexital, and thiopental are considered barbiturates. Murrell JC, "Pre-anaesthetic medication and sedation," in Duke-Novakovski T, de Vries M, Seymour C, BSAVA Manual of Canine and Feline Anaesthesia and Analgesia, ed 3, British Small Animal Veterinary Association, 2016.

77. a Because there are several mechanisms by which pain is produced, it is often helpful to use more than one type of analgesic to relieve pain. Multimodal therapy (also known as combination or balanced analgesia) may be more successful than treatment with any single agent because pain perception is affected at several points along the pain pathway and different mechanisms are targeted. For example, it has been shown in human patients that the use of piroxicam (an NSAID) and buprenorphine (an opioid) together provides analgesia that is superior to that with use of either agent alone. The concurrent use of NSAIDs with opioids may allow a 20%–50% reduction in the opioid dose. Thomas J, Phillip L, Anesthesia and Analgesia for Veterinary Technicians, ed 5, Elsevier, 2017.

78. b Methadone is a pure mu agonist opioid. Midazolam, zolazepam, and diazepam are all benzodiazepines. Murrell JC, "Pre-anaesthetic medication and sedation," in Duke-Novakovski T, de Vries M, Seymour C, BSAVA Manual of Canine and Feline Anaesthesia and Analgesia, ed 3, British Small Animal Veterinary Association, 2016.

79. c Telazol is a proprietary combination of zolazepam and tiletamine at a ratio of 1:1. This combination can produce sedation or general anesthesia in dogs and cats. The other listed combinations are not available as a commercially prepared product. Murrell JC, "Pre-anaesthetic medication and sedation," in Duke-Novakovski T, de Vries M, Seymour C, BSAVA Manual of Canine and Feline Anaesthesia and Analgesia, ed 3, British Small Animal Veterinary Association, 2016.

80. c Using several analgesic drugs, each with a different mechanism of action, is called multimodal therapy. This results in lower doses, which increases safety. Transduction agents: nonsteroidal anti-inflammatory agents (NSAIDs), opioids, local anesthetics, corticosteroids. Transmission agents: local anesthetics, alpha-2 agonists. Modulation: local anesthetics, NSAIDs, opioids, alpha-2 agonists, ketamine, tricyclic antidepressants, anticonvulsants. Perception agents: opioids, sedatives, general anesthetics. Therefore, using morphine, ketamine, and lidocaine is the best option. Thomas J, Phillip L, Anesthesia and Analgesia for Veterinary Technicians, ed 5, Elsevier, 2017.

81. a Alfaxalone is a neuroactive steroid molecule that produces hypnosis and muscle relaxation by enhancing the inhibitory effect of GABA on the GABA receptor chloride channel complex. Telazol, propofol, and etomidate do not function as a neuroactive steroid and instead are nonbarbiturate injectable induction agents. Murrell JC, "Pre-anaesthetic medication and sedation," in Duke-Novakovski T, de Vries M, Seymour C, BSAVA Manual of Canine and Feline Anaesthesia and Analgesia, ed 3, British Small Animal Veterinary Association, 2016.

82. b Before a drug is excreted, it is often metabolized (or biotransformed) and this occurs most often in the liver. The lungs, however, are responsible for metabolizing inhalant anesthetic drugs via the alveoli. The skin as well as the eyes can absorb and metabolize drugs topically. Pang D, "Inhalant Anaesthetic Agents," in Duke-Novakovski T, de Vries M, Seymour C, BSAVA Manual of Canine and Feline Anaesthesia and Analgesia, ed 3, British Small Animal Veterinary Association, 2016.

83. d Providing analgesia before tissue injury is called preemptive analgesia. Preemptive analgesia is most commonly achieved by adding an analgesic to the premedication before anesthetizing a patient for surgery. Preemptive analgesia also helps to prevent wind-up, which, through changes in the CNS from central sensitization, can lead to pain that lasts longer than anticipated and is more difficult to manage. Premedication involves an anesthetic agent or adjunct administered during the preanesthetic period to provide one or more of a variety of desired effects, including analgesia, sedation, and muscle relaxation. Local analgesia is a loss of sensation in a small area of the body produced by administration of a local anesthetic agent in proximity to the area of interest. Multimodal analgesia is the treatment of pain with analgesics that target two or more types of pain receptors. Thomas J, Phillip L, Anesthesia and Analgesia for Veterinary Technicians, ed 5, Elsevier, 2017.

84. c Hydromorphone is the only drug in the list that identifies as an opioid agonist, which is a good choice for patients that are in moderate to severe pain. Naloxone is the opposite and considered an opioid antagonist, which means it has no analgesic activity. Butorphanol is one of the opioids known as opioid agonists–antagonists. This means they are mu receptor antagonists but also kappa receptor agonists. Because they are not full mu receptor agonists like morphine and hydromorphone, they should be considered weak analgesics. Muir WW, "Physiology and Pathophysiology of Pain," in Gaynor JS, Muir WW (eds), Handbook of Veterinary Pain Management, ed 2, Elsevier, 2009; McNerney T, "Surgical Pain Management," Shaffran ME, Goldberg N (eds), Pain Management for Veterinary Technicians and Nurses, ed 1, Wiley Blackwell, 2014.

85. d Fentanyl is often used in CRI form because of its short duration of action. Peak analgesic effects are seen approximately 5 minutes after IV injection lasting approximately 30 minutes. Buprenorphine and morphine can be used in constant rate infusions; however, their duration of action is much longer, ranging anywhere from 2 to 6 hours depending on the route of administration. Ketamine is often used in conjunction with lidocaine and morphine in CRIs. Kerr C, "Pain management I: systemic analgesics in in Duke-Novakovski T, de Vries M, Seymour C, BSAVA Manual of Canine and Feline Anaesthesia and Analgesia, ed 3, British Small Animal Veterinary Association, 2016.

86. c Renal failure is not an effect of opioid administration, although it is recommended not to use opioids when a patient is experiencing renal insufficiency because the patient will take longer to recover. Vomiting, dysphoria, and respiratory depression are all known effects of opioids. Thomas J, Phillip L, Anesthesia and Analgesia for Veterinary Technicians, ed 5, Elsevier, 2017.

87. c Surgical anesthesia refers to the specific stage in general anesthesia in which there is a sufficient degree of analgesia and muscle relaxation to allow surgery to be performed without patient pain or movement. Local anesthesia is a loss of sensation in a small area of the body produced by administration of a local anesthetic. Sedation is drug-induced CNS depression and drowsiness that vary in intensity from light to deep. Thomas J, Phillip L, Anesthesia and Analgesia for Veterinary Technicians, ed 5, Elsevier, 2017.

88. c The buccal mucosal bleeding time is an in-house test that can be used in patients that are suspected of having clotting disorders and may be at high risk of intraoperative bleeding. A blood glucose measurement is an important piece of information before surgery, telling us about the patient's glucose level and whether they may need supplementation intraoperatively. A urine specific gravity will give information about the ability to concentrate urine and therefore kidney function and the Schirmer tear test will test a patient's tear formation, which is not important for patients suspected of having a clotting disorder. Thomas J, Phillip L, Anesthesia and Analgesia for Veterinary Technicians, ed 5, Elsevier, 2017.

89. c The clinical effects of NSAIDs stem chiefly from their inhibition of prostaglandin synthesis. Prostaglandins (often abbreviated PAGEs) are a group of extremely potent chemicals that are normally present in all body tissues and are involved in the mediation of pain and inflammation after tissue injury. Thomas J, Phillip L, Anesthesia and Analgesia for Veterinary Technicians, ed 5, Elsevier, 2017.

90. c Drugs given before general anesthesia are referred to as preanesthetic agents. Drugs used to induce general anesthesia are induction agents and those used to maintain general anesthesia are termed *maintenance agents*. Postanesthetic medications are given after the period of general anesthesia to maintain analgesia in the postsurgical period. Thomas J, Phillip L, Anesthesia and Analgesia for Veterinary Technicians, ed 5, Elsevier, 2017.

91. a Dexmedetomidine is the most commonly used alpha-2 agonist in dogs and cats. In horses the most widely used alpha-2 agonist is detomidine. Xylazine is an alpha-2 agonist; however, it has more side effects and adverse reactions than dexmedetomidine and its use is on the decline because safer formulations such as dexmedetomidine have become available. Morphine is an opioid not an alpha-2 agonist. Thomas J, Phillip L, Anesthesia and Analgesia for Veterinary Technicians, ed 5, Elsevier, 2017.

92. d Respiratory depression is not a known side effect of NSAID administration. Liver and kidney damage as well as gastrointestinal ulcers are often seen in patients receiving NSAIDS. Thomas J, Phillip L, Anesthesia and Analgesia for Veterinary Technicians, ed 5, Elsevier, 2017.

93. b These side effects are most commonly observed with use of propofol. Alfaxalone and thiopental use may cause some signs of excitement. Thomas J, Phillip L, Anesthesia and Analgesia for Veterinary Technicians, ed 5, Elsevier, 2017.

94. a When the tank valve is opened, the gauge indicates the gas pressure inside the tank. This gauge must be checked before commencement of any procedure to ensure that enough gas remains in the tank to complete it safely. The pressure in a full oxygen tank is about 2200 psi (about 15,000 kPa). A reading of 1100 psi indicates the tank is approximately half full and therefore contains approximately 330 L of oxygen. Thomas J, Phillip L, Anesthesia and Analgesia for Veterinary Technicians, ed 5, Elsevier, 2017.

95. d All of the listed statements are true when it comes to isoflurane. A precision vaporizer is used to administer isoflurane. Isoflurane has no analgesic properties, therefore adequate analgesic must be administered. Isoflurane is stable at room temperature and no preservative is necessary. Thomas J, Phillip L, Anesthesia and Analgesia for Veterinary Technicians, ed 5, Elsevier, 2017.

96. c Nitrous oxide (N_2O) is present in liquid and gas. Thomas J, Phillip L, Anesthesia and Analgesia for Veterinary Technicians, ed 5, Elsevier, 2017.

97. a The lingual artery is located in the tongue and cannot be used for arterial catheter placement. All remaining choices are good locations for an arterial catheter. Auricular arteries are particularly useful in long-eared dogs such as basset hounds. Critical patients with blood pressure abnormalities can benefit from direct blood pressure monitoring with an arterial line. Takada S, "Intravenous Access," in Bryant S, Anesthesia for Veterinary Technicians, ed 1, Wiley-Blackwell, 2010.

98. c Hypothermia decreases the requirement for general anesthesia. Because hypothermia slows metabolism, the patient does not need as much drug as it would at normal temperatures. Conversely, hyperthermic patients can have an increased metabolism, which can increase the rate of drug metabolism. Hypoventilation and hypotension can be of concern under anesthesia; however, they do not directly affect the depth of anesthesia. Rather, they are a result of the patient being at a plane of anesthesia that is too deep. Levensaler A, "Monitoring: Pulse Oximetry, Temperature and Hands On," in Bryant S, Anesthesia for Veterinary Technicians, ed 1, Wiley-Blackwell, 2010, p. 98.

99. b Turning the valve knob to the left opens the flowmeter and the flow of oxygen is then adjusted to the appropriate level for the patient. All flowmeters have a ball or rotor indicator that rises to a height proportional to the flow of gas. The scale on the cylinder indicates the gas flow. The meter is read at the center of a ball indicator or the top of a rotor indicator. The oxygen tank pressure gauge shows how much oxygen is in the tank. The pressure manometer is a gauge that indicates the pressure of the gases within the breathing circuit and by extension the pressure in the animal's airways and lungs. The vaporizer converts liquid inhalant anesthetic and mixes it with the carrier gases. Thomas J, Phillip L, Anesthesia and Analgesia for Veterinary Technicians, ed 5, Elsevier, 2017.

100. d Circulating warm water blankets, convective warm air devices, and commercially available bubble wrap are considered safe ways to warm a patient under anesthesia. Radiant heat from the heat lamp; however, can overheat tissues and can burn through equipment such as breathing circuits. Levensaler A, "Monitoring: Pulse Oximetry, Temperature, and Hands-on," in Bryant S, Anesthesia for Veterinary Technicians, ed 1, Wiley-Blackwell, 2010, p. 99.

101. d All of the listed parameters are useful tools in monitoring a patient recovering from anesthesia. It is important to monitor the patient's temperature until it returns to normal and to provide supplemental heat as needed. In addition, if a patient had a procedure that was thought to be painful, the patient should be monitored for signs of pain and analgesics should be administered as needed. In some patients (such as patients who underwent splenectomy and or GDV procedures), continuous ECG monitoring can be helpful to alert the technician to any arrhythmias that may develop. Cheyne M, "Recovery of the Anesthetic Patient," in Bryant S, Anesthesia for Veterinary Technicians, ed 1, Wiley-Blackwell, 2010, p. 163.

102. b Ideally the bag should hold a volume of at least 60 mL/kg of patient weight (six times the patient's VT), but this is not always practical or necessary. From a practical perspective, the bag should contain enough gas to fill the patient's lungs during an inhalation but should not be so large as to prevent visualization of respiratory movements. Thomas J, Phillip L, Anesthesia and Analgesia for Veterinary Technicians, ed 5, Elsevier, 2017.

103. a If a patient regurgitates, it is important to remove the regurgitation and lavage the esophagus as soon as possible with saline. Gastric contents are highly acidic and can damage the lining of the esophagus and oral cavity. You should not feed the patient a meal because they would probably not be able to function properly enough to eat and you would have to ensure they did not choke. You should also not place the patient on a gas anesthetic because this would be counterintuitive to what you are trying to achieve (the patient waking from anesthesia). Cheyne M, "Recovery of the Anesthetic Patient," in Bryant S, Anesthesia for Veterinary Technicians, ed 1, Wiley-Blackwell, 2010, p. 165.

104. b The main function of the pop-off valve is to allow excess carrier and anesthetic gases to exit from the breathing circuit and enter the scavenging system. By venting excess gas, the pop-off valve prevents the buildup of excessive pressure or volume of gases within the circuit. If allowed to occur, this excess pressure could damage the animal's lungs by causing the alveoli to overdistend and rupture. Excess intrathoracic pressure also dramatically decreases return of blood to the heart, resulting in severely decreased cardiac output. The vaporizer is responsible for vaporizing the anesthetic liquid. The unidirectional valve keeps the oxygen flowing in one direction only. The CO_2 absorbent canister prevents waste gases from re-entering the vaporizer. Thomas J, Phillip L, Anesthesia and Analgesia for Veterinary Technicians, ed 5, Elsevier, 2017.

105. d Drugs given before general anesthesia are referred to as preanesthetic agents. Drugs used to induce general anesthesia are induction agents and those used to maintain general anesthesia are termed *maintenance agents*. Postanesthetic medications are given after the period of general anesthesia to maintain analgesia in the postsurgical period. Thomas J, Phillip L, Anesthesia and Analgesia for Veterinary Technicians, ed 5, Elsevier, 2017.

106. a Of the drugs listed, only acepromazine is a phenothiazine tranquilizer commonly used for patients experiencing stress during recovery. Diazepam and midazolam are benzodiazepines and morphine is an opioid analgesic. Murrell JC, "Pre-anaesthetic medication and sedation," in Duke Novakovski T, de Vries M, Seymour C, BSAVA Manual of Canine and

Feline Anaesthesia and Analgesia, ed 3, British Small Animal Veterinary Association, 2016.

107. d The pressure manometer should read 0–2 cm of water when the patient is breathing spontaneously. It should read no more than 20 cm of water (15 mmHg) in small animals or 40 cm of water (30 mmHg) in large animals when positive-pressure assisted or controlled ventilation is provided, unless the chest cavity is open, in which case the pressure can be somewhat higher. Excessive pressure in the circuit can result in dyspnea, lung damage, or pneumothorax. Therefore, the pressure must be watched closely during any anesthetic procedure. Thomas J, Phillip L, Anesthesia and Analgesia for Veterinary Technicians, ed 5, Elsevier, 2017.

108. d Dexmedetomidine is the only drug listed that functions as a sedative and analgesic. Acepromazine, midazolam, and diazepam are all anxiolytic drugs that provide calming and sedation but no analgesia. Murrell JC, "Pre-anaesthetic medication and sedation," in Duke-Novakovski T, de Vries M, Seymour C, BSAVA Manual of Canine and Feline Anaesthesia and Analgesia, ed 3, British Small Animal Veterinary Association, 2016.

109. b Benzodiazepines do not have analgesic properties. They reduce skeletal muscle spasm and produce sedation through depression of the limbic system. Dexmedetomidine and opioids methadone and morphine do provide analgesia. Murrell JC, "Pre-anaesthetic medication and sedation," in Duke-Novakovski T, de Vries M, Seymour C, BSAVA Manual of Canine and Feline Anaesthesia and Analgesia, ed 3, British Small Animal Veterinary Association, 2016.

110. d Non-rebreathing systems require relatively high flow rates per unit body weight during all periods of general anesthesia (induction, maintenance, and recovery) because the removal of carbon dioxide from the circuit is dependent on fresh gas flow, which must be sufficient to ensure that there is minimal rebreathing of exhaled gases. Therefore, close attention must be given to the selection of an appropriate flow rate. Recommended rates are based on body weight and the Mapleson classification of the circuit. Because these systems are generally used for patients weighing less than 7 kg, maximum rates listed are based on this body weight. With Mapleson A systems (Magill circuit), modified Mapleson A systems (Lack circuit), and modified Mapleson D systems (Bain coaxial circuit), carrier gas flow should be near the RMV (200 mL/kg/min). This equals about 0.5–1.5 L/min depending on patient size. Thomas J, Phillip L, Anesthesia and Analgesia for Veterinary Technicians, ed 5, Elsevier, 2017.

111. a Atelectasis refers to a diminished volume or a lack of air in part or all of a lung lobe. Hypoxia is defined as impaired oxygen delivery because of systemic delivery issues. Functional residual capacity describes the amount of air left in the lungs after normal ventilation. The FRC is important to the veterinary anesthetist because during apnea it is the reservoir to supply oxygen to the blood. Tidal volume is the volume of air that moves in and out of the patient during a full respiratory cycle. Slowiak C, "Ventilation Techniques in Small Animal Patients," in Bryant S, Anesthesia for Veterinary Technicians, ed 1, Wiley-Blackwell, 2010, p. 188-189.

112. a Spraying the endotracheal tube with lidocaine will not help prevent laryngospasm. Laryngospasm is a reflex closure of the laryngeal cartilage, which results in airway obstruction. Spraying the larynx with a local anesthetic, ensuring the patient is adequately anesthetized, and using a gentle intubation technique can prevent laryngospasms. McMillan S, "Anesthetic Complications and Emergencies," in Bryant S, Anesthesia for Veterinary Technicians, ed 1, Wiley-Blackwell, 2010, p. 171.

113. c An air intake valve is present on some machines either as a separate part or incorporated into the inspiratory unidirectional valve or the pop-off valve. This valve admits room air to the circuit in the event that negative pressure (a partial vacuum) is detected in the breathing circuit, a situation indicated by a collapsed reservoir bag. If a partial vacuum develops, the patient will be unable to fill its lungs and will develop hypoxemia because of inadequate oxygen levels. This may happen when the machine is incorrectly assembled or when an active scavenging system is exerting excessive suction. Negative pressure may also develop in the circuit if the oxygen flow rate is too low or if the tank runs out of oxygen. The air intake valve ensures that the patient always receives some oxygen by admitting room air (which contains 21% oxygen) into the circuit. Even though this situation is not ideal, it is preferable that the patient breathes room air rather than none at all, as would be the case if the air intake valve were not present. Whether nitrous oxide is being used or not, a negative pressure relief valve should be present on the machine and allow room air into the circuit if negative pressure is determined. The scavenging system and carbon dioxide absorber have nothing to do with the negative pressure relief valve. Thomas J, Phillip L, Anesthesia and Analgesia for Veterinary Technicians, ed 5, Elsevier, 2017.

114. a PVC or silicon tubes are a better choice because they are clear and an occlusion can be seen easily. They are also softer and more flexible (less likely to crack) than the red rubber tubes. They are also easier to clean and the red rubber tubes are much harder to properly disinfect, thus causing cross contamination between patients. Red rubber catheters are an adequate length to provide anesthesia to the patient; however, for all of the previous reasons listed, they should not be used in today's veterinary practice. Palmer D, "Airway Maintenance," in Bryant S, Anesthesia for Veterinary Technicians, ed 1, Wiley-Blackwell, 2010, p. 57.

115. b The volume of a normal breath (tidal volume) is approximately 10–15 mL/kg body weight. Thomas J, Phillip L, Anesthesia and Analgesia for Veterinary Technicians, ed 5, Elsevier, 2017.

116. b The flowmeter reduces the pressure of the gas in the intermediate-pressure line from about 50 psi (about 345 kPa) to 15 psi (about 100 kPa). Thomas J, Phillip L, Anesthesia and Analgesia for Veterinary Technicians, ed 5, Elsevier, 2017.

117. d All of these options are patients that can benefit from a laryngeal mask airway. In all of these species, endotracheal intubation may be difficult and a laryngeal mask airway can be easier to place as an alternative that still provides an airtight seal. Palmer D, "Airway Maintenance," in Bryant S, Anesthesia for Veterinary Technicians, ed 1, Wiley-Blackwell, 2010, p. 59.

118. b The function of a laryngoscope is to facilitate endotracheal intubation by allowing direct visualization of the opening to the trachea. Anesthetic gases are delivered via an endotracheal tube. A laryngoscope is not used to obtain tissue samples or to cover the esophagus and prevent regurgitation during surgery. Palmer D, "Airway Maintenance," in Bryant S, Anesthesia for Veterinary Technicians, ed 1, Wiley-Blackwell, 2010, p. 61.

119. d Chronic exposure to nitrous oxide has been associated with increased risk of neurologic disease; a study of female dental assistants exposed to high levels of nitrous oxide showed them to have a 1.7- to 2.8-fold increase in the incidence of neurologic disease compared with the normal population. Dentists and dental assistants exposed to high levels of waste nitrous oxide reported muscle weakness, tingling sensations, and numbness. Isoflurane is not associated with these specific reproductive effects. Halothane and methoxyflurane are no longer used. Thomas J, Phillip L, Anesthesia and Analgesia for Veterinary Technicians, ed 5, Elsevier, 2017.

120. d Anesthetic gases and oxygen are delivered via an endotracheal tube. The function of a laryngoscope is to facilitate endotracheal intubation by allowing direct visualization of the opening to the trachea. An endotracheal tube is not used to obtain tissue samples or to cover the esophagus and prevent regurgitation after surgery. Palmer D, "Airway Maintenance," in Bryant S, Anesthesia for Veterinary Technicians, ed 1, Wiley-Blackwell, 2010, p. 61.

121. c A laryngoscope that has a straight blade is called a Miller laryngoscope. This is in contrast to the laryngoscopes that have a curved blade, which are known as Macintosh. Murphy, Cole, and Magill are all names used to describe different types of endotracheal tubes, not laryngoscopes. Palmer D, "Airway Maintenance," in Bryant S, Anesthesia for Veterinary Technicians, ed 1, Wiley-Blackwell, 2010, p. 61.

122. a Silicone tubes are the only ETs approved for sterilization in an autoclave using steam. Red rubber and PVC tubes must be gas sterilized with ethylene oxide or hydrogen peroxide gas plasma because they break down in the presence of extreme heat. Palmer D, "Airway Maintenance," in Bryant S, Anesthesia for Veterinary Technicians, ed 1, Wiley-Blackwell, 2010, p. 69.

123. b NIOSH recommends that the concentration of any volatile gas anesthetic (including halothane, methoxyflurane, and isoflurane) not exceed 2 ppm when used alone and not exceed 0.5 ppm when used with nitrous oxide. It is also suggested the nitrous oxide concentration not exceed 25 ppm. Thomas J, Phillip L, Anesthesia and Analgesia for Veterinary Technicians, ed 5, Elsevier, 2017.

124. c Any anesthetic machine must perform four functions: deliver oxygen, deliver anesthetic, remove carbon dioxide, and remove waste gas. An anesthetic machine will not remove oxygen. Coleman D, Latshaw H, "Anesthesia Equipment," in Bryant S, Anesthesia for Veterinary Technicians, ed 1, Wiley-Blackwell, 2010, p. 71.

125. b The MAC value in horses is 1.31%. MAC is minimum alveolar concentration. MAC is the lowest percentage of anesthetic at which 50% of a population of patients will show no response to a painful stimulus. Thomas J, Phillip L, Anesthesia and Analgesia for Veterinary Technicians, ed 5, Elsevier, 2017.

126. b The function of the flush valve within the anesthetic circuit is to deliver a burst of pure oxygen into the breathing system. The flowmeter is responsible for delivering oxygen to the system at a specific rate in liters per minute. To shut off the oxygen supply the flowmeter should be turned to zero. There is no way to flush anesthetic gas quickly through the system; instead, anesthetic concentration can be increased by increasing the percentage on the vaporizer. Coleman D, Latshaw H, "Anesthesia Equipment" in Bryant S, Anesthesia for Veterinary Technicians, ed 1, Wiley-Blackwell, 2010, p. 73.

127. b Clinic employees can inexpensively monitor waste gas levels by using detector tubes or badges. Badges may detect only one chemical, such as halothane, isoflurane, or nitrous oxide, or may be sensitive to all halogenated anesthetics. The badges (called passive dosimeters) are uncapped at the beginning of the exposure period and then worn by personnel in the surgical preparation room, operating room, or recovery area for a timed period when anesthetic gases are being used (usually an exposure time of 2–8 hours is chosen). Alternatively, the badge may be placed in a room for area monitoring. After exposure, the badge is recapped and returned to the supplier (usually an industrial health and safety supply house or a company specializing in OSHA compliance) for analysis. Results are given as a time-weighted average in parts per million. A radiation monitor has nothing to do with anesthesia monitoring and regular preventive maintenance does not detect waste anesthetic gases. Smelling gas is dangerous to the anesthetist, because when the odor is detected, maximum exposure levels have been exceeded. Thomas J, Phillip L, Anesthesia and Analgesia for Veterinary Technicians, ed 5, Elsevier, 2017.

128. a The numbers on the vaporizer dial indicate the concentration (in percent) delivered at the output of the vaporizer. Depth of anesthesia is determined by assessing the patient, not the vaporizer setting. The flow of oxygen through the system is determined by the setting on the flowmeter. The amount of liquid anesthetic left in the reservoir is observed by looking at the reservoir window. Coleman D, Latshaw H, "Anesthesia Equipment," in Bryant S, Anesthesia for Veterinary Technicians, ed 1, Wiley-Blackwell, 2010, p. 73.

129. a Low-pressure tests should be performed before use of the machine each day. Thomas J, Phillip L, Anesthesia and Analgesia for Veterinary Technicians, ed 5, Elsevier, 2017.

130. d The universal F circuit is made of an inspiratory tube running within an expiratory tube for the purpose of aiding in the warming and humidification of inspired gases. All of the other systems listed are non-rebreathing circuits. The universal F circuit is a rebreathing system. Coleman D, Latshaw H, "Anesthesia Equipment," in Bryant S, Anesthesia for Veterinary Technicians, ed 1, Wiley-Blackwell, 2010, p. 81.

131. a A normal capillary refill time in veterinary patients is 1–2 seconds. A prolonged capillary refill time of 3–4 seconds or 10 seconds can indicate dehydration and low cardiac output. A capillary refill time of less than 1 second can indicate vasodilation with good perfusion or high blood pressure. Thomas J, Phillip L, Anesthesia and Analgesia for Veterinary Technicians, ed 5, Elsevier, 2017.

132. c If a large cylinder must be moved to another location, a handcart should be used; do not drag or roll the cylinder. Thomas J, Phillip L, Anesthesia and Analgesia for Veterinary Technicians, ed 5, Elsevier, 2017.

133. a Pale mucous membranes may be caused by vasoconstriction resulting from pain, decreased cardiac output, blood loss, hypoxia, and decreased circulating red blood cells. Anesthetic agents can affect mucous membrane color. Hypertension does not cause pale mucous membranes. Levensaler A, "Monitoring: Pulse Oximetry, Temperature, and Hands-On," in Bryant S, Anesthesia for Veterinary Technicians, ed 1, Wiley-Blackwell, 2010, p. 102.

134. c It is advised that all rooms in which anesthetic gases are released have at least 15 air changes per hour. Anything less is too few air changes; anything greater is inefficient. Thomas J, Phillip L, Anesthesia and Analgesia for Veterinary Technicians, ed 5, Elsevier, 2017.

135. b Palpable arteries in dogs and cats include femoral, lingual, dorsal pedal, digital, and buccal artery. Articular arteries are not acceptable for palpating peripheral pulses. Articular arteries do not exist. Levensaler A, "Monitoring: Pulse Oximetry, Temperature, and Hands-On," in Bryant S, Anesthesia for Veterinary Technicians, ed 1, Wiley-Blackwell, 2010, p. 102.

136. b If proper equipment, techniques, and procedures are used, it is possible to reduce waste gas exposure to a level well below the NIOSH standards. This can be achieved through several means, including using a gas scavenging system, testing equipment for leaks, and using techniques and procedures that minimize exposure to waste gas. Using uncuffed endotracheal tubes allows gas to leak and increases risk of aspiration to the patient. Using masks or chambers also increases waste anesthetic exposure to team members. High fresh gas flows can be efficient when a scavenger system is in place; however, it alone will not reduce the amount of waste anesthetic gases. Thomas J, Phillip L, Anesthesia and Analgesia for Veterinary Technicians, ed 5, Elsevier, 2017.

137. c A Doppler device is used to measure the systolic blood pressure and is most accurate when the systolic pressure is within normal limits and the patient has good peripheral perfusion. A thermometer is used to measure temperature, a pulse oximeter is used to measure patient oxygenation, and a capnogram is used to measure end tidal carbon dioxide. Reuss-Lamky H, "Monitoring Blood Pressure and End Tidal CO_2 in the Anesthetized Patient," in Bryant S, Anesthesia for Veterinary Technicians, ed 1, Wiley-Blackwell, 2010, p. 111.

138. d One easy way to do a low-pressure test is to close the pop-off valve and place one hand (or preferably a stopper) over the Y-piece. This closes off all avenues of gas escape from the machine. The oxygen tank is turned on and the flowmeter is adjusted to supply a flow rate of 2 L/min. The reservoir bag will gradually fill with oxygen. When the bag is full and tight, the flow rate is reduced to 200 mL/min or less. The anesthetist should be able to squeeze the bag with significant pressure without causing escape of air from the bag (it remains tight and full). If the anesthetist is able to push air out of the bag, a leak is present, or the pop-off valve or Y-piece is not completely occluded. The circuit should maintain a pressure of 30 cm (as indicated by the pressure manometer) for 30 seconds during the test at a flowmeter setting of 200 mL/min. Thomas J, Phillip L, Anesthesia and Analgesia for Veterinary Technicians. ed 5, Elsevier, 2017.

139. b A clean soft cloth that is moistened with mild soap and water is all that is usually necessary for cleaning most devices. The use of alcohol and bleach should be avoided because surface damage may occur. Reuss-Lamky H, "Monitoring Blood Pressure and End Tidal CO_2 in the Anesthetized Patient," in Bryant S, Anesthesia for Veterinary Technicians, ed 1, Wiley-Blackwell, 2010, p. 111.

140. b As an induction agent is given, the patient passes through stage I and as it loses consciousness, it enters stage II. The loss of consciousness marks the border between these stages. As the anesthetic depth increases, the patient then enters stage III, the period of surgical anesthesia. The loss of spontaneous muscle movement marks the border between stages II and III. If the depth continues to increase, the patient will enter stage IV. The loss of all reflexes, widely dilated, unresponsive pupils, flaccid muscle tone, and cardiopulmonary collapse mark this stage, which, if not aggressively managed, is closely followed by cardiopulmonary arrest and death of the patient. As the animal passes through each stage, there is a progressive decrease in pain perception, motor coordination, consciousness, reflex responses, muscle tone, and eventually cardiopulmonary and respiratory function. Apnea and hypothermia should be avoided with any stage of anesthesia. Tachycardia is not seen when using anesthesia. Thomas J, Phillip L, Anesthesia and Analgesia for Veterinary Technicians, ed 5, Elsevier, 2017.

141. a Functional residual capacity describes the amount of air left in the lungs after normal ventilation. The FRC is important to the veterinary anesthetist because during apnea it is the reservoir to supply oxygen to the blood. Atelectasis refers to a diminished volume or a lack of air in part or all of a lung lobe. Hypoxia is defined as impaired oxygen delivery because of systemic delivery issues. Tidal volume is the volume of air that moves in and out of the patient during a full respiratory cycle. Slowiak C, "Ventilation Techniques in Small Animal Patients," in Bryant S, Anesthesia for Veterinary Technicians, ed 1, Wiley-Blackwell, 2010, p. 188-189.

142. d All of the listed examples would be reasons a patient may need controlled ventilation, either manually or mechanically. Slowiak C, "Ventilation Techniques in Small Animal Patients," in Bryant S, Anesthesia for Veterinary Technicians, ed 1, Wiley-Blackwell, 2010, p. 189.

143. b During stage III, which is subdivided into four planes, the patient is unconscious and progresses gradually from light to deep surgical anesthesia. Plane 2 is suitable for most surgical procedures. Stage III, plane 1 is inadequate to perform surgery. Stage III, plane 3 is considered to be excessively deep for most surgical procedures. Stage III, plane 4 indicates anesthetic overdose. Thomas J, Phillip L, Anesthesia and Analgesia for Veterinary Technicians, ed 5, Elsevier, 2017.

144. d Bucking the ventilator is an expression used when an animal is trying to breathe against the set respiratory rhythm and volume being delivered by the mechanical ventilator. Checking, pulling, and pushing are not terms used in conjunction with the mechanical ventilator. Slowiak C, "Ventilation Techniques in Small Animal Patients," in Bryant S, Anesthesia for Veterinary Technicians, ed 1, Wiley-Blackwell, 2010, p. 193.

145. c Midazolam is a benzodiazepine tranquilizer that has sedative and calming effects. Midazolam has no analgesic properties. Butorphanol and morphine are opioid drugs that provide some sedation and analgesia and dexmedetomidine is an alpha-2 agonist that induces both sedation and analgesia. Robbins S, "Pre-medication and Sedation Drugs," in Bryant S, Anesthesia for Veterinary Technicians, ed 1, Wiley-Blackwell, 2010, p. 193. 137-138.

146. b During stage II, also known as the excitement stage, the patient loses voluntary control and breathing becomes irregular. This stage is usually characterized by involuntary reactions in the form of vocalizing, struggling, or paddling. In stage I, the patient begins to lose consciousness. This stage is usually characterized by fear, excitement, disorientation, and struggling. The HR and RR increase and the patient may pant, urinate, or defecate. A patient in stage I is typically difficult to handle. Near the end of stage I, the patient loses the ability to stand and becomes recumbent. Stage III is suitable for surgical procedures. Thomas J, Phillip L, Anesthesia and Analgesia for Veterinary Technicians, ed 5, Elsevier, 2017.

147. a *Catalepsy* is the term that describes a state in which patients are in a trance-like state and unaware of their surroundings. Catalepsy or dissociative anesthesia is often seen with the use of cyclohexamines such as ketamine and tiletamine. Animals that are sleeping or sedated are still easily aroused and often aware of their surroundings when stimulated; therefore, this is not true of animals in a cataleptic state. Nystagmus refers to a rhythmic or oscillating motion of the eyes that is commonly seen during recovery of patients with cyclohexamines. Fuehrer L, "Induction Drugs," in Bryant S, Anesthesia for Veterinary Technicians, ed 1, Wiley-Blackwell, 2010, p. 145.

148. c Anatomic dead space includes the bronchi, trachea, larynx, pharynx, and nasal cavity. If room air was present in a breathing circuit, a leak would be present. Air within the digestive tract would indicate the esophagus was intubated instead of the trachea. Air is supposed to be in the alveoli, but it is not anatomic dead space. Thomas J, Phillip L, Anesthesia and Analgesia for Veterinary Technicians, ed 5, Elsevier, 2017.

149. b Slow IV administration is the technique that helps to minimize the occurrence of respiratory depression when using propofol as an induction agent. Propofol should not be administered SQ or IM but only as an intravenous injection. This injection should be slow to minimize side effects. A fast push of propofol IV can cause respiratory depression, apnea, and hypotension. Fuehrer L, "Induction Drugs," in Bryant S, Anesthesia for Veterinary Technicians, ed 1, Wiley-Blackwell, 2010, p. 149.

150. d All of the patients are good candidates for etomidate as the induction drug. Etomidate causes no changes to heart rate, blood pressure, or cardiac output. It also has very little fetal depressant agents. Fuehrer L, "Induction Drugs," in Bryant S, Anesthesia for Veterinary Technicians, ed 1, Wiley-Blackwell, 2010, p. 149.

151. a Owing to the extreme variability of size, large dogs tend to have lower rates, whereas small dogs and puppies have higher rates. Minimum HR for large breed dogs under anesthesia is 60 bpm. Thomas J, Phillip L, Anesthesia and Analgesia for Veterinary Technicians, ed 5, Elsevier, 2017.

152. b Alpha-2 agonists produce sedation, analgesia, and muscle relaxation. They often also produce a refractory bradycardia (decreased heart rate), not an increased heart rate. Thomas J, Phillip L, Anesthesia and Analgesia for Veterinary Technicians, ed 5, Elsevier, 2017.

153. b A patient with less than 6 bpm or greater than 20 bpm should be reported to the veterinarian. Thomas J, Phillip L, Anesthesia and Analgesia for Veterinary Technicians, ed 5, Elsevier, 2017.

154. a Alpha-2 agonists cause initial peripheral vasoconstriction, which in turn causes pale mucous membranes and cold extremities. During this period of vasoconstriction, patients will often be normotensive or even hypertensive. Alpha-2 agonists do produce a decreased hepatic blood flow, but it does not contribute to the pale mucous membranes and cold extremities. Hypothermia and hypoglycemia are not often associated with the initial phase of alpha-2 administration. Thomas J, Phillip L, Anesthesia and Analgesia for Veterinary Technicians, ed 5, Elsevier, 2017.

155. b Ketamine can cause an increase in heart rate, blood pressure, and myocardial oxygen consumption. Therefore, it should not be used in patients with hypertrophic cardiomyopathy, congestive heart failure, or unstable patients in shock. Hypotrophic cardiomyopathy does not exist and healthy patients can receive ketamine without concern. Unless the patient is experiencing another condition besides panosteitis, the patient is normally healthy enough to receive ketamine because it has no effect on bones. Albino M, "Analgesic Pharmacology," Shaffran ME, Goldberg N (eds), Pain Management for Veterinary Technicians and Nurses, ed 1, Wiley Blackwell, 2014; Plumb DC, Veterinary Drug Handbook, ed 7, Wiley Blackwell, 2011.

156. b An increase in the RR is called tachypnea. An increase in respiratory depth (tidal volume) is known as hyperventilation. Hypoventilation is a decrease in respiratory depth and a decrease in RR is bradypnea. Thomas J, Phillip L, Anesthesia and Analgesia for Veterinary Technicians, ed 5, Elsevier, 2017.
157. b Of the listed opioids, morphine has been shown to have the highest likelihood of causing vomiting in cats. Lerche P, Thomas JA. Anesthesia and Analgesia for Veterinary Technicians. ed 5, Elsevier, 2017.
158. b Saturation below 90% indicates the need for therapy. During oxygen administration, oxygen saturation should be greater than 95%. Saturation below 85% (hypoxemia) for longer than 30 seconds indicates a medical emergency. Thomas J, Phillip L, Anesthesia and Analgesia for Veterinary Technicians, ed 5, Elsevier, 017.
159. a Capnography provides a picture of how well the patient is ventilating and how efficient the gas exchange is when a patient is on mechanical ventilation. A pulse oximeter only measures the oxygen saturation, not the exchange of oxygen for carbon dioxide. Blood pressure and ECG can be affected by inadequate ventilation; however, they do not measure the efficiency of gas exchange in the patient receiving positive-pressure ventilation via a ventilator. Slowiak C, "Ventilation Techniques in Small Animal Patients," in Bryant S, Anesthesia for Veterinary Technicians, ed 1, Wiley-Blackwell, 2010, p. 194.
160. d All of the options listed are potential reasons an ophthalmology patient may have increased IOP. The main goal for the patient undergoing an ophthalmic procedure is to maintain or lower intraocular pressure. An increase in IOP can cause permanent loss of vision or even globe rupture in some patients. Lockhead K "Anesthesia for Ophthalmology Patients," in Bryant S, Anesthesia for Veterinary Technicians, ed 1, Wiley-Blackwell, 2010, p. 195.
161. b Temperatures <32°C (89.6°F) cause dangerous CNS depression and changes in heart function. Body temperatures in the range of 32°C to 34°C (89.6°F to 93.2°F) prolong anesthetic recovery and significantly decrease the dose of anesthetic agents required to maintain surgical anesthesia by slowing the rate at which liver enzymes metabolize the drugs. IV fluids being administered to surgical patients should be warmed, especially if the patient is already hypothermic. Circulating warm water blankets set at 45°C (approximately 111°F) can cause hyperthermia. Thomas J, Phillip L, Anesthesia and Analgesia for Veterinary Technicians, ed 5, Elsevier, 2017.
162. d Masking or boxing a patient should be avoided because the struggling and excitement often associated with these methods can cause an increase in intraocular pressure. Alfaxalone, propofol, and etomidate are good choices for induction of the ophthalmology patient. Lockhead K, "Anesthesia for Ophthalmology Patients," in Bryant S, Anesthesia for Veterinary Technicians, ed 1, Wiley-Blackwell, 2010, p. 196.
163. a Nystagmus is commonly seen in horses during certain planes of anesthesia. Fast nystagmus occurs in very light anesthesia and gradually slows as the anesthetic depth increases. Very slow nystagmus may still be present as a roving eye during medium ruminants. Small animals rarely show nystagmus under anesthesia. Thomas J, Phillip L, Anesthesia and Analgesia for Veterinary Technicians, . ed 5, Elsevier, 2017.
164. c Nitrous oxide is contraindicated in ocular procedures where air may be injected into a chamber of the closed eye because nitrous oxide will diffuse into the bubble of air and increase IOP. Isoflurane, sevoflurane, and desflurane are all acceptable anesthetic agents. Lockhead K, "Anesthesia for Ophthalmology Patients," in Bryant S, Anesthesia for Veterinary Technicians, ed 1, Wiley-Blackwell, 2010, p. 196.
165. c Pale mucous membranes indicate intraoperative blood loss, anemia from any cause, or poor capillary perfusion (as may occur with vasoconstriction, excessive anesthetic depth, or prolonged anesthesia). Acidosis would not necessarily produce visible signs. Hypotension might be indicated by weakness and hypertension may be indicated by red gums and sclera. Thomas J, Phillip L, Anesthesia and Analgesia for Veterinary Technicians, ed 5, Elsevier, 2017.
166. c Neuromuscular blocking agents are commonly used for ophthalmology patients to prevent movement of the eye during the procedure and to keep the eye in a central position. They do not provide analgesia or sedation; therefore, drugs such as opioids, benzodiazepines, and alpha-2 agonists are analgesics and sedatives that can be used to provide appropriate analgesia and sedation. Lockhead K, "Anesthesia for Ophthalmology Patients," in Bryant S, Anesthesia for Veterinary Technicians, ed 1, Wiley-Blackwell, 2010, p. 198.
167. a A retrobulbar block is commonly used to desensitize nerves and add additional analgesia to an intraocular or enucleation procedure. A sacrococcygeal block provides desensitization to the tail and anus, a circumferential nerve block is commonly used for declaw procedures, and an epidural is used to desensitize the lower limbs. An epidural can also be placed higher for surgery involving the cranial abdomen. Lockhead K, "Anesthesia for Ophthalmology Patients," in Bryant S, Anesthesia for Veterinary Technicians, ed 1, Wiley-Blackwell, 2010, p. 198.
168. c With increasing depth of anesthesia, the resistance to movement of the jaw will progressively decrease and the anal orifice will progressively increase in size. Tone generally is marked in light anesthesia, moderate in medium anesthesia, and flaccid in deep anesthesia. The palpebral reflex (blink reflex) is a blink in response to a light tap on the medial or lateral canthus of the eye and can be seen with a light plane of anesthesia. Irregular respiration would also indicate a light plane of anesthesia (whereas apnea would indicate a deep plane of anesthesia). The size of the pupil also varies with anesthetic depth; pupils are dilated (mydriatic) during stage II anesthesia, are normal or constricted (miotic) during light surgical anesthesia, progressively dilate as anesthetic depth increases, and are widely dilated during deep anesthesia. Thomas J, Phillip L, Anesthesia and Analgesia for Veterinary Technicians, ed 5, Elsevier, 2017.
169. a Topical anesthesia is a loss of sensation in a small area of the body produced by administration of a local

anesthetic directly to a body surface such as the eyes or skin. Epidural anesthesia is when local anesthetic is used to provide pain control and loss of sensation to the rear quarters and pelvic region. Surgical anesthesia refers to the specific stage within general anesthesia in which there is a sufficient degree of analgesia and muscle relaxation to allow surgery to be performed without patient pain or movement. Thomas J, Phillip L, Anesthesia and Analgesia for Veterinary Technicians, ed 5, Elsevier, 2017.

170. b Inhalation is initiated by the respiratory center in the brain and is normally triggered by an increased level of carbon dioxide in the arterial blood ($PaCO_2$). As $PaCO_2$ rises above a threshold level (approximately 40 mmHg), the respiratory center initiates the active inspiratory phase by stimulating the intercostal muscles and diaphragm to move, expanding the thorax. Therefore, insufficient levels of carbon dioxide would not stimulate the respiratory phase. Thomas J, Phillip L, Anesthesia and Analgesia for Veterinary Technicians, ed 5, Elsevier, 2017.

171. b Hypertrophic cardiomyopathy is the most common form of heart disease seen in cats. Dilated cardiomyopathy and mitral valve insufficiency are more commonly seem in canine patients versus feline. Low blood pressure can be seen in either species as a result of disease process or medications. Curtis-Uhle W, Waddell K, "Anesthesia for Patients with Cardiac Disease," in Bryant S, Anesthesia for Veterinary Technicians, ed 1, Wiley-Blackwell, 2010, p. 205.

172. c Hypertrophic cardiomyopathy patients should avoid stress, tachycardia, and tachyarrhythmia. Of the drugs listed, atropine is an anticholinergic used to increase heart rate. This is contraindicated in patients with hypertrophic cardiomyopathy. Curtis-Uhle W, Waddell K, "Anesthesia for Patients with Cardiac Disease," in Bryant S, Anesthesia for Veterinary Technicians, ed 1, Wiley-Blackwell, 2010, p. 209.

173. b Normal VT in the awakened animal is 10–15 mL/kg. Thomas J, Phillip L, Anesthesia and Analgesia for Veterinary Technicians, ed 5, Elsevier, 2017.

174. d All of the factors listed cause an increase in intracranial pressure, which may be detrimental to neurosurgical patients. LoMastro E, "Small Animal Patients with Head Trauma," in Bryant S, Anesthesia for Veterinary Technicians, ed 1, Wiley-Blackwell, 2010.

175. d Sensory neurons are affected by even small amounts of local anesthetic, provided the drug is deposited in proximity to the neuron. Motor and autonomic neurons are also sensitive to the effect of local anesthetics. Autonomic neurons convey impulses between the brain and the blood vessels and internal organs (including the heart). Thomas J, Phillip L, Anesthesia and Analgesia for Veterinary Technicians, ed 5, Elsevier, 2017.

176. a Controlled hyperventilation is a common way to manage intracranial pressure and therefore it reduces brain size during neurosurgery. Hypoventilation, ketamine CRI, and placing the patient in a head down position have been shown to increase intracranial pressure. Ketamine should be avoided because it will cause an increase in ICP and patients should be placed at a slight incline with the head level slightly above the heart level. LoMastro E, "Small Animal Patients with Head Trauma," in Bryant S, Anesthesia for Veterinary Technicians, ed 1, Wiley-Blackwell, 2010, p. 221.

177. b Inhalant anesthetics increase cerebral blood flow and therefore increase intracranial pressure. LoMastro E, "Small Animal Patients with Head Trauma," in Bryant S, Anesthesia for Veterinary Technicians, ed 1, Wiley-Blackwell, 2010, p. 221.

178. b Local anesthetics result in antagonism, or blockade, of sodium channels. When the sodium channels of a neuron are blocked, the neuron cannot generate electrical impulses. Local anesthetics do not affect the brain and although they block impulse transmission, they do not do so in the spinal cord. Thomas J, Phillip L, Anesthesia and Analgesia for Veterinary Technicians, ed 5, Elsevier, 2017.

179. d Remifentanil has the shortest duration of action (10–15 minutes), thus making it the most attractive for patients requiring neurological examinations. The infusion can be discontinued and shortly after a neurological exam can be performed with the assurance that any abnormal neurological signs are not attributed to opioid-induced sedation or dysphoria. Morphine, methadone, and fentanyl have a longer duration of action. Liss D, Spelts K, "Analgesia for Emergency and Critical Care Patients," Shaffran ME, Goldberg N (eds), Pain Management for Veterinary Technicians and Nurses, ed 1, Wiley Blackwell, 2014.

180. a Methadone is unlikely to produce vomiting when compared with the higher incidence of vomiting/nausea seen with morphine and hydromorphone. Midazolam is not an opioid but a benzodiazepine. Liss D, Spelts K, "Analgesia for Emergency and Critical Care Patients," Shaffran ME, Goldberg N (eds), Pain Management for Veterinary Technicians and Nurses, ed 1, Wiley Blackwell, 2014.

181. d In cats the spinal cord extends caudally, as far as S1. Thomas J, Phillip L, Anesthesia and Analgesia for Veterinary Technicians, . ed 5, Elsevier, 2017.

182. d Mannitol is the only listed drug that is effective at reducing brain edema and intracranial pressure. All of the other agents cause an increase in intracranial pressure (ICP). LoMastro E, "Small Animal Patients with Head Trauma," in Bryant S, Anesthesia for Veterinary Technicians, ed 1, Wiley-Blackwell, 2010, p. 223.

183. c The dose of lidocaine given subcutaneously to dogs, cows, and horses should not exceed 10 mg/kg and in cats should not exceed 4 mg/kg to avoid systemic toxicity. Thomas J, Phillip L, Anesthesia and Analgesia for Veterinary Technicians, ed 5, Elsevier, 2017.

184. c All of the choices cause increased cerebral blood flow and intracranial pressure. However, nitrous oxide causes the most dramatic increase in cerebral blood flow and intracranial pressure. LoMastro E, "Small Animal Patients with Head Trauma," in Bryant S, Anesthesia for Veterinary Technicians, ed 1, Wiley-Blackwell, 2010, p. 223.

185. b *Insulinoma* is the term used for a tumor of the pancreas that results in excessive insulin production, leading to hypoglycemia. Pancreatitis is inflammation of the pancreas, diabetes is caused by a deficiency of insulin, and hyperglycemia (an increase in blood glucose levels) is often seen with diabetes. Holland S, "Anesthesia for Patients with Endocrine Disease," in Bryant S, Anesthesia for Veterinary Technicians, ed 1, Wiley-Blackwell, 2010, p. 239.

186. c Because VT is reduced, the alveoli do not expand as fully as normal on inspiration. The alveoli in some sections of the lung, particularly those that are lower in the animal's body, may partially collapse (a condition called atelectasis). Excess fluid in the respiratory system is known as pleural effusion. Apnea is the absence of breathing. Bronchial constriction can be seen in asthma, a common chronic inflammatory disease of the airways characterized by variable and recurring symptoms, reversible airflow obstruction, and bronchospasm. Thomas J, Phillip L, Anesthesia and Analgesia for Veterinary Technicians, ed 5, Elsevier, 2017.

187. a Depolarizing agents, such as succinylcholine, cause a single surge of activity at the neuromuscular junction, which is followed by a period in which the muscle end plate is refractory to further stimulation. Animals given these agents may show spontaneous muscle twitching followed by paralysis. Succinylcholine has a fast onset (20 seconds) but a short duration of effect and is useful for rapid intubation. Potential adverse effects of succinylcholine include hyperkalemia and cardiac arrhythmias. Nondepolarizing agents, such as gallamine, pancuronium, atracurium besylate, and cisatracurium, act by blocking the receptors at the end plates. As their classification suggests, they do not cause an initial surge of activity at the neuromuscular junction and spontaneous muscle movements are not seen. Potential adverse effects of these agents include histamine release, hypotension or hypertension, tachycardia, and ventricular arrhythmias. Thomas J, Phillip L, Anesthesia and Analgesia for Veterinary Technicians, . ed 5, Elsevier, 2017.

188. c Surgical removal is the treatment of choice for an insulinoma. Antibiotics and antifungal drugs will not help to heal or shrink the tumor. A patient should not be started on insulin therapy because the insulinoma is already producing more insulin than the body needs. Holland S "Anesthesia for Patients with Endocrine Disease," in Bryant S, Anesthesia for Veterinary Technicians, ed 1, Wiley-Blackwell, 2010, p. 240.

189. a Dexmedetomidine is known to cause increasing glucose and then a subsequent decrease in insulin that can last several hours. Morphine and fentanyl are opioids, which cause little to no effect on the patient's glucose. The same is true for the inhalant anesthetic isoflurane. Holland S "Anesthesia for Patients with Endocrine Disease," in Bryant S, Anesthesia for Veterinary Technicians, ed 1, Wiley-Blackwell, 2010, p. 240.

190. c Regardless of the agent used, only voluntary (skeletal) muscles are affected. These agents do not affect the involuntary muscles, including cardiac muscle and the smooth muscle of the intestine and bladder. Skeletal muscles are affected in a predictable order: facial and neck paralysis is seen first, followed by paralysis of the tail, limbs, and abdominal muscles. The intercostal muscles and diaphragm are affected last. Thomas J, Phillip L, Anesthesia and Analgesia for Veterinary Technicians, ed 5, Elsevier, 2017.

191. d Many anesthetic agents have a narrow margin of safety between therapeutic and toxic doses. The incorrect administration of drugs may have serious or even fatal consequences and may arise from the confusion between syringes drawn up for two different patients. This involves either a failure to label the syringes or a failure to read the labels correctly. The technician must discard both syringes, label new syringes, and draw up new medication. Thomas J, Phillip L, Anesthesia and Analgesia for Veterinary Technicians, ed 5, Elsevier, 2017.

192. b Nonsteroidal anti-inflammatory drugs should be avoided in patients with renal disease. These drugs can cause a decrease in renal blood flow. Opioids, anticholinergics, and inhalant anesthetics do not significantly affect renal function at therapeutic doses. Cooley K, "Patients with Renal Disease," in Bryant S, Anesthesia for Veterinary Technicians, ed 1, Wiley-Blackwell, 2010, p. 254.

193. d Alanine aminotransferase (ALT) and alkaline phosphatase are laboratory values commonly used to evaluate liver function before an anesthetic event. Glucose and fructosamine would be commonly checked in diabetic patients, creatinine would commonly be used to determine kidney function, and PCV and total protein would be used to check hydration status. Carter H, "Anesthesia for Patients with Liver Disease," in Bryant S, Anesthesia for Veterinary Technicians, ed 1, Wiley-Blackwell, 2010, p. 257.

194. a It is important to be able to recognize when the machine is no longer delivering oxygen to the patient. If the oxygen flowmeter reads zero, the patient is not receiving any oxygen, regardless of the oxygen tank pressure. Occasionally when the oxygen tank is nearly empty, the oxygen tank pressure gauge reads zero, but the flowmeter indicates some oxygen flow. Even though the tank is still delivering a small amount of oxygen, loss of oxygen pressure is imminent and the tank must be changed immediately. Disconnect the patient from the circuit, connect the new tank, and then reconnect the patient to the anesthetic machine. Allowing the patient to breathe room air is unacceptable because no anesthetic will be delivered to the patient. The patient does not need to be resuscitated with the Ambu bag because it's breathing had not stopped. Switching to an injectable anesthetic would only be an option if no oxygen was available. Thomas J, Phillip L, Anesthesia and Analgesia for Veterinary Technicians, ed 5, Elsevier, 2017.

195. a Alpha-2 adrenergic agonists are not commonly used in pediatric patients because of their main side effect of bradycardia. Because pediatric patients are dependent on heart rate for cardiac output, bradycardia can be detrimental in these patients. Opioids and benzodiazepines do not commonly cause a significant change in heart rate when used at proper doses. Anticholinergics are actually preferred in pediatric patients to maintain heart rate. Farry T, Anesthesia for Pediatric Patients," in Bryant S, Anesthesia for Veterinary Technicians, ed 1, Wiley-Blackwell, 2010, p. 271.

196. d Chamber induction with isoflurane is the least suitable choice compared with injectable methods. This is because of the side effects of chamber induction (stress, cardiac compromise) and the waste gas exposure of the staff. McNerney T, "Surgical Pain Management," Shaffran ME, Goldberg N (eds), Pain Management for Veterinary Technicians and Nurses, ed 1, Wiley Blackwell, 2014.

197. b After arrest occurs, permanent brain damage may result if oxygen delivery to the brain is not reestablished within 4 minutes by either cardiopulmonary resuscitation (CPR) or restoration of cardiac function. Thomas J, Phillip L, Anesthesia and Analgesia for Veterinary Technicians, ed 5, Elsevier, 2017.

198. a The non-rebreathing system uses a higher flow of oxygen to lower resistance to breathing and minimize apparatus dead space. A rebreathing system uses lower fresh gas flow rates but also increases dead space and some rebreathing of CO_2 can occur. A ventilator must be used with caution as the small tidal volumes of these patients increase their risk for barotrauma. Farry T, "Anesthesia for Pediatric Patients," in Bryant S, Anesthesia for Veterinary Technicians, ed 1, Wiley-Blackwell, 2010.

199. c Plasma-Lyte 148 is an example of a crystalloid. Hetastarch, dextran, and plasma are examples of colloids. Colloids contain large molecular weight substances that act as expanders of the intravascular space. Beiter C, "Fluid Therapy and Blood Products," in Bryant S, Anesthesia for Veterinary Technicians, ed 1, Wiley-Blackwell, 2010, p. 125.

200. b Occasionally an anesthetist inadvertently leaves the pop-off valve in a closed position. If the pop-off valve is closed and the oxygen flow rate is greater than the patient's oxygen requirement, pressure within the circuit will rapidly rise. This can happen with use of a closed system in which the oxygen flow rate has inadvertently been set higher than the metabolic oxygen consumption (approximately 10 mL/kg/min). As pressure rises in the circuit, the reservoir bag will expand, as will the patient's lungs. This prevents exhalation and also decreases the venous return to the heart. This in turn may decrease cardiac output, cause blood pressure to fall rapidly, and can lead to death within a short time unless recognized and corrected. If the flow rate starts to drop, oxygen is not flowing to the anesthetic machine, but it is not a pop-off valve issue. If the anesthetist can smell isoflurane, there is probably a leak, but this is not related to the pop-off valve. A patient waking up from anesthesia is most probably a result of an inadequate vaporizer setting or empty vaporizer and is not a pop-off valve issue. Thomas J, Phillip L, Anesthesia and Analgesia for Veterinary Technicians, ed 5, Elsevier, 2017.

201. c Hetastarch should be used with caution in the patient with blood clotting abnormalities because it can interfere with clotting factor VIII and von Willebrand factor. Plasma-Lyte, lactated Ringer's, and Normosol-R are all crystalloids, which are considered benign at normal doses. Beiter C, "Fluid Therapy and Blood Products," in Bryant S, Anesthesia for Veterinary Technicians, ed 1, Wiley-Blackwell, 2010, p. 124.

202. b If possible, the anesthetist should preoxygenate brachycephalic patients for 5 minutes before induction. Gently restraining the animal and administering oxygen through a facemask can do this. This procedure helps maintain adequate blood oxygen levels and gives the animal an extra margin of safety during the induction period that follows. The use of dexmedetomidine as part of the anesthetic protocol is not the best choice because it can cause dyspnea in brachycephalic patients. Chamber induction is not advised and is considered dangerous. Chamber induction does not allow the patient to be monitored, releases waste gases into the atmosphere, and stresses the patient. A laryngeal mask airway is unnecessary if preoxygenation occurs. Thomas J, Phillip L, Anesthesia and Analgesia for Veterinary Technicians, ed 5, Elsevier, 2017.

203. a Normal 0.9% saline is not considered a balanced solution because it does not have a fluid composition that closely resembles the patient's extracellular fluid. Beiter C, "Fluid Therapy and Blood Products," in Bryant S, Anesthesia for Veterinary Technicians, ed 1, Wiley-Blackwell, 2010, p. 124.

204. b A tidal volume is the volume of gas exhaled in one breath. An approximate value is 10–20 mL/kg. Therefore, 40 kg×10–20 mL = 400–800 mL. Hughes L, "Breathing Systems and Ancillary Equipment," in Duke-Novakovski T, de Vries M, Seymour C, BSAVA Manual of Canine and Feline Anaesthesia and Analgesia, ed 3, British Small Animal Veterinary Association, 2016.

205. c The veterinarian and anesthetist should ensure that anesthetic agents that depress the myocardium or that exacerbate arrhythmias (e.g., alpha-2 agonists and halothane) are avoided as much as possible in these animals. Therefore, xylazine should be avoided in these patients. Opioid agents, lidocaine, diazepam, isoflurane, or sevoflurane have the advantage of relative lack of toxicity to the heart. Thomas J, Phillip L, Anesthesia and Analgesia for Veterinary Technicians, . ed 5, Elsevier, 2017.

206. a Minute volume refers to the sum of all gas volumes exhaled in 1 minute. It is calculated as a multiple of tidal volume and respiration rate. Hughes L, "Breathing Systems and Ancillary Equipment," in Duke-Novakovski T, de Vries M, Seymour C, BSAVA Manual of Canine and Feline Anaesthesia and Analgesia, ed 3, British Small Animal Veterinary Association, 2016.

207. b Acepromazine is an antagonist at alpha-1 adrenoreceptors. This causes a peripheral vasodilation, resulting in decreased temperature and overall blood pressure. For this reason acepromazine should be avoided in patients with cardiovascular instability or in shock such as a patient recently hit by a car. Murrell JC, "Pre-anaesthetic medication and sedation," in Duke-Novakovski T, de Vries M, Seymour C, BSAVA Manual of Canine and Feline Anaesthesia and Analgesia, ed 3, British Small Animal Veterinary Association, 2016.

208. b Tachypnea (rapid respirations) must be differentiated from dyspnea, in which respiratory distress is present. Tachypnea may arise at any time during anesthesia and may be disconcerting to the anesthetist. It is particularly common during procedures using opioids. Tachypnea may also be seen if anesthetic depth is inadequate, in which case it is often accompanied by tachycardia and spontaneous movement. Paradoxically, tachypnea may also occur in deep anesthesia as a response to low blood oxygen and high blood carbon dioxide levels. Tachypnea is also seen in hyperthermic patients, including animals with malignant hyperthermia. Ketamine will not cause tachypnea, but rather apneustic breathing. Thomas J, Phillip L, Anesthesia and Analgesia for Veterinary Technicians, ed 5, Elsevier, 2017.

209. c Vaporizer settings are percentages (%) and not L/min (as oxygen is). The sevoflurane vaporizer should be set at 2.5% to 4%. Thomas J, Phillip L, Anesthesia and Analgesia for Veterinary Technicians, ed 5, Elsevier, 2017.

210. d All of the listed drugs are examples of alpha-2 adrenoreceptor agonists except yohimbine, which is an alpha-2 antagonist. Therefore, it is used as a reversal for drugs such as xylazine and medetomidine. Murrell JC, “Pre-anaesthetic medication and sedation,” in Duke-Novakovski T, de Vries M, Seymour C, BSAVA Manual of Canine and Feline Anaesthesia and Analgesia, ed 3, British Small Animal Veterinary Association, 2016.

211. a To induce general anesthesia by the IV route, a volume of the agent to be administered is calculated on the basis of a prescribed dose and drawn into a syringe. The agent is then injected directly into the vein or into a winged-infusion set or indwelling catheter to effect anesthetization until the patient can be intubated or until the patient is at an adequate plane of anesthesia for completion of the planned procedure. The term *to effect* means that only the amount of injectable anesthetic necessary to produce unconsciousness is given, rather than administering the entire dose calculated on a milligram per kilogram basis. This technique is necessary because the amount of drug needed to induce or maintain anesthesia cannot be accurately predicted for a given patient and most anesthetic agents have narrow therapeutic indices. Thomas J, Phillip L, Anesthesia and Analgesia for Veterinary Technicians, ed 5, Elsevier, 2017.

212. b Before a drug is excreted, it is often metabolized (or biotransformed) and this occurs most often in the liver. The skin, eyes, and intestines can absorb drugs but not metabolize. Phillip L, Anesthesia and Analgesia for Veterinary Technicians, ed 5, Elsevier, 2017.

213. a Sedation is a drug-induced CNS depression and drowsiness that varies in intensity from light to deep. Surgical anesthesia refers to the specific stage within general anesthesia in which there is a sufficient degree of analgesia and muscle relaxation to allow surgery to be performed without patient pain or movement. Local anesthesia is a loss of sensation in a small area of the body produced by administration of a local anesthetic. Thomas J, Phillip L, Anesthesia and Analgesia for Veterinary Technicians, ed 5, Elsevier, 2017.

214. d Because of the solubility of propofol, it should only be administered via the intravenous route. Thomas J, Phillip L, Anesthesia and Analgesia for Veterinary Technicians, ed 5, Elsevier, 2017.

215. d Circulating warm water blankets, convective warm air devices, and commercially available bubble wrap are considered safe ways to warm a patient in the recovery period. Electric heating blankets, however, can overheat tissues and burn the recovering patient that may not be able to move away from the heat source. Levensaler A, “Monitoring: Pulse Oximetry, Temperature, and Hands-on,” in Bryant S, Anesthesia for Veterinary Technicians, ed 1, Wiley-Blackwell, 2010, p. 99.

216. b Hypoxia is defined as impaired oxygen delivery because of systemic delivery issues. Atelectasis refers to a diminished volume or a lack of air in part or all of a lung lobe. Functional residual capacity describes the amount of air left in the lungs after normal ventilation. The FRC is important to the veterinary anesthetist because during apnea it is the reservoir to supply oxygen to the blood. Tidal volume is the volume of air that moves in and out of the patient during a full respiratory cycle. Slowiak C, “Ventilation Techniques in Small Animal Patients,” in Bryant S, Anesthesia for Veterinary Technicians, ed 1, Wiley-Blackwell, 2010, p. 188-189.

217. b Alfaxalone is a neuroactive steroid used as a common injectable anesthetic induction agent. Pentobarbital is a barbiturate. Midazolam is a benzodiazepine often used as a skeletal muscle relaxant and adjunct to other injectable anesthetic induction drugs. Propofol is a non-barbiturate ultra–short-acting injectable anesthetic. Thomas J, Phillip L, Anesthesia and Analgesia for Veterinary Technicians, ed 5, Elsevier, 2017.

218. a Persons working in environments with a high level of waste gas have reported symptoms such as fatigue, headache, drowsiness, nausea, depression, and irritability. Although these symptoms usually resolve spontaneously when the affected person leaves the area, the frequent occurrence of these symptoms may indicate that excessive levels of waste gas are present and that a potential for long-term toxicity exists. Thomas J, Phillip L, Anesthesia and Analgesia for Veterinary Technicians, ed 5, Elsevier, 2017.

219. a An endotracheal tube of the correct diameter and length will improve efficiency of gas exchange by reducing the amount of anatomic dead space. Anatomic dead space is composed of the portions of the breathing passages that contain air but in which no gas exchange can occur (i.e., the mouth, nasal passages, pharynx, trachea, and bronchi). With the anatomic dead space minimized, the endotracheal tube ensures that a larger proportion of the gas delivered to the patient reaches the exchange surface in the alveoli. Thomas J, Phillip L, Anesthesia and Analgesia for Veterinary Technicians, ed 5, Elsevier, 2017.

220. c Long-term inhalation of air polluted with waste gas may be associated with serious health problems, including reproductive disorders, liver and kidney damage, bone marrow abnormalities, and chronic nervous system dysfunction. Although current evidence suggests that the risk of these disorders is not high in normal veterinary practice settings, every person working in an environment in which waste gas is present should be informed of the potential for adverse health effects. Thomas J, Phillip L, Anesthesia and Analgesia for Veterinary Technicians, ed 5, Elsevier, 2017.

221. b Check that the motion of the unidirectional valves coincides with breathing. The inhalation valve should open as the patient inhales and the exhalation valve should open when the patient exhales. A patient that coughs can indicate correct placement of the ET in the trachea. The manometer would indicate pressure only if the patient is being ventilated. Palpating firm structures in the neck does not indicate the ET has been placed in the esophagus. Thomas J, Phillip L, Anesthesia and Analgesia for Veterinary Technicians, ed 5, Elsevier, 2017.

222. d Using inhalant gas only will not decrease but increase the amount of waste anesthetic gases in the surgical suite. If proper equipment, techniques, and procedures are used, it is possible to reduce waste gas exposure to a level well below the NIOSH standards. This can be achieved through several means, including using a gas scavenging system, testing equipment for leaks, and using techniques and procedures that minimize exposure to waste gas. Thomas J, Phillip L, Anesthesia and Analgesia for Veterinary Technicians, ed 5, Elsevier, 2017.

223. c In dogs, return of the swallowing reflex is the most appropriate time to remove the tube because this reflex will help protect the animal from pulmonary aspiration if vomiting occurs during recovery. The ET would not be removed from the patient immediately after turning off the vaporizer because the patient will not have a swallow reflex. In addition, gases will leak into the recovery room versus being exhaled and scavenged in the anesthetic machine. Removing the ET 10 minutes after the vaporizer has been turned off decreases the risk of waste anesthetic gases but does not take into consideration whether the patient has swallow reflexes. Thomas J, Phillip L, Anesthesia and Analgesia for Veterinary Technicians, ed 5, Elsevier, 2017.

224. b An active system uses suction created by a vacuum pump or fan to draw gas into the scavenger, whereas a passive system uses the positive pressure of the gas in the anesthetic machine to push gas into the scavenger. The most commonly used type of passive system discharges waste gas to the outdoors through a hole in the wall. This system is best suited for rooms adjacent to the exterior of the building and is ineffective for interior rooms where the distance to the outlet is more than 20 feet (7 m). Thomas J, Phillip L, Anesthesia and Analgesia for Veterinary Technicians, ed 5, Elsevier, 2017.

225. b A recovering patient should be turned every 10–15 minutes to prevent pooling of blood in the dependent lung and tissues, a condition called hypostatic congestion. When the intubated patient is turned from one side to another, the breathing circuit must be briefly detached from the endotracheal tube and the head and neck should be turned as a single unit to minimize the risk of tracheal damage by the tube. Thomas J, Phillip L, Anesthesia and Analgesia for Veterinary Technicians, ed 5, Elsevier, 2017.

226. b Non-rebreathing systems do not use a chemical absorbent to remove carbon dioxide; therefore, high gas flow rates are required to eliminate carbon dioxide buildup. Increasing the gas flow rate exacerbates hypothermia and dries the respiratory tract. Reduced resistance to breathing, reduced mechanical dead space, and no soda lime requirements are all considered advantages of the non-rebreathing system. Latshaw H, Coleman D, "Anesthesia Equipment," in Bryant S, Anesthesia for Veterinary Technicians, ed 1, Wiley-Blackwell, 2010.

227. d IV induction with an ultra–short-acting agent and maintenance with an inhalant have dynamic elements, including rapid induction, good control over both increases and decreases in anesthetic depth, and a relatively rapid recovery. IM induction is too slow. IV induction with an ultra–short-acting agent and maintenance with bolus injections of the same will have a swinging anesthetic effect, yielding low control. Inhalant induction can take too long and can have risky side effects, including the escape of waste anesthetic gases. Thomas J, Phillip L, Anesthesia and Analgesia for Veterinary Technicians, ed 5, Elsevier, 2017.

228. a In the event of an emergency, the largest-gauge intravenous catheter should be placed so that fluids can be rapidly delivered by bolus. The smallest catheter possible could inadequately deliver fluids to the patient and catheters are not placed in critically ill patients only. Catheters should never be left in patients when they are not needed and if they are in place in critically ill patients, they should be replaced at least every 3 days. Takada S, "Intravenous Access," in Bryant S, Anesthesia for Veterinary Technicians, ed 1, Wiley-Blackwell, 2010.

229. c Pulse oximetry is a noninvasive measurement of the saturation of hemoglobin with oxygen calculated and expressed as a percentage. The pulse oximeter probe uses infrared and red light at different wavelengths to transilluminate a pulsatile arteriolar bed (nonpigmented tissue bed such as the tongue). Software in the pulse oximeter analyzes the absorption of light for both oxyhemoglobin and deoxyhemoglobin, thus creating a percentage for the ratio between the two. Pulse oximetry does not estimate respiratory rate, cardiac output, or the direct oxygen content of arterial blood. Schauvliege S "Patient Monitoring and Monitoring Equipment," in Duke-Novakovski T, de Vries M, Seymour C, BSAVA Manual of Canine and Feline Anaesthesia and Analgesia, ed 3, British Small Animal Veterinary Association, 2016.

230. a Small animal patients are restrained and anesthetized by means of a variety of techniques including general anesthesia, sedation, neuroleptanalgesia, and local and regional anesthesia. Of these options, general anesthesia is most commonly used for several reasons. The immobilization and unconsciousness associated with general anesthesia enable most procedures to be performed more quickly and safely than is possible with alternative techniques. General anesthetics also produce analgesia during the period of unconsciousness and, if used with an analgesic as part of a balanced protocol, during the preoperative and postoperative periods as well. In addition, general anesthetic procedures can be performed with readily available resources and at a reasonable cost. In dogs and cats general anesthesia is induced and maintained by using balanced protocols, exclusive use of inhalants, intramuscular (IM) protocols, and total intravenous (IV) techniques. Thomas J, Phillip L, Anesthesia and Analgesia for Veterinary Technicians, . ed 5, Elsevier, 2017.

231. c In both the United States and the United Kingdom, nitrous oxide cylinders are blue. In the United States, oxygen cylinders are green, medical air is yellow, and carbon dioxide is gray. Alibhai H, "The anaesthetic machine and vaporizers," in Duke-Novakovski T, de Vries M, Seymour C, BSAVA Manual of Canine and Feline Anaesthesia and Analgesia, ed 3, British Small Animal Veterinary Association, 2016.

232. d Active scavenging is the most effective way to scavenge all waste anesthetic gases and reduce overall staff exposure. Passive scavenging via activated charcoal devices only absorbs volatile anesthetics such as isoflurane, sevoflurane, and halothane. Activated charcoal does not scavenge nitrous oxide. Hughes L, "Breathing Systems and Ancillary Equipment," in Duke-Novakovski T, de Vries M, Seymour C, BSAVA Manual of Canine and Feline Anaesthesia and Analgesia, ed 3, British Small Animal Veterinary Association, 2016.

233. c An 18-kg dog would use a 9.5- to 10-mm ET tube. A smaller tube would allow waste anesthetic gases to escape and the patient could potentially aspirate. A larger tube could damage the trachea. Thomas J, Phillip L, Anesthesia and Analgesia for Veterinary Technicians, ed 5, Elsevier, 2017.

234. c Of the species listed, cats have a predisposition to laryngospasm. This most commonly occurs when intubation is attempted in patients that are not adequately anesthetized. Lidocaine is used to help prevent laryngospasm. Palmer D, "Airway Maintenance," in Bryant S, Anesthesia for Veterinary Technicians, ed 1, Wiley-Blackwell, 2010.

235. b Injecting air while applying pressure for the reservoir bag ensures that you do not overinflate the cuff. This method allows you to inject only the amount of air that is needed to provide a seal. Each patient requires a different amount of air injected into the cuff because this is based on how the endotracheal tube fits into the trachea. Palmer D, "Airway Maintenance," in Bryant S, Anesthesia for Veterinary Technicians, ed 1, Wiley-Blackwell, 2010.

236. b When properly maintained, an endotracheal tube helps to maintain an open airway, decreasing the likelihood of airway obstruction caused by patient position, collapse of pharyngeal tissues, entry of foreign material, and decreasing dead space. Because of the importance of maintaining a patent airway, it is customary to leave the tube in place throughout anesthesia and into the recovery period, until the animal regains the swallowing reflex. Although the ET allows the anesthetist to monitor the patient more closely, that is an indirect benefit, not direct. The ET does not prevent reflex tachycardia. Thomas J, Phillip L, Anesthesia and Analgesia for Veterinary Technicians, ed 5, Elsevier, 2017.

237. c Topical anesthetics such as lidocaine block sensation. Applying a small amount of local anesthetic to the arytenoids anesthetizes the area and helps prevent laryngospasm. Using a stylet or stiffer endotracheal tube without lidocaine will probably make the problem worse and potentially damage tissue. Palmer D, "Airway Maintenance," in Bryant S, Anesthesia for Veterinary Technicians, ed 1, Wiley-Blackwell, 2010.

238. b Brachycephalic breeds such as pugs often have stenotic nares, hypoplastic tracheas, and redundant tissues in the oropharyngeal region. Brachycephalic patients should not be extubated until they are fully awake and can hold their head up and maintain a free airway. Extubation is generally most successful when the patient is kept in sternal recumbency with the head and neck extended. It is also a good idea to have induction drugs and an additional endotracheal tube available in the event that the patient obstructs during recovery. Palmer D, "Airway Maintenance," in Bryant S, Anesthesia for Veterinary Technicians, ed 1, Wiley-Blackwell, 2010.

239. c The anesthetic record serves as the literal witness to significant events and physiological changes that occur during the anesthetic period. It is a legal document that must be kept in the patient's medical record. Reflexes do not need to be monitored during the anesthetic period because they do not directly correlate with overall well-being under anesthesia. Mucous membrane color, capillary refill time, heart and respiratory rates, and pulse quality and strength are important vital signs used to monitor and assess patients under general anesthesia. Dulong H, "Records and Record Keeping," in Bryant S, Anesthesia for Veterinary Technicians, ed 1, Wiley-Blackwell, 2010.

240. b Complications of improper intubation include the overinflation of the cuff or too large a tube diameter, causing necrosis of the tracheal mucosa. The correct-sized tube and proper inflation decrease dead space. Intubation with a normal-length tube will not allow the intubation of alveoli and atelectasis cannot occur, because this is the collapse of a portion or all of a lung (or both lungs). Thomas J, Phillip L, Anesthesia and Analgesia for Veterinary Technicians, ed 5, Elsevier, 2017.

241. b The anesthetic record is a legal document that is subject to subpoena. Countless disciplinary actions are brought against veterinary professionals every year. Maintaining timely, neat, complete, and organized anesthetic records can help avoid unnecessary lawsuits. This can be obtained by recording vital signs and observations every 5 minutes. Dulong H, "Records and Record Keeping," in Bryant S, Anesthesia for Veterinary Technicians, ed 1, Wiley-Blackwell, 2010.

242. c Brachycephalic breeds are predisposed to airway obstruction during the perianesthetic and postanesthetic periods because of stenotic nares, hypoplastic trachea, and redundant tissue in the oropharyngeal region. Palmer D, "Airway Maintenance," in Bryant S, Anesthesia for Veterinary Technicians, ed 1, Wiley-Blackwell, 2010.

243. c If one lung is diseased, place the healthy side up whenever possible to maximize oxygen exchange. A patient must be monitored more frequently than every 30 minutes. Patients should never be placed on electric heating pads because they cannot move away from the heat source and are at an increased risk of thermal burns. Tilting the surgery table so that the patient's head is down gives the surgeon easier access to some abdominal organs, particularly the uterus and ovaries. However, the anesthetist should be aware that more than a 15-degree elevation of the caudal aspect of the body may cause the abdominal organs to compress the diaphragm, which may compromise heart and lung function. Thomas J, Phillip L, Anesthesia and Analgesia for Veterinary Technicians, ed 5, Elsevier, 2017.

244. a Placing an indwelling catheter into an artery does direct blood pressure monitoring. This technique gives the anesthetist the ability to see continuous blood pressure in real time. Indirect monitoring is done by using a Doppler, cuff and sphygmomanometer, or via oscillometric methods. Central venous pressure is used to monitor fluid load via a central line. Peripheral venous pressure is similar to central venous pressure but is not commonly used in clinical practice. Reuss-Lamky HL, "Monitoring Blood Pressure and End-Tidal CO_2 in the Anesthetized Patient," in Bryant S, Anesthesia for Veterinary Technicians, ed 1, Wiley-Blackwell, 2010.

245. e The length of the recovery period depends on many factors. The length of the anesthetic period: as a general rule, the longer the patient is under anesthesia, the longer the expected recovery. The condition of the patient: lengthy recoveries are seen in animals that have almost any debilitating disease (particularly liver and kidney disease). The type of anesthetic given and the route of administration: lengthy recoveries are more common if an injectable agent is given intramuscularly rather than intravenously. The patient's temperature: hypothermic patients are slow to metabolize and excrete anesthetic drugs. The breed of the patient: certain canine breeds (e.g., greyhounds, salukis, Afghan hounds, whippets, and Russian wolfhounds) are slow to recover from certain anesthetic agents, especially barbiturates. Thomas J, Phillip L, Anesthesia and Analgesia for Veterinary Technicians, ed 5, Elsevier, 2017.

246. d Arterial blood gas analysis is the most accurate way to measure respiratory function and effectiveness. Depth of chest movements, respiratory rate, and air movement, even when within normal ranges, do not equate to effective respiration. Keefe J, "Introduction to Monitoring the ECG and Blood Gasses," in Bryant S, Anesthesia for Veterinary Technicians, ed 1, Wiley-Blackwell, 2010.

247. c An animal should never have a seizure while recovering from anesthesia. An animal recovering from general anesthesia gradually progresses back through the anesthetic stages and planes. As the animal moves from deep to moderate to light anesthesia, vital signs and reflexes change in predictable ways. The heart rate, respiratory rate, and respiratory volume begin to increase. After assuming a ventromedial position, the eyeballs move back to a central position. Reflex responses return and muscle tone strengthens. The animal may shiver, swallow, chew, or attempt to lick. Shortly after swallowing reflexes return, the animal will normally show signs of consciousness, including voluntary movement of the head or limbs and possibly vocalization. While passing through stage II, some patients may exhibit a variety of alarming signs including head-bobbing, delirium, hyperventilation, head-thrashing, and rapid limb paddling, especially if not premedicated. Occasionally a patient may attempt to stand and fall or may appear blind and bump into the sides of the cage. Some patients (particularly those recovering from ketamine anesthesia) may chew at their paws or claw their faces. Animals showing these signs of a rough or stormy recovery usually return to normal within a short time, but steps must be taken to prevent self-trauma or disruption of the surgical wound. Administration of preanesthetic medications before the procedure often prevents or moderates these signs, but additional tranquilization or administration of analgesics during the postoperative period may be necessary in these patients. Thomas J, Phillip L, Anesthesia and Analgesia for Veterinary Technicians, ed 5, Elsevier, 2017.

248. b ALT (alanine aminotransferase) screens for liver function, whereas BUN, creatinine, and a urinalysis analyze various aspects of renal function. Dupre J, "The Preanesthetic Workup," in Bryant S, Anesthesia for Veterinary Technicians, ed 1, Wiley-Blackwell, 2010.

249. c Leak testing, weighing the charcoal canister, and filling the vaporizer should be done before any procedure that will require anesthesia. The vaporizer is only calibrated annually or if a problem is noted. Latshaw H, Coleman D, "Anesthesia Equipment," in Bryant S, Anesthesia for Veterinary Technicians, ed 1, Wiley-Blackwell, 2010.

250. a Oxygen should be administered via the endotracheal tube at a rate of 50–100 mL/kg/min (0.5–1 L/10 kg body weight up to a maximum of 5 L/min) for 5 minutes after discontinuation of the anesthetic or until the animal swallows. This route of administration allows waste anesthetic gases to be scavenged and gives the anesthetist the ability to bag the patient during recovery to help reinflate collapsed alveoli. A patient recovering should never be left alone in a cage, especially when intubated. Patients should be turned every 15 minutes, not every 45 minutes. The patient should always be monitored for temperature to see what actions should be taken. Rarely do patients become hyperthermic. Thomas J, Phillip L, Anesthesia and Analgesia for Veterinary Technicians, ed 5, Elsevier, 2017.

251. a ASA status ranges for I–V where an ASA I is a healthy patient with minimal risk. An ASA II is a patient with slight to mild systemic changes and is at slight risk. An ASA III is a patient with system changes and some clinical alterations and is at moderate risk. An ASA IV is a patient with moderate to severe pre-existing disease and is at high risk. Last, an ASA V is a patient that is so severely compromised that it is unlikely to make it through surgery. This patient is at extreme risk. Dupre J, "Preanesthetic Workup," in Bryant S, Anesthesia for Veterinary Technicians, ed 1, Wiley-Blackwell, 2010.

252. b Treatment for hypotension can include a myriad of treatments including decreasing the vaporizer setting, giving a fluid bolus, increasing the heart rate if needed, and starting a positive inotropic drug such as a dopamine constant rate infusion. Inhalants are potent vasodilators; therefore increasing the anesthetic gas will probably make hypotension worse. Increasing the oxygen flow rate and ventilating the patient will not help treat hypotension. McMillan S, "Anesthetic Complications and Emergencies," in Bryant S, Anesthesia for Veterinary Technicians, ed 1, Wiley-Blackwell, 2010.

253. c If the procedure lasts for a considerable period, the horse may develop nasal congestion, which could lead to respiratory obstruction. To avoid this, the head should be held up in a neutral position. If the horse is placed in stocks, crossties can be used for this purpose. Horses cannot be intubated (and hooked to an anesthesia machine) during standing chemical restraint. When a horse is lying on its back or laterally, the risk of myopathy or neuropathy increases. Hypoxemia is not a complication of standing chemical restraint. Thomas J, Phillip L, Anesthesia and Analgesia for Veterinary Technicians, ed 5, Elsevier, 2017.

254. b To ensure the airway is properly protected, patients should not be extubated until the swallow reflex has returned. Waiting too long can lead to the patient biting through the tube. Dogs and cats cannot vocalize if they are intubated properly. Palmer D, "Airway Maintenance," in Bryant S, Anesthesia for Veterinary Technicians, ed 1, Wiley-Blackwell, 2010.

255. a The most common site for epidural injections in dogs is at the lumbosacral junction (L7 and S1). The spinal cord in dogs ends at vertebra L6. The epidural space surrounds the spinal cord and meninges. Patients can be placed in either sternal or lateral recumbency for drug administration. Duke-Novakovski T, "Pain management II: local and regional anaesthetic techniques," in Duke-Novakovski T, de Vries M, Seymour C, BSAVA Manual of Canine and Feline Anaesthesia and Analgesia, ed 3, British Small Animal Veterinary Association, 2016.

256. a It is also possible that external stimuli in an environment unfamiliar to the horse may result in the excitement, even if the horse initially appeared to be adequately sedated with acepromazine or an alpha-2 agonist. If this occurs, the horse should be given time to calm down (decrease external stimuli, refrain from trying to move the horse into the induction area) before proceeding. The horse should not be restrained by using ropes because this will cause the horse to panic. Acepromazine is a tranquilizer, not an induction agent. Ketamine is used in combination with other agents, not alone. Thomas J, Phillip L, Anesthesia and Analgesia for Veterinary Technicians, ed 5, Elsevier, 2017.

257. c Epidural anesthesia and analgesia are used to provide either a complete sensory blockade or pain relief for surgeries most commonly associated with the caudal half of the body, such as abdominal surgeries and various orthopedic procedures. Duke-Novakovski T, "Pain management II: local and regional anaesthetic techniques," in Duke-Novakovski T, de Vries M, Seymour C, BSAVA Manual of Canine and Feline Anaesthesia and Analgesia, ed 3, British Small Animal Veterinary Association, 2016.

258. b It is important to ensure that the horse's muscles and prominent nerves are protected when it is placed on a surgical table or surface. The anesthetist should make sure that muscle groups are well-supported and do not rest on hard surfaces during anesthesia to prevent myopathies and neuropathies. Positions do not help decrease the risk of the remaining options. Thomas J, Phillip L, Anesthesia and Analgesia for Veterinary Technicians, ed 5, Elsevier, 2017.

259. d Propofol is a short-acting hypnotic injectable anesthetic used in multiple species on veterinary patients. Propofol is highly lipid-soluble and is an oil-in-water emulsion that is a good medium for bacteria. Alfaxalone is an example of a neuroactive steroid anesthetic. Thiopental is an example of an ultra–short-acting barbiturate and examples of common dissociatives include ketamine and Telazol. Kastner S, in Duke-Novakovski T, de Vries M, Seymour C, BSAVA Manual of Canine and Feline Anaesthesia and Analgesia, ed 3, British Small Animal Veterinary Association, 2016. "Injectable anaesthetics,"

260. a This use of acepromazine in patients with epilepsy or in patients with an increased risk for convulsions is somewhat controversial. There are limited data suggesting that acepromazine decreases the seizure threshold. Acepromazine can be used in Dobermans, aggressive patients, and in older dogs when appropriate. Murrell JC, "Pre-anaesthetic medication and sedation," in Duke-Novakovski T, de Vries M, Seymour C, BSAVA Manual of Canine and Feline Anaesthesia and Analgesia, ed 3, British Small Animal Veterinary Association, 2016.

261. d Opioids can produce respiratory depression, decreased heart rate, and varying degrees of analgesia on the basis of the drug administered. Excitement is not a normal or common side effect of opioids in canine patients. Murrell JC, "Pre-anaesthetic medication and sedation," in Duke-Novakovski T, de Vries M, Seymour C, BSAVA Manual of Canine and Feline Anaesthesia and Analgesia, ed 3, British Small Animal Veterinary Association, 2016.

262. a Guaifenesin (GG; previously known as glyceryl guaiacolate ether or GGE) is a noncontrolled muscle relaxant that is commonly given to large animals to increase muscle relaxation, facilitate intubation, and ease induction and recovery. It does not provide analgesia or sedation. Thomas J, Phillip L, Anesthesia and Analgesia for Veterinary Technicians, ed 5, Elsevier, 2017.

263. a The oxygen flush valve receives oxygen directly from the pipeline or gas cylinder and bypasses the vaporizer completely. This valve allows the anesthetist to flush fresh oxygen into the circuit if needed. Because the valve flushes fresh air into the breathing system and bypasses the vaporizer, the anesthetic concentration will not increase. The oxygen flush valve does not cause the animal to breathe more deeply and it will not keep the reservoir bag deflated. Alibhai H, "The anaesthetic machine and vaporizers," in Duke-Novakovski T, de Vries M, Seymour C, BSAVA Manual of Canine and

Feline Anaesthesia and Analgesia, ed 3, British Small Animal Veterinary Association, 2016.

264. a The flow rate for a semi-closed circle system is generally calculated at 22–44 mL/kg/min. Using a semi-closed circle system is less economical compared with low-flow or closed systems, but it does allow quicker changes in anesthetic concentration because of the higher flow rates. Latshaw H, Coleman D, Anesthesia Equipment," in Bryant S, Anesthesia for Veterinary Technicians, ed 1, Wiley-Blackwell, 2010.

265. c This technique is limited to use in young foals, particularly those that are sick or those that will tolerate nasotracheal intubation. Thomas J, Phillip L, Anesthesia and Analgesia for Veterinary Technicians, ed 5, Elsevier, 2017.

266. d All anesthetic machines delivering inhalant gases need to have a scavenging system. Inhalant gases such as sevoflurane and isoflurane can be properly scavenged by using either passive or active scavenge techniques. Blood pressure and respiratory monitors are recommended but are not part of an inhalant anesthetic machine. Not all anesthetic machines have nitrous oxide. Latshaw H, Coleman D, "Anesthesia Equipment," in Bryant S, Anesthesia for Veterinary Technicians, ed 1, Wiley-Blackwell, 2010.

267. d Non-brachycephalic feline breeds can generally be extubated when the swallowing reflex returns because the anatomy of the oropharyngeal area is normal. Extubating when the swallow reflex returns helps to ensure that the endotracheal tube will not be damaged or bitten in half. Palmer D, "Airway Maintenance," in Bryant S, Anesthesia for Veterinary Technicians, ed 1, Wiley-Blackwell, 2010.

268. a Intubation in horses is performed blindly. This means that the anesthetist does not directly visualize the larynx but instead passes the tube more by feel. The oral and oropharyngeal anatomy of horses make blind intubation relatively easy. The horse's head is extended, the tongue is gently pulled to the side of the mouth, and a mouth gag or speculum is placed. Unlike in other species, it is uncommon for the tube to pass into the esophagus. It is advised to rinse the equine patient's mouth before intubation because horses may retain food in the cheek pouch area. Thomas J, Phillip L, Anesthesia and Analgesia for Veterinary Technicians, ed 5, Elsevier, 2017.

269. b The endotracheal tube is best secured by using either tie gauze or IV tubing. Using material that has too much stretch can lead to extubation (rubber band). The tube should be secured whenever the patient is intubated. The breed will often dictate how the tube is secured. Cats and brachycephalic animals need to have the tube secured behind the ears because of the shape of the face. Palmer D, "Airway Maintenance," in Bryant S, Anesthesia for Veterinary Technicians, ed 1, Wiley-Blackwell, 2010.

270. a Hypoventilation is defined as reduced minute volume because of a reduction in tidal volume and respiratory rate. This combination leads to hypercarbia (increased CO_2 levels) and potentially hypoxemia. Hypercarbia causes depression of the CNS when left untreated. McMillan S, "Anesthetic Complications and Emergencies," in Bryant S, Anesthesia for Veterinary Technicians, ed 1, Wiley-Blackwell, 2010.

271. d Compared with other species, horses are more likely to develop hypoxemia, hypoventilation, and hypotension during maintenance of anesthesia, particularly when inhalant agents are used. Thomas J, Phillip L, Anesthesia and Analgesia for Veterinary Technicians, ed 5, Elsevier, 2017.

272. c Patients that have impaired respiratory function should be induced by using methods allowing for rapid intubation. Drugs used in these cases should have a very quick onset of action. Chamber or mask induction is extremely risky in these patients because of slow induction times, the potential restraint required, and the anxiety caused for smelling the anesthetic gas. Isoflurane does not have any impact on the liver or gastrointestinal tract. Although isoflurane does affect cardiac function, it is not as significant as the respiratory tract. Bryant S, "Anesthesia for Thoracotomies and Respiratory-Challenged Patients," in Bryant S, Anesthesia for Veterinary Technicians, ed 1, Wiley-Blackwell, 2010.

273. b The liver in dogs and horses metabolizes ketamine and the metabolites of the drugs are excreted in the urine. In cats, ketamine is excreted largely unchanged by the kidney and should be avoided in feline patients with primary renal disease. Cooley K, "Anesthesia for Patients with Renal Disease," in Bryant S, Anesthesia for Veterinary Technicians, ed 1, Wiley-Blackwell, 2010.

274. c Dobutamine, a positive inotrope, is commonly used to treat hypotension in horses. Positive inotropes may cause arrhythmias and the ECG should therefore be closely monitored during infusion of dobutamine. Dextrose is used during fluid therapy and digoxin would be used to treat cardiac issues. Doxycycline is an antibiotic. Thomas J, Phillip L, Anesthesia and Analgesia for Veterinary Technicians, ed 5, Elsevier, 2017.

275. a PaO_2 is the partial pressure of oxygen. The "a" indicates the sample has been measured by using arterial blood. The partial pressure of oxygen should be five times the percentage of oxygen being delivered to the patient. For example, a patient breathing 100% oxygen and ventilating properly should have a PaO_2 of 500 mmHg. $PaCO_2$ is the partial pressure of carbon dioxide. Again the "a" indicates the sample has been measured by using arterial blood. The normal range for PaCO2 in a patient ventilating properly is 35–45 mmHg. Keefe J, "Introduction to Monitoring: Monitoring the ECG and Blood Gasses," in Bryant S, Anesthesia for Veterinary Technicians, ed 1, Wiley-Blackwell, 2010.

276. b In the United States, the approximate volume of oxygen in a full E cylinder is 650 liters. Alibhai H, "The anaesthetic machine and vaporizers," in Duke-Novakovski T, de Vries M, Seymour C, BSAVA Manual of Canine and Feline Anaesthesia and Analgesia, ed 3, British Small Animal Veterinary Association, 2016.

277. c In the United States, the approximate volume of oxygen in a full H cylinder is 6900 L. Latshaw H, Coleman D, "Anesthesia Equipment," in Bryant S,

Anesthesia for Veterinary Technicians, ed 1, Wiley-Blackwell, 2010.

278. d Horses have a psychological need to stand up shortly after awakening from anesthesia and this makes recovery particularly dangerous. Some steps can be taken to minimize injury to the horse and anesthetist, but there is a high incidence of complications from anesthetic recovery in horses and clients should be informed of the risks. Thomas J, Phillip L, Anesthesia and Analgesia for Veterinary Technicians, ed 5, Elsevier, 2017.

279. d In dogs and cats, epidural analgesia and anesthesia are most commonly administered between vertebral bodies L7 and S1. In large ruminants such as cattle, epidural analgesia and anesthesia are most commonly administered between the first and second coccygeal vertebrae. Because of many potential complications associated with general anesthesia in large ruminants, epidurals are commonly administered as an adjunct for analgesia and a complete blockade of pain. Kaiser-Klinger S, "Ruminant Anesthesia," in Bryant S, Anesthesia for Veterinary Technicians, ed 1, Wiley-Blackwell, 2010.

280. b During the postanesthetic period, the horse should be observed for any signs of neuropathy (e.g., facial nerve paralysis–drooping eyelid and lip on the affected side; radial nerve paralysis–inability to fully extend affected forelimb), myopathy (hard, swollen muscles, stiff and painful gait), or colic (rolling, kicking at the abdomen). Therefore, although signs for neuropathy and colic should be observed, those are not clinical symptoms presented in the question. Nephropathy would be a kidney issue and is not applicable to the question. Thomas J, Phillip L, Anesthesia and Analgesia for Veterinary Technicians, ed 5, Elsevier, 2017.

281. c Low-flow anesthesia is calculated at 2–7 mL/kg/min but is often estimated at 10 mL/kg/min to account for variations in age, temperature, metabolic rate, etc. Low-flow anesthesia is economical, causes less atmospheric pollution, and safe when done correctly. Low-flow anesthesia involves providing just enough fresh gas flow for cellular metabolism. Hughes L, "Breathing Systems and Ancillary Equipment," in Duke-Novakovski T, de Vries M, Seymour C, BSAVA Manual of Canine and Feline Anaesthesia and Analgesia, ed 3, British Small Animal Veterinary Association, 2016.

282. d Placing a capnometer between the endotracheal tube and the breathing circuit gives a continuous estimate of the partial pressure of carbon dioxide in the arterial blood. To obtain a true and direct reading of carbon dioxide in the arterial blood, an arterial blood gas sample must be analyzed. Pulse oximetry is a noninvasive measurement of the saturation of hemoglobin with oxygen. Direct arterial blood pressure is used to obtain continuous blood pressure via a catheter placed directly into an artery and attached to a transducer. Central venous pressure is obtained by using a centrally placed venous catheter attached to a transducer. Schauvliege S "Patient Monitoring and Monitoring Equipment," in Duke-Novakovski T, de Vries M, Seymour C, BSAVA Manual of Canine and Feline Anaesthesia and Analgesia, ed 3, British Small Animal Veterinary Association, 2016.

283. b Ruminants are very sensitive to xylazine, requiring 1/10 the dose that horses do. Thomas J, Phillip L, Anesthesia and Analgesia for Veterinary Technicians, ed 5, Elsevier, 2017.

284. b Neutral pH ranges between 7.35 and 7.45. A pH greater than 7.45 is called alkalemia. A pH less than 7.35 is called acidemia. Hypoxemia is low blood oxygen and hyponatremia is low sodium. Schauvliege S, "Patient Monitoring and Monitoring Equipment," in Duke-Novakovski T, de Vries M, Seymour C, BSAVA Manual of Canine and Feline Anaesthesia and Analgesia, ed 3, British Small Animal Veterinary Association, 2016.

285. a Normal mean arterial blood pressure in dogs and cats ranges from approximately 60 mmHg to 120 mmHg. When mean arterial blood pressure drops to <60 mmHg, blood flow to the major organs is compromised. This results in inadequate oxygen delivery to the tissues and a buildup of lactic acid in the blood. This is a prime example of why monitoring blood pressure is so important in the anesthetized patient. Schauvliege S, "Patient Monitoring and Monitoring Equipment," in Duke-Novakovski T, de Vries M, Seymour C, BSAVA Manual of Canine and Feline Anaesthesia and Analgesia, ed 3, British Small Animal Veterinary Association, 2016.

286. c Alpha-2 adrenoceptor agonist would be given to cattle to premedicate. Either xylazine (0.05–0.1 mg/kg IV or 0.05–0.2 mg/kg IM) or detomidine (0.01–0.03 mg/kg IV) can be administered. Anticholinergic drugs are not used to premedicate ruminants because they do not reduce salivation but instead cause the saliva to become thick and ropy. Local anesthetics and inhalant anesthesia are not a preanesthetic. Thomas J, Phillip L, Anesthesia and Analgesia for Veterinary Technicians, ed 5, Elsevier, 2017.

287. d CVP is used to estimate fluid load and to some extent changes in cardiac function. Using the jugular, femoral, or saphenous vessels, a catheter is aseptically placed. The tip of the catheter is placed into the vena cava. Normal ranges vary from 3–8 cm H_2O. Low numbers indicate volume under load and hypovolemia. Increased numbers indicate fluid overload. Single numbers are poor indicators for fluid status; therefore, CVP should be observed continuously throughout the anesthetic period. Schauvliege S "Patient Monitoring and Monitoring Equipment," in Duke-Novakovski T, de Vries M, Seymour C, BSAVA Manual of Canine and Feline Anaesthesia and Analgesia, ed 3, British Small Animal Veterinary Association, 2016.

288. b A double drip is a 500-mL bag of 5% dextrose in water containing 5% guaifenesin, to which 5 mL of ketamine has been added. Thomas J, Phillip L, Anesthesia and Analgesia for Veterinary Technicians, ed 5, Elsevier, 2017.

289. b Most opioids can be administered via the IV route without many negative side effects. The exceptions are morphine and meperidine. These drugs produce mast cell degranulation, histamine release, and a potential significant decrease in arterial blood pressure. If morphine is given via IV, it should be titrated very slowly. Kerr C, "Pain management I: systemic analgesics in in Duke-Novakovski T, de Vries M, Seymour C, BSAVA Manual of Canine and Feline Anaesthesia and Analgesia, ed 3, British Small Animal Veterinary Association, 2016.

290. d Butorphanol is a mixed agonist/antagonist opioid with agonist activity at the kappa receptor and antagonist activity at the mu receptor. In dogs and cats, butorphanol is a poor analgesic. Buprenorphine is a partial mu agonist with a high affinity for the mu receptor. It has better analgesic effects compared with butorphanol. Although buprenorphine is long-lasting, it is not as powerful an analgesic as a full mu opioid. Dexmedetomidine is not an opioid; it is an alpha-2 agonist with some analgesic properties. Hydromorphone is a full mu agonist opioid and provides excellent analgesia. Kerr C, "Pain management I: systemic analgesics in in Duke-Novakovski T, de Vries M, Seymour C, BSAVA Manual of Canine and Feline Anaesthesia and Analgesia, ed 3, British Small Animal Veterinary Association, 2016.

291. c Adult cattle are intubated manually by using a blind technique. The tube must be lubricated well with the animal's saliva or KY jelly before intubation. The question asks which statement is true regarding intubation; therefore, the facemask is not applicable. Thomas J, Phillip L, Anesthesia and Analgesia for Veterinary Technicians, ed 5, Elsevier, 2017.

292. a Methadone is a full mu agonist opioid. Full mu opioids provide the most profound level of analgesia in dogs and cats. Midazolam is a benzodiazepine and does not have any analgesic properties. Ketamine is a dissociative anesthetic that provides analgesia for somatic pain but is not a good analgesic for visceral pain. Buprenorphine is a partial mu agonist with a high affinity for the mu receptor. It has better analgesic effects compared with butorphanol. Kerr C, "Pain management I: systemic analgesics in in Duke-Novakovski T, de Vries M, Seymour C, BSAVA Manual of Canine and Feline Anaesthesia and Analgesia, ed 3, British Small Animal Veterinary Association, 2016.

293. c Ocular changes such as miosis in dogs and mydriasis in cats occurs after administration of mu agonist opioids. Miosis can affect ocular surgery and mydriasis can impair normal vision, leading to light sensitivity. Kerr C, "Pain management I: systemic analgesics in in Duke-Novakovski T, de Vries M, Seymour C, BSAVA Manual of Canine and Feline Anaesthesia and Analgesia, ed 3, British Small Animal Veterinary Association, 2016.

294. a The administration of nitrous oxide (N_2O) is not recommended in ruminants because of its potential for producing bloat and diffusion hypoxia. Nitrous oxide is relatively insoluble in the blood in comparison with oxygen and inhalant anesthetics and diffuses rapidly into gas-filled compartments such as the rumen. Halothane, isoflurane, and sevoflurane in oxygen can be safely used in cattle, sheep, and goats, and isoflurane and sevoflurane are suitable and safe in swine because they are not likely to cause malignant hyperthermia. Fubini SL, Ducharme N, Farm Animal Surgery, Saunders, 2004.

295. d Flumazenil reverses benzodiazepines such as diazepam and midazolam. Remifentanil is an ultra–short-acting full mu opioid used as constant rate infusions for analgesia and balanced anesthesia. Atipamezole is an alpha-2 antagonist and is used to reverse dexmedetomidine. Naloxone is an opioid antagonist and reverses the effects of full mu opioids such as morphine, hydromorphone, oxymorphone, fentanyl, methadone, and meperidine. Kerr C, "Pain management I: systemic analgesics in in Duke-Novakovski T, de Vries M, Seymour C, BSAVA Manual of Canine and Feline Anaesthesia and Analgesia, ed 3, British Small Animal Veterinary Association, 2016.

296. a NSAIDs reduce renal blood flow and are metabolized by the liver; therefore, these drugs are contraindicated in patients with renal and hepatic impairment as well as in patients that are dehydrated or hypovolemic. NAIDs can affect clotting; therefore, they should be avoided in patients with known coagulopathies. Pulmonary disease should not preclude a patient from using NSAIDs if they are otherwise healthy. Kerr C, "Pain management I: systemic analgesics in in Duke-Novakovski T, de Vries M, Seymour C, BSAVA Manual of Canine and Feline Anaesthesia and Analgesia, ed 3, British Small Animal Veterinary Association, 2016.

297. c All ruminants should be positioned for surgery with the mouth lower than the pharynx to allow drainage of saliva and any regurgitated material from the mouth, preventing buildup in the pharynx, which could lead to aspiration in recovery. Hyperventilation, hypotension, and hypoxemia can occur with the head in any position. Thomas J, Phillip L, Anesthesia and Analgesia for Veterinary Technicians, ed 5, Elsevier, 2017.

298. b The infraorbital nerve runs through the infraorbital foramen. Blocking this nerve provides a loss of sensation to the rostral portion of the maxilla. This nerve block is ideal for extractions and surgery of the rostral maxilla. To provide a loss of sensation to the rostral mandible, the mental foramen is used as a landmark to block the mandibular nerve. Blocking the inferior alveolar nerve blocks sensation to the tongue and the lower dental arcade. Last, blocking the maxillary nerve blocks sensation to the upper dental arcade and hard palate. Using an anesthetic such as lidocaine or bupivacaine performs a local block. Duke-Novakovski T, "Pain management II: local and regional anaesthetic techniques," in Duke-Novakovski T, de Vries M, Seymour C, BSAVA Manual of Canine and Feline Anaesthesia and Analgesia, ed 3, British Small Animal Veterinary Association, 2016.

299. a Support or prop the patient in sternal recumbency with the mouth lower than the pharynx. This allows eructation (the oral ejection of gas or air from the stomach; this is a normal activity for ruminants who void gases, principally methane, produced by fermentation in the rumen) as the patient regains consciousness, as well as drainage of saliva and/or regurgitus that may have accumulated during anesthesia. Thomas J, Phillip L, Anesthesia and Analgesia for Veterinary Technicians, ed 5, Elsevier, 2017.

300. b Lidocaine has duration of action of 1–2 hours, whereas bupivacaine has duration of action of about 4–6 hours.

Epidural morphine has duration of action of 12–24 hours. Because of the extent of this surgical repair and the time frame, both bupivacaine and morphine are used. Duke-Novakovski T, "Pain management II: local and regional anaesthetic techniques," in Duke-Novakovski T, de Vries M, Seymour C, BSAVA Manual of Canine and Feline Anaesthesia and Analgesia, ed 3, British Small Animal Veterinary Association, 2016.

301. d Anatomic differences, particularly in swine, make it extremely difficult to perform endotracheal intubation in small ruminants and swine without the use of a speculum, laryngoscope, and endotracheal tube stylet. An epiglotoscope does not exist. Thomas J, Phillip L, Anesthesia and Analgesia for Veterinary Technicians, ed 5, Elsevier, 2017.

302. b In dogs, the spinal cord ends at the level of the 6th lumbar vertebra. It is important to understand the anatomy to help ensure proper epidural placement. Duke-Novakovski T, "Pain management II: local and regional anaesthetic techniques," in Duke-Novakovski T, de Vries M, Seymour C, BSAVA Manual of Canine and Feline Anaesthesia and Analgesia, ed 3, British Small Animal Veterinary Association, 2016.

303. c In cats, the spinal cord ends at the level of L7. This is important because the possibility for intrathecal injection is much higher compared with the dog. Duke-Novakovski T, "Pain management II: local and regional anaesthetic techniques," in Duke-Novakovski T, de Vries M, Seymour C, BSAVA Manual of Canine and Feline Anaesthesia and Analgesia, ed 3, British Small Animal Veterinary Association, 2016.

304. d Sedative drugs are most commonly administered by IM injection in pigs owing to the lack of easily accessible peripheral veins and the presence of a thick layer of subcutaneous fat, which makes IM administration of drugs difficult without the use of needles that are at least 1½ inches long. In addition to being unable to administer IV drugs because of the challenge of accessible peripheral veins, the same applies when trying to obtain samples for preanesthetic blood work; it can cause extreme stress to the animal and handler. Oscillometric blood pressure monitors do not work well in pigs. Pigs are not sensitive to alpha-2 agonists. Thomas J, Phillip L, Anesthesia and Analgesia for Veterinary Technicians, ed 5, Elsevier, 2017.

305. c Administering epidural injections in patients with skin infections and septicemia can potentially introduce bacteria into the epidural space or CSF. Administering an epidural in a patient with a coagulopathy can introduce bleeding into the epidural space and area surrounding the spinal cord. Duke-Novakovski T, "Pain management II: local and regional anaesthetic techniques," in Duke-Novakovski T, de Vries M, Seymour C, BSAVA Manual of Canine and Feline Anaesthesia and Analgesia, ed 3, British Small Animal Veterinary Association, 2016.

306. c A neuroleptanalgesic includes an opioid and a tranquilizer used in combination together to achieve profound sedation. Common combinations include an opioid with either acepromazine or a benzodiazepine such as diazepam or midazolam. Etomidate and atropine are not considered opioids or tranquilizers. Murrell JC, "Pre-anaesthetic medication and sedation," in Duke-Novakovski T, de Vries M, Seymour C, BSAVA Manual of Canine and Feline Anaesthesia and Analgesia, ed 3, British Small Animal Veterinary Association, 2016.

307. a Porcine stress syndrome, also known as malignant hyperthermia, has been associated with anesthesia, particularly inhalant anesthetics. This metabolic condition occurs in affected animals because of a mutation in one of the genes that control calcium metabolism in the muscle. Signs include muscle rigidity, rapid rise in temperature, hypercapnia, hyperkalemia, and death. Treatment includes immediate termination of all anesthetic drugs, delivery of oxygen at high flow rates, and treatment with dantrolene. Thomas J, Phillip L, Anesthesia and Analgesia for Veterinary Technicians, ed 5, Elsevier, 2017.

308. b Synthetic colloids include hetastarch, Hexstend, and VetStarch. Synthetic colloids are made up of larger molecules that act as volume expanders and stay in the vascular space longer than crystalloids. Plasma is a natural colloid and not a synthetic colloid, but it acts in the same manner and contains clotting factors. Lactated Ringer's solution and normal saline are crystalloids. Auckburally A, "Fluid Therapy and Blood Transfusion," in Duke-Novakovski T, de Vries M, Seymour C, BSAVA Manual of Canine and Feline Anaesthesia and Analgesia, ed 3, British Small Animal Veterinary Association, 2016.

309. b Atropine is frequently used for this purpose, but in rabbits it is often relatively ineffective because many animals have high levels of atropinase (an atropine-like substance). It is therefore advisable to use glycopyrrolate in rabbits. Atropine does not cause bradycardia; rather it increases heart rate. Thomas J, Phillip L, Anesthesia and Analgesia for Veterinary Technicians, ed 5, Elsevier, 2017.

310. b The age and breed of the patient do not play a role in whether a blood transfusion is given (unless species-specific blood is not available). The type of procedure plays a huge role in the need for transfusion. A simple fracture repair is unlikely to need a transfusion, whereas a patient undergoing a hepatectomy is more likely to lose large amounts of blood. Patients with a low hematocrit and/or hemoglobin also aids in making the decision to transfuse. Auckburally A, "Fluid Therapy and Blood Transfusion," in Duke-Novakovski T, de Vries M, Seymour C, BSAVA Manual of Canine and Feline Anaesthesia and Analgesia, ed 3, British Small Animal Veterinary Association, 2016.

311. a Because the heart rate often exceeds 250 beats per minute (bpm) in many of these animals, it is not possible to assess the heart rate accurately. Problems can also arise when an electrocardiograph is used, because many instruments have an upper heart rate limit of 250 or 300 bpm and may also be unable to detect the low-amplitude signals generated in small rodents. Dark fur does not cause reading complications; however, dark skin may inhibit readings. Respiratory rates have nothing to do with pulse oximetry. Thomas J, Phillip L,

Anesthesia and Analgesia for Veterinary Technicians, ed 5, Elsevier, 2017.

312. d Increasing intraocular pressure during eye surgery can be detrimental to the patient. Most drugs either do not affect intraocular pressure or they actually reduce it. Ketamine is one of the main drugs commonly used for anesthesia that increases intraocular pressure. Jolliffe C, "Ophthalmic surgery," in Duke-Novakovski T, de Vries M, Seymour C, BSAVA Manual of Canine and Feline Anaesthesia and Analgesia, ed 3, British Small Animal Veterinary Association, 2016.

313. b Ocular reflexes are not as useful in small mammals as in dogs and cats. With most anesthetic regimens, the position of the eye remains fixed in rodents and the palpebral (blink) reflex may still be present at surgical planes of anesthesia. Thomas J, Phillip L, Anesthesia and Analgesia for Veterinary Technicians, ed 5, Elsevier, 2017.

314. a Propofol does not contribute to the increase in intracranial pressure and actually increases seizure threshold. Ketamine may increase intracranial pressure because of muscle rigidity and an increase in sympathetic tone. Morphine and hydromorphone can cause vomiting after administration. Vomiting increases intracranial pressure. Leece E, "Neurological Disease," in Duke-Novakovski T, de Vries M, Seymour C, BSAVA Manual of Canine and Feline Anaesthesia and Analgesia, ed 3, British Small Animal Veterinary Association, 2016.

315. d Both yohimbine and atipamezole have been used for the reversal purpose in small mammals, allowing a faster recovery. Atipamezole is preferable because it has fewer side effects. It can be given through the subcutaneous, intraperitoneal, intramuscular, and intravenous routes. Rodents do not have much body fat; therefore, it cannot be readily absorbed from the fat. Dexmedetomidine combined with ketamine is injected, not administered orally. Dexmedetomidine combined with ketamine does not promote gut motility and does not decrease inappetence postoperatively. Rabbits and small mammals may stop eating and drinking when experiencing pain. Thomas J, Phillip L, Anesthesia and Analgesia for Veterinary Technicians, ed 5, Elsevier, 2017.

316. c Because neonatal and pediatric animals have a large fleshy tongue and a narrowed upper airway, they are at increased risk of airway obstruction; thus, they should be intubated for general anesthetic procedures (even when short). Masking these patients may also interfere with their ability to breathe normally. Rigotti C, Brearley J, "Anaesthesia for paediatric and geriatric patients," in Duke-Novakovski T, de Vries M, Seymour C, BSAVA Manual of Canine and Feline Anaesthesia and Analgesia, ed 3, British Small Animal Veterinary Association, 2016.

317. b Average adult mouse blood volume is 2.5 mL. Thomas J, Phillip L, Anesthesia and Analgesia for Veterinary Technicians, ed 5, Elsevier, 2017.

318. b Propofol induction yields a better neonate outcome. Although propofol crosses the placenta, maternal levels of propofol are much higher than the neonates, suggesting some sort of placental barrier effect. Midazolam has rapid placental transfer with quick fetal uptake and long elimination times. Dexmedetomidine increases neonate mortality probably because of a reduction in uterine perfusion. Acepromazine is metabolized via the liver; therefore, elimination time is generally very slow in the underdeveloped neonatal liver. Acepromazine also causes vasodilation, which can be detrimental in newborns. Claude A, Meyer R, "Anaesthesia for Caesarean Section and for the pregnant patient," in Duke-Novakovski T, de Vries M, Seymour C, BSAVA Manual of Canine and Feline Anaesthesia and Analgesia, ed 3, British Small Animal Veterinary Association, 2016.

319. b The heart pumps blood around the body, with the veins carrying blood to the heart and the arteries carrying blood away from the heart. Bryant S, "Review of Cardiovascular and Respiratory Physiology," in Bryant S, Anesthesia for Veterinary Technicians, ed 1, Wiley-Blackwell, 2010.

320. c All fluids should be warmed to body temperature before administration. Fluids can be given SQ or IV; therefore, orally is not the only option. In addition, they can be given anytime, not just postoperatively. Thomas J, Phillip L, Anesthesia and Analgesia for Veterinary Technicians, ed 5, Elsevier, 2017.

321. c The P wave represents atrial depolarization. A wave of depolarization spreads from the SA node throughout the atria. The QRS complex represents ventricular depolarization. Ventricular repolarization is represented by the T wave. Bryant S, "Review of Cardiovascular and Respiratory Physiology," in Bryant S, Anesthesia for Veterinary Technicians, ed 1, Wiley-Blackwell, 2010.

322. b Ventricular repolarization is represented by the T wave. The P wave represents atrial depolarization. A wave of depolarization spreads from the SA node throughout the atria. The QRS complex represents ventricular depolarization. Bryant S, "Review of Cardiovascular and Respiratory Physiology," in Bryant S, Anesthesia for Veterinary Technicians, ed 1, Wiley-Blackwell, 2010.

323. b With smaller rabbits, it is advisable to use low dead space pediatric connectors to attach the endotracheal tube to the breathing circuit. Low dead space T-piece systems designed for use in humans are also useful. Rabbits are not allergic to latex; however, plastic is a more common component. A non-rebreathing circuit does not use soda lime. Thomas J, Phillip L, Anesthesia and Analgesia for Veterinary Technicians, ed 5, Elsevier, 2017.

324. a The QRS complex represents ventricular depolarization. Ventricular repolarization is represented by the T wave. The P wave represents atrial depolarization. A wave of depolarization spreads from the SA node throughout the atria. Bryant S, "Review of Cardiovascular and Respiratory Physiology," in Bryant S, Anesthesia for Veterinary Technicians, ed 1, Wiley-Blackwell, 2010.

325. c Because the commonly used opioids will potentiate the actions of injectable anesthetic agents, their preoperative administration could lead to inadvertent anesthetic overdose. Because of the limited information available concerning the degree of interaction between injectable anesthetics and opioids, it is safer in this case to administer opioid analgesics at the end of the operation in small rodents because the depth of anesthesia is becoming lighter. Local anesthetics are not likely to be given postoperatively. All of the morphine-like drugs that can be used in dogs and cats can also be used in small mammals but often have a shorter duration of action in these species; they do not cause severe respiratory depression. NSAIDs (particularly the more potent NSAIDs such as carprofen, ketoprofen, and meloxicam) can provide very effective pain relief in small mammals. Thomas J, Phillip L, Anesthesia and Analgesia for Veterinary Technicians, ed 5, Elsevier, 2017.

326. c Blood pressure is measured in mmHg. Systolic pressure is the pressure measured when the left ventricle fully contracts. Diastolic pressure is measured when the left ventricle relaxes. Bryant S, "Review of Cardiovascular and Respiratory Physiology," in Bryant S, Anesthesia for Veterinary Technicians, ed 1, Wiley-Blackwell, 2010.

327. a Tidal volume is calculated by using the calculation: Weight (kg) × 10–20 mL/kg; therefore, 20 kg × 10–20 = 200 to 400 mL/kg. Bryant S, "Review of Cardiovascular and Respiratory Physiology," in Bryant S, Anesthesia for Veterinary Technicians, ed 1, Wiley-Blackwell, 2010.

328. a Rabbits and small mammals may stop eating and drinking when experiencing pain. This can be difficult to detect if food is provided ad libitum, but the subsequent loss in body weight can easily be monitored. This is one of the easiest ways of following a small mammal's progress after surgery or during treatment of any disease condition. The inappetence caused by pain is a serious problem in small mammals, because failure to drink can rapidly lead to significant dehydration and lack of food intake can predispose to the development of hypoglycemia in small rodents. In rabbits, guinea pigs, and chinchillas, disturbances in food intake can lead to the development of life-threatening gastrointestinal disturbances. Porphyrin staining does not occur in rabbits and when painful, rabbits will not groom themselves. Rabbits in pain will have a much slower recovery than those in which pain is controlled. Thomas J, Phillip L, Anesthesia and Analgesia for Veterinary Technicians, ed 5, Elsevier, 2017.

329. a The Doberman is predisposed to clotting disorders often because of a decrease in von Willebrand factor. Ideally, a von Willebrand test should be performed as well as coagulation panel. A buccal mucosal bleeding time may also be useful before anesthetic induction. Labradors, Chihuahuas, and domestic short-haired cats are not predisposed to the von Willebrand factor. Dupre J, "The Preanesthetic Workup," in Bryant S, Anesthesia for Veterinary Technicians, ed 1, Wiley-Blackwell, 2010.

330. c The arteries commonly used to palpate pulse in dogs are the femoral, tibial, dorsopedal, palmar digital, lingual, and caudal arteries. The auricular artery is often too small to palpate a good pulse and is most often used in rabbits. Thomas J, Phillip L, Anesthesia and Analgesia for Veterinary Technicians, ed 5, Elsevier, 2017.

331. d A pulse oximeter is a monitoring device used to estimate the percentage oxygen saturation of hemoglobin (SpO_2) by measuring subtle differences in light absorption. Obtaining pulse pressure requires feeling the pulse at an artery. PaO_2 is a blood gas value and measures partial pressure of oxygen in the blood. Direct blood pressure monitoring will obtain an arterial blood pressure. Thomas J, Phillip L, Anesthesia and Analgesia for Veterinary Technicians, ed 5, Elsevier, 2017.

332. c The American Society of Anesthesiologists has compiled a classification system that helps the anesthetist determine a risk category for each patient undergoing anesthesia. ASA I: Minimal risk to healthy patient. ASA II: Slight risk with slight to mild systemic changes. ASA III: Moderate risk with systemic changes and some clinical alterations. ASA IV: High risk with pre-existing disease; surgical intervention may preserve life. ASA V: Extreme risk where the patient has little chance of survival with or without surgery. E: denotes an emergency for any type of case. Dupre J, "The Preanesthetic Workup," in Bryant S, Anesthesia for Veterinary Technicians, ed 1, Wiley-Blackwell, 2010.

333. d There is 1 mg in 1 µg. It is important for technicians to be able to convert between grams, milligrams, and micrograms. The concentrations of some anesthetic drugs are labeled in micrograms. Many constant rate infusions are given in µg/kg/min. Johnston S, "Mathematics for the Veterinary Anesthetist," in Bryant S, Anesthesia for Veterinary Technicians, ed 1, Wiley-Blackwell, 2010.

334. d Technicians should be able to convert easily between a percent solution and mg/mL. This will enable proper administration of the drug. 2% mathematically means 2 g/100 mL or 2000 mg/100 mL, which = 20 mg/1 mL. Johnston S, "Mathematics for the Veterinary Anesthetist," in Bryant S, Anesthesia for Veterinary Technicians, ed 1, Wiley-Blackwell, 2010.

335. b Xylazine does not have anti-inflammatory, antiemetic, or anesthetic properties. Alpha-2 adrenoceptor agonists (also written as alpha-2 agonists or α2-agonists) are a group of noncontrolled agents used alone and in combination with other anesthetics and adjuncts in both large and small animal patients for sedation, analgesia, and muscle relaxation. They are commonly administered before minor procedures such as radiography, wound treatment, or bandaging and are subsequently reversed with an alpha-2 adrenoceptor antagonist. Thomas J, Phillip L, Anesthesia and Analgesia for Veterinary Technicians, ed 5, Elsevier, 2017.

336. a Releasing your thumb before releasing the pressure in the circuit can create a vacuum effect, causing some of the carbon dioxide absorbent to be sucked into the circuit. Carbon dioxide absorbent in the circuit can flow into the patient's airway, causing extreme irritation. Warren C, "Preanesthetic Preparation," in Bryant S, Anesthesia for Veterinary Technicians, ed 1, Wiley-Blackwell, 2010.

337. c Fresh absorbent should be soft and crumble easily. Old and exhausted absorbent will be hard and very dry. Used absorbent changes to a violet color during use. Absorbent should be changed after there is a color change equaling about ⅔ of the canister. Warren C, "Preanesthetic Preparation," in Bryant S, Anesthesia for Veterinary Technicians, ed 1, Wiley-Blackwell, 2010.

338. d Checking the endotracheal tube for malfunction and leaks before use is important to help prevent anesthetic gas leakage and the potential for aspiration. Leaving the cuff inflated for 5–10 minutes will generally be enough time to identify any slow leaks in the cuff. Warren C, "Preanesthetic Preparation," in Bryant S, Anesthesia for Veterinary Technicians, ed 1, Wiley-Blackwell, 2010.

339. c The label for detomidine is for horse use only, not cattle, dogs, or cats. Detomidine is used in horses to produce sedation, analgesia, and muscle relaxation. This drug is similar to xylazine, producing similar beneficial and adverse effects, but it has approximately twice the duration of action. It is commonly administered with butorphanol to produce standing sedation. It is also used to provide analgesia for colic pain. Thomas J, Phillip L, Anesthesia and Analgesia for Veterinary Technicians, ed 5, Elsevier, 2017.

340. a Arterial catheters provide constant and accurate direct blood pressure measurement. They also provide access to quick blood collection for sampling including the ability to analyze blood gases. Central venous pressure is obtained by placing a central catheter (generally via the jugular vein). The tip of the catheter sits near the right atrium. Warren C, "Preanesthetic Preparation," in Bryant S, Anesthesia for Veterinary Technicians, ed 1, Wiley-Blackwell, 2010.

341. d Hypothermia can cause many detrimental side effects including but not limited to MAC reduction, decreased tissue perfusion because of vasoconstriction, bradycardia, poor healing postoperatively, poor coagulation, and a reduced response to drug administration. Hypertension is not caused by hypothermia. Warren C, "Preanesthetic Preparation," in Bryant S, Anesthesia for Veterinary Technicians, ed 1, Wiley-Blackwell, 2010.

342. b Butorphanol is not diuretic, anesthetic, or anti-inflammatory in composition. A synthetic opioid with agonist and antagonist properties, butorphanol was first used in veterinary medicine as a cough suppressant. Butorphanol is widely used as a preanesthetic or sedative (at a dose of 0.1–0.4 mg/kg SC or IM or in mixtures with dexmedetomidine or acepromazine) and is also an effective postoperative analgesic for mild-to-moderate visceral pain. Thomas J, Phillip L, Anesthesia and Analgesia for Veterinary Technicians, ed 5, Elsevier, 2017.

343. c There are many benefits to intubating a patient for general anesthesia. Intubation allows complete control of the airway including helping to prevent aspiration of mucus, blood, food, etc. The endotracheal tube allows positive-pressure ventilation, oxygen and inhalants to be delivered closer to the lungs, and use of lower oxygen flow rates compared with a mask. Endotracheal tubes also help prevent waste gas exposure to the staff because they decrease anatomic dead space compared with a facemask. Palmer D, "Airway Maintenance," in Bryant S, Anesthesia for Veterinary Technicians, ed 1, Wiley-Blackwell, 2010.

344. d Low-volume high-pressure endotracheal tubes (red rubber tubes) require only small volumes of air to form a complete seal. Unfortunately, the cuff is under high pressure, which can cause tracheal necrosis with time. Palmer D, "Airway Maintenance," in Bryant S, Anesthesia for Veterinary Technicians, ed 1, Wiley-Blackwell, 2010.

345. c Diazepam is an ideal drug for use in the cardiovascular-compromised patient. In patients with impaired renal or hepatic function, recovery may be significantly prolonged as a result of the metabolic requirements of diazepam. At therapeutic doses, benzodiazepines have few effects on the cardiovascular and respiratory systems and therefore have a high margin of safety. Heart rate, blood pressure, and cardiac output are minimally affected. This property makes them particularly useful for anesthesia of high-risk and geriatric animals. Thomas J, Phillip L, Anesthesia and Analgesia for Veterinary Technicians, ed 5, Elsevier, 2017.

346. a According to the Hagen–Poiseuille law, if the diameter of the airway is reduced, the resistance to gas flow will increase by a factor of four. Palmer D, "Airway Maintenance," in Bryant S, Anesthesia for Veterinary Technicians, ed 1, Wiley-Blackwell, 2010.

347. c Preoxygenation can help prevent hypoxemia during the induction period. A period of 3–5 minutes is suggested for most patients. Palmer D, "Airway Maintenance," in Bryant S, Anesthesia for Veterinary Technicians, ed 1, Wiley-Blackwell, 2010.

348. d Xylazine is not labeled for cattle but is labeled for dogs, cats, and horses. Xylazine has been available for several decades and is the first widely used alpha-2 agonist in both large and small animal species. It is supplied as a 2% solution (20 mg/mL) for small animal use and as a 10% solution (100 mg/mL) for equine use. Thomas J, Phillip L, Anesthesia and Analgesia for Veterinary Technicians, ed 5, Elsevier, 2017.

349. d The capnograph measures expired carbon dioxide. If the machine reads zero, there is a malfunction with the machine, the patient is not breathing (apnea or dead), or the patient is not intubated within the trachea. Inserting the tube too far, increasing the oxygen flow rate, or the patient being in a light plane of anesthesia does not yield a zero reading on the capnograph. Palmer D, "Airway Maintenance," in Bryant S, Anesthesia for Veterinary Technicians, ed 1, Wiley-Blackwell, 2010.

350. a The two main tanks used in veterinary hospitals include the E tank and H tank. The E tank is the small tank that attaches to the anesthesia machine and the H tank is much larger and generally located remotely from the machine. Latshaw H, Coleman D, "Anesthesia Equipment," in Bryant S, Anesthesia for Veterinary Technicians, ed 1, Wiley-Blackwell, 2010.

351. b Guaifenesin is not a diuretic. It does not provide analgesia and does not have anesthetic properties when used alone. Guaifenesin is a muscle relaxant drug used with other general anesthetics in horses and cattle. Guaifenesin (GG) (previously known as glycerol guaiacolate ether or GGE) is a noncontrolled muscle relaxant that is commonly given to large animals to increase muscle relaxation, facilitate intubation, and ease induction and recovery. Thomas J, Phillip L, Anesthesia and Analgesia for Veterinary Technicians, ed 5, Elsevier, 2017.

352. c Low-flow anesthetic rates are greater than the patient's oxygen consumption rate at 4–7 mL/kg/min but less than 22 mL/kg/min, which is the lower limit of flow for semi-closed systems. Latshaw H, Coleman D, "Anesthesia Equipment," in Bryant S, Anesthesia for Veterinary Technicians, ed 1, Wiley-Blackwell, 2010.

353. a High flow rates are required for non-rebreathing circuits because these systems do not use a CO_2 absorbent such as those used in rebreathing systems. High flow rates actually cool patients and remove more humidity from the respiratory track. Latshaw H, Coleman D, "Anesthesia Equipment," in Bryant S, Anesthesia for Veterinary Technicians, ed 1, Wiley-Blackwell, 2010.

354. b Lead II is the most commonly used ECG lead in veterinary patients under general anesthesia. Keefe J, "Introduction to Monitoring: Monitoring the ECG and Blood Gasses," in Bryant S, Anesthesia for Veterinary Technicians, ed 1, Wiley-Blackwell, 2010.

355. d Sinus tachycardia is described as a regular beat with normal morphology and often defined as greater than 200 beats per minute in cats, greater than 180 beats per minute in small dogs, and greater than 160 beats per minute in large dogs. Keefe J, "Introduction to Monitoring: Monitoring the ECG and Blood Gasses," in Bryant S, Anesthesia for Veterinary Technicians, ed 1, Wiley-Blackwell, 2010.

356. a Neither butorphanol nor xylazine causes CNS excitement. For several decades xylazine has been frequently used alone or in various combinations with ketamine, opioids, and other agents in dogs, cats, and other small animals. The combination of xylazine and butorphanol provides greater analgesia and muscle relaxation, with the effects of both drugs being enhanced. One benefit of this combination is that the dose of each drug is reduced, minimizing side effects and maximizing therapeutic effects. Thomas J, Phillip L, Anesthesia and Analgesia for Veterinary Technicians, ed 5, Elsevier, 2017.

357. b Glycopyrrolate is an anticholinergic used to increase heart rate. This drug is similar to atropine. Alfaxalone and ketamine are injectable anesthetics and doxapram is most often used as a respiratory stimulant. Keefe J, "Introduction to Monitoring: Monitoring the ECG and Blood Gasses," in Bryant S, Anesthesia for Veterinary Technicians, ed 1, Wiley-Blackwell, 2010.

358. a The ECG shows a prolonged P-R interval when first-degree AV block is present. The rhythm will otherwise show a normal, regular rhythm with normal morphology. Second-degree AV block is defined as a P wave without the presence of QRS complex to follow it. Third-degree AV is identified when the P wave and QRS complex occur completely independently of each other. AV dissociation is a rhythm where the ventricular rate is the same or faster than the atrial rate. Keefe J, "Introduction to Monitoring: Monitoring the ECG and Blood Gasses," in Bryant S, Anesthesia for Veterinary Technicians, ed 1, Wiley-Blackwell, 2010.

359. b Although acepromazine and diazepam are tranquilizers and xylazine is a sedative, the potency is a measure of drug activity expressed in terms of the amount required to produce an effect of given intensity. Detomidine is used in horses to produce sedation, analgesia, and muscle relaxation. This drug is similar to xylazine, producing similar beneficial and adverse effects, but it has approximately twice the duration of action. It is commonly given with butorphanol to produce standing sedation. It is also used to provide analgesia for colic. Detomidine is a much more potent sedative on a volume-per-volume basis. Thomas J, Phillip L, Anesthesia and Analgesia for Veterinary Technicians, ed 5, Elsevier, 2017.

360. b Second-degree AV block is defined as a P wave without the presence of QRS complex to follow it. This arrhythmia is generally treated with atropine. The ECG will show a prolonged P-R interval when first-degree AV block is present. Third-degree AV is identified when the P wave and QRS complex occur completely independently of each other. AV dissociation is a rhythm where the ventricular rate is the same or faster than the atrial rate. Keefe J, "Introduction to Monitoring: Monitoring the ECG and Blood Gasses," in Bryant S, Anesthesia for Veterinary Technicians, ed 1, Wiley-Blackwell, 2010.

361. c Diazepam is a benzodiazepine, butorphanol is an opioid agonist/antagonist, and flunixin meglumine is an NSAID, none of which causes hypotension. Acepromazine is an alpha-blocker with significant potential to produce hypotension. The hypotension produced by acepromazine is dose-dependent and more pronounced in frightened or excited patients. In animals receiving isoflurane, a significant drop in blood pressure (as much as 20%–30%) occurs. This contributes to intraoperative hypotension commonly seen in patients given this combination. Thomas J, Phillip L, Anesthesia and Analgesia for Veterinary Technicians, ed 5, Elsevier, 2017.

362. c Ventricular tachycardia is defined as more than three VPCs in a row. This rhythm is fast and irregular and has wide and bizarre QRS complexes. Third-degree AV is identified when the P wave and QRS complex occur completely independent of each other. Atrial premature complexes are premature beats originating from the atria. The beats look the same, but they come too early. Sinus bradycardia is identified as a normal-looking rhythm on the ECG, but the heart rate is too slow. Keefe J, "Introduction to Monitoring: Monitoring the ECG and Blood Gasses," in Bryant S, Anesthesia for Veterinary Technicians, ed 1, Wiley-Blackwell, 2010.

363. d A ventricular premature complex is defined as a contraction originating from the ventricle that occurred sooner than it should have. This rhythm produces a heartbeat with a pulse deficit. The pulse deficit occurs because of a lack of blood filling the ventricle. Atrial premature complexes are premature beats originating from the atria. The beats look the same, but they come too early. Ventricular fibrillation is identified by chaotic electrical activity. The ECG strip has no definable pattern. Atrial fibrillation is commonly referred to as "shoes in a dryer" rhythm. The ECG strip will show a fast, irregular rhythm without discernible P waves. The baseline is undulating or looks like the teeth on a saw blade. Keefe J, "Introduction to Monitoring: Monitoring the ECG and Blood Gasses," in Bryant S, Anesthesia for Veterinary Technicians, ed 1, Wiley-Blackwell, 2010.

364. c Telazol does not contain ketamine, xylazine, or diazepam. Tiletamine hydrochloride, another dissociative agent, is combined with the benzodiazepine zolazepam in a proprietary product called Telazol. This product is administered intravenously or intramuscularly, alone or in combination with other agents, to produce sedation and anesthesia. Thomas J, Phillip L, Anesthesia and Analgesia for Veterinary Technicians, ed 5, Elsevier, 2017.

365. c AV block is commonly seen in patients administered alpha-2 agonists such as dexmedetomidine. Other causes of AV block include hyperkalemia, cardiac disease, and high vagal tone (commonly occurs in brachycephalic dogs). Bradycardia can be observed after administration of propofol and alfaxalone and an increase in heart rate after ketamine administration. Keefe J, "Introduction to Monitoring: Monitoring the ECG and Blood Gasses," in Bryant S, Anesthesia for Veterinary Technicians, ed 1, Wiley-Blackwell, 2010.

366. d Acepromazine, diazepam, and isoflurane are all agents that cross the placental barrier. Neuromuscular-blocking agents are highly ionized and have high molecular weights, minimizing placental transfer. Neuromuscular blocking agents provide abdominal muscle relaxation and are not transferred across the placenta to the fetus. Thomas J, Phillip L, Anesthesia and Analgesia for Veterinary Technicians, ed 5, Elsevier, 2017.

367. a Lidocaine is not only a local anesthetic but also an antiarrhythmic drug. Treatment of VPCs is indicated when there are more than 15 per minute with a drop in blood pressure. In dogs, a 1–2 mg/kg bolus of lidocaine is generally administered and a constant rate infusion is started at 25–80 μg/kg/min when necessary. Lidocaine is used with caution in cats because their central nervous system is very sensitive to the systemic effects. Keefe J, "Introduction to Monitoring: Monitoring the ECG and Blood Gasses," in Bryant S, Anesthesia for Veterinary Technicians, ed 1, Wiley-Blackwell, 2010.

368. d Phenobarbital, thiopental, and pentobarbital are all barbiturates. Propofol is an ultra–short-acting nonbarbiturate injectable anesthetic with a wide margin of safety and is given intravenously for induction and short-term maintenance of general anesthesia in small animals, small ruminants, exotic animals, and neonates of any domestic species. Thomas J, Phillip L, Anesthesia and Analgesia for Veterinary Technicians, ed 5, Elsevier, 2017.

369. d There are many causes of VPCs that include hypoxia, pain, GDV, administration of barbiturate and halothane (not available in United States), reperfusion injury, hypercarbia, and excitement/fear. Anemia does not cause VPCs. Keefe J, "Introduction to Monitoring: Monitoring the ECG and Blood Gasses," in Bryant S, Anesthesia for Veterinary Technicians, ed 1, Wiley-Blackwell, 2010.

370. b Glycopyrrolate has a longer duration of action than atropine. Glycopyrrolate is a newer synthetic quaternary ammonium compound that is slightly less likely to induce cardiac arrhythmias, suppresses salivation more effectively than atropine, and only minimally crosses the placental barrier in pregnant animals. Thomas J, Phillip L, Anesthesia and Analgesia for Veterinary Technicians, ed 5, Elsevier, 2017.

371. a Patients being maintained on 100% oxygen should have oxygen saturation via pulse oximetry of 95%–100%. Decreased oxygen saturation can indicate hypoxia, severe shock, anemia, or vasoconstriction. Levensaler A, "Monitoring: Pulse Oximetry, Temperature, and Hands-On," in Bryant S, Anesthesia for Veterinary Technicians, ed 1, Wiley-Blackwell, 2010.

372. d Alpha-2 agonists such as dexmedetomidine cause vasoconstriction. Constricted vessels can cause low reading on the pulse oximeter. Opioids such as fentanyl and hydromorphone and dissociatives such as ketamine do not cause vasoconstriction. Levensaler A, "Monitoring: Pulse Oximetry, Temperature, and Hands-On," in Bryant S, Anesthesia for Veterinary Technicians, ed 1, Wiley-Blackwell, 2010.

373. c Hypothermia has severe potential side effects including impaired platelet function, death, reduced anesthetic requirements, prolonged recovery, electrocardiographic changes, increases in fibrinolysis, and decreased activity of the pathways of coagulation. Anemia is not caused by hypothermia. Levensaler A, "Monitoring: Pulse Oximetry, Temperature, and Hands-On," in Bryant S, Anesthesia for Veterinary Technicians, ed 1, Wiley-Blackwell, 2010.

374. b Palpebral reflex is absent in most species under a deeper plane of anesthesia. Swallowing and withdrawal reflexes are present in patients that are lightly anesthetized but are not present in deeper planes of anesthesia. The corneal reflex should always be present in patients under anesthesia. Levensaler A, "Monitoring: Pulse Oximetry, Temperature, and Hands-On," in Bryant S, Anesthesia for Veterinary Technicians, ed 1, Wiley-Blackwell, 2010.

375. c Normal capillary refill time is less than 1–2 seconds. CRT is an easy way to help assess tissue perfusion and cardiac output. Levensaler A, "Monitoring: Pulse Oximetry, Temperature, and Hands-On," in Bryant S, Anesthesia for Veterinary Technicians, ed 1, Wiley-Blackwell, 2010.

376. c Atropine prevents bradycardia, which is often associated with anesthesia and surgery and routinely causes the heart rate to increase. It is not species dependent. Thomas J, Phillip L, Anesthesia and Analgesia for Veterinary Technicians, ed 5, Elsevier, 2017.

377. d Drugs causing vasoconstriction often cause the mucous membranes to become pale. This is caused by the constriction of the vessels and capillaries. Although the mucous membranes are pale, the hemodynamic status is often still okay. Red mucous membranes are often caused by septic shock. Blue or cyanotic mucous membranes are caused by hypoxemia and pink mucous membranes are normal. Levensaler A, "Monitoring: Pulse Oximetry, Temperature, and Hands-On," in Bryant S, Anesthesia for Veterinary Technicians, ed 1, Wiley-Blackwell, 2010.

378. b Opioids are not anesthetics or anti-inflammatories and they are not antihistamines. Opioids have long been considered to be the most effective agents for the treatment of pain. Thomas J, Phillip L, Anesthesia and Analgesia for Veterinary Technicians, ed 5, Elsevier, 2017.

379. b Xylazine produces a short period of analgesia; acepromazine does not provide any analgesia. Neither product is an anti-inflammatory or has antiemetic properties. Thomas J, Phillip L, Anesthesia and Analgesia for Veterinary Technicians, ed 5, Elsevier, 2017.

380. a Atropine will not cause excitement, slow the heart rate, or increase salivation; however, anticholinergics (atropine) inhibit intestinal peristalsis. This can cause gut stasis and colic in horses and bloat in ruminants (even at clinical doses). Therefore, use of these agents should be avoided in these species. Thomas J, Phillip L, Anesthesia and Analgesia for Veterinary Technicians, ed 5, Elsevier, 2017.

381. b Glycopyrrolate, xylazine, and diazepam do not cause penile prolapse, whereas acepromazine has been reported to cause prolapse of the penis in horses and other large animals. This can lead to injury and subsequent permanent paralysis of the retractor penis muscle. For this reason, some veterinarians choose not to use acepromazine in breeding stallions. Thomas J, Phillip L, Anesthesia and Analgesia for Veterinary Technicians, ed 5, Elsevier, 2017.

382. a Drugs causing vasodilation often cause the mucous membranes to become pink. This is caused by the dilation of the vessels and capillaries. Although the mucous membranes are pink, the cardiac output and blood pressure may be decreased. Drugs causing vasoconstriction often cause the mucous membranes to become pale. Red mucous membranes are often caused by septic shock. Blue or cyanotic mucous membranes are caused by hypoxemia and pale mucous membranes are caused by anemia, vasoconstriction, or hypovolemic shock. Levensaler A, "Monitoring: Pulse Oximetry, Temperature, and Hands-On," in Bryant S, Anesthesia for Veterinary Technicians, ed 1, Wiley-Blackwell, 2010.

383. a Atropine is an anticholinergic, pancuronium is a neuromuscular blocking agent, and droperidol is a sedative. The opioid antagonist naloxone hydrochloride is commonly used to reverse the CNS and respiratory depression caused by administration of opioid agonists, partial agonists, or agonist–antagonists. Thomas J, Phillip L, Anesthesia and Analgesia for Veterinary Technicians, ed 5, Elsevier, 2017.

384. d Inappropriate cuff size is the leading cause of inaccurate blood pressure readings. The width of the cuff should be approximately 30% of the circumference of the leg in cats. A circumference that is larger or smaller leads to inappropriate readings. Reuss-Lamky HL, "Monitoring Blood Pressure and End-Tidal CO_2 in the Anesthetized Patient," in Bryant S, Anesthesia for Veterinary Technicians, ed 1, Wiley-Blackwell, 2010.

385. b The Doppler probe must be placed over an artery. The probe picks up the sound of the red blood cells circulating through the arteries. The probe works when placed over a vein, capillary bed, or onto mucous membranes. Reuss-Lamky HL, "Monitoring Blood Pressure and End-Tidal CO_2 in the Anesthetized Patient," in Bryant S, Anesthesia for Veterinary Technicians, ed 1, Wiley-Blackwell, 2010.

386. b Depressant preanesthetic medication will not shorten recovery time, leave the recovery time unaltered, nor necessitate increasing the dose of induction agent. The veterinarian should examine animals experiencing prolonged recovery from anesthesia. There are many possible reasons why a patient may be slow to recover; including impaired renal or hepatic function, hypothermia, individual susceptibility to a particular anesthetic, breed variations (particularly in sighthounds), or the presence of a disorder such as shock or hemorrhage. Excessive anesthetic depth or prolonged anesthesia may also result in delayed recovery. Use of certain agents (including intramuscular ketamine or repeated injections of barbiturates) may be associated with prolonged recovery even in healthy animals. In cats, it is known that hypothermia in itself can cause significant delay in recovery even if all other organs are functioning properly. Thomas J, Phillip L, Anesthesia and Analgesia for Veterinary Technicians, ed 5, Elsevier, 2017.

387. d Oscillometric blood pressure monitoring is not considered accurate in patients weighing <5 kg. Reuss-Lamky HL, "Monitoring Blood Pressure and End-Tidal CO_2 in the Anesthetized Patient," in Bryant S, Anesthesia for Veterinary Technicians, ed 1, Wiley-Blackwell, 2010.

388. b Capnography reads how much carbon dioxide is exhaled from the lungs. The capnograph mouthpiece is placed between the endotracheal tube and breathing circuit. Normal end-tidal carbon dioxide ($ETCO_2$) ranges between 35 and 45 mmHg in mammals. Low $ETCO_2$ can indicate hyperventilation, light plane of anesthesia, or an impending cardiac arrest. High $ETCO_2$ can indicate hypoventilation or a deep plane of anesthesia. A reading of zero can indicate death, apnea, or an esophageal intubation. Capnography is a good tool to help assess effectiveness of CPR. The ECG is only used to assess rate and rhythm of the heart. Central venous pressure is used to assess fluid load, and arterial blood gas assessment is used to assess acid-base status and ventilation in patients. Arterial blood gas assessment is not noninvasive. Reuss-Lamky HL, "Monitoring Blood Pressure and End-Tidal CO_2 in the Anesthetized Patient," in Bryant S, Anesthesia for Veterinary Technicians, ed 1, Wiley-Blackwell, 2010.

389. c Butorphanol is an opioid, detomidine is an alpha-2 agonist, and pentazocine is an opioid. Yohimbine is primarily used to reverse sedative and cardiovascular effects of xylazine in dogs, cats, horses, and exotic species. Thomas J, Phillip L, Anesthesia and Analgesia for Veterinary Technicians, ed 5, Elsevier, 2017.

390. a Mechanical dead space is caused by equipment such as a long endotracheal tube or the monitor itself. Air in the nasal passages, trachea, and mouth is referred to as anatomic dead space. Reuss-Lamky HL, "Monitoring Blood Pressure and End-Tidal CO_2 in the Anesthetized Patient," in Bryant S, Anesthesia for Veterinary Technicians, ed 1, Wiley-Blackwell, 2010.

391. d Hetastarch is a colloid. Colloids have large molecular weight substances that stay in the vascular space longer than crystalloids. Lactated Ringer's solution, Plasma-Lyte, and 0.9% saline are considered crystalloids. These fluids have smaller molecules and do not stay in the vascular space for long periods. Beiter C, "Fluid Therapy and Blood Products," in Bryant S, Anesthesia for Veterinary Technicians, ed 1, Wiley-Blackwell, 2010.

392. c Diazepam by itself has no analgesic properties; it does not cause hypnosis or vomiting. Diazepam, a benzodiazepine, has the following effects: antianxiety and calming only in old or ill patients, anticonvulsant activity, skeletal muscle relaxation, and appetite stimulation in cats and ruminants. Thomas J, Phillip L, Anesthesia and Analgesia for Veterinary Technicians, ed 5, Elsevier, 2017.

393. a Epinephrine does not decrease heart rate or blood pressure and does not reverse acepromazine. The adrenergic (sympathetic) effects of epinephrine increase the heart rate. Epinephrine is the drug most commonly used for initial treatment of cardiac arrest. The currently recommended dose is 1 mL/10 kg; thus, 0.5 mL for cats, 1 mL for small dogs, 2 mL for medium-sized dogs, and 3 mL for large dogs all drawn from a 1:1000 solution. Epinephrine is administered every 3–5 minutes. Thomas J, Phillip L, Anesthesia and Analgesia for Veterinary Technicians, ed 5, Elsevier, 2017.

394. b Nitrous oxide does not increase inhalation anesthetic required, it does not slow the induction process, and it does have an effect on the time or amount of anesthetic required. When used with other agents, nitrous oxide (N_2O) speeds induction and recovery and provides additional analgesia. Nitrous oxide also reduces the MAC (and therefore the vaporizer setting) of other anesthetics by 20%–30%. This reduces the risk of adverse effects on the cardiovascular, pulmonary, and other systems. Thomas J, Phillip L, Anesthesia and Analgesia for Veterinary Technicians, ed 5, Elsevier, 2017.

395. c Isotonic fluids include crystalloids such as lactated Ringer's solution, 0.9% saline, Normosol-R, and Plasma-Lyte 148. Hypertonic fluids have a higher osmolarity than extracellular fluids and hypotonic fluids have a lower osmolarity than extracellular fluids. Beiter C, "Fluid Therapy and Blood Products," in Bryant S, Anesthesia for Veterinary Technicians, ed 1, Wiley-Blackwell, 2010.

396. d All of these fluids are considered crystalloids, but 0.9% saline is unbalanced, whereas the others are balanced solutions. Unbalanced solutions do not have a fluid composition that closely resembles the extracellular fluid. Beiter C, "Fluid Therapy and Blood Products," in Bryant S, Anesthesia for Veterinary Technicians, ed 1, Wiley-Blackwell, 2010.

397. a N_2O does not increase oxygenation, slow induction time, or prolong recovery time. The use of N_2O in an anesthetic machine limits the amount of O_2 that is delivered to the patient to the extent that N_2O replaces O_2 in the circuit. Because the minimal amount of N_2O necessary to achieve analgesic effects is 50% (and values of 60%–67% are recommended), the use of this agent decreases the amount of O_2 delivered to the patient by the same amount (50%–67%). Therefore, the patient breathing N_2O should be monitored closely for adequate oxygenation with a pulse oximeter or blood gas analysis. Patients should also be monitored closely for cyanosis and cardiac arrhythmias. Because of the risk of hypoxemia, animals with pre-existing lung disease are poor candidates for N_2O anesthesia. For all patients, care should also be taken when adjusting the flowmeter of the anesthetic machine to avoid confusing O_2 controls with those for N_2O. Thomas J, Phillip L, Anesthesia and Analgesia for Veterinary Technicians, ed 5, Elsevier, 2017.

398. b Hextend and hetastarch are synthetic colloids. Whole blood is considered a natural colloid. Plasma-Lyte 148 is a crystalloid. Colloids have large molecular weight substances that stay in the vascular space longer than crystalloids. Beiter C, "Fluid Therapy and Blood Products," in Bryant S, Anesthesia for Veterinary Technicians, ed 1, Wiley-Blackwell, 2010.

399. a Sensible losses are those from urine output. Fecal waste and loss of fluid via the skin and respiratory tract are insensible losses. Beiter C, "Fluid Therapy and Blood Products," in Bryant S, Anesthesia for Veterinary Technicians, ed 1, Wiley-Blackwell, 2010.

400. c A 2% solution contains 2 g of solute (drug) in 100 mL of solvent (water); 2 g = 2000 mg, so there are 2000 mg of drug per 100 mL, or 20 mg per 1 mL (20 mg/mL). The term *percent concentration* may be used when w/v, w/w, or v/v concentrations are described. Percent (percentage) means parts of solute per 100 parts of the solution. Percent w/v means the number of grams of solute in 100 mL of solution, percent w/w describes the number of grams of solute in 100 g of solution, and v/v expresses the number of milliliters of solute in 100 mL of the solution. Wanamaker BP, Applied Pharmacology for Veterinary Technicians, ed 4, Saunders Company, 2008.

401. b Regardless of the type of blood product, products must be given within 4 hours to avoid contamination. This means within 4 hours after collection of whole blood, defrosting fresh frozen plasma, or puncturing a collection bag of RBCs. Beiter C, "Fluid Therapy and Blood Products," in Bryant S, Anesthesia for Veterinary Technicians, ed 1, Wiley-Blackwell, 2010.

402. c Dissociative anesthetics such as ketamine do not affect the respiratory system in the same way as most other anesthetics. Respiratory rate and tidal volume may change, but respiratory depression is usually insignificant at usual doses. At higher doses, animals exhibit apneustic respiration, a breathing pattern in which there is a pause for several seconds at the end of the inspiratory phase, followed by a short, quick expiratory phase. These animals appear to hold their breath. Pentobarbital and thiamylal are both barbiturates and do not cause unusual respirations. Guaifenesin is a muscle relaxant and does not affect respiration. Thomas J, Phillip L, Anesthesia and Analgesia for Veterinary Technicians, ed 5, Elsevier, 2017.

403. b 5% = 50 mg/mL; 180 mL = 9000 mg/150 kg = 60 mg/kg. The term *percent concentration* may be used when w/v, w/w, or v/v concentrations are described. Percent (percentage) means parts of solute per 100 parts of the solution. Percent w/v means the number of grams of solute in 100 mL of solution, percent w/w describes the number of grams of solute in 100 g of solution, and v/v expresses the number of milliliters of solute in 100 mL of the solution. Wanamaker BP, Applied Pharmacology for Veterinary Technicians, ed 4, Saunders, 2008.

404. d Benzodiazepines are extremely safe tranquilizers that have little effect on the cardiovascular system. In some cases, however, excitation can occur in young, healthy animals. Opioids are analgesics that often cause sedation and not excitation. Dissociates such as ketamine and Telazol are injectable anesthetics used for sedation and induction. These drugs are not considered tranquilizers. Alpha-2 agonists cause moderate to severe sedation and do not cause excitation. Robbins S, "Premedication and Sedation Drugs," in Bryant S, Anesthesia for Veterinary Technicians, ed 1, Wiley-Blackwell, 2010.

405. b Atropine is an anticholinergic that increases heart rate and decreases secretions. It has a quick onset of action and is short-acting. Because atropine increases heart rate, it should not be given to patients that are tachycardic. Methadone and morphine are opioids that generally cause sedation and offer excellent analgesia. These drugs actually decrease heart rate. Midazolam is a benzodiazepine tranquilizer that does not affect the cardiovascular system. Robbins S, "Premedication and Sedation Drugs," in Bryant S, Anesthesia for Veterinary Technicians, ed 1, Wiley-Blackwell, 2010.

406. c Local anesthetic agents have long been used to allow surgical procedures to be performed in conscious animals, but their use in preventing or treating postoperative pain is relatively recent. The presence of local anesthetic blocks sodium channels, which prevents transduction and transmission of noxious stimuli into nerve impulses peripherally (local blocks) as well as centrally (if administered by epidural). Therefore, lidocaine is an excellent caudal analgesic. Caudal epidural lidocaine can be used in a cesarean section; however, it will not prevent movement by itself. Thomas J, Phillip L, Anesthesia and Analgesia for Veterinary Technicians, ed 5, Elsevier, 2017.

407. a Unlike midazolam, which is water soluble, diazepam is highly protein-bound and mixed in a carrier solution of propylene glycol. Because of its insoluble nature, diazepam should not be mixed with most other drugs and uptake is often variable if administered via the IM and SQ routes. Robbins S, "Premedication and Sedation Drugs," in Bryant S, Anesthesia for Veterinary Technicians, ed 1, Wiley-Blackwell, 2010.

408. d Butorphanol is a kappa agonist and mu antagonist. Mammals have primarily mu pain receptors in the brain; therefore, a mu agonist opioid is needed to provide pain relief. Butorphanol is a mu antagonist and therefore does not provide adequate pain control for moderate to severe pain. Full mu opioids such as methadone, morphine, and hydromorphone are most appropriate for orthopedic pain. Robbins S, "Premedication and Sedation Drugs," in Bryant S, Anesthesia for Veterinary Technicians, ed 1, Wiley-Blackwell, 2010.

409. d Masks allow the anesthetist to administer oxygen rapidly to a fully conscious patient, sedated patient, or anesthetized patient that cannot be intubated or when tube placement is delayed. Masks have several disadvantages, however, because they do not maintain an open airway as ET tubes do and airway obstruction is therefore possible, particularly in brachycephalic breed animals and other patients prone to obstruction. There is no protection against pulmonary aspiration as there is with a tube and the anesthetist is not able to ventilate the patient when necessary. Therefore, masks should only be used in calm dogs and cats and only as a last resort to anesthetic induction. Thomas J, Phillip L, Anesthesia and Analgesia for Veterinary Technicians, ed 5, Elsevier, 2017.

410. d Naloxone is a mu antagonist, which means that it reverses the effects of full mu opioids, including the analgesic properties. Flumazenil reverses the effects of benzodiazepines. Atipamezole reverses the effects of alpha-2 agonists and alfaxalone is a neurosteroid injectable anesthetic. Robbins S, "Premedication and Sedation Drugs," in Bryant S, Anesthesia for Veterinary Technicians, ed 1, Wiley-Blackwell, 2010.

411. b Buprenorphine is a partial agonist opioid. It provides analgesia for mild to moderate pain. It has a very strong affinity for the mu receptor and will actually replace or kick a full mu opioid off the receptor. Butorphanol is a mixed agonist opioid that acts on the kappa receptor and antagonizes the mu receptor. Butorphanol provides analgesia for only mild pain. Morphine is a full mu agonist opioid used for mild to severe pain. Naloxone is a mu antagonist used to reverse the effects of mu opioids. Robbins S, "Premedication and Sedation Drugs," in Bryant S, Anesthesia for Veterinary Technicians, ed 1, Wiley-Blackwell, 2010.

412. b Atropine does not increase salivation but rather decreases it. It can also cause mydriasis and tachycardia and can decrease GI motility. Thomas J, Phillip L, Anesthesia and Analgesia for Veterinary Technicians, ed 5, Elsevier, 2017.

413. d Morphine can be given safely IV, but it must be given very slowly. Quick administration of morphine can lead to histamine release that in turn can cause severe hypotension. Hydromorphone, butorphanol, and buprenorphine do not cause histamine release when given via any route. Robbins S, "Premedication and Sedation Drugs," in Bryant S, Anesthesia for Veterinary Technicians, ed 1, Wiley-Blackwell, 2010.

414. d Ketamine is a cyclohexamine dissociative anesthetic. It increases heart rate and blood pressure by indirect sympathetic stimulation. The jaw tone is increased, palpebral reflexes are intact, and the eyes stay central. Propofol is an oil-in-water emulsion that has potent respiratory effects, can cause transient hypotension, and decreases cardiac contractility. Fentanyl is a full mu opioid that can be used as an induction agent or in a CRI. It is among the safest drugs used in the oldest, youngest, and sickest patients. The most common side effect is bradycardia. Alfaxalone is a neurosteroid injectable induction agent with properties similar to that of propofol. Fuehrer L, "Induction Drugs," in Bryant S, Anesthesia for Veterinary Technicians, ed 1, Wiley-Blackwell, 2010.

415. b 60 kg × 0.1 = 6 mg. The maximum dose is still 4 mg. The quantity of drug to be delivered to a patient is called the dose. A dosage rate expressed in milligrams per kilogram (or milligrams per pound) is multiplied by the animal's weight in kilograms (or pounds) to determine the dose. The dose is then divided by the amount (concentration) of the drug in the pharmaceutical form (tablet, solution, and so forth) to determine the actual amount of the pharmaceutical form to be administered. The formula for dosage calculation, which should be committed to memory, is as follows: Dose = Animal's weight × dosage rate ÷ concentration of drug. Wanamaker, Boyce P. Applied Pharmacology for Veterinary Technicians, ed 4, Saunders, 2008.

416. b Ketamine is a dissociative anesthetic agent. Ketamine has a quick onset of action and induces CNS depression, which leads to a dissociative state. Propofol is a short-acting hypnotic phenol anesthetic. Alfaxalone is a progesterone derivative neuroactive steroid that produces hypnosis and muscle relaxation by enhancing inhibitory effects of GABA in the brain. Etomidate is a fast-acting hypnotic agent classified as an imidazole derivative. Kastner SBR, "Intravenous Anesthetics," in Seymour C, Duke-Novakovski T, BSAVA Manual of Canine and Feline Anesthesia and Analgesia, ed 2, British Small Animal Veterinary Association, 2007.

417. c You must worry about the dosage of anesthetics. You must be concerned about even small doses because many are dose-dependent. The more anesthetic agents that are administered, the greater is the adverse effect. Major effects and adverse effects of halogenated inhalation anesthetics are as follows: dose-related CNS depression, vasodilation, decreased cardiac output and blood pressure, and dose-dependent respiratory depression (including apnea). Thomas J, Phillip L, Anesthesia and Analgesia for Veterinary Technicians, ed 5, Elsevier, 2017.

418. a Propofol can cause longer recoveries in cats given a CRI longer than 30 minutes and Heinz body formation, lethargy, vomiting, diarrhea, and anorexia when given several times throughout consecutive days. Midazolam is a benzodiazepine and is safe to give over consecutive days when needed. Ketamine should be avoided in cats with renal disease because of active metabolites in the urine. Alfaxalone is a neurosteroid injectable induction agent. Alfaxalone is a better option for CRI administration and small boluses can be given safely over consecutive days. Fuehrer L, "Induction Drugs," in Bryant S, Anesthesia for Veterinary Technicians, ed 1, Wiley-Blackwell, 2010.

419. b Ketamine is excreted via the kidneys as the active metabolite norketamine in cats. Propofol, alfaxalone, and fentanyl are not affected by renal insufficiency and can be used in cats with renal failure. Fuehrer L, "Induction Drugs," in Bryant S, Anesthesia for Veterinary Technicians, ed 1, Wiley-Blackwell, 2010.

420. c Age, temperature, stress, drugs, disease process, species, and circadian rhythm all affect MAC. The sex of the animal does not affect MAC in any way. MAC is also not affected by the intensity of stimulation or the length of the procedure. Fornes S, "Inhalant Anesthetics," in Bryant S, Anesthesia for Veterinary Technicians, ed 1, Wiley-Blackwell, 2010.

421. b Vapor pressure is important because it is indicative of the type of vaporizer that is needed for a specific type of inhalant. The vapor pressure of isoflurane and sevoflurane is >30% at room temperature; therefore, these gases must be used in a precision vaporizer. Sublimation, evaporation, and deposition have nothing to do with anesthesia. *Sublimation* is the term used for a substance going from a solid to a gas phase while skipping the liquid phase. Deposition is the opposite, with the gas progressing straight to a liquid. Fornes S, "Inhalant Anesthetics," in Bryant S, Anesthesia for Veterinary Technicians, ed 1, Wiley-Blackwell, 2010.

422. d The lower the solubility of the anesthetic, the more rapid gas anesthetics will go from the alveoli into the blood. Low solubility causes because the gas will quickly distribute from the alveoli into rapid induction in the blood. Fornes S, "Inhalant Anesthetics," in Bryant S, Anesthesia for Veterinary Technicians, ed 1, Wiley-Blackwell, 2010.

423. b The primary method of excretion of inhalant anesthetics is via respiration, not hepatic metabolism. Fornes S, "Inhalant Anesthetics," in Bryant S, Anesthesia for Veterinary Technicians, ed 1, Wiley-Blackwell, 2010.

424. a MAC is the minimum alveolar concentration. The MAC value varies by species, temperature, drugs given, age, disease status, etc. MAC is the concentration of anesthetic that produces anesthesia in 50% of patients that are given noxious stimuli. It is important to know these values for the species you are working with because it helps decide where to start setting the vaporizer settings. Fornes S, "Inhalant Anesthetics," in Bryant S, Anesthesia for Veterinary Technicians, ed 1, Wiley-Blackwell, 2010.

425. b MAC is the minimum alveolar concentration. The MAC value varies by species, temperature, drugs given, age, disease status, etc. MAC is the concentration of anesthetic that produces anesthesia in 50% of patients that are given noxious stimuli. It is important to know these values for the species you are working with because it helps decide where to start setting the vaporizer settings. Fornes S, "Inhalant Anesthetics," in Bryant S, Anesthesia for Veterinary Technicians, ed 1, Wiley-Blackwell, 2010.

426. c MAC is the minimum alveolar concentration. The MAC value varies by species, temperature, drugs given, age, disease status, etc. MAC is the concentration of anesthetic that produces anesthesia in 50% of patients that are given noxious stimuli. It is important to know these values for the species you are working with because it helps decide where to start setting the vaporizer settings. Fornes S, "Inhalant Anesthetics," in Bryant S, Anesthesia for Veterinary Technicians, ed 1, Wiley-Blackwell, 2010.

427. a MAC is the minimum alveolar concentration. The MAC value varies by species, temperature, drugs given, age, disease status, etc. MAC is the concentration of anesthetic that produces anesthesia in 50% of patients that are given noxious stimuli. It is important to know these values for the species you are working with because it helps decide where to start setting the vaporizer settings. Fornes S, "Inhalant Anesthetics," in Bryant S, Anesthesia for Veterinary Technicians, ed 1, Wiley-Blackwell, 2010.

428. c The solubility coefficient of an inhaled anesthetic is affected by increases and decreases in body temperature. When a patient becomes hypothermic, the inhalant becomes more soluble in the cooled blood. When an inhalant is more soluble, less is needed to keep the patient in a surgical plane of anesthesia. The opposite is true for hyperthermic patients. Fornes S, "Inhalant Anesthetics," in Bryant S, Anesthesia for Veterinary Technicians, ed 1, Wiley-Blackwell, 2010.

429. a Isoflurane is twice as soluble as sevoflurane. Halothane is twice as soluble as isoflurane. Sevoflurane is twice as soluble as desflurane. The lower the solubility of an anesthetic, the more rapidly the inhalant will go from the alveoli and dissolve into the blood. Inhalants with a higher solubility take longer to become effective and to be metabolized. For example, isoflurane is twice as soluble as sevoflurane, and in turn it takes longer for induction and recovery compared with sevoflurane. Fornes S, "Inhalant Anesthetics," in Bryant S, Anesthesia for Veterinary Technicians, ed 1, Wiley-Blackwell, 2010.

430. d Nitrous oxide is housed in a compressed gas cylinder and does not need to be vaporized for delivery. A regulator similar to oxygen is used. The other inhalants listed use a precision vaporizer for delivery to the patient. Fornes S, "Inhalant Anesthetics," in Bryant S, Anesthesia for Veterinary Technicians, ed 1, Wiley-Blackwell, 2010.

431. c Inhalant anesthetics cause a dose-dependent vasodilation, which often leads to hypotension. Fentanyl (opioid), thiopental (barbiturate), and midazolam (benzodiazepine) do not cause dose-dependent vasodilation. Fornes S, "Inhalant Anesthetics," in Bryant S, Anesthesia for Veterinary Technicians, ed 1, Wiley-Blackwell, 2010.

432. a Patients that are hypothermic have slower recovery times. Hyperthermia, reproductive status, and sex of the patient do not contribute to prolonged recovery times. Other contributing factors to prolonged recovery time are drug protocol, disease status, and age. Cheyne M, "Recovery of the Anesthetic Patient," in Bryant S, Anesthesia for Veterinary Technicians, ed 1, Wiley-Blackwell, 2010.

433. c Ideally, patients recovering from anesthesia should have vital signs monitored every 15–20 minutes. This helps ensure recovery is moving in the correct direction and the temperature is returning to normal. More critical patients often need continuous monitoring during this time. Cheyne M, "Recovery of the Anesthetic Patient," in Bryant S, Anesthesia for Veterinary Technicians, ed 1, Wiley-Blackwell, 2010.

434. b Respiratory acidosis is caused by a buildup of CO_2 and not hyperventilation or too little CO_2. Normal breathing is termed *eupnea* and will not cause respiratory acidosis. McMillan S, "Anesthetic Complications and Emergencies," in Bryant S, Anesthesia for Veterinary Technicians, ed 1, Wiley-Blackwell, 2010.

435. b Hypercarbia is too much CO_2. Endotracheal tubes that are obstructed do not allow exhalation and thus CO_2 increasing. A plugged endotracheal tube also causes hypoxia and dyspnea and potentially respiratory arrest is not corrected. Eupnea is normal breathing, aspiration of gastric contents has nothing to do with endotracheal tube obstruction, and respiratory acidosis is most often caused by overventilation or hyperventilation. McMillan S, "Anesthetic Complications and Emergencies," in Bryant S, Anesthesia for Veterinary Technicians, ed 1, Wiley-Blackwell, 2010.

436. a Benzodiazepines such as midazolam can cause excitation in some healthy patients. The other drugs do not. When using a benzodiazepine during induction, it is suggested that the other injectable agent is provided, followed by the benzodiazepine. Excitation is much less likely when, for example, a small dose of propofol or ketamine has been administered first. McMillan S, "Anesthetic Complications and Emergencies," in Bryant S, Anesthesia for Veterinary Technicians, ed 1, Wiley-Blackwell, 2010.

437. b Apnea is one of the most common side effects of administering propofol too quickly. Other side effects include cyanosis and transient hypotension. Tachycardia, hypertension, and hypothermia are not side effects of a propofol induction. McMillan S, "Anesthetic Complications and Emergencies," in Bryant S, Anesthesia for Veterinary Technicians, ed 1, Wiley-Blackwell, 2010.

438. b Airway obstruction can occur at any time, but it is most likely to occur during the preanesthetic and recovery periods when the patient has been administered drugs and the airway is not protected with an endotracheal tube. McMillan S, "Anesthetic Complications and Emergencies," in Bryant S, Anesthesia for Veterinary Technicians, ed 1, Wiley-Blackwell, 2010.

439. c Laryngospasm is most often observed in cats during endotracheal intubation. Lidocaine is a local anesthetic that acts by anesthetizing the glottis and thus helping with endotracheal tube placement. Methadone, isoflurane, and diazepam do not have a direct effect on the laryngeal tissue. McMillan S, "Anesthetic Complications and Emergencies," in Bryant S, Anesthesia for Veterinary Technicians, ed 1, Wiley-Blackwell, 2010.

440. a Hypoventilation is caused by a decreased respiratory rate or reduction in tidal volume, thus reducing minute volume. Dyspnea is defined as difficulty in breathing, disordered or inadequate breathing, or uncomfortable awareness of breathing. Tachypnea is an increase in respiratory rate, whereas hyperventilation is an increase in respiratory rate and depth. McMillan S, "Anesthetic Complications and Emergencies," in Bryant S, Anesthesia for Veterinary Technicians, ed 1, Wiley-Blackwell, 2010.

441. a Hyperthermia generally increases respiratory rate, not decreases it. All other answers contribute to hypoventilation. Other processes that contribute include pain when the thorax is expanded, pleural space disease, diaphragmatic hernia, hypothermia, cervical disease, severe hypotension, and anesthetic overdose. McMillan S, "Anesthetic Complications and Emergencies," in Bryant S, Anesthesia for Veterinary Technicians, ed 1, Wiley-Blackwell, 2010.

442. d Hypothermia does not contribute to hyperventilation, but pyrexia (fever) and hyperthermia do. Inadequate anesthetic depth, pain, hypoxia, overventilation, and surgical stimulation all contribute. McMillan S, "Anesthetic Complications and Emergencies," in Bryant S, Anesthesia for Veterinary Technicians, ed 1, Wiley-Blackwell, 2010.

443. b The lowest acceptable mean arterial blood pressure in small animals such as dogs and cats is 60 mmHg and 70 mmHg should really be the lowest aimed for. When the mean arterial blood pressure drops to <60 mmHg, blood is shunted away from the major organs to help sustain basic life support. This can lead to organ failure in the future. McMillan S, "Anesthetic Complications and Emergencies," in Bryant S, Anesthesia for Veterinary Technicians, ed 1, Wiley-Blackwell, 2010.

444. b Cardiopulmonary arrest is a sudden cessation of functional ventilation and systemic perfusion. This results in reduced oxygen delivery to tissues with decreased removal of CO_2. Bradycardia is defined as a slow heart rate. Ventricular tachycardia is an abnormally fast heart rate with three or more abnormal heart beats in a row. Hypercapnia is too much CO_2. During cardiopulmonary arrest, the heart is not beating or not beating well and little to no CO_2 is being created. McMillan S, "Anesthetic Complications and Emergencies," in Bryant S, Anesthesia for Veterinary Technicians, ed 1, Wiley-Blackwell, 2010.

445. d Studies indicated that there is only a 3-minute window of opportunity to restore cerebral perfusion after cardiopulmonary arrest before irreversible neurological damage will occur. McMillan S, "Anesthetic Complications and Emergencies," in Bryant S, Anesthesia for Veterinary Technicians, ed 1, Wiley-Blackwell, 2010.

446. d Central venous catheters are ideal because of the proximity to the heart. The peripheral vessels are next because it is convenient and most anesthetized patients already have a catheter in place. Injections given in the peripheral vessels should be flushed with at least a few milliliters of saline to help advance the drugs. Intraosseous administration is the third choice. This is a good option when vessel administration is not possible. Intratracheal administration is last on this list. Because this is not given directly into the vessel or medullary cavity, a much larger dose needs to be given. McMillan S, "Anesthetic Complications and Emergencies," in Bryant S, Anesthesia for Veterinary Technicians, ed 1, Wiley-Blackwell, 2010.

447. a Epinephrine is a mixed adrenergic agonist and a catecholamine. It is most often used as a first-line drug during CPCR for severe bradycardia including asystole. Epinephrine has alpha-2 agonist effects, which causes vasoconstriction. This vasoconstriction increases coronary and cerebral perfusion. McMillan S, "Anesthetic Complications and Emergencies," in Bryant S, Anesthesia for Veterinary Technicians, ed 1, Wiley-Blackwell, 2010.

448. b Lidocaine is a local anesthetic and antiarrhythmic. This drug is often used to treat ventricular tachycardia, atrial fibrillation, refractory ventricular fibrillation, and some forms of supraventricular tachycardia. Thiopental is a barbiturate injectable anesthetic. Alfaxalone is a neurosteroid injectable anesthetic and dopamine is a positive inotrope used most commonly to treat hypotension. McMillan S, "Anesthetic Complications and Emergencies," in Bryant S, Anesthesia for Veterinary Technicians, ed 1, Wiley-Blackwell, 2010.

449. d Atropine is an anticholinergic parasympatholytic drug used to treat vagally induced bradycardia. Atropine reduces the effects of parasympathetic stimulation and cholinergic responses. Atropine increases heart rate, often increasing blood pressure, and increases systemic vascular resistance. Lidocaine is a local anesthetic and antiarrhythmic. This drug is often used to treat ventricular tachycardia, atrial fibrillation, refractory ventricular fibrillation, and some forms of supraventricular tachycardia. Alfaxalone is a neurosteroid injectable anesthetic and dobutamine is a positive inotrope used most commonly to treat hypotension. McMillan S, "Anesthetic Complications and Emergencies," in Bryant S, Anesthesia for Veterinary Technicians, ed 1, Wiley-Blackwell, 2010.

450. c The electrocardiogram (ECG) is the only way to monitor both the heart rate and rhythm. The capnograph only measures respiratory rate and end-tidal CO2. The Doppler provides an audible heart rate and the pulse oximeter gives heart rate and percentage of oxygen saturation. McMillan S, "Anesthetic Complications and Emergencies," in Bryant S, Anesthesia for Veterinary Technicians, ed 1, Wiley-Blackwell, 2010.

451. c Alcohol is flammable and can cause the patient to catch fire if defibrillation is performed. Alcohol can cool a patient, but not with the small amounts people generally use on ECG clips. Alcohol in small amounts does not usually cause skin irritation. McMillan S, "Anesthetic Complications and Emergencies," in Bryant S, Anesthesia for Veterinary Technicians, ed 1, Wiley-Blackwell, 2010.

452. b Multimodal anesthesia is defined as a protocol that uses multiple agents in an effort to decrease the dose of each agent and thus decrease the negative side effects of the anesthetic drugs. Multimodal anesthesia is very beneficial because it generally provides MAC reduction while providing additional analgesia. Drugs used in multimodal anesthesia come from various different categories such as opioids, inhalants, alpha-2 agonists, etc. Curtis-Uhle Wendy, Waddell KW, "Anesthesia for Patients with Cardiac Disease," in Bryant S, Anesthesia for Veterinary Technicians, ed 1, Wiley-Blackwell, 2010.

453. c Preoxygenation before induction can increase the alveolar oxygen concentration and thus increase the amount of oxygen transported by hemoglobin. This is beneficial for patients during the period before intubation. Although not ideal in all patients, preoxygenation is most effective when using a mask with a fitted diaphragm. Curtis-Uhle Wendy, Waddell KW, "Anesthesia for Patients with Cardiac Disease," in Bryant S, Anesthesia for Veterinary Technicians, ed 1, Wiley-Blackwell, 2010.

454. b If the heart cannot effectively pump blood, it cannot meet metabolic needs. The kidney, liver, and respiratory system are not actively involved in moving blood around the body. Curtis-Uhle Wendy, Waddell KW, "Anesthesia for Patients with Cardiac Disease," in Bryant S, Anesthesia for Veterinary Technicians, ed 1, Wiley-Blackwell, 2010.

455. d Peak inspiratory pressure between 15 and 20 cm H_2O will most often provide adequate ventilation when normal lung tissue is present. Low peak inspiratory pressure may not be large enough to help provide adequate ventilation and increased peak inspiratory pressures can lead to trauma. Higher pressures may be needed to provide appropriate tidal volumes in patients that have diaphragmatic hernias, are obese, or are in some positions required for surgery. Bryant S, "Respiratory-Challenges Patients," Anesthesia for Veterinary Technicians, ed 1, Wiley-Blackwell, 2010.

456. b In most patients the respiratory rate on a ventilator can be set between 8 and 12 breaths per minute. Some patients may require more or less. A capnograph will help evaluate adequate ventilation. Bryant S, "Respiratory-Challenges Patients," Anesthesia for Veterinary Technicians, ed 1, Wiley-Blackwell, 2010.

457. a An intact thoracic cavity is under negative pressure. Without negative pressure, the lungs would not be able to expand and contract properly. If the thorax is opened via surgery or from trauma, the negative pressure is lost, leading to a pneumothorax. The lungs cannot expand and contract on their own and assistance with ventilation is necessary. Bryant S, "Respiratory-Challenges Patients," Anesthesia for Veterinary Technicians, ed 1, Wiley-Blackwell, 2010.

458. d Surprisingly, a loss of 70%–75% of renal function must occur before it is present on a chemistry panel. There is not one single test that is used to diagnose renal disease; therefore, BUN and creatinine are used in conjunction with a physical examination and history. Patients with renal disease often require a larger volume of fluids during the perianesthetic and postanesthetic periods. Cooley K, "Anesthesia for Patients with Renal Disease," in Bryant S, Anesthesia for Veterinary Technicians, ed 1, Wiley-Blackwell, 2010.

459. a In cats, ketamine is eliminated virtually unchanged by the kidney. This can lead to extremely prolonged recoveries from anesthesia. Propofol, hydromorphone, and isoflurane are safe drugs to use in patients with renal disease because they do not have a direct effect on the kidneys. Cooley K, "Anesthesia for Patients with Renal Disease," in Bryant S, Anesthesia for Veterinary Technicians, ed 1, Wiley-Blackwell, 2010.

460. d The liver is the one organ that handles the metabolism and clearance of most anesthetic drugs. The pancreas does not play a role in metabolism of anesthetic drugs. The kidneys primarily handle the excretion of drugs from the body and the lungs play a role in clearance for drugs such as inhalants and propofol. Carter H, "Anesthesia for Patients with Liver Disease," in Bryant S, Anesthesia for Veterinary Technicians, ed 1, Wiley-Blackwell, 2010.

461. a If drugs cannot bind properly, they are metabolized less efficiently and more slowly. This can lead to prolonged recoveries or overdose of drugs. BUN, creatinine, and PCV do not affect these factors. Carter H, "Anesthesia for Patients with Liver Disease," in Bryant S, Anesthesia for Veterinary Technicians, ed 1, Wiley-Blackwell, 2010.

462. d There are many disadvantages to using heavy sedation and general anesthesia in most ruminants, although it is required under some circumstances. Regurgitation and excess salivation can lead to aspiration; therefore, light sedation and a standing technique that uses ropes, chutes, and local blocks are generally used. Kaiser-Klinger S, "Ruminant Anesthesia," in Bryant S, Anesthesia for Veterinary Technicians, ed 1, Wiley-Blackwell, 2010.

463. d Rumen contents are less likely to be regurgitated when food is withheld for 24 hours before anesthetic induction. Water is generally withheld for 6–12 hours. Kaiser-Klinger S, "Ruminant Anesthesia," in Bryant S, Anesthesia for Veterinary Technicians, ed 1, Wiley-Blackwell, 2010.

464. c This position helps to keep excessive saliva and regurgitation from pooling in the proximal esophagus and mouth. The saliva/regurgitation that pools will drain easily because of the position of the head. Kaiser-Klinger S, "Ruminant Anesthesia," in Bryant S, Anesthesia for Veterinary Technicians, ed 1, Wiley-Blackwell, 2010.

465. b The cornual nerve has several branches. Only a few branches of the cornual nerve supply the lateral and caudal parts of the horn. The branches of the lacrimal and infratrochlear nerves must be blocked to provide adequate analgesia. The auriculopalpebral nerve block is used to aid in the examination and surgery of the eye. This block does not provide analgesia but prevents the lid from closing. The peroneal block is used for providing anesthesia to the hind limb below the hock. The digital block is used for providing anesthesia to the digits. Kaiser-Klinger S, "Ruminant Anesthesia," in Bryant S, Anesthesia for Veterinary Technicians, ed 1, Wiley-Blackwell, 2010.

466. a An epidural block is used to provide anesthesia/analgesia for procedures involving the flank, abdomen, inguinal, and perineal regions. The caudal block is used primarily for obstetric procedures of the vagina and vulva or for tail docking. The peroneal block is used for providing anesthesia to the hind limb below the hock. The cornual block is used for dehorning procedures. Kaiser-Klinger

S, "Ruminant Anesthesia," in Bryant S, Anesthesia for Veterinary Technicians, ed 1, Wiley-Blackwell, 2010.

467. b Hypertension is not caused by an overdose or improper administration of local anesthetics into the epidural space. Hypotension can be a negative side effect as well as seizures, paralysis of the respiratory tract, muscle spasm and contraction, and hypothermia. The side effects occur because of placement of drugs into the incorrect area, leading to blockade of the wrong nerve(s). Full cardiovascular collapse can occur with overdose. Kaiser-Klinger S, "Ruminant Anesthesia," in Bryant S, Anesthesia for Veterinary Technicians, ed 1, Wiley-Blackwell, 2010.

468. d Animals that will be slaughtered for food should not be given any sedatives or tranquilizers. These drugs can be used in traditional food animals if they are not going to be slaughtered. Kaiser-Klinger S, "Ruminant Anesthesia," in Bryant S, Anesthesia for Veterinary Technicians, ed 1, Wiley-Blackwell, 2010.

469. d Anticholinergics are generally not suggested for use in ruminants unless there is a true need. Drugs such as atropine and glycopyrrolate increase the viscosity of saliva without decreasing the amount. This makes it harder to drain the saliva from the oropharynx. Kaiser-Klinger S, "Ruminant Anesthesia," in Bryant S, Anesthesia for Veterinary Technicians, ed 1, Wiley-Blackwell, 2010.

470. a The jugular vein is the largest and most easily accessible vessel in the cow. The cephalic and saphenous veins are more commonly used in smaller ruminants such as sheep and goats. The auricular vein located on the pinna is not generally the first choice in most species. Kaiser-Klinger S, "Ruminant Anesthesia," in Bryant S, Anesthesia for Veterinary Technicians, ed 1, Wiley-Blackwell, 2010.

471. d Yohimbine is an alpha-2 antagonist used to reverse xylazine. Flumazenil reverses benzodiazepines. Naloxone reverses mu agonist opioids and dexmedetomidine is another alpha-2 agonist and is not a reversal agent. Nann LE, "Equine Anesthesia," in Bryant S, Anesthesia for Veterinary Technicians, ed 1, Wiley-Blackwell, 2010.

472. b Knowing the MAC of the species you are working with is extremely important. This is the starting point for setting the vaporizer. Many different things such as disease status, age, temperature, drug protocol, and ASA status affect MAC. Nann LE, "Equine Anesthesia," in Bryant S, Anesthesia for Veterinary Technicians, ed 1, Wiley-Blackwell, 2010.

473. c Heart rate is not a good indicator of anesthetic depth. The heart rate does not generally significantly increase or decrease with a deep or light plane of anesthesia. The swallow reflex, respiratory rate and depth, lateral nystagmus, palpebral reflex, arterial blood pressure, corneal reflex, anal tone, ocular position, and muscular relaxation can all be used to assess the plane of anesthesia because they increase or decrease with anesthetic depth. Nann LE, "Equine Anesthesia," in Bryant S, Anesthesia for Veterinary Technicians, ed 1, Wiley-Blackwell, 2010.

474. b Blood gas analysis is the gold standard technique used to assess ventilation in any animal under anesthesia. This measures the actual oxygen and carbon dioxide content of the arterial blood. Mucous membrane color can give an idea of ventilation, but a patient can still have pink mucous membranes yet not be ventilated properly. The $ETCO_2$ is a good estimate of ventilation, but it is not as accurate as blood gas analysis. Pulse oximetry measures oxygen saturation and not ventilation status. Nann LE, "Equine Anesthesia," in Bryant S, Anesthesia for Veterinary Technicians, ed 1, Wiley-Blackwell, 2010.

475. b Using a flow rate in the 10–15 mL/kg/min range helps wash out nitrogen and CO_2 in the respiratory tract and rapidly fills the bag and circuit with anesthetic gas. Higher flows are fine but are more wasteful. Lower flows can lead to more time necessary for filling the circuit with anesthetic gases. Nann LE, "Equine Anesthesia," in Bryant S, Anesthesia for Veterinary Technicians, ed 1, Wiley-Blackwell, 2010.

476. c Lower flow rates are more economical and conserve the amount of oxygen and inhalant used. There is also less environmental contamination when lower flows are used. Using this lower range still meets the metabolic needs of the patient. Nann LE, "Equine Anesthesia," in Bryant S, Anesthesia for Veterinary Technicians, ed 1, Wiley-Blackwell, 2010.

477. d Hypoxemia can occur if the patient is not able to oxygenate properly. Anesthetic drugs cause hypoventilation. This can lead to poor ventilation and oxygenation. Administering higher percentages of oxygen helps prevent problems such as hypoxemia. Hypertension, hyperthermia, and apnea are not direct potential problems caused by using room air during anesthesia. Nann LE, "Equine Anesthesia," in Bryant S, Anesthesia for Veterinary Technicians, ed 1, Wiley-Blackwell, 2010.

478. d Giving two types of NSAIDs at the same time or administering an NSAID with a corticosteroid can cause an increased risk of GI ulceration. It does not increase the risk of liver or renal failure and the drugs do not cancel out the therapeutic effects of each other. Spelts K, Gaynor J, "Pain Management Strategies," in Bryant S, Anesthesia for Veterinary Technicians, ed 1, Wiley-Blackwell, 2010.

479. c Tramadol is a synthetic, centrally acting analgesic. It is not a true opioid, but its metabolites bind to mu receptors and cause opioid-like effects. Hydromorphone and meperidine are full mu opioids and deracoxib is an NSAID. Spelts K, Gaynor J, "Pain Management Strategies," in Bryant S, Anesthesia for Veterinary Technicians, ed 1, Wiley-Blackwell, 2010.

480. b Central neuronal hypersensitization or wind-up pain occurs when the dorsal horn of the spinal cord is bombarded with the transmission of noxious stimuli. N-methyl-D-aspartate (NMDA) receptors within the dorsal horn are activated and amplify the signal of pain to the brain. Using drugs that are NMDA agonists can help reduce wind-up pain. Ketamine is also an NMDA antagonist. Spelts K, Gaynor J, "Pain Management Strategies," in Bryant S, Anesthesia for Veterinary Technicians, ed 1, Wiley-Blackwell, 2010.

481. a Chronic pain occurs because of a persistent stimulus such as osteoarthritis or profound dental disease. The other examples are of acute pain. Spelts K, Gaynor J, "Pain Management Strategies," in Bryant S, Anesthesia for Veterinary Technicians, ed 1, Wiley-Blackwell, 2010.

482. b Maladaptive pain occurs when the body's central processing has gone awry. This results from damage to the peripheral and/or central nervous system or when the CNS is not processing pain properly. Maladaptive pain occurs from chronic pain and not acute pain such as a fresh laceration. Spelts K, Gaynor J, "Pain Management Strategies," in Bryant S, Anesthesia for Veterinary Technicians, ed 1, Wiley-Blackwell, 2010.

483. b Acute pain lasts anywhere from hours to about 1 month and dissipates as the initial source of pain resolves, that is, a laceration heals. The other examples fit under long-term chronic pain. Spelts K, Gaynor J, "Pain Management Strategies," in Bryant S, Anesthesia for Veterinary Technicians, ed 1, Wiley-Blackwell, 2010.

484. a Adaptive pain ranges from mild to severe and is acute in nature. As the source of the pain heals, the pain dissipates. Maladaptive pain, chronic pain, and neuropathic pain are all associated with long-term painful stimuli and are not acute in nature. Spelts K, Gaynor J, "Pain Management Strategies," in Bryant S, Anesthesia for Veterinary Technicians, ed 1, Wiley-Blackwell, 2010.

485. c Alpha-2 agonists such as dexmedetomidine cause a severe decrease in cardiac output as well as a decrease in tissue perfusion and oxygenation. Although these drugs are great sedatives, they should not be used in patients that are compromised. Morphine (opioid), meloxicam (NSAID), and ketamine (dissociative) do not severely impact cardiac output. Spelts K, Gaynor J, "Pain Management Strategies," in Bryant S, Anesthesia for Veterinary Technicians, ed 1, Wiley-Blackwell, 2010.

486. d Methadone does not generally induce vomiting. Morphine induces vomiting in a majority of the patients that receive it preoperatively. Hydromorphone and fentanyl may cause vomiting after administration. Spelts K, Gaynor J, "Pain Management Strategies," in Bryant S, Anesthesia for Veterinary Technicians, ed 1, Wiley-Blackwell, 2010.

487. d Local anesthetics such as lidocaine and bupivacaine are the only drugs that cause a complete and total loss of sensation of pain. These drugs block the transmission of pain from an injury or surgery site to the spinal cord. Local anesthetics help prevent the formation of wind-up pain. Spelts K, Gaynor J, "Pain Management Strategies," in Bryant S, Anesthesia for Veterinary Technicians, ed 1, Wiley-Blackwell, 2010.

488. d A 4- to 10-day washout period is suggested when switching from one NSAID to another. This will help reduce the occurrence of GI ulceration. Spelts K, Gaynor J, "Pain Management Strategies," in Bryant S, Anesthesia for Veterinary Technicians, ed 1, Wiley-Blackwell, 2010.

489. d Adjuncts for pain management include weight loss, laser therapy, physical rehabilitation, and stem-cell therapy. Spelts K, Gaynor J, "Pain Management Strategies," in Bryant S, Anesthesia for Veterinary Technicians, ed 1, Wiley-Blackwell, 2010.

490. b There are many signs of pain that include but are not limited to dilated pupils, decreased (not increased) grooming, lack of appetite, licking the wound or surgery site, aggression, rapid shallow breathing, trembling, shivering, limping or unwillingness to walk, restlessness, and increased respiratory rate, heart rate, and blood pressure. Lockhead K, "Pain Assessment," in Bryant S, Anesthesia for Veterinary Technicians, ed 1, Wiley-Blackwell, 2010.

491. b The International Association for the Study of Pain has described pain as an unpleasant sensory and emotional experience that individuals have when they perceive actual or potential tissue damage to their body. Dysphoria is often experienced after opioid administration. Dysphoric patients will often whine, howl, and act agitated. It is sometimes difficult to differentiate between pain and dysphoria. Anxiety is a feeling of nervousness, whereas aggression is shown by excessive barking, nipping, lunging, and biting. DeGouff L, "Basic Physiology of Pain," in Bryant S, Anesthesia for Veterinary Technicians, ed 1, Wiley-Blackwell, 2010.

492. a Visceral pain is characterized by dull, diffuse, achy pain and is caused by a disease process in the internal organs such as the bladder, liver, kidneys, spleen, and intestines. Deep burning sensations, throbbing pain, and superficial pain are considered somatic pain. Somatic pain occurs in the mucous membranes, skin, and subcutaneous tissues. DeGouff L, "Basic Physiology of Pain," in Bryant S, Anesthesia for Veterinary Technicians, ed 1, Wiley-Blackwell, 2010.

493. b Acute pain is a protective pain because it serves as a warning. For example, a thermal burn warns that something is hot and that it should not be touched again. Chronic pain serves no biological purpose and issues with chronic pain cause neuropathic and wind-up pain. DeGouff L, "Basic Physiology of Pain," in Bryant S, Anesthesia for Veterinary Technicians, ed 1, Wiley-Blackwell, 2010.

494. d Visceral pain is characterized by dull, diffuse, achy pain and is caused by a disease process in the internal organs such as the bladder, liver, kidneys, spleen, and intestines. Deep burning sensations, throbbing pain, and superficial pain are considered somatic pains. Somatic pain occurs in the mucous membranes, skin, and subcutaneous tissues. DeGouff L, "Basic Physiology of Pain," in Bryant S, Anesthesia for Veterinary Technicians, ed 1, Wiley-Blackwell, 2010.

495. d Butorphanol is a kappa agonist drug that attaches to and provides pain relief on the kappa receptor. This would provide better analgesia in cases where there were more kappa receptors present. Morphine, oxymorphone, and hydromorphone are all mu receptor opioids. DeGouff L, "Basic Physiology of Pain," in Bryant S, Anesthesia for Veterinary Technicians, ed 1, Wiley-Blackwell, 2010.

496. d Ferrets have a fast metabolism; therefore, the fasting period is fairly short. Fasting for 4–6 hours provides enough time to clear the GI tract and helps prevent excessive vomiting and regurgitation. Fasting longer than 6 hours is not recommended because of the high metabolic rate. Stowell J, "Anesthesia for Small Exotics:

Ferrets, Rodents, and Rabbits," in Bryant S, Anesthesia for Veterinary Technicians, ed 1, Wiley-Blackwell, 2010.

497. c The caudal lumbar muscles are large and an easy site for IM administration of drugs. The muscles of the forelimbs are very small and not often used for drug administration. The forelimbs can be used, but care should be taken to not damage the sciatic nerve. IV drugs can be given via any vein, but this is not common in ferrets. Stowell J, "Anesthesia for Small Exotics: Ferrets, Rodents, and Rabbits," in Bryant S, Anesthesia for Veterinary Technicians, ed 1, Wiley-Blackwell, 2010.

498. b Lidocaine is a local anesthetic that helps prevent laryngospasm. Lidocaine has a fast onset of action and short duration of action. Drugs such as ketamine, alfaxalone, and propofol do not increase or decrease laryngospasms and unlike lidocaine, they are not given directly onto the glottis. Stowell J, "Anesthesia for Small Exotics: Ferrets, Rodents, and Rabbits," in Bryant S, Anesthesia for Veterinary Technicians, ed 1, Wiley-Blackwell, 2010.

499. a Placing an IO catheter into the greater trochanter of the femur is the most common site in rats. The tibia, fibula, and radius are too small. Stowell J, "Anesthesia for Small Exotics: Ferrets, Rodents, and Rabbits," in Bryant S, Anesthesia for Veterinary Technicians, ed 1, Wiley-Blackwell, 2010.

500. b Signs of hypovolemic shock include tachycardia, hypotension, prolonged capillary refill time, and pale mucous membranes. Hyperthermia, light plane of anesthesia, and hypocapnia do not cause this combination of symptoms. The first line of treatment for hypovolemic shock includes a fluid bolus. Gilkey A, "Anesthesia for Non-Trauma Emergency Patients," in Bryant S, Anesthesia for Veterinary Technicians, ed 1, Wiley-Blackwell, 2010.

501. b The 0.9% sodium chloride does not contain potassium. Patients with hyperkalemia have increased potassium; therefore, using a maintenance fluid without added potassium is often ideal. D5W is 5% dextrose in water. This is not a fluid used for maintenance therapy. Gilkey A, "Anesthesia for Non-Trauma Emergency Patients," in Bryant S, Anesthesia for Veterinary Technicians, ed 1, Wiley-Blackwell, 2010.

502. b Sodium bicarbonate is used to increase blood pH. It is generally administered in a separate syringe and given via a syringe pump for several minutes. Dopamine is a positive inotrope used to help increase blood pressure. Etomidate is an IV induction agent used primarily in cardiovascular compromised patients. Doxapram is a respiratory stimulant. Gilkey A, "Anesthesia for Non-Trauma Emergency Patients," in Bryant S, Anesthesia for Veterinary Technicians, ed 1, Wiley-Blackwell, 2010.

503. a A large-bore catheter allows for a large bolus of fluids to be administered at a given time. The jugular is ideal because this is the large vessel and is closest to the heart. Cephalic is fine, too. The auricular vein is not generally used in dogs unless there is no other option. The jugular allows fluids and emergency drugs to become effective more quickly than the peripheral vessels. Gilkey A, "Anesthesia for Non-Trauma Emergency Patients," in Bryant S, Anesthesia for Veterinary Technicians, ed 1, Wiley-Blackwell, 2010.

504. d Morphine induces vomiting in most patients. Vomiting should be avoided in those presenting with a GDV. Hydromorphone may induce vomiting, but it is variable. Methadone and fentanyl generally do not induce vomiting. Gilkey A, "Anesthesia for Non-Trauma Emergency Patients," in Bryant S, Anesthesia for Veterinary Technicians, ed 1, Wiley-Blackwell, 2010.

505. d Pain, electrolyte imbalances, arrhythmias, regurgitation, shock, hypoxemia, and inadequate myocardial perfusion are just some of the potential problems caused by a GDV. Severe blood loss is not anticipated for this type of surgery. Gilkey A, "Anesthesia for Non-Trauma Emergency Patients," in Bryant S, Anesthesia for Veterinary Technicians, ed 1, Wiley-Blackwell, 2010.

506. b Airway obstructions are not generally severely painful and hypovolemic shock is not something expected with this case unless there is another underlying disease process. Aspiration can occur with any anesthetic case. This patient is not at an increased risk for aspiration. A major concern on recovery is airway obstruction as a result of swelling from the foreign body. Gilkey A, "Anesthesia for Non-Trauma Emergency Patients," in Bryant S, Anesthesia for Veterinary Technicians, ed 1, Wiley-Blackwell, 2010.

507. b A myelogram is performed to help diagnose intervertebral disk disease. With the patient under anesthesia, contrast is injected into the subarachnoid space. This can cause seizures in some patients. Elevating the head can help reduce seizures. Bleeding, hyperthermia, and pain are not expected for this procedure. Gilkey A, "Anesthesia for Non-Trauma Emergency Patients," in Bryant S, Anesthesia for Veterinary Technicians, ed 1, Wiley-Blackwell, 2010.

508. d Patients that have been unable to urinate generally present with electrolyte imbalances including increased potassium. A patient with widened QRS complexes and absent P waves is usually hyperkalemic. Inducing anesthesia in this patient can easily lead to cardiac arrest. Hypernatremia, hypophosphatemia, and hyperchloremia are not generally associated with this type of cardiac rhythm. Gilkey A, "Anesthesia for Non-Trauma Emergency Patients," in Bryant S, Anesthesia for Veterinary Technicians, ed 1, Wiley-Blackwell, 2010.

509. c This patient is compromised and probably in great deal of pain. Any drug protocol with butorphanol and buprenorphine is not going to provide enough analgesia. Because this patient is compromised, dexmedetomidine is probably not an ideal choice. Choosing a protocol that includes a neuroleptanalgesic (opioid + tranquilizer) is probably the safest; therefore midazolam and methadone are appropriate. Waddell KW, "Emergency Trauma Patients," in Bryant S, Anesthesia for Veterinary Technicians, ed 1, Wiley-Blackwell, 2010.

510. a Because this patient is compromised, the best induction protocol would include either an opioid such as fentanyl and a benzodiazepine or etomidate and a benzodiazepine. These drugs have little effect on the cardiovascular system. Propofol causes hypotension and decreases cardiac contractility. This is not ideal in a compromised patient. Masking a patient should never occur unless there is no other option. This would be especially stressful for a patient that was in a recent house fire presenting with dyspnea. Waddell KW, "Emergency Trauma Patients," in Bryant S, Anesthesia for Veterinary Technicians, ed 1, Wiley-Blackwell, 2010.

511. b Midazolam is a class IV controlled substance that acts as an anxiolytic, muscle relaxant, hypnotic, and anticonvulsant. Propofol is not controlled and is an oil-in-water fast-acting injectable induction agent. Fentanyl is a full mu opioid and is a class II controlled substance. Thiopental is a short-acting barbiturate and is not currently available in the United States. Waddell KW, "Emergency Trauma Patients," in Bryant S, Anesthesia for Veterinary Technicians, ed 1, Wiley-Blackwell, 2010.

512. d Posttraumatic pulmonary lesions can continue to worsen for 24–36 hours. It is imperative that radiographs are used to monitor any potential damage. The anesthetist must be aware of this potential because the act of manual or mechanical ventilation can lead to further damage, including pneumothorax. Waddell KW, "Emergency Trauma Patients," in Bryant S, Anesthesia for Veterinary Technicians, ed 1, Wiley-Blackwell, 2010.

513. b Full-term bitches are at high risk of regurgitation and aspiration during the perianesthetic period; because of this, mask induction is not recommended. The PCV and PP are decreased, not increased, in these patients, and the USG is increased, not decreased. Norkus CL, "Cesarean Section Techniques," in Bryant S, Anesthesia for Veterinary Technicians, ed 1, Wiley-Blackwell, 2010.

514. c Doxapram is a respiratory stimulant that has traditionally been used to stimulate breathing in neonates after emerging from the uterus. It is no longer recommended because it increases cerebral oxygen demand. Dobutamine and dopamine are positive inotrope drugs used primarily to support blood pressure. Naloxone is a mu antagonist drug that reverses the effects of mu opioids. This is commonly given in neonates after a cesarean section. Norkus CL, "Cesarean Section Techniques," in Bryant S, Anesthesia for Veterinary Technicians, ed 1, Wiley-Blackwell, 2010.

515. a Epidurals can provide additional analgesia, thus helping reduce the amount of system opioids and inhalant anesthetics needed. Constant rate infusions such as morphine and ketamine should be avoided when the neonates are still in the uterus because these drugs cross the placental barrier. Bier blocks are used for procedures primarily of the forelimb and do not help with analgesia/anesthesia in the cesarean section patient. Norkus CL, "Cesarean Section Techniques," in Bryant S, Anesthesia for Veterinary Technicians, ed 1, Wiley-Blackwell, 2010.

516. c The avian trachea is made up of complete tracheal rings that lack elasticity. Because the tracheal rings do not expand, a cuffed endotracheal tube can cause extensive damage and pressure necrosis lesions. Longley, LA, "Avian Anesthesia," Anesthesia of Exotic Pets," ed 1, Elsevier, 2008.

517. b The syrinx is responsible for sound generation in birds. The syrinx lies beyond the tracheal bifurcation, making it possible for vocalization during intubation. The choana is the large opening at the roof of the mouth that opens into the respiratory system. Birds do not have a larynx. The opercula are small projections housed just inside the nares. Longley, LA, "Avian Anesthesia," Anesthesia of Exotic Pets," ed 1, Elsevier, 2008.

518. d The femur and humerus are pneumatic (air filled) in the avian patient. This is important because pneumatic bones have a direct connection to the respiratory system. Intraosseous catheters should not be placed into pneumatic bones because fluids and drugs administered via the catheter can easily drown the patient. Longley, LA, "Avian Anesthesia," Anesthesia of Exotic Pets," ed 1, Elsevier, 2008.

519. c The palatal ostium is an anatomic structure causing the opening between the oral cavity and the opening to the trachea to be very small. Visualization is difficult and the tissues surrounding the glottis can be easily damaged, causing laryngeal edema. Laryngeal edema can lead to respiratory distress or arrest. Quesenberry KE, Donnelly TM, Mans C, "Biology, Husbandry, and Clinical Techniques of Guinea Pigs and Chinchillas," Ferrets, Rabbits, and Rodents, ed 3, Saunders, 2012.

520. c Rabbits are the only species on this list that can be nasally intubated. Ferrets, chinchillas, and guinea pigs are too small for nasal intubation. Longley, LA, "Rabbit Anesthesia," Anesthesia of Exotic Pets," ed 1, Elsevier, 2008.

521. c Fifty to 150 mL/min of gas is sampled with sidestream capnography. Spelts K, Gaynor J, "Monitoring Blood Pressure and End-Tidal CO2 in the Anesthetized Patient," in Bryant S, Anesthesia for Veterinary Technicians, ed 1, Wiley-Blackwell, 2010.

522. c The pectoral muscle is the largest muscle group in the bird. Injections should be given lateral to the keel bone in the event of necrosis. Birds also have a renal portal system. Blood from the caudal portion of the body may pass through the kidneys before passing through the heart and absorbing systemically. If this happens, undiluted drugs may filter into the kidneys. This is why the quadriceps and gastrocnemius muscles are not used. The biceps are generally very small and are therefore avoided. Longley, LA, "Avian Anesthesia," Anesthesia of Exotic Pets," ed 1, Elsevier, 2008.

523. a MS-222 is the most commonly used drug to induce and maintain anesthesia in fish and amphibians. Tricaine methanesulfonate (MS-222) is a powder that is weighed out and added to a calculated volume of water. It is buffered with baking soda. Drugs such as propofol, isoflurane, and ketamine are not commonly used in these species. Longley, LA, "Amphibian Anesthesia," Anesthesia of Exotic Pets," ed 1, Elsevier, 2008.

524. b The ventral abdominal vein is the easiest and largest vessel for blood sampling in a small frog. The cephalic and saphenous vessels are not used in frogs. The lingual venous plexus is used in larger species. Longley, LA, "Amphibian Anesthesia," Anesthesia of Exotic Pets," ed 1, Elsevier, 2008.

525. c Opioids, such as Morphine, can reduce heart rate, but this is easily treated with an anticholinergic such as atropine or glycopyrrolate. Midazolam and lidocaine do not decrease heart rate. Farry T, "Anesthesia for Pediatric Patients," in Bryant S, Anesthesia for Veterinary Technicians, ed 1, Wiley-Blackwell, 2010.

526. c All non-crocodilian reptiles have a three-chambered heart consisting of two atria and one ventricle. Longley, LA, "Reptile Anesthesia," Anesthesia of Exotic Pets," ed 1, Elsevier, 2008.

527. b Bradycardia in the pediatric patient can greatly affect cardiac output and blood pressure. Pediatric patients rely on heart rate to maintain a normal blood pressure. Tachycardia, apnea, and hyperthermia do not profoundly affect cardiac output or blood pressure. Farry T, "Anesthesia for Pediatric Patients," in Bryant S, Anesthesia for Veterinary Technicians, ed 1, Wiley-Blackwell, 2010.

528. a Pediatric patients are highly dependent on heart rate to maintain a normal cardiac output and blood pressure. Body temperature, systemic vascular resistance, myocardial oxygen consumption, pulmonary reserve, glycogen storage, and hepatic flow are not dependent on heart rate. Farry T, "Anesthesia for Pediatric Patients," in Bryant S, Anesthesia for Veterinary Technicians, ed 1, Wiley-Blackwell, 2010.

529. c Renal and hepatic systems are not fully developed in pediatric patients. Drug doses often need to be reduced because of slow metabolism, biotransformation, and excretion of drugs. Drugs often show exaggerated effects and prolonged duration of action in this population. Pediatric patients are not prone to hyperglycemia; they are prone to hypoglycemia and oxygen consumption is only about 2–3 times higher than that of adults. Farry T, "Anesthesia for Pediatric Patients," in Bryant S, Anesthesia for Veterinary Technicians, ed 1, Wiley-Blackwell, 2010.

530. b The rib cage of pediatric patients is more pliable compared with adults and can lead to less efficient ventilation as well as respiratory fatigue. Farry T, "Anesthesia for Pediatric Patients," in Bryant S, Anesthesia for Veterinary Technicians, ed 1, Wiley-Blackwell, 2010.

531. d Unweaned puppies and kittens should not be fasted before anesthesia. These patients are at high risk of hypoglycemia and dehydration. Farry T, "Anesthesia for Pediatric Patients," in Bryant S, Anesthesia for Veterinary Technicians, ed 1, Wiley-Blackwell, 2010.

532. a Pediatric patients older than 6 weeks should only be fasted for a maximum of 3 hours before anesthetic induction. These patients are at high risk of hypoglycemia and dehydration. Farry T, "Anesthesia for Pediatric Patients," in Bryant S, Anesthesia for Veterinary Technicians, ed 1, Wiley-Blackwell, 2010.

533. a Withholding water is unnecessary in these patients. Pediatric patients older than 6 weeks should only be fasted for a maximum of 3 hours before anesthetic induction. Neonatal patients should not be fasted at all. Farry T, "Anesthesia for Pediatric Patients," in Bryant S, Anesthesia for Veterinary Technicians, ed 1, Wiley-Blackwell, 2010.

534. c The minimal baseline laboratory tests evaluated in a pediatric patient should include PCV, TP, and blood glucose, although a full CBC and biochemistry panel can be evaluated if clinical findings indicate full blood work. Farry T, "Anesthesia for Pediatric Patients," in Bryant S, Anesthesia for Veterinary Technicians, ed 1, Wiley-Blackwell, 2010.

535. d Dexmedetomidine is contraindicated in these patients because of the common side effects. Midazolam and morphine have little effect on cardiac contractility. Opioids can reduce heart rate, but this is easily treated with an anticholinergic such as atropine or glycopyrrolate. Bradycardia in pediatric patients is not ideal because blood pressure is dependent on heart rate. Farry T, "Anesthesia for Pediatric Patients," in Bryant S, Anesthesia for Veterinary Technicians, ed 1, Wiley-Blackwell, 2010.

536. a Shivering leads to an increase in oxygen demands by up to 300%. Supplemental oxygen is suggested for all patients recovering from anesthesia and especially for those that are hypothermic. Farry T, "Anesthesia for Pediatric Patients," in Bryant S, Anesthesia for Veterinary Technicians, ed 1, Wiley-Blackwell, 2010.

537. c Peak airway pressure should range between 15 and 20 cm H_2O. Increased pressures can lead to barotrauma. Farry T, "Anesthesia for Pediatric Patients," in Bryant S, Anesthesia for Veterinary Technicians, ed 1, Wiley-Blackwell, 2010.

538. d Direct blood pressure monitoring is the gold standard for any patient regardless of age. Cannulating an artery and measuring blood pressure is the only method that provides real-time, second-by-second measurements and monitoring. Doppler and oscillometric methods can be used, but the Doppler is more accurate in smaller patients. Palpation of the pulse is not suggested for monitoring blood pressure. Farry T, "Anesthesia for Pediatric Patients," in Bryant S, Anesthesia for Veterinary Technicians, ed 1, Wiley-Blackwell, 2010.

539. a Fasting is generally kept to a minimum because of the fact that geriatric patients are prone to hypoglycemia. Eight hours is enough time for food to be digested without worrying about excessive reductions in blood glucose. Farry T, "Anesthesia for Geriatric Patients," in Bryant S, Anesthesia for Veterinary Technicians, ed 1, Wiley-Blackwell, 2010.

540. a Acepromazine is a commonly used tranquilizer that does not provide analgesia and is not reversible. Diazepam is a benzodiazepine tranquilizer that is reversible by using flumazenil. Methadone is a mu opioid agonist and is reversible by using naloxone. Dexmedetomidine is an alpha-2 agonist that provides some analgesia and moderate sedation. Using atipamezole reverses this drug. Farry T, "Anesthesia for Geriatric Patients," in Bryant S, Anesthesia for Veterinary Technicians, ed 1, Wiley-Blackwell, 2010.

541. c Opioids and benzodiazepines such as fentanyl and midazolam are among the safest anesthetic drugs for geriatric patients. Alfaxalone has a wide safety margin producing minimal respiratory depression and is rapidly metabolized by the liver. Etomidate should not be used in patients with impaired adrenocortical function because it can suppress and inhibit adrenocortical function. Farry T, "Anesthesia for Geriatric Patients," in Bryant S, Anesthesia for Veterinary Technicians, ed 1, Wiley-Blackwell, 2010.

542. c Balanced anesthesia is the process of using various drugs to achieve multiple different effects such as analgesia, sedation, amnesia, and muscle relaxation. Drugs administered into the epidural space before surgery can aid in MAC reduction and analgesia during and after surgery. Regional anesthesia is the infiltration of a local anesthetic to block the sensation of pain to a specific targeted area. A premedication drug is any drug that is used before anesthetic induction. Drugs can include the use of opioids, benzodiazepines, anticholinergics, dissociatives, and/or alpha-2 agonists. Devey JJ, "Anesthesia in the Critically Ill or Injured Patient," in Battaglia AM, Steele AM, Small Animal Emergency and Critical Care for Veterinary Technicians, ed 3, Elsevier, 2015.

543. c Blood pressure cuffs that are too large will give an artificially low reading, whereas cuffs that are too tight will yield an artificially high reading. Devey JJ, "Anesthesia in the Critically Ill or Injured Patient," in Battaglia AM, Steele AM, Small Animal Emergency and Critical Care for Veterinary Technicians, ed 3, Elsevier, 2015.

544. a Vital signs such as heart and respiratory rates, blood pressure, oxygen saturation, and end-tidal carbon dioxide should all be monitored and recorded. Mucous membrane color, eye position, and jaw tone should be observed but not necessarily recorded. Temperature is often recorded every 15 minutes, even when continuously monitored. Devey JJ, "Anesthesia in the Critically Ill or Injured Patient," in Battaglia AM, Steele AM, Small Animal Emergency and Critical Care for Veterinary Technicians, ed 3, Elsevier, 2015.

545. d The primary signs of hypotension include vasoconstriction, poor pulses, increasing heart rate, deepening of anesthetic depth, and decreasing $ETCO_2$. As the patient becomes hypotensive, the heart rate increases and the vessels constrict to try to maintain normal blood flow. The pulse is often poor because the pressure is low. The $ETCO_2$ decreases because of a decrease in cardiac output. Devey JJ, "Anesthesia in the Critically Ill or Injured Patient," in Battaglia AM, Steele AM, Small Animal Emergency and Critical Care for Veterinary Technicians, ed 3, Elsevier, 2015.

546. a The two most common causes of hypotension are hypovolemia and the administration of anesthetic drugs. Hyperthermia, toxemia, hypercarbia, and increased central venous pressure are not considered primary causes of hypotension. Cardiac arrhythmias in rare cases can lead to hypotension and opioid administration can cause bradycardia that in turn can contribute to hypotension. Devey JJ, "Anesthesia in the Critically Ill or Injured Patient," in Battaglia AM, Steele AM, Small Animal Emergency and Critical Care for Veterinary Technicians, ed 3, Elsevier, 2015.

547. b The common signs of pain include vocalization, increased heart rate, inappetence, increased temperature, increased respiratory rate, increased blood pressure, trembling, chewing or licking at the painful area, and changes in normal posture and movements. Shaffran N, "Pain Assessment and Treatment," in Battaglia AM, Steele AM, Small Animal Emergency and Critical Care for Veterinary Technicians, ed 3, Elsevier, 2015.

548. d Buprenorphine is the only drug listed where studies have shown that it is effective when administered via the transmucosal route in cats. Shaffran N, "Pain Assessment and Treatment," in Battaglia AM, Steele AM, Small Animal Emergency and Critical Care for Veterinary Technicians, ed 3, Elsevier, 2015.

549. a Ketamine is an NMDA receptor antagonist. Using ketamine as an adjunct analgesic may help this patient by blocking sensitization of neurons in the spinal cord. Shaffran N, "Pain Assessment and Treatment," in Battaglia AM, Steele AM, Small Animal Emergency and Critical Care for Veterinary Technicians, ed 3, Elsevier, 2015.

550. c Lidocaine can be administered as a single injection to provide regional anesthesia or it can be given as a constant rate infusion. Cats are particularly sensitive to lidocaine when given as a constant-rate infusion because of the potential for severe cardiovascular collapse and toxicity. Signs of toxicity include muscle tremors, seizures, nausea, vomiting, and cardiovascular collapse. Morphine, dexmedetomidine, and ketamine do not cause these potential effects when administered to cats. Shaffran N, "Pain Assessment and Treatment," in Battaglia AM, Steele AM, Small Animal Emergency and Critical Care for Veterinary Technicians, ed 3, Elsevier, 2015.

551. d Slowly titrating naloxone to effect will help reverse the dysphoria caused by the opioids the patient had been administered. Giving micro doses of naloxone to effect removes the dysphoria but does not affect the analgesic properties of the drug. Administering more opioids could make the patient worse if you are dealing with dysphoria and not pain. Holding the patient will probably cause more stress to the staff and patient and injury could occur. Inducing anesthesia and trying to recover the patient again will probably yield the same results. Shaffran N, "Pain Assessment and Treatment," in Battaglia AM, Steele AM, Small Animal Emergency and Critical Care for Veterinary Technicians, ed 3, Elsevier, 2015.

552. c A CRI allows delivery of a continuous low dose of a drug. Giving a CRI is advantageous because the peaks and valleys of giving an intermittent bolus are avoided; therefore, the patient experiences constant pain control rather than analgesia that varies with time. Shaffran N, "Pain Assessment and Treatment," in Battaglia AM, Steele AM, Small Animal Emergency and Critical Care for Veterinary Technicians, ed 3, Elsevier, 2015.

553. a Epidural anesthesia and analgesia are generally used for procedures caudal to the ribs. Shaffran N, "Pain Assessment and Treatment," in Battaglia AM, Steele AM, Small Animal Emergency and Critical Care for Veterinary Technicians, ed 3, Elsevier, 2015.

554. b An antagonist blocks a particular opioid receptor. An example of an opioid antagonist is naloxone. It blocks the mu pain receptor and does not allow mu opioids to attach to the receptor. An agonist is a drug that attaches to the receptor. COX-1 and COX-2 inhibition are associated with NSAID administration and have nothing to do with opioid receptors. Shaffran N, "Pain Assessment and Treatment," in Battaglia AM, Steele AM, Small Animal Emergency and Critical Care for Veterinary Technicians, ed 3, Elsevier, 2015.

555. d Anesthesia should provide immobilization, amnesia, and pain relief for the patient. There should never be a standard, black-and-white anesthetic protocol. Each protocol should be tailored for the individual animal. Devey JJ, "Anesthesia in the Critically Ill or Injured Patient," in Battaglia AM, Steele AM, Small Animal Emergency and Critical Care for Veterinary Technicians, ed 3, Elsevier, 2015.

556. b Propofol causes Heinz body formation in cats when administered as either multiple boluses or over a few consecutive days. Ideally, propofol should not be used as a CRI in cats unless the time frame is short, for example less than 30 minutes. The other drugs listed do not cause Heinz body formation. Alfaxalone is probably a better choice for a CRI in cats. Devey JJ, "Anesthesia in the Critically Ill or Injured Patient," in Battaglia AM, Steele AM, Small Animal Emergency and Critical Care for Veterinary Technicians, ed 3, Elsevier, 2015.

557. c Jaw tone is the best guide for anesthetic depth. There should always be some jaw tone present in the anesthetized animal. When jaw tone is absent, the patient is too deep. Toe pinch and palpebral reflex are generally not present in a surgical plane of anesthesia. Blood pressure is not a good indicator of depth. Hypotension can still be present when the patient is under a light plane of anesthesia. Devey JJ, "Anesthesia in the Critically Ill or Injured Patient," in Battaglia AM, Steele AM, Small Animal Emergency and Critical Care for Veterinary Technicians, ed 3, Elsevier, 2015.

558. d Low-flow anesthesia can only be used with a rebreathing circuit. Devey JJ, "Anesthesia in the Critically Ill or Injured Patient," in Battaglia AM, Steele AM, Small Animal Emergency and Critical Care for Veterinary Technicians, ed 3, Elsevier, 2015.

559. d Overventilation can cause a decrease in preload that leads to a decrease in blood pressure and cardiac output. Overventilation does not lower core body temperature. Devey JJ, "Anesthesia in the Critically Ill or Injured Patient," in Battaglia AM, Steele AM, Small Animal Emergency and Critical Care for Veterinary Technicians, ed 3, Elsevier, 2015.

560. a Keeping the container sealed helps prevent absorption of carbon dioxide from the environment. It also helps prevent moisture loss and the color indicator from becoming deactivated. High temperatures do not affect absorbents in a sealed container, but freezing temperatures can be harmful because the moisture will expand the absorbent and cause the granules to fragment. Absorbents are a respiratory irritant and are caustic to the skin. Dorsch JA, Dorsch SE, "The Circle System," Understanding Anesthesia Equipment, ed 5, Wolters Kluwer Health, 2008.

561. c Unidirectional valves are also called flutter valves, one-way valves, directional valves, dome valves, flap valves, nonreturn valves, and inspiratory or expiratory valves. These valves ensure proper directional gas flow to the anesthetic patient. The other answers are incorrect. Dorsch JA, Dorsch SE, "The Circle System," Understanding Anesthesia Equipment, ed 5, Wolters Kluwer Health, 2008.

562. b A respirometer measures the ventilatory volume for each breath given to the patient. A capnograph is needed to measure $ETCO_2$. The respiratory rate is counted either manually or via a multiparameter machine. Moisture is not generally measured in the breathing circuit. Dorsch JA, Dorsch SE, "The Circle System," Understanding Anesthesia Equipment, ed 5, Wolters Kluwer Health, 2008.

563. a Mapleson systems are non-rebreathing systems. These systems do not have unidirectional valves as do those seen in circle systems. There are no carbon dioxide absorbents present; therefore, fresh gas flows need to be increased to wash out the waste gases. This makes the system less economical compared with circle systems. Dorsch JA, Dorsch SE, "Mapleson Breathing Systems," Understanding Anesthesia Equipment, ed 5, Wolters Kluwer Health, 2008.

564. d The PISS is a safety system that only allows cylinders to operate if they are placed in the correct yoke. Without the proper fit, the gas will not be able to be delivered to the patient. This prevents delivery of the wrong gas to a patient under anesthesia. Dorsch JA, Dorsch SE, "Anesthesia Machines and Breathing Systems," Understanding Anesthesia Equipment, ed 5, Wolters Kluwer Health, 2008.

565. c If there are two vaporizers on one machine, for example, sevoflurane and isoflurane, the vaporizer interlock device prevents both from accidently turning on. Dangerously high percentages of inhalants can be delivered to the patient when both are accidently turned on. Dorsch JA, Dorsch SE, "Anesthesia Machines and Breathing Systems," Understanding Anesthesia Equipment, ed 5, Wolters Kluwer Health, 2008.

566. d A capnograph that does not return to baseline is indicative of rebreathing carbon dioxide. Several things, including lack of oxygen being delivered to the patient, exhausted absorbent, or a damaged flutter valve, can cause this. Hyperventilation will show a decreased reading on the capnograph, whereas hypoventilation will show an increased reading. When esophageal intubation occurs, the capnograph will show a reading of zero with no waveform present. Dorsch JA, Dorsch SE, "Monitoring Devices," Understanding Anesthesia Equipment, ed 5, Wolters Kluwer Health, 2008.

567. d Carbon dioxide analysis allows assessment of ventilation, circulation, equipment malfunction, patient-related anesthetic problems, and metabolism. Core body temperature cannot be analyzed. Dorsch JA, Dorsch SE, "Anesthesia Machines and Breathing Systems," Understanding Anesthesia Equipment, ed 5, Wolters Kluwer Health, 2008.

568. b The common gas outlet connects anesthetic machine to the breathing systems, ventilator, or oxygen supply device. The other answers listed are incorrect. Alibhai H, "The Anaesthetic Machine and Vaporizers," in Duke-Novakovski T, de Vries M, Seymour C, BSAVA Manual of Canine and Feline Anaesthesia and Analgesia, ed 3, British Small Animal Veterinary Association, 2016.

569. a The oxygen flush is initiated by pressing a button. Oxygen is delivered at a high flow of 30–70 L/min at a pressure of 400 kPa. Flushing oxygen with a patient attached should be performed with caution. Because of the high flow, patients are at risk of barotrauma. Alibhai H, "The Anaesthetic Machine and Vaporizers," in Duke-Novakovski T, de Vries M, Seymour C, BSAVA Manual of Canine and Feline Anaesthesia and Analgesia, ed 3, British Small Animal Veterinary Association, 2016.

570. b Apparatus dead space is the volume of the breathing system occupied by gases that are rebreathed without any change in composition. Tidal volume is the volume of air inspired and expired in a single breath. Peak inspiratory pressure is the highest level of pressure applied to the lungs during inspiration. Minute volume is the sum of all gas volumes exhaled in one minute. Hughes L, "Breathing Systems and Ancillary Equipment," in Duke-Novakovski T, de Vries M, Seymour C, BSAVA Manual of Canine and Feline Anaesthesia and Analgesia, ed 3, British Small Animal Veterinary Association, 2016.

571. a Ketamine increases intraocular pressure. Raising pressure can potentially cause vitreous prolapse and retinal detachment. Propofol, diazepam, and alfaxalone do not affect intraocular pressure. Jolliffe C, "Ophthalmic Surgery," in Duke-Novakovski T, de Vries M, Seymour C, BSAVA Manual of Canine and Feline Anaesthesia and Analgesia, ed 3, British Small Animal Veterinary Association, 2016.

572. d Morphine, dexmedetomidine, and hydromorphone can cause gagging and vomiting. Drugs that cause emesis should be avoided in patients where raised intraocular and intracranial pressures are concerns. Methadone is one of the few opioids that does not cause vomiting in the majority of patients. Jolliffe C, "Ophthalmic Surgery," in Duke-Novakovski T, de Vries M, Seymour C, BSAVA Manual of Canine and Feline Anaesthesia and Analgesia, ed 3, British Small Animal Veterinary Association, 2016.

573. c Severe bradycardia, arrhythmias, or cardiac arrest can occur when pressure is applied to the globe or when it is surgically manipulated. This reaction is called the oculocardiac reflex and is treated with an anticholinergic. Jolliffe C, "Ophthalmic Surgery," in Duke-Novakovski T, de Vries M, Seymour C, BSAVA Manual of Canine and Feline Anaesthesia and Analgesia, ed 3, British Small Animal Veterinary Association, 2016.

574. b Pupil dilation after opioid administration in cats is normal and expected. In dogs, miosis, or constriction of the pupils, occurs. Meiosis and mitosis have nothing to do with the eye. These terms relate to cell division. Jolliffe C, "Ophthalmic Surgery," in Duke-Novakovski T, de Vries M, Seymour C, BSAVA Manual of Canine and Feline Anaesthesia and Analgesia, ed 3, British Small Animal Veterinary Association, 2016.

575. c It is important to know what is normal before you understand what is abnormal for a particular species. The average, normal blood volume in the dog is 80–90 mL/kg. After you know the normal blood volume and estimate the percentage blood loss, you can calculate volume deficits by using the equation VD = BV × % blood loss, in which VD = volume deficit and BV = blood volume. Auckburally A, "Fluid Therapy and Blood Transfusion," in Duke-Novakovski T, de Vries M, Seymour C, BSAVA Manual of Canine and Feline Anaesthesia and Analgesia, ed 3, British Small Animal Veterinary Association, 2016.

576. b Different solutions are used for different purposes. Fluids such as lactated Ringer's solution and 0.9% saline are isotonic. The administration of these fluids does not produce a change in osmotic pressure and there is no fluid shift between compartments. Hypotonic fluids are those that have fewer particles compared with plasma. Hypotonic fluids decrease osmotic pressure. Hypertonic fluids have more particles compared with plasma and increase osmotic pressure. When given, fluids are drawn into the intravascular space from the interstitial space. Buffered solutions are solutions that resist changes in pH when small quantities of an acid or base are added. This has nothing to do with types of systemic fluids given to a patient. Auckburally A, "Fluid Therapy and Blood Transfusion," in Duke-Novakovski T, de Vries M, Seymour C, BSAVA Manual of Canine and Feline Anaesthesia and Analgesia, ed 3, British Small Animal Veterinary Association, 2016.

577. b Blocking the lower dental arcade is best done via the inferior alveolar nerve. When done correctly, blocking the inferior alveolar nerve can provide local anesthesia to the tongue, lower dental arcade, and chin. The infraorbital block provides anesthesia to the rostral maxilla. The auriculotemporal block is a good way to provide pain relief to the pinna and ear canal. An RUMM block is used for patients having surgery on the limb distal to the elbow. RUMM stands for radial, ulnar, median, and musculocutaneous nerves. Duke-Novakovski T, " Pain Management II: Local and Regional Anaesthetic Techniques" in Duke-Novakovski T, de Vries M, Seymour C, BSAVA Manual of Canine and Feline Anaesthesia and Analgesia, ed 3, British Small Animal Veterinary Association, 2016.

578. a Local anesthetics are the only drugs that can provide complete loss of sensation when administered correctly. The other drugs listed do not cause complete loss of pain sensation and they do not act by inhibiting the voltage-gated sodium channels within a nerve. Duke-Novakovski T, " Pain Management II: Local and Regional Anaesthetic Techniques" in Duke-Novakovski T, de Vries M, Seymour C, BSAVA Manual of Canine and Feline Anaesthesia and Analgesia, ed 3, British Small Animal Veterinary Association, 2016.

579. c Local blockades are the only way to provide a complete loss of sensation when performed correctly. Patients with rib fractures or those undergoing a lateral thoracotomy benefit from intercostal blocks. A RUMM block is used for procedures distal to the elbow. Epidural blocks are primarily performed for abdominal and orthopedic procedures in the caudal half of the body. Paravertebral blocks are used for forelimb surgery. Duke-Novakovski T, " Pain Management II:

Local and Regional Anaesthetic Techniques" in Duke-Novakovski T, de Vries M, Seymour C, BSAVA Manual of Canine and Feline Anaesthesia and Analgesia, ed 3, British Small Animal Veterinary Association, 2016.

580. d Acepromazine does not cause respiratory depression when administered at the proper clinical doses. It does, however, decrease body temperature because of peripheral vasodilation. Acepromazine has antiarrhythmic properties that result from its activity at the alpha-1 adrenoreceptors. Acepromazine also has antiemetic properties. This is most evident when it is given before opioid administration. Murrell J, "Premedication and Sedation," in Duke-Novakovski T, de Vries M, Seymour C, BSAVA Manual of Canine and Feline Anaesthesia and Analgesia, ed 3, British Small Animal Veterinary Association, 2016.

581. b Benzodiazepines do not produce a great deal of sedation when given as a sole agent in healthy dogs and cats. This class of drugs works best when combined with other drugs such as opioids. Acepromazine, dexmedetomidine, and morphine all produce sedation when administered alone. Murrell J, "Premedication and Sedation," in Duke-Novakovski T, de Vries M, Seymour C, BSAVA Manual of Canine and Feline Anaesthesia and Analgesia, ed 3, British Small Animal Veterinary Association, 2016.

582. a It is important to know what is normal before you understand what is abnormal for a particular species. The average, normal blood volume in the cat is 60–70 mL/kg. After you know the normal blood volume and estimate the percent blood loss, you can calculate volume deficits by using the equation VD = BV × % blood loss, in which VD = volume deficit and BV = blood volume. Auckburally A, "Fluid Therapy and Blood Transfusion," in Duke-Novakovski T, de Vries M, Seymour C, BSAVA Manual of Canine and Feline Anaesthesia and Analgesia, ed 3, British Small Animal Veterinary Association, 2016.

583. d Placing pressure on the jugular vein can cause an increase in intracranial pressure. Leashes should not be placed around the necks of dogs with suspected intracranial disease or trauma and the jugular vein should not be used for sample collection. Keeping the head slightly elevated helps decrease intracranial pressure. Mannitol increases blood volume and oxygen delivery to the brain, resulting in vasoconstriction and a decrease in intracranial pressure. Keeping the $ETCO_2$ in the low-normal range around 35 mmHg helps prevent intracranial pressure from increasing. Leece E, "Neurological Disease," in Duke-Novakovski T, de Vries M, Seymour C, BSAVA Manual of Canine and Feline Anaesthesia and Analgesia, ed 3, British Small Animal Veterinary Association, 2016.

584. c Palpating a peripheral pulse (most often the femoral) assesses adequate cardiac massage. When effective chest compressions are performed, a palpable pulse is produced and the mucous membranes become pink. The ECG may not be completely normal after cardiac arrest, especially if ischemia has occurred. Heart rate varies by species and size of the animal; therefore, a set heart rate of 60 beats per minute is not a good way to measure adequate cardiac massage. End-tidal CO_2 is often not normal during adequate cardiac massage. McMillan S, "Anesthetic Complications and Emergencies," in Bryant S, Anesthesia for Veterinary Technicians, ed 1, Wiley-Blackwell, 2010.

585. c Nitrous oxide alone cannot be used to anesthetize a patient fully because of the high MAC value in dogs and cats. Because of this, it must be used with another inhalant anesthetic. Nitrous oxide is most commonly used at 50%–65%. Using within this percentage range helps facilitate appropriate anesthetic depth without using higher concentrations of the volatile gases that have more cardiopulmonary depressant effects. The maximum percentage of nitrous oxide is capped at 65% to allow adequate inspired oxygen levels. Inspired oxygen should be kept >30%. Pang D, "Inhalant Anaesthetic Agents," in Duke-Novakovski T, de Vries M, Seymour C, BSAVA Manual of Canine and Feline Anaesthesia and Analgesia, ed 3, British Small Animal Veterinary Association, 2016.

586. b It is recommended that the nitrous oxide is terminated 5–10 minutes before recovery and oxygen should be provided during the recovery period. This will help prevent diffusion hypoxia caused by the rapid outpouring of nitrous oxide into the alveoli after it has been discontinued. This rapid accumulation of nitrous oxide can dilute oxygen levels within the alveoli and cause hypoxemia. Biotransformation, solubility, and inflammation have nothing to do with how a patient recovers from anesthesia after using nitrous oxide. Pang D, "Inhalant Anaesthetic Agents," in Duke-Novakovski T, de Vries M, Seymour C, BSAVA Manual of Canine and Feline Anaesthesia and Analgesia, ed 3, British Small Animal Veterinary Association, 2016.

587. b Local anesthetics work by blocking the generation and conduction of nerve impulses by inhibiting voltage-gated sodium channels in neuronal membranes. Local anesthetics are the only drugs that provide a complete blockade of pain when administered correctly. Local anesthetics do not cause a release of inhibitory neurotransmitters. They also do not work by acting on GABA receptors and they do not block the release of catecholamines. Duke-Novakovski T, " Pain Management II: Local and Regional Anaesthetic Techniques" in Duke-Novakovski T, de Vries M, Seymour C, BSAVA Manual of Canine and Feline Anaesthesia and Analgesia, ed 3, British Small Animal Veterinary Association, 2016.

588. b Brachycephalic dogs have small, stenotic nares, redundant tissue in the oropharyngeal areas, and small, hypoplastic tracheas; therefore they need to remain intubated much longer to help avoid airway obstruction on recovery. Non-brachycephalic breeds can generally be extubated when the swallowing reflex returns because the previously mentioned anatomy is normal. Palpebral reflex generally returns before the swallowing reflex. The eye position is also often central (normal) before the swallowing reflex returns. Patients can also have voluntary movement of the limbs without the swallowing reflex being present. The swallowing reflex must be present before extubation to help prevent problems. Bryant S, "Anesthesia for

Thoracotomies and Respiratory-Challenged Patients," Anesthesia for Veterinary Technicians, ed 1, Wiley-Blackwell, 2010.

589. b Alpha-2 adrenergic agonists such as dexmedetomidine, medetomidine, and xylazine require extensive hepatic metabolism and have dose-related negative effects on the cardiovascular, respiratory, and central nervous systems. This class of drugs is best avoided in geriatric patients when possible. Atropine is generally safe for geriatric patients when given at appropriate doses. Isoflurane can cause negative effects such as dose-dependent vasodilation in any patient under anesthesia regardless of age. These negative side effects can be counteracted with decreasing the percentage administered, giving a fluid bolus when needed for hypotension, including other drugs to reduce MAC, and/or adding in a positive inotrope or vasopressor. Midazolam is one of the safest drugs that can be used in the sickest, oldest, and youngest patients. Farry T, "Anesthesia for Geriatric Patients," in Bryant S, Anesthesia for Veterinary Technicians, ed 1, Wiley-Blackwell, 2010.

590. b Normal capillary refill time (CRT) is approximately 1–2 seconds in dogs and cats. Anesthetic agents and hemodynamic status contribute to a decreased CRT. Prolonged CRT should be taken seriously in the anesthetized patient because it suggests reduced cardiac output and/or poor tissue perfusion. Renal failure does not directly cause an increase in CRT. Hypertension is an increase in blood pressure and does not increase CRT. Hyperventilation or increased ventilation does not increase CRT either. Levensaler A, "Monitoring Pulse Oximetry, Temperature, and Hands-On," in Bryant S, Anesthesia for Veterinary Technicians, ed 1, Wiley-Blackwell, 2010.

591. c Normal urinary output is important because it can be used as an assessment for cardiovascular status and overall renal perfusion. Renal perfusion can be reduced because of cardiovascular disease/failure, hypovolemia, and shock. Liver and pulmonary function does not affect urinary output. Ventilation status or rate does not affect urinary output. Central venous pressure does not directly affect urinary output. Schauvliege S "Patient Monitoring and Monitoring Equipment," in Duke-Novakovski T, de Vries M, Seymour C, BSAVA Manual of Canine and Feline Anaesthesia and Analgesia, ed 3, British Small Animal Veterinary Association, 2016.

592. b Cardiac output in pediatric patients is primarily heart-rate dependent. A decreased heart rate decreases the cardiac output; therefore, it is important to keep the rate normal during anesthesia. The heart has a lot of noncontractile tissue and low vascular compliance. Stroke volume is fixed and increases in preload and afterload are not well-tolerated. Cardiac output is not dependent on fluid rate, respiratory rate, or the quality of the pulse produced. Rigotti C, Brearley J, "Anaesthesia for paediatric and geriatric patients," in Duke-Novakovski T, de Vries M, Seymour C, BSAVA Manual of Canine and Feline Anaesthesia and Analgesia, ed 3, British Small Animal Veterinary Association, 2016.

593. d A closed pop-off valve increases the risk of barotrauma and leads to cardiac arrest. Excessive peak inspiratory pressure when the patient is being ventilated can cause barotrauma. Patients that have severe collapse of the lung during anesthesia can experience barotrauma during the process of trying to reinflate the lung. There is a wide safety margin for ventilation rates in animals undergoing anesthesia. As long as the peak inspiratory pressure and tidal volume are within normal limits, increased ventilation rates are safe. Egger C, "Anesthetic Complications, Accidents and Emergencies," in Duke-Novakovski T, de Vries M, Seymour C, BSAVA Manual of Canine and Feline Anaesthesia and Analgesia, ed 3, British Small Animal Veterinary Association, 2016.

594. a The SA node is the natural pacemaker of the heart and controls the rate of contractions of the heart muscle. The atrioventricular node coordinates the top portion of the heart. It also connects the atrial and ventricular chambers of the heart via the heart's electrical conduction system. The Purkinje fibers create synchronized contractions of the ventricles and are essential in maintaining consistent rhythm. The bundle of His is a collection of specialized cells that transmit electrical impulses from the AV node to the apex. Bryant S, " Review of Cardiovascular and Respiratory Physiology," Anesthesia for Veterinary Technicians, ed 1, Wiley-Blackwell, 2010.

595. b Spirometers are used to measure tidal volume and minute volume. Spirometers will show whether ventilation falls within an acceptable range, but they do not indicate whether gas exchange is appropriate. Respiratory rate can be measured visually or via multiparameter monitors or capnographs. Respiratory effort can be estimated visually. *Pulmonary ventilation* is another term for breathing. Gas exchange is best measured by using blood gas analysis. Central venous pressure is measured by using a transducer attached to a multiparameter monitor or via a water manometer. Mechanical dead space is the volume of gas rebreathed as a result of a mechanical device, for example placing a capnograph adaptor onto the endotracheal tube. Mechanical dead space can be calculated when necessary. Schauvliege S "Patient Monitoring and Monitoring Equipment," in Duke-Novakovski T, de Vries M, Seymour C, BSAVA Manual of Canine and Feline Anaesthesia and Analgesia, ed 3, British Small Animal Veterinary Association, 2016.

596. a Low pH values indicate acidosis. High pH values indicate alkalosis. As CO_2 increases, pH decreases, and as CO_2 decreases, pH increases. This is very important when monitoring ventilation and acid-base status of patients. Ketoacidosis and ketoalkalosis are presentations occurring in the diabetic patient. With diabetic ketoacidosis, the animal is not producing enough insulin; therefore, fat is broken down as an alternate fuel source. Toxic acids called ketones build up in the bloodstream. This is an emergent state that must be treated. Untreated diabetic ketoacidosis can lead to death. Ketoalkalosis is rare in the diabetic patient but is caused by vomiting and the loss of electrolytes. Randels-Thorpe A, "Introduction to Acid-Bas and

Electrolytes" in Randles-Thorp A, Liss D Acid-Base and Electrolyte Handbook for Veterinary Technicians, ed 1 Wiley-Blackwell, 2016.

597. d Anticholinergics are generally not recommended for use in ruminants unless there is a true need. Drugs such as atropine and glycopyrrolate increase the viscosity of saliva without decreasing the amount. This makes it harder to drain the saliva from the oropharynx. Kaiser-Klinger S, "Ruminant Anesthesia," in Bryant S, Anesthesia for Veterinary Technicians, ed 1, Wiley-Blackwell, 2010.

SECTION 12

1. a D5W is a hypotonic fluid and is least useful. It is oxidized to CO_2 and H_2O, providing free water, and it should be used in the face of a free-water deficit or hypernatremia. Plasma-Lyte 48 is an isotonic crystalloid and will provide rapid intravascular volume expansion. Hypertonic saline is a hypertonic crystalloid and Hetastarch is a colloid. Both will expand vascular volume and are useful for patients that will not tolerate a large volume of fluids (head trauma, heart failure). Bassert JM, Thomas JA, McCurnin's Clinical Textbook for Veterinary Technicians, ed 9, Elsevier, 2017, p. 820-821.

2. a Diazepam is a benzodiazepine and is considered the drug of choice to treat seizures in both dogs and cats. It is considered a first-line drug, whereas pentobarbital and levetiracetam are second-line drugs. Phenobarbital is a maintenance drug and is not used as an emergency treatment for status epilepticus. Silverstein D, Hopper K, Small Animal Critical Care Medicine, ed 2, Saunders, 2014, p. 429-430.

3. c A tension pneumothorax occurs when air is able to enter the pleural space but is unable to escape (it has been compared to a one-way valve that allows air in, but air is not able to exit). Pressure builds up in the pleural space and after that pressure becomes greater than atmospheric pressure, the patient is unable to expand the lungs. A tension pneumothorax will not resolve without a thoracocentesis to remove air from the pleural space. Battaglia AM, Small Animal Emergency and Critical Care for Veterinary Technicians ed 3, Elsevier, 2015, p. 266.

4. b Hydrocarbons, such as fuels, solvents, etc., are life-threatening because of the possibility of aspiration pneumonia. Aspiration can occur when the substance is ingested or when the patient vomits. Because of this risk, inducing emesis is contraindicated. The less viscous (thinner) a hydrocarbon, the more likely it is to be aspirated. The lungs are very vulnerable to hydrocarbons, and aspiration <1 mL can lead to death. Emesis is beneficial when a patient has ingested organophosphates (pesticides, insecticides), salicylates (aspirin), and anticholinergics (commonly found in medications). Peterson ME, Talcott PA, Small Animal Toxicology, ed 3, Elsevier, 2012, p. 74.

5. b Septic shock occurs when there is circulatory failure secondary to sepsis. Early in septic shock, there is a hyperdynamic response (tachycardia, vasodilation, fever, and bounding pulses) causing hyperemic (red) mucous membranes. Icteric (yellow) mucous membranes are caused by an excessive amount of bilirubin in the blood. Bilirubin increases with liver disease or the breakdown of RBCs. Pale mucous membranes are seen when there is vasoconstriction or a decrease in perfusion (both of which decrease blood flow to the membranes) or anemia. Cyanosis (blue mucous membranes) is seen when hemoglobin is not carrying oxygen. This deoxygenated hemoglobin causes blood to be blue. To detect cyanosis, there must be >5 g/dL of deoxygenated hemoglobin present in the blood (5 g/dL is equivalent to a PCV of 15%). Cyanosis is not detectable in a patient that is severely anemic and it cannot be relied on to indicate hypoxemia. Bassert JM, Thomas JA, McCurnin's Clinical Textbook for Veterinary Technicians, ed 9, Elsevier, 2017, p. 847.

6. c Propofol does not cross the placental barrier and so is the safest induction agent in regard to the fetuses. Etomidate crosses the placental barrier but is eliminated quickly, therefore it may be a good second choice if the bitch cannot tolerate propofol. Diazepam and thiopental cross the placental barrier and have adverse effects on the neonates. Thomas J, Lerche P, Anesthesia and Analgesia for Veterinary Technicians, ed 5, Mosby, 2016, p. 73, 83.

7. a The most common cause of feline aortic thromboembolism is cardiomyopathy. The turbulent blood flow seen with cardiomyopathy causes the formation of thrombi. This clot (or pieces of a clot) breaks free, travels through the circulatory system, and becomes lodged in the distal aorta where it causes an aortic thromboembolism. This is commonly known as a saddle thrombosis and causes the loss of the use of one, or both, hind limbs. Common clinical signs include acute loss of motor in the hind legs, loss of femoral and/or dorsal pedal pulses, and cyanotic pads or toenail beds. Because it is cardiac in origin, the liver, renal, and respiratory systems do not apply. Bassert JM, Thomas JA, McCurnin's Clinical Textbook for Veterinary Technicians, ed 9, Elsevier, 2017, p. 642-643; Battaglia AM, Small Animal Emergency and Critical Care for Veterinary Technicians ed 3, Elsevier, 2015, p. 315-316.

8. d Mannitol is an osmotic diuretic that decreases intracranial pressure by reducing blood viscosity. This allows an increase in blood flow (and thus an increase in oxygen delivery) to the brain and causes a decrease in the water content of the brain as well. Atropine is an anticholinergic used to treat bradycardia, as a preanesthetic, or as an antidote for organophosphate toxicity. Diazepam is a benzodiazepine used for sedation, muscle relaxation, or treatment of seizure activity. Dexamethasone is a glucocorticoid that is often used to decrease inflammation. However, it is contraindicated in head trauma and should never be administered as frequently as every 4–6 hours. Battaglia AM, Small Animal Emergency and Critical Care for Veterinary Technicians ed 3, Elsevier, 2015, p. 428-429.

9. a The most life-threatening problem should be treated first. In this scenario, the dyspneic patient should be seen first. Respiratory distress or dyspnea can quickly worsen and may even turn into respiratory arrest. It is always treated first. Proptosis, laceration, and dystocia can be serious emergencies but are not immediately life-threatening conditions. Bassert JM, Thomas JA, McCurnin's Clinical Textbook for Veterinary Technicians, ed 8, Elsevier, 2014, p. 908-911.

10. c First-intention healing occurs when the edges of a wound are brought together and closed with sutures or staples. This can be performed in the case of a laceration. A degloving wound is usually too extensive to close without performing daily bandage changes for several days until the tissue has developed a bed of granulation tissue. After this has occurred, the wound can be closed. This is referred to as third-intention healing. An abscess or puncture wound can be cleaned and flushed and then left to heal with no closure, which is known as second-intention healing. Aspinall V, "Table 8.1," Clinical Procedures in Veterinary Nursing, ed 3, Butterworth-Heinemann, 2014; Sirois M, Principles and Practice of Veterinary Technology, ed 4, Elsevier, 2016, p. 300.

11. c Intravenous administration is the most effective route of delivery, with a catheter in the jugular vein being most desirable. Intracardiac delivery should be avoided because of the possibility of causing cardiac arrhythmias or damage to the heart and lungs. Medication administered through the e-tube (intratracheal) is appropriate, but it is not as effective as intravenous administration. It is important to keep in mind that sodium bicarbonate cannot be administered via the trachea. The intraosseous route is another possibility in small animals; however, this route is inaccessible in larger animals and is contraindicated in those with sepsis or when there is an infection present in the area of the insertion site. Silverstein D, Hopper K, Small Animal Critical Care Medicine, ed 1, Saunders, 2009, p. 16-18.

12. c Current recommendations from RECOVER (Reassessment Campaign on Veterinary Resuscitation) are for chest compressions to be performed at a rate of 100–120 (compressions per minute) on any size, age, or species. Battaglia AM, Small Animal Emergency and Critical Care for Veterinary Technicians ed 3, Elsevier, 2015, p. 237.

13. c Pressure applied at the area adjacent and ventral to the mandible allows control of maxillary blood flow and hemorrhage to the head. The temporomandibular joint is the area where the jaw hinges and applying pressure to this area does not stop hemorrhage to the head. By applying pressure to one or both jugular grooves, you will prevent venous drainage from the head and may actually cause an increase in hemorrhage. This may also increase intracranial pressure, which should be avoided in any patient with possible head trauma. Battaglia AM, Small Animal Emergency and Critical Care for Veterinary Technicians ed 3, Elsevier, 2015, p. 258-259.

14. b In cases in which large volumes of fluids are contraindicated (head trauma, congestive heart failure), hypertonic saline provides intravascular volume expansion with a small volume. Hypertonic saline pulls fluid from the interstitial space into the vascular space. Because dehydrated patients are already deficient in fluid in the interstitial space, and hypertonic saline pulls fluid from here, it will worsen dehydration and should not be used in these patients. DiBartola SP, Fluid, Electrolyte, and Acid-Base Disorders in Small Animal Practice, ed 4, Elsevier, 2012, p. 568.; Battaglia AM, Small Animal Emergency and Critical Care for Veterinary Technicians ed 3, Elsevier, 2015, p. 229-230.

15. c Cranial nerve X is the vagus nerve. Stimulation of this nerve increases vagal tone, causing bradycardia. Cranial nerve I is the olfactory nerve, which transmits smell. Cranial nerve XII is the hypoglossal nerve, which controls the tongue and geniohyoid muscles. Cranial nerve IV is the trochlear nerve, which controls the dorsal oblique muscles of the eye. Stimulation of these last three nerves does not cause bradycardia. Battaglia AM, Small Animal Emergency and Critical Care for Veterinary Technicians ed 3, Elsevier, 2015, p. 178.

16. b Epistaxis (blood coming from the nose) can indicate head trauma or hemorrhage in the respiratory tract. If this occurs, the patient should be allowed to breathe through his mouth or to pant. Tying the mouth shut will prevent this. The Good Samaritan should be told to watch for aggression, apply pressure to any wounds (if possible), and transport the dog on a board (again, if possible). Battaglia AM, Small Animal Emergency and Critical Care for Veterinary Medicine, ed 2, Elsevier, 2007, p. 350.

17. a The CVP measures the heart's ability to pump the blood that returns from the body. The higher the CVP, the less able the heart is to pump the blood forward. Although the normal CVP varies dependent on the patient's condition, a healthy, normally hydrated patient has a CVP between 0 and 5 cm H_2O. A CVP of 5–10 cm H_2O indicates borderline hypervolemia, whereas a CVP >10 cm H_2O indicates fluid overload. Ford RB, Mazzaferro EM, Kirk and Bistner's Handbook of Veterinary Procedures and Emergency Treatment, ed 9, Elsevier, 2012 p. 30-31.

18. b Normal urine output of a patient on intravenous fluids is 1–2 mL/kg/h. Urine output <0.5 mL/kg/h is considered anuria. Urine output between 0.5 mL/kg/h and 1 mL/kg/h is considered oliguria. Urine output greater than 2 mL/kg/h is considered polyuria. Battaglia AM, Small Animal Emergency and Critical Care for Veterinary Technicians ed 3, Elsevier, 2015, p. 256-257.

19. a The CVP measures the right ventricular end-diastolic pressure and the heart's ability to pump blood forward. Anything that decreases this ability also increases the CVP. Cardiogenic shock occurs when there is a decrease in contractility of the heart. This decrease in contractility prevents the heart from pumping blood forward. In this type of shock, the CVP is elevated. Hypovolemic shock is supported by a decrease in the CVP, because the decrease in vascular volume decreases the right ventricular end-diastolic pressure. Distributive shock is a result of an inability of the body to cause vasoconstriction in response to a decrease in blood volume or tissue perfusion. In this case, the CVP may be normal (if the blood volume is normal) or decreased (if the blood volume is low). Septic shock also causes vasodilation and the CVP will be normal because the heart is still able to pump blood forward. DiBartola SP, Fluid, Electrolyte, and Acid-Base Disorders in Small Animal Practice, ed 4, Elsevier, 2012, p. 559-561.

20. d Septic shock occurs when sepsis has caused hypotension that is unresponsive to fluid therapy. Hypoglycemia occurs because inflammatory mediators, hypotension, and hypovolemia all combine to cause a decreased intake, decreased production, and increased use of glucose. Hypoglycemia is rarely seen with anaphylactic, cardiogenic, or neurogenic shock unless there is an underlying cause. Ford RB, Mazzaferro EM, Kirk and Bistner's Handbook of Veterinary Procedures and Emergency Treatment, ed 9, Elsevier, 2012, p. 279-280; Silverstein D, Hopper K, Small Animal Critical Care Medicine, ed 1, Saunders, 2009, p. 298, 461.

21. d This is the classic presentation of a dog or cat with Schiff-Sherrington posture. Extension of the thoracic limbs and pelvic limbs that are flexed (instead of flaccid) indicates a decerebellate posture. These patients also exhibit normal mentation but are not able to walk when placed on the ground. A decerebrate posture is indicated by extension of all four limbs and the patient is stuporous or comatose. Opisthotonus is flexion of the head and neck, often resembling a patient with tetanus. Bassert JM, Thomas JA, McCurnin's Clinical Textbook for Veterinary Technicians, ed 9, Elsevier, 2017, p. 843-844.

22. d Damage to T3–L3 causes Schiff-Sherrington posture. A lesion at C6 causes hyperflexion in all four limbs. A lesion at C6–T2 causes hyperflexion of the pelvic limbs and a lesion at T1–T3 causes Horner's syndrome. Bassert JM, Thomas JA, McCurnin's Clinical Textbook for Veterinary Technicians, ed 9, Elsevier, 2017, p. 844.

23. a Prostaglandins are involved in causing pain and inflammation associated with tissue injury. NSAIDs inactivate cyclooxygenase (COX), preventing the production of prostaglandins; therefore, NSAIDs are known as anti-prostaglandins. There are no such things as neoprostaglandins, pro-prostaglandins, or prostaglandoids. Thomas JA, Lerche P, Anesthesia and Analgesia for Veterinary Technicians, ed 4, Mosby, 2011, p. 223.

24. a Colloids contain large molecules that remain in the intravascular space for a longer period than crystalloids. Hetastarch is a synthetic colloid. Lactated Ringer's, Normosol-R, and Plasma-Lyte are all crystalloids. These consist of smaller molecules that only stay in the vascular space for a short period. Thomas J, Lerche P, Anesthesia and Analgesia for Veterinary Technicians, ed 5, Mosby, 2016, p. 36-39.

25. b Defibrillation is used when the patient is in ventricular fibrillation. The goal is to stop the fibrillation of the ventricles by causing them to depolarize. The normal conduction system will then take over and the cells will repolarize normally (and in a uniform manner). Battaglia AM, Small Animal Emergency and Critical Care for Veterinary Technicians ed 3, Elsevier, 2015, p. 242.

26. a Shock is defined as insufficient oxygen delivery to the tissues that results in the inability to meet the needs of the cells, which in turn causes insufficient intracellular energy production. This decrease in oxygen delivery is not always a result of a decrease in blood flow but is sometimes caused by decreased oxygenation of the blood or the inability of RBCs to offload oxygen in the tissues. Damage to the cells and the detection of a decrease in oxygen delivery causes the commonly seen clinical signs of tachycardia, tachypnea, and hypotension. Hyperthermia is rarely seen in shock. DiBartola SP, Fluid, Electrolyte, and Acid-Base Disorders in Small Animal Practice, ed 4, Elsevier, 2012, p. 557.

27. c When the stomach distends, it puts pressure on the caudal vena cava, portal vein, and splenic veins. This causes a decrease in blood flow to the caudal vena cava, which in turn causes a decrease in venous return to the heart. Cardiac output decreases as does the blood pressure. A GDV does not cause obstruction of the femoral vein, gastroduodenal vein, or renal vein. Battaglia AM, Small Animal Emergency and Critical Care for Veterinary Technicians ed 3, Elsevier, 2015, p. 343.

28. d Insulin is measured in international units (IU). This is true regardless of the type of insulin. The concentration is measured as Units/mL. U-40 insulin will contain 40 Units/mL whereas U-100 insulin contains 100 Units/mL. It is always important to double check the insulin syringe in use (U-40 syringes must be used with U-40 insulin and U-100 syringes must be used with U-100 insulin). Microliters and milliliters are both measurements of the volume whereas milligrams is a measurement of the concentration. Wanamaker BP, Massey KL, Applied Pharmacology for Veterinary Technicians, ed 5, Saunders, 2014, p. 32.

29. d It can take ≤60 minutes to deliver a fetus, during which time a veterinary technician may see maximum straining for as long as 30 minutes. Dystocia is defined as active straining for >60 minutes without the delivery of a fetus, no straining for >4 hours when fetuses are present, weak contractions lasting >2 hours, or a case in which the mother or fetuses are showing signs of stress. Battaglia AM, Small Animal Emergency and Critical Care for Veterinary Technicians ed 3, Elsevier, 2015, p. 394.

30. b Approaching the patient from the lateral direction (from the side) allows you to monitor the patient's response and to note any signs of fear or aggression. It also allows the patient to be aware of your approach and to sniff your offered hand (palm down, fingers bent). Approaching them from caudally (from the back) or rostrally (from the front) may startle or scare the patient, causing it to bite or try to escape. Sheldon CC, Sonsthagen J, Topel TF, Animal Restraint for Veterinary Professionals, ed 2, Elsevier, Mosby, 2016, p. 68.

31. c Topical steroids should not be used if there is a disruption of the cornea (corneal ulcer) because they inhibit healing and often make the ulceration worse. Flushing the eye is recommended to remove any toxin and sedation may be required when performing an ocular examination. Analgesia should always be provided. Antibiotics (either topical or systemic) are also necessary to prevent or to treat infection. Ford RB, Mazzaferro EM, Kirk and Bistner's Handbook of Veterinary Procedures and Emergency Treatment, ed 9, Elsevier, 2012, p. 197-198.

32. d As more time passes, less toxin will be recovered. It is best to induce emesis within 1 hour and it is not recommended after 4 hours. Hydrogen peroxide, although effective, is not recommended for use in cats because of the possibility for hemorrhagic gastroenteritis. Salt is not recommended because it will cause hypernatremia. Syrup of ipecac has multiple side effects including bloody diarrhea, muscle weakness, and cardiac arrhythmias. Battaglia AM, Small Animal

Emergency and Critical Care for Veterinary Technicians ed 3, Elsevier, 2015, p. 434-435.

33. c Eclampsia (puerperal tetany) is a result of hypocalcemia (which causes muscle tremors and hyperthermia). Eclampsia can occur early or late in pregnancy as well as after parturition. A large fetal mass is not necessary. Endotoxins are not present during pregnancy unless the fetuses die and are not delivered. If this were the case, an elevated temperature would result because of the infection. Bassert JM, Thomas JA, McCurnin's Clinical Textbook for Veterinary Technicians ed 8, Elsevier, 2014, p. 700.

34. c A nasal oxygen catheter should be measured from the tip of the nose to the medial canthus of the eye. If the patient is panting, a nasopharyngeal catheter can be placed. This is placed in the same way as a nasal cannula, but it is measured from the tip of the nose to the ramus of the mandible. Measuring to the pharynx or thoracic inlet will not place the nasal cannula in an appropriate place for oxygen delivery. Because of the differences in anatomy and the length of the nose, there is no standard measurement for a nasal cannula. Ford RB, Mazzaferro EM, Kirk and Bistner's Handbook of Veterinary Procedures and Emergency Treatment, ed 9, Elsevier, 2012, p. 47.

35. c The first and most important advice for the owner is to disconnect the plug from the wall, stopping the flow of electricity. There is no indication the cat has arrested, therefore CPR is not needed. Placing the cat in a carrier and bringing it into the clinic should be done as soon as possible, but only after the lamp has been unplugged. It is important to know the amperage of the lamp because its amperage, not its voltage, determines the extent of injury. Silverstein D, Hopper K, Small Animal Critical Care Medicine, ed 1, Saunders, 2009, p. 687.

36. b The femoral artery is easy to find and is the most common artery for assessing the pulse. If the animal is too nervous to allow the femoral artery to be palpated, the dorsal pedal artery can be used instead. There are no jugular, carpal, or tarsal arteries. Battaglia AM, Small Animal Emergency and Critical Care for Veterinary Medicine, ed 2, Elsevier, 2007, p. 66.

37. b Small dogs normally have a heart rate ≤160 beats/min. When in the veterinary practice, these dogs might become nervous, causing their heart rates to elevate to 175 beats/min. A heart rate >250, even in a nervous, small-breed dog, is a concern. Bassert JM, Thomas JA, McCurnin's Clinical Textbook for Veterinary Technicians, ed 9, Elsevier, 2017, p. 214.

38. d A pulse deficit is exactly as the term describes: a deficit in pulses. To detect a pulse deficit you must auscultate the heart and palpate the pulse at the same time. When the heart beats, the pulse should occur at the same time or be slightly delayed. If you hear a heartbeat and do not feel a pulse, this is a pulse deficit. This occurs because there is little to no stroke volume associated with cardiac contraction. Ford RB, Mazzaferro EM, Kirk and Bistner's Handbook of Veterinary Procedures and Emergency Treatment, ed 9, Elsevier, 2012, p. 317.

39. b A normal sinus arrhythmia occurs when the heart rate increases with inspiration and decreases with expiration. This is caused by a change of the pressure in the thoracic cavity causing a mild vagal response, which decreases the heart rate. This is a normal finding in dogs, horses, and cattle, but it is rare in cats. Thomas J, Lerche P, Anesthesia and Analgesia for Veterinary Technicians, ed 5, Mosby, 2016, p. 22.

40. b Dyspnea is defined as difficult or labored breathing. Hyperpnea is an increased depth and rate of respirations, whereas orthopnea is the inability to breathe while lying down (often seen in patients in severe respiratory distress). Tachypnea is defined as an increased respiration rate. Ford RB, Mazzaferro EM, Kirk and Bistner's Handbook of Veterinary Procedures and Emergency Treatment, ed 9, Elsevier, 2012, p. 316.

41. b An 18-gauge needle is too large for a cockatiel, kitten, or rat. Of the patients listed, it is most appropriate for the Labrador retriever. Sirois M, Principles and Practice of Veterinary Technology, ed 4, Elsevier, 2016, p. 613-614.

42. d An intraperitoneal injection should be performed 2–3 inches cranial to the umbilicus on the midline; any other area increases the risk of hitting a major organ. This procedure is not performed often because of the risk of lacerating or puncturing an organ or causing peritonitis; it is most useful in neonates or for peritoneal lavage. Bassert JM, Thomas JA, McCurnin's Clinical Textbook for Veterinary Technicians, ed 9, Elsevier, 2017, p. 556.

43. c Flushing a large fluid bolus, placing the fluid in the pharyngeal area, or forcing the patient to swallow may cause choking or aspiration of the liquid. Small amounts of fluid should be introduced between the cheek and teeth and the patient should be allowed to swallow of its own accord. Bassert JM, Thomas JA, McCurnin's Clinical Textbook for Veterinary Technicians, ed 9, Elsevier, 2017, p. 543-544.

44. a The lateral aspect of the neck is the best area to assess skin turgor. The other areas listed either do not have enough loose skin or have skin that is too thin to provide an accurate response. Bassert JM, Thomas JA, McCurnin's Clinical Textbook for Veterinary Technicians, ed 9, Elsevier, 2017, p. 237.

45. b Knuckling is a neurological abnormality. It occurs when a patient walks on the dorsal aspect of the paw or hoof; therefore, cardiac, respiratory, and urinary do not apply. De Lahunta A, Glass E, Veterinary Neuroanatomy and Clinical Neurology, ed 3, Saunders, 2009, p. 228.

46. b Hyperkalemia causes cardiac arrest by decreasing the ability of the heart to depolarize as well as repolarize. Supplementation should never exceed 0.5 mEq/kg/h. Potassium does not play a direct role in respiratory function, therefore hyperkalemia will not directly cause respiratory arrest. The body does not respond to hyperkalemia by increasing urine production (polyuria) or thirst (polydipsia). Bassert JM, Thomas JA, McCurnin's Clinical Textbook for Veterinary Technicians, ed 9, Elsevier, 2017, p. 870.

47. d Potassium should only be administered intravenously or subcutaneously. Subcutaneous potassium should not exceed 35 mEq/L to avoid discomfort, whereas intravenous potassium that exceeds 60 mEq/L causes sclerosis of peripheral veins. If the patient requires a higher dose of potassium, a central catheter should be placed. Intramuscular administration of potassium is very painful. DiBartola SP, Fluid, Electrolyte, and Acid-Base Disorders in Small Animal Practice, ed 4, Elsevier, 2012, p. 107.

48. d Any patient that has experienced trauma will benefit from fluid therapy (unless it is contraindicated because of an underlying disease). Pulmonary edema and cerebral edema will worsen with fluid therapy. Pitting of the soft tissues can be a clinical sign of fluid overload. Swelling secondary to trauma is not related to fluid overload and does not indicate that the patient is at risk of fluid overload. Battaglia AM, Small Animal Emergency and Critical Care for Veterinary Medicine, ed 2, Elsevier, 2007, p. 50, 66.

49. d The easiest and least expensive method for monitoring fluid therapy is by weight. One liter of fluids weighs 1 kg. Acute weight loss or gain (over several hours or days) while in the hospital is likely to be caused by a loss or gain of fluids because it takes longer to lose body mass. After the patient is hydrated, the weight should remain relatively the same. The CVP, PCV/TP, and UOP require invasive and costly procedures (placement of a central line for the CVP, venipuncture for the PCV/TP, and placement of a urinary catheter for the UOP). These are excellent ways to monitor fluid therapy, but monitoring the weight is the easiest. Bassert JM, Thomas JA, McCurnin's Clinical Textbook for Veterinary Technicians, ed 9, Elsevier, 2017, p. 829-830.

50. a One of the clinical signs of fluid overload is chemosis, which is swelling of the conjunctiva, secondary to edema. The lens, pupil, and nictitating membrane are not affected by fluid overload, therefore changes will not be seen in these areas. Bassert JM, Thomas JA, McCurnin's Clinical Textbook for Veterinary Technicians, ed 9, Elsevier, 2017, p. 830.

51. c Cerebral edema is a contraindication for rapid infusion of crystalloids, which will move into the brain tissue, worsening the edema. Hypertonic saline can be used in patients that require rapid fluid therapy but are unable to tolerate large volumes. Patients suffering from renal failure, severe dehydration, or shock can benefit from rapid fluid replacement. Silverstein D, Hopper K, Small Animal Critical Care Medicine, ed 1, Saunders, 2009, p. 273.

52. d VetStarch is considered a colloid, whereas LRS, Normosol-R, and sodium chloride are considered crystalloids. Bassert JM, Thomas JA, McCurnin's Clinical Textbook for Veterinary Technicians, ed 9, Elsevier, 2017, p. 820-821.

53. d Isotonic fluids cause the least amount of discomfort and also cause fewer complications (cellulitis, infection, or necrosis secondary to infection). Hypertonic and hypotonic fluids are irritating when administered subcutaneously. Colloids should not be given subcutaneously. DiBartola SP, Fluid, Electrolyte, and Acid-Base Disorders in Small Animal Practice, ed 4, Elsevier, 2012, p. 351.

54. a Intraosseous fluids can be administered as rapidly as intravenous fluids and they will enter the circulation as quickly via the bone marrow sinusoids and medullary cavity. Intraperitoneal fluids are absorbed quickly but not as quickly as IO. Patients that require large amounts of fluids rapidly are unlikely to be able to consume anything orally (they may be limited by nausea or vomiting). There is a maximum amount of subcutaneous fluids that can be administered, as well as a limit to how quickly the fluids can be absorbed. Bassert JM, Thomas JA, McCurnin's Clinical Textbook for Veterinary Technicians, ed 9, Elsevier, 2017, p. 547.

55. c Fluid therapy is warranted in hypovolemic, distributive, and obstructive shock. Because of the possibility of causing a patient to go into heart failure, fluids should be used with caution in patients with cardiogenic shock. Battaglia AM, Small Animal Emergency and Critical Care for Veterinary Technicians ed 3, Elsevier, 2015, p. 223-225.

56. c The ABCs of the primary survey should be followed. A = airway, B = breathing, and C = circulation. The respiratory system should always be evaluated first. The patient's airway should be assessed for obstruction along with respiratory rate, effort, and pattern. The cardiac, neurologic, and urinary systems should be evaluated after the respiratory system. Silverstein D, Hopper K, Small Animal Critical Care Medicine, ed 1, Saunders, 2009, p. 7-8.

57. c Immersing the area in lukewarm water will allow the ice crystals that have formed in the tissue to dissolve. Massaging the area will actually cause tissue damage as the crystals move around in the tissue. Immersing the area in hot water may cause scalding, whereas rubbing the area with snow will cause tissue damage (and may enhance the frostbite). Ford RB, Mazzaferro EM, Kirk and Bistner's Handbook of Veterinary Procedures and Emergency Treatment, ed 9, Elsevier, 2012, p. 144.

58. b Direct pressure is the most effective way to control hemorrhage while avoiding further trauma to the tissues. Clamping the wound with a hemostat is painful and may cause damage to the area. Tourniquets are effective on extremities; however, cutting off blood flow to the rest of the limb causes further damage. Silver nitrate is painful as well as messy, it will be difficult to clean the wound, and it may cause contamination. Battaglia AM, Small Animal Emergency and Critical Care for Veterinary Technicians ed 3, Elsevier, 2015, p. 258-259.

59. d The heart rate, respiratory rate, and capillary refill time will allow you to determine whether the patient is stable or critical. A weight is eventually necessary but can be obtained after the patient is deemed stable or becomes stable. Battaglia AM, Small Animal Emergency and Critical Care for Veterinary Technicians ed 3, Elsevier, 2015, p. 12-14.

60. c A patient in the early stages of shock compensates for fluid loss and decreased oxygen delivery with an increase in heart rate. This maintains blood flow to the heart and brain. In the later stages of shock, the patient is no longer able to compensate and the heart rate decreases. Battaglia AM, Small Animal Emergency and Critical Care for Veterinary Technicians ed 3, Elsevier, 2015, p. 226-227.

61. d Hemorrhagic shock is caused by the loss of blood. The body responds with peripheral vasoconstriction, which decreases blood flow to the mucous membranes, causing them to be pale or white. Cyanotic mucous membranes are seen when the hemoglobin is no longer carrying oxygen. Because hemoglobin must be present at a concentration greater than 5 g/dL (PCV of 15%), it is unlikely that you will be able to detect cyanosis in a patient in hemorrhagic shock because the hemoglobin/PCV will fall below these levels. Hyperemic mucous membranes are evident in patients that are in a hyperdynamic state (vasodilation allowing blood to move to the periphery, causing the bright red mucous membranes). A patient who is anemic because of hemorrhage responds to the blood loss with vasoconstriction and the mucous membranes are therefore not hyperemic. Icteric mucous membranes result from the breakdown of red blood cells and are not seen in patients experiencing hemorrhage. Hemorrhagic shock is caused by the loss of blood. Silverstein D, Hopper K, Small Animal Critical Care Medicine, ed 1, Saunders, 2009, p. 2-3.

62. c 5 g/dL of hemoglobin is required to detect cyanosis. This correlates with a PCV/TP of 15%. If there is less than this, there is not enough deoxygenated hemoglobin present to detect the blue color associated with cyanosis. Battaglia AM, Small Animal Emergency and Critical Care for Veterinary Technicians ed 3, Elsevier, 2015, p. 254.

63. b Triage is defined as the prioritization of patients, with the most critical patient being seen first. The most critical patient, or the one who is more likely to die first, is the dog in respiratory distress. The other patients have non–life-threatening conditions and can be seen afterward. Silverstein D, Hopper K, Small Animal Critical Care Medicine, ed 1, Saunders, 2009, p. 5.

64. d Petechiation is the presence of small spots of hemorrhage and can be seen anywhere on the body. This is caused by thrombocytopenia. Hemoglobinemia and myoglobinemia will not cause petechiae and methemoglobinemia causes brown mucous membranes. Summers A, Common Diseases of Companion Animals, ed 4, Elsevier, 2019, p. 91.

65. c Compensatory shock is the stage of shock in which the patient is able to compensate for a loss of intravascular fluid. The body compensates with tachycardia and peripheral vasoconstriction, both of which aid in maintaining normal blood pressure. Vasoconstriction also causes the extremities to be cool. Peripheral vasoconstriction causes the capillary refill time to be normal to prolonged, because the blood flow to that area is decreased. Silverstein D, Hopper K, Small Animal Critical Care Medicine, ed 1, Saunders, 2009, p. 41-42.

66. b Triage is defined as the prioritization of patients, with the most critical patient being seen first. The most critical patient, or the one who is more likely to die first, is the dog with acute gastric dilatation volvulus. The other patients are stable, do not have conditions that are immediately life-threatening, and can be seen after the first dog is more stable. Bassert JM, Thomas JA, McCurnin's Clinical Textbook for Veterinary Technicians ed 8, Elsevier, p. 908.

67. a Green or black vulvar discharge is normal during parturition and it is therefore not an indication of dystocia. Dystocia is considered when there is active straining for >60 minutes without delivering a fetus, no straining for >4 hours when fetuses are present, weak contractions lasting >2 hours, or if the mother or fetuses are showing signs of stress. A pup or kitten should not take longer than 5 minutes to move through the birth canal. Profuse hemorrhage from the vulva is also a sign of dystocia. Battaglia AM, Small Animal Emergency and Critical Care for Veterinary Technicians ed 3, Elsevier, 2015, p. 394.

68. d Although diarrhea may occur, unproductive vomiting, hypersalivation, and abdominal distention are all classic clinical signs of GDV. Battaglia AM, Small Animal Emergency and Critical Care for Veterinary Technicians ed 3, Elsevier, 2015, p. 343.

69. d Crackles are heard when the alveoli that have collapsed pop open. This is indicative of pulmonary edema (fluid within the lungs), which will cause a collapse of the alveoli. If pleural effusion (fluid between the lungs and chest wall) is present, it will muffle the lung sounds. Fluid will fall and be present in the ventral chest, causing decreased lung sounds ventrally. A pneumothorax (air between the lugs and chest wall) also causes muffled lung sounds. Because air rises, lung sounds will decrease dorsally. Asthma causes wheezing. Silverstein D, Hopper K, Small Animal Critical Care Medicine, ed 1, Saunders, 2009, p. 124-126; Bassert JM, Thomas JA, McCurnin's Clinical Textbook for Veterinary Technicians ed 8, Elsevier, p. 218-219.

70. b Cats straining to urinate are often mistaken by owners as straining to defecate. If these owners call, they should be advised to bring the cat to the hospital immediately. The cat should be evaluated for a urinary obstruction as soon as it presents. Cats suffering from peritonitis or intestinal obstruction are generally experiencing pain in the abdomen and may exhibit vomiting, but they do not appear to be straining to urinate or defecate in the litter box. Cats with an upper respiratory viral infection will present with sneezing and discharge from the eyes and nose. Battaglia AM, Small Animal Emergency and Critical Care for Veterinary Technicians ed 3, Elsevier, 2015, p. 374-375.

71. c A diaphragmatic hernia occurs when the contents of the abdominal cavity appear within the thoracic cavity. This prevents expansion of the lungs and increases respiratory distress. Emergency treatment includes elevating the cranial half of the body in an attempt to cause the abdominal organs to slide back into the abdomen. If the caudal half of the body is elevated, the organs will put more pressure on the lungs, causing the breathing to become even more labored. Bassert JM, Thomas JA, McCurnin's Clinical Textbook for Veterinary Technicians ed 9, Elsevier, p. 1172-1173.

72. d If the patient can feel pain, it should respond by moving away (withdrawal) from the pain while vocalizing. If the patient withdraws its foot and does not vocalize, this is considered a reflex and does not indicate the perception of pain. The patient will not kick, because the first instinct is to move away from the pain. Ford RB, Mazzaferro EM, Kirk and Bistner's Handbook of Veterinary Procedures and Emergency Treatment, ed 9, Elsevier, 2012, p. 188.

73. a Cardiopulmonary arrest is the cessation of spontaneous and effective ventilation and perfusion. Signs include dilation of the pupils, lack of a femoral pulse, and/or agonal breathing. Although alert animals can arrest in the near future, this is not a sign of cardiopulmonary arrest. Ford RB, Mazzaferro EM, Kirk and Bistner's Handbook of Veterinary Procedures and Emergency Treatment, ed 9, Elsevier, 2012, p. 110-111.

74. a Although any of these choices might be the cause, the force required to cause pelvic fractures is also enough to rupture the urinary bladder. Renal failure, an obstruction secondary to urethral calculi, or severe dehydration should all be ruled out if the urinary bladder is intact. Battaglia AM, Small Animal Emergency and Critical Care for Veterinary Technicians ed 3, Elsevier, 2015, p. 265-266.

75. a Anticoagulant rodenticides are vitamin K antagonists and cause a deficiency in clotting factors II, VII, IX, and X. Ethylene glycol causes renal failure, strychnine causes tremors, ataxia, and seizures, and organophosphates cause SLUD signs, including salivation, lacrimation, urination, and defecation. Peterson ME, Talcott PA, Small Animal Toxicology, ed 2, Elsevier, 2006, p. 705, 945-946, and 1078-1079.

76. b Status epilepticus is defined as continuous seizure activity or seizures occurring close together with no return to a normal mentation between each seizure. Seizures can cause hyperthermia, hypoxia, and neurological damage, making status epilepticus a life-threatening condition. Seizures can occur at any age, although the causes can change as the animal ages. Acepromazine is contraindicated in animals with a history of seizure activity and should be used with caution, if used at all. Status epilepticus is unlikely to resolve spontaneously. Battaglia AM, Small Animal Emergency and Critical Care for Veterinary Medicine, ed 2, Elsevier, 2007, p. 174.

77. c Clinical signs caused by organophosphates fall into three categories, with the patient starting at the first and eventually reaching the third (without treatment): First category: Muscarinic can be remembered by the mnemonic DUMBELS (defecation, urination, myosis, bradycardia, emesis, lacrimation [b], and salivation [d]). Second category: Nicotinic (tremors, stiffness, ataxia, and paralysis). Third category: CSN signs (depression, hyperactivity, anxiety, and coma). Organophosphate poisoning causes myosis, not mydriasis. Peterson ME, Talcott PA, Small Animal Toxicology, ed 2, Elsevier, 2006, p. 945-946.

78. b A normal capillary refill time is 1–2 seconds. Less than 1 second indicates vasodilation or a hemodynamic state, whereas anything longer than 2.5 seconds indicates shock. Bassert JM, Thomas JA, McCurnin's Clinical Textbook for Veterinary Technicians ed 9, Elsevier, p. 219.

79. a Animals that have suffered trauma should be seen immediately, even if they appear normal. There is the possibility they have suffered internal damage that will not be evident to the owner. Waiting until the next day may be detrimental to the pet. Because technicians are not allowed to diagnosis patients, a technician should not examine the patient to decide whether it needs to be seen by a veterinarian. Bassert JM, Thomas JA, McCurnin's Clinical Textbook for Veterinary Technicians ed 9, Elsevier, p. 841-842.

80. a Motor oil contains petroleum. Because of the high risk of aspiration, emesis is contraindicated with the ingestion of petroleum products. The puppy should be brought in to the clinic as soon as possible. Peterson ME, Talcott PA, Small Animal Toxicology, ed 2, Elsevier, 2006, p. 993-994.

81. b Sugar-free gum often contains xylitol, which is toxic to dogs and can cause hypoglycemia within 30–60 minutes of ingestion; it also has the potential to cause liver failure. Although it is not ideal to have an owner induce emesis at home (because of the possibility of damage to the esophagus and stomach with hydrogen peroxide and the risk of aspiration), the dog is 90 minutes from your clinic and, in this case, it would be beneficial to instruct the owner to induce emesis before leaving for the hospital. Even if emesis is induced right away it is unlikely that all of the toxin will be removed from the stomach. The dog can still suffer the ill effects of the toxin and treatment should begin immediately to avoid hypoglycemia and liver failure. Peterson ME, Talcott PA, Small Animal Toxicology, ed 2, Elsevier, 2006, p. 128-129, 241.

82. c Based on the history of diabetes and receiving insulin, despite not eating all day, it is likely that the seizure is secondary to hypoglycemia. Corn syrup, Karo syrup, or honey can be placed on the gums to increase the blood glucose. Because this is a temporary fix, the cat should be brought to the clinic right away instead of being observed at home. Another dose of insulin will drop the glucose further, causing hypoglycemic coma and death. Silverstein D, Hopper K, Small Animal Critical Care Medicine, ed 1, Saunders, 2009, p. 298.

83. b The most important treatment for topical toxins is to bathe the animal to remove as much toxin as possible. The kitten should be bathed at home (with Dawn dish soap if possible) and seen by a veterinarian as soon as possible. Knowing that the kitten has been exposed to a toxin, it is not appropriate to tell the owner to observe the kitten at home. Acetaminophen should never be administered to a cat and medications should never be recommended without a veterinarian's approval. Emesis is not required because the kitten did not orally ingest the toxin. Peterson ME, Talcott PA, Small Animal Toxicology, ed 2, Elsevier, 2006, p. 57-58.

84. d Strings should never be removed because of the high likelihood of trauma to the GI tract. Cutting the string will prevent possible removal by the veterinarian, whereas inducing emesis or giving laxatives may cause the string to move or might cause damage to the GI tract. The cat should be brought in immediately for an examination and possible surgery. Ford RB, Mazzaferro EM, Kirk and Bistner's Handbook of Veterinary Procedures and Emergency Treatment, ed 9, Elsevier, 2012, p. 161-162.

85. c Fish hooks often require sedation for removal. Because of this, the owner should not be told to remove the fish hook at home. In addition, a veterinarian should see the dog as soon as possible, before the dog causes trauma by pawing at his face. Fish hooks may dissolve in fish but this is not the case in dogs or cats and a fish hook will not fall out spontaneously. A technician should not advise the owner to administer medications at home without the veterinarian's recommendation. Summers A, Common Diseases of Companion Animals, ed 4, Elsevier, 2019, p. 25.

86. b If strikethrough occurs before the laceration is repaired, the bandage should not be removed. Rather, a second bandage should be placed over the original bandage to avoid disturbing any clots that are forming or have already formed. If there is strikethrough, the bleeding is excessive and the laceration should be repaired. Battaglia AM, Small Animal Emergency and Critical Care for Veterinary Technicians ed 3, Elsevier, 2015, p. 258.

87. b Chest compressions are the most important aspect of CPR. Before leaving for the hospital, chest compressions should be started. Meanwhile the dog should be transported to the hospital as soon as possible, even if the dog seems to recover. Battaglia AM, Small Animal Emergency and Critical Care for Veterinary Technicians ed 3, Elsevier, 2015, p. 237.

88. c Patients with a suspected spinal injury should be transported lying on a flat, stable surface. If they are allowed to sit, stand, or move around, they can cause further trauma to the spine. Ford RB, Mazzaferro EM, Kirk and Bistner's Handbook of Veterinary Procedures and Emergency Treatment, ed 9, Elsevier, 2012, p. 274.

89. d The patient should be kept quiet (imitating bed rest in a kennel) to avoid worsening the potential hernia. Because treatment should be started immediately, the owner should not be told to wait. Summers A, Common Diseases of Companion Animals, ed 3, Elsevier, 2014, p. 211.

90. c A laryngoscope, intravenous catheter, and Ambu bag may all be necessary in an emergency. An otoscope is used to examine the ear canal and should not be necessary in an emergency. Bassert JM, Thomas JA, McCurnin's Clinical Textbook for Veterinary Technicians ed 9, Elsevier, p. 846.

91. d An upper airway obstruction must be removed as soon as possible and can be accomplished with the Heimlich maneuver. If the foreign body is not quickly dislodged, a tracheostomy must be performed. Placing the patient in an oxygen cage or placing a nasal cannula will not help the animal to breathe. The presence of the ball will prevent the passing of an endotracheal tube. Ford RB, Mazzaferro EM, Kirk and Bistner's Handbook of Veterinary Procedures and Emergency Treatment, ed 9, Elsevier, 2012, p. 257.

92. c Agonal respirations are a sign that the animal has entered cardiopulmonary arrest. CPR should be initiated and as much fluid suctioned from the airway as possible. Intravenous fluids should not be administered to an animal that has possible cardiac disease (as indicated by the frothy fluid). Administering furosemide and then placing the animal in oxygen will not address the cardiorespiratory arrest. A tracheostomy is not indicated because the airway is not obstructed and you should be able to intubate the patient. Battaglia AM, Small Animal Emergency and Critical Care for Veterinary Technicians ed 3, Elsevier, 2015, p. 236-237.

93. a An intraosseous catheter can be placed in the medullary cavity of the femur. Fluids should not be infused into an artery and the patient would not tolerate a catheter in the lingual (tongue) vein. In a patient of this size, an ear vein would not be accessible. Battaglia AM, Small Animal Emergency and Critical Care for Veterinary Technicians ed 3, Elsevier, 2015, p. 56-57.

94. c Although intraperitoneal is the least desirable route of administration for fluids (because of the slow absorption, risk for damage to an organ, and risk for infection), it is the best of the options listed here. Blood products should not be administered subcutaneously, intramuscularly, or by mouth. Sirois M, Principles and Practice of Veterinary Technology, ed 3, Elsevier, 2011, p. 422-423 .

95. b Material used for a muzzle should be made of a soft material. A metal chain will cause trauma to the patient. Rope, pantyhose, and a necktie are all soft materials that are effective as well as safe for the patient. Sirois M, Principles and Practice of Veterinary Technology, ed 4, Elsevier, 2016, p. 523.

96. a Apomorphine is a medical drug that is not found outside a veterinary clinic. Syrup of ipecac, hydrogen peroxide, and salt are all readily available in any grocery store. Wanamaker BP, Massey KL, Applied Pharmacology for Veterinary Technicians, ed 5, Saunders, 2014, p. 154.

97. a Gastric dilatation volvulus (GDV) occurs when the stomach distends and then rotates. This prevents the animal from being able to vomit; therefore, the induction of emesis is contraindicated. An intravenous catheter should be placed to treat shock. Decompression of the stomach is a very important part of emergency treatment for GDV and can be accomplished by passing a gastric tube or by trocharization of the stomach (placing a needle through the body wall into the stomach to allow for the release of air). Silverstein D, Hopper K, Small Animal Critical Care Medicine, ed 1, Saunders, 2009, p. 586.

98. c Applying a warm compress causes vasodilation, which increases bleeding in epistaxis patients. Epistaxis may result from a number of things, including trauma, rodenticide ingestion, presence of a foreign body, or neoplasia. Keeping the patient quiet (with or without sedation), placing epinephrine in the nares (causing vasoconstriction), and the administration of fresh frozen plasma (to replace clotting factors) will all assist in decreasing the bleeding. Ford RB, Mazzaferro EM, Kirk and Bistner's Handbook of Veterinary Procedures and Emergency Treatment, ed 9, Elsevier, 2012, p. 257.

99. c When placing a stomach tube, a roll of tape can be used to prevent the patient from biting the tube. The tube should be measured from the nose to the 13th rib and fluid should be injected into the tube to confirm placement in the stomach. If the tube is measured to the thoracic inlet, the risk of aspiration increases. Bassert JM, Thomas JA, McCurnin's Clinical Textbook for Veterinary Technicians ed 8, Elsevier, p. 587-588.

100. a An endotracheal tube, nasal oxygen catheter, and tracheostomy tube all deliver oxygen to the airway, whereas a chest tube delivers oxygen to the pleural space, causing a pneumothorax. Battaglia AM, Small Animal Emergency and Critical Care for Veterinary Technicians ed 3, Elsevier, 2015, p. 135-131.

101. a The elevated temperature associated with heatstroke is the main cause of mortality in these patients. Cooling will decrease morbidity and mortality. Control of infection, providing oxygen, and pain management are each important factors, but cooling is most important. Silverstein D, Hopper K, Small Animal Critical Care Medicine, ed 1, Saunders, 2009, p. 24-25.

102. d Applying a warm compress causes the penis to swell more, making it difficult to replace in the sheath. Applying hypertonic saline to the penis will pull fluid from the tissue, causing it to shrink. Cleaning and lubricating the penis will make it easier to replace in the sheath. Battaglia AM, Small Animal Emergency and Critical Care for Veterinary Medicine, ed 2, Elsevier, 2007, p. 328.

103. d Radiographs are required; however, this is considered a diagnostic, whereas the other listed options are considered treatments. Bassert JM, Thomas JA, McCurnin's Clinical Textbook for Veterinary Technicians ed 9, Elsevier, p. 845-846.

104. c A dog having a seizure may hurt itself if allowed to fall against a wall or table. Making sure it does not come into contact with anything and hurt itself is most important. Grasping the tongue is not safe and will likely result in a bite. A dog experiencing a seizure will not be able to take any oral medications and intravenous fluids will not treat the seizure. Battaglia AM, Small Animal Emergency and Critical Care for Veterinary Medicine, ed 2, Elsevier, 2007, p. 355.

105. a Trying to replace the globe will only cause further trauma and may result in the owner being bitten. If possible, the owner should apply lubricant to keep the globe moist, cover it (a disposable cup works well for this), or place an e-collar to prevent further damage, and then bring the dog to the veterinarian as soon as possible. Ford RB, Mazzaferro EM, Kirk and Bistner's Handbook of Veterinary Procedures and Emergency Treatment, ed 9, Elsevier, 2012, p. 201.

106. b A penetrating wound from a BB pellet may not appear to have caused much damage and you may be inclined to recommend that the owner observe the dog at home and bring it in if necessary or when convenient. However, the pellet may have caused significant internal damage that is not obvious when looking at the dog and the owner should be advised to bring the dog in right away. Silverstein D, Hopper K, Small Animal Critical Care Medicine, ed 1, Saunders, 2009, p. 665.

107. d Initial treatment should address the immediate, life-threatening problem. In this case, that is the presence of a pneumothorax. Providing oxygen, performing a thoracocentesis, and covering the wound should all be performed before taking radiographs (which is a diagnostic, not a treatment). Bassert JM, Thomas JA, McCurnin's Clinical Textbook for Veterinary Technicians ed 9, Elsevier, p. 848-849.

108. b Occasionally the cat is so ill that sedation is not necessary and may even cause the cat to enter cardiopulmonary arrest. If the obstruction is because of a mucous plug at the tip of the penis, massaging the tip of the penis may remove the plug, allowing the cat to urinate, but this is not always possible. A urinary obstruction is life-threatening because of the elevation in potassium that occurs if the obstruction is not relieved. Battaglia AM, Small Animal Emergency and Critical Care for Veterinary Technicians ed 3, Elsevier, 2015, p. 374-377.

109. c Oxytocin is a hormone used to increase uterine contraction and is not used in neonates. Cleaning the nose and mouth, rubbing the neonate to stimulate breathing, and ligating the umbilical cord are all standard procedures during a cesarean section. Bassert JM, Thomas JA, McCurnin's Clinical Textbook for Veterinary Technicians ed 9, Elsevier, p. 1167-1168.

110. c The sooner emesis is induced, the greater the amount of material that will be removed from the stomach. Up to 75% of material will be removed if emesis is induced within the first 30 minutes and ≤60% if induced within the first hour. Emesis is minimally effective at 4 hours and it is of little value beyond that. Peterson ME, Talcott PA, Small Animal Toxicology, ed 2, Elsevier, 2006, p. 128-129.

111. b Remember the CABs of CPR: circulation, airway, and breathing. An animal in cardiopulmonary arrest does not require analgesia and this would actually make resuscitation efforts more difficult. If the patient has received analgesia, it should be reversed. Bassert JM, Thomas JA, McCurnin's Clinical Textbook for Veterinary Technicians, ed 8, Elsevier, p. 921-922.

112. b Respirations should be delivered at a rate of 8–12 breaths per minute, regardless of the size of the patient. Faster than this will cause hyperventilation and hypocapnia. A decrease in carbon dioxide will cause vasoconstriction and a decrease in blood flow and oxygen delivery to the brain. Bassert JM, Thomas JA, McCurnin's Clinical Textbook for Veterinary Technicians, ed 9, Elsevier, p. 853.

113. d When shock first occurs, the body compensates (compensatory shock) for the decrease in oxygen delivery to the tissues with an increase in heart rate (tachycardia) and vasoconstriction, which will maintain a normal blood pressure and will maintain oxygen delivery to the tissues. The body is unable to maintain this response and eventually will no longer be able to compensate (decompensatory shock) and the heart rate will decrease along with the blood pressure. Eventually the patient will go into end-stage decompensatory shock and the bradycardia that results will not respond to atropine. Vasodilation, an increase in the capillary refill time, and hypothermia are all signs of decompensatory shock. It is very difficult to recover from this stage of shock and most patients will enter respiratory or cardiac arrest. Ford RM, Mazzaferro EM, Kirk and Bistner's Handbook of Veterinary Procedures and Emergency Care, ed 8, Elsevier, 2006, p. 894.

114. c The central venous pressure measures pressure in the heart, indicates the heart's ability to pump the blood that has returned from the body, and helps guide fluid therapy. If the CVP is low, the patient is probably hypovolemic and requires additional fluid therapy. If the CVP is high, the patient is hypervolemic and may be fluid overloaded. Temperature, oxygenation, and pain will indirectly affect the heart; however, the CVP is not used to guide rewarming, oxygen therapy, or pain management. Bassert JM, Thomas JA, McCurnin's Clinical Textbook for Veterinary Technicians, ed 9, Elsevier, p. 829.

115. a The sclera is a fibrous tissue covering the eye and is not a mucous membrane. The gingiva, lining of the vulva, and prepuce are all mucous membranes and can be used to assess mucous membrane color. Colville T, Bassert JM, Clinical Anatomy and Physiology for Veterinary Technicians, ed 2, Mosby, 2008, p. 351.

116. d Mucous membrane moisture, skin turgor, heart rate, pulses, capillary refill time, packed-cell/total protein, and ocular position can all be used to assess dehydration. Nasal discharge can be associated with many diseases and is not a good indicator of dehydration. Battaglia AM, Small Animal Emergency and Critical Care for Veterinary Technicians, ed 3, Elsevier, 2015, p. 63-64.

117. a Maintenance = 66 mL/kg/day = 66 mL × 20 kg = 1320 mL/day Dehydration = 20 kg × 0.08 = 1.6 L or 1600 mL 1600 + 1320 = 2920 mL in 24 h. Lake T, Green N, Essential Calculations for Veterinary Technicians, ed 2, Elsevier, 2009, p. 91-93.

118. b Do not let this question fool you. It includes the percentage dehydration but does not ask for that to be included in the fluid rate. Also note that it provides the maintenance rate of 66 mL/kg/day but asks you to calculate two times the daily maintenance rate. 32 kg × 66 mL/kg/day = 2112 mL/day; 2112 mL/day/24 h = 88 mL/h; 88 mL/h × 2 = 176 mL/h. Lake T, Green N, Essential Calculations for Veterinary Nurses and Technicians, ed 2, Elsevier, 2009, p. 91-93.

119. c Patients with a coagulopathy or suspect coagulopathy, such as that seen in a patient with thrombocytopenia, should not have blood drawn from the jugular vein because bleeding would be difficult to control. Vomiting, pancreatitis, and renal failure are unlikely to cause bleeding. Silverstein D, Hopper K, Small Animal Critical Care Medicine, ed 1, Saunders, 2009, p. 862.

120. d Basic life support includes intubation, ventilation, and chest compressions. Medications are included in advanced life support along with EKG, defibrillation, and intravenous fluids. Battaglia AM, Small Animal Emergency and Critical Care for Veterinary Technicians, ed 3, Elsevier, 2015, p. 237-240.

121. b Six parameters can be used to assess perfusion: mucous membrane color, capillary refill time, pulse quality, heart rate, mentation, and temperature of extremities. The rectal temperature is not a good indicator of perfusion because the patient may be febrile. Creedon JMB, Davis H, Advanced Monitoring and Procedures for Small Animal Emergency and Critical Care, ed 1, Wiley-Blackwell, 2012, p. 8-9.

122. b A patient in respiratory arrest always takes precedence over any other emergency, including a dog with a penetrating abdominal wound, intestinal foreign body, or a GDV. Bassert JM, Thomas JA, McCurnin's Clinical Textbook for Veterinary Technicians, ed 8, Elsevier, p. 908.

123. c Incorrectly treating hyperthermia can be detrimental to the patient. There are several different causes (true fever, heatstroke, exercise, tetany, metabolic disturbances) and each is treated differently. The duration of the hyperthermia can be detrimental and plays a role in prognosis; however, the cause must first be determined. The breed and age of the patient are insignificant when deciding treatment (unless they contribute to the cause of the hyperthermia). Silverstein D, Hopper K, Small Animal Critical Care Medicine, ed 1, Saunders, 2009, p. 22-24.

124. d When administering a drug via the endotracheal tube, the amount can be as much as 10 times the intravenous dose. This should be diluted with 5–10 mL of sterile saline. Battaglia AM, Small Animal Emergency and Critical Care for Veterinary Technicians, ed 3, Elsevier, 2015, p. 242.

125. b A distended abdomen, restlessness, and nonproductive vomiting are classic signs of GDV. This dog should be seen as soon as possible and the owner should not be told to wait for any reason. Inducing vomiting is contraindicated in a GDV. Bassert JM, Thomas JA, McCurnin's Clinical Textbook for Veterinary Technicians, ed 9, Elsevier, p. 1156.

126. c Marijuana (*Cannabis sativa*) causes all of these clinical signs and dribbling urine is considered a classic sign of marijuana toxicity. A patient that ingested chocolate will be hyperexcited and tachycardic. Grapes cause renal failure, but the patient will not exhibit any clinical signs for several days. Xylitol causes hypoglycemia almost immediately and liver failure in a few days. The patient may present obtunded if the blood glucose is low enough. Ford RB, Mazzaferro EM, Kirk and Bistner's Handbook of Veterinary Procedures and Emergency Treatment, ed 9, Elsevier, 2012, p. 241-242.

127. d Providing medication is never recommended without speaking to the veterinarian first. The patient may be taking other medications that would make aspirin a contraindication. In addition, it is illegal for a veterinary technician to prescribe medications. As long as the remaining recommendations do not put the client at risk, they would be deemed appropriate. Wanamaker BP, Massey KL, Applied Pharmacology for Veterinary Technicians, ed 4, Saunders, 2009, p. 302-303.

128. a An intraosseous catheter should not be placed in septic patients because of the risk of worsening a life-threatening infection. Intraosseous catheters are an excellent option for young or debilitated patients in which intravenous access is not possible. In addition, this type of catheter allows rapid access to the circulatory system and any medication that is administered intravenously can also be given through an intraosseous catheter. Bassert JM, Thomas JA, McCurnin's Clinical Textbook for Veterinary Technicians, ed 9, Elsevier, p. 556.

129. a Intravenous administration of fluids and medications is always preferred. A critically ill animal will not be able to take anything orally and dehydration or peripheral vasoconstriction prevents the absorption of subcutaneous fluids. Intramuscular injections must be provided in small volumes to avoid pain. DiBartola SP, Fluid, Electrolyte, and Acid-Base Disorders in Small Animal Practice, ed 4, Elsevier, 2012, p. 352.

130. b Lactated Ringer's solution is the only crystalloid listed. Packed red blood cells, hetastarch, and oxyglobin are all colloids. Bassert JM, Thomas JA, McCurnin's Clinical Textbook for Veterinary Technicians, ed 9, Elsevier, p. 820-821.

131. b Whole blood provides red blood cells, platelets, and coagulation factors. A patient with hemorrhage secondary to anticoagulant rodenticide ingestion requires whole blood to replace lost coagulation factors. Patients with anemia resulting from an autoimmune disease, those suffering hemorrhage during surgery, or those suffering from anemia because of trauma only require red blood cells. They should not require replacement of platelets or coagulation factors. Battaglia AM, Small Animal Emergency and Critical Care for Veterinary Technicians, ed 3, Elsevier, 2015, p. 79-80.

132. a Enteral nutrition is always preferred because it keeps the gastrointestinal tract healthy by providing enterocytes with nutrition. Partial and total parenteral nutrition are provided intravenously and should be used if the patient will not eat and if a feeding tube cannot be placed. Feeding per rectum is not a viable option because the nutrients will not be absorbed. Case LP, Daristotle L, Hayek MG, Raasch MF, Canine and Feline Nutrition, ed 3, Mosby, 2011, p. 485-485.

133. a Although any of these choices can signal a transfusion reaction, fever is the most common clinical sign. Battaglia AM, Small Animal Emergency and Critical Care for Veterinary Technicians, ed 3, Elsevier, 2015, p. 100-102.

134. c The normal blood pH of a dog is 7.4. Anything lower than 7.4 is considered acidic whereas anything higher than 7.4 is considered alkalotic. Bassert JM, Thomas JA, McCurnin's Clinical Textbook for Veterinary Technicians, ed 9, Elsevier, p. 845.

135. a The inability to urinate prevents the patient from excreting potassium. The potassium will be reabsorbed back into the blood, causing hyperkalemia. Sodium, calcium, and chloride are not normally excreted in the urine and are therefore not elevated when there is a urethral obstruction. Bassert JM, Thomas JA, McCurnin's Clinical Textbook for Veterinary Technicians, ed 9, Elsevier, p. 860.

136. d An esophageal stethoscope is inserted into the esophagus (to the 5th rib) in an anesthetized patient to monitor the heart rate during anesthesia. A conventional stethoscope, electrocardiograph monitor, and manual palpation of the pulse rate can be used on a patient that is awake. Thomas JA, Lerche P, Anesthesia and Analgesia for Veterinary Technicians, ed 4, Mosby, 2011, p. 145.

137. c Noninvasive monitoring is achieved without invading the body. A tympanic thermometer, stethoscope, and EKG are all noninvasive measures. Monitoring blood pressure with an arterial catheter requires placement of an arterial catheter, which is an invasive procedure. Muir WW, Hubble JAE, Handbook of Veterinary Anesthesia, ed 5, Elsevier, 2013, p. 256-257.

138. c Gaining intravenous access and being prepared to provide oxygen via an oxygen mask or through an endotracheal tube after intubation are all high priorities when treating a critical patient. Warming the patient is important (and should soon follow the other options); however, it is the lowest priority and can wait until the others have been accomplished. Silverstein D, Hopper K, Small Animal Critical Care Medicine, ed 1, Saunders, 2009, p. 5-8.

139. b Fasciculations are irregular, involuntary muscular movements. Tremors are also involuntary movements but are regular. Dyskinesia is any involuntary movement, whereas myoclonus is a sudden contraction of a muscle with immediate relaxation. Lorenz MB, Coates J, Kent M, Handbook of Veterinary Neurology, ed 5, Elsevier, 2011, p. 308-309.

140. d In a dehydrated patient, a crystalloid is the correct fluid choice. This type of fluid moves out into the interstitial space, which is where the fluid deficit is located, in a dehydrated patient. The remaining options are colloids and will draw more fluid out of the interstitial space, enhancing the dehydration. Battaglia AM, Small Animal Emergency and Critical Care for Veterinary Technicians, ed 3, Elsevier, 2015, p. 69.

141. d Hemoglobin is normally in a ferrous state ($Fe2+$), which allows the hemoglobin to carry oxygen. Methemoglobin is hemoglobin that has been oxidized to the ferric form ($Fe3+$). This gives the blood a brown color and also causes the mucous membranes to become brown. Anemia causes the mucous membranes to be pale or white, whereas bilirubinemia causes yellow mucous membranes. Hyperthermia may cause the mucous membranes to be bright red. Battaglia AM, Small Animal Emergency and Critical Care for Veterinary Technicians, ed 3, Elsevier, 2015, p. 285.

142. d Organophosphates cause classic SLUD signs: salivation, lacrimation, urination, and defecation. Grapes and lilies cause renal disease and clinical signs may not be seen for several days. Acetaminophen causes liver disease in dogs and methemoglobinemia in cats, neither of which cause these clinical signs. Battaglia AM, Small Animal Emergency and Critical Care for Veterinary Technicians, ed 3, Elsevier, 2015, p. 442.

143. a The primary layer contacts the wound, whereas the secondary layer provides padding. The tertiary layer covers the bandage and keeps it clean. Bandages do not normally include a quaternary layer. Sirois M, Principles and Practice of Veterinary Technology, ed 4, Elsevier, 2016, p. 308-310.

144. c When the core body temperature reaches 107°F, the body is no longer able to meet the increasing oxygen demands of the cells. Permanent organ damage occurs and the temperature must be lowered as soon as possible. Silverstein D, Hopper K, Small Animal Critical Care Medicine, ed 1, Saunders, 2009, p. 25.

145. c The most common clinical signs of hypoadrenocorticism (Addison's disease) are waxing and waning, including lethargy, decreased appetite, weight loss, weakness, and vomiting. Electrolyte changes include hyponatremia and hyperkalemia with a Na:K ratio of $<27:1$ (normal is 27:1–40:1). This patient's Na:K ratio is 15.4. The changes in electrolytes are a result of a decrease in aldosterone and cortisol, causing an increase in sodium excretion and a decrease in potassium excretion. A patient experiencing diabetes insipidus will have an increased water intake and an increase in urine output. A diabetic ketoacidosis patient does not have waxing and waning clinical signs. Although this patient will have changes in its blood work, hyponatremia and hyperkalemia are not classic signs for this disease. A patient experiencing a thyroid storm is more likely to experience hypokalemia. Battaglia AM, Small Animal Emergency and Critical Care for Veterinary Technicians, ed 3, Elsevier, 2015, p. 356-357.

146. a *Bordetella bronchiseptica* causes kennel cough. *Clostridium tetani* is responsible for tetanus, *Neospora caninum* causes neurological disease, and *Toxoplasmosis gondii* is seen in cats. Battaglia AM, Small Animal Emergency and Critical Care for Veterinary Medicine, ed 2, Elsevier, 2007, p. 171-177.

147. b Phenobarbital can cause hepatotoxicity and should therefore not be used in patients that already have liver disease. Levetiracetam, potassium bromide, and propofol are safe for use in patients with liver disease. Wanamaker BP, Massey KL, Applied Pharmacology for Veterinary Technicians, ed 5, Saunders, 2015, p. 88; Bassert JM, Thomas JA, McCurnin's Clinical Textbook for Veterinary Technicians, ed 9, Elsevier, p. 971-972.

148. c Because this wound has just occurred (is not old or infected) and was caused by trauma, it is considered a contaminated wound. A clean wound is aseptic, such as an incision for surgery. A clean-contaminated wound is also a surgical wound but it enters a hollow viscus (such as the stomach or bladder). A contaminated wound is caused by trauma or is a surgical incision into a contaminated area (such as the colon). A dirty-infected wound is an old, infected wound or is caused by perforated viscera (such as a perforated intestine). Bassert JM, Thomas JA, McCurnin's Clinical Textbook for Veterinary Technicians, ed 9, Elsevier, p. 921.

149. b Regular insulin has an immediate onset of action, is short lasting, and should be used for an insulin CRI. NPH, glargine, and PZI are all long-acting insulins used for the maintenance of diabetes. Battaglia AM, Small Animal Emergency and Critical Care for Veterinary Technicians, ed 3, Elsevier, 2015, p. 352-353.

150. b Magnesium is an important cofactor for the ATPase pump, which is responsible for moving potassium in and out of cells. When magnesium is low, potassium is unable to move into cells and an excessive amount of potassium is lost through the kidneys. Sodium and calcium are also affected by magnesium, but they do not have any effect on potassium. Chloride does not affect potassium levels. Silverstein D, Hopper K, Small Animal Critical Care Medicine, ed 1, Saunders, 2009, p. 240-242; DiBartola SP, Fluid, Electrolyte, and Acid-Base Disorders in Small Animal Practice, ed 4, Elsevier, 2012, p. 218-219.

151. a Potassium plays an important role in maintaining the normal resting membrane potential in muscle cells. Hypokalemia will result in muscular weakness with ventroflexion being a classical clinical sign of hypokalemia in cats. Hyponatremia causes neurological signs such as seizures and coma. Hypocalcemia causes muscle tremors and cramping, whereas hypomagnesemia causes cardiac arrhythmias. Bassert JM, Thomas JA, McCurnin's Clinical Textbook for Veterinary Technicians, ed 9, Elsevier, p. 286.

152. a The level of carbon dioxide in the arterial blood controls the depth and rate of breathing. As the carbon dioxide levels increase, a feedback mechanism increases the rate or depth of respirations. As the carbon dioxide levels decrease, the rate or depth of respirations decrease. Oxygen and humidity do not control the depth and rate of respirations. Bassert JM, Thomas JA, McCurnin's Clinical Textbook for Veterinary Technicians, ed 9, Elsevier, p. 842.

153. d Anticoagulant rodenticides cause a depletion of vitamin K-dependent coagulation factors. Factor VII is depleted first, causing an elevation in the PT. The aPTT will not be prolonged until factors II, IX, and X are depleted, which takes longer. The BMBT tests primary homeostasis (platelet function and response of the bleeding vessel) and will not increase with ingestion of an anticoagulant rodenticide. The ACT checks the time it takes for fibrin to form a clot and it may be elevated but is not diagnostic for this toxin. Silverstein D, Hopper K, Small Animal Critical Care Medicine, ed 1, Saunders, 2009, p. 317.

154. c A decrease in perfusion causes a decrease in oxygen delivery to the tissues. When this occurs, the cells must switch from aerobic metabolism to anaerobic metabolism. A byproduct of anaerobic metabolism is lactic acid, which causes an elevation in blood lactate levels. Creatinine, glucose, and sodium might also be elevated in this patient, but the elevation is more likely related to dehydration instead of perfusion. Bassert JM, Thomas JA, McCurnin's Clinical Textbook for Veterinary Technicians, ed 9, Elsevier, p. 829.

155. b An increase in the blood lactate indicates an increase in lactic acid. Because this is an acid, it causes the blood to be more acidic and a decrease in the pH would be seen. Bassert JM, Thomas JA, McCurnin's Clinical Textbook for Veterinary Technicians, ed 8, Elsevier, p. 913.

156. d Ketoacetone is not a ketone. Acetone, acetoacetate, and beta-hydroxybutyrate are all ketones. Bassert JM, Thomas JA, McCurnin's Clinical Textbook for Veterinary Technicians, ed 9, Elsevier, p. 400.

157. c The goal of oxygen therapy is to decrease hypoxemia by increasing the oxygen content in the blood, to decrease the work of breathing (preventing the patient from tiring and going into respiratory arrest), and to decrease the work of the myocardium (preventing the patient from entering cardiac arrest). An improvement in mentation may be seen but is not a goal of oxygen therapy. Wingfield WE, Veterinary Emergency Medicine Secrets, ed 2, Hanley & Belfus, p. 18.

158. c The blood in the ventricles causes the myocardial fibers to stretch. The more these fibers stretch, the stronger the contraction of the heart (akin to stretching a rubber band; the more it is stretched, the further it will travel). The amount of stretch on the heart is called the preload. The afterload is the amount of force or pressure the heart has to push against (or the pressure required to open the aortic valve) to expel blood from the ventricles. Contractility is how strongly the heart is able to contract and resistance refers to the resistance in the blood vessels. Battaglia AM, Small Animal Emergency and Critical Care for Veterinary Medicine, ed 1, Saunders, 2001, p. 180.

159. c These clinical signs all point toward pericardial effusion. This occurs when the pericardial sac surrounding the heart fills with blood. This prevents the heart from beating effectively, causing collapse. Inspiration changes the pressure in the thoracic cavity and causes blood to flow into the right side of the heart, decreasing pulse pressure. With each beat the heart changes position in the pericardial sac, causing the height of the QRS wave to change height. Pneumothorax, heart failure, and hypovolemia may cause one of these clinical signs but not all. Battaglia AM, Small Animal Emergency and Critical Care for Veterinary Technicians, ed 3, Elsevier, 2015, p. 356-314-315.

160. a Prothrombin time measures coagulation factors I (fibrinogen), II (prothrombin), V, VII, and X. Battaglia AM, Small Animal Emergency and Critical Care for Veterinary Technicians, ed 3, Elsevier, 2015, p. 356-279-280.

161. c A mean arterial pressure of 60 mmHg (or a systolic of 90 mmHg) is required to maintain adequate perfusion to vital organs. A mean arterial pressure of 70 mmHg is adequate but should be monitored closely and action should be taken if it continues to decrease. Silverstein D, Hopper K, Small Animal Critical Care Medicine, ed 1, Saunders, 2009, p. 708-709.

162. a Bromethalin causes cerebral edema, therefore causing neurological signs. An easy way to remember this is that the word contains "meth" (meaning methamphetamine), which can have neurological effects in people. The other rodenticides listed are all anticoagulant rodenticides and cause clinical signs associated with hemorrhage. Bassert JM, Thomas JA, McCurnin's Clinical Textbook for Veterinary Technicians, ed 9, Elsevier, p. 912.

163. a This breathing pattern is known as Cheyne-Stokes and is caused by an interruption in the regulation of breathing via carbon dioxide levels. Kussmaul's breathing is a deep, regular breathing pattern. Paradoxical breathing occurs when there is a disruption in the chest wall (such as a segment of broken ribs). This section of the chest wall will move in the opposite direction compared with the rest of the chest wall. Orthopnea refers to a position instead of a pattern. The patient will sit or stand with the neck stretched out and elbows rotated away from the body in an attempt to decrease airway resistance and to make breathing easier. This is an indication that the patient is tiring and should be watched closely for respiratory arrest. Bassert JM, Thomas JA, McCurnin's Clinical Textbook for Veterinary Technicians, ed 9, Elsevier, p. 842.

164. c Signs of tick paralysis usually appear 7 days after the tick has attached. After the tick is removed, clinical signs will start to resolve in 24 hours and will completely resolve in 72 hours. Silverstein D, Hopper K, Small Animal Critical Care Medicine, ed 1, Saunders, 2009, p. 139.

165. b Hypoglycemia is a common finding in septic patients. This has several causes, including decreased intake by the patient, decreased production by the liver because of hepatic dysfunction, and increased consumption by cells. Hypoglycemia in sepsis is not caused by an increase in insulin. Silverstein D, Hopper K, Small Animal Critical Care Medicine, ed 1, Saunders, 2009, p. 298.

166. b Misoprostol is a prostaglandin used to decrease secretion of hydrogen in the stomach as well as to increase the production of mucus and bicarbonate. These elements act to decrease or prevent the formation of ulcers. This medication can also cause abortion in pregnant patients and people and it should therefore not be used in pregnant patients. Owners should be cautioned and instructed to wear gloves when handling. Wanamaker BP, Massey KL, Applied Pharmacology for Veterinary Technicians, ed 5, Saunders, 2014, p. 159-160.

167. a A Doppler is a piece of equipment that is used to measure blood pressure. Central venous pressure is measured with a manometer, SpO_2 is measured with a pulse oximeter, and end-tidal CO_2 is measured with a capnograph. Aspinall V, Clinical Procedures in Veterinary Nursing, ed 3, Butterworth-Heinemann, 2014, p. 118.

168. b An increase in intraocular pressure (IOP) is diagnostic for glaucoma. This is caused by an increase in the fluid in the eye, which increases the intraocular pressure, causing damage to the optic nerve and, if not treated, blindness. Uveitis is caused by inflammation of the uvea and can cause either an increase or a decrease in IOP. Ulcerative keratitis (or corneal ulcers) does not cause an increase in IOP. Blepharitis is swelling of the eyelids and is usually secondary to irritation, allergies, or a viral or bacterial infection. Blepharitis does not cause an increase in IOP. Summers A, Common Diseases of Companion Animals, ed 4, Elsevier, 2019, p. 80-81.

169. d Blepharospasm (squinting) is caused by irritation to the eye. Intraocular pressure, lacrimation, and ocular discharge are all clinical signs (not causes) of ocular disease. Summers A, Common Diseases of Companion Animals, ed 4, Elsevier, 2019, p. 367-368.

170. a The most common cause of hypercalcemia (in dogs) is neoplasia. Pregnancy most commonly causes hypocalcemia, whereas vomiting and diarrhea do not directly cause hypercalcemia. Bassert JM, Thomas JA, McCurnin's Clinical Textbook for Veterinary Technicians, ed 9, Elsevier, p. 726.

171. b Normal mentation in a patient is BAR (bright, alert, responsive) or QAR (quiet, alert, responsive). As mentation decreases, the patient progresses from quiet to obtunded (a decrease in responsiveness to its environment), to stuporous (only responsive to painful stimuli), and finally the patient becomes comatose (unresponsive to any stimuli). Silverstein D, Hopper K, Small Animal Critical Care Medicine, ed 1, Saunders, 2009, p. 34.

172. c High-rise syndrome refers to an animal (most commonly a cat) that falls from a great height. After the cat passes seven stories, it reaches terminal velocity and the vestibular system is no longer stimulated. At this point the cat becomes more horizontal, which spreads the impact over a larger area, decreasing the possibility of a life-threatening injury. Silverstein D, Hopper K, Small Animal Critical Care Medicine, ed 1, Saunders, 2009, p. 665.

173. a The end-tidal CO_2 is a valuable monitoring tool during anesthesia and CPR. The end-tidal CO_2 should be 2–5 mmHg less than the $PaCO_2$. This should allow you to monitor the animal's ventilation (which is indicated by the CO_2) without needing to perform a blood gas. Thomas J, Lerche P, Anesthesia and Analgesia for Veterinary Technicians, ed 5, Mosby, 2016, p. 195.

174. c The cardiorespiratory arrest was most probably caused by air in the fluid line. A bolus of air can be trapped in the vein or heart, causing an obstruction. This is also called an air embolus and can be deadly. An intravenous catheter that is not patent will only cause an obstruction of the flow of fluid or will cause pain. A high fluid rate will cause fluid overload and could eventually cause death, but this would not occur so quickly. It is unlikely that a young, healthy patient has an underlying disease that would cause sudden death. Silverstein D, Hopper K, Small Animal Critical Care Medicine, ed 1, Saunders, 2009, p. 744.

175. d Feline panleukopenia is caused by the parvovirus and can be diagnosed with a canine parvovirus snap test. Changes may be seen on the complete blood count, electrolyte panel, and blood gas, but these will not be specifically diagnostic for panleukopenia. Bassert JM, Thomas JA, McCurnin's Clinical Textbook for Veterinary Technicians, ed 8, Elsevier, p. 270.

176. b An activated partial thromboplastin time tests coagulation factors I (fibrinogen), II (prothrombin), V, and VIII–XII. Bonagura JD, Twedt DC, Kirk's Current Veterinary Therapy XV, Elsevier, 2014, p. 288.

177. c CPP is the pressure inside the cranial vault and is controlled by tissue and fluid within the space. CPP = MAP - ICP. As the intracranial pressure increases, the mean arterial pressure must also increase to maintain the cerebral perfusion pressure and blood flow (and thus oxygen delivery) to the brain. Silverstein D, Hopper K, Small Animal Critical Care Medicine, ed 1, Saunders, 2009, p. 883.

178. b Type II hypersensitivity occurs when antibodies attack normal cells. Type I hypersensitivity is related to mast cells and causes clinical signs related to allergies. A type III hypersensitivity is caused by the combination of antibodies and antigens. When this occurs, immune complexes are formed and cause inflammation. Type IV hypersensitivity is a delayed response to some sort of irritant. Tizard IR, Veterinary Immunology, ed 9, Elsevier, 2013, p. 346.

179. b The current that flows through the body is equal to the amperage, which is a function of voltage/resistance. Resistance decreases with wet tissue (including mucous membranes) and decreases with dry tissue. Therefore, the wetter the tissue, the more damage that is done. A dry animal will not experience as much of a shock unless it chews the cord and the cord comes in contact with the mucous membranes. Shaving the animal will not make any difference in regard to resistance. Wearing metal tags may increase damage if the electrical charge comes directly in contact with the tags. Silverstein D, Hopper K, Small Animal Critical Care Medicine, ed 1, Saunders, 2009, p. 687.

180. c Beta-hydroxybutyrate is the most prominent ketone seen in ketoacidosis. The urine ketone strip reacts with acetoacetate instead of beta-hydroxybutyrate. Beta-hydroxybutyrate can be detected in the serum, which is a more sensitive measurement than urine. Silverstein D, Hopper K, Small Animal Critical Care Medicine, ed 1, Saunders, 2009, p. 289.

181. b A patient with a flail chest should be placed with the affected side down. This will help stabilize the flail segment as well as allow the unaffected, healthy lung to expand. Placing the patient with the affected side up will prevent the healthy side from expanding fully and the patient will not be willing to expand the affected side, which will decrease his oxygenation. A dyspneic patient should never be placed in dorsal recumbency. Placing the dog in sternal recumbency will allow the lungs to expand but will not stabilize the affected area. Silverstein D, Hopper K, Small Animal Critical Care Medicine, ed 1, Saunders, 2009, p. 139.

182. d Because metoclopramide is a prokinetic drug that increases gastrointestinal motility, it should not be used in a patient with a gastrointestinal obstruction. Many postoperative patients benefit from metoclopramide as do patients with pancreatitis. Papich MG, Saunders Handbook of Veterinary Drugs: Small and Large Animal, ed 4, Elsevier, 2015, p. 520-521.

183. c A pericardiocentesis is performed on the right side of the chest to avoid damage to the lungs and the coronary arteries. The chest should be shaved and surgically prepped from the 3rd to the 7th ribs. Silverstein D, Hopper K, Small Animal Critical Care Medicine, ed 1, Saunders, 2009, p. 182-183.

184. b When a patient's temperature drops to 83°F–86°F, it has a decrease in cardiac function causing the patient to become comatose and develop cardiac arrhythmias and muscular rigidity. The patient goes into cardiac arrest when its temperature is below 83°F. Between 86°F and 93°F, the patient becomes stuporous and bradycardic, and at 93°F–98°F, the patient is still alert, tachycardic, and shivers in response to the hypothermia. Matthews KA, Veterinary Emergency and Critical Care Manual, ed 2, Lifelearn, 2006, p. 291.

185. c Tumor lysis syndrome can be evident after a patient receives chemotherapy for a highly responsive neoplasia (such as lymphoma). This can occur within a few hours or it might not happen for several days after receiving chemotherapy. The breakdown of the cancer cells causes a release of cellular contents that causes vomiting, diarrhea, depression, and signs of shock (pale mucous membranes, prolonged CRT, and bradycardia). Signs of extravasation are local and are seen at the site of the injection. Heart failure is not usually associated with chemotherapy and sterile hemorrhagic cystitis is associated with bloody urine. Bassert JM, Thomas JA, McCurnin's Clinical Textbook for Veterinary Technicians, ed 9, Elsevier, p. 742.

186. a As soon as the extravasation occurs, injection of the medication should stop immediately. When extravasation does occur, it is recommended to try to withdraw as much medication as possible back through the intravenous catheter. The area should be infiltrated with saline, dexamethasone sodium phosphate, and sodium bicarbonate around the site. In addition, a warm compress should be applied to help increase circulation to the area. Silverstein DC, Hopper K, Small Animal Critical Care Medicine, ed 2, Elsevier, 2015, p. 909-910.

187. c Stroke volume (the amount of blood pumped from the heart with one contraction) is determined by the preload, afterload, and contractility. Heart rate does not determine stroke volume. Battaglia AM, Small

Animal Emergency and Critical Care for Veterinary Technicians, ed 3, Elsevier, 2015, p. 303.

188. c One of the most common problems associated with chemotherapy is myelosuppression, which manifests itself through acute vomiting, diarrhea, and fever. A complete blood count shows neutropenia resulting from suppression of the white blood cells. Monocytosis is an increase in monocytes and is not seen with chemotherapy. Anemia and thrombocytopenia are also not commonly associated with chemotherapy. Bonagura JD, Twedt DC, Kirk's Current Veterinary Therapy XV, Elsevier, 2014, p. 330-331.

189. d The weakness, collapse, and quick recovery indicate syncope. This is secondary to heart disease and is caused by a lack of blood flow (and therefore oxygen delivery) to the brain. If the dog had a seizure, he would have had a postictal period and would not have returned to normality as quickly. Anaphylaxis may have occurred quickly and resulted in collapse, but the dog would have not recovered without medical care. The same can be said about cardiac arrest. Bassert JM, Thomas JA, McCurnin's Clinical Textbook for Veterinary Technicians, ed 8, Elsevier, p. 686.

190. d The history and clinical signs indicate tetanus. This is caused by *Clostridium tetani*, which gains access to the body through open wounds. The bacteria produce tetanospasmin, a toxin that prevents the release of neurotransmitters that inhibit the firing of neurons. When this occurs, these neurons fire uncontrollably, causing the muscles to become stiff and the patient is unable to relax. Seizure activity, bromethalin toxicity, and botulism do not cause these classic clinical signs. Battaglia AM, Small Animal Emergency and Critical Care for Veterinary Medicine, ed 2, Elsevier, 2007, p. 177.

191. a Myasthenia gravis is often associated with megaesophagus. Another common complaint is weakness associated with exercise that resolves with rest, which is caused by a neuromuscular transmission disorder. In the acquired form, antibodies are produced that attack the acetylcholine neurotransmitters. In the congenital form, there is a lack of neurotransmitters. A myopathy is associated with muscle stiffness instead of weakness. Polyradiculoneuritis is associated with weakness that starts in the hind legs and moves forward. This is also known as coonhound paralysis and is seen after a dog has been exposed to saliva from a raccoon (and is therefore not associated with megaesophagus). Tick paralysis does not resolve until the tick is removed; therefore the patient would not recover with rest. Bassert JM, Thomas JA, McCurnin's Clinical Textbook for Veterinary Technicians, ed 9, Elsevier, p. 656.

192. a A patient with an increased inspiratory effort probably has an upper airway obstruction. This may be the result of a foreign body, brachycephalic disease, or swelling secondary to an allergic reaction. An increased expiratory effort is associated with lower airway disease. Lung disease can be indicated by an overall increased respiratory rate and effort, whereas pleural space disease is associated with a shallow, rapid respiratory pattern. Ford RB, Mazzaferro EM, Kirk and Bistner's Handbook of Veterinary Procedures and Emergency Treatment, ed 9, Elsevier, 2012, p. 256.

193. b Abdominal effusion associated with trauma may be blood or urine. If the fluid is clear, a uroabdomen can be confirmed by comparing the potassium of the abdominal effusion with the potassium of the serum. A uroabdomen is confirmed if the ratio of the abdominal fluid potassium and serum potassium is 1.9:1. A uroabdomen can also be confirmed by comparing the creatinine of the abdominal effusion with the serum creatinine. If there is a 2:1 ratio (fluid: serum), a uroabdomen is confirmed. A hemoabdomen would be confirmed by the presence of blood in the abdomen. Peritonitis may cause mild abdominal effusion, but the fluid does not contain creatinine. The fluid seen in a septic abdomen contains white blood cells and bacteria. Silverstein D, Hopper K, Small Animal Critical Care Medicine, ed 1, Saunders, 2009, p. 673.

194. d A release of endotoxin secondary to pyometra causes a decrease in the ability of the renal tubules to concentrate urine, which causes the patient to experience polyuria and polydipsia. Being febrile does not increase thirst and the release of prostaglandins does not cause polyuria/polydipsia. Dehydration does not cause polyuria/polydipsia. Ford RB, Mazzaferro EM, Kirk and Bistner's Handbook of Veterinary Procedures and Emergency Treatment, ed 9, Elsevier, 2012, p. 134-135.

195. d The preferred antidote for ethylene glycol toxicity is 4-methylpraole. Ethanol can be used if 4-methylprazole is unavailable. Ethylene glycol is metabolized by alcohol dehydrogenase into glycolaldehyde, which in turn is oxidized into the toxic components of ethylene glycol. 4-methylpyrazole prevents the metabolism of ethylene glycol through the inhibition of alcohol dehydrogenase. Calcium EDTA is used as an antidote for zinc poisoning. Deferoxamine is used in iron toxicity, whereas acetylcysteine is the antidote for acetaminophen toxicity. Battaglia AM, Small Animal Emergency and Critical Care for Veterinary Technicians, ed 3, Elsevier, 2015, p. 446-47.

196. b When obtaining an EKG, the patient should be placed in right lateral recumbency (unless the patient does not tolerate this position). This position provides the most accurate reading. Bassert JM, Thomas JA, McCurnin's Clinical Textbook for Veterinary Technicians, ed 9, Elsevier, p. 860-861.

197. b The P wave indicates depolarization of the atria. Repolarization of the atria is hidden within the QRS complex and is rarely seen. The QRS complex indicates depolarization of the ventricles, whereas repolarization is indicated by the T wave. Bassert JM, Thomas JA, McCurnin's Clinical Textbook for Veterinary Technicians, ed 9, Elsevier, p. 864.

198. b When the EKG indicates that a patient no longer has a heartbeat, you should immediately auscultate the heart. You should not start CPR until cardiorespiratory arrest is confirmed. You should never assume the monitoring equipment is incorrect, but should always confirm what it is indicating. If you auscultate a heartbeat, you can adjust the EKG leads. Thomas JA, Lerche P,

Anesthesia and Analgesia for Veterinary Technicians, ed 4, Mosby, 2011, p. 151.

199. a The transducer should be placed at the level of the heart. Any other location will provide inaccurate readings. Silverstein D, Hopper K, Small Animal Critical Care Medicine, ed 1, Saunders, 2009, p. 861.

200. b The pulse pressure (the pressure that allows you to feel a patient's pulse) is the difference between the systolic and diastolic pressures. If these numbers are close together, the pulse will not be as strong, and if they are further apart, the pulse will be stronger. Central venous pressure is the pressure in the right atrium, mean arterial pressure is the overall pressure of the cardiac cycle, and the blood pressure includes the systolic, diastolic, and mean arterial pressures. Bassert JM, Thomas JA, McCurnin's Clinical Textbook for Veterinary Technicians, ed 9, Elsevier, p. 214.

201. d The central venous pressure measures the pressure at the right atrium and the zero on the manometer should therefore be level with the right atrium. If it is held higher than the right atrium, the water level in the manometer will drop and provide a falsely low reading. If it is held too low, the water level in the manometer will rise and give a falsely elevated reading. Silverstein D, Hopper K, Small Animal Critical Care Medicine, ed 1, Saunders, 2009, p. 862.

202. d The expected PaO_2 of a patient that is breathing room-air should be five times the fraction of inspired oxygen. The concentration of oxygen of room-air is 21%. 21×5 is roughly 100 mmHg. If the patient is on 100% oxygen, the expected PaO_2 would be 500 mmHg. Bassert JM, Thomas JA, McCurnin's Clinical Textbook for Veterinary Technicians, ed 8, Elsevier, p. 921.

203. a A temporary tracheostomy tube is placed in the area of the 2nd to 4th tracheal rings. To keep the site clean and free of hair, a large area should be shaved. It is recommended to shave from the mandible to the manubrium and the area should be wide enough to encompass each jugular vein. Creedon JMB, Davis H, Advanced Monitoring and Procedures for Small Animal Emergency and Critical Care, ed 1, Wiley-Blackwell, 2012, p. 308-309.

204. c To access the area for tracheostomy placement easily, the patient should be positioned dorsally with the legs pulled caudally. It would be difficult to access the trachea if the patient was in lateral recumbency and pulling the legs cranially would obscure the area. Creedon JMB, Davis H, Advanced Monitoring and Procedures for Small Animal Emergency and Critical Care, ed 1, Wiley-Blackwell, 2012, p. 308.

205. a The veins, nerves, and arteries are on the caudal side of the rib and to avoid hitting them, the needle should be inserted (with the bevel up) on the cranial side of the rib. After the needle is inserted into the chest, it is angled down so that the needle is lying against the chest wall and the bevel is facing the lungs. This decreases the likelihood of lacerating lung tissue. Bassert JM, Thomas JA, McCurnin's Clinical Textbook for Veterinary Technicians, ed 9, Elsevier, p. 566-567.

206. c When performing a diagnostic peritoneal lavage, 20 mL/kg of sterile saline is infused into the abdomen. The patient should be gently rotated to allow the fluid to move around in the abdomen and then it is removed. Creedon JMB, Davis H, Advanced Monitoring and Procedures for Small Animal Emergency and Critical Care, ed 1, Wiley-Blackwell, 2012, p. 308.

207. b When preparing placement of a nasogastric tube, it should be measured from the nares to the last rib. This will ensure that the tube is in the stomach. Measuring to the thoracic inlet, 5th rib, or 10th rib places the tube in the esophagus and fails to place (or remove) anything from the stomach. It also increases the risk of aspiration. Silverstein D, Hopper K, Small Animal Critical Care Medicine, ed 1, Saunders, 2009, p. 586.

208. d Studies have shown that washing hands between patients is the best way to prevent or reduce nosocomial infections. Barrier nursing and cleaning the facility are also important, but they fall behind handwashing. Administering antibiotics before an infection is present is not advised, because it can cause resistant bacteria. Creedon JMB, Davis H, Advanced Monitoring and Procedures for Small Animal Emergency and Critical Care, ed 1, Wiley-Blackwell, 2012, p. 697.

209. c Mannitol crystalizes and should be infused with a filter to ensure any crystals present are not injected into the patient. Cerenia, enrofloxacin, and propofol will not crystalize; therefore, a filter is not required. Silverstein D, Hopper K, Small Animal Critical Care Medicine, ed 1, Saunders, 2009, p. 428.

210. b Calculate the mg required/day and then break it down to mg/h: $10\ \text{kg} \times 2\ \text{mg/kg/day} = 20\ \text{mg/day}$ $20\ \text{mg/day}/24\ \text{h} = 0.83\ \text{mg/h}$. Calculate how many hours the fluid bag will last: $1000\ \text{mL}/100\ \text{mL} = 10\ \text{h}$. Calculate how many mg are required to last the same amount of time: $10\ \text{h} \times 0.83\ \text{mg/h} = 8.3\ \text{mg}/1000\ \text{mL}$. Calculate the mL required: $8.3\ \text{mg}/5\ \text{mg/mL} = 1.7\ \text{mL}$ metoclopramide. Lake T, Green N, Essential Calculations for Veterinary Nurses and Technicians, ed 2, Elsevier, 2009, p. 99-105.

211. c Skin that is yellow/black is considered a deep partial-thickness burn. It will have decreased sensation because the nerves are damaged. A superficial burn is also known as a first-degree burn. The skin will be red, dry, and painful. A superficial burn with partial thickness is considered a second-degree burn. The skin will still have hair present and there will be leakage of plasma from the area. A full-thickness burn is considered a third-degree burn. This will affect the muscle, tendon, and bone. The skin will be leathery and will have no sensation. Silverstein D, Hopper K, Small Animal Critical Care Medicine, ed 1, Saunders, 2009, p. 683; Creedon JMB, Davis H, Advanced Monitoring and Procedures for Small Animal Emergency and Critical Care, ed 1, Wiley-Blackwell, 2012, p. 779.

212. c During heatstroke, the peripheral veins vasodilate. This allows the blood to move to the periphery and be cooled through radiation. Ice and cold water should be avoided. These cause peripheral vasoconstriction, preventing cooling via convection as well as shunting the blood to vital organs, causing irreversible damage. A fan takes advantage of cooling through convection, whereas intravenous fluids increase blood flow to the periphery, which increases cooling. Tepid water applied to the skin increases cooling while avoiding vasoconstriction. Ford RB, Mazzaferro EM, Kirk and Bistner's Handbook of Veterinary Procedures and Emergency Treatment, ed 9, Elsevier, 2012, p. 145-146.

213. c When a mistake is made, a line should be drawn through it so that it is still legible. The mistake should be initialed and the correct information entered. If the mistake is scratched out or blacked out, it will be illegible. A mistake should be written in pen so that it cannot be erased. Prendergast H, Front Office Management for the Veterinary Team, ed 2, Saunders, 2019, p. 152.

214. a An acute, severe upper airway obstruction (such as seen in a choking episode) causes a decrease in the intrathoracic pressure because the patient is breathing against an obstruction. This causes an increase in pulmonary arterial pressure, which forces fluid across the capillary wall into the alveoli, resulting in a noncardiogenic pulmonary edema. King LG, Textbook of Respiratory Disease in Dogs and Cats, ed 1, Saunders, 2003, p. 283.

215. b Central vestibular disease includes causes found within the brain. These include neoplasia, infection, and inflammation. Peripheral vestibular disease includes causes found outside the brain. These include otitis interna and otitis media. Battaglia AM, Small Animal Emergency and Critical Care for Veterinary Technicians, ed 3, Elsevier, 2015, p. 420-423.

216. a A Robert Jones bandage is used to stabilize fractures distal to the elbow and is most appropriate for this fracture. An Elmer sling is used to stabilize the hip, whereas a Velpeau sling is used to stabilize the shoulder. A spica splint is also used to stabilize the shoulder as well as the forelimb. Bassert JM, Thomas JA, McCurnin's Clinical Textbook for Veterinary Technicians, ed 9, Elsevier, p. 928-929.

217. a Because of the location of the esophagus, the left side of the neck is preferred. An esophagostomy tube is a feeding tube placed through the neck and into the esophagus, therefore it will not be placed through the abdomen. Bassert JM, Thomas JA, McCurnin's Clinical Textbook for Veterinary Technicians, ed 9, Elsevier, p. 311-312.

218. a Cryoprecipitate contains von Willebrand factor, factor VIII, fibrinogen, and fibronectin and it would therefore be appropriate in this patient. Fresh whole blood contains red blood cells, white blood cells, proteins, and coagulation factors, whereas packed red blood cells contain red blood cells. Fresh frozen plasma contains albumin and coagulation factors. Battaglia AM, Small Animal Emergency and Critical Care for Veterinary Technicians, ed 3, Elsevier, 2015, p. 81-82.

219. b Antibodies against red blood cells develop within 5–7 days of receiving a transfusion. For this reason, if it has been 5 days, a crossmatch should be performed before a second transfusion is attempted. If it has not been 5 days and an additional transfusion is required, a crossmatch is not required, although some doctors will order one anyway. Bassert JM, Thomas JA, McCurnin's Clinical Textbook for Veterinary Technicians, ed 8, Elsevier, p. 136.

220. c Heating wood pulp and then washing it in inorganic acids produces activated charcoal. After it is dry, the particles are activated with acid or steam, producing a product that contains a very large surface area. A total of 1 g of activated charcoal contains 1000 m^2 of surface area, which is why it is so effective when used to prevent absorption of toxins. Peterson ME, Talcott PA, Small Animal Toxicology, ed 2, Elsevier, 2006, p. 136.

221. a When hypernatremia occurs, fluid is pulled out of the cell in an attempt to equalize the concentration of sodium. This causes the cells to shrink and, in response, the body produces idiogenic osmoles, which prevent fluid from being pulled out of the cells. This does not occur with hyperkalemia, hyperchloremia, or hyponatremia. Silverstein D, Hopper K, Small Animal Critical Care Medicine, ed 1, Saunders, 2009, p. 226.

222. d A pulse oximeter is unable to detect abnormal hemoglobin (such as carboxyhemoglobin or methemoglobin); therefore, the machine will show a normal pulse oxygen value. Silverstein D, Hopper K, Small Animal Critical Care Medicine, ed 1, Saunders, 2009, p. 882.

223. c The activated clotting time measures the function of intrinsic and common pathways. The activated partial thromboplastin time tests the intrinsic pathway whereas the prothrombin time tests the extrinsic pathway. The buccal mucosal bleeding time checks platelet function. It shows the amount of time it takes for platelets to be activated and to form a primary platelet plug. Ford RB, Mazzaferro EM, Kirk and Bistner's Handbook of Veterinary Procedures and Emergency Treatment, ed 9, Elsevier, 2012, p. 489-490.

224. b *Clostridium tetani* is responsible for tetanus. *Bordetella bronchiseptica* causes kennel cough. *Neospora caninum* causes neurological disease. *Toxoplasmosis gondii* is seen in cats. Silverstein DC, Hopper K. Small Animal Critical Care Medicine, ed. 1, Elsevier; 2009, p. 427-428.

225. a Atropine is an anticholinergic used to treat bradycardia, as a preanesthetic, or as an antidote for organophosphate toxicity. Mannitol is an osmotic diuretic that decreases intracranial pressure by reducing blood viscosity. This allows an increase in blood flow (and thus an increase in oxygen delivery) to the brain and it causes a decrease in the water content of the brain as well. Diazepam is a benzodiazepine used for sedation, muscle relaxation, or treatment of seizure activity. Dexamethasone is a glucocorticoid that is often used to decrease inflammation. Silverstein DC, Hopper K. Small Animal Critical Care Medicine, ed. 1, Elsevier; 2009, p. 427-428.

SECTION 13

1. c Communicating directly with the clinician about particular concerns shows the veterinarian that the technician is aware of pain and assessment. It also provides the clinician with information if medication changes are necessary. Although monitoring urine and fecal output is important, unless it has direct bearing on a particular case it would not be the best answer to this question. Veterinary technicians cannot change ineffective medication without input from the attending clinician. It is important that the veterinary technician sees the animal receive the medication directly and this should therefore not be passed off to someone else. Goldberg ME, Chapter 22, "Pain Management," in Tighe MM, Brown M, Mosby's Comprehensive Review for Veterinary Technicians, ed 5, Elsevier/Mosby, 2020, p. 496

2. b Resentment of being handled, aggression, and abnormal posture are all three characteristics of pain in cats. Sleeping continuously, overeating, and attention-seeking behaviors are not indicative of pain. Hyperactivity, pupillary enlargement, and tail swishing combined would not necessarily indicate pain. Hypotension, hypocapnia, hypopnea, and bradycardia are not signs of pain; increased heart rate, increased respiratory rate, and dilated pupils would be expected instead. Goldberg ME, Chapter 22, "Pain Management," in Tighe MM, Brown M, Mosby's Comprehensive Review for Veterinary Technicians, ed 5, Elsevier/Mosby, 2020, p. 497, 499.
3. a A pain assessment should be completed every 4–6 hours. Assessment every 30 minutes to 1 hour is not needed unless the time period is within the immediate postoperative period. Assessing every 8 and 12–24 hours is not often enough. Goldberg ME, Chapter 22, "Pain Management," in Tighe MM, Brown M, Mosby's Comprehensive Review for Veterinary Technicians, ed 5, Elsevier/Mosby, 2020, p. 500.
4. b Speaking in low tones and interacting with the animal makes the patient feel better, but behaviors will resume when the interaction stops (this will show that the patient has pain and is not dysphoric). Placing the patient on comfortable blankets will not relieve an animal with dysphoria; it would be comforting, but it will not stop dysphoric behavior. Moving the animal to a different ward would help; again this shows that the patient can be comforted, but it will not stop dysphoric behavior. Automatically reversing the analgesic medication is reserved. Goldberg ME, Chapter 22, "Pain Management," in Tighe MM, Brown M, Mosby's Comprehensive Review for Veterinary Technicians, ed 5, Elsevier/Mosby, 2020, p. 500.
5. c Pain is the 4th Vital Sign as set forth by the 2015 AAHA-AAFP Pain Management Guidelines. Epstein ME, Rodan I, Griffenhagen G, et al. 2015 AAHA/AAFP Pain Management Guidelines for Dogs and Cats, Journal of Feline Medicine and Surgery (2015) 17, 251-272.
6. a Nociception is defined as the activity in the peripheral pathway that transmits and processes the information about the stimulus to the brain. Adaptive acute pain is a normal response to tissue damage. Pain without apparent biological value that has persisted beyond the normal tissue healing time of (approximately) 3 months is defined as chronic maladaptive pain. Allodynia is defined as any stimuli to the affected area that would normally be innocuous, which becomes noxious. Goldberg ME, Chapter 22, "Pain Management," in Tighe MM, Brown M, Mosby's Comprehensive Review for Veterinary Technicians, ed 5, Elsevier/Mosby, 2020, p. 501.
7. a The correct sequence of the pain pathway is transduction, transmission, modulation, and perception. Goldberg ME, Chapter 22, "Pain Management," in Tighe MM, Brown M, Mosby's Comprehensive Review for Veterinary Technicians, ed 5, Elsevier/Mosby, 2020, p. 501-502.
8. d Wind-up is described as the perceived increase in pain intensity with time when a given painful stimulus is delivered repeatedly above a critical rate. An increase in the excitability of spinal neurons, mediated in part by the activation of NMDA receptors in dorsal horn neurons, is defined as central sensitization. Peripheral sensitization occurs when tissue inflammation leads to the release of a complex array of chemical mediators, resulting in reduced nociceptor thresholds. Brief trauma or noxious stimuli are described as phase 1 of chronic maladaptive pain. Goldberg ME, Chapter 22, "Pain Management," in Tighe MM, Brown M, Mosby's Comprehensive Review for Veterinary Technicians, ed 5, Elsevier/Mosby, 2020, p. 503.
9. c Morphine is an opioid agonist, whereas butorphanol and buprenorphine are partial agonists, and naloxone is an antagonist. Goldberg ME, Chapter 22, "Pain Management," in Tighe MM, Brown M, Mosby's Comprehensive Review for Veterinary Technicians, ed 5, Elsevier/Mosby, 2020, p. 506.
10. d Prostaglandins play an important role in mammalian renal physiology. The production of endorphins and leukotrienes does not involve prostaglandins, nor is it involved in mammalian cardiovascular physiology. Goldberg ME. Chapter 22, "Pain Management," in Tighe MM, Brown M (eds), Mosby's Comprehensive Review for Veterinary Technicians, ed 5, Elsevier/Mosby, 2020, p. 508.
11. a Ketamine is a NMDA antagonist. Lidocaine is a sodium channel blocker, meperidine is considered an opioid, and dexmedetomidine is an alpha-2 adrenoceptor agonist. Goldberg ME, Chapter 22, "Pain Management," in Tighe MM, Brown M, Mosby's Comprehensive Review for Veterinary Technicians, ed 5, Elsevier/Mosby, 2020, p. 510.
12. c Gabapentin in an antiepileptic drug. Corticosteroids, such as prednisolone, have powerful anti-inflammatory and immunosuppressive effects. Sodium channel blockers are agents that impair conduction of sodium ions and they include drugs such as lidocaine or bupivacaine. Nutraceuticals are medications such as glucosamine and chondroitin. Goldberg ME, Chapter 22, "Pain Management," in Tighe MM, Brown M, Mosby's Comprehensive Review for Veterinary Technicians, ed 5, Elsevier/Mosby, 2020, p. 512.
13. b EMLA cream is a eutectic mixture of local anesthetics (lidocaine and prilocaine) applied topically, which produces anesthesia to a maximum depth of 5 mm, is applied to the skin, and is left in place for at least 1 hour. Buprenorphine is administered either by injection or as a transmucosal agent. Bupivacaine is only administered by injection. Fentanyl is administered via injection or transdermal patch. Goldberg ME, Chapter 22, "Pain Management," in Tighe MM, Brown M, Mosby's Comprehensive Review for Veterinary Technicians, ed 5, Elsevier/Mosby, 2020, p. 513.
14. b Intratesticular blocks are excellent for canine and feline orchiectomies. Intratesticular blocks can be used in many species and veterinary patients, not just for large animal patients. They do not require the use

of a vaporizer because injectable anesthetics are used. Goldberg ME, Chapter 22, "Pain Management," in Tighe MM, Brown M, Mosby's Comprehensive Review for Veterinary Technicians, ed 5, Elsevier/Mosby, 2020, p. 517.

15. d Veterinary technicians should never leave patients on CRI for long periods unobserved. Benefits of CRIs include providing a more stable plane of analgesia with less incidence of breakthrough pain, providing a greater control over drug administration. CRIs allow a lower dose of drug to be delivered at any given time, resulting in a lower incidence of dose-related side effects. Goldberg ME, Chapter 22, "Pain Management," in Tighe MM, Brown M, Mosby's Comprehensive Review for Veterinary Technicians, ed 5, Elsevier/Mosby, 2020, p. 518.

16. a Massage is an example of manual therapy. Effleurage technique is a type of massage and physical modalities involve the use of light, heat, sound, water, and electrotherapies. Therapeutic exercise is not a form of massage because massage does not involve the use of the animal's movement. Goldberg ME, Chapter 22, "Pain Management," in Tighe MM, Brown M, Mosby's Comprehensive Review for Veterinary Technicians, ed 5, Elsevier/Mosby, 2020, p. 520.

17. b Cryotherapy decreases the production of pain mediators, leading to analgesia. Cryotherapy does not decrease metabolism and it is certainly not recommended in treating or preventing hyperthermia. If cryotherapy is used post injury, it must be applied within the first 48 hours. Goldberg ME, Chapter 22, "Pain Management,"in Tighe MM, Brown M, Mosby's Comprehensive Review for Veterinary Technicians, ed 5, Elsevier/Mosby, 2020, p. 522.

18. c Myofascial trigger points are painful areas of soft tissues that include motor and sensory dysfunction, thus preventing self-release. Muscle does not contain a point at which a reflex can be elicited. Transcutaneous electrical nerve stimulation (TENS) applies high-frequency current to the skin. Acupuncture is the technique in which needles are used to pierce the skin at certain points to bring about a physiologic change to treat or prevent disease. Goldberg ME, Chapter 22, "Pain Management," in Tighe MM, Brown M, Mosby's Comprehensive Review for Veterinary Technicians, ed 5, Elsevier/Mosby, 2020, p. 523.

19. d Viscera are defined as any internal body organ that is enclosed within a cavity. Osteosarcoma is not part of the viscera, whereas the pancreas and intestinal tract are. Therefore pancreatitis, gastroenteritis, and bowel ischemia are examples of visceral pain. Goldberg ME, Chapter 22, "Pain Management," in Tighe MM, Brown M, Mosby's Comprehensive Review for Veterinary Technicians, ed 5, Elsevier/Mosby, 2020, p. 504.

20. b Osteoarthritis, IVDD, and cancer all produce chronic pain. GDV is an acute pain condition, therefore negating the choices of lymphoma, diabetes, and GDV. Respiratory infections, cardiac disease, and hypertension are conditions that do not always produce pain, and blocked cats, broken legs, and bronchitis are examples of acute pain. Goldberg ME, Chapter 22, "Pain Management," in Tighe MM, Brown M, Mosby's Comprehensive Review for Veterinary Technicians, ed 5, Elsevier/Mosby, 2020, p. 505.

21. c Human neonatal and pediatric nurses and veterinary technicians share the position of patient advocate, providing a voice for their patients and attending to their perceived needs. Orthopedic, psychiatric, emergency, and critical care nurses do not necessarily encompass pain management in their daily routines. Shaffran N, "Pain management: the veterinary technician's perspective," Vet Clin North Am Small Anim Pract, 38(6):1415-1428, 2008.

22. b Knowledge of the physiology of pain and the pharmacology of analgesics is essential for communication. Optimally, the veterinarian regards the technician as an integral member of the pain-management team. The skilled technician is a source of vital information required to choose and administer appropriate analgesics. Knowing each other's routines and what is regularly done for patients is incorrect, because each case is handled on an individual basis. Although attaining the CVPP from IVAPM is a worthy goal, it is not necessary for good pain-management practice. Veterinary technicians are not just robots and must be capable of making educated judgment calls to report to the veterinarian; therefore, this knowledge is an essential skill. Shaffran N, "Pain management: the veterinary technician's perspective," Vet Clin North Am Small Anim Pract, 38(6):1416, 2008.

23. a Certain breeds do vocalize and appear more sensitive to pain whereas others seem to remain stoic in the face of pain, therefore the skilled technician factors this knowledge into his or her pain assessments. Dogs and cats have differences in expressions and although a grimace scale has not been developed, this is not a reason not to consider these expressions in pain management decisions. Shaffran N, "Pain management: the veterinary technician's perspective," Vet Clin North Am Small Anim Pract, 38(6):1416, 2008.

24. d The veterinary technician assesses pain, differentiates pain from stress, and monitors for drug effects (in addition, treating, if applicable). Goldberg ME, Chapter 22, "Pain Management," in Tighe MM, Brown M, Mosby's Comprehensive Review for Veterinary Technicians, ed 5, Elsevier/Mosby, 2020, p. 496.

25. c Speaking can temporarily soothe most animals experiencing mild to moderate pain. Animals that are dysphoric or delirious because of opioid overdose rarely respond to soothing interaction or to light palpation of the painful area. Thrashing and yowling alone does not prove dysphoria, because many times, when spoken to or touched, the painful animal will calm down until it is alone again. The claustrophobic animal generally weaves in the cage or tries to escape by digging or chewing on the bars. Shaffran N, "Pain Management: The Veterinary Technician's Perspective," in Mathews KA, The Veterinary Clinics of North America: Small Animal Practice: Update on Pain Management, Saunders/Elsevier 2008, p. 1423.

26. c Panting, anorexia, and depression are very common behaviors seen in dogs experiencing pain. Although vocalization is seen in painful dogs, increased appetite is not (more commonly, decreased appetite is seen). Playful actions, excessive licking, and increased attention to activities occurring in the environment are behavioral signs of a dog that is not experiencing pain. Wiese AJ, Chapter 5, "Assessing Pain," in Muir WW, Gaynor JS, Handbook of Veterinary Pain Management, ed 3, Elsevier/Mosby, 2015, p. 67-81.

27. c Dogs and cats that willingly stretch their abdominal muscles are not in pain. Dogs experiencing pain have a decreased appetite, are more aggressive, and exhibit less social interaction. Mathews K, Kronen P, Lascelles D, et al. WSAVA Guidelines for Recognition, Assessment and Treatment of Pain, Journal of Small Animal Practice, Volume 55, 2014, E10-E68.

28. c Multidimensional pain scales yield better interobserver agreement than unidimensional pain scales because they take into account the various dimensions of pain. Physiological parameters, such as heart rate and blood pressure, are only one criterion and are therefore considered unidimensional. Visual analog scales (VAS) are also considered unidimensional. Much more than vocalization and serum cortisol levels are involved in multidimensional pain scales and this selection is therefore considered incorrect. Wiese AJ, "Assessing Pain," in Muir WW, Gaynor JS, Handbook of Veterinary Pain Management, ed 2, Elsevier/Mosby, 2009, p. 88-89. Karas, Alicia, "Pain, Anxiety, or Dysphoria-How to Tell? A Video Assessment Lab" , 2011, https://www.acvs.org/files/proceeding.

29. c Reduced jumping to higher places is one of the primary signs of pain in cats with degenerative joint disease or osteoarthritis. A common, normal behavior of cats is to hide from company and to sleep all day and these are therefore not necessarily signs of pain. Eating fewer meals is not specifically a sign of pain because it can be a symptom of many conditions. Robertson S, "Managing pain in feline patients," Veterinary Clinics of North America: Small Animal Practice, 38(6), 2008, p. 1269.

30. a The observer's subjective opinion and physiologic signs can be described using a pain scale, such as a visual analog scale. A force plate gait analysis measures lameness for scoring and is therefore not applicable solely to pain. A health-related quality-of-life instrument not only takes pain into account but also includes parameters such as mobility and daily functioning. Serum cortisol levels are only a physiologic way to evaluate whether the patient is stressed or not. Shaffran N, "Pain Management: The Veterinary Technician's Perspective," in Mathews KA, The Veterinary Clinics of North America: Small Animal Practice: Update on Pain Management, Saunders/Elsevier, 2008, p. 1419.

31. d A low pain score does not indicate that analgesic therapy is sufficient, even in an animal exhibiting some questionable behaviors, because some patients are stoic. Pain scales should encourage routine evaluation of hospitalized animals. In addition, they can be used to determine whether analgesic therapy should be discontinued and effective analgesic therapy should result in an animal with a low pain score. Muir WW, Gaynor JS. Handbook of Veterinary Pain Management, ed 3, Elsevier/Mosby, 2015 p. 86.

32. d Basal cell tumors do not induce pain attributed to old age. Spondylosis, intervertebral disc disease, and osteoarthritis can induce pain and are most commonly a result of old age. Epstein ME, Rodan I, Griffenhagen G, et al. 2015 AAHA/AAFP Pain Management Guidelines for Dogs and Cats, Journal of Feline Medicine and Surgery (2015) 17, 251-272.

33. b For an animal with chronic pain, a minimum of every 3 months has been the acceptable period for assessment of blood-work values and patient response to medication. A postoperative period refers to acute pain, as does a patient suffering from a traumatic injury. Yearly evaluation for pain is unacceptable because the patient may then experience pain for some time before reassessment. Epstein ME, Rodan I, Griffenhagen G, et al. 2015 AAHA/AAFP Pain Management Guidelines for Dogs and Cats, Journal of Feline Medicine and Surgery (2015) 17, 251-272.

34. a Because pain scales are mainly subjective, they cannot provide absolute evidence. But they can be an aid to providing treatment in any medical or surgical case. Therefore they do not provide concrete evidence, nor do they support legal documentation. Happy faces should not be used in patient charts. Muir WW, Gaynor JS, Handbook of Veterinary Pain Management, ed 3, Elsevier/Mosby, 2015, p.83.

35. b Subjective scoring system (SSS) is based on the amount of pain an observer thinks the animal will experience for any given procedure. Preemptive scoring systems assign a degree of pain (none, mild, moderate, severe) based on the procedure performed and the amount of tissue trauma involved. A visual analog scale, simple descriptive scale, and numerical rating scale are all types of a subjective scoring system. Mathews K, Kronen P, Lascelles D, et al. WSAVA Guidelines for Recognition, Assessment and Treatment of Pain, Journal of Small Animal Practice, Volume 55, 2014, E10-E68.

36. c The University of Melbourne Pain Scale is based on behavioral and physiologic responses and it includes multiple descriptors in six categories of parameters or behaviors related to pain. Therefore hematological values and physiologic responses are inaccurate. Australia does not have regulations in place to scale pain. Muir WW, Gaynor JS, Handbook of Veterinary Pain Management, ed 3, Elsevier/Mosby, 2015, p. 87.

37. c The newest version of the Colorado State University Veterinary Medical Center Acute Pain Scales for dogs or cats have numbers, drawings and descriptions of various stages of pain that are easy to use in a clinical setting. Muir WW, Gaynor JS, Handbook of Veterinary Pain Management, ed 3, Elsevier/Mosby, 2015, p. 90-91.

38. b The mental nerve block provides analgesia to the lower lip and incisors on the ipsilateral side. The maxillary nerve block is used to provide anesthesia/analgesia to the ipsilateral maxilla, including the teeth, hard and soft palate, and nasal passage. The infraorbital block is used to provide anesthesia/analgesia to the upper lip and nose, dorsal aspect of the nasal cavity, and skin ventral to the infraorbital foramen. The mandibular nerve block provides anesthesia of the ipsilateral incisors, canine tooth, premolars, molars, and skin and mucosa of the chin and lower lip. Muir WW, Gaynor JS, Handbook of Veterinary Pain Management, ed 3, Elsevier/Mosby, 2015, p. 234-235.

39. d Lidocaine patches have been used to provide analgesia for skin abrasions, lacerations, and severe local skin irritations and itching (hot spots). Goldberg ME, Chapter 22, "Pain Management," in Tighe MM and Brown M, Mosby's Comprehensive Review for Veterinary Technicians, ed 5, Elsevier/Mosby, 2020, p. 511.
40. d The MILA soaker catheter (MILA, Erlanger, KY) has a reservoir that gradually discharges the local anesthetic into the catheter, bathing the tissues in the area into which it has been applied. Goldberg ME, Chapter 22, "Pain Management," in Tighe MM, Brown M, Mosby's Comprehensive Review for Veterinary Technicians, ed 5, Elsevier/Mosby, 2020, p. 519-520.
41. b The interpleural block is used to provide analgesia and anesthesia related to thoracic and cranial abdominal pain, especially pain related to pancreatitis. Local anesthetic cannot be used for heart pain because injection would cause the heart to have local ischemia. The colon and kidneys are located in the lower abdomen and this block would therefore not be deemed appropriate. Muir WW, Gaynor JS, Handbook of Veterinary Pain Management, ed 3, Elsevier/Mosby, 2015, p. 246.
42. c A brachial plexus block is used to provide anesthesia distal to the elbow. An interpleural block or intercostal block can provide analgesia for the thorax. A forefoot block provides analgesia for declawing of the front feet. A Bier's block can provide analgesia proximal to the elbow if a tourniquet is placed proximal to the elbow. Muir WW, Gaynor JS, Handbook of Veterinary Pain Management, ed 3, Elsevier/Mosby, 2015, p. 238.
43. b The sciatic nerve block will result in anesthesia of the stifle (partial) and the structures distal to it. The femoral nerve block is excellent for surgery of distal femur, stifle, and distal limb. The brachial plexus block is used for portions distal to the elbow. The epidural block and sacrococcygeal block are useful at the epidural and intercoccygeal space. Mary Ellen Goldberg (2017) Be the pain-attacking offensive midfielder – local anaesthetic blocks every practice can utilise, Veterinary Nursing Journal, 32:11, 329-338.
44. d Local or regional anesthesia can be accomplished with the Bier's block by injecting a large volume of dilute local anesthetic intravenously into an extremity isolated by a tourniquet from the rest of the circulation. The tissue distal to the tourniquet is blocked. Baer's, Bayer's, and Byer's are incorrectly spelled, and are therefore not the best choices. Goldberg ME, Chapter 22, "Pain Management," in Tighe MM and Brown M, Mosby's Comprehensive Review for Veterinary Technicians, ed 5, Elsevier/Mosby, 2020, p. 513.
45. a Most epidural injections in dogs and cats are performed at the L–S space. The spinal cord usually ends at the last lumbar vertebra (L7) in dogs. Muir WW, Gaynor JS, Handbook of Veterinary Pain Management, ed 3, Elsevier/Mosby, 2015, p. 258.
46. d Successful acupuncture neuromodulation and acupuncture analgesia depend on accurate identification of the structures responsible for generating pain and adequate stimulation of these structures. All remaining statements are true of acupuncture. Alvarez L, Chapter 18 "Acupuncture," in Muir WW, Gaynor JS, Handbook of Veterinary Pain Management, ed 3, Elsevier/Mosby, 2015, p. 265-379.
47. c Acupuncture points and channels follow neurovascular pathways. Acupuncture treats pain by inducing neuromodulation along peripheral, central, and autonomic pathways through the use of thin, sterile needles. Veterinary manual therapy includes a variety of manipulative techniques, ranging from high-velocity, low-amplitude chiropractic thrusts to less-invasive measures such as massage and soft-tissue therapy. Although some herbs and diluted substances in homeopathic remedies are used to treat pain, they do not involve the use of needles for treatment. Alvarez L, Chapter 18 ACUPUNCTURE, in Muir WW, Gaynor JS, Handbook of Veterinary Pain Management, ed 3, Elsevier/Mosby, 2015, p. 265-379.
48. d Contraindications of acupuncture include excessive patient movement or aggression that prohibit safe and effective treatment, pregnancy, sepsis, severe bleeding abnormalities, spinal or joint instability local to the treatment site, and tumor or infection at the site of desired needling. Alvarez L, Chapter 18 "Acupuncture," in Muir WW, Gaynor JS, Handbook of Veterinary Pain Management, ed 3, Elsevier/Mosby, 2015, p. 265-379.
49. a Identifying myofascial pain entails palpating for taut bands and trigger points encased within the myofascial fabric. Myofascial pain specifically relates to trigger points and therefore does not apply to swollen segments of muscle, nodules of infection, or nerve bundles. Conarton L. "Myofascial Trigger Point Therapy," in Goldberg ME, Shaffran N, Pain Management for Veterinary Technicians and Nurses, John Wiley & Sons, 2015, p. 318-322.
50. c Capsaicin activates transient receptor potential variant 1 (TRPV1) receptors in sensory nerves. It is derived from chili peppers and responsible for their hot taste. White willow bark, devil's claw and ginger are herbs that have COX inhibition. Muir WW, Gaynor JS, Handbook of Veterinary Pain Management, ed 3, Elsevier/Mosby, 2015, p. 136.
51. d All therapies listed are complementary and alternative medicines. Goldberg ME, Shaffran N, Pain Management for Veterinary Technicians and Nurses, ed 1, Wiley Blackwell, 2015, p. 138.
52. c Cold temperatures raise the activation threshold of tissue nociceptors. Unless the temperature is below 0°F, reflexes are not affected. Cold temperatures cause blood vessels to constrict, reducing the nerve conduction velocity of pain nerves. This effect is considered linear until 10°C, when neural transmission is blocked. Muir WW, Gaynor JS, Handbook of Veterinary Pain Management, ed 3, Elsevier/Mosby, 2015, p. 384.
53. d Cryotherapy is best applied during the acute inflammatory phase of tissue healing and after exercise to minimize any inflammatory response. Cryotherapy is effective in reducing pain, particularly acute postoperative pain. Muir WW, Gaynor JS, Handbook of Veterinary Pain Management, ed 3, Elsevier/Mosby, 2015, p. 384.
54. d Cold therapy should not be used in patients with generalized or localized vascular compromise or that

possess an impaired thermoregulatory capacity. If there is a history of frostbite to the area, further cold application is contraindicated. Observe for signs of frostbite during and after cryotherapy application. A patient that has a large percentage of body fat is not of concern because the cold has little chance of reaching the affected muscles. Muir WW, Gaynor JS, Handbook of Veterinary Pain Management, ed 3, Elsevier/Mosby, 2015, p. 384.

55. a The primary benefit of cryokinetics is to facilitate the patient's ability to perform pain-free exercise as long as the level of exercise remains below levels that cause further injury. If an animal is experiencing hyperthermia, IV fluids and emergency care may be needed in addition to cool compresses. Patients that are in pain should not be competing in athletic events. Muir WW, Gaynor JS, Handbook of Veterinary Pain Management, ed 3, Elsevier/Mosby, 2015, p. 385.

56. b Near the end of a 20-minute treatment, the skin may normally be erythematous, but pale or white skin is an indication that cold-induced tissue damage might be occurring. Therefore, circulation is not restored and normal. External heat creams or rubs can cause the skin to become red temporarily. If melanin is needed, a dietary supplement is added to the feeding regime; however, it would not show up on external skin. Muir WW, Gaynor JS, Handbook of Veterinary Pain Management, ed 3, Elsevier/Mosby, 2015, p. 385.

57. d Ice packs, cold immersion bath, and ice massage are also examples of cryotherapy. Muir WW, Gaynor JS, Handbook of Veterinary Pain Management, ed 3, Elsevier/Mosby, 2015, p. 385-386.

58. c Heat therapy is indicated for patients with chronic pain, especially pain resulting from muscle spasm. Heat is also beneficial for patients in which stretching is indicated to help enhance collagen extensibility. Muir WW, Gaynor JS, Handbook of Veterinary Pain Management, ed 3, Elsevier/Mosby, 2015, p. 386-389.

59. c Joint mobility treatment consists of ROM and stretching exercises. Muir WW, Gaynor JS, Handbook of Veterinary Pain Management, ed 3, Elsevier/Mosby, 2015, p. 391-394.

60. d The patient's position is very important because the animal should be placed in lateral recumbency with the affected limb supported and elevated for treatment. Treatment should be performed in a quiet, comfortable area, and a muzzle may be needed for initial treatments. Muir WW, Gaynor JS, Handbook of Veterinary Pain Management, ed 3, Elsevier/Mosby, 2015, p. 392-393.

61. b The target tissue for lengthening a muscle that is contracted is the muscle belly, not the tendon, ligament, or joint capsule. When working with a joint capsule, range of motion is targeted. A tendon and ligament can only be lengthened with a surgical procedure. Muir WW, Gaynor JS, Handbook of Veterinary Pain Management, ed 3, Elsevier/Mosby, 2015, p. 393.

62. d Swimming or walking in water results in greater flexion of joints and greater ROM. Other activities that may be performed include walking in snow, sand, or tall grass, and crawling through a play tunnel. Climbing stairs may increase joint excursion while also increasing strength. Muir WW, Gaynor JS, Handbook of Veterinary Pain Management, ed 3, Elsevier/Mosby, 2015, p. 394.

63. a Pulling or carrying weight is a method of increasing the force that muscles must use and encourages muscle strengthening. Cavaletti rails, treadmill walking, and wheelbarrowing are great therapeutic exercises. Muir WW, Gaynor JS, Handbook of Veterinary Pain Management, ed 3, Elsevier/Mosby, 2015, p. 394-400.

64. b Transcutaneous electrical nerve stimulation (TENS) is a form of neuromuscular electrical stimulation (NMES). LLLT is laser therapy; an EEG is a measurement of brain electrical activity. An EMG is a measurement of muscle activity. Muir WW, Gyanor JS, Handbook of Veterinary Pain Management, ed 3, Elsevier/Mosby, 2015, p. 404.

65. c Contraindications for TENS include high-intensity stimulation directly over the heart, animals with pacemakers, animals with seizure disorders, over infected areas or neoplasms, over the carotid sinus, or over the trunk during pregnancy. Patients recovering from cruciate ligament reconstruction, orthopedic injury, or experiencing osteoarthritis may actually benefit from therapy with TENS. Muir WW, Gyanor JS, Handbook of Veterinary Pain Management, ed 3, Elsevier/Mosby, 2015, p. 404.

66. d Low-level laser should not be applied over malignancies or areas suspected of cancer. The goal of LLLT is not to stimulate malignant cells, causing them to proliferate and increase in number. LLLT can be used over muscle trigger points, acupuncture points, and with osteoarthritis of muscle spasms. Muir WW, Gaynor JS, Handbook of Veterinary Pain Management, ed 3, Elsevier/Mosby, 2015, p. 406.

67. d Effleurage, petrissage and trigger point therapy are all massage techniques. Muir WW, Gaynor JS, Handbook of Veterinary Pain Management, ed 3, Elsevier/Mosby, 2015, p. 391.

68. b ESWT may be beneficial to patients with chronic OA of the major joints, especially if they cannot tolerate NSAIDs or other forms of treatment. ESWT involves the application of high-energy, high-amplitude acoustic pressure waves to tissues, which would never be used when a patient is pregnant because it could damage the fetus. Neoplastic joint disease, infectious arthritis, and diskospondylitis should not be treated with ESWT because of the risk of spreading the disease process with treatment. Shock waves should not be delivered over the lung field, brain, heart, major blood vessels, nerves, neoplasms, or a gravid uterus. Muir WW, Gaynor JS, Handbook of Veterinary Pain Management, ed 3, Elsevier/Mosby, 2015, p. 408-411.

69. c A goniometer is used to measure PRM. Initial goniometry measurements can provide information needed to decide on the rehabilitation exercises and modalities for use and to measure the effectiveness of the interventions. Calipers are used to measure tumor sizes and a slide rule is used in mathematics. An oliometer is another name for a Gulick tape measure. Muir WW, Gaynor JS, Handbook of Veterinary Pain Management, ed 3, Elsevier/Mosby, 2015, p. 423.

70. a Caution must be used when a patient has plastic or metal implants because the reflection may cause more intense heating, leading to burns or discomfort. Indications for therapeutic ultrasound can include decreased pain, accelerated wound healing, and an increase in the patient's ROM. Muir WW, Gaynor JS, Handbook of Veterinary Pain Management, ed 3, Elsevier/Mosby, 2015, p. 412-413.

71. d Phototherapy can be used for soft tissue injuries such as sprains, strains, and tendinitis, osteoarthritis, chronic pain, wound management of ulcers, pressure sores, burns, skin infections, and healing of incision sites. Kirkby Shaw K, Brown L, Chapter 15, "Modalities Part 2: Laser Therapy," in Goldberg ME, Tomlinson JE, Physical Rehabilitation for Veterinary Technicians and Nurses, Wiley Blackwell, 2018, p. 231-240.

72. c Aquatic therapy is contraindicated in feline patients experiencing cardiac dysfunction, respiratory dysfunction, surface infection, severe peripheral vascular disease, or diarrhea. Aquatic therapy is indicated for cats experiencing muscle weakness, osteoarthritis, or for geriatric care. Kirkby Shaw K, Brown L, Chapter 15, "Modalities Part 2: Laser Therapy," in Goldberg ME, Tomlinson JE, Physical Rehabilitation for Veterinary Technicians and Nurses, Wiley Blackwell, 2018, p. 231-240.

73. c A balance board is an example of a proprioception exercise. A jump rope is not used in cat rehabilitation and swimming is used to increase muscle strength and lung capacity. Massage stimulates nociception in the skin and muscles and relaxes the patient. Goldberg ME, Tomlinson JE, Physical Rehabilitation for Veterinary Technicians and Nurses, Wiley Blackwell, 2018, p. 302.

74. c The American Animal Hospital Association's standards require that pain be included in every veterinary patient assessment regardless of a presenting complaint. NAVTA, ACVAA, and AVMA do not have standards in place requiring a pain assessment. Goldberg ME, Shaffran N, Pain Management for Veterinary Technicians and Nurses, ed 1, Wiley Blackwell, 2014, p. 15.

75. b Because pain promotes inflammation and wound healing is delayed, the patient is negatively affected. Pain does not have an effect on cataract formation, nor does it induce or increase susceptibility to viral diseases. Although the client's refusal to pay for medications to alleviate pain affects the patient negatively, it has no direct correlation to the patient itself. Goldberg ME, Shaffran N, Pain Management for Veterinary Technicians and Nurses, ed 1, Wiley Blackwell, 2014, p. 15.

76. d There are many examples of pain scales. Each scale has advantages and limitations. Regardless of the scale used, it is important to choose one system for use by the entire veterinary team. Goldberg ME, Shaffran N, Pain Management for Veterinary Technicians and Nurses, ed 1, Wiley Blackwell, 2014, p. 16.

77. a Minor surgeries, such as abscess repair, are considered minimally painful. Moderate pain can be induced from castrations, whereas severe pain occurs with a thoracotomy. A laminectomy produces extremely severe pain. Goldberg ME, Shaffran N, Pain Management for Veterinary Technicians and Nurses, ed 1, Wiley Blackwell, 2014, p. 16.

78. b Moderate surgeries, such as ovariohysterectomies or castrations, are considered to produce moderate pain. Abscess repair is considered minimally painful, whereas severe pain is achieved with a thoracotomy. A laminectomy produces extremely severe pain. Goldberg ME, Shaffran N, Pain Management for Veterinary Technicians and Nurses, ed 1, Wiley Blackwell, 2014, p. 16.

79. c Major surgeries, such as thoracotomies or exploratory laparotomies, are considered to produce severe pain. A ripped toenail may produce mild pain and a castration produces moderate pain. A laminectomy produces severe pain. Goldberg ME, Shaffran N, Pain Management for Veterinary Technicians and Nurses, ed 1, Wiley Blackwell, 2014, p. 16.

80. a The observer's subjective opinion as well as physiological signs can be described using a pain scale such as a visual analog scale (VAS). The Glasgow Composite Pain Scale is an objective example. Goldberg ME, Shaffran N, Pain Management for Veterinary Technicians and Nurses, ed 1, Wiley Blackwell, 2014, p. 16.

81. b The Colorado State Canine and Feline Pain Scales fall under the subjective pain scale category, whereas the Glasgow Composite Pain Scale is an objective category. Goldberg ME, Shaffran N, Pain Management for Veterinary Technicians and Nurses, ed 1, Wiley Blackwell, 2014, p. 17.

82. c The Glasgow Pain Scoring System is one of the more frequently used advanced pain scales and is considered state of the art. A pain scale should ideally be multidimensional, with several aspects of pain intensity and pain-related disability included; in addition it should question the dynamic aspects of pain. The Glasgow CPS is thought to be multidimensional. The Colorado State Canine and Feline Pain Scales fall under the subjective pain-scale category. The scales use an observational period and a hands-on evaluation of the patient in an easy-to-use format. The disadvantage of this scale is the lack of validation by clinical studies that compare it with other scales. A scale that you create yourself, although easy to use, is not a validated pain scale, nor is it a client-specific outcome scale. A self-created scale is best used for the client at home to report to the veterinarian. Goldberg ME, Shaffran N, Pain Management for Veterinary Technicians and Nurses, ed 1, Wiley Blackwell, 2014, p. 17.

83. d A pain score should be provided to a client every time the pain score is assessed. The record may help the client more accurately assess the pet's quality of life when end of life is imminent. Goldberg ME, Shaffran N, Pain Management for Veterinary Technicians and Nurses, ed 1, Wiley Blackwell, 2014, p. 19.

84. d The pain state in the horse is a multidimensional experience. Pain can be exhibited though changes in behavior, emotion, or physiologic parameters. Goldberg ME, Shaffran N, Pain Management for Veterinary Technicians and Nurses, ed 1, Wiley Blackwell, 2014, p. 22.

85. b Maladaptive pain is in response to damage already done to peripheral tissue or the nervous system. Physiologic pain is a protective response by the CNS to warn the individual after a noxious stimulus occurs to prevent tissue damage and is also referred to as pain. Peripheral pain does not exist. Goldberg ME, Shaffran N, Pain Management for Veterinary Technicians and Nurses, ed 1, Wiley Blackwell, 2014, p. 22.

86. d Inflammatory pain can involve visceral or somatic pain; visceral pain involves the thorax and abdomen, whereas somatic pain involves muscles, joints, skin, and the periosteum of the bones. Goldberg ME, Shaffran N, Pain Management for Veterinary Technicians and Nurses, ed 1, Wiley Blackwell, 2014, p. 22.

87. c The most common types of pain in horses are orthopedic pain and abdominal/colic pain. Orthopedic pain typically presents as lameness and can include pain of the joints, tendon/ligaments, long bones, and back pain. Lameness is a result of the horse trying to avoid the painful area by compensating on the other limbs. Sometimes the behaviors associated with pain can be nonspecific or can correlate with a specific location such as the abdomen, limb, foot, head, mouth, or castration site. Goldberg ME, Shaffran N, Pain Management for Veterinary Technicians and Nurses, ed 1, Wiley Blackwell, 2014, p. 22.

88. d All of the answers are validated pain scales that exist for horses. Goldberg ME, Shaffran N, Pain Management for Veterinary Technicians and Nurses, ed 1, Wiley Blackwell, 2014, p. 24-25.

89. d A cow may experience depression and appear dull. In addition, grinding teeth, lack of appetite, and standing with one foot behind the other may be exhibited. Goldberg ME, Shaffran N, Pain Management for Veterinary Technicians and Nurses, ed 1, Wiley Blackwell, 2014, p. 26.

90. b Sheep often only show subtle signs of pain, whereas goats are intolerant of painful procedures. Goats will often bleat, whereas sheep may only exhibit tachypnea, inappetence, grinding of teeth, immobility, or abnormal gait. Goldberg ME, Shaffran N, Pain Management for Veterinary Technicians and Nurses, ed 1, Wiley Blackwell, 2014, p. 27.

91. d Pig vocalization and the lack of normal social behavior may be helpful indicators of a pig in pain. Pigs normally squeal and attempt to escape when handled; however, these reactions may be accentuated when the animal is in pain. Squealing is also characteristic when painful areas are palpated. Goldberg ME, Shaffran N, Pain Management for Veterinary Technicians and Nurses, ed 1, Wiley Blackwell, 2014, p. 27.

92. d First, local anesthetics produce true analgesia resulting in the complete absence of pain for the duration of the block. Second, long-term (chronic) pain states may be diminished or eliminated. Third, these drugs are nonscheduled agents, therefore there is no cumbersome paperwork or special license required. Goldberg ME, Shaffran N, Pain Management for Veterinary Technicians and Nurses, ed 1, Wiley Blackwell, 2014, p. 67.

93. d The potential systemic side effects of local anesthetics involve the central nervous system and cardiovascular system. Other potential side effects include the development of methemoglobinemia, nerve and skeletal muscle toxicities, and allergic reactions, including hypersensitivity or anaphylactic responses. Goldberg ME, Shaffran N, Pain Management for Veterinary Technicians and Nurses, ed 1, Wiley Blackwell, 2014, p. 67.

94. c Circumferential ring blocks are used for onychectomy procedures. A leg block and foot block do not exist. Brachial plexus blocks are used at the site of the brachial plexus junction near the shoulder and foreleg. Goldberg ME, Shaffran N, Pain Management for Veterinary Technicians and Nurses, ed 1, Wiley Blackwell, 2014, p. 68.

95. d All of the listed blocks are considered dental blocks except the retrobulbar block, which is an ophthalmic block. Goldberg ME, Shaffran N, Pain Management for Veterinary Technicians and Nurses, ed 1, Wiley Blackwell, 2014, p. 68-71.

96. b An incisional block can be used before surgical incision or after surgery and before skin closure. A sacrococcygeal block is an excellent block to use on a cat that has urinary blockage. A mental nerve block is a dental block. A Bier's block is an intravenous regional analgesic technique that involves a limb and the use of a tourniquet. Goldberg ME, Shaffran N, Pain Management for Veterinary Technicians and Nurses, ed 1, Wiley Blackwell, 2014, p. 72.

97. d The ribs serve as bony landmarks unless the patient is severely obese. The sternum is positioned too ventral for an intercostal block, whereas the thoracic vertebrae are too dorsal for this block. The humerus is located on the forelegs and is therefore insignificant to the ribs. Goldberg ME, Shaffran N, Pain Management for Veterinary Technicians and Nurses, ed 1, Wiley Blackwell, 2014, p. 73.

98. d The advantages of an interpleural block instead of an intercostal nerve block include the ease of administration, the ability to re-dose easily, and the ability to provide analgesia following median sternotomy. Goldberg ME, Shaffran N, Pain Management for Veterinary Technicians and Nurses, ed 1, Wiley Blackwell, 2014, p. 74.

99. a An intratesticular block is extremely easy to perform and provides <8 hours of postoperative pain relief for companion animals, large animals, and exotic patients undergoing castration by anesthetizing the spermatic cord. Indications for an epidural include intra- and postoperative analgesia for hindquarter surgeries in dogs and cats (e.g., tail amputation, anal–rectal surgeries, tibial–femoral fractures, total hip replacement, cruciate ligament repair), exploratory laparotomy, cesarean section, and surgical procedures caudal to the region of the twelfth or thirteenth ribs. An intra-articular block is placed between joint spaces. An interpleural block technique provides anesthesia to the thoracic as well as cranial abdominal nerves (which enter the spinal cord at the level of the thorax). Goldberg ME, Shaffran N, Pain Management for Veterinary Technicians and Nurses, ed 1, Wiley Blackwell, 2014, p. 75, 81, 83, 84.

100. b The sacrococcygeal block is an excellent technique to use when unblocking cats with urethral obstruction. Indications for an epidural include intra- and postoperative analgesia for hindquarter surgeries in dogs and cats (e.g., tail amputation, anal–rectal surgeries, tibial–femoral fractures, total hip replacement, cruciate ligament repair), exploratory laparotomy, cesarean section, and surgical procedures caudal to the region of the twelfth or thirteenth ribs. Pelvic and penile blocks do not exist. Goldberg ME, Shaffran N, Pain Management for Veterinary Technicians and Nurses, ed 1, Wiley Blackwell, 2014, p. 76-77.

101. c An epidural is in the spinal column, most often the lumbosacral area. A TECA procedure is a total ear canal ablation and is therefore not applicable to an epidermal. Cesarean sections, tibial–femoral fractures, and cruciate repairs would all benefit from an epidural block. Goldberg ME, Shaffran N, Pain Management for Veterinary Technicians and Nurses, ed 1, Wiley Blackwell, 2014, p. 77-78.

102. a Needles that can be used in an epidural block are the spinal needle (Quincke needle, 22- or 20-gauge, 1.5–3.5 inches, depending on patient size) or Tuohy needle (22–18-gauge). A butterfly catheter needle is used to draw blood. A 16-gauge IV catheter is a large needle used to place an IV catheter. An auto-vac needle is used for drawing blood. Goldberg ME, Shaffran N, Pain Management for Veterinary Technicians and Nurses, ed 1, Wiley Blackwell, 2014, p. 77.

103. d Caudal epidural analgesia in horses can be used for procedures such as amputation of the tail, rectovaginal fistula repairs, Caslick's closure (operation for pneumovagina), prolapsed rectum, urethrostomy, and anal, perineal, vulvar, and bladder procedures. Goldberg ME, Shaffran N, Pain Management for Veterinary Technicians and Nurses, ed 1, Wiley Blackwell, 2014, p. 82.

104. b Goats do not tolerate pain associated with minor surgical procedures and can die of shock if adequate analgesia is not provided. The exact cause of this shock is not known; it is believed to be a reaction to intense fear or fright from a combination of restraint and pain. Goats do not faint from pain. Goats vocalize but do not roll from pain. Goats do not become lame from pain unless it is related specifically to a foot or leg. Goldberg ME, Shaffran N, Pain Management for Veterinary Technicians and Nurses, ed 1, Wiley Blackwell, 2014, p. 84.

105. a Dehorning has been delayed until a time when the horn must be surgically removed. In these cases, local anesthesia and a good analgesic plan are necessary. The block used is the cornual nerve block. The application of epidural analgesics is necessary in surgery of the caudal reproductive and GI tracts (e.g., cervical lacerations, rectal prolapse) and in cases of reproductive emergencies. A facial nerve block would not block the entire horn in cattle. A disbudding nerve block does not exist. Goldberg ME, Shaffran N, Pain Management for Veterinary Technicians and Nurses, ed 1, Wiley Blackwell, 2014, p. 84-86.

106. d Epidurals can be performed in ruminants, pigs, and camelids. Goldberg ME, Shaffran N, Pain Management for Veterinary Technicians and Nurses, ed 1, Wiley Blackwell, 2014, p. 86-90.

107. d Decreased pain and inflammation are managed with multimodal analgesics, nutritional supplements, and PRT modalities. PRT can help to maintain or increase joint ROM and flexibility. Strength is maintained or increased through therapeutic exercise. Goldberg ME, Shaffran N, Pain Management for Veterinary Technicians and Nurses, ed 1, Wiley Blackwell, 2014, p. 296.

108. a Massage can decrease muscle spasms and increase local blood flow and lymphatic flow. Although the patient may enjoy a massage, the animal will not reach a state of nirvana as described by humans. Massage includes direct physiological effects and can be performed on canine companions. Goldberg ME, Shaffran N, Pain Management for Veterinary Technicians and Nurses, ed 1, Wiley Blackwell, 2014, p. 297.

109. d Thermotherapy includes heat and cold. Heat is used to decrease pain and to increase tissue extensibility. Cold therapy can help reduce pain by causing vasoconstriction, which can help decrease pressure on nociceptors. Cold is commonly used for acute injury or after surgery in the first 48 hours. Cold can decrease hemorrhage, control spasm, and be used after exercise to reduce pain and edema. Laser therapy affects tissues by activating enzymes that trigger biochemical reactions that reduce pain and inflammation and that promote healing (also known as the process of photobiostimulation). Goldberg ME, Shaffran N, Pain Management for Veterinary Technicians and Nurses, ed 1, Wiley Blackwell, 2014, p. 297.

110. c Swimming can be challenging and should be slowly introduced depending on patient functional level, fitness, endurance, and tolerance. Swimming or walking in water should be started gradually with short sessions. Patients that have no fitness level cannot tolerate an arduous exercise program. Swimming several times a day immediately could cause the patient to collapse. Incisions should be allowed to heal before starting water therapy. Goldberg ME, Shaffran N, Pain Management for Veterinary Technicians and Nurses, ed 1, Wiley Blackwell, 2014, p. 304.

111. a TCVM is categorized into five branches that include diet and food, exercise Qigong, Tui-Na, acupuncture, and herbal medicine. Yin-yang theory maintains that everything is essentially composed of two opposing, yet complementary, pairs of opposites. Eight principles are the subdivisions of yin and yang, classifying the patterns of disharmony. Five elements principles can describe the nature of zang-fu organs, the inter-relationships between the organs, and the relationship between the animal body and the natural world. The five elements are wood, fire, earth, water, and metal. Zang-fu physiology classifies organs to help understand and treat disease. The organ systems are interconnected with both physiological and mental/emotional functions. Zang-fu physiology includes heart, blood, spleen, lung, and kidney. Goldberg ME, Shaffran N, Pain Management for Veterinary Technicians and Nurses, ed 1, Wiley Blackwell, 2014, p. 309.

112. c Electrical stimulation is often used at select acupuncture points to increase the duration of effect. Acupuncture at a higher frequency (80–200 Hz) stimulates dynorphins, enkephalins, serotonin, norepinephrine, and gamma-aminobutyric acid (GABA) providing long-term pain relief. Moxibustion uses a burning herbal stick to stimulate and warm acupuncture points. Gold beads or threads are occasionally implanted at an acupuncture point for a permanent effect. Goldberg ME, Shaffran N, Pain Management for Veterinary Technicians and Nurses, ed 1, Wiley Blackwell, 2014, p. 313.

113. b An MTrP is a hyperirritable spot in skeletal muscle that is associated with a hypersensitive palpable nodule in a taut band. The spot is tender when pressed and can give rise to characteristic referred pain, motor dysfunction, and autonomic phenomena. MTrPs are known to cause decreased range of motion, muscle weakness, and dysfunction, and they may create future postural problems because of functional changes in gait patterns. MTrPs within a taut band may be located near the origin/insertion or belly of the muscle being examined. They are often described as a knot or nodule, with the consistency of a firm or hard spot in the already tight band of muscle fiber(s). In animal patients, a jump sign is a reaction the patient may have to pain elicited during palpation of MTrPs. The MTrP is not a muscle spasm. Goldberg ME, Shaffran N, Pain Management for Veterinary Technicians and Nurses, ed 1, Wiley Blackwell, 2014, p. 317.

114. a In animal patients, a jump sign is a reaction the patient may have to pain elicited during palpation of MTrPs. The jump sign has nothing to do with how high the animal can physically jump. The jump sign is not what occurs when a patient is surprised. The jump sign is not referring to the patient jumping because of an injection. Goldberg ME, Shaffran N, Pain Management for Veterinary Technicians and Nurses, ed 1, Wiley Blackwell, 2014, p. 318.

115. d For those practices in which the technician has first contact with the client and patient, it is the technician who takes the preliminary history and conducts the initial examination and pain assessment, reporting the findings to the chiropractor before the adjustment begins. During the adjustment, the technician provides restraint of the chiropractic patient as needed, as well as stabilization for specific adjustments. Goldberg ME, Shaffran N, Pain Management for Veterinary Technicians and Nurses, ed 1, Wiley Blackwell, 2014, p. 327.

116. c Obesity can be defined as an increase in fat tissue mass sufficient to contribute to disease; therefore 10% or 20% is negligible. Goldberg ME, Shaffran N, Pain Management for Veterinary Technicians and Nurses, ed 1, Wiley Blackwell, 2014, p. 286.

117. d Obesity has been linked with a number of disease conditions as well as with a reduced life span. Dogs and cats weighing 10%–19% more than the optimal weight for their breeds are considered overweight; those weighing 20% or more above the optimum weight are considered obese. Goldberg ME, Shaffran N, Pain Management for Veterinary Technicians and Nurses, ed 1, Wiley Blackwell, 2014, p. 286.

118. a Obesity is a risk factor for OA and the most common traumatic cause of OA in dogs is ruptured cruciate ligaments. Overweight/obese dogs are two to three times more likely to rupture cruciate ligaments compared with normal-weight dogs. For many owners, understanding the correlation between maintaining their dog at a healthy weight and decreasing the risk of disease might be a powerful motivator. Torn Achilles, hip dysplasia, and phalangeal fractures are not the most common traumatic causes of OA in dogs. Goldberg ME, Shaffran N, Pain Management for Veterinary Technicians and Nurses, ed 1, Wiley Blackwell, 2014, p. 287.

119. b Pain suppresses the immune response, predisposing to infection or sepsis and increasing hospitalization time and cost. The remaining statements are true regarding the negative effects of pain. Goldberg ME, Shaffran N, Pain Management for Veterinary Technicians and Nurses, ed 1, Wiley Blackwell, 2014, p. 15.

120. a In cats, DHA, rather than EPA (in dogs), inhibits the aggrecanase enzymes responsible for cartilage degradation. Arachidonic acid is a polyunsaturated omega-6 fatty acid that does not participate in cartilage degradation in cats. Methionine does not inhibit aggrecanase. Goldberg ME, Shaffran N, Pain Management for Veterinary Technicians and Nurses, ed 1, Wiley Blackwell, 2014, p. 291.

121. c Porphyrin staining in rodents is a red hematoporphyrin exudate, which may encircle the eye. Therefore it is not hair standing on end or the color of cage litter resulting from urine. Goldberg ME, Shaffran N, Pain Management for Veterinary Technicians and Nurses, ed 1, Wiley Blackwell, 2014, p. 217.

122. a Pain in rabbits is usually characterized by a reduction in food and water intake (and thus weight loss and dehydration) and limited movement. Teeth grinding (bruxism) can be a sign of pain but is not the most common. Squinted eyes can be a sign of pain but not closed eyes. Lateral recumbency would indicate a severely ill rabbit. Goldberg ME, Shaffran N, Pain Management for Veterinary Technicians and Nurses, ed 1, Wiley Blackwell, 2014, p. 223.

123. a The most likely causes of pain in ferrets are arthritis, cancer, or dental problems. Dystocia is not common in ferrets because most are altered before being released to the public for sale. Ear mites could cause intense itching, but not pain. Albinism in ferrets is a result of recessive genes and has nothing to do with pain. Goldberg ME, Shaffran N, Pain Management for Veterinary Technicians and Nurses, ed 1, Wiley Blackwell, 2014, p. 235.

124. c Birds with chronic or overwhelming pain more often display conservation-withdrawal responses, perhaps in an attempt to minimize further pain that struggling might induce and to avoid attracting the attention of potential predators. Birds do not weave in their cages because of pain. They are not known for coprophagia. Birds can be aggressive, but this is not a primary sign of pain. Goldberg ME, Shaffran N, Pain Management for Veterinary Technicians and Nurses, ed 1, Wiley Blackwell, 2014, p. 242.

125. c Chronic pain can cause immobility or stinting of the area and some animals might become aggressive if handling or manipulation is attempted. Signs of acute pain include withdrawal of painful limbs (e.g., in chelonians and lizards), escape behavior, avoidance, restlessness, aggression, and increased respiratory rate. In some cases, florid displays of pain can be seen with biting or scratching of the region in question and vocalization. Goldberg ME, Shaffran N, Pain Management for Veterinary Technicians and Nurses, ed 1, Wiley Blackwell, 2014, p. 249.

126. a Signs of pain in fish can include anorexia, abnormal swimming behavior, attempting to jump out of water, rapid opercular movements, clamped fins, pale or darkened color, and hiding. All others are abnormal behaviors but they may not necessarily indicate pain. Goldberg ME, Shaffran N, Pain Management for Veterinary Technicians and Nurses, ed 1, Wiley Blackwell, 2014, p. 253-255.

127. d Oxygen consumption increases (not decreases) during the initial onset of pain. Vasoconstriction, increased myocardial workload, and an increase in sympathetic tone are all physiological changes that occur during the initial onset of pain. Goldberg ME, Shaffran N, Pain Management for Veterinary Technicians and Nurses, ed 1, Wiley Blackwell, 2014.

128. b Pain itself is described in terms of a noxious stimulus, meaning the damaging or potentially tissue-damaging stimulus. Sensory neurons are responsible for the changing of the nervous system based on the environment. A toxic overdose of a drug is termed an *overdose toxicity*. A nitrous oxide reaction is a false term. Muir WW, Gaynor JS, "Nociception and Pain Mechanisms," Handbook of Veterinary Pain Management, ed 3, Elsevier/Mosby, 2015.

129. b The term *afferent* is used to describe a painful stimulus that is moving toward the central nervous system. In contrast, the term *efferent* refers to signals moving away from the spinal cord. Signals do not travel toward the area of inflammation; they travel outward from it to alert the central nervous system. Muir WW, Gaynor JS, "Nociception and Pain Mechanisms," Handbook of Veterinary Pain Management, ed 3, Elsevier/Mosby, 2015.

130. c The minimal stimulus required to elicit a transmittable electrical signal from a peripheral sensory receptor is called its threshold. By contrast, the action potential is the transformation of environmental stimuli into electrical signals. Polymodal nociceptors participate to modulate the transmission of pain information via descending fibers from the brain. These fibers act through different interneurons to block the transmission of information from the nociceptors to secondary neurons. Muir WW, Gaynor JS, "Nociception and Pain Mechanisms," Handbook of Veterinary Pain Management, ed 3, Elsevier/Mosby, 2015.

131. a A-delta and C fibers are necessary for the detection of all pain sensations, whereas A-beta fibers are responsible for conducting harmless information. Interleukins and substance P are inflammatory mediators of pain, not sensory nerve fibers. Nociceptors transmit painful stimuli. Todd AJ, "Neuronal circuitry for pain processing in the dorsal horn," Nature Reviews Neuroscience, 11(12), 2010, p. 823-826.

132. d The A-delta receptors are activated by thermal or mechanical stimulation and produce short-lived, discriminative, sharp pain. C fibers are associated with a slower burning type of pain. A-beta fibers are responsible for conducting harmless information. Histamine is an inflammatory neurotransmitter. Muir WW, Gaynor JS, "Nociception and Pain Mechanisms," Handbook of Veterinary Pain Management, ed 3, Elsevier/Mosby, 2015.

133. a The pain pathway consists of four events that take place to transmit a painful stimulus: transduction of noxious input, transmission of the signal, modulation of the sensory information, and the perception of pain. Cooley K, "Physiology of Pain," in Goldberg ME, Shaffran N, Pain Management for Veterinary Technicians and Nurses, ed 1, Wiley Blackwell, 2014.

134. c The modulation of pain involves the changing, inhibiting, or amplifying of the transmission of impulses (noxious and non-noxious) within the spinal cord. Transmission refers to the pain signal traveling to the spinal cord via afferent nerves and the perception of pain happens when the signal reaches the central nervous system. Inflammation is the biological response of body tissues to harmful stimuli. Cooley K, "Physiology of Pain," in Goldberg ME, Shaffran N, Pain Management for Veterinary Technicians and Nurses, ed 1, Wiley Blackwell, 2014.

135. c The dorsal horn of the spinal cord receives and manages sensory information from the peripheral nerves and sends that information to the brain for further processing. The actual awareness of pain is termed *perception*. Blood pressure is regulated via the sympathetic nervous system, which is controlled by the hypothalamus. Neurotransmitters are brain chemicals that communicate information. Cooley K, "Physiology of Pain," in Goldberg ME, Shaffran N, Pain Management for Veterinary Technicians and Nurses, ed 1, Wiley Blackwell, 2014.

136. b The gate control theory works by theorizing that A-beta inhibitory interneurons reduce the output of the active A-delta and C nociceptive neurons by closing a gate that would otherwise allow them to relay information to the brain. Myelin is an electrically insulating material that helps to increase the speed of signals across neurons. Melzack R, Wall PD, "Pain mechanisms: a new theory," Science, 150 (3699), 1965, p. 971-979.

137. a Pain originating from injury to the skin, muscles, joints, and deep tissues is termed *somatic pain*. Visceral pain is pain that originated from the internal organs of the thorax and abdomen. Referred pain is often associated with visceral pain whereby the sensation of pain is felt elsewhere other than the site of injury. Deep somatic pain is usually described as dull or aching. Localized pain occurs in one area. Lamont LA, Tranquilli WJ, Grimm KA, "Physiology of pain," Veterinary Clinics of North America, 30 (4), 2000, p. 703-723.

138. d The A-delta and C nerve fibers can start in the skin, but they terminate in the dorsal horn of the spinal cord. Excitatory neurotransmitters must be used for the signal to jump from the dorsal horn of the spinal cord to the brain. The hypothalamus is part of the brain. Cooley K, "Physiology of Pain," in Goldberg ME, Shaffran N, Pain Management for Veterinary Technicians and Nurses, ed 1, Wiley Blackwell, 2014.

139. a Thermoreceptors are sensitive to high and low temperatures. Mechanoreceptors are sensitive to pressure, swelling, and cutting-type injuries. Only chemoreceptors respond to the release of chemicals from damaged cells as well as external chemicals. Cooley K, "Physiology of Pain," in Goldberg ME, Shaffran N, Pain Management for Veterinary Technicians and Nurses, ed 1, Wiley Blackwell, 2014.

140. d Histamine, bradykinins, and substance P are all considered inflammatory mediators of pain. They are major ingredients in the "inflammatory soup" (the acidic mixture that stimulates and sensitizes the nociceptors to prevent further tissue damage). Estrogen is not an inflammatory mediator of pain, but it is a female steroid hormone produced by the ovaries. Muir WW, Gaynor JS, "Nociception and Pain Mechanisms," Handbook of Veterinary Pain Management, ed 3, Elsevier/Mosby, 2015.

141. b C fibers are responsible for a diffuse, burning type of pain accompanying the secondary pain felt because of inflammation and tissue injury. C fibers are smaller unmyelinated nerve fibers that have a slower conduction than A-delta fibers, which carry a short-lived, localized, sharp pain signal. A-beta nerve fibers carry nonpainful signals that convey touch, vibration, movement, and pressure. Myelinated nerve fibers carry impulses faster. Muir WW, Gaynor JS, "Nociception and Pain Mechanisms," Handbook of Veterinary Pain Management, ed 3, Elsevier/Mosby, 2015.

142. a Gray matter is separated into three zones: the dorsal horn, the ventral horn, and the intermediate zone. White matter is that part of the brain consisting of cells called axons, which connect one to the other so that nerves can communicate. Muir WW, Gaynor JS, "Nociception and Pain Mechanisms," Handbook of Veterinary Pain Management, ed 3, Elsevier/Mosby, 2015.

143. d Perception of pain is characterized by the recognition of sensory input. The somatosensory cortex is the area of the cerebrum responsible for the perception and awareness of pain. The intermediate zones of the spinal cord and the medulla oblongata help to transmit and project painful stimulations. The adrenal glands produce hormones, such as cortisol and aldosterone. Cooley K, "Physiology of Pain," in Goldberg ME, Shaffran N, Pain Management for Veterinary Technicians and Nurses, ed 1, Wiley Blackwell, 2014.

144. b Somatic pain arises from the skin and muscles and is conducted via A-delta and C fibers. Visceral pain arises from the internal organs and is conducted via C fibers only. Referred pain is when the sensation of pain is felt elsewhere other than the area of injury. Neuropathic pain arises from damage to the nervous system as a result of trauma, injury, infection, inflammation, etc. Cooley K, "Physiology of Pain," in Goldberg ME, Shaffran N, Pain Management for Veterinary Technicians and Nurses, ed 1, Wiley Blackwell, 2014.

145. d Visceral pain arises from the internal organs and is conducted via C fibers only. Referred pain is when the sensation of pain is felt elsewhere other than the area of injury. Neuropathic pain arises from damage to the nervous system as a result of trauma, injury, infection, inflammation, etc. Central sensitization involves changes in the central nervous system (CNS). Cooley K, "Physiology of Pain," in Goldberg ME, Shaffran N, Pain Management for Veterinary Technicians and Nurses, ed 1, Wiley Blackwell, 2014.

146. a Somatic pain arises from the skin and muscles and is conducted via A-delta and C fibers. Visceral pain arises from the internal organs and is conducted via C fibers only. Referred pain is when the sensation of pain is felt elsewhere besides the area of injury. Neuropathic pain arises from damage to the nervous system as a result of trauma, injury, infection, inflammation, etc. Cooley K, "Physiology of Pain," in Goldberg ME, Shaffran N, Pain Management for Veterinary Technicians and Nurses, ed 1, Wiley Blackwell, 2014.

147. b Visceral pain arises from the internal organs and is conducted via C fibers only. C fibers are responsible for the diffuse, burning type of pain accompanying the secondary pain felt because of inflammation and tissue injury. C fibers are smaller unmyelinated nerve fibers that have a slower conduction than A-delta fibers, which carry a short-lived, localized, sharp pain signal. A-beta nerve fibers carry nonpainful signals that convey touch, vibration, movement, and pressure. Myelinated nerve fibers carry impulses faster. Muir WW, Gaynor JS, "Nociception and Pain Mechanisms," Handbook of Veterinary Pain Management, ed 3, Elsevier/Mosby, 2015.

148. a C fibers are responsible for a diffuse, burning type of pain accompanying the secondary pain felt because of inflammation and tissue injury. C fibers are smaller unmyelinated nerve fibers that have a slower conduction than A-delta fibers, which carry a short-lived, localized, sharp pain signal. A-beta nerve fibers carry nonpainful signals that convey touch, vibration, movement, and pressure. Muir WW, Gaynor JS, "Nociception and Pain Mechanisms," Handbook of Veterinary Pain Management, ed 3, Elsevier/Mosby, 2015.

149. c Chronic pain persists beyond tissue healing and offers no useful biologic function or survival advantage. Chronic pain significantly alters a patient's quality of life and tends to be debilitating and poorly responsive to traditional analgesic therapy. Chronic pain is pain of a prolonged duration (days, weeks, or months). Lamont LA, Tranquilli WJ Grimm KA, "Physiology of Pain," Veterinary Clinics of North America, 30(4), 2000, p. 703-723.

150. c Chronic pain persists beyond tissue healing and offers no useful biologic function or survival advantage. Chronic pain significantly alters a patient's quality of life and tends to be debilitating and poorly responsive to traditional analgesic therapy. Chronic pain is pain of a prolonged duration (days, weeks, or months). Pain that lasts minutes or hours is considered acute pain. Lamont LA, Tranquilli WJ Grimm KA, "Physiology of Pain," Veterinary Clinics of North America, 30(4), 2000, p. 703-723.

151. b The NMDA receptor is normally blocked by magnesium and does not allow ions to pass through and generate a signal. When increased pain stimulation occurs, AMPA receptors can depolarize the membrane that dislodges the magnesium from the NMDA receptor, allowing it to respond to glutamate. Activating the NMDA receptor can lead to increased nerve transmission and increased nerve excitability. Woolf CJ, Salter MW, "Plasticity and Pain: role of the dorsal horn," in McMahon SB, Koltzeburg M, Wall & Melzack's Textbook of Pain, ed 5, Elsevier, 2006.

152. d Central sensitization is contingent on the development of peripheral sensitization and is the indirect consequence of tissue trauma and inflammation. Central sensitization can be caused by a surge of stimulation from peripheral nociceptors, also known as the wind-up of the central nervous system. Of the terms mentioned, only neuroplasticity describes the ability of neurons to change their structure and function in response to different environmental stimuli. Muir WW, Gaynor JS, "Nociception and Pain Mechanisms," Handbook of Veterinary Pain Management, ed 3, Elsevier/Mosby, 2015.

153. d By providing preemptive pain control, the veterinary team can help prevent the emergence of central sensitization and all of the negative sequelae associated with it, including nervous system reorganization and the memory of pain. Patients that have a history of injury may be more sensitive to future nociceptive input. All of the other ways that patients can be made comfortable, such as comfortable bedding and minimal restraint, help to lessen overall stress. Cooley K, "Physiology of Pain," in Goldberg ME, Shaffran N, Pain Management for Veterinary Technicians and Nurses, ed 1, Wiley Blackwell, 2014.

154. c Myelin covers the A-delta nerve fibers. This myelin helps transmit impulses more quickly across the axons and synapses of nerves. Substance P is a neurotransmitter that transmits pain impulses along the A-delta fibers. Muir WW, Gaynor JS, "Nociception and Pain Mechanisms," Handbook of Veterinary Pain Management, ed 3, Elsevier/Mosby, 2015.

155. d Myelin covers the A-delta nerve fibers. This myelin helps transmit impulses more quickly. It cannot suppress central sensitization and does not act as an inflammatory neurotransmitter. Muir WW, Gaynor JS, "Nociception and Pain Mechanisms," Handbook of Veterinary Pain Management, ed 3, Elsevier/Mosby, 2015.

156. a Histamine is an inflammatory mediator that originates from mast cells. Many inflammatory mediators can originate from damaged tissue; however, mast cells are responsible for the release of histamine. C fibers and A-delta fibers are nerve fibers. Muir WW, Gaynor JS, "Nociception and Pain Mechanisms," Handbook of Veterinary Pain Management, ed 3, Elsevier/Mosby, 2015.

157. b The area innervated by a sensory nerve fiber is the receptive field. A dermatome is the area of the skin innervated by the dorsal root. The nerve fibers that innervate the receptive field include both C fibers and A-delta fibers. Muir WW, Gaynor JS, "Nociception and Pain Mechanisms," Handbook of Veterinary Pain Management, ed 3, Elsevier/Mosby, 2015.

158. b Pharmacokinetics refers to the series of events that occur after a drug is administered to a patient. Pharmacodynamics refers to the way a particular drug affects the body. The degree to which a drug is absorbed and reaches general circulation is bioavailability. Efficacy is the degree to which the drug binds to its receptor. Albino M, "Analgesic Pharmacology," in Goldberg ME, Shaffran N, Pain Management for Veterinary Technicians and Nurses, ed 1, Wiley Blackwell, 2014.

159. a The *first-pass effect* is the term that describes the phenomenon of drug metabolism in which the concentration of a drug is greatly reduced before it reaches the systemic circulation. Pharmacokinetics refers to the series of events that occur after a drug is administered to a patient. Pharmacodynamics refers to the way a particular drug affects the body. Albino M, "Analgesic Pharmacology," in Goldberg ME, Shaffran N, Pain Management for Veterinary Technicians and Nurses, ed 1, Wiley Blackwell, 2014.

160. d The brand of syringe used to administer the medication does not play a role in how a drug is absorbed; however, the route of administration (SQ, IM, IV) and the solubility of the drug do play significant roles. The patient's temperature can also play a role in drug absorption, such as when drugs are administered topically, for example, fentanyl patches. Albino M, "Analgesic Pharmacology," in Goldberg ME, Shaffran N, Pain Management for Veterinary Technicians and Nurses, ed 1, Wiley Blackwell, 2014.

161. c Pharmacokinetics refers to the series of events that occur after a drug is administered to a patient. Pharmacodynamics refers to the way a particular drug affects the body. The degree to which a drug is absorbed and reaches general circulation is bioavailability. Efficacy is the degree to which the drug binds to its receptor. Albino M, "Analgesic Pharmacology," in Goldberg ME, Shaffran N, Pain Management for Veterinary Technicians and Nurses, ed 1, Wiley Blackwell, 2014.

162. a The most common way for a drug to be eliminated from the body is through urine excretion via the kidneys. Before a drug is excreted it is often metabolized (or biotransformed) and this most often occurs in the liver. Muir WW, Gaynor JS, "Nociception and Pain Mechanisms," Handbook of Veterinary Pain Management, ed 3, Elsevier/Mosby, 2015.

163. b Before a drug is excreted it is often metabolized (or biotransformed) and this most often occurs in the liver. The skin, as well as the eyes, can absorb drugs topically. Muir WW, Gaynor JS, "Nociception and Pain Mechanisms," Handbook of Veterinary Pain Management, ed 3, Elsevier/Mosby, 2015.

164. c The tendency of a drug to combine with an intended receptor is called affinity and the degree to which it binds to this receptor is termed *efficacy*. Efficacy refers to the maximum response achievable from a drug. Bioavailability describes when the drug is absorbed systemically and the degree to which it is absorbed. Albino M, "Analgesic Pharmacology," in Goldberg ME, Shaffran N, Pain Management for Veterinary Technicians and Nurses, ed 1, Wiley Blackwell, 2014.

165. d An agonist drug binds with a receptor but has no effect at that receptor. Agonist drugs are often used as reversal agents because of their ability to combine with a receptor, but they have no effect. Partial agonist drugs have affinity for the receptor; however, they have poor efficacy. When affinity and efficacy are both present, the drug is described as an agonist. Muir WW, Gaynor JS, "Nociception and Pain Mechanisms," Handbook of Veterinary Pain Management, ed 3, Elsevier/Mosby, 2015.

166. a Morphine is the only choice that is identified as an opioid agonist. Naloxone is the opposite and is considered an opioid antagonist. Butorphanol and nalbuphine are of the same class of opioids known as opioid agonists–antagonists. This means they are mu receptor antagonists but also kappa receptor agonists. Because they are not full mu receptor agonists similar to morphine and hydromorphone, they should be considered weak analgesics. Muir WW, Gaynor JS, "Nociception and Pain Mechanisms," Handbook of Veterinary Pain Management, ed 3, Elsevier/Mosby, 2015.

167. c Hydromorphone is the only choice that is identified as an opioid agonist, which is a good choice for patients that are in moderate to severe pain. Naloxone is the opposite and is considered an opioid antagonist, which means it has no analgesic activity. Butorphanol is one of the opioids that are known as opioid agonists–antagonists. This means that they are mu receptor antagonists but also kappa receptor agonists. Because they are not full mu receptor agonists similar to morphine and hydromorphone, they should be considered weak analgesics. Muir WW, Gaynor JS, "Nociception and Pain Mechanisms," Handbook of Veterinary Pain Management, ed 3, Elsevier/Mosby, 2015.

168. c The three well-defined opioid receptor types are as follows: kappa, mu, and delta. Gamma is not an opioid receptor type. Muir WW, Hubbell JA, Bednarski RM, Lerche P, Handbook of Veterinary Anesthesia, ed 5, Elsevier/Mosby, 2013.

169. d Opioid administration given via intravenous, intramuscular, or subcutaneous injection produces a rapid onset of action. Because of the first-pass effect, many opioids include variable systemic absorption when administered orally. Albino M, "Analgesic Pharmacology," in Goldberg ME, Shaffran N, Pain Management for Veterinary Technicians and Nurses, ed 1, Wiley Blackwell, 2014.

170. b Pure or full mu opioid agonists can elicit maximal activation of the mu receptor when they bind to it and the subsequent downstream processes produce a maximal analgesic effect. Kappa agonists such as butorphanol can produce some analgesia, although it is considered a weak analgesic when compared with a full mu agonist such as morphine. Lamont LA, Mathews KA, "Opioids, Non-steroidal anti-inflammatories and analgesic adjuvants," in Tranquilli WJ, Thurmon JC, Grimm KA, Lumb and Jones' Veterinary Anesthesia and Analgesia, ed 4, Blackwell, 2007.

171. d Fentanyl is often used in CRI form because of its short duration of action. Peak analgesic effects are seen approximately 5 minutes after IV injection, lasting approximately 30 minutes. Buprenorphine and morphine can be used in constant-rate infusions; however, their duration of action is much longer, ranging anywhere from 2 to 6 hours depending on the route of administration. Ketamine is not an opioid. Muir WW, Hubbell JA, Bednarski RM, Lerche P, Handbook of Veterinary Anesthesia, ed 5, Elsevier/Mosby, 2013.

172. b Methadone is a synthetic mu opioid agonist that is unique in that it possesses additional affinity for NMDA receptors. Methadone may decrease norepinephrine and serotonin reuptake to augment analgesia, making it useful for neuropathic or wind-up pain. Ketamine and propofol are not opioids. Morphine is an opioid; however, it does not show affinity for the NMDA receptor. Codd EE, Shank RP, Schupsky JJ, Raffa RB, "Serotonin and norepinephrine uptake inhibiting activity of centrally acting analgesics," Journal of Pharmacology and Experimental Therapeutics, 1995, p. 274.

173. a Of these, only hydromorphone has been shown to cause hyperthermia in cats. Albino M, "Analgesic Pharmacology," in Goldberg ME, Shaffran N, Pain Management for Veterinary Technicians and Nurses, ed 1, Wiley Blackwell, 2014.

174. d Of the listed drugs, only oxymorphone can be classified as an opioid. Carprofen is a nonsteroidal anti-inflammatory and amantadine and ketamine are NMDA receptor antagonists. Muir WW, Hubbell JA, Bednarski RM, Lerche P, Handbook of Veterinary Anesthesia, ed 5, Elsevier/Mosby, 2013.

175. b Naloxone hydrochloride is a pure mu opioid antagonist that reverses all opioid effects at all receptors. Conversely, morphine and hydromorphone are opioid agonists and they fully activate the mu receptors. Butorphanol is a mixed agonist–antagonist, which functions to antagonize mu receptors, but it also acts as a kappa agonist eliciting a full effect at those receptors. Albino M, "Analgesic Pharmacology," in Goldberg ME, Shaffran N, Pain Management for Veterinary Technicians and Nurses, ed 1, Wiley Blackwell, 2014.

176. c Opioid agonist–antagonist drugs such as butorphanol and nalbuphine exert mild analgesic activity by stimulating the kappa receptors that are responsible for mild visceral analgesia. Mu agonist drugs such as morphine are effective for somatic and visceral pain. Albino M, "Analgesic Pharmacology," in Goldberg ME, Shaffran N, Pain Management for Veterinary Technicians and Nurses, ed 1, Wiley Blackwell, 2014.

177. c Nonsteroidal anti-inflammatory drugs exert their analgesic activity by inhibiting the enzyme cyclooxygenase (COX). All of the other choices are characteristics of local anesthetics. Albino M, "Analgesic Pharmacology," in Goldberg ME, Shaffran N, Pain Management for Veterinary Technicians and Nurses, ed 1, Wiley Blackwell, 2014.

178. b Newer NSAIDs that selectively inhibit COX-2 are thought to produce fewer GI side effects. The COX enzymes themselves (both COX-1 and COX-2) help to facilitate the breakdown of arachidonic acid. Wannamaker BP, Massey KL, Applied Pharmacology for the Veterinary Technician, ed 3, Saunders, 2004.

179. b Certain anti-inflammatory agents have been shown to have antipyretic or fever-reducing effects. GI and renal effects are some of the negative side effects of NSAID use. Cowbell effects refers to the infamous Saturday Night Live skit in which Christopher Walken plays legendary music producer Bruce Dickinson, who states that the only thing that will reduce his fever is "more cowbell." Lamont LA, Mathews KA, "Opioids, Non-steroidal anti-inflammatories and analgesic adjuvants," in Tranquilli WJ, Thurmon JC, Grimm KA, Lumb and Jones' Veterinary Anesthesia and Analgesia, ed 4, Blackwell, 2007.

180. a Veterinary technicians cannot refill medications without the veterinarian's approval. NSAIDs commonly exert unwanted side effects in the GI, kidneys, liver and affect platelet function. Many side effects are unnoticed until they cause a real problem because of the drug being used inappropriately and without screening and follow-up. It is important for the veterinary technician to discuss these side effects with the owner and to provide follow-up care. Lascalles BD, Blikslager AT, Fox SM, Reece D, "Gastrointestinal tract perforation in dogs treated with a selective cyclooxygenase-2 inhibitor: 29 cases (2002-2003)," Journal of the American Veterinary Medical Association, 227(7), 2005, p. 1112-1117.

181. a NSAIDs are most commonly associated with adverse reactions to the GI tract (64%), renal system (21%), and liver (14%). Hampshire VA, Doddy FM, Post LO, et al, "Adverse drug event reports at the United States Food and Drug Administration Center for Veterinary Medicine," Journal of the American Veterinary Medical Association, 225, 2004, p. 533-536.

182. d Because side effects of NSAIDs are mainly GI, pet owners should be informed that if their pet vomits while taking an NSAID, the drug should be discontinued and the patient should be examined. No other drugs or treatments should be recommended without physical examination or consultation from their prescribing veterinarian. Albino M, "Analgesic Pharmacology," in Goldberg ME, Shaffran N, Pain Management for Veterinary Technicians and Nurses, ed 1, Wiley Blackwell, 2014.

183. b Although some opioids can cause GI disturbances such as nausea and vomiting, the corticosteroids are responsible for more severe GI effects when used in conjunction with NSAIDs. Corticosteroids should not be used in conjunction with NSAIDs. Local anesthetics and topical flea treatments should not cause any gastrointestinal side effects when used in conjunction with NSAIDs. Albino M, "Analgesic Pharmacology," in Goldberg ME, Shaffran N, Pain Management for Veterinary Technicians and Nurses, ed 1, Wiley Blackwell, 2014.

184. b Of the listed drugs, carprofen is a nonsteroidal anti-inflammatory. Amantadine and ketamine are NMDA receptor antagonists. Oxymorphone is an opioid. Muir WW, Hubbell JA, Bednarski RM, Lerche P, Handbook of Veterinary Anesthesia, ed 5, Elsevier/Mosby, 2013.

185. a Often patients will need to switch NSAIDs. When switching from one NSAID to another NSAID, a washout period of 3–5 days should be observed to minimize the risk of concurrent adverse effects. Starting both drugs at the same time can increase the incidence of side effects such as GI upset and bleeding. Mealey K, Common Adverse Drug reactions in Veterinary Patients, Western Veterinary Conference Proceedings, Las Vegas, NV, 2013.

186. c Acetaminophen is contraindicated in cats because of the deficient glucuronidation of acetaminophen in this species, leading to a buildup of toxic metabolites and resultant toxicity. Meloxicam, carprofen, and robenacoxib are COX-1– and COX-2–specific NSAIDs. Albino M, "Analgesic Pharmacology," in Goldberg ME, Shaffran N, Pain Management for Veterinary Technicians and Nurses, ed 1, Wiley Blackwell, 2014.

187. b Of these NSAIDs, only flunixin is labeled for use in horses and cattle. Currently carprofen and meloxicam are labeled in the United States for use in dogs only. Albino M, "Analgesic Pharmacology," in Goldberg ME, Shaffran N, Pain Management for Veterinary Technicians and Nurses, ed 1, Wiley Blackwell, 2014.

188. d Of the listed choices only piroxicam has been proven effective as an analgesic in the lower urinary tract associated with cystitis and urethritis. Plumb DC, Veterinary Drug Handbook, ed 7, Wiley-Blackwell, 2011.

189. b Local anesthetics reversibly bind sodium channels and block nerve conduction in nerve fibers. Choices a, c, and d relate to the effects of nonsteroidal anti-inflammatory drugs. Muir WW, Hubbell JA, Bednarski RM, Lerche P, Handbook of Veterinary Anesthesia, ed 5, Elsevier/Mosby, 2013.

190. b Local anesthetics produce desensitization and analgesia to skin surfaces when applied topically. To exert an effect on the other body systems listed, local anesthetics must be administered via injection either IV or epidurally. Muir WW, Hubbell JA, Bednarski RM, Lerche P, Handbook of Veterinary Anesthesia, ed 5, Elsevier/Mosby, 2013.

191. c Of all of the drugs listed, meperidine is not a local anesthetic. It is an opioid. Muir WW, Hubbell JA, Bednarski RM, Lerche P, Handbook of Veterinary Anesthesia, ed 5, Elsevier/Mosby, 2013.

192. b The potency and speed of onset of local anesthetics is directly related to the lipid solubility of the drug. The larger the lipophilic property of the local anesthetic, the more readily the anesthetic permeates the axonal nerve membranes. The brand, temperature, and volume of drug do not influence time of onset. Skarda RT, Tranquilli WW, in Tranquilli WJ, Thurmon JC, Grimm KA, Lumb and Jones' Veterinary Anesthesia and Analgesia, ed 4, Blackwell, 2007, p. 395-418.

193. d The first signs of toxicity involving local anesthetics are muscle twitching and convulsing. The other side effects listed are often seen as problems associated with NSAID use, not with local anesthetics. Skarda RT, Tranquilli WW, in Tranquilli WJ, Thurmon JC, Grimm KA, Lumb and Jones' Veterinary Anesthesia and Analgesia, ed 4, Blackwell, 2007, p. 395-418.

194. c A circumferential nerve block is commonly used to desensitize nerves and to add additional analgesia to an onychectomy procedure. A retrobulbar block is commonly used to desensitize the eye before enucleation surgery. An epidural provides desensitization to the trunk and lower extremities. A sacrococcygeal block provides desensitization to the tail, anus, penis, or vulva. Albino M, "Analgesic Pharmacology," in Goldberg ME, Shaffran N, Pain Management for Veterinary Technicians and Nurses, ed 1, Wiley Blackwell, 2014.

195. b *Regional anesthesia* is the correct term to describe the injection of a local anesthetic into the area around a peripheral nerve to block sensory and/or motor function. Although some regional anesthesia can be administered by subcutaneous injection, this term does not adequately describe what is happening (blocking sensory and motor function). Other listed techniques describe various ways to deliver local anesthetics, either in the subarachnoid space with spinal anesthesia or to the skin or mucous membranes via topical anesthesia. Albino M, "Analgesic Pharmacology," in Goldberg ME, Shaffran N, Pain Management for Veterinary Technicians and Nurses, ed 1, Wiley Blackwell, 2014.

196. a *Spinal anesthesia* is the correct term to describe the injection of a local anesthetic into the cerebrospinal fluid to block sensory and/or motor function. Other listed techniques describe various ways to deliver local anesthetics, either in the epidural space via epidural anesthesia or to the skin or mucous membranes via topical anesthesia. *Regional anesthesia* is the correct term to describe the injection of a local anesthetic into the area around a peripheral nerve to block sensory and/or motor function. Albino M, "Analgesic Pharmacology," in Goldberg ME, Shaffran N, Pain Management for Veterinary Technicians and Nurses, ed 1, Wiley Blackwell, 2014.

197. d A diffusion or wound catheter can be beneficial in many types of situations such as limb amputations, total ear canal ablations, and radical mastectomies. Specific dental blocks are used for tooth extractions Albino M, "Analgesic Pharmacology," in Goldberg ME, Shaffran N, Pain Management for Veterinary Technicians and Nurses, ed 1, Wiley Blackwell, 2014.

198. b Lidocaine is available in combination with epinephrine to prolong duration of action via vasoconstriction. Dexmedetomidine can also sometimes be added to a local anesthetic to provide peripheral vasoconstriction and to prolong the duration of action; however, at this time a lidocaine–dexmedetomidine combination is not commercially available in contrast with lidocaine + epinephrine. Albino M, "Analgesic Pharmacology," in Goldberg ME, Shaffran N, Pain Management for Veterinary Technicians and Nurses, ed 1, Wiley Blackwell, 2014.

199. a EMLA cream is most often used to facilitate IV catheter placement. It is applied topically. EMLA cream should not be applied to the mucous membranes or eyes; however, other topical anesthetic formulations are available for these purposes. Albino M, "Analgesic Pharmacology," in Goldberg ME, Shaffran N, Pain Management for Veterinary Technicians and Nurses, ed 1, Wiley Blackwell, 2014; Plumb DC, Veterinary Drug Handbook, ed 7, Wiley-Blackwell, 2011.

200. c Intercostal nerve blocks provide analgesia to the surgical area in the thoracic wall. This allows improved ventilation by minimizing pain during respiration as the animal recovers. The other nerve blocks mentioned do not block nerves associated with the thoracic cavity. Mental nerve blocks are used to desensitize the cranial lower jaw, infraorbital nerve blocks desensitize the cranial maxilla, and a retrobulbar block is used for ocular procedures. Ko J, Inoue T, "Local anesthetic agents and anesthetic technique," in Ko, Jeff, Small Animal Anesthesia and Pain Management: A Color Handbook, Manson, 2013, p. 252-254, 259-260.

201. c Mepivacaine is useful in veterinary medicine because it does not sting on injection. It is approved for use in dogs and horses and it has a moderate duration of action (2–4 hours). It is not metabolized in the lungs; however, it is metabolized in the liver and excreted by the kidneys. Albino M, "Analgesic Pharmacology," in Goldberg ME, Shaffran N, Pain Management for Veterinary Technicians and Nurses, ed 1, Wiley Blackwell, 2014; Plumb DC, Veterinary Drug Handbook, ed 7, Wiley-Blackwell, 2011.

202. d Of the drugs listed, acepromazine is the only one that is not an alpha-2 agonist. Acepromazine is considered a phenothiazine tranquilizer. Muir WW, Hubbell JA, Bednarski RM, Lerche P, Handbook of Veterinary Anesthesia, ed 5, Elsevier/Mosby, 2013.

203. d Administering the antagonist atipamezole can effectively reverse the drug dexmedetomidine. The other drugs listed are all examples of drugs within the alpha-2 agonist class. Muir WW, Hubbell JA, Bednarski RM, Lerche P, Handbook of Veterinary Anesthesia, ed 5, Elsevier/Mosby, 2013.

204. b Alpha-2 agonists produce sedation, analgesia, and muscle relaxation. They often also produce a refractory bradycardia (decreased heart rate), not an increased heart rate. Muir WW, Hubbell JA, Bednarski RM, Lerche P, Handbook of Veterinary Anesthesia, ed 5, Elsevier/Mosby, 2013.

205. a Alpha-2 agonists cause initial peripheral vasoconstriction, which in turn causes pale mucous membranes and cold extremities. During this period of vasoconstriction, patients will often be normotensive or even hypertensive. Alpha-2 agonists produce a decreased hepatic blood flow, but this does not contribute to the pale mucous membranes and cold extremities. Hypothermia and hypoglycemia are not often associated with the initial phase of alpha-2 administration. Muir WW, Hubbell JA, Bednarski RM, Lerche P, Handbook of Veterinary Anesthesia, ed 5, Elsevier/Mosby, 2013.

206. b In contrast to the sedation and analgesic effects of alpha-2 receptors, alpha-1 receptors produce arousal, excitement, and increased locomotor activity. Albino M, "Analgesic Pharmacology," in Goldberg ME, Shaffran N, Pain Management for Veterinary Technicians and Nurses, ed 1, Wiley Blackwell, 2014; Plumb DC, Veterinary Drug Handbook, ed 7, Wiley-Blackwell, 2011.

207. a Xylazine possesses a high affinity for alpha-1, therefore the unwanted side effects of arousal, excitement, and increased locomotor activity are seen when using this drug compared with medetomidine and dexmedetomidine, which are highly selective for the alpha-2 receptor. Atipamezole is the reversal (antagonist) for the alpha-2 agonists. Albino M, "Analgesic Pharmacology," in Goldberg ME, Shaffran N, Pain Management for Veterinary Technicians and Nurses, ed 1, Wiley Blackwell, 2014; Plumb DC, Veterinary Drug Handbook, ed 7, Wiley-Blackwell, 2011.

208. c Alpha-2s are rapidly absorbed after IV, IM, SQ, or transmucosal administration. The transdermal route is not commonly used to administer alpha-2s. Albino M, "Analgesic Pharmacology," in Goldberg ME, Shaffran N, Pain Management for Veterinary Technicians and Nurses, ed 1, Wiley Blackwell, 2014; Plumb DC, Veterinary Drug Handbook, ed 7, Wiley-Blackwell, 2011.

209. d Alpha-2 agonists can cause first- and second-degree AV block, but complete AV block is uncommon. Ventricular bradycardia and even ventricular tachycardia can occur following pronounced sinus bradycardia. Muir WW, Hubbell JA, Bednarski RM, Lerche P, Handbook of Veterinary Anesthesia, ed 5, Elsevier/Mosby, 2013.

210. a Transient hypoinsulinemia and hyperglycemia have been reported in several species sedated with xylazine and other alpha-2 agonists. They suppress insulin release by stimulating receptors in the pancreas. Because of this, alpha-2 agonists should be used with caution or not at all in patients with diabetes. Vasoconstriction, bradycardia, and decreased hepatic blood flow are also evident; however, these specific side effects are not of major concern in the diabetic patient. Plumb DC, Veterinary Drug Handbook, ed 7, Wiley-Blackwell, 2011.

211. c Of the listed drugs, all choices are alpha-2 agonists similar to xylazine; however, yohimbine is an alpha-2 antagonist used to reverse the effects of xylazine. Plumb DC, Veterinary Drug Handbook, ed 7, Wiley-Blackwell, 2011.

212. c NMDA receptor antagonists include the drugs ketamine, amantadine, and memantine. The opioid methadone is also thought to have activity at the NMDA receptor as well as being a mu opioid agonist. Hydromorphone is an agonist at the mu opioid receptor. Plumb DC, Veterinary Drug Handbook, ed 7, Wiley-Blackwell, 2011.

213. d Ketamine is used in many ways as part of a multimodal analgesic plan to help reduce wind-up. Ketamine can be administered via CRI, epidural and can even be combined with opioids in premedication. Ketamine is not commonly given orally after surgery. Plumb DC, Veterinary Drug Handbook, ed 7, Wiley-Blackwell, 2011.

214. d Ketamine can cause an increase in heart rate, blood pressure, and myocardial oxygen consumption. It should therefore not be used in patients with hypertrophic cardiomyopathy, with congestive heart failure, or in unstable patients suffering from shock. Albino M, "Analgesic Pharmacology," in Goldberg ME, Shaffran N, Pain Management for Veterinary Technicians and Nurses, ed 1, Wiley Blackwell, 2014; Plumb DC, Veterinary Drug Handbook, ed 7, Wiley-Blackwell, 2011.

215. c Amantadine is the only drug listed that is a human antiviral drug currently used in veterinary patients for its NMDA receptor antagonist properties. The other listed drugs are opioids. Plumb DC, Veterinary Drug Handbook, ed 7, Wiley-Blackwell, 2011.

216. b Of the listed drug classes, although NSAIDs and opioids are important in managing pain, only the NMDA receptor antagonist drugs have been shown to be efficacious in the management of neuropathic pain in animals suffering from hyperalgesia and allodynia. Antibiotics are not used for pain management. Albino M, "Analgesic Pharmacology," in Goldberg ME, Shaffran N, Pain Management for Veterinary Technicians and Nurses, ed 1, Wiley Blackwell, 2014; Plumb DC, Veterinary Drug Handbook, ed 7, Wiley-Blackwell, 2011.

217. b Serotonin syndrome has been shown to occur when patients who are on SSRIs or MAOI drugs are given tramadol. This is most likely because of tramadol's effect inhibiting neuronal reuptake of norepinephrine and serotonin. Serotonin syndrome is not often associated with antibiotics, opioids, or anticholinergics. Albino M, "Analgesic Pharmacology," in Goldberg ME, Shaffran N, Pain Management for Veterinary Technicians and Nurses, ed 1, Wiley Blackwell, 2014; Plumb DC, Veterinary Drug Handbook, ed 7, Wiley-Blackwell, 2011.

218. a Gabapentin is used to help alleviate the symptoms of neuropathic pain, which can often be described as burning, lancing, or a pins-and-needles sensation. Burning and lancing pain is more likely to respond to gabapentin than is dull and aching pain. Muir WW, Gaynor JS, "Alternative Drug and Novel Therapies" Handbook of Veterinary Pain Management, ed 3, Elsevier/Mosby, 2015.

219. a Gabapentin has been shown especially useful for patients experiencing osteoarthritis pain, especially when used in combination with NSAIDs. The other drugs listed are not analgesics and are not often combined with gabapentin. Muir WW, Gaynor JS, "Alternative Drug and Novel Therapies" Handbook of Veterinary Pain Management, ed 3, Elsevier/Mosby, 2015.

220. d Of the drugs listed, only amitriptyline has been shown to provide relief of pain associated with chronic cystitis. The other drugs mentioned are all antibiotics. Muir WW, Gaynor JS, "Alternative Drug and Novel Therapies" Handbook of Veterinary Pain Management, ed 3, Elsevier/Mosby, 2015.

221. b Gabapentin is often administered to cats before they undergo limb amputation or declaw surgery to help prevent neuropathic pain and to lessen the chances of chronic pain developing. Although carprofen reduces inflammation before surgery, it is not used for neuropathic pain and is not currently labeled for use in cats in the United States. Cefazolin and glucose are not used to prevent or to treat pain. Muir WW, Gaynor JS, "Alternative Drug and Novel Therapies", Handbook of Veterinary Pain Management, ed 3, Elsevier/Mosby, 2015.

222. d Tricyclic antidepressants are contraindicated in patients with seizure disorders because these agents may lower the seizure threshold. Amitriptyline is actually quite useful for senior patients who may have mobility issues because of chronic pain from osteoarthritis. There is currently no contraindication for diabetic patients. Albino M, "Analgesic Pharmacology," in Goldberg ME, Shaffran N, Pain Management for Veterinary Technicians and Nurses, ed 1, Wiley Blackwell, 2014; Plumb DC, Veterinary Drug Handbook, ed 7, Wiley-Blackwell, 2011.

223. a Maropitant has been shown useful in reducing not only opioid-related nausea and vomiting but also the MAC of anesthetic gases needed when administered preoperatively. Carprofen is an anti-inflammatory and has not been shown to reduce nausea and vomiting. Morphine and hydromorphone are opioids and often a main side effect of their use is nausea and vomiting. Laird JMA, Olivar T, Roza C, et al., "Deficits in visceral pain and hyperalgesia of mice with a disruption of the tachykinin NK1 receptor gene," Neuroscience, 98, 2000, p. 345-352.

224. a Multimodal analgesia involves combining different drug classes acting on different pain pathways. Although some take-home medications and constant-rate infusions can involve different drug classes, the term *multimodal analgesia* is the combination of different drug classes acting on different pain pathways. Muir WW, Gaynor JS, Handbook of Veterinary Pain Management, ed 3, Elsevier/Mosby, 2015, p. 341.

225. b Because morphine has a strong tendency to cause physical dependency or addiction in humans, it is classified as a schedule II drug in the United States and Canada. An example of a schedule III drug is buprenorphine and a schedule I example is heroin. Lerche P, Thomas JA, Anesthesia and Analgesia for Veterinary Technicians, ed 4, Elsevier, 2011.

226. b Of the opioids, methadone has the lowest likelihood of causing vomiting in cats. All other opioids may cause a higher incidence of nausea and vomiting. Lerche P, Thomas JA, Anesthesia and Analgesia for Veterinary Technicians, ed 4, Elsevier, 2011.

227. d Of the drugs listed, fentanyl is most commonly given as a transdermal patch for patients needing a stronger mu opioid in the postoperative period. Lidocaine is also often provided via a transdermal patch; however, lidocaine is not an opioid drug. In veterinary patients morphine is most commonly administered by injection and carprofen is given by either oral administration or injection. Lerche P, Thomas JA, Anesthesia and Analgesia for Veterinary Technicians, ed 4, Elsevier, 2011.

228. d When transdermal fentanyl patches are heated, they can release excessive amounts of fentanyl, causing sedation, dysphoria, and sometimes even an overdose. Lerche P, Thomas JA, Anesthesia and Analgesia for Veterinary Technicians, ed 4, Elsevier, 2011.

229. a Morphine is the opioid most commonly used for epidural analgesia. Buprenorphine can be used; however, it is less potent than morphine because it is a partial agonist. Lidocaine and bupivacaine are local anesthetics and, although they are commonly used as epidural analgesics, they are not opioids. Lerche P, Thomas JA, Anesthesia and Analgesia for Veterinary Technicians, ed 4, Elsevier, 2011.

230. c Of the common take-home analgesics listed, all (acepromazine, fentanyl patch, and tramadol) can be used in the feline patient except Tylenol with codeine. Acetaminophen (Tylenol) can be toxic to cats. Lerche P, Thomas JA, Anesthesia and Analgesia for Veterinary Technicians, ed 4, Elsevier, 2011.

231. c Premedication refers to the administration (SC, IM, or IV) of anesthetic and analgesic agents and adjuncts (sedatives or tranquilizers) to calm and prepare the patient for anesthetic induction. Induction refers to the administration of a drug or combination of drugs at the beginning of an anesthetic that results in a state of general anesthesia. Recovery is the period after general anesthesia when anesthetic agents are being cleared from the body. McNerney T, "Surgical Pain Management," in Goldberg ME, Shaffran N, Pain Management for Veterinary Technicians and Nurses, ed 1, Wiley Blackwell, 2014.

232. d Of the mentioned induction methods, chamber induction with isoflurane is the least suitable choice compared with injectable methods. This is because of the side effects of chamber induction and the waste gas exposure of the staff. All of the other mentioned induction methods (propofol, ketamine/diazepam mixture, and alfaxalone) are acceptable, with fewer overall side effects than chamber or mask induction. McNerney T, "Surgical Pain Management," in Goldberg ME, Shaffran N, Pain Management for Veterinary Technicians and Nurses, ed 1, Wiley Blackwell, 2014.

233. b Visceral pain describes the type of pain that will be experienced from any surgery of the reproductive tract that involves manipulation of organs such as the uterus and ovaries. Somatic pain will be a component of the entire surgery because the skin incision will probably contribute to somatic pain. If this pain is not treated properly, it can lead to a condition known as wind-up or central sensitization. Wind-up pain refers to pain that results as a consequence of a previously painful event or stimulus that was not treated effectively. McNerney T, "Surgical Pain Management," in Goldberg ME, Shaffran N, Pain Management for Veterinary Technicians and Nurses, ed 1, Wiley Blackwell, 2014.

234. a Of the opioids listed, hydromorphone is the most desirable choice because it is a pure mu opioid agonist and provides the best level of pain control when compared with butorphanol and buprenorphine. Midazolam is not an opioid analgesic. McNerney T, "Surgical Pain Management," in Goldberg ME, Shaffran N, Pain Management for Veterinary Technicians and Nurses, ed 1, Wiley Blackwell, 2014.

235. b Intratesticular blocks can be particularly useful in providing <8 hours of pain control by anesthetizing the spermatic cord. Ovarian ligament blocks are indicated for patients undergoing ovariohysterectomy. Infraorbital nerve blocks and maxillary nerve blocks are useful in patients undergoing dentistry. Moses L, www.MSPCA.org, 2013. (Accessed 6 May 2014).

236. c Although most technicians tend to increase the percentage of inhalant anesthetic, a faster and more beneficial practice is to administer additional analgesics via IV catheter. If the patient is responding to surgical stimulation, additional analgesics are necessary, usually via an injection of an opioid. If the technician chooses to do nothing or to reduce the percentage of inhalant anesthesia, the patient would likely awaken from anesthesia, become aware of its surroundings, and suffer pain and psychological harm. McNerney T, "Surgical Pain Management," in Goldberg ME, Shaffran N, Pain Management for Veterinary Technicians and Nurses, ed 1, Wiley Blackwell, 2014.

237. a If your patient begins responding to surgical stimulation under anesthesia and you choose to increase the inhalant percentage, you must also increase the fresh gas flow to ensure the patient receives the percentage dialed on the vaporizer in a timely manner. This is known as the concept of time constants. Starting constant rate infusions and performing local blocks will lower the minimum alveolar concentration of inhalant anesthetic required but will not directly affect the percentage dialed on the vaporizer. Lerche P, Thomas JA, Anesthesia and Analgesia for Veterinary Technicians, ed 4, Elsevier, 2011.

238. c Of the listed surgeries, cataract removal surgery would most likely involve the use of a neuromuscular blocking agent because the procedure requires the eye to be in a central position. Neuromuscular blocking agents are not routinely used with the other surgeries mentioned. McNerney T, "Surgical Pain Management," in Goldberg ME, Shaffran N, Pain Management for Veterinary Technicians and Nurses, ed 1, Wiley Blackwell, 2014.

239. b An initial loading dose of 2 mg/kg IV lidocaine should be administered to achieve therapeutic blood levels before initiating a lidocaine CRI. A loading dose is always recommended before starting a constant rate infusion of lidocaine. Plumb DC, Veterinary Drug Handbook, ed 7, Wiley-Blackwell, 2011.

240. a In large skin incisions such as radical mastectomies, a wound diffusion catheter can be used to provide <72 hours of continuous analgesia. The other blocks listed provide anywhere from 4 to 8 hours of analgesics. McNerney T, "Surgical Pain Management," in Goldberg ME, Shaffran N, Pain Management for Veterinary Technicians and Nurses, ed 1, Wiley Blackwell, 2014.

241. d The patient presenting for a thoracotomy with fractured ribs or trauma can benefit from preemptive analgesics because they will help to create a more consistent breathing pattern and will improve patient ventilation. In addition, patients that cannot ventilate well are anxious and decompensate with aggressive restraint. Bryant S, "Anesthesia for Thoracotomies and Respiratory Challenged Patients," Anesthesia for Veterinary Technicians, Wiley-Blackwell, 2011, p. 227-238.

242. a The analgesia provided by intercostal nerve blocks provides superior analgesia and improved postoperative ventilation for the thoracotomy patient. Intratesticular blocks are for providing anesthesia/analgesia to the testicles, whereas infraorbital and maxillary nerve blocks are for dentistry procedures. Thompson SE, Johnson JM, "Analgesia in dogs after intercostal thoracotomy: A comparison of morphine, selective intercostal nerve blocks, and intrapleural regional anesthesia with bupivacaine," Veterinary Surgery, 20, 1991, p. 73-77.

243. d The technician placing retrobulbar blocks must be familiar with the anatomy of the eye, because risks such as hemorrhage, perforation of the globe, and damage to the optic nerve can occur with an improperly placed retrobulbar nerve block. Guliano EA, "Regional anesthesia as an adjunct for eyelid surgery in dogs," Topics in Companion Animal Medicine, 23, 2008, p. 51-56.

244. a Dexmedetomidine is the only one of the mentioned drugs that is labeled as both a sedative an analgesic. Dexmedetomidine is useful in the postoperative period because it can be provided in a low dose of 1 μg/kg/IV and still exert effects. The other drugs listed (propofol, diazepam, and midazolam) are all sedatives and are not labeled as analgesics. McNerney T, "Surgical Pain Management," in Goldberg ME, Shaffran N, Pain Management for Veterinary Technicians and Nurses, ed 1, Wiley Blackwell, 2014.

245. d Of the therapies mentioned, low-level laser therapy can help with pain and wound healing, icing can help with inflammation, and massage can aid with lowering edema and pain. McNerney T, "Surgical Pain Management," in Goldberg ME, Shaffran N, Pain Management for Veterinary Technicians and Nurses, ed 1, Wiley Blackwell, 2014; Moore et al, "The effect of Infra-Red Diode Radiation on the Duration and Severity of Post-Operative Pain: A Double Blind Trial," Laser Therapy 4, 1992.

246. a Of all of the available opioids, methadone is unlikely to produce vomiting when compared with the higher incidence of vomiting/nausea seen with morphine and hydromorphone. Midazolam is not an opioid but a benzodiazepine. Liss D, Spelts K, "Analgesia for Emergency and Critical Care Patients," in Goldberg ME, Shaffran N, Pain Management for Veterinary Technicians and Nurses, ed 1, Wiley Blackwell, 2014.

247. d Of the listed opioids, remifentanil has the shortest duration of action (10–15 minutes), thus making it the most attractive for patients requiring neurological examinations. The infusion can be discontinued and shortly after a neurologic examination can be performed with the assurance that any abnormal neurological signs are not attributed to opioid-induced sedation or dysphoria. Fentanyl is also thought to have a shorter duration of action around 30 minutes whereas the effects of morphine and methadone can last 2–4 hours. Liss D, Spelts K, "Analgesia for Emergency and Critical Care Patients," in Goldberg ME, Shaffran N, Pain Management for Veterinary Technicians and Nurses, ed 1, Wiley Blackwell, 2014.

248. d Epidurals should not be performed in patients with a coagulation disorder (DIC, thrombocytopenia, and von Willebrand's disease) because of the risk of hemorrhage into the epidural space if an epidural venous sinus vessel is inadvertently perforated during needle placement. Diabetic patients usually have no contraindication to epidurals and patients with hind-limb trauma can receive epidurals as long as the spinal column and epidural space are not damaged. Liss D, Spelts K, "Analgesia for Emergency and Critical Care Patients," in Goldberg ME, Shaffran N, Pain Management for Veterinary Technicians and Nurses, ed 1, Wiley Blackwell, 2014.

249. c Patients that are hospitalized long term can benefit from being kept in a physiologic position of head-elevated sternal recumbency. Having the patient in left or right lateral recumbency for too long can result in pressure points on areas such as the hips and elbows. Patients that spend long periods standing might experience pain or anxiety. Liss D, Spelts K, "Analgesia for Emergency and Critical Care Patients," in Goldberg ME, Shaffran N, Pain Management for Veterinary Technicians and Nurses, ed 1, Wiley Blackwell, 2014.

250. a Chronic pain is often divided into two categories: nociceptive pain (caused by activation of nociceptors) and neuropathic pain (pain caused by direct damage to or indirect alteration of the nervous system). The other types of pain listed can each contribute to chronic pain; however, they fall into the two categories of nociceptive pain and neuropathic pain. Norkus C, "Chronic Pain Management for the Companion Animal," in Goldberg ME, Shaffran N, Pain Management for Veterinary Technicians and Nurses, ed 1, Wiley Blackwell, 2014.

251. b Of the drug classes listed, bisphosphonates is the drug class used for patients with osteosarcoma, which acts by preventing loss of bone mass. Although opioids, gabapentinoids, and neurokinin-1 inhibitors all function to control some pain, bisphosphonates are the only drug class that functions to prevent loss of bone mass. Norkus C, "Chronic Pain Management for the Companion Animal," in Goldberg ME, Shaffran N, Pain Management for Veterinary Technicians and Nurses, ed 1, Wiley Blackwell, 2014.

252. c Of the drugs listed, capsaicin has been used as a topical analgesic adjunct. Capsaicin ointment is applied to a painful area and activates the TrpV1. Prolonged TrpV1 activation results in receptor desensitization, which leads to substance-P depletion and ultimately to alleviation of pain. The other medications listed (gabapentin, amantadine, and bisphosphonates) are commonly administered orally. Norkus C, "Chronic Pain Management for the Companion Animal," in Goldberg ME, Shaffran N, Pain Management for Veterinary Technicians and Nurses, ed 1, Wiley Blackwell, 2014.

253. d All of the choices are ways that pet owners can keep dogs comfortable when they are experiencing chronic pain from osteoarthritis. When patients are overweight, it creates more stress on joints that are already painful. Animals with painful joints benefit from soft padded areas to lie down and light low-impact regular exercise can be beneficial. Norkus C, "Chronic Pain Management for the Companion Animal," in Goldberg ME, Shaffran N, Pain Management for Veterinary Technicians and Nurses, ed 1, Wiley Blackwell, 2014.

254. a Substance P is a neurotransmitter that plays a role in the process of pain perception as well as in the vomiting reflex. Although prolonged TrpV1 activation results in receptor desensitization, which leads to substance-P depletion and ultimate alleviation of pain, it is not involved with the vomiting reflex. Epinephrine and norepinephrine are not involved with substance P or the vomiting receptors; these are our fight-or-flight hormones. Norkus C, "Chronic Pain Management for the Companion Animal," in Goldberg ME, Shaffran N, Pain Management for Veterinary Technicians and Nurses, ed 1, Wiley Blackwell, 2014.

255. c Maropitant is an NK-1 receptor antagonist and it works to block NK-1 receptors and subsequent activation of substance P. Bisphosphonates are the drug class used for patients with osteosarcoma, which acts by preventing loss of bone mass. Gabapentin and amantadine both function to suppress neuropathic pain and to prevent the wind-up phenomenon that leads to central sensitization and allodynia. Norkus C, "Chronic Pain Management for the Companion Animal," in Goldberg ME, Shaffran N, Pain Management for Veterinary Technicians and Nurses, ed 1, Wiley Blackwell, 2014; Lerche P, Thomas JA, Anesthesia and Analgesia for Veterinary Technicians, ed 4, Elsevier, 2011.

256. a Of the inhalant anesthetic agents, only nitrous oxide is thought to contain weak analgesic properties via its NMDA receptor antagonist properties. It should be noted that these are weak analgesic properties and nitrous oxide should never be used as a sole analgesic. Isoflurane and sevoflurane function only as anesthetic agents and they have no analgesic properties. Plumb DC, Veterinary Drug Handbook, ed 7, Wiley-Blackwell, 2011; Norkus C, "Chronic Pain Management for the Companion Animal," in Goldberg ME, Shaffran N, Pain Management for Veterinary Technicians and Nurses, ed 1, Wiley Blackwell, 2014.

257. b Corticosteroids are often used for their powerful anti-inflammatory effects and they play a role in chronic pain management in companion animals. Corticosteroids act as anti-inflammatory agents by blocking prostaglandins and leukotrienes. Corticosteroids do not exert effects at opioid receptors or at NMDA receptors. They are also not known for their antinausea properties. Norkus C, "Chronic Pain Management for the Companion Animal," in Goldberg ME, Shaffran N, Pain Management for Veterinary Technicians and Nurses, ed 1, Wiley Blackwell, 2014.

258. b The most beneficial wavelength for pain management is 810–980 nm. Flaherty MJ, Rehabilitation Therapy in Perioperative Pain Management, Veterinary Clinics of North America: Small Animal Practice, 2019, Nov 49(6) p. 1143-1156.

259. c Health-related quality of life (HRQL) is concerned with those aspects of QOL that change as a result of ill health and medical interventions. Consequently, HRQL is the subjective evaluation of circumstances including an altered health state and related interventions. Reid J, Wiseman-Orr ML, et al. Chapter 6 Health-Related Quality of Life Measurement, Muir WW, Gaynor JS, Handbook of Veterinary Pain Management, ed 3, Elsevier/Mosby, 2015, p. 98.

260. d In feline practice, all of these areas are used to evaluate pain in cats. These combined steps make a complete assessment of acute pain in cats. Steagall PV, Monteiro BP, Acute Pain in Cats: Recent advances in clinical assessment. Journal of Feline Medicine and Surgery (2019) 21, p. 25-34.

261. a The Client Specific Outcome Measures (CSOM) is an instrument that was originally developed for dogs and subsequently applied in cats. The CSOM has been used in some studies for its ongoing validation. Monteiro BP, Steagall PV, Chronic Pain in Cats: Recent advances in Clinical Assessment, Journal of Feline Medicine and Surgery (2019) 21, p. 601-614.

262. b The first step in the establishment of neuropathic pain is development of a lesion somewhere within the somatosensory system. The initiating stimulus is typically associated with nociceptive pain. Under normal circumstances, noxious stimuli diminish as healing occurs and the experience of nociceptive pain decreases over time. Moore SA (2016) Managing Neuropathic Pain in Dogs. Front. Vet. Sci. 3:12.

SECTION 14

1. c Moistened kibble or a more natural diet can help decrease dental abrasions in ferrets. This is likely because a kibble diet is low in moisture and is very crunchy. Chewing on wire cages can contribute to dental abrasions. Ferrets are obligate carnivores and should not be given vegetables. Annual periodontal treatments will help with overall dental disease but not with dental abrasions caused by a pelleted diet. Hoefer HL, Fox JG, Bell JA, "Gastrointestinal Disease," in Quesenberry K, Carpenter JW, Ferrets, Rabbits, and Rodents, ed 3, Saunders, 2012.
2. d MRI and CT are not the correct modalities for looking at GI transit time. To evaluate transit time, you could use radiographs, but this does not show movement in real time. The only modality used for real-time evaluation is fluoroscopy. Hoefer HL, Fox JG, Bell JA, "Gastrointestinal Disease," in Quesenberry K, Carpenter JW, Ferrets, Rabbits, and Rodents, ed 3, Saunders, 2012.
3. b Ibuprofen toxicity can cause ataxia, coma, and tremors. Arrhythmias, vomiting, drooling, and heart failure are not common signs of ibuprofen toxicity. Antinoff N, Giovanella CJ, "Musculoskeletal and Neurologic Diseases," in Quesenberry K, Carpenter JW, Ferrets, Rabbits, and Rodents, ed 3, Saunders, 2012.
4. a Canine distemper virus is most commonly transmitted by aerosol exposure but can also be spread by direct contact with conjunctival and nasal exudates, urine, feces, skin, and sometimes fomites. The incubation period in ferrets is generally 7 to 10 days. The disease spreads by viremia after it is in the body and it is almost always fatal. Influenza B has a low pathogenicity and is primarily passed via aerosol droplets. It is not necessarily fatal. *Pneumocystis carinii* is pneumonia caused by a yeast-like organism. Cryptococcosis is caused by a fungus and can be fatal. Barron HW, Rosenthal KL, "Respiratory Diseases," in Quesenberry K, Carpenter JW, Ferrets, Rabbits, and Rodents, ed 3, Saunders, 2012.
5. b Ferret physique is tube-like. The heart is located in the caudal thorax, which is much more caudal in comparison with other mammals. Morrisey JK, Kraus MS, "Cardiovascular and Other Diseases," in Quesenberry K, Carpenter JW, Ferrets, Rabbits, and Rodents, ed 3, Saunders, 2012.
6. d Vestibular signs in the ferret include head tilt, ataxia, circling, and loss of proprioception. Antinoff N Giovanella CJ, "Musculoskeletal and Neurologic Diseases," in Quesenberry K, Carpenter JW, Ferrets, Rabbits, and Rodents, ed 3, Saunders, 2012.
7. b Around 50% of the total lymphoid tissue in rabbits is found in the GI tract. Lymphoid tissue is distributed throughout various other organ systems but is not as large a percentage. Vella D, Donnelly TM, "Basic Anatomy, Physiology, and Husbandry," in Quesenberry K, Carpenter JW, Ferrets, Rabbits, and Rodents, ed 3, Saunders, 2012.
8. a *Encephalitozoon cuniculi* is an extremely common disease, causing a neurological disease seen in pet rabbits. *Baylisascaris procyonis* is a species of roundworm found in raccoons and it is zoonotic. *Toxoplasma gondii* is an intracellular protozoan that causes toxoplasmosis. *Pasteurella multocida* is a Gram-negative coccobacillus commonly found in rabbits. Rabbits with *Pasteurella multocida* are often said to have snuffles. Taylor DK, Lee V, Mook D, Huerkamp MJ, "Rabbits," in Ballard B, Cheek R, Exotic Animal Medicine for the Veterinary Technician, ed 3, Wiley-Blackwell, 2017.
9. d To diagnose syncope in any species, you need to be able to see the rhythm of the heart in real time. The ECG is the only diagnostic tool that provides a graphic representation of the rhythm. CT and thoracic radiographs show the size and shape of the heart. The echocardiogram is excellent for measurement as well as for evaluating function. Huston SM, Ming-Show LP, Quesenberry KE, Pilny AA, "Cardiovascular Disease, Lymphoproliferatvie Disorders, and Thymomas," in Quesenberry K, Carpenter JW, Ferrets, Rabbits, and Rodents, ed 3, Saunders, 2012.
10. a This patient probably has septic mastitis because it is presenting with a fever, anorexia, depression, and lethargy. GI stasis would not cause a fever, nor would cellulitis or nonseptic cystic mastitis. Klaphake E, Paul-Murphy J, "Disorders of the Reproductive and Urinary Systems," in Quesenberry K, Carpenter JW, Ferrets, Rabbits, and Rodents, ed 3, Saunders, 2012.
11. b *Treponema paraluiscuniculi* is the spirochete responsible for rabbit syphilis. Transmission occurs via venereal contact between rabbits. CBC, ELISA, and PCR testing do not aid in the diagnosis of this disease. Klaphake E, Paul-Murphy J, "Disorders of the Reproductive and Urinary Systems," in Quesenberry K, Carpenter JW, Ferrets, Rabbits, and Rodents, ed 3, Saunders, 2012.
12. c GI neoplasia does not present as an ingesta-filled stomach with large amounts of gas in the intestines. This is only seen with GI stasis. Patients with acute GI dilation present with an air-filled or fluid-filled stomach, whereas a GI obstruction exhibits a fluid-filled or ingesta-filled stomach but intestines that are not gas filled. Oglesbee BL, Jenkins JR, "Gastrointestinal Diseases," in Quesenberry K, Carpenter JW, Ferrets, Rabbits, and Rodents, ed 3, Saunders, 2012.
13. a Porphyrin pigments fluoresce under a Wood's lamp but hemoglobin does not. Urinary tests and microscopic examinations do not diagnose porphyrins, but they might indicate the presence of blood. Klaphake E Paul-Murphy J, "Disorders of the Reproductive and Urinary Systems," in Quesenberry K, Carpenter JW, Ferrets, Rabbits, and Rodents, ed 3, Saunders, 2012.
14. b Pregnancy toxemia generally occurs during the last week of gestation. This is the same time that nest-building behavior begins. The exact cause of pregnancy toxemia is unknown. Stress, obesity, low-calorie intake, and environmental changes contribute to toxemia. Klaphake

E Paul-Murphy J, "Disorders of the Reproductive and Urinary Systems," in Quesenberry K, Carpenter JW, Ferrets, Rabbits, and Rodents, ed 3, Saunders, 2012.

15. c *Clostridium difficile* is the most common bacteria associated with enterotoxemia in the guinea pig. Guinea pigs have primarily Gram-positive GI flora and are very sensitive to antibiotics such as penicillin, ampicillin, clindamycin, and lincomycin. Other bacteria can cause issues when the wrong antibiotics are given, but generally not to the extent of *Clostridium difficile*. Oglesbee BL, Jenkins JR, "Gastrointestinal Diseases," in Quesenberry K, Carpenter JW, Ferrets, Rabbits, and Rodents, ed 3, Saunders, 2012.

16. d *Bordetella bronchiseptica* is one of the most common etiologic agents and it causes bacterial pneumonia in guinea pigs. Poor husbandry and increased humidity contribute to bacterial pneumonia. *Demodex caviae*, *Trixacarus caviae*, and *Gyropus ovalis* are parasites that do not contribute to bacterial pneumonia. Murray J, Crane M, "Guinea Pigs," in Ballard B, Cheek R, Exotic Animal Medicine for the Veterinary Technician, ed 3, Wiley-Blackwell, 2017.

17. c Penile fur rings are accumulations of fur and smegma around the base of the penis. Fur rings are found in single-housed males as well as breeding males. Diagnosis is made on physical examination generally after the patient presents for excessive grooming, straining to urinate, repeatedly cleaning the penis, and production of several small spots of urine in the litter box. Renal failure, urinary calculi, and a urinary tract infection do not present with excessive grooming or cleaning of the penis. Mans C, Donnelly TM, "Disease Problems of Chinchillas," in Quesenberry K, Carpenter JW, Ferrets, Rabbits, and Rodents, ed 3, Saunders, 2012.

18. a Common fur mites in pet mice include *Myobia musculi*, *Myocoptes musculinus*, and *Radfordia affinis*. Dermatophytes and contact dermatitis from bedding can cause alopecia but this is not as common as fur mites. Endoparasites do not generally lead to dermatitis or alopecia. Brown C, Donnelly TM, "Disease Problems of Small Rodents," in Quesenberry K, Carpenter JW, Ferrets, Rabbits, and Rodents, ed 3, Saunders, 2012.

19. b Lean diet, low body weight, and handling of the mother and young can lead to cannibalism. Decreased ambient temperature, not increased ambient temperature, also contributes to cannibalism of young. Brown C, Donnelly TM, "Disease Problems of Small Rodents," in Quesenberry K, Carpenter JW, Ferrets, Rabbits, and Rodents, ed 3, Saunders, 2012.

20. d Sugar gliders in captivity often suffer from malnutrition. Without the proper balance of ingested calcium, vitamin D, and phosphorus, calcium cannot be absorbed properly, leading to hypocalcemia. Ness RD, "Sugar Gliders," in Quesenberry K, Carpenter JW, Ferrets, Rabbits, and Rodents, ed 3, Saunders, 2012.

21. b Hepatic lipidosis is common in hedgehogs. Although these animals can experience acute renal failure, bacterial pneumonia, and glomerulosclerosis, these diseases are not as common and do not cause diarrhea or icterus. Ivey E, Carpenter JW, "African Hedgehogs," in Quesenberry K, Carpenter JW, Ferrets, Rabbits, and Rodents, ed 3, Saunders, 2012.

22. d Peripheral vessels are small and only used for very small volume samples. The jugular vein is most commonly used for CBC and chemistry sample collection. The cranial vena cava can be used, but there is a much higher risk of cardiac puncture. Ivey E, Carpenter JW, "African Hedgehogs," in Quesenberry K, Carpenter JW, Ferrets, Rabbits, and Rodents, ed 3, Saunders, 2012.

23. b These clinical findings are indicative of hypovitaminosis A. This is commonly found in birds fed an all-seed diet. Hypovitaminosis C is not a common finding in avian patients. Hypocalcemia is most commonly found in African grey parrots on all-seed diets. Candidiasis is caused by *Candida albicans*, not a poor diet. Signs for candidiasis include delayed crop emptying, white plaques in the oral cavity, and regurgitation. . Greenacre CB, Gerhardt L, "Psittacines and Passerines," in Ballard B, Cheek R, Exotic Animal Medicine for the Veterinary Technician, ed 3, Wiley-Blackwell, 2017.

24. a The avian kidney produces both urine and urates. Because uric acid (urates) is a main component of nitrogenous waste, uric acid best represents renal function in birds. Greenacre CB, Gerhardt L, "Psittacines and Passerines," in Ballard B, Cheek R, Exotic Animal Medicine for the Veterinary Technician, ed 3, Wiley-Blackwell, 2017.

25. c UV-B light is required for the metabolism of vitamin D3 and calcium. UV-A light is required for the regulation of behavior and appetite. Feeding a proper diet regulates calcium, magnesium, and other vitamins/minerals. Calcium cannot be absorbed properly without vitamin D3. Wilson B, "Lizards," in Ballard B, Cheek R, Exotic Animal Medicine for the Veterinary Technician, ed 3, Wiley-Blackwell, 2017.

26. a Reptiles do not have a loop of Henle in their urinary system. Reptiles have a much slower metabolism and synthesis of water. Drinking water and then reabsorbing it from the cloaca and bladder, if present, accomplishes homeostasis. Cheek R, Crane M, "Snakes," in Ballard B, Cheek R, Exotic Animal Medicine for the Veterinary Technician, ed 3, Wiley-Blackwell, 2017.

27. b Autotomy is the natural predatory response that reptiles use to escape potential predation. Dysecdysis is the act of improper shedding of the skin, generally as a result of poor husbandry. Amputation is not a correct term because this is an automatic physiologic response resulting from perceived danger and not from actual trauma or surgery. Autolysis is defined as self-digestion. Wilson B, "Lizards," in Ballard B, Cheek R, Exotic Animal Medicine for the Veterinary Technician, ed 3, Wiley-Blackwell, 2017.

28. b The Doppler is the most commonly used piece of equipment for obtaining a heart rate. The stethoscope does not work well in most reptiles because of the shell or thick scales. The pulse is generally impossible to palpate. An ultrasound would work well, but it is not practical. Cheek R, Crane M, "Snakes," in Ballard B, Cheek R, Exotic Animal Medicine for the Veterinary Technician, ed 3, Wiley-Blackwell, 2017.

29. d The caudal tail vein is the most common vein used for blood collection in lizards. The jugular vein can be used, but a cut-down may be necessary and lymphatic fluid contamination is possible. The cephalic vein is also possible, but it is very small and is also a blind stick. The ventral abdominal vein is not practical, it is a blind stick, and it is difficult to provide hemostasis. Wilson B, "Lizards," in Ballard B, Cheek R, Exotic Animal Medicine for the Veterinary Technician, ed 3, Wiley-Blackwell, 2017.

30. a In reptilian patients, the approximate circulating blood volume is between 5% and 8% of the body weight. Bounous DL, "Avian and Reptile Hematology," in Ballard B, Cheek R, Exotic Animal Medicine for the Veterinary Technician, ed 3, Wiley-Blackwell, 2017.

31. c In avian patients, the approximate circulating blood volume is 10% of the body weight. Bounous DL, "Avian and Reptile Hematology, "in Ballard B, Cheek R, Exotic Animal Medicine for the Veterinary Technician, ed 3, Wiley-Blackwell, 2017.

32. d These signs are indicative of a snake preparing to shed. These are normal signs. The dermis is sensitive during this time; patients about to shed should therefore not be handled unless absolutely necessary. Patients with fungal dermatoses and contact dermatitis do not generally show sudden aggression or a blue-opaque coloration of the skin and eyes. Patients with paramyxovirus show neurologic and respiratory signs. Cheek R, Crane M, "Snakes," in Ballard B, Cheek R, Exotic Animal Medicine for the Veterinary Technician, ed 3, Wiley-Blackwell, 2017.

33. a Oral examinations in snakes are often performed at the end of the PE because of the potential stress it can cause. To help avoid trauma to the teeth and jaw, a soft plastic spatula is most often used to open the mouth. Cheek R, Crane M, "Snakes," in Ballard B, Cheek R, Exotic Animal Medicine for the Veterinary Technician, ed 3, Wiley-Blackwell, 2017.

34. b The heart and caudal tail vein are the two most common sites for venipuncture in the snake. The lateral or ventral approach can be used for the caudal tail vein. The ventral abdominal vein is not an option in snakes. Cheek R, Crane M, "Snakes," in Ballard B, Cheek R, Exotic Animal Medicine for the Veterinary Technician, ed 3, Wiley-Blackwell, 2017.

35. d The scutes are formed from keratinized epithelium. Rivera S, "Chelonians," in Ballard B, Cheek R, Exotic Animal Medicine for the Veterinary Technician, ed 3, Wiley-Blackwell, 2017.

36. c Reptiles and birds do not have diaphragms. The thorax and abdominal cavities are not separated; therefore the single cavity is referred to as a coelomic cavity. Rivera S, "Chelonians," in Ballard B, Cheek R, Exotic Animal Medicine for the Veterinary Technician, ed 3, Wiley-Blackwell, 2017.

37. b The plastron (bottom shell) is usually concave in most male species because it is used to help mount the female during mating. Rivera S, "Chelonians," in Ballard B, Cheek R, Exotic Animal Medicine for the Veterinary Technician, ed 3, Wiley-Blackwell, 2017.

38. c Gout is common in reptiles and is generally caused by improper diet and husbandry. Hypovitaminosis A causes aural abscesses to form. Surgical intervention is required to remove the abscesses and a diet change is a must. Hypocalcemia often causes seizures and is corrected by diet and husbandry adjustments. Metabolic bone disease is caused by poor husbandry and improper calcium-to-phosphorus ratio. Rivera S, "Chelonians," in Ballard B, Cheek R, Exotic Animal Medicine for the Veterinary Technician, ed 3, Wiley-Blackwell, 2017.

39. d These are signs of dystocia. Dystocia is common in the tortoise, especially in those with poor husbandry and underlying metabolic disease. This is easily diagnosed with radiographs. A GI foreign body and internal parasites would not present with bloody discharge. Hypervitaminosis A presents with flaky skin or sloughing. Rivera S, "Chelonians," in Ballard B, Cheek R, Exotic Animal Medicine for the Veterinary Technician, ed 3, Wiley-Blackwell, 2017.

40. c A complete radiographic series includes the anterior-posterior, dorsoventral, and lateral views. Turtles and tortoises do not have diaphragms; therefore they should not be placed on their backs. A horizontal beam is suggested for the lateral and anterior-posterior views. This decreases artifact of visceral organs falling into the lung cavity. The anterior-posterior view is used to assess the lungs. Rivera S, "Chelonians," in Ballard B, Cheek R, Exotic Animal Medicine for the Veterinary Technician, ed 3, Wiley-Blackwell, 2017.

41. a About 90% of parrot feces are Gram-positive. Gram-negative feces are common in raptors and waterfowl. Little to no bacteria are common in passerines. Any deviations from feces that are primarily Gram-positive indicate infection. Greenacre CB, Gerhardt L, "Psittacines and Passerines," in Ballard B, Cheek R, Exotic Animal Medicine for the Veterinary Technician, ed 3, Wiley-Blackwell, 2017.

42. d Cockatiels are small birds. The jugular vessel is the largest vein available for blood collection. The medial metatarsal vessels are too small and birds do not have a cephalic vein. The cutaneous ulnar vessels might be used in some cases for a small sample, but they are too small for large-volume blood collection. Greenacre CB, Gerhardt L, "Psittacines and Passerines," in Ballard B, Cheek R, Exotic Animal Medicine for the Veterinary Technician, ed 3, Wiley-Blackwell, 2017.

43. b If it is safe to remove 10% of the blood volume in a healthy bird, then 10 mL of blood can be taken from a 1-kg macaw. To calculate this, you would use the following formula: $1 \text{ kg} \times 0.01 = 0.010 \text{ L}$ or 10 mL. Greenacre CB, Gerhardt L, "Psittacines and Passerines," in Ballard B, Cheek R, Exotic Animal Medicine for the Veterinary Technician, ed 3, Wiley-Blackwell, 2017.

44. a The pectoral muscles are large and are part of the easiest muscle group to use for injection of medications in the avian patient. The biceps could be used, but they are very small in most birds. The epaxial muscles are also small. The quadriceps is in a larger muscle group, but it is located caudal to the kidneys. Birds have a reniportal system. Drugs administered below the kidneys are absorbed into the blood stream and are potentially filtered directly to the kidneys without systemic uptake. How this affects most drugs is poorly understood and therefore it is best avoided when possible. Greenacre CB, Gerhardt L, "Psittacines and Passerines," in Ballard B, Cheek R, Exotic Animal Medicine for the Veterinary Technician, ed 3, Wiley-Blackwell, 2017.

45. c The figure-8 bandage is used to immobilize the radius, ulna, and the distal wing bones. This bandage does not stabilize the humerus unless an additional wrap is placed around the body. Greenacre CB, Gerhardt L, "Psittacines and Passerines," in Ballard B, Cheek R, Exotic Animal Medicine for the Veterinary Technician, ed 3, Wiley-Blackwell, 2017.

46. d The jugular vein is the largest vessel and it is easiest to obtain a larger volume of blood from there. The peripheral vessels are very small and are primarily used for IV catheterization, not blood collection. The auricular veins are not accessible in the chinchilla. Schuller A, Ballard B, "Chinchillas," in Ballard B, Cheek R, Exotic Animal Medicine for the Veterinary Technician, ed 3, Wiley-Blackwell, 2017.

47. c The cephalic and jugular veins are possible, but a surgical cut down must be performed before catheterization. The cephalic vein is also very small even in large lizards. The femoral vein is not really used in lizards. The caudal tail vein is the most common site for IV catheter placement in lizards. Nugent-Deal J, "Avian and Exotic Emergencies," in Battaglia AM, Steele AM, Small Animal Emergency and Critical Care for Veterinary Technicians, ed 3, Elsevier, 2015.

48. b Seizures, tremors, anorexia, kyphosis, pliable or thickened bones, and fractures are all signs of metabolic bone disease (MBD). MBD is caused by poor husbandry, improper lighting/temperature, and diet, primarily an imbalance in the calcium-to-phosphorus ratio. Hypercalcemia and hypervitaminosis A do not cause these symptoms and are uncommon in lizards. Gout is caused by poor husbandry and diet, but it causes swelling in the joints and extreme pain resulting from the buildup of uric acid. Nugent-Deal J, "Avian and Exotic Emergencies," in Battaglia AM, Steele AM, Small Animal Emergency and Critical Care for Veterinary Technicians, ed 3, Elsevier, 2015.

49. d Basic blood work may be indicated based on other clinical findings or if it has not been analyzed for a while. Computed tomography (CT) can be performed, but this is not a first-line diagnostic. Radiographs can be easily obtained in most snakes and can help rule out a potential foreign body. Nugent-Deal J, "Avian and Exotic Emergencies," in Battaglia AM, Steele AM, Small Animal Emergency and Critical Care for Veterinary Technicians, ed 3, Elsevier, 2015.

50. c It is estimated that about 30%–50% of rabbits have endogenous atropinase enzymes that block the effectiveness of the drug. This is not present in the other species. Nugent-Deal J, "Avian and Exotic Emergencies," in Battaglia AM, Steele AM, Small Animal Emergency and Critical Care for Veterinary Technicians, ed 3, Elsevier, 2015.

51. b The mucous membranes in birds are very dry and assessing the saliva is therefore not appropriate. The quality of the feathers has nothing to do with current hydration status. The capillary refill time is difficult to assess in birds; using venous refill time is therefore the easiest and most effective way to assess hydration. Depressing the cutaneous ulnar vein assesses venous refill time. It should refill instantly. If it does not, the patient is dehydrated. Nugent-Deal J, "Avian and Exotic Emergencies," in Battaglia AM, Steele AM, Small Animal Emergency and Critical Care for Veterinary Technicians, ed 3, Elsevier, 2015.

52. d In most avian species, the femur and humerus are pneumatized. Pneumatic bones have a direct connection to the respiratory system. Placing an intraosseous catheter is contraindicated in pneumatic bones. Nugent-Deal J, "Avian and Exotic Emergencies," in Battaglia AM, Steele AM, Small Animal Emergency and Critical Care for Veterinary Technicians, ed 3, Elsevier, 2015.

53. b Approximately 5% of the body weight can be tube fed to avian patients at one time. For example, a 100-g cockatiel can be tube fed about 5 mL of food. Nugent-Deal J, "Avian and Exotic Emergencies," in Battaglia AM, Steele AM, Small Animal Emergency and Critical Care for Veterinary Technicians, ed 3, Elsevier, 2015.

54. a The standard daily maintenance fluid for avian patients is 50–60 mL/kg/day. Most commonly this is given subcutaneously but can also be administered via the IV or IO routes. Nugent-Deal J, "Avian and Exotic Emergencies," in Battaglia AM, Steele AM, Small Animal Emergency and Critical Care for Veterinary Technicians, ed 3, Elsevier, 2015.

55. c Lead and zinc are the two most common metals that cause toxicity after ingestion and birds left unattended easily consume them. Lead is commonly found in costume jewelry, solder, batteries, lead-based paint, and linoleum. Zinc is commonly found in galvanized wire, pennies minted after 1982, wire clips, and Monopoly pieces. Nugent-Deal J, "Avian and Exotic Emergencies," in Battaglia AM, Steele AM, Small Animal Emergency and Critical Care for Veterinary Technicians, ed 3, Elsevier, 2015.

56. b These signs are indicative of zinc toxicity, especially because this bird has been chewing on a galvanized wired cage. Iron and copper toxicity are very uncommon in birds. Lead toxicity shows signs of lethargy, regurgitation, diarrhea, ataxia, wing droop, and leg paresis. Nugent-Deal J, "Avian and Exotic Emergencies," in Battaglia AM, Steele AM, Small Animal Emergency and Critical Care for Veterinary Technicians, ed 3, Elsevier, 2015.

57. c The pupil in birds and reptiles is composed of striated skeletal muscle. These species have voluntary control over constriction and dilation of the pupil. Because of this, a pupillary light reflex may not be present on physical examination. Nugent-Deal J, "Avian and Exotic Emergencies," in Battaglia AM, Steele AM, Small Animal Emergency and Critical Care for Veterinary Technicians, ed 3, Elsevier, 2015.

58. b Malnutrition, breeding, and bacterial infections are not considered common causes of penile prolapse in the chinchilla. Penile prolapse is generally caused by fur accumulation around the base of the penis. Fur rings can be found in both breeding and nonbreeding males and can occur anytime throughout the year. The penis should be examined during the PE. Fur accumulation can be removed using saline, lubricant, and a swab to pull the fur away gently. Nugent-Deal J, "Avian and Exotic Emergencies," in Battaglia AM, Steele AM, Small Animal Emergency and Critical Care for Veterinary Technicians, ed 3, Elsevier, 2015.

59. c GI stasis is not common in hamsters and, if present, diarrhea would be an unexpected finding. Diarrhea is also not generally present with cystic calculi or dental disease. Straining to urinate and anorexia would be expected with cystic calculi and dental disease, respectively. Nugent-Deal J, "Avian and Exotic Emergencies," in Battaglia AM, Steele AM, Small Animal Emergency and Critical Care for Veterinary Technicians, ed 3, Elsevier, 2015.

60. c The pain is described as moderate to severe. Full mu opioids such as hydromorphone and fentanyl would be the best choice to treat moderate-to-severe pain in this patient. Buprenorphine is a partial mu agonist opioid. This drug is best used for mild-to-moderate pain. Butorphanol is a kappa agonist opioid that is best used for sedation and mild analgesia. Nugent-Deal J, "Avian and Exotic Emergencies," in Battaglia AM, Steele AM, Small Animal Emergency and Critical Care for Veterinary Technicians, ed 3, Elsevier, 2015.

61. b These are the most common signs of dental disease in a rabbit, chinchilla, and guinea pig. Trichobezoars are hairballs. These are much less common than once believed and when present, they act as a GI foreign body or blockage. *Pasteurella multocida* is a common bacterium of the upper respiratory tract. This is found most often in rabbits. Cystic ovaries will often cause abdominal pain and anorexia. Nugent-Deal J, "Avian and Exotic Emergencies," in Battaglia AM, Steele AM, Small Animal Emergency and Critical Care for Veterinary Technicians, ed 3, Elsevier, 2015.

62. a Uterine adenocarcinoma is common in unspayed female rabbits older than 4 years. Clinical signs include hematuria, frank blood at the end of urination, depression, anorexia, and dehydration. The other neoplasms are not very common in rabbits. Nugent-Deal J, "Avian and Exotic Emergencies," in Battaglia AM, Steele AM, Small Animal Emergency and Critical Care for Veterinary Technicians, ed 3, Elsevier, 2015.

63. a *Pasteurella multocida* is the most common bacteria of the upper airway causing these clinical signs. Bacterial enteritis causes GI signs, whereas allergic dermatitis causes clinical signs related to the skin. Pneumonia most commonly affects the lower airway and pulmonary system. Nugent-Deal J, "Avian and Exotic Emergencies," in Battaglia AM, Steele AM, Small Animal Emergency and Critical Care for Veterinary Technicians, ed 3, Elsevier, 2015.

64. d The peripheral vessels are small and will probably not yield enough blood needed for transfusion. You cannot draw blood from the auricular vessels in ferrets. The cranial vena cava is the largest vessel that will yield the most blood in the shortest amount of time. Nugent-Deal J, "Avian and Exotic Emergencies," in Battaglia AM, Steele AM, Small Animal Emergency and Critical Care for Veterinary Technicians, ed 3, Elsevier, 2015.

65. b The choana is the opening at the roof of the mouth that connects the trachea to the sinuses and the nares. The choanal slit is located on the roof of the mouth and has many sharp papillae protruding from it. Nugent-Deal J, "Avian and Exotic Emergencies," in Battaglia AM, Steele AM, Small Animal Emergency and Critical Care for Veterinary Technicians, ed 3, Elsevier, 2015.

66. d The other bones listed are not pneumatic in most species of birds. Pneumatic bones are filled with air and have a direct connection to the respiratory system. Nugent-Deal J, "Avian and Exotic Emergencies," in Battaglia AM, Steele AM, Small Animal Emergency and Critical Care for Veterinary Technicians, ed 3, Elsevier, 2015.

67. d Hematoma formation is not a complication of IO catheterization because the catheter is placed into the bone and not into a vessel. Nugent-Deal J, "Avian and Exotic Emergencies," in Battaglia AM, Steele AM, Small Animal Emergency and Critical Care for Veterinary Technicians, ed 3, Elsevier, 2015.

68. c The wing web and areas over the back can be used, but the largest area to administer fluids in avian patients is in the inguinal area. Nugent-Deal J, "Avian and Exotic Emergencies," in Battaglia AM, Steele AM, Small Animal Emergency and Critical Care for Veterinary Technicians, ed 3, Elsevier, 2015.

69. a Myotoxins are common in foods such as seeds, peanuts, pellets, and millet. In severe cases, acute death can occur. Moldy peanuts are not associated with *Salmonella*, *Escherichia coli*, or *Clostridium difficile*. Nugent-Deal J, "Avian and Exotic Emergencies," in Battaglia AM, Steele AM, Small Animal Emergency and Critical Care for Veterinary Technicians, ed 3, Elsevier, 2015.

70. c Air sac cannulas are tubes that can be placed into the caudal thoracic and abdominal air sacs. This allows the bird to bypass breathing out of the mouth and to breathe through the cannula. The cervicocephalic and clavicular air sacs are located near the neck and are not used for air sac cannulation. Nugent-Deal J, "Avian and Exotic Emergencies," in Battaglia AM, Steele AM, Small Animal Emergency and Critical Care for Veterinary Technicians, ed 3, Elsevier, 2015.

71. d External parasites can cause alopecia but it would not be uniform. An insulinoma generally presents with severe hypoglycemia and potential seizures. Green slime disease is also known as coronaviral diarrhea syndrome. Patients can present with severe, green, mucoid diarrhea, anorexia, weakness, dehydration, and emaciation. Classic ferret adrenal disease presents with alopecia at the tail tip, symmetrical alopecia along the trunk of the body, intense pruritus, and an enlarged vulva. Nugent-Deal J, "Avian and Exotic Emergencies," in Battaglia AM, Steele AM, Small Animal Emergency and Critical Care for Veterinary Technicians, ed 3, Elsevier, 2015.

72. c A CBC and chemistry panel could be beneficial to examine overall health status but will not specifically diagnose a foreign body. MRI is great for looking at soft tissue but is not a diagnostic normally used for a GI foreign body. Radiographs and ultrasound are the two most commonly used modalities for diagnosing a foreign body. Nugent-Deal J, "Avian and Exotic Emergencies," in Battaglia AM, Steele AM, Small Animal Emergency and Critical Care for Veterinary Technicians, ed 3, Elsevier, 2015.

73. a Odontomas are common causes of upper respiratory disease in captive prairie dogs. Odontomas are caused by inflammation of the periodontal bone generally because of trauma or dental disease. Chronic inflammation leads to narrowing of nasal passages. This is diagnosed via radiographs and physical examination. Treatment consists of removal of the affected teeth and debridement of abnormal tissue. Rivera S, "Prairie Dogs," in Ballard B, Cheek R, Exotic Animal Medicine for the Veterinary Technician, ed 3, Wiley-Blackwell, 2017.

74. c The jugular vein is the largest vessel that is most easily assessable in most patients (although it can be difficult in obese animals). The lateral saphenous and cephalic vessels can be used, but the peripheral veins tend to be small and often do not yield enough blood for a full CBC and chemistry panel. The caudal tail vein is not generally used. Rivera S, "Prairie Dogs," in Ballard B, Cheek R, Exotic Animal Medicine for the Veterinary Technician, ed 3, Wiley-Blackwell, 2017.

75. a The jugular vein, cranial vena cava, and medial tibial artery are the most commonly used vessels for collection of larger blood samples. The cephalic, lateral saphenous, femoral, ventral coccygeal, and lateral tail veins can be used for blood sampling but do not often yield enough blood for a full CBC and chemistry panel. Rivera S, "Sugar Gliders," in Ballard B, Cheek R, Exotic Animal Medicine for the Veterinary Technician, ed 3, Wiley-Blackwell, 2017.

76. c Most diseases in exotic species are caused by improper husbandry. Nutritional osteodystrophy is one of the most common diseases seen in captive sugar gliders. The most common presenting complaint is an acute onset of hind limb paresis or paralysis. This disease is caused by feeding a diet low in calcium and vitamin D3. Obesity and lymphoid neoplasia are common, but they do not cause an acute onset of hind limb paresis or paralysis. Cardiomyopathy is not a common disease in sugar gliders. Rivera S, "Sugar Gliders," in Ballard B, Cheek R, Exotic Animal Medicine for the Veterinary Technician, ed 3, Wiley-Blackwell, 2017.

77. d The sugar glider is the only species listed that is considered arboreal. Providing branches and climbing areas is essential for captive animals. The prairie dog, chinchilla, and guinea pig are all ground-dwelling animals. Rivera S, "Sugar Gliders," in Ballard B, Cheek R, Exotic Animal Medicine for the Veterinary Technician, ed 3, Wiley-Blackwell, 2017.

78. d The sugar glider is the only mammal listed that has a cloaca similar to that seen in a bird or reptile. Rivera S, "Sugar Gliders," in Ballard B, Cheek R, Exotic Animal Medicine for the Veterinary Technician, ed 3, Wiley-Blackwell, 2017.

79. a Sugar gliders eat nectar and sap in the wild. In captivity, they should be fed a diet of insects, small invertebrates, fruits, sugar-glider pelleted diet, commercial insectivore diet, and nectar. Chicken is not a normal part of the captive diet. Rivera S, "Sugar Gliders," in Ballard B, Cheek R, Exotic Animal Medicine for the Veterinary Technician, ed 3, Wiley-Blackwell, 2017.

80. d Pet skunks are vaccinated against rabies, feline panleukopenia, and canine distemper. Skunks are not vaccinated against parvovirus disease. Rivera S, "Skunks," in Ballard B, Cheek R, Exotic Animal Medicine for the Veterinary Technician, ed 3, Wiley-Blackwell, 2017.

81. c These signs are most commonly associated with cardiomyopathy. Signs such as anorexia, weight loss, and lethargy are very generalized and can occur with several different diseases. The key to heart disease is the dyspnea, coughing, ascites, and exercise intolerance. Cardiomyopathy is diagnosed via radiographs, echocardiogram, and ECG. Rivera S, "Skunks," in Ballard B, Cheek R, Exotic Animal Medicine for the Veterinary Technician, ed 3, Wiley-Blackwell, 2017.

82. a Hedgehogs are insectivores with a captive diet often consisting of crickets, mealworms, grasshoppers, snails, slugs, pinkie mice, and frogs. A small amount of fruit can also be offered. Many feed mixes include high-quality pelleted diets. Schuller A, Jones MD, "Hedgehogs," in Ballard B, Cheek R, Exotic Animal Medicine for the Veterinary Technician, ed 3, Wiley-Blackwell, 2017.

83. b This strange behavior is called self-anointing and is associated with smells and seeing other small animals. This can be often be mistaken for a seizure, but this is normal hedgehog behavior. Schuller A, Jones MD, "Hedgehogs," in Ballard B, Cheek R, Exotic Animal Medicine for the Veterinary Technician, ed 3, Wiley-Blackwell, 2017.

84. d Vessels commonly used in hedgehogs include the femoral, cephalic, jugular, and cranial vena cava. The peripheral vessels are small, making it difficult to obtain larger sample volumes. The jugular and cranial vena cava are the best options for collection of a full CBC and chemistry panel. Schuller A, Jones MD, "Hedgehogs," in Ballard B, Cheek R, Exotic Animal Medicine for the Veterinary Technician, ed 3, Wiley-Blackwell, 2017.

85. a These symptoms describe wobbling hedgehog syndrome. This disease generally occurs between 18 and 24 months of age. It starts in the hind legs and ascends to the head. This can take weeks to months. There is no treatment or known etiologic treatment. Neoplasia and nephritis would not generally cause symptoms that include progressive ataxia and paralysis. Schuller A, Jones MD, "Hedgehogs," in Ballard B, Cheek R, Exotic Animal Medicine for the Veterinary Technician, ed 3, Wiley-Blackwell, 2017.

86. a *Clostridium piliforme* causes Tyzzer's disease. This disease is a hepatoenteric, infectious, and fatal in the hamster and gerbil. Mice and rats that contract the disease are able to overcome it. Clinical signs include sudden death, listlessness, poor/rough hair coat, and weight loss. Stress and infected bedding contribute to infection. Romagnano A, "Mice, Rats, Gerbils, and Hamsters," in Ballard B, Cheek R, Exotic Animal Medicine for the Veterinary Technician, ed 3, Wiley-Blackwell, 2017.

87. d Captive rabbits are rarely affected, but when present, tularemia will cause an acute and febrile condition. Tularemia is often spread to humans by contact with wild rabbits. Gloves and hand washing greatly reduce the spread of the disease from rabbits to humans. Taylor DK, Lee V, Mook D, Huerkamp MJ, "Rabbits," in Ballard B, Cheek R, Exotic Animal Medicine for the Veterinary Technician, ed 3, Wiley-Blackwell, 2017.

88. d The crop is an outpouching of the esophagus. The crop is also called the ingluvies. The crop stores food until it passes into the proventriculus. The proventriculus is the glandular stomach. The food then passes from the proventriculus into the gizzard. The gizzard is also called the ventriculus. Greenacre CB, Gerhardt L, "Psittacines and Passerines," in Ballard B, Cheek R, Exotic Animal Medicine for the Veterinary Technician, ed 3, Wiley-Blackwell, 2017.

89. c Pterylae are the areas where feathers lie on the body. Apterylae are featherless areas. Rectrices and remiges are tail and wing feathers, respectively. Barbules are parts of the feather that help keep the feather pulled together neatly. Greenacre CB, Gerhardt L, "Psittacines and Passerines," in Ballard B, Cheek R, Exotic Animal Medicine for the Veterinary Technician, ed 3, Wiley-Blackwell, 2017.

90. a The keel is part of the sternum and serves as the attachment for the pectoral muscles. The pygostyle is the fusion of the caudal vertebrae where the tail muscle attaches. The notarium is the fusion of the first thoracic vertebrae. The synsacrum is the fusion of the caudal thoracic, lumbar, sacral, and caudal vertebrae. Greenacre CB, Gerhardt L, "Psittacines and Passerines," in Ballard B, Cheek R, Exotic Animal Medicine for the Veterinary Technician, ed 3, Wiley-Blackwell, 2017.

91. a The operculum is an anatomical structure that helps prevent the inhalation of foreign material into the respiratory system. The operculum sits just inside the nares. Longley LA, "Avian Anesthesia," Anesthesia of Exotic Pets, ed 1, Saunders-Elsevier, 2008.

92. c Unlike mammals, the larynx does not produce sound in the avian patient. The syrinx is responsible for sound production. The glottis is the opening to the trachea and the infraorbital sinus communicates with the nasal passages and has nothing to do with sound production. Longley LA, "Avian Anesthesia," Anesthesia of Exotic Pets, ed 1, Saunders-Elsevier, 2008.

93. a Unlike mammals, birds and reptiles do not have an epiglottis. This makes them extremely easy to intubate. Longley LA, "Avian Anesthesia," Anesthesia of Exotic Pets, ed 1, Saunders-Elsevier, 2008.

94. b The cloaca is the final holding area for feces, urine/urates, and eggs before being expelled from the body through the vent. The choana is the opening at the roof of the mouth that leads into the upper respiratory system. The cecum is part of the gastrointestinal tract. Longley LA, "Avian Anesthesia," Anesthesia of Exotic Pets, ed 1, Saunders-Elsevier, 2008.

95. c Similar to dogs and cats, the liver sits below the heart. In the case of birds, there is no diaphragm separating the two structures. The kidneys are located near the pelvis. The cecum and pancreas are located within the coelomic cavity and are not near the heart. Longley LA, "Avian Anesthesia," Anesthesia of Exotic Pets, Saunders-Elsevier, 2008.

96. d All-seed diets are high in fat and lack adequate amounts of vitamin A. Hypovitaminosis A leads to immune-suppression and epithelial abnormalities, including squamous metaplasia. Longley LA, "Avian Anesthesia," Anesthesia of Exotic Pets, Saunders-Elsevier, 2008.

97. b Although lethargy and inappetence can be seen with almost any disease, green feces and urates paired with poor feather quality and abnormal beak and nails are highly indicative of liver disease. Longley LA, "Avian Anesthesia," Anesthesia of Exotic Pets, Saunders-Elsevier, 2008.

98. d The major respiratory organs in fish are the gills. Gas exchange, nitrogenous waste excretion, acid-base balance, and osmotic control all take place here. Fiddes M, "Fish Anesthesia," in Longley LA, Anesthesia of Exotic Pets, ed 1, Saunders-Elsevier, 2008.

99. b The cardiovascular system is fairly simple in fish. The heart consists of two chambers with four distinct regions. Fiddes M, "Fish Anesthesia," in Longley LA, Anesthesia of Exotic Pets, ed 1, Saunders-Elsevier, 2008.

100. d The POTZ is the normal temperature zone where a species thrives. This zone is extremely important for normal daily functions such as drug metabolism, digestion, healing, and reproduction. Longley LA, "Reptile Anesthesia," in Longley LA, Anesthesia of Exotic Pets, ed 1, Saunders-Elsevier, 2008.

101. a The term *gravid* is used in reptiles that carry and lay eggs (oviparous). Reptiles that are ovoviviparous or viviparous are termed pregnant because they have embryos present. Wilson B, "Lizards," in Ballard B, Cheek R, Exotic Animal Medicine for the Veterinary Technician, ed 3, Wiley-Blackwell, 2017.

102. d Chromatophores are specific to the chameleon and anole species. These specialized cells allow color change in the skin. The other cells have nothing to do with reflecting light or changing the color of the skin. Heterophils and azurophils are types of white blood cells. Wilson B, "Lizards," in Ballard B, Cheek R, Exotic Animal Medicine for the Veterinary Technician, ed 3, Wiley-Blackwell, 2017.

103. c Pleurodont teeth have no root and are attached to the jaw. Elodont teeth increase in length throughout life. Hypsodont teeth are teeth and cusps that are elongated. Monophyodont is defined as only one set of teeth throughout life. Monophyodonts do not have deciduous teeth. Wilson B, "Lizards," in Ballard B, Cheek R, Exotic Animal Medicine for the Veterinary Technician, ed 3, Wiley-Blackwell, 2017.

104. a Large femoral pores are common in many male species of lizard including the green iguana. Large femoral pores are only indicative of maleness. Wilson B, "Lizards," in Ballard B, Cheek R, Exotic Animal Medicine for the Veterinary Technician, ed 3, Wiley-Blackwell, 2017.

105. b Lizards have internal paired hemipenes that are housed in a diverticulum at the proximal tail. The testicles are internal. Wilson B, "Lizards," in Ballard B, Cheek R, Exotic Animal Medicine for the Veterinary Technician, ed 3, Wiley-Blackwell, 2017.

106. d The parietal eye is also known as the third eye. This is easily seen on top of the head in iguanas. The spectacle is an impermeable structure that connects the upper and lower eyelid. The Jacobson's organ is used to help track prey and potentially to detect mates or enemies. The thyroid gland secretes hormones. Wilson B, "Lizards," in Ballard B, Cheek R, Exotic Animal Medicine for the Veterinary Technician, ed 3, Wiley-Blackwell, 2017.

107. b Most disease processes are caused by improper husbandry. It is important to be aware of commonly kept species and their native environment. The Jackson's chameleon is the only listed arboreal species. The other lizards listed are terrestrial. Wilson B, "Lizards," in Ballard B, Cheek R, Exotic Animal Medicine for the Veterinary Technician, ed 3, Wiley-Blackwell, 2017.

108. c Because of diet, most carnivores do not require UV-B lighting for synthesis of vitamin D3 and absorption of calcium. The other statements are false. Wilson

B, "Lizards," in Ballard B, Cheek R, Exotic Animal Medicine for the Veterinary Technician, ed 3, Wiley-Blackwell, 2017.

109. d Carnivorous lizards do not require UV-B light for absorption of calcium and synthesis of vitamin D3, but insectivorous, herbivorous, and omnivorous lizards do. Wilson B, "Lizards," in Ballard B, Cheek R, Exotic Animal Medicine for the Veterinary Technician, ed 3, Wiley-Blackwell, 2017.

110. a Lizards have a poor sense of detecting conductive heat. Burns are common when they lie directly on a heat source, therefore everything should be placed outside the cage or out of reach of the animal. Wilson B, "Lizards," in Ballard B, Cheek R, Exotic Animal Medicine for the Veterinary Technician, ed 3, Wiley-Blackwell, 2017.

111. b Nervous animals or those not adjusted to living in a glass or plastic terrarium will often rub and bump into the walls, causing abrasions on the rostrum. Although fungal infections and trauma can cause lesions, this is not common or specific to the rostrum. Wilson B, "Lizards," in Ballard B, Cheek R, Exotic Animal Medicine for the Veterinary Technician, ed 3, Wiley-Blackwell, 2017.

112. c Fungal and bacterial infections are not common complications after dysecdysis occurs. Some species eat the shed skin, but this does not cause constipation. Extremity necrosis, especially of the toes or tail tip, is common and causes constriction, acting as a rubber band. When this happens, amputation is often necessary. Wilson B, "Lizards," in Ballard B, Cheek R, Exotic Animal Medicine for the Veterinary Technician, ed 3, Wiley-Blackwell, 2017.

113. d Prolapse of the cloaca can be caused by reproductive, digestive, and excretory disorders. Septicemia does not affect the cloaca or surrounding tissues. Wilson B, "Lizards," in Ballard B, Cheek R, Exotic Animal Medicine for the Veterinary Technician, ed 3, Wiley-Blackwell, 2017.

114. a Gout is caused by diets high in purines. This is most common in the herbivorous lizard. Gout is an excessive buildup of uric acid in the blood that crystalizes and precipitates into the tissues. Swelling and pain is often noted around the joints. Diets high in purines do not lead to heart failure, liver failure, or salmonellosis. Wilson B, "Lizards," in Ballard B, Cheek R, Exotic Animal Medicine for the Veterinary Technician, ed 3, Wiley-Blackwell, 2017.

115. b It is suggested that ferrets are vaccinated against rabies and canine distemper. Ferrets can have severe reactions to the canine distemper vaccine and a ferret-safe vaccine should therefore be administered. Roman C, Hadley T, "Ferrets," in Ballard B, Cheek R, Exotic Animal Medicine for the Veterinary Technician, ed 3, Wiley-Blackwell, 2017.

116. d The average life span in domestic ferrets is approximately 5–7 years. Roman C, Hadley T, "Ferrets," in Ballard B, Cheek R, Exotic Animal Medicine for the Veterinary Technician, ed 3, Wiley-Blackwell, 2017.

117. d The radius, ulna, and fibula are too small to use for IO catheter placement. The femur is the largest and easiest bone to use in most mammals including the ferret. Roman C, Hadley T, "Ferrets," in Ballard B, Cheek R, Exotic Animal Medicine for the Veterinary Technician, ed 3, Wiley-Blackwell, 2017.

118. b The predominant white blood cells in the rabbit are lymphocytes and heterophils. Heterophils in the rabbit are equivalent to neutrophils. Taylor DK, Lee V, Mook D, Huerkamp MJ, "Rabbits," in Ballard B, Cheek R, Exotic Animal Medicine for the Veterinary Technician, ed 3, Wiley-Blackwell, 2017.

119. c The cat skeleton is approximately 13% of the total body weight, whereas in rabbits it is only 8%. Because of the large muscular legs in rabbits, the lumbar spine is at a great risk of fracture compared with most other mammals. Taylor DK, Lee V, Mook D, Huerkamp MJ, "Rabbits," in Ballard B, Cheek R, Exotic Animal Medicine for the Veterinary Technician, ed 3, Wiley-Blackwell, 2017.

120. a Cecotropes are the soft feces that are excreted and then consumed. Consumption is important because it allows additional digestion of nutrients. Taylor DK, Lee V, Mook D, Huerkamp MJ, "Rabbits," in Ballard B, Cheek R, Exotic Animal Medicine for the Veterinary Technician, ed 3, Wiley-Blackwell, 2017.

121. c A large part of a rabbit's diet should consist of hay and dark leafy greens with a small amount of pellets. The type of hay and pellets depends on the life stage. Different hays have various mineral and nutritional values. Hay is important to help maintain a healthy weight, wear teeth properly, and maintain good GI health. Taylor DK, Lee V, Mook D, Huerkamp MJ, "Rabbits," in Ballard B, Cheek R, Exotic Animal Medicine for the Veterinary Technician, ed 3, Wiley-Blackwell, 2017.

122. d The skull is placed in lateral recumbency and then rotated about 10 to 20 degrees to the left and to the right to obtain oblique films. These views allow separation of the mandible and maxilla, therefore providing a better view of the tooth roots. Taylor DK, Lee V, Mook D, Huerkamp MJ, "Rabbits," in Ballard B, Cheek R, Exotic Animal Medicine for the Veterinary Technician, ed 3, Wiley-Blackwell, 2017.

123. a Rabbits do not vocalize when in pain but do show other signs such as bruxism, anorexia, and reduced activity and grooming. Taylor DK, Lee V, Mook D, Huerkamp MJ, "Rabbits," in Ballard B, Cheek R, Exotic Animal Medicine for the Veterinary Technician, ed 3, Wiley-Blackwell, 2017.

124. c Female rabbits are referred to as does. A jill and a hob are female and male ferrets, respectively. A bitch is an intact female dog. Taylor DK, Lee V, Mook D, Huerkamp MJ, "Rabbits," in Ballard B, Cheek R, Exotic Animal Medicine for the Veterinary Technician, ed 3, Wiley-Blackwell, 2017.

125. a Male rabbits are referred to as bucks. A hob is a male ferret. A tom is a male cat. A colt is a male horse. Taylor DK, Lee V, Mook D, Huerkamp MJ, "Rabbits," in Ballard B, Cheek R, Exotic Animal Medicine for the Veterinary Technician, ed 3, Wiley-Blackwell, 2017.

126. c The average gestational period for domestic rabbits is between 31 and 32 days. Taylor DK, Lee V, Mook D, Huerkamp MJ, "Rabbits," in Ballard B, Cheek R, Exotic

Animal Medicine for the Veterinary Technician, ed 3, Wiley-Blackwell, 2017.

127. a The normal rectal temperature range in rabbits is greater than that in dogs and cats. Taylor DK, Lee V, Mook D, Huerkamp MJ, "Rabbits," in Ballard B, Cheek R, Exotic Animal Medicine for the Veterinary Technician, ed 3, Wiley-Blackwell, 2017.

128. b PCV is important to memorize if you are treating different species. Each species has its own range. You must know the normal before you can know the abnormal. Taylor DK, Lee V, Mook D, Huerkamp MJ, "Rabbits," in Ballard B, Cheek R, Exotic Animal Medicine for the Veterinary Technician, ed 3, Wiley-Blackwell, 2017.

129. a A rat's incisors grow continuously throughout life, but the molars do not. In rabbits, chinchillas, and guinea pigs, all teeth grow continuously throughout life. Romagnano A, "Mice, Rats, Gerbils, and Hamsters," in Ballard B, Cheek R, Exotic Animal Medicine for the Veterinary Technician, ed 3, Wiley-Blackwell, 2017.

130. b There are up to 90 hairs per follicle in a chinchilla's coat. This helps keep it warm in its native environment of the Andes Mountains. Chinchillas should not be bathed with water. Offering a dust bath daily will help keep the coat and skin healthy. The other answers are not used for maintaining coat and skin quality. Schuller A, Ballard B, "Chinchillas," in Ballard B, Cheek R, Exotic Animal Medicine for the Veterinary Technician, ed 3, Wiley-Blackwell, 2017.

131. d Nonaromatic shavings such as aspen, newspaper, and recycled newspaper products can all be used for bedding. Aromatic shavings such as pine and cedar should not be used. These shavings can cause respiratory irritation. Schuller A, Ballard B, "Chinchillas," in Ballard B, Cheek R, Exotic Animal Medicine for the Veterinary Technician, ed 3, Wiley-Blackwell, 2017.

132. c Back fractures are common in rabbits, but not chinchillas. Dental disease, heat stroke, and choke are all very common. The teeth grow continuously throughout life, therefore uncorrected malocclusion can lead to dental disease. Chinchillas are native to cool climates, therefore heat stroke is common when exposed to temperature >80°F and in environments with high humidity. Chinchillas cannot vomit; therefore choke can occur when objects become stuck in the esophagus. Schuller A, Ballard B, "Chinchillas," in Ballard B, Cheek R, Exotic Animal Medicine for the Veterinary Technician, ed 3, Wiley-Blackwell, 2017.

133. a The normal weight of an adult chinchilla ranges between 400 g and 600 g. Schuller A, Ballard B, "Chinchillas," in Ballard B, Cheek R, Exotic Animal Medicine for the Veterinary Technician, ed 3, Wiley-Blackwell, 2017.

134. b Female guinea pigs are referred to as sows. A hen is a female chicken. A queen is a female cat. A doe is a female rabbit. Murray J, Crane M, "Guinea Pigs," in Ballard B, Cheek R, Exotic Animal Medicine for the Veterinary Technician, ed 3, Wiley-Blackwell, 2017.

135. c These are classic signs of pododermatitis. Obesity, wire-bottom cages, and unsanitary environments often cause this disease. Gout, vitamin C deficiency, and bacterial infections do not cause the plantar thinning and ulceration. Murray J, Crane M, "Guinea Pigs," in Ballard B, Cheek R, Exotic Animal Medicine for the Veterinary Technician, ed 3, Wiley-Blackwell, 2017.

136. b Fur slip is a natural predatory response found in chinchillas to help escape danger. If they are frightened, large amounts of fur can be released during scruffing. Schuller A, Ballard B, "Chinchillas," in Ballard B, Cheek R, Exotic Animal Medicine for the Veterinary Technician, ed 3, Wiley-Blackwell, 2017.

137. a Discharge from the ears is not a common symptom of dental disease. Drooling, anorexia, overgrooming, crusting on front legs, decreased fecal output, dehydration, and pain are just some of the signs and symptoms of dental disease. Schuller A, Ballard B, "Chinchillas," in Ballard B, Cheek R, Exotic Animal Medicine for the Veterinary Technician, ed 3, Wiley-Blackwell, 2017.

138. b Ferrets are obligate carnivores. A ferret's diet should consist of meat-based protein and not greens or vegetables. Nugent-Deal J, "Avian and Exotic Emergencies," in Battaglia AM, Steele AM, Small Animal Emergency and Critical Care for Veterinary Technicians, ed 3, Elsevier, 2015.

139. d Rabbits exhibit a unique reproductive tract with a duplex uterus and two cervices. Taylor DK, Lee V, Mook D, Huerkamp MJ, "Rabbits," in Ballard B, Cheek R, Exotic Animal Medicine for the Veterinary Technician, ed 3, Wiley-Blackwell, 2017.

140. a Ferrets are obligate carnivores. A balanced diet consists of 30%–40% protein and 15%–30% fat. Roman C, Hadley T, "Ferrets," in Ballard B, Cheek R, Exotic Animal Medicine for the Veterinary Technician, ed 3, Wiley-Blackwell, 2017.

141. a The outermost feathers of the wing are the primary feathers. These are the only feathers that should be trimmed as part of the avian wing trim. Trims vary based on bird type. Heavy-bodied birds such as Amazon parrots should have conservative trims (2–5 feathers). This prevents falling and fracturing the keel bone. Light-bodied birds such as cockatiels probably need 8–10 feathers trimmed to help prevent flying. The secondary, tertiary, and tail feathers should not be trimmed. Poor trims can lead to feather picking. Greenacre CB, Gerhardt L, "Psittacines and Passerines," in Ballard B, Cheek R, Exotic Animal Medicine for the Veterinary Technician, ed 3, Wiley-Blackwell, 2017.

142. d Obesity, diets low in vitamin A, and improper perch surfaces all lead to plantar thinning and can cause pododermatitis. Psittacine beak and feather disease affect the feather and beak quality and growth. This disease is often fatal. Parrots with this disease are predisposed to secondary bacterial, viral, and fungal infections. Greenacre CB, Gerhardt L, "Psittacines and Passerines," in Ballard B, Cheek R, Exotic Animal Medicine for the Veterinary Technician, ed 3, Wiley-Blackwell, 2017.

143. d These signs are typical of avian chlamydophila virus. Avian chlamydophila is highly contagious to people, causing flu-like symptoms. Diagnosis is made by radiographs, which often show splenomegaly and potentially show hepatomegaly. CBC shows a heterophilic, monocytic leukocytosis with a nonregenerative anemia. PCR testing can confirm diagnosis. Patients with proventricular dilation disease present in poor health with crop stasis and chronic regurgitation. Psittacine beak and feather disease affects the overall beak and feather quality. Papillomatosis causes wart-like masses along the GI tract, cloaca, and oropharynx. Greenacre CB, Gerhardt L, "Psittacines and Passerines," in Ballard B, Cheek R, Exotic Animal Medicine for the Veterinary Technician, ed 3, Wiley-Blackwell, 2017.

144. b The heterophil is functionally similar to the neutrophil and is generally the most numerous in bird blood. Eosinophils, basophils, and lymphocytes are present in avian blood smears, although eosinophils and basophils are rare. Bounous DL, "Avian and Reptile Hematology," in Ballard B, Cheek R, Exotic Animal Medicine for the Veterinary Technician, ed 3, Wiley-Blackwell, 2017.

145. d Azurophils are unique in that they are only found in reptiles. Bounous DL, "Avian and Reptile Hematology," in Ballard B, Cheek R, Exotic Animal Medicine for the Veterinary Technician, ed 3, Wiley-Blackwell, 2017.

146. d Predisposing factors leading to dystocia include poor environmental conditions, metabolic disease, and improper husbandry. Clinical signs include anorexia, lethargy, straining, and bloody discharge. Rivera S, "Chelonians," in Ballard B, Cheek R, Exotic Animal Medicine for the Veterinary Technician, ed 3, Wiley-Blackwell, 2017.

147. a The upper shell is called the carapace and the lower shell is called the plastron. Epiplastral, endoplastral, hypoplastral, and xiphiplastral relate to bones found in the plastron. Rivera S, "Chelonians," in Ballard B, Cheek R, Exotic Animal Medicine for the Veterinary Technician, ed 3, Wiley-Blackwell, 2017.

148. b The heart is generally located in the cranial ¼ of the body. Locations just below the base of the skull or 2 inches below the skull are not correct because these indicators vary with the length of the patient. Cheek R, Crane M, "Snakes," in Ballard B, Cheek R, Exotic Animal Medicine for the Veterinary Technician, ed 3, Wiley-Blackwell, 2017.

149. c Most species of snakes have a right lung and a vestigial or nonfunctioning left lung. The right lung runs at least ½ the length of the body. In many species, the posterior ⅓ of the lung is an air sac. Cheek R, Crane M, "Snakes," in Ballard B, Cheek R, Exotic Animal Medicine for the Veterinary Technician, ed 3, Wiley-Blackwell, 2017.

150. c Gravel and corncob bedding are detrimental when ingested, leading to GI foreign bodies and impaction. These substrates are also abrasive and can cause skin irritation or wounds. Corncob bedding can become moldy fairly easily when wet. The other beddings listed are safe, easy to clean or dispose of, and do not cause physical harm to the patient. Cheek R, Crane M, "Snakes," in Ballard B, Cheek R, Exotic Animal Medicine for the Veterinary Technician, ed 3, Wiley-Blackwell, 2017.